a LANGE medical book

CURRENT Diagnosis & Treatment in Family Medicine

second edition

Jeannette E. South-Paul, MD
Andrew W. Mathieson Professor and Chair
Department of Family Medicine
University of Pittsburgh School of Medicine
Pittsburgh, Pennsylvania

Samuel C. Matheny, MD, MPH
Professor and Nicholas J. Pisacano, MD, Chair of Family Medicine
Department of Family and Community Medicine
University of Kentucky College of Medicine
Lexington, Kentucky

Evelyn L. Lewis, MD, MA
Director, Healthcare Policy
Pfizer, Inc.
Bowie, Maryland
Adjunct Associate Professor
Departments of Family Medicine and Medical and Clinical Psychology
Uniformed Services University of the Health Sciences
Bethesda, Maryland

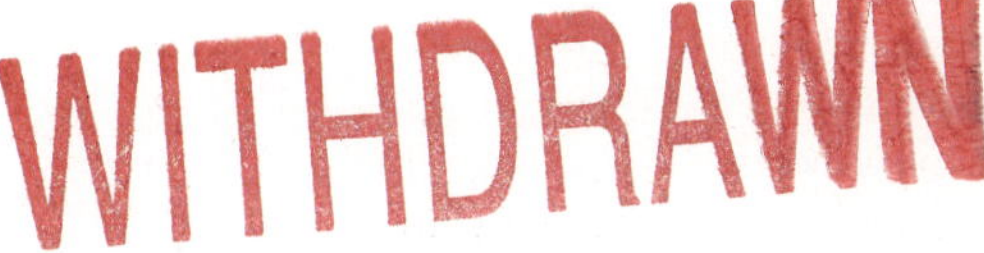

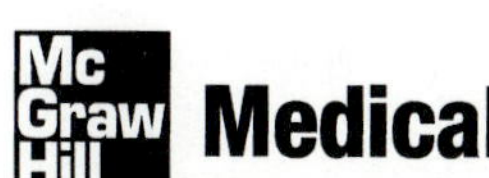

New York Chicago San Francisco Lisbon London Madrid Mexico City
New Delhi San Juan Seoul Singapore Sydney Toronto

The McGraw-Hill Companies

Current Diagnosis & Treatment in Family Medicine, Second Edition

1 2 3 4 5 6 7 8 9 0 DOC/DOC 0 9 8 7

ISBN 9780071461535
MHID 0-07-146153-1
ISSN 1548-2189

Notice

Medicine is an ever-changing science. As new research and clinical experience broaden our knowledge, changes in treatment and drug therapy are required. The authors and the publisher of this work have checked with sources believed to be reliable in their efforts to provide information that is complete and generally in accord with the standards accepted at the time of publication. However, in view of the possibility of human error or changes in medical sciences, neither the authors nor the publisher nor any other party who has been involved in the preparation or publication of this work warrants that the information contained herein is in every respect accurate or complete, and they disclaim all responsibility for any errors or omissions or for the results obtained from use of the information contained in this work. Readers are encouraged to confirm the information contained herein with other sources. For example and in particular, readers are advised to check the product information sheet included in the package of each drug they plan to administer to be certain that the information contained in this work is accurate and that changes have not been made in the recommended dose or in the contraindications for administration. This recommendation is of particular importance in connection with new or infrequently used drugs.

This book was set in Adobe Garamond by Silverchair Science & Communications, Inc.
The editors were James F. Shanahan and Harriet Lebowitz.
The production supervisor was Phil Galea and Thomas G. Kowalczyk.
The illustration manager was Armen Ovsepyan.
Project management was provided by Silverchair Science & Communications, Inc.
The designer was Eve Siegel.
Cover design: Mary McKeon
RR Donnelley was printer and binder.

This book is printed on acid-free paper.

INTERNATIONAL EDITION ISBN 9780071287395, MHID 0-07-128739-6

We would like to dedicate this book
to all family physicians who deliver care in austere environments,
especially our colleagues in uniform, and the families that support them.

Jeannette E. South-Paul, MD
Samuel C. Matheny, MD, MPH
Evelyn L. Lewis, MD, MA

Contents

SECTION III: ADULTS

SECTION VI: PSYCHOSOCIAL DISORDERS

SECTION VII: PHYSICIAN–PATIENT ISSUES

Authors

Ya'aqov Abrams, MD
Assistant Professor of Family Medicine, University of Pittsburgh, Pittsburgh, Pennsylvania
abramsym@upmc.edu
Pharmacogenomics

Sheila Ann B. Alas, MD
Chief Resident, University of Pittsburgh Medical Center, Family Medicine Residency Program, Pittsburgh, Pennsylvania
Sheila_alas@hotmail.com
Common Geriatric Problems

Pamela Allweiss, MD, MSPH
Assistant Professor, University of Kentucky, Lexington, Kentucky
pallweiss@alltel.net
Endocrine disorders

Nicole T. Ansani, PharmD
Associate Director, Drug Information Center; Assistant Professor, Department of Pharmacy and Therapeutics, University of Pittsburgh School of Pharmacy, Pennsylvania
ansanint@msx.upmc.edu
Pharmacotherapeutics

Thomas D. Armsey, MD
Midlands Orthopaedics, P.A., Columbia, South Carolina
Common Upper & Lower Extremity Fractures

Cindy Barter, MD
Clinical Faculty, Lehigh Valley Hospital Family Medicine Residency Program, Allentown, Pennsylvania
cindy.barter@lvh.com
Abdominal Pain

Daphne P. Bicket, MD, MLS
University of Pittsburgh Medical Center, McKeesport Family Medicine Residency Program, McKeesport, Pennsylvania
bicketdp@upmc.edu
Common Geriatric Problems

Marian Block, MD
Department of Family Medicine, West Penn Hospital, Pittsburgh, Pennsylvania
mblock@wpahs.org
Communication

Deborah J. Bostock, MD
Assistant Professor, Department of Family Medicine, Uniformed Services University of the Health Sciences, Bethesda, Maryland
Elder Abuse

Anne S. Boyd, MD
Director, Primary Care Sports Medicine Fellowship Program, UPMC St. Margaret, Assistant Clinical Professor, University of Pittsburgh School of Medicine, Department of Family Medicine, Pittsburgh, Pennsylvania
boydas@upmc.edu
Acute Musculoskeletal Complaints

Susan C. Brunsell, MD
Assistant Residency Director, Georgetown University/ Providence Hospital Family Medicine Residency Program, Washington DC
suemd@earthlink.net
Contraception

Peter J. Carek, MD, MS
Residency Program Director, Professor Department of Family Medicine, Medical University of South Carolina, Charleston, South Carolina
carekpj@musc.edu
Endocrine Disorders

Robert J. Carr, MD
Medical Director, Primary Care of Southbury, Southbury, Connecticut
robber.carr@charter.net
Urinary Incontinence

Ronald A. Chez, MD
Formerly Deputy Director, Samueli Institute, Corona del Mar, California
rchez@siib.org
Complementary & Alternative Medicine

C. Randall Clinch, DO, MA
Associate Professor, Department of Family & Community Medicine, Wake Forest University School of Medicine, Winston-Salem, North Carolina
crclinch@wfubmc.edu
Headache

Tracey D. Conti, MD
Faculty, University of Pittsburgh Medical Center McKeesport, Family Medicine Residency Program, McKeesport, Pennsylvania
tconti@pitt.edu
Breast-feeding & Infant Nutrition

Kathleen A. Culhane-Pera, MD, MA
Associate Medical Director, West Side Community Health Services, St. Paul, Minnesota
kathiecp@yahoo.com
Cultural Competence

Essam Demian, MD, MRCOG
Clinical Assistant Professor, Department of Family Medicine, University of Pittsburgh School of Medicine, Pittsburgh, Pennsylvania
demiane@upmc.edu
Preconception Care

Laura Dunne, MD
Orthopedic Associates of Allentown, Allentown, Pennsylvania
lauradunne@aol.com
Abdominal Pain

William Elder, PhD
Associate Professor, Department of Family and Community Medicine, University of Kentucky, Lexington, Kentucky
welder@email.uky.edu
Personality Disorders
Somatoform Symptoms & Disorders

Patricia Evans, MD, MA
Program Director, Georgetown University-Providence Hospital, Family Medicine Residency
evansp@georgetown.edu
Vaginal Bleeding

W. Gregory Feero, MD, PhD
Chief, Genomic Healthcare Branch, National Human Genome Research Institute, National Institutes of Health, Bethesda, Maryland
feerow@mail.nih.gov
Genetics for Family Physicians

Deborah Auer Flomenhoft, MD
Assitant Professor of Internal Medicine and Pediatrics, Division of Gastroenterology, University of Kentucky College of Medicine, Lexington, Kentucky
drflom0@email.uky.edu
Failure to Thrive

Ronald M. Glick, MD
Assistant Professor of Psychiatry, Physical Medicine and Rehabilitation and Family Medicine, Pittsburgh, Pennsylvania
glickrm@upmc.edu
Chronic Pain Management

Marisela Gomez, MD, PhD, MPH
Depression in Diverse Populations

Wanda Gonsalves, MD
Associate Professor, Department of Family Medicine, Medical University of South Carolina, Charleston, South Carolina
gonsalvw@musc.edu
Oral Health

Terence L. Gutgsell, MD
Medical Director, Hospice of the Bluegrass, Lexington, Kentucky; Medical Director, Palliative Care Center of the Bluegrass, Lexington, Kentucky
lestug@hospicebg.com
Hospice & Palliative Medicine

Garry W. K. Ho, MD
UCU Fairfax Family Practice Sports Medicine Center, Fairfax, Virginia
gho@ffpcs.com
Neck Pain

Robert G. Hosey, MD
Associate Professor, Department of Family and Community Medicine, University of Kentucky, Lexington, Kentucky
rhosey@email.uky.edu
Common Upper & Lower Extremity Fractures

Thomas M. Howard, MD
Program Director, UCU Fairfax Family Practice Sports Medicine Fellowship, Fairfax,Virginia
thoward@ffpcs.com
Neck Pain

William J. Hueston, MD
Department of Family Medicine, Medical University of South Carolina, Charleston
huestowj@musc.edu
Respiratory Problems
Endocrine Disorders

Andrew Hyland, PhD
Roswell Park Cancer Institute, Department of Health, Buffalo, New York
andrew.hyland@roswellpark.org
Tobacco Cessation

Bruce E. Johnson, MD
Professor of Medicine, Director-Division of General Internal Medicine at East Carolina University, Greenville, North Carolina
johnsonbru@mail.ecu.edu
Arthritis: Osteoarthritis, Gout, & Rheumatoid Arthritis

Wayne B. Jonas, MD
Director, Samueli Institute, Alexandria, Virginia
wjonas@siib.org
Complementary & Alternative Medicine

Peter J. Katsufrakis, MD, MBA
Associate Vice President, Post-Graduate and Developmental Activities National Board of Medical Examiners, Philadelphia, Pennsylvania
pkatsu@hsc.usc.edu
Adolescent Sexuality
Sexually Transmitted Diseases
Caring for Gay, Lesbian, Bisexual, & Transgender Patients

Shersten Killip, MD, MPH
Assistant Professor, Department of Family and Community Medicine, University of Kentucky, Lexington, Kentucky
skill2@email.uky.edu
Urinary Tract Infections

Sanford R. Kimmel, MD
Professor, University of Toldeo College of Medicine, Toledo, Ohio
sanfordkimmel@utoledo.edu
Routine Childhood Vaccines

Michael King, MD, MPH
Assistant Professor, Department of Family and Community Medicine, College of Medicine, University of Kentucky, Lexington, Kentucky
Mrking02@uky.edu
Heart Failure

Kenneth L. Kirsh, PhD
Assistant Professor, Pharmacy Practice and Science, University of Kentucky College of Pharmacy, Clinical Psychologist, The Pain Treatment Center of the Bluegrass, Lexington, Kentucky
klkirsh@uky.edu
Hospice & Palliative Medicine

Mark A. Knox, MD
Clinical Associate Professor, University of Pittsburgh School of Medicine, Department of Family Medicine, Pittsburgh, Pennsylvania
knoxma@upmc.edu
Common Infections in Children
Skin Diseases in Infants & Children

Matthew Krasowaki, MD, PhD
Assistant Professor, Department of Pathology, University of Pittsburgh, Pennsylvania
krasowskim@upmc.edu
Pharmacogenomics

Mary V. Krueger, DO, MPH, MAJ, MC, USA
Assistant Professor, Uniformed Services University o f the Health Sciences, Bethesda, Maryland
mary.krueger@us.army.mil
Menstrual Disorders

Nancy Levine, MD
Vice-Chair, Western Pennsylvania Hospital, Associate Professor, Temple University School of Medicine, Pittsburgh, Pennsylvania
nlevine@wpahs.org
Communication

Evelyn L. Lewis, MD, MA
Medical Director, Healthcare Policy, Pfizer, Inc., Bowie, Maryland; Adjunct Associate Professor, Departments of Family Medicine and Medical and Clinical Psychology, Uniformed Services University of the Health Sciences, Bethesda, Maryland
elewis@usuhs.mil
Eating Disorders
Health & Health Care Disparities

Jamee H. Lucas, MD, FAAFP
Associate Professor, University of South Carolina SOM Palmetto Health Family Medicine Residency, Columbia, South Carolina
jamee.lucas@palmettohealth.org
Anxiety Disorders

Charles W. Mackett III, MD
Executive Vice Chair, Department of Family Medicine, University of Pittsburgh Medical Center, Pittsburgh, Pennsylvania
mackettcw@upmc.edu
Adult Sexual Dysfunction

Kiame J. Mahaniah, MD
Associate Residency Director, Greater Lawrence Family Medicine Residency, Lawrence, Massachusetts
kmahaniah@glfhc.org
Anemia

Martin C. Mahoney, MD, PhD, FAAFP
Associate Professor of Oncology, Roswell Park Cancer Institute, Buffalo, New York, Associate Professor, Department of Family Medicine, State University of New York at Buffalo, Buffalo, New York
martin.mahoney@roswellpark.org
Neonatal Hyperbilirubinemia
Tobacco Cessation

Robert Mallin, MD
Associate Professor, Department of Family Medicine, Medical University of South Carolina, Charleston
mallinr@musc.edu
Substance Use Disorders

Crystal March, MD
Depression in Older Patients

Dawn A. Marcus, MD
Associate Professor, Department of Anesthesiology, University of Pittsburgh Medical Center, Pennsylvania
marcusd@anes.upmc.edu
Chronic Pain Management

William H. Markle, MD, FAAFP, DTM&H
Clinical Associate Professor Family Medicine, university of Pittsburgh School of Medicine, Director Family medicine Residency, UPMC McKeesport, McKeesport, Pennsylvania
marklew@upmc.edu
Travel Medicine

Ronica A. Martinez, MD
Sports Medicine M.D. Primary Care Sports Medicine, Woodland Hills California
Ronica_ellini@hotmail.com
Acute Musculoskeletal Complaints

Samuel C. Matheny, MD, MPH
Professor and Nicholas J. Pisacano, MD, Chair of Family Medicine, Department of Family and Community Medicine, University of Kentucky College of Medicine, Lexington, Kentucky
matheny@email.uky.edu
Hepatobiliary Disorders

Rodrick McKinlay, MD
Rocky Mountain Associated Physicians, Salt Lake City, Utah
Hepatobiliary Disorders

Bonnie Meyer, DMin,
Hospice & Palliative Medicine

Philip J. Michels, PhD
Professor and Director, Division of Behavioral Medicine Department of Family and Preventive Medicine, University of South Carolina School of Medicine, Columbia, South Carolina
phil.michels@palmettohealth.org
Anxiety Disorders

Donald B. Middleton, MD
Professor, Department of Family Medicine, University of Pittsburgh School of Medicine, UPMC St. Margaret, Pittsburgh, Pennsylvania
middletondb@upmc.edu
Well Child Care
Routine Childhood Vaccines
Seizures

T.A. Miller, MD
Director, Graduate Medical Education, Naval Medical Education and Training Command, Bethesda, Maryland
Adult Sexual Dysfunction

Christine M. Mueller, DO
Postdoctoral Cancer Genetics Research Fellow, Clinical Genetics Branch, Division of Cancer Epidemiology and Genetics, National Cancer Institute, National Institutes of Health, Department of Health and Human Services, Rockville, Maryland
muellerc@mail.nih.gov
Genetics for Family Physicians

David A. Nikovits, MD
Sports Medicine Physician, Omni HealthCare, Palm Bay, Florida
Common Upper & Lower Extremity Fractures

Margaret R. H. Nusbaum, DO, MPH
Associate Professor, Department of Family Medicine, University of North Carolina, Chapel Hill
margaret_nusbaum@med.unc.edu
Adolescent Sexuality
Sexually Transmitted Diseases
Adult Sexual Dysfunction

Francis G. O'Connor, MD, MPH, COL, MC, USA
Associate Professor of Family Medicine; Medical Director, USUHS Consortium for Health and Military Performance (CHAMP), Uniformed Services University of the Health Sciences, Bethesda, Maryland
foconnor@usuhs.mil
Low Back Pain

Maureen O'Hara Padden, MD, MPH, FAAFP
Deputy Chief of Staff, Navy Medicine National Capital Area, Bethesda, Maryland
mopadden@navmednca.med.navy.mill
Hypertension

Steven D. Passik, PhD
Associate Attending Psychologist, Psychiatry and Behavioral Sciences, Memorial Sloan Kettering Cancer Center, New York, New York
passiks@mskcc.org
Hospice & Palliative Medicine

Sonia Patten, PhD
Visiting Assistant Professor, Department of Anthropology, Macalester College, St. Paul, Minnesota
patten@macalester.edu
Cultural Competence

Hahn X. Pham, MD
Associate Medical Director, Hospice of the Bluegrass, Lexington, Kentucky
Hospice & Palliative Medicine

Brian A. Primack, MD, EdM
Assistant Professor, Departments of Medicine and Pediatrics, School of Medicine, University of Pittsburgh, Pittsburgh, Pennsylvania
primackba@upmc.edu
Anemia

Annelle B. Primm, MD, MPH
Director, Minority and National Affairs, American Psychiatric Association, Arlington, Virginia
Depression in Diverse Populations

Goutham Rao, MD
Assistant Professor, Department of Family Medicine, University of Pittsburgh School of Medicine, Pennsylvania
raog@upmc.edu
Movement Disorders

Brian V. Reamy, MD, COL, USAF, MC
Associate Professor & Chair, Department of Family Medicine, Uniformed Services University, Bethesda, Maryland
breamy@usuhs.mil
Dyslipidemias

Charles F. Reynolds III, MD
UPMC Professor of Geriatric Psychiatry, University of Pittsburgh School of Medicine, Pittsburgh, Pennsylvania
reynoldscf@msx.upmc.edu
Depression in Older Patients

Richard E. Rodenberg, Jr., MD
Columbus Children's Hospital, Ohio State University Medical Center, Columbus, Ohio
rerodenb@yahoo.com
Heart Failure
Common Upper & Lower Extremity Fractures

Richie-Ann G. Rodriguez, MD
University of Pittsburgh Medical Center Family Medicine Residency Program, McKeesport Pennsylvania
Richie_ann@yahoo.com
Common Geriatric Problems

Jo Ann Rosenfeld, MD
Assistant Professor, Department of Medicine, The Johns Hopkins Univeristy School of Medicine, Baltimore, Maryland
jrosenfe@jhmi.edu
Evaluation of Breast Lumps

Tracy Sbrocco, PhD
Associate Professor, Department of Medical and Clinical Psychology, Uniformed Services University of the Health Sciences, Bethesda, Maryland
tsbrocco@usuhs.mil
Eating Disorders

Robert W. Smith, MD, MBA
Vice Chair for Education, Department of Family Medicine, University of Pittsburgh, Pittsburgh, Pennsylania
smithrw@upmc.edu
Interpersonal Violence

Melissa A. Somma, PharmD, CDE
Assistant Professor of Pharmacy & Therapeutics, University of Pittsburgh School of Pharmacy, Pittsburgh, Pennsylvania
soma@pitt.edu
Pharmacotherapeutics

Jeannette E. South-Paul, MD
Andrew W. Mathieson Professor and Chair
Department of Family Medicine
University of Pittsburgh School of Medicine, Pittsburgh, Pennsylvania
southpaulj@upmc.edu
Osteoporosis
Health & Health Care Disparities

Sukanya Srinivasan, MD, MPH
Private Practice, Penn Plum Family Medicine, Pittsburgh, Pennsylvania
srinivasans@upmc.edu
Well Child Care

Sharm Steadman, PharmD
Anxiety Disorders

Mark B. Stephens, MD, MS, FAAFP
Associate Program Director, Naval Hospital Camp Lejeune Family Medicine Residency, Associate Professor of Family Medicine, Uniformed Services University, Camp Lejeune, North Carolina
mstephens@usuhs.mil
Physical Activity in Adolescents

Bernhard K. Stepke, MD, PhD, LCDR, MC, USN
Navel Hospital Camp Pendleton, Camp Pendleton, California
Bernhard.stepke@med.navy.mil
Hypertension

William S. Sykora, MD, COL, USAF, MC
Assistant Dean for Curriculum, Assistant Professor of Family Medicine, Uniformed Services University of the Health Sciences, Bethesda, Maryland
wsykora@usuhs.mil
Disruptive Behavioral Disorders in Children

Andrew B. Symons, MD, MS
Assistant Professor of Family Medicine, State University of New York at Buffalo, Buffalo, New York
symons@buffalo.edu
Neonatal Hyperbilirubinemia

Belinda Vail, MD
Associate Professor, Residency Director and Vice Chair, Department of Family Medicine, University of Kansas School of Medicine, Kansas City, Kansas
bvail@kumc.edu
Diabetes Mellitus

Jacqueline S. Weaver-Agostoni, DO, MPH
Faculty, University of Pittsburgh Department of Family Medicine, UPMC Shadyside Hospital, Pittsburgh Pennsylvania
Jackie.weaver@gmail.com
Acute Coronary Syndrome

Charles W. Webb, DO, FAAFP, CAQ Sports Medicine
Assistant Professor, Department of Family Medicine, Oregon Health & Science University, Portland, Oregon
webbo18@aol.com
Low Back Pain

Sherri Weisenfluh, LCSW
Associate vice-President of Counseling Service, Hospice of the Bluegrass, Lexington, Kentucky
sweisenfluh@hospicebg.com
Hospice & Palliative Medicine

Alan L. Williams, MD
Staff Physician, National Institute of Health, Occupational Medical Service, Bethesda, Maryland
jackdoodle@comcast.net
Hearing & Vision Impairment in the Elderly

Cynthia M. Williams, DO. MA, FAACP
Assistant Professor Family Medicine, Uniformed Services University of the Health Sciences, Fellow, Pain and Palliative Care, National Institutes of Health
williamscm@cc.nih.gov
Healthy Aging
Elder Abuse

Pamela M. Williams, MD
Assistant Professor, Department of Family Medicine, Uniformed Services University of the Health Sciences Bethesda, Maryland
pawilliams@usuhs.mil
Hearing & Vision Impairment in the Elderly

Calvin L. Wilson, MD
Associate Professor, Department of Family Medicine, University of Colorado at Denver and Health Sciences Center, Denver, Colorado
Cal.wilson@uchsc.edu
Travel Medicine

Stephen A. Wilson, MD
Assistant Director, UPMC St. Margaret Family Medicine Residency, Associate Director UPMC St. Margaret Faculty Development Fellowship, Clinical Associate Professor, University of Pittsburgh, Department of Family Medicine, Pittsburgh, Pennsylvania
wilsons2@upmc.edu
Acute Coronary Syndrome

Kimberly A. Workowski, MD, FACP
Emory University, Department of Infectious Diseases, CDC Division of STD Prevention, Atlanta Georgia
kworkow@emory.edu
Sexually Transmitted Diseases

Yagin Xia, MD, MHPE
Department of Family Medicine, University of Pittsburgh School of Medicine, Assistant Professor, UPMC, Pittsburgh, Pennsylvania
xiaxy@upmc.edu
Movement Disorders

Richard Kent Zimmerman, MD, MPH
Professor, Department of Family Medicine and Clinical Epidemiology, University of Pittsburgh, Pittsburgh, Pennsylvania
zimmer@pitt.edu
Childhood Vaccines

Preface

Current Diagnosis & Treatment in Family Medicine is the second edition of this single-source reference for house staff and practicing family physicians who provide comprehensive and continuous care of individuals of both sexes throughout the lifespan. The text is organized according to the developmental lifespan, beginning with childhood and adolescence, encompassing a focus on the reproductive years, and progressing through adulthood and the mature, senior years.

OUTSTANDING FEATURES

- Evidence-based recommendations
- Culturally related aspects of each condition
- Conservative and pharmacologic therapies
- Complementary and alternative therapies when relevant
- Suggestions for collaborations with other health care providers
- Attention to the mental and behavioral health of patients as solitary as well as comorbid conditions
- Recognition of impact of illness on the family
- Patient education information
- End-of-life issues

INTENDED AUDIENCE

Primary care trainees and practicing physicians will find this text a useful resource for common conditions seen in ambulatory practice. Detailed information in tabular and text format provides a ready reference for selecting diagnostic procedures and recommending treatments. Advanced practice nurses and physician's assistants will also find the approach provided here a practical and complete first resource for both diagnosed and undifferentiated conditions and an aid in continuing management.

Unlike smaller medical manuals that focus on urgent, one-time approaches to a particular presenting complaint or condition, this text was envisioned as a resource for clinicians who practice continuity of care and have established a longitudinal, therapeutic relationship with their patients. Consequently, recommendations are made for immediate as well as subsequent clinical encounters.

ACKNOWLEDGMENTS

We wish to thank our many contributing authors for their diligence in creating complete, practical, and readable discussions of the many conditions seen on a daily basis in the average family medicine and primary care practice. Furthermore, the vision and support of our editors at McGraw-Hill for creating this new resource for primary care have been outstanding and critical to its completion.

Jeannette E. South-Paul, MD
Samuel C. Matheny, MD, MPH
Evelyn L. Lewis, MD, MA

SECTION I
Infancy & Childhood

Well Child Care 1

Sukanya Srinivasan, MD, MPH, & Donald B. Middleton, MD

ESSENTIALS OF WELL CHILD CARE

Caring for children is an integral and enjoyable part of family medicine. The provision of comprehensive well child care is one cornerstone of the distinction between the family physician and other medical specialists. Periodic examinations of children allow the family physician to build a strong foundation for continuity of care with entire families and their communities.

Better nutrition and broader immunization coverage have significantly improved the health of US children, but other serious childhood health problems persist. Inadequate or delayed prenatal care, childhood obesity, and poor management of developmental delay are examples of critical issues that need to be addressed. Barriers to health care such as insufficient health literacy and societal problems such as poverty compound these issues. Armed with preventive care expertise, primary care practitioners play pivotal roles as advocates for improving children's health.

The components of routine well child care include the following:

- Interval history taking.
- Complete physical examination.
- Relevant screening tests.
- Developmental assessment.
- Tracking of growth parameters.
- Anticipatory guidance about child-rearing issues.
- Administration of recommended immunizations.

The underlying purpose is to identify concerns about a child's physical and psychological development and to intervene with early preventive treatment. Family physicians need to comfortably identify common normal variants as well as abnormal findings that may require referral.

The advised schedule of visits for routine well child checkups (Table 1–1) provides ample opportunities to observe the child and family at critical junctures during development and melds with the Advisory Committee on Immunization Practice's (ACIP) recommended timetable of immunizations. However, any encounter, even for an acute illness, is an opportunity to update health screening, provide anticipatory guidance, and administer immunizations. Recognized problems such as growth delay can necessitate additional checkups for more intense follow-up. Supplemental visits may also be required if the child is adopted or living with surrogate parents; is at high risk for medical disorders as suggested by the pregnancy, delivery, or neonatal history; exhibits psychological disorders as suggested by speech delay, persistent temper tantrums, or poor school performance; if the family is socially or economically disadvantaged; or if the parents request or require additional education or guidance.

GENERAL APPROACH

A general principle for well child examinations is to perform maneuvers from least to most invasive, but some parts of the examination are best accomplished when the infant is quiet so may be done "out of order." Clinicians should first make observations about the child-parent(s) interaction, obtain an interval history, and then perform a direct examination of the child, reserving the use of any specialized instruments until the end. Although most of the communications and decisions about the child's

Table 1–1. Proposed schedule of routine well care visits.

Newborn examination within 24 h of birth and prior to discharge from hospital	
2–4 weeks	$2^1/_2$ years[1]
2 months	3 years
4 months	4 years
6 months	5 years
9 months	6 years
12 months	8 years
15 months	10 years
18 months	
24 months	
Annually, between ages of 11 and 21 years	

[1]Well child check at 30 months ($2^1/_2$ years) is highly recommended but not yet in general practice.

Source: Green M, Palfrey JS, eds.: *Bright Futures: Guidelines for Health Supervision of Infants, Children, and Adolescents*, 2nd ed, revised. National Center for Education in Maternal and Child Health, Health Resources and Services Administration, 2002.

health are typically between the physician and the parents, clinicians should attempt to communicate directly with the patient to gauge whether his or her growth is developmentally appropriate and to develop familiarity over time directly with the patient. Patient-physician communication is particularly important during adolescence to gain the patient's trust and to assess comprehension and compliance.

A child's medical record must be kept meticulously. Parents should be encouraged to maintain their own record, especially for immunizations and growth, for each child. A checklist-based system is an efficient way to ensure completeness in physical and developmental examinations. A table or flow sheet, which can be updated on an ongoing basis, is helpful for tracking immunizations and screening tests. Finally, standardized growth charts from the Centers for Disease Control and Prevention (CDC) to track the child's weight, height, and head circumference and body-mass index (BMI) after age 3 years are a concise way to identify any worrisome trends.

Centers for Disease Control and Prevention: *2000 CDC Growth Charts: United States.* Available at: http://www.cdc.gov/growthcharts/.

Dinkevich E, Ozuah PO: Well-child care: Effectiveness of current recommendations. Clin Pediatr 2002;41:211. [PMID: 12041716].

Green M, Palfrey JS (editors). *Bright Futures, Guidelines for Health Supervision of Infants, Children, and Adolescents,* 2nd ed, revised. National Center for Education in Maternal and Child Health, Health Resources and Services Administration, 2002.

Middleton DB, Schroeder M: *Well Child Care: Reference Guide of the American Board of Family Practice,* 8th ed. American Board of Family Practice, 2000.

HEALTH MAINTENANCE & DISEASE PREVENTION

Well child care ideally begins in the preconception period. During a routine or specific preconception office visit, family physicians can discuss ways for patients to optimize their health in anticipation of bearing children. Prospective parents should be counseled about tobacco and alcohol cessation; appropriate nutrition, including 0.4 mg of folic acid daily for all women of childbearing age; and prevention of congenital infections such as rubella (immunization) or toxoplasmosis (avoidance of kittens and litter boxes). Ideally, expectant parents will plan to have the family physician perform the delivery or at least have a prenatal visit to review pertinent family and genetic history and office policies and procedures. Physicians can also gather information at this visit about how the parents are preparing for the child's arrival and discuss plans for feeding and child care.

A mother's decision about feeding her infant, often made long before the child is born, is based largely on cultural beliefs and value judgments rather than medical knowledge. The prenatal visit is a good opportunity to promote breast-feeding once again to the parents, emphasizing the health benefits for both mother and infant. With this background, the first newborn visit can then be dedicated to providing parents with specific guidance about child care.

A systematic approach to preventive care and anticipatory guidance allows family physicians to provide the caregivers with appropriate and timely advice. Topics for discussion include nutrition, development, safety, behavior, elimination, sleep, play, and oral health.

Nutrition (see also Chapter 4)

During the newborn period, all mothers should be strongly encouraged to breast-feed their infants. A widely accepted goal is exclusive breast-feeding for the first 6 months of life. Vitamin D supplement (400 units/day) may be indicated for some breast-fed children. Family doctors can initiate a "baby-friendly" office by providing information about lactation consultants, instructing staff to avoid giving formula samples or literature from formula companies, and providing a private room in the office for breast-feeding mothers.

The mother who chooses to bottle-feed her newborn has several choices in formulas but should not use cow's milk, because of the risk of anemia. Commercial formulas are typically fortified with iron and vitamin D. Some are also supplemented with fatty acids such as docosahexaenoic acid (DHA) and arachidonic acid (ARA), theoretically but not proven to promote nervous system development. Soy or lactose-free formulas can be used when medically necessary or as the parents wish.

An appropriate weight gain is 1 ounce/day during the first 6 months of life and 0.5 ounce/day during the next 6 months. This weight gain requires a caloric intake of 120 kcal/kg/day during the first 6 months and 100 kcal/kg/day thereafter. Caregivers need to be questioned at every visit about the amount and duration of the child's feedings. Initially, the child should be fed on demand, when caregivers note signs of hunger such as soft, suckling noises, hand-to-mouth movements, or rooting movements. Breast-fed infants typically feed every 2–3 hours for 10–15 minutes on each breast. Formula-fed infants typically feed every 3–4 hours, ingesting approximately 1.5–3 ounces.

Partly because the work of feeding is much less with a rubber nipple on a bottle, children who are given formula can easily be overfed, leading to emesis and perhaps a misdiagnosis of reflux. If interval weight gain is excessive, parents should be cautioned against inadvertent overfeeding. Once the child's eating patterns become more established, parents can learn to use alternative measures to comfort a crying child, instead of offering a feeding.

Solid foods such as cereals or strained, pureed baby foods such as vegetables and fruits are introduced at 4–6 months of age when the infant can support his or her head and the tongue extrusion reflex has extinguished. Delaying introduction of solid foods until this time appears to limit the incidence of food sensitivities. The child can also continue breast- or bottle-feeding, limited to 32 ounces/day, because the solids now provide additional calories. Around 1 year of age when the infant can drink from a cup, bottle-feeding should be discontinued to protect teeth from caries. No specified optimum age exists for weaning a child from breast-feeding, and the decision to stop is based on each individual family's needs. Small toddlers can tolerate soft adult foods such as yogurt and mashed potatoes. A well-developed pincer grasp allows children to self-feed finger foods. With the eruption of primary teeth at 8–12 months of age, children may try foods such as soft rice or pastas.

With toddlers, mealtimes can be a source of both pleasure and anxiety as children become "finicky." The normal child may exhibit specific food preferences or be disinterested in eating. A child's appropriate growth rate and developmental milestones should reassure frustrated parents. Coping strategies include offering small portions of preferred items first and offering limited food choices. After weaning, ingestion of whole or 2% cow's milk may promote nervous system development. Parents should be encouraged to eat as a family so toddlers have role models for healthy eating and develop appropriate social behaviors during mealtimes.

By school age, children need to have a variety of table foods in their diet. A well-balanced diet with appropriate table foods and low-fat milk may be difficult to maintain because children can make their own food choices at home and at school. Vitamin or mineral supplementation can be considered. Parents should minimize the availability and consumption of "junk" food. Childhood obesity is an alarming concern: studies show a prevalence of nearly 15% among US children aged 6 years and older. Furthermore, childhood onset of obesity increases the severity of obesity in adults. Physicians need to intervene early so that eating and activity patterns can be modified with the cooperation of caregivers. Plotting the BMI after age 3 years can serve as an impetus to parents to better control their child's diet. Food should not be used as a reward. Increasing physical activity and minimizing television watching are additional prevention strategies. Often, the clinician may need to refer the entire family to a weight-loss program, including behavioral modification and nutritional counseling.

American Academy of Family Physicians. *Position Paper on Breastfeeding*. Available at: http://www.aafp.org/policy/x1641.xml.

Kleinman RE, ed: *Pediatric Nutrition Handbook,* 5th ed. American Academy of Pediatrics, 2004.

Kramer MS, Kakuma R: Optimal duration of exclusive breast-feeding. Cochrane Database Syst Rev 2002;(1):CD003517. [PMID: 11869667]

Lawrence RA: Breastfeeding: Benefits, risks and alternatives. Curr Opin Obstet Gynecol 2000;12:519. [PMID: 11128416]

Middleton DB, Srinivasan S: Healthy newborn. In: *FP Essentials,* Edition No. 291, AAFP Home Study. American Academy of Family Physicians, August 2003:1–76.

Oddy WH: Breastfeeding protects against illness and infection in infants and children: A review of the evidence. Breastfeed Rev 2001;9:11. [PMID: 11550600]

Oken E, Lightdale JR: Updates in pediatric nutrition. Curr Opin Pediatr 2001;13:280. [PMID: 11389365]

Development & Behavior

Watching a newborn develop from a dependent being to a communicative child with a unique personality is an amazing process that caregivers and clinicians can actively promote. Unfortunately, physicians fail to initially identify over 50% of developmental problems, even though screening tools are available. Table 1–2 shows a brief list of red flags in developmental milestones. Because the period of most active development occurs during the first 2 years, clinicians must ensure that a developmental assessment is performed and documented periodically during this time. Major developmental problems, such as cerebral palsy and mental retardation, are often identified at birth or present in the first 6–8 months of life. These conditions can be associated with a chromosomal abnormality. Referral to a pediatric developmental specialist for a definitive diagnosis and long-term care is usually appropriate.

Table 1–2. Developmental "red flags."[1]

Age (months)	Clinical Observation
2	Not turning toward sights or sounds
4–5	No social smiling or cooing
8–9	Not reaching for objects or reciprocating emotions/expressions
12	No signs of expression or immitative sound exchange with caregivers
18	No signs of complex problem-solving interactions (following 2-step directions)
24	Not using words to get needs met
36–48	No signs of using logical ideas with caregivers or pretend play with toys

[1]Serious emotional difficulties in parents or family members at any time warrant full evaluation.

Source: Brazelton TB, Greenspan SH: *The Irreducible Needs of Children: What Every Child Must Have to Grow, Learn, and Flourish.* Perseus Publishing, 2001.

Table 1–3 contrasts the prevalence of some common development abnormalities.

Table 1–4 lists several useful developmental screening tests. Although commonly held to be the gold standard, the Denver Developmental Screening Test–revised (DDST II) requires trained personnel about 20–30 minutes of office time to administer. Proper use is therefore not widespread in practice. The Parents' Evaluation of Developmental Status (PEDS) questionnaire or Ages and Stages program may be of more practical use.

Development tests screen children who are apparently normal, confirm any concerns the clinician may have uncovered, and offer a way to monitor children at high risk for developmental delay. The clinician or parents may note specific problems in fine motor, gross motor, language, or social skill development that also need further evaluation. Shortened, customized lists of developmental milestones that may result in some increased recognition of delays should not replace periodic use of validated developmental assessment tests. To enhance normal development, parents are encouraged to read to their children on a regular basis, limit television altogether in toddlers and to no more than 2 hours daily for older children, and directly engage in age-appropriate stimulating activities. The physician should question parents about any concerns regarding their child's development at every office visit.

Table 1–3. Prevalence of developmental disorders.

Disorder	Cases per 1000
Attention-deficit/hyperactivity disorder	75–150
Learning disabilities	75
Behavioral disorders	60–130
Mental retardation	25
Autism spectrum disorders	2–5
Cerebral palsy	2–3
Hearing impairment	0.8–2
Visual impairment	0.3–0.6

Adapted, with permission, from Levy SE, Hyman SL: Pediatric assessment of the child with developmental delay. Pediatr Clin North Am 1993;40:465.

Many factors influence temperament, the way a child experiences and reacts to the environment (eg, with passive observation or excessive activity). Genetic influences, physical health, and psychosocial environment all contribute to the formation of a child's temperament or behavioral style. Just like physical attributes, temperaments differ from child to child but many variants in behavior are still deemed normal. Clinicians should discuss the child's temperament with his or her caregivers to guide future understanding and management of behavior and discipline.

Toddlers develop independence and autonomy, accomplishing important tasks such as self-feeding, language acquisition, learning to fall asleep alone, and toilet training. Older children incorporate previously gained skills into preparation for scholastic achievement. At about age 3 years, children are typically enrolled in preschool, where their social skills are enhanced through interaction with others and where they become accustomed to a group learning situation. As children near kindergarten age, developmental skills testing to assess readiness for formal education may assuage concerned parents.

An inability to concentrate, follow directions, or pay attention to the same degree as their peers prevents some children from succeeding at this task. Attention-deficit/hyperactivity disorder (ADHD) is the most common mental diagnosis in children and is characterized by inattention, hyperactivity, and impulsivity (see Chapter 8). The prevalence in school-aged children is estimated to be between 8% and 10%. ADHD occurs two to four times more commonly among boys than girls. Family history of ADHD, history of premature birth, traumatic brain injury, exposure to toxic substances, nervous system infection, and in utero exposure to alcohol and other substances are all possible risk factors. Stimulant medications and behavioral interventions are the major effective treatments. The symptoms of ADHD sometimes overlap with learning disabilities such as dyslexia and dyscalculia and behavioral and emotional problems such as depression, anxiety, or post-traumatic stress disorder. For example, children who have learning disabilities may seem inatten-

Table 1–4. Developmental screening tests.

Test	Age	Time (min)	Source
Office Administered			
Denver II	0–6 y	30	http://www.denverii.com
Early Screening Inventory—Revised	3–6 y	15	http://www.pearsonearlylearning.com
Early Language Milestone (ELM)	0–3 y	5–10	http://www.proedinc.com
Clinical Adaptive Test (CAT)/Clinical Linguistic and Auditory Milestone Scale (CLAMS)	0–3 y	15	http://www.kennedykreiger.org
Parent Administered			
Ages & Stages Questionnaires (ASQ)	4–60 mo (every 4 mo)	15	http://www.pbrookes.com
Parents' Evaluation of Development Status (PEDS)	0–8 y	< 5	http://www.pedstest.com
Behavioral Screening			
Eyberg Child Behavior Inventory (ECBI; parents)/ Sutte Eyberg Student Behavior Inventory Revised (SESBI-R; teachers)	2–16 y	5	http://www.parinc.com
Screening for School Dysfunction			
Safety Word Inventory and Literacy Screener (SWILS)	6–14 y	5	http://www.pedstest.com/files/SWILS.pdf

tive as a result of inability to understand new information. Other considerations include medical conditions such as hearing or visual impairment, diabetes mellitus, asthma, fetal alcohol syndrome, sleep disorder, autism spectrum disorder, and seizure disorder.

Carter AS et al: Assessment of young children's social-emotional development and psychopathology: Recent advances and recommendations for practice. J Child Psychol Psychiatry 2004; 45:109. [PMID: 14959805]

Clinical practice guideline: Diagnosis and evaluation of the child with attention-deficit/hyperactivity disorder. American Academy of Pediatrics. Pediatrics 2000;105:1158. [PMID: 10836893]

Crosby AG et al, eds: *About Children: An Authoritative Resource on the State of Childhood Today*. American Academy of Pediatrics, 2005. Available at: http://www.aap/org/AboutChildren.

Elimination

Regular patterns for voiding and defecation provide reassurance that the child is developing appropriately. Newborn infants are expected to void within 24 hours of birth. An infant urinates approximately 6–8 times a day. Parents may count diapers in the first few weeks to confirm adequate feeding. The older child usually voids 4–6 times daily. Changes in voiding frequency indicate the child's hydration status, especially when the child is ill.

Routine circumcision of male infants is not currently recommended so parents who are considering circumcision require additional guidance. A circumcised male has a decreased incidence of urinary tract infections (OR 3–5) and a decreased risk of phimosis and squamous cell carcinoma of the penis. However, some clinicians raise concerns about bleeding, infection, pain of the procedure, or damage to the genitalia (incidence of 0.2–0.6%). Therefore, the decision about circumcision is based on the parents' personal preferences and cultural influences.

The procedure is usually performed after the second day of life, on a physiologically stable infant. Contraindications include ambiguous genitalia, hypospadias, HIV, and any overriding medical conditions. The denuded mucosa of the phallus appears raw for the first week post-procedure, exuding a small amount of serosanguineous drainage on the diaper. Infection occurs in less than 1% of cases. Mild soap and water washes are the best method of cleansing the area. By the 2-week checkup, the phallus should be completely healed with a scar below the corona radiata. The parents should note whether the infant's urinary stream is straight and forceful.

Newborns are expected to pass black, tarry meconium stools within the first 24 hours of life. Failure to pass stool in that period necessitates a workup for Hirschsprung disease (aganglionic colon) or imperforate anus. Later on the consistency of the stool is usually semisolid and soft, with a yellow-green seedy appearance. Breast-fed infants typically stool after each feeding, but some defecate only two or three times a day. Bottle-fed infants generally have a lower frequency of stooling.

Occasionally, some infants may have only one stool every 2 or 3 days without discomfort. If the child seems to be grunting forcefully with defecation or is passing extremely hard stools, treatment with lubricants can be advised. Any appearance of blood in the stools is abnormal and warrants investigation. Anal fissure is common.

With the introduction of solid foods, stool becomes more solid and malodorous. Increased dietary intake of certain fruits, vegetables, and water often relieves constipation. Treatment of mild to moderate constipation may include the use of karo syrup mixed in with feedings (1–2 teaspoonfuls in 2 ounces of milk) or psyllium seed or mineral oil (15–30 mL) for older children. Children who are severely constipated may require referral to a gastroenterologist.

After the second year of age, the child may start toilet training for both urination and defecation. Monitoring the child's intake and output ensures that the behavioral challenges of continence do not lead to retention or constipation.

Lerman SE, Liao JC: Neonatal circumcision. Pediatr Clin North Am 2001;48:1539. [PMID: 11732129]

Oral Health

As other health outcomes improve, the poor state of oral health in children is now emerging as a major area of concern. Tooth decay remains one of the most common chronic diseases of childhood, even more common than asthma. Medically and developmentally compromised children and children from low-income families are at highest risk, and affected children remain at higher risk for cavities throughout their childhood and adulthood. To minimize the incidence of early childhood caries, children should not be put to sleep with a bottle or by breast-feeding. Parents should also be discouraged from inappropriately using the bottle or "sippy" cup as a pacifier. Dietary sugars along with cariogenic bacteria, most often acquired from the mother, lead to accelerated decay in the toddler's primary teeth.

Current recommendations encourage an initial oral evaluation to establish a dental home before the first birthday, within 6 months of the eruption of the first primary tooth, often around 6–9 months of age. Children should continue with regular biannual dental appointments thereafter. Primary prevention includes provision of a diet high in calcium and prescription of fluoride supplementation for those with an unfluoridated water supply (< 0.6 ppm). Once primary teeth erupt, parents should use a soft-bristled brush or washcloth with water to clean the teeth at least daily. Infants should drink from a cup and be weaned from the bottle at around 12–14 months of age. Pacifiers and thumb sucking are best limited after teeth have erupted. All children, toddler to school age, need limits on the intake of high-sugar drinks, especially between meals. (For further discussion and recommendations relating to oral health, see Chapter 45.)

Sanchez OM, Childers NK: Anticipatory guidance in infant oral health: Rationale and recommendations. Am Fam Physician 2000;61:115. [PMID: 10643953]

Sonis A, Zaragoza S: Dental health for the pediatrician. Curr Opin Pediatr 2001;13:289. [PMID: 11389366]

CLINICAL FEATURES

History & Physical Examination

The prenatal and neonatal records should be reviewed for gestational age at birth; any abnormal maternal obstetric laboratory tests; maternal illnesses such as diabetes, preeclampsia, depression, or infections that occurred during the pregnancy; maternal use of drugs or exposure to teratogens; date of birth; mode of delivery; Apgar scores at 1 and 5 minutes; and birth weight, length, and head circumference. A social history should include the family structure (caregivers, siblings, etc) and socioeconomic status.

A physical examination of the newborn should include:

- General observation: Evidence of birth trauma, dysmorphic facies, resting muscle tone, respiratory rate, skin discolorations, or rashes.
- Head, ears, eyes, nose, and throat (HEENT) examination: Mobile sutures, open fontanelles, bilateral retinal red reflexes, clarity of lens, nasal patency, absence of cleft palate or lip, and palpation of clavicles to rule out fracture.
- Cardiovascular examination: Cardiac murmurs, peripheral pulses, capillary refill, and the presence of cyanosis.
- Pulmonary examination: Use of accessory muscles and auscultation of breath sounds.
- Abdominal examination: Masses, distention, and the presence of bowel sounds.
- Extremity examination: Number and abnormalities of digits and toes, and screening for congenital dislocation of the hips using Ortolani and Barlow maneuvers.
- Genitourinary examination: Genitalia and anus.
- Neurologic examination: Presence of newborn reflexes (ie, rooting, grasping, sucking, stepping, and Moro).

A brief developmental assessment using the Clinical Neonatal Behavioral Assessment System (CLNBAS), a neurobehavioral assessment, in the presence of the parents can educate them about the capacities of their new child. The CLNBAS consists of 18 behavioral and reflex items designed to examine newborn physiologic and motor states that have an impact parents' caregiving in relation to sleep, feeding, crying, and consolability. Although the CLNBAS is not a formal screening tool for developmental delay, it may identify infants at risk for future problems. Furthermore, parents obtain valuable information regarding their infant's individuality and temperament, which can enable them to adjust care to better suit the infant's needs. All newborn infants should be placed on their backs to sleep to reduce the risk of sudden infant death syndrome.

Interval well child visits provide a valuable opportunity to track the child's physical and developmental progress. A comprehensive interval history and physical examination is important at each encounter, even if the parents do not report concerns. The child's weight (completely undressed), length, and head circumference (until 3 years of age) are measured at each visit. When plotted on standard CDC growth charts, a child's rate of growth will usually follow one percentile (25th, 50th, etc) from birth through school age. A child can appropriately cross percentiles upward (eg, a premature infant who then "catches up") or inappropriately (eg, a child who becomes obese). Any child who drops more than two percentiles over any period of time may be diagnosed with failure to thrive (see Chapter 2).

By 15 months of age, children experience stranger anxiety and are much less likely to be cooperative. Clinicians can minimize the child's adverse reactions by approaching the child slowly and performing the examination while the child is in the parent's arms, going from least to most invasive task. Touching the child's shoe first and then gradually moving up to the chest while distracting with a toy or otoscope light is often helpful. After the first year of life, the pace of the infant's growth begins to plateau. At the 15- to 18-month visit, the infant most likely will be mobile and may want to stand on the table during the examination. The child may become engaged if the clinician asks questions about where to do the examination or which body part to examine first.

Comprehensive examinations should continue annually from ages 2 to 6 years, concentrating primarily on the child's psychological and intellectual development. Beginning at 3 years of age, the child's blood pressure is measured and BMI is plotted. Eye examinations for strabismus allow early treatment. By age 4 or 5 years, documentation of visual acuity should be attempted. Hearing, often tested at birth, is informally evaluated until the age of 5 years, when audiometry should be attempted. At least 75% of speech in 3-year-olds should be intelligible. Speech delay should trigger referral. Physicians need to assess gait, spinal alignment, and injuries, looking particularly for signs of child abuse or neglect. Table 1–5 highlights the important components of the physical examination at each age.

Bordley WC et al: Improving preventive service delivery through office systems. Pediatrics 2001;108:E41. [PMID: 11533359]

DeVito GA Jr, Angelo W: Well child care: Ages 2 months to 2 years. In: *FP Essentials,* Edition No. 312, AAFP Home Study. American Academy of Family Physicians, May 2005:1–81.

Table 1–5. Highlights of physical examination by age.

Age of Child	Components of Examination
2 weeks	Presence of bilateral red reflex Auscultation of the heart for murmurs Palpation of the abdomen for masses Ortolani/Barlow maneuvers for hip dislocation Assessment of overall muscle tone Reattainment of birth weight
2 months	Observation of anatomic abnormalities or congenital malformations (effects of birth trauma resolved by this point) Auscultation of the heart for murmurs
4–6 months	Complete musculoskeletal examination (neck control, evidence of torticollis) Ortolani/Barlow maneuvers for hip dislocation (limited abduction, asymmetric buttock creases) Metatarsus adductus Vision assessment (conjugate gaze, symmetric light reflex, visual tracking of an object to 180°) Bilateral descent of testes
9 months	Pattern and degree of tooth eruption Assessment of muscle tone Presence of bilateral pincer grasp Observation of crawling behavior
12 months	Range of motion of the hips, rotation and leg alignment Bilateral descent of the testes
15–18 months	Cover test for strabismus Signs of dental caries Gait assessment Any evidence of injuries

Screening Laboratory Tests

Every state requires newborns to undergo serologic screening for inborn errors of metabolism. Requirements vary from state to state. The most commonly screened diseases along with their biochemical markers are listed in Table 1–6. Some institutions routinely screen newborns for hearing loss, but the US Preventive Services Task Force has not recommended for or against universal screening (level I recommendation).

Screening for anemia with finger stick hemoglobin levels begins between the ages of 9 and 12 months. Due to the high prevalence of iron deficiency anemia in toddlers, repeat screenings has been recommended approximately 6 months after the first screening. Measurement of hemoglobin or hematocrit levels alone detects only those patients

Table 1–6. Commonly screened components of newborn screening panels.[1]

Diseases Screened	Incidence of Disease in Live Births
Congenital hypothyroidism	1:4000
Duchenne muscular dystrophy	1:4500
Congenital adrenal hyperplasia	1:10,000–1:18,000
Phenylketonuria	1:14,000
Galactosemia	1:30,000
Cystic fibrosis	1:44,000–1:80,000 (depending on population)
Biotinidase deficiency	1:60,000

[1]Screening panel requirements vary in each state.
Source: Newborn Screening Fact Sheets. American Academy of Pediatrics Policy Statement. http://www.aap.org/policy/01565.html.

with iron levels low enough to become anemic. For this reason, some authorities recommend screening by ferritin levels or red cell distribution width (RDW) to identify iron deficiency earlier. A positive screening test is an indication for a therapeutic trial of iron to establish a diagnosis of iron deficiency. Thalassemia minor is the major differential consideration. A sickle cell screen is indicated in all African-American children.

Annual lead screening begins at age 9 months to 1 year if the child is considered to be at high risk. Risk factors include exposure to chipping or peeling paint in buildings built before 1950, frequent contact with an adult who may have significant lead exposure, having a sibling who is being treated for a high lead level, and location of the home near an industrial setting likely to release lead fumes. Many agencies require a one-time universal lead screening at 1 year of age.

Tuberculosis screening using a purified protein derivative (PPD) is offered to high-risk children at 1 year of age. Routine testing of children without risk factors is not indicated. Children require testing if they have had contact with persons with confirmed or suspected cases of infectious tuberculosis, if they have emigrated from endemic countries such as those in Asia or the Middle East, or if they have any clinical or radiographic findings suggestive of tuberculosis. HIV-infected children need to have PPD tests annually. Children at risk due to exposure to high-risk adults (HIV positive, homeless, institutionalized, etc) are retested every 2–3 years. Children without specific risk factors but who live in high-prevalence communities may be retested twice: once at ages 4–6 years and again at ages 11–12 years.

A cholesterol level may be obtained after age 2 years if the child has a notable family history of early coronary artery disease. The National Cholesterol Education Program (NCEP) recommends screening in a child with a parent who has a total cholesterol of 240 mg/dL or greater or a parent or grandparent with onset of cardiovascular disease before age 55 years. Clinical evaluation and management of the child are to be initiated if the low-density lipoprotein (LDL) cholesterol level is 130 mg/dL or greater.

Although formal audiometry and visual acuity testing can begin as early as age 3 years, failure to meet informal developmental milestones should trigger earlier referral. A screening urinalysis is not indicated.

Guide to Clinical Preventive Services, 3rd ed, 2000–2003. Report of the US Preventive Services Task Force. Available at: http://www. ahcpr.gov/clinic/cps3dix.htm.

Kohli-Kumar M: Screening for anemia in children: AAP recommendations—a critique. Pediatrics 2001;108:E56. [PMID: 11533374]

Kronn DF et al: Management of hypercholesterolemia in childhood and adolescence. Heart Dis 2000;2:348. [PMID: 11728281]

CONCERNS IN NORMALLY DEVELOPING CHILDREN

A wide variation exists in the spectrum of child behavior, with the majority of these behaviors considered normal if the child is growing normally and meeting developmental milestones. Anticipatory guidance regarding variations from ideal behavior can be very helpful and reassuring to caregivers when their child exhibits such characteristics. Selected behavioral issues that are commonly encountered include infantile colic, temper tantrums, and reluctant toilet training.

Infantile Colic

Colic is a term often used to describe an infant who is difficult to manage or fussy despite being otherwise healthy. Colic may be defined as 3 or more hours of uncontrollable crying or fussing at least three times a week for at least 3 weeks. Other symptoms include facial expressions of pain or discomfort, pulling up of the legs, passing flatus, fussiness with eating, and difficulty falling or staying asleep. Symptoms classically worsen during the evening hours. Because the diagnosis depends on parental report, the incidence of colic varies from 5% to 20%. It occurs equally in both sexes.

The underlying cause of colic is unknown, but organic pathology is present in less than 5% of the cases. Possible etiologies include an immature digestive system sensitive to certain food proteins, an immature nervous system sensitive to external stimuli, or a mismatch of the infant's temperament and those of caregivers. Feeding method is probably unrelated to incidence, which peaks around 3–4 weeks of age. Clinicians can provide reassurance to caregivers of children with colic by informing them that colicky children continue to eat and gain weight appropriately, despite the prolonged periods of crying, and that the syndrome is self-limited and usually dissipates once the child reaches 3–4 months of age. Colic has no known long-term consequences; therefore, the main problem for caregivers is to cope with anxiety over the crying child. A stressed caregiver who is unable to handle the situation is at risk for abusing a child.

No definitive treatment can be offered for colic. Little evidence supports the use of simethicone or acetaminophen drops. Switching to a hypoallergenic (soy) formula is effective when the child has other symptoms suggestive of cow's milk protein allergy. Breast-feeding mothers can attempt to make changes in their diets (eg, avoidance of cruciferous vegetables such as broccoli, cabbage, etc) to see if the infant improves. Both clinicians and caregivers have proposed many "home remedies." Reducing the amount of stimulation or sometimes changing the scenery with a car ride or walk outdoors is recommended. Frequent burping, swaddling the infant, infant massage, or the use of a crib vibrator or increasing background noise from household appliances have been shown to be moderately effective. Rigorous study of these techniques is difficult, but clinicians can suggest any or all because the potential harm is minimal.

Temper Tantrums

A normal part of child development temper tantrums encompass excessive crying, screaming, kicking, thrashing, head banging, breath-holding, breaking or throwing objects, and aggression. Between the ages of 1 and 3 years, a child's growing sense of independence is in conflict with physical limitations and parental controls and hampered because of limited vocabulary and inability to express feelings or experiences. This power struggle sets the stage for the expression of anger and frustration through a temper tantrum. Tantrums can follow minor frustrations, occur for no obvious reason, and are mostly self-limited. A child's tendency toward impulsivity or impatience or a delay in the development of motor skills or cognitive deficits, and parental inconsistency—excessive restrictiveness, overindulgence, or overreaction—may increase the incidence of tantrums. Tantrums that produce a desired effect have an increased likelihood of recurrence.

As much as possible, parents should provide a predictable home environment. Consistency in routines and rules will help the child know what to expect. Parents should prepare the child for transitions from one activity to another, offer some simple choices to satisfy the child's growing need for control, acknowledge the child's wants during a tantrum, and act calmly when handling negative behaviors to avoid reinforcement. Physical punishment is not advised.

Most importantly, ignoring attention-seeking tantrums and not giving in to the demands of the tantrum will, in time, decrease the recurrence. Children who are disruptive enough to hurt themselves or others must be removed to a safe place and given time to calm down in a nonpunitive manner. Most children learn to work out their frustrations with their own set of problem-solving and coping skills, thus terminating tantrums. Persistence of tantrums beyond age 4 or 5 years requires further investigation and usually includes referral or group education and counseling.

Toilet Training

Some indicators of readiness for toilet use include an awareness of impending urination or defecation, prolonged involuntary dryness, and the ability to walk easily, to pull clothes on and off easily, to follow instructions, to identify body parts, and to initiate simple tasks. These indicators are not likely to be present until 18–30 months of age. Once the child becomes interested in bathroom activities or in watching his or her parents use the toilet, parents should provide a potty chair. Parents can then initiate toilet training by taking the diaper off and sitting the child on the potty at a time when she or he is likely to urinate or defecate. Routine sittings on the potty at specified times, such as after meals when the gastrocolic reflex is functional, may be helpful. The child who is straining or bending at the waist may be escorted to the bathroom for a toileting trial. If the child eliminates in the potty or toilet, praise or a small reward may be given to reinforce that behavior. Stickers, storybooks, or added time with the parents can be used for motivation.

With repeated successes transitional diapers or training pants may be used until full continence is achieved. The training process may take days to months, and caregivers can expect accidents. Accidents need to be dealt with plainly; the child should not be punished or made to feel guilty or forced to sit on the toilet for prolonged periods. Significant constipation can be treated medically, because it may present a barrier to training. About 80% of children achieve success at daytime continence by 30 months of age.

As with many child-rearing issues, consistency and a nurturing environment give the child a sense of security. Training should not start too early or during times of family stress. Parents can be asked to describe specific scenarios so concrete anticipatory guidance may be given to deal with any barriers. Toilet training, as with most behavior modification, has a higher chance of success if positive achievements are rewarded and failures are not emphasized.

Table 1–7. Medical problems commonly diagnosed in childhood.

Problem	Definition	Prevalence	Risk Factors	Assessment	Treatment
Developmental dysplasia of hips	Spectrum of abnormalities that cause hip instability, ranging from dislocation to inadequate development of acetabulum	8–25 cases per 1000 births	Female gender Breech delivery Family history Possibly birth weight > 4 kg	Diagnosis: ultrasound in infants < 6 mo; x-rays > 6 mo Screening by clinical examination at well child visits is of marginal use	Abduction splints in infants < 6 mo; open or closed reduction more effective in those > 6 mo Optimal treatment remains controversial; consider orthopedic referral
Congenital heart disease	Major—large VSDs, severe valvular stenosis, cyanotic disease Minor—small VSDs mild valvular stenosis	5–8 cases per 1000 newborns, 50% with major disease and 50% with minor disease	Maternal diabetes or connective tissue disease Congenital infections (CMV, HSV, rubella, or coxsackievirus) Drugs taken during pregnancy Family history Down syndrome	Major disease presents shortly after birth Minor disease can present with murmur, tachycardia, tachypnea, pallor, peripheral pulses	Cardiology evaluation and surgical treatment options
Cryptorchidism	Testicles are absent or undescended Absence due to agenesis or vascular compromise	2–5% of full-term and 30% of premature male infants Prevalence varies geographically	Disorders of testosterone secretion Abdominal wall defects Trisomies	Increased risk of inguinal hernia, testicular torsion, infertility, and testicular cancer	Hormonal or surgical treatment, or both; can start at 6 mo of age and should be completed before 2 y
Pyloric stenosis	Hypertrophy of pylorus, with elongation and thickening; progresses to obstruction of gastric outlet	3 cases per 1000 live births	Male infants First-born infants Unconjugated hyperbilirubinemia	Diagnosis by clinical examination, ultrasound, or upper GI series Electrolyte abnormalities (metabolic alkalosis)	Surgical repair
Hypospadias	Ventral location of urethral meatus (anywhere from proximal glans to perineum)	~ 1 case per 250 male births	Advanced maternal age Maternal diabetes mellitus Caucasian ethnicity Delivery before 37 weeks' gestation	Check for other abnormalities (cryptorchidism) and rule out intersex conditions (congenital adrenal hyperplasia)	Circumcision contraindicated Urology referral, usually within 3–6 mo

Inguinal hernia	Protrusion of tissue or organ through an abnormal opening in muscle wall that normally contains it	1–5% of all newborns and 9–11% of those born prematurely	Male gender (3:1) Right side more common than left Often bilateral	Diagnosis by ultrasound Rule out incarceration and strangulation; incidence of both is highest during first year of life	Inguinal hernia repair is the most commonly performed surgical procedure in children (usually bilateral laparoscopic approach)
Childhood anemia	Hemoglobin level < 11.0 g/dL	Toddlers 1–3 y (9% iron deficient; 3% anemic)	Iron deficiency Excessive intake of cow's milk (< 16 oz/d) Thalassemia minor Lead poisoning	Rule out GI blood loss, malabsorption, and chronic inflammatory diseases	Therapeutic trial of iron supplements
Lead toxicity	Elevated blood lead levels > 10 mcg/dL (0.48 μmol/L)	1.6% among all US children[1]	Exposure to environmental lead through ingestion or inhalation Children < 6 y are susceptible to toxic effects due to immature nervous system, iron deficiency, crawling, and hand-to-mouth behavior	Confirmatory venous blood samples needed Symptoms include abdominal pain, vomiting, mental retardation, behavioral issues, developmental disorders, seizure, encephalopathy, anemia, and renal insufficiency	All children with high levels of lead need action—public health department should be notified for home inspection and environmental remediation Children with lead levels > 70 mcg/dL (3.38 μmol/L) need hospitalization for severe intoxication
Strabismus	Anomaly of ocular alignment (one or both eyes, any direction)	~ 2–4% of population	Family history Low birth weight Retinopathy of prematurity Cataract	Clinical tests: corneal light reflex, red reflex, cover test, and cover/uncover test	Child should be referred to pediatric ophthalmologist for early treatment to reduce visual loss (amblyopia)
Asthma	Chronic inflammatory disorder of airways with variable degrees of obstruction, causing cough, wheezing, and dyspnea	Most common chronic disease of childhood—prevalence of 126 cases per 1000 population; 80% develop symptoms before 5 y	Family history of asthma or allergy Exposure to secondhand smoke in infancy African–American ethnicity	Pulmonary function testing	Bronchodilators, anti-inflammatory inhalers, trigger avoidance, and education

VSD, ventricular septal defect; CMV, cytomegalovirus; HSV, herpes simplex virus; GI, gastrointestinal; y, years; mo, months.
[1]1999–2000 data.

Barlow J, Stewart-Brown S: Behavior problems and group-based parent education programs. J Dev Behav Pediatr 2000;21: 356. [PMID: 11064964]

Roberts DM et al: Infantile colic. Am Fam Physician 2004;70:735. [PMID: 15338787]

Wolraich ML, ed: *Guide to Toilet Training.* American Academy of Pediatrics, 2003.

MEDICAL PROBLEMS

Beyond the normal variations in child development, the family physician may need to identify and treat significant medical problems. Early diagnosis and referral lead to prevention of potentially serious sequelae and improved quality of life. Some of the major abnormalities detected in the young child (Table 1–7) underscore the importance of regular and thorough well child care visits with the family physician.

Centers for Disease Control and Prevention: *Managing Elevated Blood Lead Levels Among Young Children: Recommendations from the Advisory Committee on Childhood Lead Poisoning Prevention, March 2002.* Available at: http://www.cdc.gov/nceh/lead/lead.htm.

D'Agostino J: Common abdominal emergencies in children. Emerg Med Clin North Am 2002;20:139. [PMID: 11826631]

Docimo SG et al: The undescended testicle: Diagnosis and management. Am Fam Physician 2000;62:2037. [PMID: 11087186]

Hermiston ML, Mentzer WC: A practical approach to the evaluation of the anemic child. Pediatr Clin North Am 2002;49:877. [PMID: 12430617]

Kazal LA Jr: Prevention of iron deficiency in infants and toddlers. Am Fam Physician 2002;66:1217. [PMID: 12387433]

Simon JW, Kaw P: Commonly missed diagnoses in the childhood eye examination. Am Fam Physician 2001;64:623. [PMID: 11529261]

Weeks B, Friedman AH: Training pediatric residents to evaluate congenital heart disease in the current era. Pediatr Clin North Am 2004;51:1641. [PMID: 15561178]

Witt C: Detecting developmental dysplasia of the hip. Adv Neonatal Care 2003;3:65. [PMID: 12881948]

Wood, RA: Pediatric asthma. JAMA 2002;288:745. [PMID: 12169079]

Wren T: Penile and testicular disorders. Nurs Clin North Am 2004;39:319. [PMID: 15159182]

Failure to Thrive

2

Deborah Auer Flomenhoft, MD

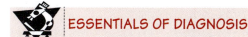

ESSENTIALS OF DIAGNOSIS

- *Persistent weight loss over time.*
- *Weight below the third percentile for age.*
- *Weight crosses two major percentiles downward over any period of time and continues to fall.*
- *Median weight for age of 76–90% (mild undernutrition), 61–75% (moderate undernutrition), or less than 61% (severe undernutrition).*
- *Most prevalent in at-risk populations least likely to have good continuity of care.*

General Considerations

Failure to thrive (FTT) is an old problem that continues to be an important entity for all practitioners who provide care to children. Growth is one of the essential tasks of childhood and is an indication of the child's general health. Growth failure may be the first symptom of serious organ dysfunction. Most frequently, however, growth failure represents inadequate caloric intake. Malnutrition during the critical period of brain growth in early childhood has been linked to delayed motor, cognitive, and social development. Developmental deficits may persist even after nutritional therapy has been instituted.

FTT was first described by Holt in 1897: he describes a group of children who suddenly "ceased to thrive" and became "wasted skeletons" when weaned after the first 4–6 weeks of life. More than 100 years later there is no consensus definition of FTT. Residents and medical students need to be familiar with several definitions of FTT. Practitioners must also recognize the limitations of each definition. Competing definitions of FTT include the following:

- **Persistent weight loss over time.** Children should steadily gain weight. Weight loss beyond the setting of an acute illness is pathologic. However, the assessment and treatment of FTT need to be addressed *before* the child has had persistent weight loss.
- **Growth failure associated with disordered behavior and development.** This old definition is useful because it reminds the practitioner of the serious sequelae associated with undernutrition. Currently, FTT is more commonly defined by anthropometric guidelines alone.
- **Weight less than the third percentile for age** is a classic definition. However, this definition includes children with genetic short stature and children whose weight transiently dips beneath the third percentile with an intercurrent illness.
- **Weight crosses two major percentiles downward over any period of time.** Thirty percent of normal children will drop two major percentiles within the first 2 years of life as their growth curve shifts to their genetic potential. These healthy children will continue to grow on the adjusted growth curve. Children with FTT do not attain a new curve, but continue to fall.

The preceding statements comprise the classic definitions, but perhaps not the most useful. An assessment of **the percentage of the child's median weight for age** is the most clinically useful definition of FTT. This quick calculation enables the clinician to assess the degree of undernutrition and plan an appropriate course of evaluation and intervention. The median weight for age is determined by the US Centers for Disease Control and Prevention (CDC) growth charts. The median should not be adjusted for race, ethnicity, or country of origin. Differences in growth that had previously been attributed to these factors are more likely due to inadequate nutrition in specific geographic or economically deprived populations. Determinations of nutritional status are as follows:

Mild undernutrition: 76–90% median weight for age. These children are in no immediate danger and may be safely observed over time.

Moderate undernutrition: 61–75% median weight for age. These children warrant immediate evaluation and intervention with close follow-up in an outpatient setting.

Severe undernutrition: less than 61% median weight for age. These children may require hospitalization for evaluation and nutritional support.

FTT is one of the most common diagnoses of early childhood in the United States. It affects all socioeconomic groups, although children living in poverty are more likely to be affected and more likely to suffer long-term sequelae. FTT comprises between 3% and 5% of all hospital admissions for children younger than 2 years. Ten percent of children living in poverty meet criteria for FTT. As many as 30% of children presenting to emergency departments for unrelated complaints can be diagnosed with FTT. This last group of children is of most concern. They are least likely to have good continuity of care and most likely to suffer additional developmental insults such as social isolation, tenuous housing situations, and neglect. Because FTT is most prevalent in at-risk populations that are least likely to have good continuity of care, it is crucial to address growth parameters at *every* visit, both sick and well. Many children with FTT may not present for well child visits: if that is the only visit at which the clinician considers growth, many opportunities for meaningful intervention may be lost.

Pathogenesis

When diagnosing FTT it is essential to consider the etiology. Historically there has been a dichotomy: organic versus nonorganic FTT. Either children had major organ dysfunction (organic) or psychosocial problems led to inadequate nutrition (nonorganic). Over the past decades FTT has been better understood as a mixed entity in which both organic disease and psychosocial factors influence each other. With this understanding, the old belief that a child who gains weight in the hospital has nonorganic FTT has been debunked.

A. Organic FTT

Organic causes are identified in 10% of children with FTT. In-hospital evaluations reveal an underlying organic etiology in about 30% of children. However, these data are misleading. More than two thirds of these children are diagnosed with gastroesophageal reflux disease (GERD). The practitioner risks one of two errors in diagnosing GERD as the source of FTT. Physiologic reflux is found in as many as 70% of infants; it may be a normal finding in an infant who is failing to thrive for other reasons. Further, undernutrition causes decreased lower esophageal segment tone, which may lead to reflux as an effect rather than a cause of FTT.

B. Nonorganic FTT

Nonorganic FTT, weight loss in which no physiologic disease is identified, constitutes 80% of cases. Historically, the responsibility for this diagnosis fell on the caregiver. Either the parent was unable to provide enough nutrition or the parent was emotionally unavailable to the infant. In either circumstance the result was unsuccessful feeding. Psychosocial stressors were thought to create a neuroendocrine milieu preventing growth even when calories were available (ie, increased cortisol and decreased insulin levels in undernourished children inhibit weight gain).

C. Mixed FTT

Most FTT is neither purely organic nor nonorganic, but rather *mixed*: there is a transaction between both physiologic and psychosocial factors that creates a vicious cycle of undernutrition. For example, a child with organic disease may initially have difficulty eating for purely physiologic reasons. However, over time, the feedings become fraught with anxiety for both parents and child and are even less successful. The child senses the parents' anxiety and eats less and more fretfully than before. The parents, afraid to overtax the "fragile" child, may not give the child the time needed to eat. They may become frustrated that they are not easily able to accomplish this most basic and essential component of care for the child. Parents of an ill child may perceive that other aspects of care are more important than feeding, such as strict adherence to a medication or therapy regimen.

Children with organic disease underlying FTT often gain weight in the hospital when fed by emotionally uninvolved parties such as nurses, volunteers, or physicians: these people do not feel that the child's difficulties represent personal failure and may be more patient. They are also not the sole providers for all of the child's needs. This happy circumstance (weight gain in the hospital) should not be mistaken for parental neglect in the home; rather, the primary care provider should pay close attention to the psychosocial stressors on the feeding dyad.

Conversely the child who seems to be failing to thrive for purely psychosocial reasons often has complicating organic issues. The undernourished child is lethargic and irritable, especially at feeding times. As previously noted, undernutrition decreases lower esophageal sphincter tone and may worsen reflux: the undernourished child is more difficult to feed and holds down fewer calories. Poor nutrition adversely affects immunity: children with FTT often have recurrent infections that increase their caloric requirements and decrease their ability to meet them.

The mixed model reminds the clinician that FTT is an interactive process involving physiologic and psychosocial elements and, more importantly, both parent and child. The child's attributes affect the relationship as surely as the parents'. A fussy child may be more difficult for a particular parent to feed. A "good" or passive infant may not elicit enough feeding. Physical characteristics also affect parent-child relationships: organic disease not only may make feeding difficult but also may engender a sense of failure or disappointment in the parent. It is crucial to remember that each child is different; parents have unique relationships with each of their children. Therefore, a parent whose first child is

Table 2–1. Causes of failure to thrive.

Decreased Caloric Intake	Increased Caloric Requirement	Impaired Utilization/Loss
Neurologic disorders	Sepsis	Inborn errors of metabolism
Structural anomalies	Trauma	Storage diseases
Injury or infection of mouth or esophagus	Burns	Pyloric stenosis
Chromosomal abnormalities	Congenital heart disease	GERD
Metabolic disease	Renal disease	Pancreatic insufficiency
Improper formula preparation	Cystic fibrosis	Brush border enzyme deficiency (after chronic diarrhea)
Inappropriate diet	Chronic infection: HIV; TB	Short bowel
Food allergies	Hyperthyroidism; malignancy	IBD; celiac disease
Anorexia	Cerebral palsy	Parasitic infection: *Giardia*
Parental/infant factors	Sickle cell disease	Chronic enteric infection
Asthma	Asthma	Diabetes mellitus; Addison's disease
BPD	BPD	Allergies

GERD, gastroesophageal reflux disease; HIV, human immunodeficiency virus; TB, tuberculosis; IBD, inflammatory bowel disease; BPD, bronchopulmonary dysplasia.

diagnosed with FTT is not doomed to repeat the cycle with the second child. Conversely, an experienced parent who has fed previous children successfully is not immune from the specter of FTT.

D. Causes of FTT

All FTT is caused by undernutrition; however, the mechanism varies. The child may have increased caloric requirements because of organic disease or have inadequate intake, either because not enough food is made available or because of mechanical difficulty in eating. Alternately, adequate calories may be provided but the child may be unable to utilize them either because nutrients cannot be absorbed across the bowel wall or because of inborn errors of metabolism (Table 2–1).

The astute clinician will note that there may be overlap between these mechanisms. For example, a child with cystic fibrosis has increased caloric requirements associated with chronic respiratory tract infections. However, shortness of breath may make it difficult for the child to eat sufficient quantities, and the associated pancreatic insufficiency limits nutrient absorption.

Prevention

FTT may be prevented by good communication between the primary care provider and the family. The practitioner should regularly assess feeding practices and growth and educate parents about appropriate age-specific diets. As a general rule, infants who are feeding successfully gain about:

- 30 g/day at 0–3 months.
- 20 g/day at 3–6 months.
- 15 g/day at 6–9 months.
- 12 g/day at 9–12 months.
- 8 g/day at 1–3 years.

In addition, growth parameters need to be recorded at every visit, sick or well. Weight should be documented for all children. Recumbent length is measured for children younger than 2 years. Height is measured for children older than 3 years. Between the ages of 2 and 3 years either height or length may be recorded. Length measurements exceed heights by an average of 1 cm. With a good growth chart in hand, the primary care provider can monitor growth and intervene early if problems arise.

Clinicians should investigate the economic stresses on families. In a family struggling with recent unemployment or underemployment, referral to a walk-in clinic or other social support programs may prevent hunger and subsequent FTT.

Clinical Findings

A. Symptoms and Signs

The importance of a complete, long-term growth curve in making the diagnosis of FTT cannot be overemphasized. Acute undernutrition manifests as "wasting"; the velocity of weight gain decreases while height velocity continues to be preserved. The result is a thin child of normal height. Chronic undernutrition manifests as "stunting"; both height and weight are affected. The child may appear proportionately small. Review of a growth curve may reveal that weight was initially affected and increase the suspicion for FTT.

B. History

The clinician's most valuable tool in the diagnosis of FTT is the history. While taking the history, health care providers have the opportunity to establish themselves as the child's advocate and the parents' support. Care must be taken not to establish an adversarial relationship with the parents. It is useful to begin by asking the parents their perception of their child's health; many parents do not recognize FTT until the clinician brings it to their attention.

The history and physical examination are more valuable than any standard battery of tests in uncovering significant organ dysfunction contributing to growth failure. For example, the child who feeds poorly may have a physical impediment to caloric intake such as cleft palate or painful dental caries. Poor suck may also raise concerns for neurologic disease. Recurrent upper or lower respiratory tract infections may suggest cystic fibrosis, HIV infection, or immunodeficiency. Sweating during feeding should prompt consideration of an underlying cardiac problem with or without cyanosis. Chronic diarrhea indicates malabsorption: chronic infection, allergic disease, celiac disease, and pancreatic insufficiency should be evaluated.

The health care provider must elicit more subtle aspects of the past medical history as well: particular attention must be paid to developmental history and intercurrent illnesses. Delay in achievement of milestones should prompt a close neurologic examination: inborn errors of metabolism and cerebral palsy can present with growth failure. A history of recurrent serious illness may be the only indicator of inborn errors of metabolism. Recurrent febrile illness without a clear source may indicate urinary tract infection. A history of snoring or sleep apnea should prompt an evaluation for tonsillar and adenoidal hypertrophy, which has been identified as a cause of FTT.

Past medical history must include a complete perinatal history. Children with lower birth weights and those with specific prenatal exposures are at higher risk for growth problems. Birth weights were below 2500 g in 40% of children with FTT versus only 7% of all births.

Low birth weights may be caused by infection, drug exposure, or other maternal and placental factors. The child with symmetric growth retardation is of particular concern. Infants exposed *in utero* to rubella, cytomegalovirus, syphilis, toxoplasmosis, or malaria are at high risk for low birth weight, decreased length, and decreased head circumference. These measurements portend poor catch-up growth potential. Short stature is often accompanied by developmental delay and mental retardation in these children.

Children with asymmetric intrauterine growth retardation (preserved head circumference) have better potential for catch-up growth and appropriate development. Fetal growth is affected by both maternal factors and exposure to toxins. Drugs of abuse such as tobacco, cocaine, and heroin have been correlated with low birth weight. Placental insufficiency caused by hypertension, preeclampsia, collagen vascular disease, or diabetes may result in an undernourished infant with decreased birth weight. And, finally, intrauterine physical factors may reduce the fetus's growth: uterine malformation, multiple gestation, and fibroids may all contribute to smaller infants.

A careful investigation of the health of the mother is warranted. Maternal HIV infection is a significant risk factor for FTT. Most children born to HIV-infected mothers have normal birth weights and lengths. However, children who are infected frequently develop FTT within the first year of life.

An examination of family members' relationships with the child and one another can uncover valuable information. Children described as "difficult" or "unpredictable" by their mothers have been noted to be slow or poor feeders by independent observers. Maternal depression and history of abuse are strong risk factors for FTT; addressing these issues is integral to establishing a functional feeding relationship between parent and child. Finally, a thorough assessment of economic supports may reveal that nutritious foods are unobtainable or difficult to access. Social financial supports are often inadequate to meet children's needs: the supplemental nutrition program for Women, Infants, and Children (WIC) provides about 26 ounces of formula per day, and food stamps provide three dollars per person per day. Tenuous housing or homelessness may make it impossible to keep appropriate foods readily available.

C. Feeding History

A careful feeding history constitutes the history of present illness; it often sheds more light on the problem than a battery of laboratory tests. When assessing an infant, it is essential to know what formula the infant is taking, what volume, and how frequently. Careful attention must be paid to the mixing of formula. Pictograms on the back of powdered formulas routinely show a single scoop of formula being added to a full bottle of water, and families that are non-English speaking or have low literacy skills may be inadvertently mixing dilute formula. In calculating caloric intake, the practitioner should remember that breast milk and formula have 20 cal/ounce. Baby foods range from 40 to 120 cal/jar: a good rule is 80 cal/4-ounce jar.

How the infant eats is as important as how much he or she eats. The examiner should ask how long it takes the infant to eat: slow eating may be associated with poor suck or decreased stamina secondary to organic dysfunction. Parental estimation of the infant's suck may also be helpful. Parents should be asked both if the infant is "spitty" and if the infant vomits frequently, as they may endorse one symptom and deny the other. The clinician should inquire about feeding techniques: bottle propping may indicate a poor parent–child relationship or an overtaxed parent.

The breast-fed infant merits special mention. The sequelae of unsuccessful breast-feeding are profound. Infants may present with severe dehydration: normal infants have been neurologically devastated and even died. Parents rarely recognize that the infant is failing to thrive. Mothers are often discharged from the hospital before their breasts are fully producing milk and may be unsure about what to expect or misinterpret their experience in the hospital as successful nursing.

The neonatal period is the most critical period in the establishment of breast-feeding. The primary care provider should educate the breast-feeding mother prior to hospital discharge. Transitional milk should be produced by day 3 or 4 and mature milk by day 10. The neonate should feed at least eight times in a 24-hour period and should not be sleeping through the night. Report of a "good baby"—that is, a newborn infant who sleeps through the night—should rouse concerns of possible dehydration. Breast-fed infants should have at least six wet diapers a day. Whereas formula-fed infants may have many stool patterns, the successful breast-fed neonate should have at least 4–6 yellow seedy stools a day. After 4 weeks of life, stool pattern may change to once a day or less.

Breast-fed neonates should be followed up within the first week of life to evaluate infant weight and feeding success. Weight loss is expected until day 5 of life. Neonates should regain their birthweight by the end of the second week of life. Any weight loss greater than 8% should elicit concern: weight loss greater than 10–12% should prompt evaluation for dehydration (ie, serum sodium). Primary care providers should ask about the infant's suck and whether the mother feels her breasts are emptied at the feeding. The successful infant should empty the mother's breast and be contented at the end of the nursing session. Breast-feeding is discussed in more detail in Chapter 4.

The evaluation of older children also requires a thorough diet history. An accurate diet history begins with a 24-hour diet recall: parents should be asked to quantify the amount their child has eaten of each food. The 24-hour recall acts as a template for a 72-hour diet diary, the most accurate assessment of intake; the first 48 hours of the diet diary are the most reliable. All intakes must be recorded, including juices, water, and snacks. The child who consumes an excessive amount of milk or juice may not have the appetite to eat more nutrient-rich foods: a child needs no more than 16–24 ounces of milk and should be limited to less than 12 ounces of juice per day.

It is as important to assess mealtime habits as the meals themselves. Activity in the household during mealtime may be distracting to young children. Television watching may preempt eating. Excessive attention to how much the child eats can increase the tension and ultimately decrease the child's intake. Most toddlers cannot sit for longer than 15 minutes: prolonging the table time in the hopes of increasing the amount eaten may only exacerbate the already fragile parent-child relationship. And although many toddlers graze throughout the day, some are unable to take in appropriate calories with this strategy.

The primary care provider should also discuss the family's beliefs about a healthy diet. Some families have dietary restrictions, either by choice or culturally, that affect growth. Many have read the dietary recommendations for a healthy adult diet, but a low-fat, low-cholesterol diet is not an appropriate diet for a toddler. Until the age of 2 years children should drink whole milk and their fats should not be limited. Only after the age of 5 years is it appropriate to move to an American Heart Association Step 1 diet. This may seem counterintuitive to many parents.

D. Physical Examination

In addition to reviewing the growth curve the clinician must complete a physical examination. Weight, length, or height measurements, as appropriate for the child's age, and head circumference are indicated for all children. Growth parameters may be roughly interpreted using the following guidelines:

- **Acute undernutrition:** low weight, normal height, normal head circumference.
- **Chronic undernutrition:** short height, normal weight for height, normal head circumference.
- **Acute or chronic undernutrition:** short height, proportionately low weight for height, normal head circumference.
- **Congenital infection or genetic disorder impairing growth:** short height, normal to low weight for height, small head circumference.

The general examination provides a wealth of information. Vital signs should be documented: bradycardia and hypotension are worrisome findings in the malnourished child and should prompt immediate hospitalization. It is important to document observations of the parent-child interaction in the physical examination: are the parent and child responsive to one another or is the child lying unattended on the examining table? In the same vein, it is useful to note both the parent's and the child's affect: parental depression has been associated with higher risk of FTT. And, as previously noted, the child's disposition is integral in shaping the parent-child relationship. Occasionally the examiner may find subtle indications of neglect such as a flat occiput, indicating that the child is left alone for long periods. However, in this day of "Back to Sleep" a flat occiput may be a normal finding.

In children who are undernourished, objective findings of their nutritional state are often present. Unlike the genetically small child, children with FTT have decreased subcutaneous fat. If undernutrition has been prolonged they will also have muscle wasting. In infants it is easier to assess muscle wasting in the calves and thighs rather than in the interosseous muscles. It is also important to remember that infants suck rather than chew; therefore, they will not have the characteristic facies of temporal wasting. Nail beds and hair should be carefully noted, because nutritional deficiencies may cause pitting or lines in the nails. Hair may be thin or brittle. Skin should be examined for scaling and cracking, which may be seen with both zinc and fatty acid deficiencies.

The physical examination should be completed with special attention directed to the organ systems of concern uncovered in the history. However, examination of some organ systems may reveal abnormalities not elicited through the history. A thorough abdominal examination is of particular importance: organomegaly in the child with FTT raises the possibility of inborn errors of metabolism and requires laboratory evaluation. The examiner should note the genitourinary examination: undescended testicles may indicate panhypopituitarism; ambiguous genitalia may indicate congenital adrenogenital hyperplasia. A careful neurologic examination may reveal subtly increased tone consistent with cerebral palsy and, therefore, increased caloric requirements. Finally, the examiner must not neglect the rectal examination: fissures and hemorrhoids can be signs of inflammatory bowel disease in young children.

Children who are undernourished have been repeatedly shown to have behavioral and cognitive delays. Unfortunately the Denver Developmental Screening Test–revised (DDST II) is an inadequate tool to assess the subtle but real delays in these children. It has been suggested that the Bayley Test may be a more sensitive tool when assessing these children. Even with nutritional and social support, behavioral and cognitive lags may not correct. Children who have suffered FTT remain sensitive to undernutrition throughout childhood: one study found a significant decrease in fluency in children with a remote history of undernutrition when they did not eat breakfast. Children with a normal nutritional history were not found to be similarly affected.

The immune system is affected by nutritional status. Children with FTT may present with recurrent mucosal infections: otitis media, sinusitis, pneumonia, and gastroenteritis. Immunoglobulin A production is extremely sensitive to undernutrition. With this in mind, the clinician must be sensitive to the growth parameters of children presenting frequently for intercurrent illness. Children with more severe malnutrition may be lymphopenic (lymphocyte count < 1500) or anergic.

Undernourished children are frequently iron deficient, even in the absence of anemia. Iron and calcium deficiencies enhance the absorption of lead. In areas in which there is any concern for lead exposure, lead levels should be assessed as part of the workup for FTT.

E. Laboratory Findings

No single battery of laboratory tests or imaging studies can be advocated in the workup of FTT. Testing should be guided by the history and physical examination. Less than 1% of "routine laboratory tests" ordered in the evaluation of FTT provide useful information for treatment or diagnosis.

Tests that had been advocated as markers of nutritional status have limitations. Albumin has an extremely long half-life (21 days) and is a poor indicator of recent undernutrition. Prealbumin, which has been touted as a marker for recent protein nutrition, is decreased in both acute inflammation and undernutrition. Retinol-binding protein reflects only the calories consumed but is unaffected by the protein content and, by extension, the quality of the diet.

Laboratory evaluation is indicated when the history and physical examination suggest underlying organic disease. Children with developmental delay and organomegaly or severe episodic illness should have a metabolic workup, including urine organic and serum amino acids: there is a 5% yield in this subset of patients. Children with a history of recurrent respiratory tract infections or diarrhea should have sweat chloride testing performed at a cystic fibrosis center. Less experienced laboratories offer unreliable results. A history of poorly defined febrile illnesses or recurrent "viral illness" may be followed up with a urinalysis, culture, and renal function to evaluate for occult urinary tract disease. In children with diarrhea it may be useful to send stool for evaluation of *Giardia* antigen, qualitative fat, white blood cell count, occult blood, ova and parasites, rotavirus, and α_1-antitrypsin. Rotavirus has been associated with prolonged gastroenteritis and FTT. Elevated α_1-antitrypsin in the stool is a marker for protein enteropathy.

Infectious diseases need to be specifically addressed. Worldwide, tuberculosis is one of the most common causes of FTT. A Mantoux test and anergy panel must be performed on any child with risk factors for tuberculosis exposure. HIV infection must also be entertained. FTT is frequently a presenting symptom of HIV infection in the infant. Testing for HIV is not legally required in prenatal assessment; thus, mothers may not know their children are at risk. Any suspicion of HIV merits testing. Less ominous infectious etiologies can also cause FTT: persistent giardiasis and rotavirus are two common infections in toddlers that cause poor growth.

Differential Diagnosis

It is essential to differentiate a small child from the child with FTT. No criterion is specific enough to exclude those who are small for other reasons. Included in the differential diagnosis of FTT are familial short stature, Turner syndrome, normal growth variant, prematurity, endocrine dysfunction, and genetic syndromes limiting growth.

Here, too, a good growth chart is of great utility. The child with FTT has a deceleration in weight first. Height velocity continues unaffected for a time. Children with familial short stature have a simultaneous change in their height and weight curves. Height velocity slows first (it can even plateau) in endocrine disorders such as hypothyroidism. The preterm infant's growth parameters need to be adjusted for gestational age: head circumference is adjusted until 18 months, weight until 24 months, and height through 40 months.

The family history is helpful in differentiating the child with FTT from the child with constitutional growth delay or familial short stature. Midparental height, which can be calculated from the family history, is a useful calculation of probable genetic potential:

- For girls: (father's height in inches – 5 + mother's height)/2 ± 2 inches.
- For boys: (mother's height in inches + 5 + father's height)/2 ± 2 inches.

If the child's current growth curve translates into an adult height that falls within the range of midparental height reassurance may be offered.

It is most difficult to differentiate the child with constitutional growth delay from the child with FTT. These children typically have reduced weight for height as do children with FTT. However, unlike children with FTT they ultimately gain both weight and height on a steady curve. Family history is often revealing in constitutional growth delay. Querying parents about the onset of their own pubertal signs may seem intrusive but often gives the clinician the information needed to reassure parents about their child's growth.

Breast-feeding infants may be growing normally and not follow the CDC growth curves. After 4–6 months their weight may decrease relative to their peers. After 12 months their weight catches up to that of age-matched formula-fed infants. However, a decrease in weight in early infancy is a symptom of unsuccessful breast-feeding and should be interpreted as FTT.

Complications

Developmental delay may persist in children with FTT well past the period of undernutrition. Studies have repeatedly shown that these children, as a group, have more behavioral and cognitive problems in school than their peers, even into adolescence. One caveat about these studies is that many defined FTT by that classic definition: growth failure associated with disordered behavior and development. These studies do not doom every child with FTT to scholastic and social failure, but the clinician must be vigilant and act as the child's advocate. Formal developmental screening is especially important in the child with a history of FTT. Intervention should be offered early rather than waiting "to see if the child catches up." Children with FTT can be successful but may need specific supports on the road to achieving that success.

Treatment

A. Nutrition

The cornerstone of therapy is nutrition. The goal of treatment is catch-up growth. Children with FTT may need 1.5–2 times the usual daily calories to achieve catch-up growth. For an infant this is roughly 150–200 cal/kg/day. There are many formulas for calculating caloric requirements: one simple estimate is:

$$\text{kcal/kg} = 120\ \text{kcal/kg} \times \text{median weight for current height/current weight (kg)}$$

It is important that this nutrition include adequate calories from protein. Children who are undernourished require 3 g protein per kg body weight per day to initiate catch-up growth and may need as much 5 g/kg. (In the literature from the developing world, some malnourished children have required as much as 12 g protein/kg/day!) High-calorie diets should continue until the child achieves an age-appropriate weight for height.

It is almost impossible for any child to take in two times the usual volume of food. Some solutions are to offer higher calorie formulas (24–30 cal/oz) to infants. For older children it is possible to replace or add higher calorie foods. Heavy cream may be substituted for milk on cereal or in cooking. Cheese may be added to vegetables. Instant breakfast drinks may be offered as snacks. It is advisable to enlist a dietician in designing a high-calorie diet for the child with FTT.

Occasionally tube feedings are indicated in the child with FTT. Some children may benefit from nighttime feedings through a nasogastric or a percutaneous endoscopic gastrostomy tube. This solution is particularly useful in children with underlying increased caloric requirements (eg, children with cystic fibrosis and cerebral palsy). Children with mechanical feeding difficulties may also require tube feeding for some period of time. The child who is primarily tube fed should have early intervention with an occupational or speech therapist. Without therapy the child may develop oral aversions or fail to develop appropriate oral-motor coordination. Both issues will worsen FTT when oral feeding is reinstituted.

Parents need to be educated at the onset of nutritional therapy. Catch-up growth is expected within the first month. However, some children may not show accelerated weight gain until after the first 2 weeks of increased nutrition. Children usually gain 1.5 times their daily expected weight gains during the catch-up phase. Children's weight improves well before their height increases; parents may expect their previously skinny child to become cherubic and even plump. This change in body habitus does not indicate overfeeding but, rather, successful therapy. It does not matter how quickly the child gains; the composition of weight gain will be 45–65% lean body mass.

B. Medications

Few medications are indicated in the treatment of FTT. Those few are nutritional supports. Children with FTT should be supplemented with iron. Zinc has also been shown to improve linear growth. It is sufficient to supplement children with a multivitamin containing zinc and iron. Vitamin D supplementation should also be considered. Vitamin D replacement is especially important in dark-skinned children and in children who are not regularly exposed to sunlight.

C. Social Support

Beyond nutritional support the importance of social support has already been alluded to. The services offered must be tailored to the family and the child. Certainly frequent visits with the primary care provider are useful: weight gain can be measured and concerns addressed. Home visits by social services have been shown to decrease hospitalizations and improve weight gain. Children with developmental delay need early assessment and intervention by the appropriate therapists.

The primary care provider plays a critical role in recognizing and assessing FTT. These seemingly simple interventions made early in childhood have lasting ramifications throughout the life span.

D. Indications for Referral or Admission

Most FTT can and should be managed by the primary care provider. A trusting relationship between the clinician and the family is an invaluable asset in the treatment of failure to thrive. Parents struggling with the diagnosis often believe that the health care system views them as neglectful. This anxiety creates barriers to open and honest communication about the child's feeding and developmental status. However, suspicions may be allayed when primary care providers enlist themselves as allies in the treatment.

The primary indication for referral is the treatment of an underlying organ dysfunction (eg, cystic fibrosis) that requires specialized care. The clinician may also wish to reevaluate the child who fails to begin catch-up growth after 1–2 months of nutritional intervention.

Most children with FTT can be managed in the outpatient setting; a few may need hospitalization at some point during their evaluation. Indications for admission at initial evaluation are bradycardia or hypotension, which are signs of severe malnutrition. Children who are less than 61% of the median weight for their age should be admitted for nutritional support. The practitioner should have a low threshold for admitting children with hypoglycemia: low serum glucose is a worrisome finding that may indicate severe malnutrition and metabolic disease.

The majority of families of children with FTT are neither abusive nor neglectful. However, if the clinician suspects abuse or neglect the child should be admitted. About 10% of children with FTT are abused; these children ultimately experience worse developmental outcomes than other children with FTT if left in the home. When abuse is documented social services must be involved.

The third group of children who may be considered for hospital admission are those who have failed to initiate catch-up growth with outpatient management. A hospital stay of several days will allow the clinician to observe feeding practices and enable the family to internalize the plan of care. Further testing for organ dysfunction may be indicated during hospitalization. It can also be a time to enlist other health professionals in the treatment plan: occupational therapists and social workers are often helpful allies in the treatment of FTT.

Frank DA, Zeisel SH: Failure to thrive. Pediatr Clin North Am 1988;35:1187. [PMID: 3059294]

Neifert MR: Prevention of breastfeeding tragedies. Pediatr Clin North Am 2001;48:273. [PMID: 11339153]

Schwartz ID: Failure to thrive: An old nemesis in the new millennium. Pediatr Rev 2000;21:257. [PMID: 10922022]

Neonatal Hyperbilirubinemia

3

Andrew B. Symons, MD, MS, & Martin C. Mahoney, MD, PhD, FAAFP

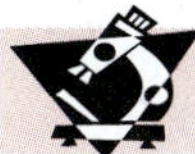

ESSENTIALS OF DIAGNOSIS

- *Visible yellowing of the skin, ocular sclera, or both are present in neonatal jaundice; however, because visual estimates of total bilirubin are prone to error, quantitative testing (serum or transcutaneous) should be completed in infants noted to be jaundiced within the first 24 hours of life.*
- *Risk of subsequent hyperbilirubinemia can be assessed by plotting serum bilirubin levels onto a nomogram; all bilirubin levels should be interpreted according to the infant's age (in hours).*

General Considerations

Nearly every infant is born with a serum bilirubin level higher than that of the normal adult. Approximately 60% of newborns are visibly jaundiced during the first week of life. The diagnostic and therapeutic challenge for the physician is to differentiate normal physiologic jaundice from pathologic jaundice, and to institute appropriate evaluation and therapy when necessary.

Table 3–1 lists several maternal and neonatal factors that increase the risk of developing severe hyperbilirubinemia among infants of 35 or more weeks' gestation. Among the most significant clinical characteristics associated with severe hyperbilirubinemia are predischarge levels in the high-risk zone on the serum bilirubin nomogram (Figure 3–1). The following factors (in order of decreasing importance) are associated with decreased risk of significant jaundice: total serum bilirubin (TSB) or transcutaneous bilirubin (TcB) level in the low-risk zone, gestational age greater than 41 weeks, exclusive bottle-feeding, black race, and discharge from the hospital after 72 hours.

Pathogenesis

A. Physiologic Jaundice

The three classifications of neonatal hyperbilirubinemia are based on the following mechanisms of accumulation: increased bilirubin load, decreased bilirubin conjugation, and impaired bilirubin excretion. In the newborn, unconjugated bilirubin is produced faster and removed more slowly than in the normal adult due to immaturity of the glucuronyl transferase enzyme system. The main source of unconjugated bilirubin is the breakdown of hemoglobin in senescent red blood cells. Newborns have an increased erythrocyte mass at birth (average hematocrit of 50% vs 33% in the adult) and a shorter life span for erythrocytes (90 days vs 120 days in the adult). The newborn cannot readily excrete unconjugated bilirubin, and much of it is reabsorbed by the intestine and returned to the enterohepatic circulation.

Increased production and decreased elimination of bilirubin lead to a *physiologic jaundice* in most normal newborns. Bilirubin is a very effective and potent antioxidant, and physiologic jaundice may provide a mechanism for protecting the newborn from oxygen free-radical injury. The average full-term white newborn experiences a peak serum bilirubin concentration of 5–6 mg/dL (86–103 μmol/L), which begins to rise after the first day of life, peaks on the third day of life, and falls to normal adult levels by days 10–12. African-American infants tend to have slightly lower peaks in serum bilirubin. In Asian infants, serum bilirubin levels rise more quickly than in white infants and tend to reach higher peaks on average (8–12 mg/dL; 135–205 μmol/L). This leads to a longer period of physiologic jaundice among Asian and Native American newborns. Preterm infants (< 37 weeks' gestation) of all races may take 4–5 days to reach peak serum bilirubin levels, and these peaks may be twice that observed among full-term infants.

B. Breast-feeding and Breast Milk Jaundice

Infants who are breast-fed may experience exaggerated bilirubin levels due to two separate phenomena associated with breast-feeding and breast milk.

Breast-fed infants may experience relative starvation in the first few days of life due to delayed release of milk by the mother or difficulties with breast-feeding. This nutritional inadequacy can result in increased enterohepatic circulation of bilirubin, leading to elevated serum bilirubin levels in the first few days of life. Termed *breast-feeding jaundice,* this finding is considered abnormal and can be overcome by offering frequent feedings (10–12 times per day) and by avoiding water supplementation in breast-fed infants.

Table 3–1. Risk factors for development of severe hyperbilirubinemia in infants of 35 or more weeks' gestation.[1]

Major Risk Factors
Predischarge TSB or TcB level in the high-risk zone (see Figure 3–1)
Jaundice observed in the first 24 h of life
Blood group incompatibility with positive direct antiglobulin test, other known hemolytic disease (eg, G6PD deficiency), elevated ETCO
Gestational age of 35–36 wk
Previous sibling who received phototherapy
Cephalohematoma or significant bruising
Exclusive breast-feeding, particularly if nursing is not going well and weight loss is excessive
East Asian race
Minor Risk Factors
Predischarge TSB or TcB level in the high intermediate-risk zone
Gestational age of 37–38 wk
Jaundice observed before discharge
Previous sibling with jaundice
Macrosomic infant of diabetic mother
Maternal age > 25 y
Male gender

TSB, total serum bilirubin; TcB, transcutaneous bilirubin; G6PD, glucose-6-phosphate dehydrogenase; ETCO, end-tidal carbon monoxide.

[1]Listed in approximate order of importance.

Reproduced, with permission, from American Academy of Pediatrics Subcommittee on Hyperbilirubinemia. Management of hyperbilirubinemia in the newborn infant 35 or more weeks of gestation. Pediatrics 2004;114:297.

Breast milk is believed to increase the enterohepatic circulation of bilirubin; however, the specific factor(s) in breast milk that are responsible for this action are unknown. For the first 5 days of life, the serum bilirubin level in breast-fed infants parallels that in non–breast-fed infants. Beginning at approximately day 6, *breast milk jaundice* occurs in breast-fed infants as serum bilirubin either rises a little for a few days or declines more slowly. Approximately two thirds of breast-fed infants may be expected to have hyperbilirubinemia from 3 weeks to 3 months of age, with as many as one third exhibiting clinical jaundice. Breast milk jaundice (unlike breast-feeding jaundice) is considered a form of normal physiologic jaundice in healthy, thriving breast-fed infants.

C. Pathologic Jaundice

Exaggerated physiologic jaundice occurs at serum bilirubin levels between 7 and 17 mg/dL (104–291 μmol/L). Bilirubin levels above 17 mg/dL in full-term infants are no longer considered physiologic, and further investigation is warranted.

The onset of jaundice within the first 24 hours of life or a rate of increase in serum bilirubin exceeding 0.5 mg/dL/h (8 μmol/L/h) is potentially pathologic and suggestive of hemolytic disease. Conjugated serum bilirubin concentrations exceeding 10% of total bilirubin or 2 mg/dL (35 μmol/L) are also not physiologic and suggest hepatobiliary disease or a general metabolic disorder.

Table 3–2 summarizes factors that may indicate that jaundice is pathologic as opposed to physiologic, warranting further evaluation. Important historical features include family history of hemolytic disease, onset of jaundice in the first 24 hours of life, a rapid rise in serum bilirubin levels, and ethnicity, as well as infant feeding patterns, stool and urine appearance, and activity levels. Clinical assessment requires careful attention to vital signs, weight loss, general appearance, pallor, and hepatosplenomegaly.

The primary concern with severe hyperbilirubinemia is the potential for neurotoxic effects as well as general cellular injury, which can occur at TSB levels exceeding 20–25 mg/dL. The term *kernicterus* refers to the yellow staining of the basal ganglia observed postmortem among infants who died with severe jaundice. (Bilirubin deposition in the basal ganglia can also be imaged using magnetic resonance techniques.) The American Academy of Pediatrics (AAP) has recommended that the term *acute bilirubin encephalopathy* be used to describe the acute manifestations of bilirubin toxicity seen in the first weeks after birth and that the term *kernicterus* be reserved for the chronic and permanent clinical sequelae of bilirubin toxicity.

Although a common complication of hyperbilirubinemia in the 1940s and 1950s due to Rh erythroblastosis fetalis and ABO hemolytic disease, kernicterus is rare today with the use of Rh immunoglobulin and with the intervention of phototherapy and exchange transfusion. With early discharge to home, however, a small resurgence of kernicterus has been observed in countries in which this complication had essentially disappeared. For instance, although no cases of kernicterus were identified in Denmark during the 20 years preceding 1994, six cases were diagnosed between 1994 and 1998. No published data on the incidence or prevalence of kernicterus in the United States are available.

Bilirubin can interfere with DNA synthesis as well as protein synthesis and protein phosphorylation. Bilirubin can also interfere with neuroexcitatory signals and impair nerve conduction, particularly in the auditory nerve. Hyperbilirubinemia may also impair cerebral glucose metabolism in the brain.

The concentration of bilirubin in the brain and the duration of exposure are important determinants of the

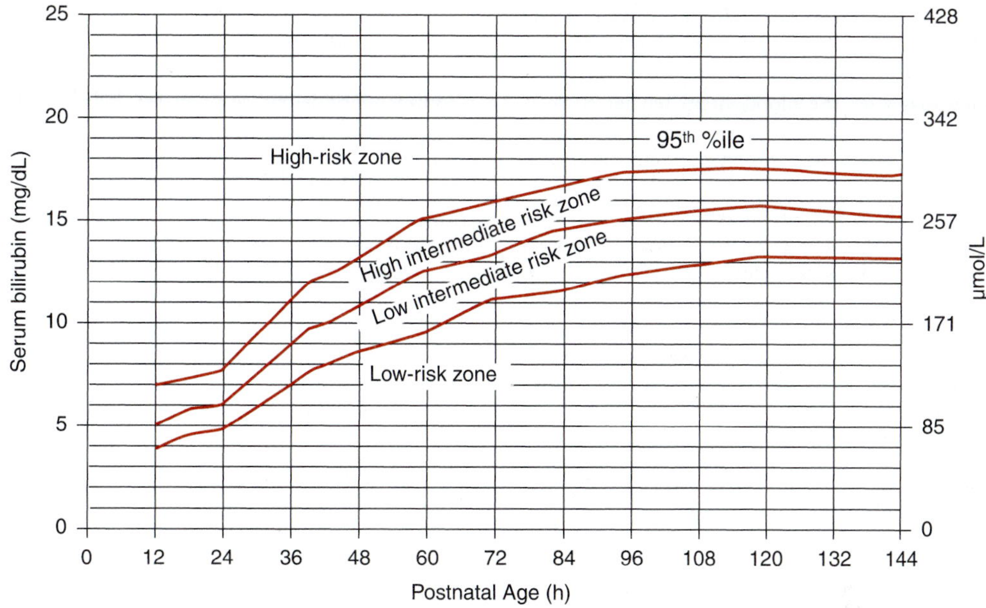

Figure 3–1. **Nomogram for designation of risk in 2840 well newborns of 36 or more weeks' gestational age with birth weight of 2000 g or more or 35 or more weeks' gestational age and birth weight of 2500 g or more based on the hour-specific serum bilirubin value.** (Reproduced, with permission, from American Academy of Pediatrics Subcommittee on Hyperbilirubinemia. Management of hyperbilirubinemia in the newborn infant 35 or more weeks of gestation. Pediatrics 2004;114:297.)

Table 3–2. Factors that may indicate a pathologic cause of jaundice among newborns.

General considerations	Family history of significant hemolytic disease Onset of jaundice before age of 24 h Rise in serum bilirubin levels of more than 0.5 mg/dL/h Pallor, hepatosplenomegaly Rapid increase in TSB level after 24–48 h (consider G6PD deficiency) Ethnicity suggestive of inherited disease (G6PD deficiency, etc) Failure of phototherapy to lower TSB level
Clinical signs suggesting possibility of other diseases (eg, sepsis, galactosemia) in which jaundice may be one manifestation	Vomiting Lethargy Poor feeding Hepatosplenomegaly Excessive weight loss Apnea Temperature instability Tachypnea
Signs of cholestatic jaundice suggesting the need to rule out biliary atresia or other causes of cholestasis	Dark urine or urine positive for bilirubin Light-colored stools Persistent jaundice of more than 3 weeks' duration

TSB, total serum bilirubin; G6PD, glucose-6-phosphate dehydrogenase.

Adapted, with permission, from American Academy of Pediatrics Subcommittee on Hyperbilirubinemia. Management of hyperbilirubinemia in the newborn infant 35 or more weeks of gestation. Pediatrics 2004;114:297.

neurotoxic effects of bilirubin. Bilirubin can enter the brain when not bound to albumin, so infants with low albumin are at increased risk of developing kernicterus. Conditions that alter the blood–brain barrier such as infection, acidosis, hypoxia, sepsis, prematurity, and hyperosmolarity may affect the entry of bilirubin into the brain.

In infants without hemolysis, serum bilirubin levels and encephalopathy do not correlate well. In infants with hemolysis, TSB levels higher than 20 mg/dL are associated with worse neurologic outcomes, although some infants with concentrations of 25 mg/dL are normal. Kernicterus was detected in 8% of infants with associated hemolysis who had TSB levels of 19–25 mg/dL, 33% of infants with levels of 25–29 mg/dL, and 73% of infants with levels of 30–40 mg/dL. It should be noted that the majority of cases of kernicterus described in recent years have been among neonates who had TSB levels higher than 30 mg/dL at the time of diagnosis, which is well above the recommended treatment thresholds of 15 or 20 mg/dL.

It is estimated that up to 15% of infants with kernicterus have no obvious neurologic signs or symptoms. In its acute form, kernicterus may present in the first 1–2 days with poor sucking, stupor, hypotonia, and seizures. During the middle of the first week, hypertonia of extensor muscles, opisthotonus (backward arching of the trunk), retrocollis (backward arching of the neck), and fever may be observed. After the first week, the infant may exhibit generalized hypertonia. Some of these changes disappear spontaneously or can be reversed with exchange transfusion. In most infants with moderate (10–20 mg/dL) to severe (> 20 mg/dL) hyperbilirubinemia, evoked neurologic responses return to normal within 6 months. A minority of infants (ranging between 6% and 23%) exhibit persistent neurologic deficits.

In its chronic form, kernicterus may present in the first year with hypotonia, active deep tendon reflexes, obligatory tonic neck reflexes, dental dysplasia, and delayed motor skills. After the first year, movement disorders, upward gaze, and sensorineural hearing loss may develop. It has been suggested that long-term effects of severe hyperbilirubinemia on intelligence quotient (IQ) are more likely in boys than in girls. Seidman and colleagues studied 1948 subjects from Hadaasah Hebrew University Medical Center in Jerusalem born in 1970–1971 and drafted into the army 17 years later and found a significantly higher risk of lowered IQ (< 85) among males with a history of TSB exceeding 20 mg/dL (OR 2.96; 95% CI 1.29–6.79).

Clinical Findings

The American Academy of Family Physicians offers no clinical policy on neonatal hyperbilirubinemia. In 2004, the AAP issued an updated practice parameter for the management of hyperbilirubinemia among newborns of 35 or more weeks' gestation. Elements of these recommendations are summarized below and can be accessed in full at http://www.aap.org.

A. Symptoms and Signs

Clinically, jaundice usually progresses from head to toe. The TSB level can be estimated by the degree of caudal extension: face, 5 mg/dL; upper chest, 10 mg/dL; abdomen, 12 mg/dL; palms and soles, more than 15 mg/dL. However, visual estimates of total bilirubin are prone to error, especially in infants with pigmented skin. TSB or TcB levels should be measured in infants who develop jaundice within the first 24 hours, and all bilirubin levels should be interpreted according to the infant's age (in hours). TcB measurement devices may provide an alternative to frequent blood draws for the accurate assessment of serum bilirubin. Unfortunately, transcutaneous measurement units are not widely available in community hospital settings.

Evaluation of infants who develop abnormal signs such as feeding difficulty, behavior changes, apnea, and temperature changes is recommended regardless of whether jaundice has been detected in order to rule out underlying disease. Clinical protocols for evaluating jaundice, with assessments to be performed no less than every 8–12 hours in the newborn nursery, should be in place.

B. Laboratory Findings

When a pathologic cause for jaundice is suspected, laboratory studies should be promptly completed:

- When jaundice is noticed within the first 24 hours, clinicians should consider a sepsis workup, evaluation for rubella and toxoplasmosis infection, assessment of fractionated serum bilirubin levels, and blood typing to rule out erythroblastosis fetalis. Results of thyroid and galactosemia testing, obtained during the newborn metabolic screening, also should be reviewed.
- If the level of conjugated bilirubin is higher than 2 mg/dL, a reason for impaired bilirubin excretion should be sought. If conjugated bilirubin is lower than 2 mg/dL, hemoglobin levels and reticulocyte counts should be evaluated. A high hemoglobin concentration indicates polycythemia whereas a low hemoglobin concentration with an abnormal reticulocyte count suggests hemolysis. If the reticulocyte count is normal, the infant must be evaluated for a nonhemolytic cause of jaundice.
- Infants with a poor response to phototherapy and those whose family history is consistent with the possibility of glucose-6-phosphate dehydrogenase (G6PD) deficiency require further testing.

Maternal prenatal testing should include ABO and Rh (D) typing and a serum screen for unusual isoimmune antibodies. If the mother has not had prenatal blood grouping, or is Rh negative, a direct Coomb's test, blood type, and Rh (D) type of the infant's cord blood should be performed. Institutions are encouraged to save cord blood for future testing, particularly when the mother's blood type is group O.

C. Neonatal Jaundice after Hospital Discharge

Follow-up should be provided to all neonates discharged less than 48 hours after birth. This evaluation by a health care professional should occur within 2–3 days of discharge.

Approximately one third of healthy breast-fed infants have persistent jaundice after 2 weeks of age. A report of dark urine or light stools should prompt a measurement of direct serum bilirubin. If the history and physical examination are normal, continued observation is appropriate. If jaundice persists beyond 3 weeks, a urine sample should be tested for bilirubin, and a measurement of total and direct serum bilirubin should be obtained.

Prediction & Prevention

Shorter hospital stays after delivery limit the time for hospital-based assessment of infant feeding, instruction about breast-feeding, and the detection of jaundice. Hyperbilirubinemia and problems related to feeding are the main reasons for hospital readmission during the first week of life. Of 29,934 infants discharged between 1988 and 1994 from a large suburban hospital in Michigan, just 0.8% were readmitted by the age of 14 days. Of those readmitted, 51% were diagnosed with hyperbilirubinemia and 31% with sepsis.

Because bilirubin levels usually peak on day 3 or 4 of life, and most newborns are discharged within 48 hours, most cases of jaundice occur at home. It is therefore important that infants be seen by a health care professional within a few days of discharge to assess for jaundice and overall well-being. This is particularly important in near-term infants (35–36 weeks' gestation) who are at particular risk for hyperbilirubinemia due to both relative hepatic immaturity and inadequate nutritional intake.

Measuring TSB before discharge and then plotting this value on a nomogram (see Figure 3–1) can be useful for predicting the risk of subsequent moderately severe hyperbilirubinemia (> 17 mg/dL) and can guide physicians in identifying neonates for whom close follow-up is warranted. Neonates in the high-risk group (95th percentile for TSB) at 18–72 hours of life had a 40% chance of developing moderately severe hyperbilirubinemia upon discharge, whereas for those in the low-risk group (40th percentile for TSB) the probability for subsequently developing moderately severe hyperbilirubinemia was zero. However, it should be noted that there are no evidence-based guidelines that endorse this approach.

Carbon monoxide is a byproduct resulting from the breakdown of heme. Measuring end-tidal carbon monoxide (ETCO) in neonates has been proposed as a potential tool for predicting the development of severe hyperbilirubinemia; however, the value of routine measurements of ETCO has been questioned. At present, ETCO measurements to assess hyperbilirubinemia are not yet validated for use in clinical settings.

Treatment

A. Suspected Pathologic Jaundice

The decision whether to intervene in cases of elevated bilirubin levels during the neonatal period is tempered by clinical judgment, and the physician team (including the family physician and consultants) is encouraged to discuss management options with the parents or guardians of the infant. Treatment decisions for both phototherapy (Figure 3–2) and exchange transfusion (Figure 3–3) are based on TSB levels. Intensive phototherapy should produce a decline in TSB of 1–2 mg/dL within 4–6 hours, and the decline should continue thereafter. If the TSB does not respond appropriately to intensive phototherapy, exchange transfusion is recommended. If levels are in the range that suggests the need for exchange transfusion (see Figure 3–3), intensive phototherapy should be attempted while preparations for exchange transfusion are made. Exchange transfusion is also recommended in infants whose TSB levels rise to exchange transfusion levels despite intensive phototherapy. In any of the preceding situations, failure of intensive phototherapy to lower the TSB level strongly suggests the presence of hemolytic disease or other pathologic processes and strongly warrants further investigation or consultation.

In infants with isoimmune hemolytic disease, administration of intravenous gamma globulin (0.5–1 g/kg over 2 hours) is recommended if the TSB is rising despite intensive phototherapy or the TSB is within 2–3 mg/dL of the exchange level. If necessary, this dose can be repeated in 12 hours.

Figure 3–2 summarizes the management strategy for hyperbilirubinemia in infants of 35 or more weeks' gestation. Management decisions regarding phototherapy (see Figure 3–2) and exchange transfusion (see Figure 3–3) are based on the infant's age, risk factors, and TSB levels.

B. Phototherapy and Exchange Transfusion

1. Phototherapy—Phototherapy involves exposing the infant to high-intensity light in the blue-green

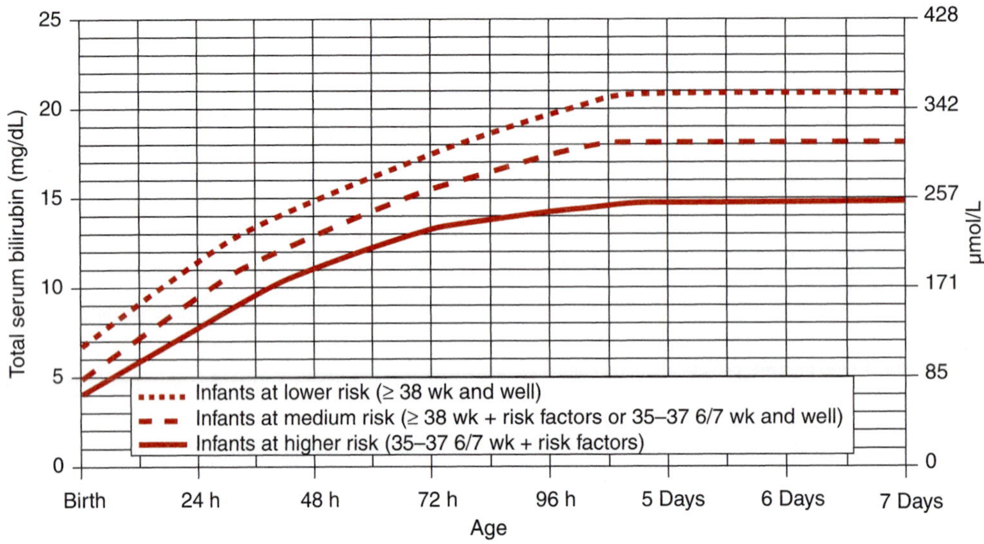

Figure 3–2. Guidelines for phototherapy in hospitalized infants of 35 or more weeks' gestation. (Reproduced, with permission, from American Academy of Pediatrics Subcommittee on Hyperbilirubinemia. Management of hyperbilirubinemia in the newborn infant 35 or more weeks of gestation. Pediatrics 2004;114:297.)

wavelengths. Light interacts with unconjugated bilirubin in the skin, converting it to less toxic photoisomers that are excreted in the bile and urine without conjugation. The efficacy of phototherapy is strongly influenced by the energy output in the blue spectrum, the spectrum of the light, and the surface area of the infant exposed to phototherapy. Phototherapy units contain several fluorescent tubes that are either freestanding or part of a radiant warming device. Fiberoptic systems have been developed that deliver light through a fiberoptic blanket. The phototherapy tubes (designated F20 T12/BB) make the infants look blue, which may

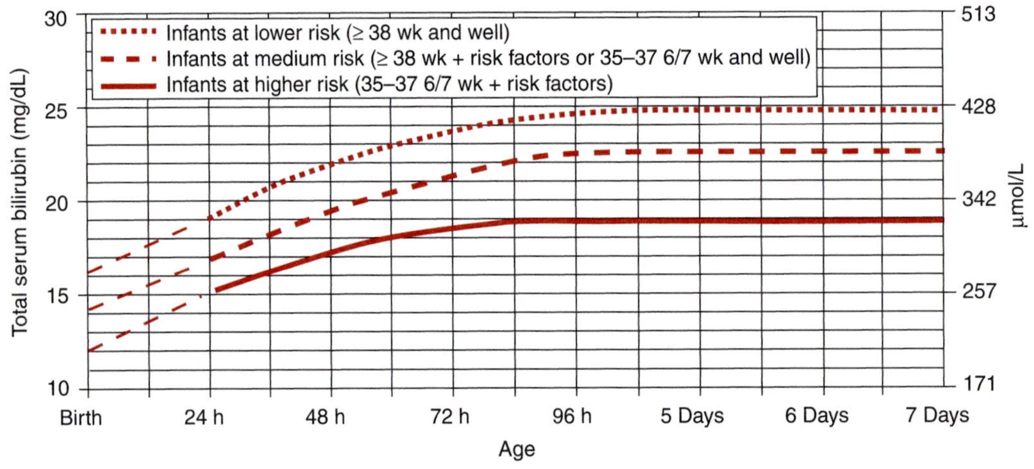

Figure 3–3. Guidelines for exchange transfusion in infants of 35 or more weeks' gestation. (Reproduced, with permission, from American Academy of Pediatrics Subcommittee on Hyperbilirubinemia. Management of hyperbilirubinemia in the newborn infant 35 or more weeks of gestation. Pediatrics 2004;114:297.)

be bothersome to health care workers and make clinical evaluation of jaundice difficult. However, this problem can be mitigated by using four special blue tubes and two daylight fluorescent tubes in the unit. Eye protection is placed on the infant, and the bank of lights is placed 15–20 cm from the infant. The infant is placed naked in a bassinet. Exposure is increased by placing a fiberoptic blanket under the infant, by placing lighting units all around the infant, or by putting a white sheet around the bassinet to serve as a reflecting surface. If slight warming of the infant is noted, the tubes can be moved away a bit. Phototherapy may be interrupted briefly for parental visits or breast-feeding.

In infants with TSB levels higher than 25 mg/dL, phototherapy should be administered continuously until a response is documented, or until exchange therapy is initiated. If the TSB is not responding to conventional phototherapy (a response is defined as a sustained reduction in total serum bilirubin of 1–2 mg/dL in 4–6 hours), the intensity should be increased by adding more lights; the intensity of the lights should also be increased while exchange transfusion is prepared. With commonly used light sources, overdose is impossible, although the infant may experience loose stools. Phototherapy is continued until the TSB level is lower than 14–15 mg/dL. The infant may be discharged after the completion of phototherapy. Rebound of total serum bilirubin following cessation of phototherapy is usually less than 1 mg/dL.

2. Exchange transfusion—Exchange transfusion rapidly removes bilirubin from the circulation. Circulating antibodies against erythrocytes are also removed. Exchange transfusion is particularly beneficial in neonates with hemolysis. One or two central catheters are placed. Small aliquots of blood (8–10 mL per pass) are removed from the infant's circulation and replaced with equal amounts of donor red cells mixed with plasma. The procedure is repeated until twice the infant's blood volume is replaced (~160–200 mL/kg). Serum electrolytes and bilirubin are measured periodically during the procedure. In some cases the procedure must be repeated to lower serum bilirubin levels sufficiently. Infusing salt-poor albumin at a dose of 1 g/kg 1–4 hours before exchange transfusion has been shown to increase the amount of bilirubin removed during the procedure.

Complications of exchange transfusion include thrombocytopenia, portal vein thrombosis, necrotizing enterocolitis, electrolyte imbalance, graft-versus-host disease, and infection. Mortality from exchange transfusion approaches 2%, and an additional 12% of infants may suffer serious complications. Therefore, exchange transfusion should be reserved for neonates who have failed intensive phototherapy and should be performed by clinicians and facilities with proper experience.

Measurement of serum albumin levels in an infant suspected of jaundice is an option, considering levels less than 3.0 g/dL as one risk for lowering the threshold for phototherapy. If exchange transfusion is being considered, the bilirubin/albumin ratio is used in conjunction with the TSB level and other factors in determining the need for exchange transfusion (see Figure 3–3).

C. Suspected Nonpathologic Jaundice

For the management of breast-feeding jaundice, interruption of breast-feeding in healthy term newborns is generally discouraged. Frequent breast-feeding sessions (at least 8–10 times in 24 hours) are advised. However, if the mother and physician wish, they may consider using supplemental formula feedings or temporarily interrupting breast-feeding and replacing it with formula feedings. Phototherapy may be initiated, depending on TSB levels.

As previously discussed, breast milk jaundice is seen initially after day 6 of life in the majority of healthy breast-fed infants between ages 3 weeks and 3 months of age. This is a form of normal physiologic jaundice.

Conclusions

Because up to 60% of all newborns are noted to be clinically jaundiced, all family physicians who care for neonates will encounter this common clinical entity. In the overwhelming majority of cases, this jaundice is entirely benign. However, it is important that the family physician recognize cases in which jaundice could represent a pathologic process or the risk for development of severe hyperbilirubinemia.

As in the treatment of other conditions such as fever in the neonate, close monitoring and surveillance are important, and strategies for assessing risk must be used. Infants who are discharged prior to 48 hours of age, particularly those who are born at less than 35 weeks' gestation, should be seen in the office within a few days of discharge to evaluate jaundice and overall clinical status.

The possibility of jaundice should be discussed with parents before hospital discharge. Parents of newborns should be assured of the generally benign nature of most cases of jaundice, especially breast-feeding jaundice and breast milk jaundice. Parental education should emphasize the need to monitor the infant for jaundice and associated symptoms such as poor feeding, lethargy, dark urine, and light-colored stools. Family physicians should encourage parents to contact the office with specific questions and concerns. An example of a parent information sheet in English and Spanish is available at http://www.aap.org/family/jaundicefaq.htm.

Agrawal VK et al: Brainstem auditory evoked response in newborns with hyperbilirubinemia. Indian Pediatr 1998;35:513. [PMID: 10216645]

AAP Subcommittee on Neonatal Hyperbilirubinemia: Neonatal jaundice and kernicterus. Pediatrics 2001;108:763. [PMID: 1153348]

American Academy of Pediatrics Subcommittee on Hyperbilirubinemia. Management of hyperbilirubinemia in the newborn infant 35 or more weeks of gestation. Pediatrics 2004;114:297. [PMID: 15231951]

Bertini G et al: Prevention of bilirubin encephalopathy. Biol Neonate 2001;79:219. [PMID: 11275655]

Bhutani VK et al: Predictive ability of a predischarge hour-specific serum bilirubin for subsequent hyperbilirubinemia in healthy term and near-term newborns. Pediatrics 1999;103:6. [PMID: 9917432]

Dennery PA et al: Drug therapy: Neonatal hyperbilirubinemia. N Engl J Med 2001;344:581. [PMID: 1127355]

Gartner LM: Neonatal jaundice. Pediatr Rev 1994;15:422. [PMID: 7824404]

Halamek LP, Stevenson DK: Neonatal jaundice and liver disease. In Fanaroff AA, Martin RJ, eds: *Neonatal-Perinatal Medicine: Diseases of the Fetus and Infant,* 7th ed, Vol 2. Mosby, 2002.

Hansen TWR: Kernicterus in term and near term infants—the specter walks again. Acta Paediatr 2000;89:1155. [PMID: 11083367]

Maisels MJ, Kring E: Transcutaneous bilirubinometry decreases the need for serum bilirubin measurements and saves money. Pediatrics 1997;99:599. [PMID:9093305]

Maisels MJ, Kring E: Length of stay, jaundice and hospital readmission. Pediatrics 1998;101:995. [PMID: 9606225]

Maisels MJ, Newman TB: Predicting hyperbilirubinemia in newborns: The importance of timing. Pediatrics 1999;103:493. [PMID: 9925847]

Moyer VA et al: Accuracy of clinical judgment in neonatal jaundice. Arch Pediatric Adolesc Med 2000;154:391. [PMID: 1076879]

Porter ML, Dennis BL: Hyperbilirubinemia in the term newborn. Am Fam Physician 2002;65:599. [PMID: 11871676]

Seidman DS et al: Neonatal hyperbilirubinemia and physical and cognitive performance at 17 years of age. Pediatrics 1991;88: 828. [PMID: 1896294]

Siberry GK, Iannone R, eds: *The Harriet Lane Handbook: A Manual for Pediatric House Officers,* 17th ed. Mosby, 2005.

Stevenson DK et al: Prediction of hyperbilirubinemia in near-term and term infants. Pediatrics 2001;108:31. [PMID: 11433051]

Valaes T: Problems with prediction of neonatal hyperbilirubinemia. Pediatrics 2001;108:175. [PMID: 11433071]

Volpe JJ: *Neonatal Neurology,* 4th ed. WB Saunders, 2001.

Breast-feeding & Infant Nutrition 4

Tracey D. Conti, MD

General Considerations

Nutrition is a critical capstone for the proper growth and development of infants. Breast-feeding of term infants by healthy mothers is the optimal mechanism for providing the caloric and nutrient needs of infants. Preterm infants can also benefit from breast milk and breast-feeding although supplementation and fortification of preterm breast milk may be required. Barring some unique circumstances, human breast milk can provide nutritional, social, and motor developmental benefits for most infants.

Despite increased emphasis on breast-feeding education, less than 65% of women choose to breast-feed their children. Of these women, only 29% and 16% are still breast-feeding at 6 months and 1 year, respectively. The Department of Health and Human Services Healthy People 2010 initiative proposes to increase these numbers to 50% and 25% for infants at 6 and 12 months, respectively. Education of practitioners as well as their patients is an integral component of this initiative.

Most women presently of childbearing age were not breast-fed and report having no maternal relatives who breast-fed their children. Because evidence clearly suggests familial influences in the development of infant feeding practices, practitioners may find it difficult to encourage breast-feeding behaviors among women with no direct familial breast-feeding experience.

Efforts to alter knowledge, attitudes, and behaviors regarding breast-feeding must effectively address the numerous psychosocial barriers. Health care providers are critical conduits for maternal and familial education. All members of the health care team, including physicians, midwives, and nurses, are valuable sources of important evidence-based information as well as psychological support for mothers in search of guidance regarding infant feeding practices. Unless health care practitioners are properly educated regarding breast-feeding practices and barriers, efforts to achieve the Healthy People 2010 objectives will remain suboptimal.

Numerous studies have shown the superiority of breast milk and the health advantages that breast-fed children have. The literature has shown that infants who are breast-fed have fewer episodes of diarrheal illness, ear infections, and allergies. There are likewise financial advantages to breast-feeding. Other somewhat controversial investigations suggest higher intelligence among breast-fed infants.

Numerous consensus recommendations advocate breast-feeding for the first 4–6 months prior to the introduction of age-appropriate solid foods and advise continued breast-feeding for the first year of life.

The American Academy of Pediatrics (AAP) Committee on Nutrition recommends breast-feeding for the first year of life with supplemental vitamin D at birth and the addition of supplemental iron at age 4 months and possible addition of fluoride at age 6 months for infants living in regions in which water is low in fluoride. Vitamin D supplementation is particularly applicable in regions with limited sunlight and for infants of mothers with decreased daily intake of cow's milk. Further recommendations include delaying introduction of cow's milk until after 1 year and delaying addition of reduced-fat milk until 2 years of age. To this end, new mothers should be encouraged to continue prenatal vitamins containing supplemental iron, calcium, and vitamin D. Supplemental solid foods should be considered at or around 6 months of age once the infant demonstrates appropriate readiness.

Anatomy of the Human Breast & Breast-feeding

Women are able to produce milk by the age they are able to bear children. There is no evidence that breast function, breast milk production, or composition is different among younger women. The principal external structures of the mature human female breast are the nipple, areola, and Montgomery tubercles. The areola is the darker part of the breast, with the nipple being the central-most structure through which milk ducts open and milk is expressed. Within the areola are Montgomery tubercles, through which sebaceous and sweat glands (Montgomery glands) open, producing lubricating substances for the nipple.

Underlying structures include mammary gland cells and contractile myoepithelial cells surrounding the gland cells (allowing for milk ejection) that produce alveoli. Milk produced within the alveoli is ejected into the milk ducts, which empty into lactiferous ducts and sinuses, in which milk is stored between breast-feeding periods.

Infant breast-feeding draws the nipple and areola into the mouth, causing elongation of the nipple. The elongated nipple is compressed between the palate and the tongue and milk is expressed less than 0.05 seconds after the nipple has elongated. Compression of the areola between the infant's gums causes expression of milk from lactiferous sinuses. Stimulation of the areola is essential for the oxytocin-mediated hormonal cascade that controls milk ejection.

Physiology of Breast-feeding

Two principal hormones—oxytocin and prolactin—controlled by the hypothalamic-pituitary axis are required for breast milk production. Oxytocin production and secretion are under the control of the posterior pituitary and are stimulated by suckling. Oxytocin production in response to suckling is intermittent and stimulates ejection ("let down") of breast milk. Oxytocin does not appear to affect breast milk production, although numerous stressors can negatively impact breast milk let down. Evidence suggests that lactogenesis may be delayed and let down reduced following stressful vaginal delivery or cesarean section.

Milk production is controlled primarily by the release of prolactin. Prolactin secretion is through a feedback loop under dopaminergic control with the primary action on prolactin receptors on mammary epithelium. Suckling likewise stimulates prolactin release. Furthermore, prolactin acts as an inhibitor of ovulation through hormonal feedback control, although breast-feeding is considered a relatively unreliable contraceptive mechanism.

Several additional hormones are required for milk production: cortisol, human growth hormone, insulin, thyroid and parathyroid hormones, and feedback inhibitor of lactation (FIL). Not entirely understood, FIL appears to act at the level of breast tissue to inhibit continued breast milk production when the breast is not completely emptied.

Milk production begins during the postpartum period with prolactin production and concomitant decreased estrogen and progesterone production following placental delivery. Milk production will persist under this hormonal control for the first several days; however, continued milk production beyond the initial 48 hours postpartum requires suckling. Although mothers will continue to produce milk between feedings once suckling has initiated the feedback loop, milk production significantly rises during breast-feeding.

Breast Milk

A. Stages of Production

Production of human breast milk among healthy mothers who deliver full-term infants occurs in three phases: colostrum, transitional milk, and mature milk. Colostrum is a thick, yellow substance produced during the first several days postpartum. Healthy mothers produce approximately 80–100 mL daily. Colostrum is rich in calcium, antibodies, minerals, proteins, potassium, and fat-soluble vitamins. This milk has immunologic qualities that are vital to the infant and it possesses gastrointestinal properties to aid in secretion of meconium. Production of colostrum is followed for the next 5–6 days with transitional milk, which provides essential components more closely resembling mature breast milk. Most women will notice a significant change evidenced by the fullness of their breasts and the change in the consistency of the milk. True milk is white and sometimes has a bluish tint. The consistency is similar to cow's milk with a sweet taste. Mature breast milk, produced beginning at or near postpartum day 10, produces key components, discussed in the next section.

Numerous factors may affect the supply of breast milk, including anxiety, medications, maternal nutritional status, sleep, exercise, breast-feeding frequency, tactile stimulation, and fluid intake. Breast-feeding mothers should be encouraged to consume generous amounts of fluids and express breast milk every 2–3 hours. The hormonal feedback loop that controls the production and release of prolactin and oxytocin is initiated by suckling or other tactile stimulation of the breast. The greater the amount of suckling or other tactile breast stimulation, the greater the milk supply.

B. Components

Mature human breast milk contains protein, carbohydrate, and fat components and provides approximately 20 kcal/ounce and 1 gram % of protein. The principal protein elements of both mature and premature breast milk are casein (40%) and whey (60%). Breast milk contains approximately 2.5 g/L of casein. Also called "curds," this protein forms calcium complexes. Higher concentrations of this protein are found in cow's milk. Whey (approximately 6.4 g/L) is a protein component composed of α-lactalbumin, lactoferrin, lysozyme, immunoglobulins, and albumin.

Free nitrogen, vital for amino acid synthesis, is also a significant component of mature breast milk and is integral for multiple biochemical pathways, including production of uric acid, urea, ammonia, and creatinine. It is also a key component of insulin and epidermal growth factor.

There are approximately 70 g/L of lactose, the primary carbohydrate in mature breast milk. Composed of galactose and glucose, the lactose concentration continues to increase throughout breast-feeding. Human milk fat likewise increases with continued breast-feeding. Mature breast milk provides approximately 40 g/L and includes triacylglycerides, phospholipids, and essential fatty acids. There is no evidence that lipid levels are not affected by maternal diet, although the type of lipids may vary.

The principal electrolytes in breast milk are sodium, potassium, magnesium, and calcium. Calcium appears to be mediated through the parathyroid hormone–related protein, which allows for mobilization of calcium stores from bone in otherwise healthy women. Bone calcium levels return to normal after termination of breast-feeding. Regulation of sodium and potassium concentrations in breast milk occurs through corticosteroids.

Iron absorption is particularly high in newborns and infants, although the relative concentration of iron in mature breast milk is low. For infants younger than 6 months of age, the concentration of iron in breast milk is sufficient and supplementation is not necessary; however, recommendations for infants older than 6 months include supplemental iron from green vegetables, meats, and iron-rich cereals. The recommended amount of supplemental elemental iron is 1 mg/kg/day. Iron is an essential component in the synthesis of hemoglobin.

Vitamin K, a lipid-soluble vitamin and important component in the clotting cascade, is routinely provided in the immediate postpartum period as a 1-mg intramuscular injection. There is evidence that oral vitamin K may produce similar benefit as well as maternal supplementation of 5 mg/day of oral vitamin K for 12 weeks following delivery.

Another lipid-soluble component, vitamin D, is essential for bone formation. Women who have limited exposure to sunlight or suboptimal vitamin D intake will produce little or no vitamin D in breast milk. The recommended daily intake of vitamin D is 400 IU/day. Practitioners must be cognizant of mothers with special diets (ie, vegetarian diets) whose low vitamin D intake might indicate a need for supplemental vitamin D.

Other elemental minerals in breast milk (eg, zinc, copper, selenium, manganese, nickel, molybdenum, and chromium) are found in trace amounts but nonetheless are essential for a multitude of biochemical processes.

C. Composition of Preterm Breast Milk

The composition of breast milk in mothers of preterm infants is different from that in mothers of term infants. This difference persists for approximately 4 weeks before the composition approaches that of term infant breast milk. The difference in preterm milk composition reflects the increased nutrient demands of preterm infants. Preterm breast milk contains higher concentrations of total and bound nitrogen, immunoglobulins, sodium, iron, chloride, and medium-chain fatty acids. However, it may not contain sufficient amounts of phosphorus, calcium, copper, and zinc. Preterm infants are more likely to require fortification with human milk fortifiers (HMFs) to correct these deficiencies.

Breast-feeding Technique

Preparation for breast-feeding should begin in the preconception period or at the first contact with the patient. Most women choose their method of feeding prior to conception. Psychosocial support and education may encourage breast-feeding among women who might not otherwise have considered it. Evidence for this strategy, however, is anecdotal and requires further investigation.

There are numerous potential supports available to women who are considering feeding behaviors. Practitioners are encouraged to identify members of the patient's support network and provide similar education to minimize the potential barriers posed by uninformed support individuals.

One commonly perceived physical barrier is nipple inversion. Women who have inverted nipples will have difficulty with the latch-on process (discussed later). Nipple shields are relatively inexpensive devices that can draw the nipple out. Manual or electric breast pumps may also be used to draw out inverted nipples, typically beginning after delivery.

Adoptive mothers represent another group with perceived potential barriers to breast-feeding. Feeding of the infant must be discussed once the decision to adopt has been made. Adoptive mothers can be medicated to simulate pregnancy and stimulate production of milk. Despite these hormonal adjuncts, these mothers sometimes will have an inadequate response and subsequent inadequate milk supply. There are several types of supplemental feeding systems that women can wear while breast-feeding that attach to the nipple to provide additional nutrition along with the breast milk.

Breast-feeding should begin immediately in the postpartum period, ideally in the first 30–40 minutes after delivery. This is easier to accomplish if the infant is left in the room with the mother before being bathed and before the newborn examination is performed. It is also safe to allow breast-feeding before administration of vitamin K and erythromycin ophthalmic ointment.

Clinical situations arise that preclude initiation of breast-feeding in the immediate postpartum period (ie, cesarean delivery, maternal perineal repair, maternal or fetal distress). In such cases breast-feeding should be initiated at the earliest time possible. Only when medically necessary should a supplemental feeding be initiated. If mothers have expressed a desire to breast-feed, the practitioner should coordinate an interim feeding plan, emphasizing that bottle feeding not be started. Acceptable alternatives include spoon, cup, or syringe feeding.

Breast-fed children commonly feed at least every 2–3 hours during the first several weeks postpartum. Infants should not be allowed to sleep through feedings; however, if necessary, feeding intervals may be increased to every 3–4 hours overnight. The production of breast milk is on a supply-demand cycle. Breast stimulation through suckling and the mechanism of breast-feeding signals the body to make more milk. When feedings are missed or breasts are not emptied effectively, the feedback loop decreases the milk supply. As the infant grows, feedings every 3–4 hours are acceptable. During growth spurts, the amount of milk needed for the rate of growth often exceeds milk production. Feeding intervals often must be adjusted to growth periods until the milk supply "catches up."

Although feeding intervals may be increased during nighttime periods, a common question becomes when to stop waking the infant for night feedings. Anecdotal evidence suggests that after the first 2 weeks postpartum, in the absence of specific nutritional concerns, the infant can determine its own overnight feeding schedule. Typically, most infants will begin to sleep through the night once they have reached approximately 10 pounds.

Positioning of the infant is critical for effective feeding in the neonatal period, allowing for optimal latch-on. In general, infant and mother should face each other in one of the following three positions: the cradle (the most common) the football, or the lay/side. The cradle hold allows the mother to hold the infant horizontally across the front of the chest. The infant's head can be on the left or right side of the mother depending on which side he or she is feeding. The infant's head should be supported with the crook of the mother's arm. The football hold is performed with the mother sitting on a bed or chair, the infant's bottom against the bed or chair and its body lying next to the mother's side, and the infant's head cradled in her hand. The side position allows the mother to lay on her left or right side with the infant lying parallel to her. Again, the infant's head is cradled in the crook of the mother's elbow. This position is ideally suited for women post–cesarean delivery as it reduces the pain associated with pressure from the infant on their incisions. It must be stressed that choice of position is based on mother and infant comfort. It is not unusual to experiment with any or all positions prior to determining the most desirable. It is likewise not uncommon to find previously undesirable positions more effective and comfortable as the infant grows and the breast-feeding experience progresses. All breast-feeding positions should allow for cradling of the infant's head with the mother's hand or elbow allowing for better head control in the latch-on stage. The infant should be placed at a height (often achieved with a pillow) appropriate for preventing awkward positioning, maximizing comfort, and encouraging latch-on.

Many of the difficulties with breast-feeding result from improper latch-on. Latch-on problems are often the source of multiple breast-feeding complaints among mothers, ranging from engorgement to sore cracked nipples. Many women discontinue breast-feeding secondary to these issues. The latch-on process is governed by primitive reflexes. Stroking the infant's cheek will cause the infant to turn toward the side on which the cheek was stroked. This reflex is useful if the infant is not looking toward the breast. Tickling the infant's bottom lip will cause his or her mouth to open wide in order to latch onto the breast. The mother should hold her breast to help position the areola to ease latch-on. It is important that the mother's fingers be behind the areola so as not to provide a physical barrier to latch-on. Once the infant's mouth is opened wide, the head should be pulled quickly to the breast. The infant's mouth should encompass the entire areola to compress the milk ducts. If this is done improperly, the infant will compress the nipple, leading to pain and eventually cracking, with minimal or no milk expression. The mother should not experience pain with breast-feeding. If this occurs the mother should break the suction by inserting a finger into the side of the infant's mouth and then latch the infant on again. This process should be repeated as many times as necessary until proper latch-on is achieved.

One issue that continually concerns parents is whether the infant is receiving adequate amounts of breast milk. Several clinical measures can be used to determine if infants are receiving enough milk. Weight is an excellent method of assessment. Pre- and postfeed measurement of an infant with a scale that is of high quality and measures to the ounce is a very accurate means of determining weight. The problem is that this type of scale is not available to most families. Weight can also be evaluated on a longer term basis. Infants should not lose more than about 8% of their birth weight after delivery and should gain this weight back in 2 weeks. Most infants with difficulties, however, will decompensate before this 2-week period. Breast-fed infants should be evaluated 2–3 days after discharge, especially if discharged prior to 48 hours postdelivery. A more convenient way to determine the adequacy of the infant's intake of milk is through clinical signs such as infant satisfaction postfeeding and bowel and bladder amounts. In most cases infants who are satisfied after feeding will fall asleep. Infants who do not receive enough milk will usually be fussy or irritable or continuously want to suck at the breast, their finger, and so on. Breast-fed infants usually will stool after most feeds but at a minimum five to six times a day. After the first couple of days, the stool should turn from meconium-like to a mustard-colored seedy type. If breast-fed infants are still passing meconium or do not have an adequate amount of stool, parents and health care team should evaluate whether they are taking in enough milk. Infants should also urinate approximately three or four times a day. This may be hard to assess with the era's superabsorbent diapers. Careful examination of the diaper should be made.

Problems Associated with Breast-feeding

An inadequate milk supply can lead to disastrous outcomes if not identified and treated. There are two types of milk inadequacies: inability to make milk and inability to keep the supply adequate. The first type of milk inadequacy is quite rare but examples include surgeries in which the milk ducts are severed or Sheehan syndrome. There is no specific treatment to initiate milk production in affected women. The inability to maintain an adequate milk supply has numerous etiologies, ranging from dietary deficiencies to engorgement. The key in preventing adverse events is early recognition and effective treatment. One of the mainstays of treatment is working with the body's own feedback loop of supply and demand to increase the supply. As more milk is needed, more milk will be produced. This is effectively done by using a breast pump. Pumping should be performed after the infant has fed.

Engorgement is caused by inadequate or ineffective emptying of the breasts. As milk builds up in the breasts they become swollen. If the condition is not relieved, the breasts can become tender and warm. Mastitis can also develop. The mainstay of treatment is emptying the breasts of milk, either by the infant or if that is not possible by mechanical means. Usually when the breast is engorged, the areola and nipple are affected and proper latch-on becomes difficult if not impossible. A warm compress may be used to help with let down, and the breast can be manually expressed enough to allow the infant to latch on. If this is not possible or is too painful the milk can be removed with an electrical breast pump. Between feedings a cold pack can be used to decrease the amount of swelling. There have been reports that chilled cabbage leaves used to line the bra can act as a cold pack that conforms to the shape of the breast and can reduce the pain and swelling. However, there is no evidence of any medicinal properties in the cabbage that affect engorgement. Mastitis, if occurring, is treated with antibiotics. Mothers can continue to breast-feed with the affected breast so care should be taken to choose an antibiotic that is safe for the infant.

Sore nipples are a common problem for breast-feeding mothers. In the first few weeks there may be some soreness associated with breast-feeding as the skin gets used to the constant moisture. There should not be pain with breast-feeding; if there is pain it is usually secondary to improper latch-on, which resolves with correction. With severe cracking there will occasionally be bleeding. Breast-feeding can be continued with mild bleeding, but if severe bleeding occurs the breast should be pumped and the milk discarded to prevent gastrointestinal upset in the infant. There are some remedies that can be used in the event of cracking. Keeping the nipples clean and dry between feedings can help prevent and heal cracking. The mother's own milk or a pure lanolin ointment can also be used as a salve. Mothers should be warned not to use herbal rubs or vitamin E because of the risk of absorption by the infant. Another cause of sore nipples is candidal infection. This usually occurs when an infant has thrush. Sometimes treating the infant will resolve the problem, but occasionally the mother will need to be treated as well. Taking the same nystatin liquid dose that the infant is using twice a day will resolve the infection. Again, keeping the nipples clean and dry can help.

Other issues with breast-feeding include medications, nutrient supplementation, and mothers returning to work. These issues are broad in scope; in fact, whole books have been dedicated to these subjects. The most important issue to understand when considering medication use during pregnancy is that limited research has been done in this area and that there is insufficient information on most medicines to advocate their use. Health care providers should try to use the safest medications possible that will allow mothers to continue breast-feeding. If this is not possible mothers should be encouraged to pump the milk and discard it to maintain the milk supply.

Nutrient supplementation is another controversial issue. Vitamin D is recommended for supplementation in either dark-skinned women or women who do not receive much sunlight. The iron found in breast milk, although in low concentrations, is highly absorbable. Infants who are breast-fed do not need additional sources of iron until they are 4–6 months old. This is the time when most children are started on cereal. Choosing an iron-fortified cereal will satisfy the additional iron requirement.

Return to work is the major reason why women discontinue breast-feeding. Planning this return from birth and pumping milk for storage help women to continue breast-feeding. Employers who provide time and a comfortable place to pump milk at work will also improve breast-feeding rates. Although the goal is to increase the number of women who begin breast-feeding and continue it throughout the first year of the infant's life, many women cannot or do not choose to breast-feed. Their decision must be supported and they must be educated on alternative methods of providing nutrition for their infant.

Vegetarian Diet

The number of Americans choosing a vegetarian diet has increased dramatically in the past decade. With these increasing numbers more research has been done in an effort to evaluate the feasibility of a vegetarian diet in infancy. A vegetarian diet is defined as a diet consisting of no meat. This definition does not encompass the variety of vegetarian diets that are consumed. A pure vegetarian or vegan consumes only plant food. In general most pure vegetarians also do not use products that result from animal cruelty such as wool, silk, and leather. Lacto-ovo vegetarians consume dairy products and eggs in addition to plants and lacto vegetarians consume only dairy products with their plant diet.

There is great variety in each of these diets and therefore great variety in the type and amount of food necessary for adequate nutrition. Milk from breast-feeding mothers who are vegetarians is adequate in all nutrients necessary for proper growth and development. Although all required nutrients can be found in any vegetarian diet, in infancy the amount necessary may be difficult to provide without supplementation. The American Dietetic association stated that a lacto-ovo vegetarian diet is recommended in infancy. If this diet is not desired by parents or is not tolerated by children then supplementation may be necessary. Vitamin B_{12}, iron, and vitamin D are nutrients that may need to be supplemented, depending on environmental factors.

Contraindications to Breast-feeding

Although considered the optimal method of providing infant nutrition during the first year of life, breast-feeding may be contraindicated in some mothers. Scenarios that may preclude breast-feeding include mothers who actively use illicit drugs such as heroin, cocaine, alcohol, and PCP; mothers with HIV infection or AIDS; and mothers receiving pharmacotherapy with agents transmitted in breast milk and contraindicated in children, particularly potent cancer agents. Some immunizations for foreign travelers and military personnel may also be contraindicated in breast-feeding mothers. Infants with galactosemia should also not breast-feed.

Infant Formulas

The historical record reveals that methods of replacing, fortifying, and delivering milk and milk substitutes date back to the Stone Age. Evidence suggests that the original infant "formulas" of the early and mid-20th century consisted of 1:1 concentrations of evaporated milk and water with supplemental cod liver oil, orange juice, and honey. As the number of working mothers steadily increased during this time, the use of infant formulas became more popular.

In the past three decades, more sophisticated neonatal medical practices have led to the development of countless infant formula preparations to meet a wide variety of clinical situations. Formulas exist as concentrates and powders that require dilution with water and as ready-to-feed preparations. Commonly, formula preparations provide 20 calories per ounce with standard dilutions of 1 ounce concentrate to 1 ounce water and 1 scoop powder formula to 2 ounces water for liquid concentrates and powders, respectively. Formulas exist as cow's milk-based, soy-based, and casein-based preparations.

A. Cow's Milk–Based Formula Preparations

This is the preferred, standard non–breast milk preparation for otherwise healthy term infants who do not breast-feed or for whom breast-feeding has been terminated prior to 1 year of age. Cow's milk–based formula closely resembles human breast milk and is composed of 20% whey and 80% casein with 50% more protein/dL than breast milk as well as iron, linoleic acid, carnitine, taurine, and nucleotides. Approximately 32 ounces will meet 100% of the recommended daily allowance (RDA) for calories, vitamins, and minerals. These formula preparations are diluted to a standard 20 calories per ounce and are typically whey-dominant protein preparations with vegetable oils and lactose. There are also multiple lactose-free preparations. Most standard formula preparations do not meet the RDA for fluoride, and exclusively formula-fed infants may require 0.25 mg/day of supplemental fluoride.

B. Soy-Based Formula Preparations

Indicated primarily for vegetarian mothers and lactose-intolerant, galactosemic, and cow's milk–allergic infants, soy-based formulas provide a protein-rich formula that contains more protein per deciliter than both breast milk and cow's milk formula preparations. Because the proteins are plant based, vitamin and mineral composition is increased to compensate for plant-based mineral antagonists while supplementing protein composition with the addition of methionine. Soy-based formulas tend to have a sweeter taste owing to a carbohydrate composition that includes sucrose and corn syrup. ProSobee, Isomil, and I-Soyalac are common soy-based preparations.

C. Casein Hydrolysate–Based Formula Preparations

This poor-tasting, expensive formula preparation is indicated principally for infants with either milk and soy-protein allergies or intolerance. Other indications include complex gastrointestinal pathologies. This formula, which contains casein-based protein and glucose, is not recommended for prolonged use in preterm infants owing to inadequate vitamin and mineral composition and proteins that may be difficult to metabolize. Standard preparations provide 20–24 calories per ounce.

D. Premature Infant Formula Preparations

Indicated for use in preterm infants of less than 1800 g birth weight, and with three times the vitamin and mineral content of standard formula preparations, these formulations provide 20–24 calories per ounce. Premature infant preparations are approximately 60% casein and 40% whey, with 1:1 concentrations of lactose and glucose as well as 1:1 concentrations of long- and medium-chain fatty acids. Commercially available preparations include Enfamil Premature with Iron, Similac Natural Care Breast Milk Fortifier, and Similac Special Care with Iron. Similac Neo-Care, designed for preterm infants weighing more than 1800 g at birth, provides 22 calories per ounce in standard dilution.

Human Milk Fortifiers for Preterm Infants

Human milk fortifiers (HMFs) are indicated for preterm infants less than 34 weeks' gestation or less than 1500 g birth weight once feeding has reached 75% full volume. HMFs are designed to supplement calories, protein, phosphorus, calcium, and other vitamins and minerals.

Enfamil-HMF is mixed to 24 calories per ounce by adding one 3.8-g packet to 25 mL of breast milk, increasing the osmolality to greater than 350 mOsm/L. Increased osmolality may enhance gastrointestinal irritability and affect tolerance. Practitioners may recommend a lower osmolality for the first 48 hours, beginning with one packet of Enfamil-HMF in 50 mL of breast milk, producing 22 calories per ounce. The maximum caloric density from this HMF is 24 calories per ounce. Practitioners may add emulsified fat blends to meet increased caloric needs.

Similac Natural Care is a liquid milk fortifier that is typically mixed in a 1:1 ratio with breast milk. Other alternatives may include feedings with breast milk and fortifier. The osmolality of Similac Natural Care is lower than that of Enfamil—280 mOsm/L. This liquid fortifier may be preferable, particularly for infants whose mothers have low milk production.

American Dietetic Association: *Nutrition Management of the Infant. Manual of Clinical Dietetics.* ADA, 1997.

Bachrach VR et al: Breastfeeding and the risk of hospitalization for respiratory disease in infancy: A meta-analysis. Arch Pediatr Adolesc Med 2003;157:237. [PMID: 12622672]

Bentley ME et al: Breastfeeding among low income, African-American women: Power, beliefs and decision making. J Nutr 2003;133:305S. [PMID: 12514315]

Chezem J et al: Breastfeeding knowledge, breastfeeding confidence, and infant feeding plans: Effects on actual feeding practices. J Obstet Gynecol Neonatal Nurs 2003;32:40. [PMID: 12570180]

Dewey KG: Is breastfeeding protective against child obesity? J Hum Lact 2003;19:9. [PMID: 12587638]

Dewey KG: Maternal and fetal stress are associated with impaired lactogenesis in humans. J Nutr 2001;131:3012S. [PMID: 11694638]

Furman L et al: The effect of maternal milk on neonatal morbidity of very low-birth-weight infants. Arch Pediatr Adolesc Med 2003;157:66. [PMID: 12517197]

Gartner LM et al, American Academy of Pediatrics Section on Breastfeeding: Breastfeeding and the use of human milk. Pediatrics 2005;115:496. [PMID: 15687461]

Greenwood K, Littlejohn P: Breastfeeding intentions and outcomes of adolescent mothers in the Starting Out program. Breastfeed Rev 2002;10:19. [PMID: 12592776]

Howard CR et al: Randomized clinical trial of pacifier use and bottle-feeding or cupfeeding and their effect on breastfeeding. Pediatrics 2003;111:511. [PMID: 12612229]

Khoury AJ et al: Improving breastfeeding knowledge, attitudes, and practices of WIC clinic staff. Public Health Rep 2002;117:453. [PMID: 12500962]

Lawrence RA, Lawrence RM: *Breastfeeding, a Guide for the Medical Profession,* 6th ed. Elsevier/Mosby, 2005.

Lovelady CA et al: Effect of exercise on immunologic factors in breast milk. Pediatrics 2003;111:E148. [PMID: 12563088]

Mikiel-Kostyra K et al: Effect of early skin-to-skin contact after delivery on duration of breast-feeding: A prospective cohort study. Acta Paediatr 2002;91:1301. [PMID: 12578285]

Mizuno K, Ueda A: The maturation and coordination of sucking, swallowing, and respiration in preterm infants. J Pediatr 2003;142:36. [PMID: 12520252]

Neville MC: Anatomy and physiology of lactation. Pediatr Clin North Am 2001;48:13. [PMID: 11236721]

Oddy WH: The impact of breastmilk on infant and child health. Breastfeed Rev 2002;10:5. [PMID: 12592775]

Pediatrician's responsibility for infant nutrition. American Academy of Pediatrics Committee on Practice and Ambulatory Medicine. Pediatrics 1997;99:749. [PMID: 9157387]

US Department of Health and Human Services. Office on Women's Health: *HHS Blueprint for Action on Breastfeeding.* DHHS, 2000.

Web Sites

American Academy of Pediatrics—"A Woman's Guide to Breastfeeding":

http://www.aap.org/family/brstguid.htm

La Leche League:

http://www.lalecheleague.org

Resources for breast-feeding products and information:

http://www.breastfeedingbasics.org

http://www.breastfeeding.hypermart.net

http://www.medela.com

Common Infections in Children 5

Mark A. Knox, MD

Infectious diseases are a major cause of disease in children. The widespread use of antibiotics has greatly reduced morbidity and mortality, but infections are still one of the most common types of problems encountered by physicians who care for children.

FEVER WITHOUT A SOURCE

General Considerations

Fever is the primary sign that indicates an infectious process in children of all ages. Other than fever, however, many children do not display signs or symptoms indicative of the underlying disease. Twenty percent of febrile children, after history and physical examination, have fever without a source of infection. The physician's dilemma is to separate children with a serious bacterial illness from those with a viral or nonserious bacterial illness. A serious bacterial illness is defined variably, but generally includes growth of a known bacterial pathogen from cerebrospinal fluid, blood, urine, or stool, as well as abscess or cellulitis and pneumonia with positive blood cultures. Children are generally divided into three groups for evaluation purposes: young children aged 3 months to 3 years, young infants aged 2–3 months, and neonates (1 month of age or younger). Young children are much more likely to show outward signs of illness, and their evaluation is much easier than that of younger infants. Neonates are a separate diagnostic group, more likely to have infections with organisms seen in the newborn period and less likely to show overt clinical signs of infection.

No officially adopted, evidence-based guidelines have been published to guide physicians in the workup and management of febrile illnesses, although several papers have been written detailing suggested guidelines based on expert opinion, group consensus, and locally performed research studies. Baraff and colleagues published a set of useful practice guidelines that are summarized in Table 5–1.

The frequency and nature of serious bacterial illness is different in the three different age groups. Neonates younger than 1 month of age are the most difficult to diagnose. The rate of serious bacterial illness in nontoxic febrile neonates has been reported to be between 8.6% and 12.6%. However, existing screening protocols lack the sensitivity and negative predictive value to identify infants at low risk for these infections. For this reason, it is generally accepted that all febrile infants younger than 1 month of age be admitted to the hospital, given a complete sepsis workup, and treated with parenteral antibiotics pending the results of the workup. Of these infants, approximately 65% have a viral infection, 13% have a serious bacterial illness, and the rest have nonbacterial gastroenteritis, aseptic meningitis, or bronchiolitis. Of the infants with serious bacterial illnesses, roughly 7% have a urinary tract infection (UTI), with *Escherichia coli* being the most common pathogen. Three percent have bacteremia, with group B *Streptococcus, Enterobacter, Listeria, Streptococcus pneumoniae, E coli, Enterococcus,* and *Klebsiella* all being found. Fewer than 2% have meningitis, usually caused by *Klebsiella, Listeria,* and group B *Streptococcus.*

In evaluating infants older than 1 month of age, it is useful to first identify which infants are at low risk for a serious bacterial illness. The criteria for low risk are being previously healthy, having no focal source of infection found on physical examination, and having a negative laboratory evaluation, defined as a white blood cell (WBC) count of 5000–15,000/mm^3, fewer than 1500 bands/mm^3, normal urinalysis, and, if diarrhea is present, fewer than 5 WBCs per high-power field in the stool. Chest radiography is included in some, but not all, sets of criteria. Lumbar puncture may be performed at the physician's discretion but should always be done if empiric antibiotics are to be used. Additional low-risk criteria are appearing nontoxic and having a good social situation with reliable follow-up. Low-risk, nontoxic-appearing infants may be treated as outpatients, with close follow-up. Most recommendations are to use empiric antibiotics, but some authors feel that antibiotics may be withheld if the infant can be followed closely. All toxic-appearing or non–low-risk infants should be hospitalized and treated with parenteral antibiotics. The risk of serious bacterial illness in toxic-appearing infants in this age group is about 17%. The

Table 5–1. Evaluation and treatment of febrile children.

Infant < 1 Month of Age	Child 3 Months to 3 Years of Age
Admit for evaluation and treatment	Toxic: admit
Infant 2–3 Months of Age	Nontoxic:
Toxic or non–low risk: admit	Temperature < 39.0°C (102.2°F):
Nontoxic, low risk:	No tests or antibiotics
Option 1	Symptomatic treatment for fever
• Blood culture	Return if fever persists > 48 h or if condition deteriorates
• Urine culture	Temperature > 39.0°C (103.1°F):
• Lumbar puncture	Urinalysis: if positive, perform culture, treat with oral third-generation cephalosporin
• Ceftriaxone, 50 mg/kg IM (1 g max)	
• Return for reevaluation within 24 h	If child has not received pneumococcal conjugate vaccine:
Option 2	• If temperature > 39.5°C, obtain WBC count
• Blood culture	• If WBC count > 15,000/mm^3, obtain blood culture, administer ceftriaxone, 50 mg/kg
• Urine culture	
• Careful observation	If Sao_2 < 95%, respiratory distress, tachypnea, rales, or temperature > 39.5°C and WBC count > 20,000, obtain chest x-ray
Low-risk criteria:	
Clinical	Symptomatic treatment for fever
• Previously healthy, term infant with uncomplicated nursery stay	Return if fever persists > 48 h or if condition deteriorates
• Nontoxic appearance	
• No focal bacterial infection on examination (except otitis media)	
Laboratory	
• WBC count 5000–15,000/mm^3, < 1500 bands/mm^3	
• Negative Gram stain of unspun urine (preferred), or negative urine leukocyte esterase and nitrite, or < 5 WBCs/hpf	
• CSF < 8 WBCs/mm^3 and negative Gram stain	

IM, intramuscular; WBC, white blood cell; HPF, high-power field; CSF, cerebrospinal fluid; Sao_2, oxygen saturation.
Adapted from Baraff L: Management of fever without source in infants and children. Ann Emerg Med 2000;36:602.

overall frequency of such infections in this age group is roughly 9% overall and 1–2% in low-risk infants, with most of the infections being UTIs, bacteremia, and bacterial enteritis. Meningitis accounts for slightly more than 1% of febrile infants.

Similar criteria may be used to evaluate children aged 3 months to 3 years. The most common serious bacterial illnesses in this group are bacteremia and UTIs. UTIs are present in nearly 5% of febrile infants younger than 12 months of age. In this group, 6–8% of girls and 2–3% of boys have UTIs. The rates are higher in those with higher temperatures. After 12 months of age, the prevalence of UTI is lower.

In this age group, the rate of bacteremia has been reported to be 3–11%, with a mean of 4.3% if the temperature is 39°C (102.2°F) or higher. The most common organisms isolated are *S pneumoniae* (85%), *Haemophilus influenzae* type b (10%), and *Neisseria meningitidis* (3%). The rate of infection with *H influenzae* has fallen dramatically since the use of the Hib vaccine has become widespread, and the rate of pneumococcal bacteremia is expected to do likewise in the near future.

Occult pneumonia is rare in febrile children who have a normal WBC count and who do not have signs of lower respiratory infection, such as cough, tachypnea, rales, or rhonchi.

As in younger infants, toxic-appearing or non–low-risk infants should be hospitalized and treated with parenteral antibiotics. The rate of serious bacterial infections in toxic-appearing children in this age group has been reported to be 10–90%, depending on the definition of toxic.

Low-risk, non–toxic-appearing children in this age group may be treated as outpatients. The use of empiric antibiotics pending culture results is left to the physician's discretion. There is general consensus that bacteremia is a risk factor for development of infectious complications, such as meningitis. However, pneumococcal bacteremia responds well to oral antibiotics, so these drugs can be used in children who appear well despite having positive blood cultures.

Clinical Findings

A. Symptoms and Signs

The most important clinical decision is to decide which infants appear toxic and therefore need more aggressive evaluation and treatment. "Toxic" is defined as a picture consistent with the sepsis syndrome: lethargy, signs of poor perfusion, marked hypoventilation or hyperventilation, or cyanosis. "Lethargy" is defined as an impaired level of consciousness as manifested by poor or absent eye contact or by failure of the child to recognize parents or to interact with people or objects in the environment.

Fever is defined as temperature of 38°C (100.4°F) or higher. Rectal measurement is the only accurate way to determine fever. A careful, complete physical examination is necessary to exclude focal signs of infection. The skin should be examined for exanthems, cellulitis, abscesses, or petechiae. Between 2% and 8% of children with fever and a petechial rash have a serious bacterial infection, most often caused by *N meningitidis.* Common childhood infections such as pharyngitis and otitis media should be sought, and a careful lung examination should be done looking for evidence of pneumonia. The abdomen should be examined for signs of peritonitis or tenderness. A musculoskeletal examination should be done looking for evidence of osteomyelitis or septic arthritis. The neurologic examination should be directed toward the level of consciousness and should look for focal neurologic deficits.

B. Laboratory and Imaging Findings

WBC count and differential, urinalysis and urine culture, blood culture, lumbar puncture with routine analysis and culture, and chest x-ray should be obtained. If the child has diarrhea, stool cultures should be evaluated.

Treatment

All infants younger than 1 month of age should be hospitalized. An appropriate antibiotic regimen includes ceftriaxone (50 mg/kg/day) with or without gentamicin. In the past, ampicillin has been used routinely to cover the possibility of *Listeria* infection. Although it appears that the frequency of infection with *Listeria* is decreasing, ampicillin may be added to this regimen if the physician chooses.

Ceftriaxone is likewise an appropriate antibiotic for hospitalized older infants and children and for infants and children treated as outpatients. In infants 2–3 months of age, a single intramuscular dose of ceftriaxone should be given. The child should be reevaluated in 18–24 hours and a second dose of ceftriaxone given. If blood cultures are found to be positive, the child should be admitted for further treatment. If the urine culture is positive and the child has a persistent fever, the child should be admitted for treatment. If the child is afebrile and well, outpatient antibiotics may be used.

Table 5–1 presents guidelines that may be useful for investigating and treating febrile children.

Baraff L: Management of fever without source in infants and children. Ann Emerg Med 2000;36:602. [PMID: 11097701]

INFECTIONS OF THE UPPER RESPIRATORY TRACT

OTITIS MEDIA

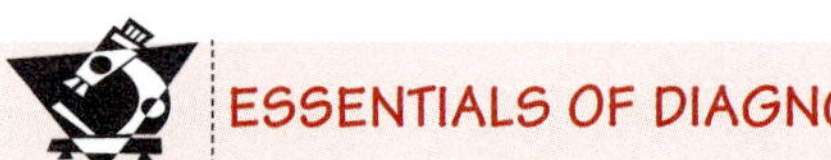

- *Preexisting upper respiratory infection (URI; 93%).*
- *Fever (25%).*
- *Ear pain (variable, depending on age).*
- *Bulging, immobile tympanic membrane that is dull gray, yellow, or red in color.*
- *Perforated tympanic membrane with purulent drainage (diagnostic).*

General Considerations

Acute otitis media (AOM) is the most common reason that children see a physician, accounting for almost 30 million physician visits each year among children younger than 1 year of age. Almost all children have at least one episode of otitis media each year, and one third have three or more episodes.

Pathogenesis

When cultures of middle ear fluid are done, *S pneumoniae* is found in about 35%, *H influenzae* in about 25%, and *Moraxella catarrhalis* in about 15%. Ten percent of effusions show more than one of these bacteria, and about 25% are sterile. Viruses are recovered in a large percentage of cases, with or without bacteria, but whether their role is causative or not remains unclear.

Prevention

There are several identified risk factors for otitis media, not all of which are easily modifiable for prevention of the disease. The chief risk factor is day care. Other risk factors include increased number of siblings in the house, exposure to tobacco smoke, pacifier use, formula feeding, and lower socioeconomic status. Children with abnormalities of the palatal architecture, such as those with cleft palate or Down syndrome, are at greatly increased risk. Widespread use of vaccines against *H influenzae* type b and *S pneumoniae* are not expected to have much impact on the disease, as the infection is generally caused by nontypeable *Haemophilus* and by strains of pneumococcus not covered by the pediatric 7-valent vaccine.

Clinical Findings

A. Symptoms and Signs

Despite the frequency with which physicians see children with otitis media, the diagnostic criteria are not standardized, and the diagnosis itself is often unclear. Otitis media most often begins with a URI, and as many as 93% of children with AOM have typical symptoms of URI. Symptoms of AOM may develop over only a few hours, or the onset may be more gradual. Ear pain is the most characteristic symptom. Younger children do not localize pain as obviously as older children. Fever is present only in about 25% and is more common in younger children. The tympanic membrane bulges and may be cloudy, yellow, or red in color. Erythema of the tympanic membrane may be caused by fever or by screaming, so this sign is of questionable reliability. The drum generally is immobile with pneumatic otoscopy or tympanometry. The infection is bilateral in half of affected children. The tympanic membrane ruptures in fewer than 5% of cases, but pus draining through a perforation is diagnostic.

Differential Diagnosis

As previously discussed, the primary illness that may be confused with AOM is acute URI. Many of the symptoms are identical, and findings in the tympanic membrane may be subtle and nondiagnostic.

Complications

Complications of otitis media fall into two main categories: suppurative and nonsuppurative. Suppurative complications may arise from direct extension of the infection into the surrounding bones or into the adjacent brain, such as mastoiditis, venous sinus thrombosis, and brain abscess. They may also arise from hematogenous spread of the bacteria from the middle ear, primarily sepsis and meningitis. The main suppurative complication is mastoiditis, which develops in about 1 in 1000 cases. Recent research shows that treatment of otitis media does not reduce the incidence of this complication. The bacteria responsible for hematogenous spread are principally *S pneumoniae* and *H influenzae.*

Nonsuppurative complications are primarily those that arise from middle ear effusion and inflammation and scarring of the structures of the middle ear. Antibiotic treatment does not influence the persistence of middle ear effusions after otitis media, nor does it have any effect on long-term hearing and language development. In summary, it appears that complications of otitis media may not be preventable by antibiotic treatment.

Treatment

Although antibiotic treatment has long been the standard of care for children with AOM, research has shown that the benefits of antibiotics are much less clear than was believed in the past. As many as 59% of children have resolution of symptoms within 24 hours without treatment, and between 80% and 85% recover in 1–7 days without antibiotics. Antibiotic treatment reduces the persistence of symptoms at 2–7 days to 7%, or about a 12% reduction.

The high spontaneous resolution rate makes comparisons of treatments difficult. Narrow-spectrum antibiotics have the same success rate as broad-spectrum antibiotics, although adverse effects, primarily gastrointestinal, are more common with the latter. High-dose amoxicillin (80 mg/kg/day) is no more effective than the standard dose (40 mg/kg/day). Single-dose intramuscular ceftriaxone (50 mg/kg) is as effective as oral antibiotics. Studies also document that a 5-day course of antibiotics is as effective as the standard 10-day course. Thus, based on numerous studies, a recommended approach is to treat children with AOM using a 5-day course of narrow-spectrum antibiotics.

Another acceptable option is withholding antibiotic treatment for 48–72 hours, treating pain as needed, and beginning antibiotic therapy if the symptoms do not resolve within this time period. This may be considered in children over the age of 2 years if the presenting illness is not severe (fever < 39°C [102.2°F] and mild or no pain). This is also an option for children between the ages of 6 months and 2 years, if the diagnosis of otitis media is uncertain and the symptoms are not severe.

It is important to note that studies have not adequately addressed the issues of treatment of children younger than 2 years of age and treatment of frequently recurrent or complicated otitis media. Physicians are left to their clinical judgment as to the best treatment for these children.

The best treatment for children with frequent recurrences of otitis media is another area of study. The best evidence is that children will only benefit from daily antibiotic prophylaxis if they have had more than three episodes in 6 months or four episodes in 1 year. The magnitude of benefit is small, with a reduction of about one episode per year. Antibiotics studied have primarily been narrow-spectrum drugs, such as erythromycin, amoxicillin, sulfisoxazole, and trimethoprim-sulfamethoxazole.

Prognosis

In general, children with otitis media recover uneventfully. The half-life of the middle ear effusion is about 4 weeks, with 10% persistence at 4 months. Repeated courses of antibiotics have no effect on these effusions and should not be used.

American Academy of Family Physicians, American Academy of Pediatrics: *Diagnosis and Management of Acute Otitis Media.* March 2004. Available at: http://www.aafp.org/online/en/home/clinical/clincalrecs/aom.html.

Takata G et al: Evidence assessment of management of acute otitis media: I. The role of antibiotics in treatment of uncomplicated otitis media. Pediatrics 2001;108:239. [PMID: 11483783]

PHARYNGITIS

Sore throat is a common problem in pediatrics, leading to millions of physician office visits each year. However, obtaining a clear diagnosis as to the cause of this problem is far from simple. The most important diagnosis to make is infection with group A β-hemolytic streptococci (GABHS), which is responsible for about 15% of cases of pharyngitis. Antibiotic treatment has only a modest effect on the course of the disease, but adequate treatment with antibiotics effectively prevents the important complication of rheumatic fever. Non-GABHS occasionally cause pharyngitis but do not lead to rheumatic fever. Viruses of many sorts cause the vast majority of cases, including some cases of exudative pharyngitis. Adenoviruses can cause pharyngoconjunctival fever, with exudative pharyngitis and conjunctivitis. Epstein-Barr virus causes infectious mononucleosis, which commonly produces other signs, such as generalized lymphadenopathy and splenomegaly, in addition to exudative pharyngitis. Herpesviruses and coxsackieviruses can cause ulcerative stomatitis and pharyngitis. Most viruses, however, cause signs and symptoms that overlap with those of GABHS. The literature contains numerous recommendations for diagnosis and treatment, but there is no clear consensus as to the most accurate or most cost-effective method for evaluation and treatment of the child with a sore throat. (For more complete discussion of pharyngitis in the child or adult, see Chapter 26.)

INFLUENZA

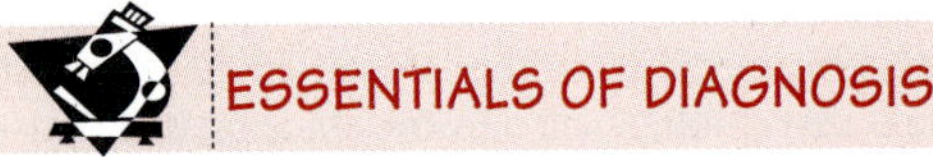

- *Nonspecific respiratory infection in infants and young children.*
- *In older children, respiratory symptoms—coryza, conjunctivitis, pharyngitis, dry cough.*
- *In older children, pronounced high fever, myalgia, headache, malaise.*

General Considerations

Influenza is a respiratory virus that causes a respiratory infection of variable severity in children. Although influenza itself is a benign, self-limited disease, its sequelae, primarily pneumonia, can cause serious illness and occasionally death.

Pathogenesis

Influenza is caused by a variety of influenza viruses. Types A and B cause epidemic illness, whereas type C produces sporadic cases of respiratory infections. Infection with influenza virus confers limited immunity that lasts several years, until the natural antigenic drift of the virus produces a pathogen that is genetically distinct enough to escape this protection. Because every virus is new for infants, the attack rate is highest in infants and young children, with between 30% and 50% showing serologic evidence of infection in a normal year.

Prevention

The most effective way to prevent influenza and its complications is to immunize people of all ages at highest risk for complications. Influenza vaccine protects against both types A and B. Recent studies show that complication rates are similar across all children, regardless of what are often considered to be risk factors, and that otherwise healthy children younger than 2 years of age, and possibly those between the ages of 2 and 4 years as well, have a higher rate of complications than older children. For this reason, routine annual immunization is now recommended for children between the ages of 6 and 59 months. Immunization of older children is optional.

Children younger than 9 years who have never been immunized against influenza should receive two doses of vaccine, 1 month apart. Children 9 years of age and older need only one dose. The unit dose for children 6–35 months of age is 0.25 mL. The unit dose for children 36 months of age and older is 0.5 mL. The vaccine must be repeated annually. The vaccine should be given in October or November, to protect children during the peak months of December through February. Peak antibody levels are achieved roughly 2 weeks after immunization (2 weeks after the second dose in vaccine-naive children).

Chemoprophylaxis with a variety of drugs is an alternative to immunization, although this option is much more expensive than the vaccine. Because strains of influenza virus most recently active in the United States have been resistant to amantadine and rimantadine, these drugs are no longer recommended for this purpose. Oseltamivir is indicated for prophylaxis in children older than 1 year, and zanamivir can be used in children older than 5 years of age. The optimal duration of treatment is not known.

Clinical Findings

A. Symptoms and Signs

Influenza viruses types A and B cause nearly identical symptoms, except that the duration of symptoms in type A infection is usually several days, whereas symptoms usually last only 2 or 3 days in type B infection. Influenza in infants and young children causes a nonspecific respiratory infection. Occasionally the fever is high enough and the child toxic enough in appearance to prompt hospitalization and workup for sepsis. In older children and adolescents, the disease presents with the abrupt onset of respiratory symptoms, such as URI symptoms, conjunctivitis, pharyngitis, and dry cough. The features that distinguish influenza from the usual URI are high fever and pronounced myalgia, headache, and malaise. The acute symptoms typically last for 2–4 days, but the cough and malaise may persist for several days longer. Physical findings are nonspecific and include pharyngitis, conjunctivitis, cervical lymphadenopathy, and occasionally rales, wheezes, or rhonchi in the lungs.

B. Special Tests

Influenza is generally diagnosed based on clinical criteria. If confirmation of infection is desired, the virus can be identified by nasopharyngeal swabs sent for viral culture.

Complications

Otitis media and pneumonia are the most common complications from influenza. Up to 25% of children develop otitis media after a documented influenza infection. Influenza causes a primary viral pneumonia, but the more serious pneumonic complications are caused by bacterial superinfection.

Treatment

Treatment of established influenza infection within 2 days of the onset of symptoms can reduce the duration of symptoms by about 1 day compared with placebo. However, no drug has been shown to reduce the incidence of serious complications following the disease. Because of resistance in recent viral strains, amantadine and rimantadine are no longer recommended. Oseltamivir can be used in children older than 1 year of age, and zanamivir can be used for children age 7 years and older. Both are given as a 5-day course. Given the cost of these medications and their inability to prevent complications, immunization is clearly a superior alternative for controlling influenza and its sequelae.

Prognosis

Influenza is ordinarily a benign self-limited disease. Morbidity and mortality are related either to postinfluenza pneumonia or to exacerbation of underlying chronic illness caused by the virus.

Advisory Committee on Immunization Practices; Smith N et al: Prevention and control of influenza: Recommendations of the Advisory Committee on Immunization Practice (ACIP). MMWR Recomm Rep 2006;55:1. [PMID: 16874296]

INFECTIONS OF THE LOWER RESPIRATORY TRACT

CROUP (ACUTE LARYNGEOTRACHEOBRONCHITIS)

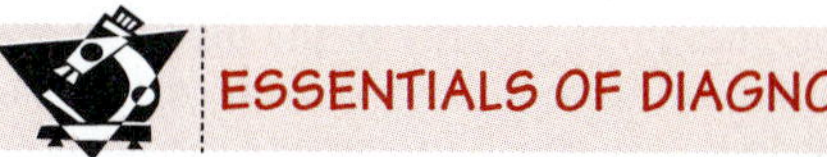

- *URI prodrome.*
- *Barking cough.*
- *Symptoms worst on first or second day, with gradual resolution.*
- *Lungs clear.*
- *Inspiratory stridor, respiratory distress, cyanosis in severe cases.*

General Considerations

Croup is a relatively common infection in children, causing between 27,000 and 62,000 hospitalizations each year. Most cases occur in the autumn and early winter, with most hospitalizations in October and February. The peak age incidence of croup is 3 months to 5 years of age.

Pathogenesis

Croup is caused by an infection of the upper airways—the larynx, trachea, and the upper levels of the bronchial tree—and obstruction of these airways caused by edema produces most of the classic symptoms of the disease. Nearly all cases of croup are caused by viruses. Parainfluenza viruses cause 75% of cases. Adenovirus and respiratory syncytial virus (RSV) cause most of the remainder, and *Mycoplasma pneumoniae* accounts for 3–4% of cases.

Clinical Findings

A. Symptoms and Signs

The symptoms of croup are usually typical, and diagnosis is not difficult. Most children present after several days of prodromal URI symptoms, which are followed by the gradual onset of a barking, "seal-like" cough. Stridor is generally mild and intermittent at first, primarily with inspiration and worse when the child is agitated. Typically, respiratory distress is only mild to moderate. In most children, this is the maximum extent of the disease. The symptoms are generally worst on the first or second day, are usually worse at night than during the day, and gradually resolve over several days. If the symptoms progress beyond this point, the child develops worsening respiratory distress, more pronounced and more constant stridor, and cyanosis.

The physical findings of croup are variable and depend on the severity of the illness. The lungs are usually clear. The degree of subcostal and intercostal retractions, the degree of stridor, and the presence of cyanosis are important clues to the severity of the illness. If the child is cyanotic and in respiratory distress, manipulation of the pharynx (eg, trying to examine the pharynx using a tongue depressor) may trigger respiratory arrest. This maneuver should therefore be avoided until the clinician is in a position to manage the child's airway by endotracheal intubation.

B. Laboratory Findings

Laboratory findings are generally minimal. The WBC count is usually normal or slightly elevated; however, counts greater than 15,000/mm^3 are seen in about 20% of children. The blood oxygen saturation may be normal or decreased, depending on the severity of the disease.

C. Imaging Studies

In a typical child with croup, the chest x-ray is normal. In 40–50% of children, anteroposterior soft-tissue x-rays of the neck show subglottic narrowing, causing the classic "steeple" sign of croup.

Differential Diagnosis

Croup must be differentiated from other respiratory illness that cause cough as the main symptom. Normally, the time course and nature of the cough are diagnostic. Spasmodic croup lacks the URI prodrome and has a more abrupt onset than typical croup. Bacterial tracheitis presents as typical croup that worsens instead of improving after a few days. Children with epiglottitis and peritonsillar abscess are acutely ill and often toxic appearing, and while they may have a cough, it is not the predominant feature of the disease. Children with bronchiolitis are usually younger than are children with croup, and their lungs show diffuse fine end-expiratory wheezes. Likewise, expiratory wheezing is a prominent feature of asthma but not of croup, which may produce prominent inspiratory stridor in children with severe disease. Children with pneumonia usually have a looser, more productive cough, they often have more focal pulmonary findings on examination, and chest x-ray often shows an infiltrate.

Complications

About 15% of children with croup experience complications of varying severity. These are usually related to extension of the infection to other parts of the respiratory tract, such as otitis media or viral pneumonia. Bacterial pneumonia is unusual, but bacterial tracheitis may occur. Children with severe croup may develop complications of hypoxemia, if this is not adequately treated. Death is unusual and generally due to laryngeal obstruction.

Treatment

Perhaps the most critical decision to make when evaluating children with croup is which patients need to be treated in the hospital and which will do well at home. Between 1.5% and 15% of children with croup are hospitalized for treatment, and of these, 1–5% require intubation and ventilation. The published croup scoring systems may be useful for research purposes, but they do not present validated criteria for determining the best course of treatment for an individual child. High fever, toxic appearance, worsening stridor, respiratory distress, cyanosis or pallor, hypoxia, and restlessness or lethargy are all symptoms of more severe disease and should prompt the physician to admit the child for inpatient treatment.

Most children with croup may be treated at home. The mainstay of treatment has long been held to be cool, moist air, although research has not confirmed the effectiveness of this treatment. Although corticosteroids have long been an accepted part of inpatient treatment, their role in outpatient management of this disease has only more recently been addressed. A single intramuscular dose of dexamethasone, 0.6 mg/kg, may be effective in reducing the severity of moderate to severe croup in patients treated at home. Because the onset of action for dexamethasone is about 6 hours, a single dose of racemic epinephrine may be given before the child is sent home. β_2-Agonist bronchodilators have not been shown to be effective.

Inpatient treatment of croup has changed little in recent years. As with home treatment, the mainstay of therapy is cool, humidified air, using a croup tent. Supplemental oxygen is used to correct hypoxemia. Racemic epinephrine has long been the mainstay of treatment for patients who do not respond to cool, moist air or who have respiratory distress. Numerous studies have confirmed its effectiveness. The drug is administered via nebulizer and face mask. It has a duration of action of 1–2 hours. Although racemic epinephrine is the drug most commonly used, L-epinephrine is equally effective, less expensive, and more widely available. Numerous studies have shown systemic dexamethasone to be effective in reducing both the severity and duration of the disease and the need for intubation. Because of its long action, the drug can be given as a single dose, which remains effective for the remainder of the course of the disease. The dose is 0.6 mg/kg, intramuscularly, and it should be given as early as possible in the course of the disease. Nebulized steroids and oral dexamethasone are more effective than placebo but less effective than intramuscular dexamethasone. Children hospitalized for treatment of croup should be observed carefully for any signs of respiratory distress. Intubation and mechanical ventilation are necessary in a small percentage of children with this disease.

Prognosis

The natural history of croup is that recurrences are common. However, as children grow, the airways grow larger and are less affected by edema, and symptoms tend to become less severe over time.

BRONCHIOLITIS

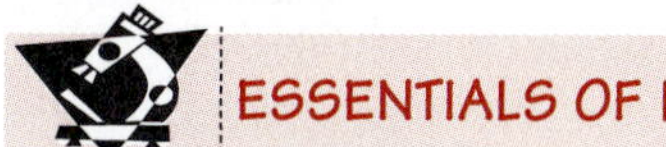

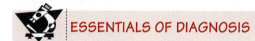

ESSENTIALS OF DIAGNOSIS

- *URI symptoms.*
- *Paroxysmal wheezy cough.*
- *Dyspnea.*
- *Tachypnea.*
- *Diffuse fine rales.*

General Considerations

Bronchiolitis is a common disease of infants, affecting up to 7% of infants and leading to hospitalization in up to 1% during the first 2 years of life. It is an infection that causes edema and obstruction of the small airways. Bronchiolitis is seen most commonly in the first 2 years of life, with a peak age of about 6 months. Older children and adults contract the same infection, but because they have larger airways, they do not experience the same degree of airway obstruction. In fact, an older sibling or a parent is often the source of the infant's infection.

Pathogenesis

Bronchiolitis is almost always viral in etiology. RSV causes more than half of cases; others are caused by parainfluenza viruses, with a few cases caused by *M pneumonia*. Pathologically, edema and accumulated cellular debris cause obstruction of small airways. This obstruction causes a ventilation-perfusion mismatch with wasted perfusion, a right-to-left shunt, and hypoxemia early in the course of the disease.

Prevention

Since 1999, palivizumab has been available in the United States for prevention of RSV disease in high-risk infants. The drug has been shown to decrease hospitalization rates among high-risk infants with and without chronic lung disease, although the death rates in the initial studies were not significantly different between the treatment and placebo groups. The decision to use this drug is based on the age of the child at the onset of RSV season and the child's medical history. The American Academy of Pediatrics recommends prophylaxis with palivizumab for children younger than 2 years of age with chronic lung disease who have required medical treatment in the preceding 6 months, for infants younger than 1 year of age who were born at 28 weeks' gestation or earlier, for infants younger than 6 months of age who were born at 29–32 weeks' gestation, and for infants younger than 6 months of age born between 32 and 35 weeks' gestation who have other risk factors for RSV infection such as day-care attendance or three or more siblings. Palivizumab is given in a dose of 15 mg/kg intramuscularly once a month beginning with the onset of the local RSV season and continuing for 4–5 months. Protective antibody levels are achieved in 66% of infants after one injection and in 86% after a second injection.

Clinical Findings

A. Symptoms and Signs

The typical course of bronchiolitis begins with the exposure of an infant to another person with a URI. The infant generally has URI symptoms for several days, with or without fever, then experiences the gradual onset of respiratory distress, with a paroxysmal wheezy cough and dyspnea. The infant may be irritable and feed poorly, but there are usually no other systemic symptoms. The temperature is often in the range of 38.5–39°C (101.3–102.2°F), although it may be subnormal to greatly elevated.

Physical examination shows the child to be tachypneic, with a respiratory rate as high as 60–80 per minute, and often in severe respiratory distress. Alar flaring, retractions, and use of accessory muscles of respiration may be evident. Examination of the lungs often shows a prolonged expiratory phase with diffuse wheezes. Diffuse fine rales at the end of expiration and the beginning of inspiration are typical findings. The lungs are often hyperinflated with shallow respirations, and breath sounds may be nearly inaudible if the obstruction is severe.

The most critical phase of bronchiolitis is the first 2–3 days of the illness. Most cases resolve in 1–3 days without much difficulty. However, in severe cases, symptoms may develop within hours and may be protracted.

B. Laboratory Findings

The laboratory finding of most utility is the oxygen saturation, which may be used to help determine the severity of respiratory distress and the need for hospitalization. If bronchiolitis is suspected, a nasopharyngeal swab may be done for RSV culture, but this has little, if any, effect on the outcome of the illness.

C. Imaging Studies

Radiography usually shows signs of hyperinflation. In about one third of children, x-rays show scattered areas of consolidation. These may represent postobstructive atelectasis or inflammation of alveoli. It may not be possible to exclude early bacterial pneumonia solely on the basis of radiographic findings.

Differential Diagnosis

An important item in the differential diagnosis of bronchiolitis is acute asthma, as there may be many similarities in history and physical examination between these two conditions. Asthma is unusual in the first year of life, and the incidence of bronchiolitis peaks at 6 months of age. The presence of one or more of the following favors the diagnosis of asthma: family history of asthma, sudden onset without a preceding URI, repeated attacks, a markedly prolonged expiratory phase of respiration, and response to one dose of epinephrine.

Complications

Bronchiolitis is ordinarily a benign disease. Complications are related to hypoxemia and are more common and more severe in children with underlying cardiac or pulmonary disease. The mortality rate is 1–2% for all infants, 3–4% in children with underlying cardiac or pulmonary disease, and 20–67% in immunocompromised children.

Treatment

Treatment of bronchiolitis is primarily supportive. The decision to hospitalize the child is clinical, based on the degree of respiratory distress. Placing the child in a tent with cool humidified oxygen both relieves hypoxemia and reduces water loss from tachypnea. Intravenous fluids may be necessary. Antibiotics and steroids are of no benefit in bronchiolitis, but antibiotics may be given if the x-ray suggests pneumonia. The role of bronchodilators is controversial. Bronchodilators are not helpful in bronchiolitis per se, but some infants with what appears to be bronchiolitis respond to these medications, suggesting a possible link between bronchiolitis and reactive airways disease. Many physicians elect to use bronchodilators for children in whom wheezing is a prominent feature of their disease. Treatment with anti-inflammatory medications such as nebulized budesonide or cromolyn sodium after an episode of bronchiolitis can reduce wheezing episodes and hospital admissions for bronchospasm. Whether such treatment is useful for all children or should be reserved only for children with clinically apparent wheezing after bronchiolitis has not been established. Despite considerable initial interest, ribavirin has not been shown to be of benefit, and it is no longer recommended for use in children with bronchiolitis.

Prognosis

There appears to be a relationship between bronchiolitis and reactive airways disease, although the exact connection is unclear. Some studies have shown an increased incidence of airway hyperreactivity that may persist for years in children who have had bronchiolitis.

PERTUSSIS

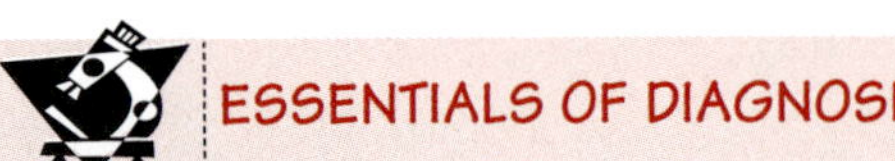

- *URI symptoms.*
- *Paroxysms of coughing, often with "whoops" on inspiration.*
- *Coughing to the point of vomiting.*
- *Dyspnea.*
- *Seizures.*

General Considerations

Pertussis is a bacterial infection that affects airways lined with ciliated epithelium. It is endemic in the general population, with epidemics occurring every 3–4 years. The disease is most common in unimmunized infants and in adults, because immunity wanes 5–10 years after the last immunization. Pertussis causes serious disease in children and mild or asymptomatic disease in adults. Infants younger than 6 months of age have greater morbidity than older children, and those under 2 months have the highest rates of pertussis-related hospitalization, pneumonia, seizures, encephalopathy, and death. Pertussis is highly contagious, with attack rates as high as 100% in susceptible individuals exposed at close range.

Pathogenesis

The most common cause of pertussis is *Bordetella pertussis,* but adenoviruses can cause a similar disease. Pathologically, the bacteria attack ciliated epithelium in the respiratory tree, where they produce toxins and other active factors. These cause inflammation and necrosis of the walls of small airways, which lead in turn to plugging of airways, bronchopneumonia, and hypoxemia.

Prevention

The key to prevention of pertussis is immunization. However, immunization does not confer complete protection, and immunized children may be asymptomatic reservoirs for infection. Of the 7288 cases reported in 1999, 27% occurred in children younger than 7 months of age (ie, in children too young to have received the full initial course of three doses of pertussis vaccine), 11% occurred in children between the ages of 1 and 4 years, and 28% were in children between the ages of 10 and 19 years. In 2006, a vaccine combining acellular pertussis vaccine with tetanus and diphtheria toxoids (Tdap) was recommended for use in children aged 11–18 years as a substitute for the adolescent tetanus-diphtheria vaccine.

Clinical Findings

A. Symptoms and Signs

Children younger than 2 years of age show the most typical symptoms of the disease. In these children, 100% have paroxysms of coughing, with 60–70% manifesting the "whoops" that give the disease its nickname of "whooping cough"; 60–80% have vomiting induced by coughing; 70–80% have dyspnea lasting more than 1 month; and 20–25% have seizures. Children older than 2 years have lower incidences of all these symptoms and a shorter duration of disease, whereas adults often have atypical symptoms. High fever is unusual in all ages.

Pertussis has an incubation period lasting 3–12 days. After that, the disease progresses through three stages, each lasting approximately 2 weeks.

1. The *catarrhal stage* is characterized by symptoms typical of a URI. The symptoms are nonspecific, and the diagnosis of pertussis is usually not considered.
2. The *paroxysmal stage* lasts 2–4 weeks, occasionally longer. During this stage, episodes of coughing increase in severity and number. The typical paroxysm is five to ten hard coughs in a single expiration, followed by the classic "whoop" as the patient inspires. The paroxysms recur until the mucus plugs causing the cough are dislodged. Coughing to the point of vomiting is common, and the diagnosis of pertussis should be considered in any patient with this symptom. The paroxysms are exhausting; the child may appear apathetic and may lose weight because he or she is too weak to eat or drink. The paroxysms may be frequent enough to cause hypoxemia, which may be severe enough to cause anoxic encephalopathy. Between the paroxysms, however, the patient may not appear otherwise especially sick.
3. During the *convalescent stage,* the paroxysms gradually decrease in frequency and number. The patient may experience a cough for several months after the disease has otherwise resolved.

The diagnosis of pertussis can usually be made in the paroxysmal stage, but it requires a certain level of suspicion. A cough lasting more than 2 weeks and associated with posttussive vomiting should prompt the physician to consider the diagnosis. There are no specific physical findings.

B. Laboratory Findings

A high WBC count (20,000–50,000/mm^3) with an absolute lymphocytosis is common but not specific to the disease. The organism can be obtained for culture or staining by a nasopharyngeal swab. The sensitivity of culture is related to the stage of the disease and is very high early in the disease, when pertussis is least suspected. Culture is about 80% sensitive during the first 2 weeks of infection, 14% after the fourth week of infection, and zero after 5 weeks. Direct fluorescent antibody staining can provide a rapid diagnosis, but it has variable sensitivity and specificity, and all suspected cases should be cultured for definitive identification. Serology is useful only for retrospective diagnosis.

Differential Diagnosis

Any illness that causes cough should be considered in the differential diagnosis. Older children and children who have been immunized against the disease may have milder, atypical symptoms, and the only clue to the disease may be the long duration of the symptoms.

Complications

Complications of pertussis are numerous and often severe. Pneumonia is the most frequent complication and is seen in almost all fatal cases. *S pneumoniae,*

Staphylococcus aureus, and oral flora are the most common organisms involved. A high fever or absolute neutrophilia in a patient with pertussis may be the only clues to a secondary bacterial infection. The cough may be severe enough to rupture alveoli and may cause interstitial and subcutaneous emphysema or pneumothorax. The cough may also cause epistaxis, melena, subconjunctival hemorrhage, spinal epidural hematoma, intracranial hemorrhage, rupture of the diaphragm, or umbilical or inguinal hernia. Inability to eat or drink may lead to dehydration or electrolyte imbalances. Seizures are usually caused by anoxia but may be caused by hyponatremia secondary to inappropriate antidiuretic hormone secretion. Finally, anoxia may be severe enough to lead to coma.

Treatment

Treatment is primarily supportive, involving hydration, pulmonary toilet, and oxygen. The decision to hospitalize the patient depends on the child's age and general condition. Essentially all children younger than 6 months of age are admitted to the hospital. Nearly all children who require ventilation are younger than 3 months of age. Older children may be admitted if they experience complications of the disease or if their families are unable to provide care at home. Infants born prematurely and those with underlying cardiac, pulmonary, or neuromuscular disorders are also at higher risk for complications.

The patient should be placed in respiratory isolation until antibiotics have been given for at least 5 days. Erythromycin given for 14 days will eliminate the bacteria from the respiratory tract within 3–4 days. Clarithromycin and azithromycin may be equally effective, if more expensive. Trimethoprim-sulfamethoxazole for 14 days may be as effective as erythromycin in clearing the organism from the nasopharynx, but whether it is as effective clinically is unknown. If antibiotics are given within 14 days of the onset of the disease, they may abort or shorten the course of the disease, but the diagnosis of pertussis is rarely made in this stage of the illness. Once the paroxysmal stage begins, erythromycin will not affect the course of the disease, although it will shorten the period of infectivity and reduce communicability. Other appropriate antibiotics should be given if pneumonia or another secondary bacterial infection is suspected. Bronchodilators and steroids are probably of no benefit, and cough suppressants are likewise not helpful.

During a pertussis epidemic, newborns should receive their first immunization at 4 weeks of age, with repeat doses given at 6, 10, and 14 weeks of age. Partially immunized children younger than 7 years of age should complete the immunization series at the minimum intervals, and completely immunized children younger than 7 should receive one booster dose, unless they have received one in the preceding 3 years. Children older than 7 years do not need further immunizations. Children who have had documented pertussis at any age are exempt from further pertussis immunizations. All contacts of patients with pertussis should be given erythromycin for 14 days after the date of their last contact with the patient. Continuous contacts of the patient (eg, parents) should be given erythromycin until the patient's cough has stopped, or until the patient has received erythromycin for 7 days.

Prognosis

The prognosis of pertussis depends primarily on the age of the patient. Mortality is rare in adults and children. With proper supportive care, the mortality rate for children younger than 6 months of age—the group at highest risk—is approximately 1%. Most mortality is due to pneumonia and cerebral anoxia.

Centers for Disease Control and Prevention (CDC): Pertussis—United States, 2001–2003. MMWR Morb Mortal Wkly Rep 2005;154(50):1283-1286. [PMID: 16371944]

PNEUMONIA

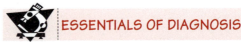

ESSENTIALS OF DIAGNOSIS

- *Fever.*
- *Acute respiratory symptoms.*
- *Radiographic evidence of parenchymal infiltrates.*

General Considerations

Pneumonia occurs more often in young children than in any other age group, with an incidence of 34–40 cases per 1000 in children younger than 5 years of age. Many definitions of pneumonia have been proposed, based on several different criteria. The criteria used in this chapter are the presence of fever, respiratory findings, and evidence of parenchymal infiltrates on chest radiography. Although accurate diagnosis of an infection as potentially serious as pneumonia is obviously desirable, there are significant obstacles to diagnostic certainty.

Pathogenesis

Viruses are a leading cause of pneumonia in children of all ages. Bacterial infections are more common in developing countries and in children with complicated infections.

Age is an important consideration in determining the potential etiology of pneumonia. Neonates younger than 20 days of age are most likely to have infections with pathogens that cause other neonatal infection syndromes, including group B streptococci, gram-negative enteric bacteria, cytomegalovirus, and *Listeria monocytogenes.*

Children between the ages of 3 weeks and 3 months may have infections caused by *Chlamydia trachomatis,* normally acquired from exposure, at the time of birth, to infection in the mother's genital tract. RSV pneumonia peaks at 2–7 months of age and is difficult to distinguish from bronchiolitis. *S pneumoniae* is probably the most common cause of bacterial pneumonia in this age group. *S aureus* is an uncommon cause of pneumonia but is associated with severe disease.

Respiratory viruses of many types are the most common cause of pneumonia in children between the ages of 4 months and 4 years. *S pneumoniae* and nontypeable *H influenzae* are common bacterial causes. *M pneumoniae* mainly affects older children in this age group. Tuberculosis should be considered in children who live in areas of high tuberculosis prevalence.

M pneumoniae is the most common cause of pneumonia in children aged 5–15 years. *Chlamydia pneumoniae* has long been thought to be an important cause of pneumonia in these children, but its role is open to question, given a high rate of recovery of this organism from asymptomatic children. *Pneumococcus* is the most likely cause of lobar pneumonia. As in younger children, tuberculosis should be considered in areas of high prevalence.

Prevention

The only significantly effective form of prevention is immunization. With widespread immunization in the United States, pneumonia caused by *H influenzae* type b has become uncommon, and infections caused by *S pneumoniae* are likewise expected to soon become unusual.

Clinical Findings

A. Symptoms and Signs

Perhaps that most confounding problem in diagnosis of pneumonia is that the symptoms and signs of pneumonia overlap significantly, and indeed are often identical to, those of other cough-producing illnesses, such as those discussed previously. Young infants are particularly likely to have nonspecific signs and symptoms. Assessing the sensitivity and specificity of signs is complicated by the lack of a true gold standard for diagnosis. Tachypnea is an important finding. This is defined by a respiratory rate greater than 60 per minute in infants younger than 2 months, greater than 50 in infants aged 2–12 months, and greater than 40 in children older than 12 months of age. Evidence of increased work of breathing, such as subcostal or intercostal retractions, nasal flaring, and grunting, may indicate more severe disease. Auscultatory findings are variable and include decreased breath sounds, wheezes, rhonchi, and crackles. The absence of these various pulmonary findings is helpful in predicting that a child will not have pneumonia, but the presence of these is only moderately predictive of the presence of pneumonia.

B. Laboratory Findings

Laboratory findings are generally not helpful in the diagnosis of pneumonia. A WBC count greater than 17,000/mm^3 indicates a higher likelihood of bacteremia, although blood cultures are rarely positive except in complicated infections, and oxygen desaturation indicates more severe disease. Sputum culture is the most accurate way to ascertain the cause of the infection, although obtaining a sputum sample from a child is obviously problematic.

C. Imaging Studies

A positive chest radiograph is generally considered to be diagnostic evidence of pneumonia. In children, however, radiographic patterns of respiratory infections are highly variable and may not be helpful in differentiating pneumonia from bronchiolitis, or bacterial disease from infection with viruses or atypical organisms. In infants especially, bacterial pneumonia may produce infiltrates that range from lobar consolidation to interstitial infiltrates.

Differential Diagnosis

The differential diagnosis of pneumonia includes all the previously discussed illness in which dyspnea and cough are prominent features of the disease.

Treatment

The appropriate treatment of childhood pneumonia depends on the age of the child and on the physician's clinical judgment as to how sick the child is. Neonates should all be treated as inpatients. Infants aged 3 weeks to 3 months may be treated as outpatients if they are not febrile or hypoxemic and do not appear toxic or have an alveolar infiltrate or a large pleural effusion. Older infants and children may be treated as outpatients if they do not appear seriously ill.

The choice of antibiotics depends on the age of the child and the most likely cause of infection. Neonates should be treated with ampicillin and gentamicin, with or without cefotaxime, as appropriate for a neonatal sepsis syndrome. Macrolides are appropriate first choices for children 3 weeks to 3 months and 5–15 years of age. All macrolides are equally effective. Doxycycline may be used in children older than 8 years. Children who are ill enough to require inpatient treatment should be treated with erythromycin, either orally or intravenously, plus either cefotaxime or cefuroxime.

In children between 4 months and 4 years of age, treatment may be withheld if a viral infection is considered to be the most likely cause. Otherwise, high-dose amoxicillin is the appropriate first-line treatment. For children sick enough to require hospitalization, intravenous ampicillin is appropriate. For children who appear septic or who have alveolar infiltrates or large pleural effusions, cefotaxime or cefuroxime should be used.

An important caveat in choosing an antibiotic is the consideration of the likelihood that the child has an infection with *S pneumoniae.* If this is thought to be likely, knowledge of local antibiotic resistance patterns is important. A growing rise in macrolide resistance is paralleling the rise in penicillin resistance in some parts of the United States, with important implications for antibiotic selection.

Prognosis

Worldwide, pneumonia is an important cause of death in children. In developed countries, however, the death rate for childhood pneumonia has dropped dramatically with the development of antibiotics.

McIntosh K: Community-acquired pneumonia in children. N Engl J Med 2002;346:429. [PMID: 11832532]

OTHER VIRAL INFECTIONS

INFECTIOUS MONONUCLEOSIS

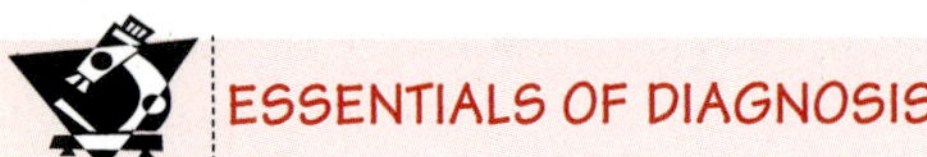

- *Fever.*
- *Pharyngitis.*
- *Generalized lymphadenopathy.*

General Considerations

Infectious mononucleosis is a clinical syndrome usually caused by Epstein-Barr virus (EBV). Although ordinarily a benign illness, it has several important, if unusual complications.

Pathogenesis

Although EBV is by far the most common cause of mononucleosis, 5–10% of mononucleosis-like illnesses are caused by cytomegalovirus, *Toxoplasma gondii,* or a variety of other viruses. EBV infects 95% of the world's population. It is transmitted in oral secretions by kissing and saliva-to-saliva transmission, as is common in children. The virus is shed for up to 6 months after the acute infection and then intermittently for the life of the person. Most infants and young children have inapparent infections or infections that are indistinguishable from other childhood respiratory infections. In developed countries, about one third of infections occur in adolescence or early adulthood, and of those infected, about one half develop clinically apparent disease.

The infection begins in the cells of the oral cavity, then spreads to adjacent salivary glands and lymphoid tissue. Eventually the virus infects the entire reticuloendothelial system, including the liver and spleen.

Prevention

Because the virus is ubiquitous and is shed intermittently by nearly every adult, there is no effective prevention for this illness.

Clinical Findings

A. Symptoms and Signs

In adolescents, the incubation period is 30–50 days, but it may be shorter in younger children. There is often a 1–2 week prodromal period of nonspecific respiratory symptoms, including fever and sore throat. Typical symptoms include fever, sore throat, myalgia, headache, nausea, and abdominal pain.

Physical findings include pharyngitis, often with exudative tonsillitis and palatal petechiae similar to streptococcal pharyngitis. Lymphadenopathy is seen in 90% of cases, most often in the anterior and posterior cervical chains and less often in the axillary and inguinal chains. Epitrochlear adenopathy is a highly suggestive finding. Splenomegaly is found in about 50% of cases and hepatomegaly in 10–25%. Symptomatic hepatitis, with or without jaundice, may occur but is unusual. Various rashes, most often maculopapular, are seen in less than half of patients, but nearly all patients develop a rash if they are given ampicillin or amoxicillin.

B. Laboratory Findings

At the onset of the illness, the WBC count is usually elevated to 12,000–25,000/mm^3; 50–70% of these cells are lymphocytes and 20–40% are atypical lymphocytes. Fifty to 80% of patients have elevated hepatic transaminases, but jaundice occurs in only about 5%.

The most commonly performed diagnostic test is the Monospot test. The diagnosis may be confused by the fact that this test is often negative during the first week of symptoms. It should only be used in adolescents, as it has a sensitivity of less than 50% in children younger than 14 years of age.

C. Imaging Studies

No imaging studies are routinely useful in this illness. Ultrasound shows splenomegaly more accurately than physical examination but is usually performed only to assess the risk of splenic rupture in patients who are active in sports.

Differential Diagnosis

Streptococcal pharyngitis is the chief illness in the differential diagnosis. This may coexist with mononucleosis, or the child with mononucleosis may be a carrier of *Streptococcus,* so a positive throat culture does not definitively rule out mononucleosis. Likewise, a negative Monospot test in the first several days of the illness does not rule out mononucleosis. Lymphadenopathy associated with mononucleosis is usually more generalized than that associated with streptococcal infections.

Complications

Mononucleosis is normally a benign illness. The most serious complication is spontaneous splenic rupture. This occurs in fewer than 0.5% of patients, usually during the second week of the illness. The risk of splenic rupture with trauma is elevated, and all patients with this illness should avoid contact sports for 1 month. Those with documented splenomegaly should not return to sports until resolution has been confirmed by ultrasound.

Other complications are unusual and include rare cases of airway obstruction (< 5%), symptomatic hepatitis (rare), and a variety of neurologic complications (1–5%), including meningitis, encephalitis, and cranial, autonomic, or peripheral neuritides. Hemolytic anemia may occur in about 3% of cases. Aplastic anemia is rare. Mild neutropenia and thrombocytopenia are common early in the disease, but severe cytopenias are rare.

Treatment

Treatment is generally symptomatic. Steroids speed recovery, but because most patients recover uneventfully, these should be used only for severe or complicated cases. Accepted indications for the use of steroids include impending airway obstruction, severe hemolytic anemia, severe thrombocytopenia, and persistent severe disease.

Prognosis

Symptoms typically last 2–4 weeks. Relapses may occur for 6 months to 1 year.

Papesch M, Watkins R: Epstein-Barr virus infectious mononucleosis. Clin Otolaryngol Allied Sci 2001;26:3. [PMID: 11298158]

GASTROENTERITIS

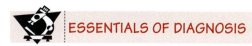

- *Diarrhea.*
- *Vomiting may be present or absent.*

General Considerations

Diarrheal diseases are among the most common illnesses and perhaps the leading cause of death among children worldwide. It is estimated that there are 1 billion illnesses and 3–5 million deaths from these illnesses each year. In the United States, there are an estimated 20–35 million cases of diarrhea annually, with 2–4 million visits to physicians and over 200,000 hospitalizations but only 400–500 deaths. Gastroenteritis may be caused by any of a large number of viruses, bacteria, or parasites. Most infections are caused by ingestion of contaminated food or water.

Pathogenesis

Four families of viruses can cause gastroenteritis. All are spread easily through fecal-oral contact, and many are associated with localized outbreaks in hospitals, daycare centers, and schools. Rotavirus is a common cause of gastroenteritis during winter months. It primarily affects children between 3 months and 2 years of age, and by age 4 or 5 years, nearly all children have serologic evidence of infection. Norwalk virus is the most common cause of gastroenteritis among older children and, along with astroviruses and enteric adenoviruses, causes year-round, often localized outbreaks of disease.

Bacteria may cause either inflammatory or noninflammatory diarrhea. Common causes of inflammatory diarrhea are *Campylobacter jejuni,* enteroinvasive or enterohemorrhagic *E coli, Salmonella* species, *Shigella* species, and *Yersinia enterocolitica.* Noninflammatory diarrhea may be caused by enteropathogenic or enterotoxigenic *E coli* or by *Vibrio cholerae.*

The most common parasitic cause of diarrhea in the United States is *Giardia lamblia.* Numerous other parasites, including protozoa and various types of roundworms and flatworms, may cause diarrhea. Most parasitic infections cause chronic diarrhea and are beyond the scope of this chapter.

Prevention

The most effective prevention measure is for children to have access to uncontaminated food and water. Careful hand washing and good sanitation practices also help prevent the spread of infection among children. An increased rate of breast-feeding has been shown to decrease the incidence of gastroenteritis among all children in small communities.

In 2006, the Advisory Committee on Immunization Practices recommended that the new oral rotavirus vaccine be given to all children at 2, 4, and 6 months of age. This immunization schedule has been shown to be effective for two seasons after administration, but no studies have been done to establish whether it is effective for longer. It should be noted that, unlike the initial rotavirus vaccine, which was withdrawn from the market, the new vaccine has not been shown to be associated with an increased rate of intussusception.

Clinical Findings

A. Symptoms and Signs

The cardinal sign of gastroenteritis is diarrhea, with or without vomiting. Systemic symptoms and signs may include fever and malaise. Fever and severe abdominal pain are more common with inflammatory diarrhea. The estimated degree of dehydration should be established before beginning treatment.

In most children with viral gastroenteritis, fever and vomiting last less than 2–3 days, although diarrhea may persist up to 5–7 days. Most cases of diarrhea caused by food-borne toxins last 1–2 days. Many, but not all bacterial infections persist for longer periods of time.

B. Laboratory Findings

Most children with gastroenteritis from any cause have a short-lived illness, and the cause of the infection is rarely ascertained. Stool cultures for bacteria and examination for parasites should be done if the stool is positive for blood or leukocytes, if diarrhea persists for more than 1 week, or if the patient is immunocompromised. The presence of fecal leukocytes indicates an inflammatory infection, although not all such infections produce a positive test. Blood indicates a hemorrhagic or inflammatory infection. In a child who appears significantly dehydrated, serum electrolytes should be tested, especially if the child is hospitalized for fluid therapy.

Complications

Diarrheal diseases are for the most part benign, self-limited infections. Mortality is primarily caused by dehydration, shock, and circulatory collapse. Bacterial pathogens may spread to remote sites and cause meningitis, pneumonia, and other infections. *E coli* O157:H7 may cause hemolytic-uremic syndrome.

Treatment

The keys to treatment of gastroenteritis are rehydration, or avoidance of dehydration, and early refeeding. Children who are severely (> 10%) dehydrated or who appear toxic or seriously ill should be admitted to the hospital for rehydration and treatment. Otherwise, children may be managed at home. Vomiting is the chief obstacle to rehydration or maintenance of hydration. Children who are vomiting should be given frequent (every 1–2 minutes) very small amounts (5 mL) of rehydration solution to avoid provoking further attacks of emesis. The idea that the gastrointestinal tract should be rested for a time by avoiding oral intake has been disproved.

Children who have diarrhea but who are not dehydrated should continue on whatever age-appropriate foods they were taking before the illness. In those who are dehydrated but not severely so, oral rehydration has been shown to be the preferred method of rehydration. Juices, water flavored with drink mix, and sports drinks do not have the recommended concentrations of carbohydrates and electrolytes and should be avoided. The World Health Organization or UNICEF reduced-osmolarity rehydration solution is the preferred therapy. Children who are mildly (3–5%) dehydrated should be given 50 mL/kg of solution, plus replacement of ongoing losses from stool or emesis, over each 4-hour period. Children who are moderately (6–9%) dehydrated should be given 100 mL/kg, plus losses, over each 4-hour period. Refeeding with age-appropriate foods should begin as soon as the child is interested in eating. The classic BRAT (bananas, rice cereal, applesauce, toast) diet is lacking in calories, protein, and fat and is no longer recommended.

Therapy with antidiarrheal and antiemetic medications has been shown to have minimal effect on the volume of diarrhea. Additionally, these drugs have an unacceptably high rate of side effects, and their use is not recommended.

Even when diagnosed, many bacterial infections do not require treatment. All *Campylobacter* (erythromycin) and *Shigella* (trimethoprim-sulfamethoxazole or cephalosporin) infections should be treated. Infections with *Salmonella* should not be treated with antibiotics unless the child is younger than 3 months of age or has evidence of bacteremia or disseminated infection. Ampicillin, chloramphenicol, trimethoprim-sulfamethoxazole, and cefotaxime are appropriate choices. Treatment of *E coli* O157:H7 infection does not reduce the severity of the illness and may increase the likelihood of hemolytic-uremic syndrome. Other *E coli* infections should be treated only if they are severe or prolonged.

Giardia infections should be treated with metronidazole or quinacrine.

Prognosis

With proper rehydration and refeeding, morbidity and mortality from viral gastroenteritis is minimal. Morbidity and mortality from bacterial infections is dependent on the virulence of the organism and complications from distant spread or remote effects, such as hemolytic-uremic syndrome.

URINARY TRACT INFECTIONS

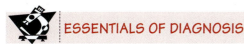

- *Common bacterial cause of febrile illness in young children.*
- *Symptoms often lacking or nonspecific in young children.*
- *Urinalysis not always reliable, need culture for accurate diagnosis.*

General Considerations

Urinary tract infections (UTIs) are the most common serious bacterial infection in children younger than 2 years of age. Among febrile young children, between 3% and 5% have a UTI, and among infants younger than 8 weeks of age, UTIs account for approximately 7.5% of febrile illnesses. UTI may be a marker for urinary tract anomalies in young children. It is generally believed that UTIs may lead to renal scarring, which may cause hypertension and renal insufficiency later in life.

Pathogenesis

In the first 8–12 weeks of life, some UTIs may be caused by hematogenous spread of bacteria from a remote source. Otherwise, the infections are caused by bacteria ascending the urethra into the bladder. From the bladder, bacteria may ascend the ureters to cause pyelonephritis.

The most common pathogens responsible for UTIs are enteric bacteria. *E coli* is found in 70–90% of infections. *Pseudomonas aeruginosa* is the most common nonenteric gram-negative pathogen, and *Enterococcus* species are the most common gram-positive organisms seen. Group B *Streptococcus* is occasionally found in neonates. *S aureus* is rarely seen in children who do not have indwelling catheters and suggests seeding from a distant focus, such as renal abscess, osteomyelitis, or endocarditis. The most important factors in prevalence of UTI are the patient's age and gender. In newborns, preterm infants are several times more likely to have a UTI than full-term infants. Until the age of 3 months, boys are more likely to be infected than girls, but thereafter infections in girls predominate for the rest of childhood. The usual age at which children experience a first symptomatic infection is 1–5 years. In this age group girls are 10–20 times more likely to have a UTI than boys.

Clinical Findings

A. Symptoms and Signs

Among children younger than 2 years of age, symptoms are often lacking or nonspecific. Parents may become suspicious if the child appears to be in pain while urinating, but otherwise fever may be the only presenting complaint. Among children who have developed language skills, typical UTI symptoms, such as dysuria, urgency, and urinary frequency, may be seen. Fever is the only reliable clinical sign distinguishing upper tract infection (pyelonephritis) from lower tract infection (cystitis).

B. Laboratory Findings

To be reliable, urine for analysis must be collected by catheterization or by suprapubic aspiration. Urine collected in an adhesive collection bag is too often contaminated by skin flora to be useful.

Positive findings on urinalysis are positive dipstick tests for leukocyte esterase or nitrite or the microscopic finding of pyuria (> 5 WBCs per high-power field). However, urinalysis in young children is not sensitive enough to stand alone as a diagnostic test, and urine culture is needed for accurate diagnosis. The bacterial colony count that defines a UTI varies by collection method and by gender. In a specimen collected by suprapubic aspiration, the finding of any gram-negative organisms or of more than 10^3 gram-positive organisms indicates a 99% probability of UTI. In catheter-obtained specimens, more than 10^5 bacteria indicates a 95% probability of UTI and 10^4–10^5 is considered suspicious. The numbers are similar for clean-voided urine specimens, although in boys, more than 10^4 bacteria indicates a probable UTI.

Blood cultures should be done as part of the workup of a young infant with fever without an apparent source. Blood cultures are unlikely to be positive in children older than 2 months. Even when blood cultures are positive, they will show the same organism as the urine culture, and they contribute little if anything to the diagnosis.

C. Imaging Studies

The goal of imaging is to diagnose the presence of vesicoureteral reflux (VUR) and other urinary tract anomalies that are associated with a high rate of recurrent infections. Shortly after finishing treatment for a first UTI, children should have a voiding cystourethrogram (VCUG), either with x-ray contrast dye or with a radionuclide tracer. Renal ultrasonography will show other structural abnormalities and may be considered in addition to the VCUG. VUR is found in 30–50% of children after a first UTI, and other anomalies, such as posterior urethral valves (in boys) or duplication of the collecting system, are found in a small number of children.

Although all boys with a first UTI should receive a full diagnostic workup, as girls grow from toddlers to school age, the likelihood of significant findings decreases. There is no clear guidance from the literature as to the age after which a girl with a first UTI should be subjected to an expensive, uncomfortable, and potentially traumatic investigation.

Differential Diagnosis

UTI should be considered in any child who presents with a febrile illness in whom the cause of the fever cannot be readily ascertained by physical examination.

Complications

Acute complications of UTI include sepsis, renal abscess, and disseminated infection, including meningitis. Recurrent pyelonephritis can cause renal scarring, which can lead to hypertension or renal insufficiency later in life.

Treatment

A. Acute Infection

Infants younger than 2 months with UTI should be hospitalized and treated with intravenous antibiotics as indicated for sepsis until cultures identify the causative organism and the best antibiotic for treatment. Infants 2 months to 2 years of age may be treated as outpatients with oral antibiotics unless they appear toxic, are dehydrated, or are unable to retain oral intake. Older children can usually be treated as outpatients unless they appear seriously ill. The initial choice of antibiotic may be a sulfonamide, trimethoprim-sulfamethoxazole, or a cephalosporin. Resistance of *E coli* to ampicillin is widespread enough in the United States to make ampicillin or amoxicillin a poor choice for initial therapy. Nitrofurantoin, which is excreted in the urine but does not reach therapeutic blood levels, should not be used to treat febrile children with a UTI. In general, the duration of treatment should be 7–10 days. Some authorities recommend 14 days of treatment, but there are no data comparing 10 days to 14 days of treatment.

If the child responds clinically to treatment within 2 days, no further immediate follow-up is needed (eg, reculture of the urine or immediate imaging studies). If the child is not improving after 2 days of treatment, the urine should be recultured and renal ultrasonography should be performed immediately.

Once treatment of a first infection has been completed, the child should be continued on either full or prophylactic doses of antibiotics until imaging studies have been completed. Appropriate prophylactic antibiotics include trimethoprim-sulfamethoxazole, sulfisoxazole, and nitrofurantoin.

B. Prevention of Recurrent Infection

Prevention of long-term sequelae focuses on prevention of recurrent infection. This, in turn, involves correction, if possible, of associated urinary tract abnormalities. Widespread use of prenatal ultrasonography has led to the identification of infants with intrauterine hydronephrosis. In many boys with VUR, renal scarring is thought to be congenital, whereas in girls it is more highly associated with recurrent infection. The degree of VUR is important in determining appropriate treatment. Mild VUR generally improves over time as the bladder enlarges and the length of the submucosal tunnel through which the ureter passes increases. More severe degrees of reflux are unlikely to improve and more often require surgical correction. Posterior urethral valves and ureterovesical obstruction also require surgical intervention.

In children with structurally normal urinary tracts, treatment of chronic constipation has been shown to decrease the recurrence of UTI, as has behavioral correction of voiding dysfunction associated with incomplete emptying of the bladder. Improving hygiene, especially in girls, has not been shown to decrease UTI rates. Based on retrospective studies, circumcision of boys has been claimed to be associated with decreased UTI rates, but there are no randomized controlled trials investigating this idea.

For some children with recurrent UTIs, long-term prophylactic antibiotic treatment may be effective in reducing the frequency of infections. However, there are no clear guidelines as to when this treatment should be considered.

Bachur R, Harper M: Reliability of the urinalysis for predicting urinary tract infections in young febrile children. Arch Pediatr Adolesc Med 2001;155:60. [PMID: 11177064]

Pitetti R, Choi S: Utility of blood cultures in febrile children with UTI. Am J Emerg Med 2002;20:271. [PMID: 12098170]

Schlager T: Urinary tract infections in children younger than 5 years of age: Epidemiology, diagnosis, treatment, outcomes, and prevention. Paediatr Drugs 2001;3:219. [PMID: 11310718]

Skin Diseases in Infants & Children 6

Mark A. Knox, MD

INFECTIONS OF THE SKIN

IMPETIGO

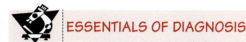

ESSENTIALS OF DIAGNOSIS

- *Nonbullous—yellowish crusted plaques.*
- *Bullous—bullae, with minimal surrounding erythema, rupture to leave a shallow ulcer.*

General Considerations

Impetigo is a bacterial infection of the skin. More than 70% of cases are of the nonbullous variety.

Pathogenesis

Most cases of nonbullous impetigo are caused by *Staphylococcus aureus*. Group A β-hemolytic streptococci are found in some cases. Coagulase-positive *S aureus* is the cause of bullous impetigo. Impetigo can develop in traumatized skin, or the bacteria can spread to intact skin from its reservoir in the nose.

Clinical Findings

Nonbullous impetigo usually starts as a small vesicle or pustule, followed by the classic small (< 2 cm) honey-colored crusted plaque. The infection may be spread to other parts of the body by fingers or clothing. There is usually little surrounding erythema, itching occurs occasionally, and pain is usually absent. Regionally lymphadenopathy is seen in most patients. Without treatment, the lesions resolve without scarring in 2 weeks.

Bullous impetigo is usually seen in infants and young children. Lesions begin on intact skin on almost any part of the body. Flaccid, thin-roofed vesicles develop, which rupture to form shallow ulcers.

Differential Diagnosis

Nonbullous impetigo is unique in appearance. Bullous impetigo is similar in appearance to pemphigus and bullous pemphigoid. Growth of staphylococci from fluid in a bulla confirms the diagnosis.

Complications

Cellulitis follows about 10% of cases of nonbullous impetigo but rarely follows bullous impetigo. Either type may rarely lead to septicemia, septic arthritis, or osteomyelitis. Scarlet fever and post-streptococcal glomerulonephritis, but not rheumatic fever, may follow streptococcal impetigo.

Treatment

Localized disease may be treated with mupirocin ointment. Patients with widespread lesions or evidence of cellulitis should be treated with systemic antibiotics effective against staphylococci and streptococci.

FUNGAL INFECTIONS

General Considerations

Fungal infections of the skin and skin structures may be generally grouped into three categories: dermatophyte infections, other tinea infections, and candidal infections.

Pathogenesis

Dermatophytoses are caused by a group of related fungal species—primarily *Microsporum*, *Trichophyton*, and *Epidermophyton* species—that require keratin for growth and can invade hair, nails, and the stratum corneum of the skin. Some of these organisms are spread from person to person, some from animals to people, and some infect people from the soil. Other fungi can also cause skin disease, such as *Malassezia furfur* in tinea versicolor. Finally, *Candida albicans*, a common resident of the gastrointestinal tract, can cause diaper dermatitis and thrush.

Clinical Findings

A. Symptoms and Signs

1. Dermatophytoses—

a. Tinea Corporis—Infection of the skin produces one or more characteristic gradually spreading lesions with an erythematous raised border and central areas that are generally scaly but relatively clearer and less indurated than the margins of the lesions. The central clearing helps to differentiate these lesions from those of psoriasis. Small lesions may resemble those of nummular eczema. The lesions may have a somewhat serpiginous border, but they are usually more or less round in shape, hence the common name of "ringworm." They can range in size from one to several centimeters.

b. Tinea Capitis—Fungal infection of the scalp and hair is the most common dermatophytosis in children. This presents as areas of alopecia with more or less regular borders. Typically, the hair shafts break off a few millimeters from the skin surface, distinguishing this from alopecia areata. The infection may also produce a sterile inflammatory mass in the scalp, called a *kerion,* which may be confused with a bacterial infection.

2. Nondermatophyte Infections—

a. Tinea Versicolor—Tinea versicolor is normally seen in adolescents and adults. The causative organism, *M furfur*, is part of the normal skin flora. The infection most often becomes evident during warm weather, when new lesions develop. A warm, humid environment, excessive sweating, and genetic susceptibility are important factors for developing this infection. Because treatment does not eradicate the fungus from the skin, it often recurs annually, during the summer months, in susceptible individuals. The lesions are characteristically scaly macules, usually reddish brown in light-skinned people but often hyper- or hypopigmented in people of color. They can be found almost anywhere on the body but are seen most commonly on the torso. The lesions are rarely pruritic. The individual lesions may enlarge and coalesce to form larger lesions with irregular borders.

3. Candidal Infections—

a. Thrush—Thrush is a common oral infection in infants. Isolated incidents of this disease are common in immunocompetent infants, but recurrent infections in infants or infections in children and adolescents may indicate an underlying immune deficiency. The infection presents as thick white plaques on the tongue and buccal mucosa. These can be scraped off only with difficulty, revealing an erythematous base.

b. Candidal Diaper Dermatitis—This infection is most common in infants aged 2–4 months. *Candida* is a common colonist of the gastrointestinal tract, and infants with diaper dermatitis should be examined for signs of thrush. The fungus does not ordinarily invade the skin, but the warm, humid environment of the diaper area provides an ideal medium for growth. The infection is characterized by an intensely erythematous plaque with a sharply demarcated border. Advancing from the border are numerous satellite papules, which enlarge and coalesce to enlarge the affected area.

B. Special Tests

Dermatophyte and other tinea infections are usually diagnosed clinically. Examination of potassium hydroxide preparations of scrapings from the affected area, which show hyphae, confirms the diagnosis. Fungal cultures may be helpful when the diagnosis is suspected but cannot otherwise be confirmed. Diagnosis of candidal infections is generally made by clinical findings.

Treatment

Tinea corporis is treated with topical antifungal medications. Nystatin, miconazole, clotrimazole, ketoconazole, and terbinafine creams are all effective. Rarely, widespread infection requires systemic therapy.

Topical therapy is ineffective in tinea capitis. The gold standard for treatment has long been griseofulvin, but because of the 6-week duration of therapy required, other treatments of shorter duration are becoming more popular. Fluconazole, itraconazole, and terbinafine can be given for 2 weeks, with an additional week of treatment if the response is incomplete. Ketoconazole is not recommended, due to rare incidents of hepatotoxicity.

Tinea versicolor can be treated with topical selenium sulfide lotion or any of the previously listed topical creams. In older children, systemic treatment can also be given, either with ketoconazole or itraconazole for 5 days.

Candidal infections are most often treated with nystatin. Diaper dermatitis responds well to topical nystatin cream. If intense inflammation is present, topical steroids for a few days may be helpful. Thrush is usually treated with nystatin suspension. Up to 2 weeks may be needed for complete resolution of the infection. In resistant cases, the mouth may be painted with gentian violet.

Prognosis

All these infections in immunocompetent children respond well to treatment. However, left untreated, they can cause widespread and significant skin disease.

Gupta AK et al: Therapeutic options for the treatment of tinea capitis caused by Trichophyton species: Griseofulvin versus the new oral antifungal agents, terbinafine, itraconazole, and fluconazole. Pediatr Dermatol 2001;18:433. [PMID: 11737692]

PARASITIC INFESTATIONS

SCABIES

ESSENTIALS OF DIAGNOSIS

- *Intense pruritus.*
- *Small erythematous papules.*
- *Burrows are pathognomonic but may not be seen.*

Pathogenesis

Scabies is a common infestation caused by the mite *Sarcoptes scabiei*. The disease is acquired by physical contact with an infected person. Transmission of the disease by contact with infested linens or clothing is less common, because the mites can only live off the body for 2–3 days. The female mite burrows between the superficial and deeper layers of the epidermis, laying eggs and depositing feces as she goes along. After 4–5 weeks, her egg laying is complete, and she dies in the burrow. The eggs hatch, releasing larvae which move to the skin surface, molt into nymphs, mature to adults, mate, and begin the cycle again. Pruritus is caused by an allergic reaction to mite antigens.

Clinical Findings

A. Symptoms and Signs

Diagnosis is based primarily on clinical suspicion, as physical findings are highly variable and the disease can mimic a wide variety of skin conditions. The classic early symptom is intense pruritus. The usual finding is 1- to 2-mm erythematous papules, often in a linear pattern. The finding of burrows connecting the papules is diagnostic but is not always seen. In infants, the disease may involve the entire body—including the face, scalp, palms, and soles—and pustules and vesicles are common. In older children and adolescents, the lesions are most often seen in the interdigital spaces, wrist flexors, umbilicus, groin, and genitalia. Severe infestation may produce widespread crusted lesions.

B. Special Tests

Potassium hydroxide preparations of skin scrapings may show entire mites, eggs, or fecal pellets. However, success in finding these is limited and a negative examination does not rule out the disease.

Treatment

Permethrin cream, applied to the entire body (excluding the face in older children) is the preferred treatment. Recently, good results have been reported from a single oral dose of ivermectin, with no adverse reactions. Treatment will kill mites and eliminate the risk of contagion within 24 hours. However, pruritus may continue for several days to 2 weeks after treatment. The entire family should be treated at the same time, and all clothing and bedding should be washed.

del Mar Saez-De-Ocariz M et al: Treatment of 18 children with scabies or cutaneous larva migrans using ivermectin. Clin Exp Dermatol 2002;27:264. [PMID: 12139665]

LICE (PEDICULOSIS)

ESSENTIALS OF DIAGNOSIS

- *Pruritus.*
- *Visualization of lice on the body or nits in hair.*

Pathogenesis

Three varieties of lice cause human disease. *Pediculus humanus corporis* causes infestations on the body, and *Pediculus humanus capitis* causes infestation on the head. *Phthirus pubis*, or crab lice, infests the pubic area. All are spread by physical contact, either with an infested person or with clothing, towels, or hairbrushes that have been in recent contact with an infested person. Symptoms are caused by an allergic reaction to louse antigens that develops after a period of sensitization. Body lice can be a vector for other disease, such as typhus, trench fever, and relapsing fever. Infestation with pubic lice is highly correlated with infection by other sexually transmitted diseases. Nits are the eggs of the louse. They are cemented to hairs, are usually less than 1 mm in length, and are translucent. Body lice lay their nits in the seams of clothing. The nits can remain viable for up to 1 month and will hatch when exposed to body heat when the clothing is worn again.

Prevention

Body lice are associated primarily with poor hygiene and can be prevented by regular bathing and washing of clothing and bedding. There are no specific measures for prevention of infestation by other types of lice.

Clinical Findings

The cardinal symptom of louse infestation is pruritus, which develops as the person becomes sensitized. Excoriations in the infested area are common. The lice themselves can usually be seen easily. Head and pubic lice are easily seen, but body lice are only present on the body when feeding.

Treatment

Permethrin cream, applied for 8–12 hours, is the treatment of choice for body lice. Clothing and bedding should be washed, because exposure to hot water will kill the nits. Permethrin cream rinse is used to treat head and pubic lice. Thorough combing with a fine-toothed nit comb after treatment for head lice is useful in removing nits and reducing the probability of reinfestation.

INFECTIOUS DISEASES WITH SKIN MANIFESTATIONS

BACTERIAL INFECTIONS

Scarlet Fever (Scarlatina)

ESSENTIALS OF DIAGNOSIS

- *Symptoms of streptococcal pharyngitis.*
- *"Sandpaper" rash.*
- *Circumoral pallor.*
- *"Strawberry" tongue (red or white).*

General Considerations

Scarlet fever is an infection caused by certain strains of group A streptococci. The infection most commonly begins as a typical streptococcal pharyngitis, but it can also follow streptococcal cellulitis or infection of wounds or burns.

Clinical Findings

The classic feature of scarlet fever is the rash. It develops 12–48 hours after the onset of pharyngitis symptoms, usually beginning in the neck, axillae, and groin and becoming generalized within 24 hours. The rash is a fine, faintly erythematous exanthem that is often more easily felt than seen, giving it the name of "sandpaper" rash. The rash itself is usually not present on the face, but there is often flushing of the face except for the area around the mouth (circumoral pallor). The tongue is often erythematous and swollen. In the early stages of the disease, the tongue may have swollen papillae protruding through a white coating (white "strawberry" tongue). Later in the illness, the coating desquamates, leaving the tongue red and the papillae swollen (red "strawberry" tongue). After about 1 week, desquamation begins on the face and progresses downward over the body, finally involving the hands and feet.

Differential Diagnosis

Kawasaki disease and any of the viral exanthems may be confused with scarlet fever.

Complications

Scarlet fever is generally a benign disease. In severe cases, bacteremia and sepsis may occur, and rheumatic fever may follow an untreated infection. Glomerulonephritis may also be a sequel.

Treatment

Treatment of scarlet fever is no different from treatment of the primary streptococcal infection.

VIRAL INFECTIONS

1. Roseola (Exanthem Subitum)

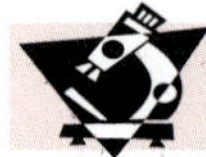

ESSENTIALS OF DIAGNOSIS

- *Sudden onset of high fever.*
- *No diagnostic signs.*
- *Development of rash as fever breaks after 3–4 days.*

Pathogenesis

Human herpesvirus 6 (HHV 6) causes the vast majority of cases of clinical roseola, although other viruses cause some cases, as well. It is rare in infants younger than 3 months and in children older than 2 years of age; most cases occur in infants between the ages of 6 and 12 months. Infections occur year round.

Clinical Findings

A. Symptoms and Signs

The hallmark of roseola is the abrupt onset of high fever, often 39.4–41.1°C (103–106°F). Febrile seizures occur in up to one third of patients. Despite the high fever, children usually look relatively well. Mild signs of upper respiratory infection may be seen, but there are no diagnostic signs. After 3–4 days, the fever breaks suddenly, followed by the appearance of a rash. This is usually a macular or maculopapular rash that starts on the trunk and spreads to the arms and neck and then often to the face and legs. The rash resolves within 3 days, but it may be more transient.

B. Laboratory Findings

Laboratory findings are usually normal.

Differential Diagnosis

In the early stages of the disease, many children with high fever and seizures are admitted to the hospital for workup of suspected meningitis or sepsis. After the rash appears, the diagnosis is obvious in retrospect.

Complications

Rare cases of encephalitis or fulminant hepatitis have been reported.

Treatment & Prognosis

Treatment is entirely symptomatic. Unless the patient develops one of the rare complications listed earlier, roseola is a benign, self-limited infection.

2. Varicella (Chickenpox)

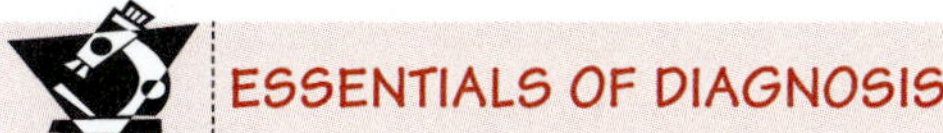

ESSENTIALS OF DIAGNOSIS

- *Prodrome of upper respiratory–like symptoms.*
- *Rash consists of small vesicles on erythematous base.*
- *Vesicles rupture with crusting.*

General Considerations

Approximately 90% of adults in the United States have serologic evidence of varicella infection, whether they have had clinically apparent disease or not.

Pathogenesis

The varicella-zoster virus is a herpesvirus. After resolution of the initial infection, the virus produces a latent infection in the dorsal root ganglia. Reactivation produces herpes zoster (shingles).

Prevention

Childhood immunization should prevent most disease. The vaccine is given as a single dose between 12 and 18 months of age with a booster between 4 and 6 years of age. Varicella-zoster immune globulin can help prevent infection in immunocompromised children, nonimmune pregnant women who are exposed to the virus, and newborns exposed to maternal varicella.

Clinical Findings

The usual incubation period of varicella is about 14 days. Most children experience a prodromal phase of upper respiratory–like symptoms for 1–2 days before the onset of the rash. Fever is usually moderate. Almost all infected children will develop a rash. The extent of the rash is highly variable. Lesions usually begin on the trunk or head but eventually can involve the entire body. The classic lesion is a pruritic erythematous macule that develops a clear central vesicle. After 1–2 days, the vesicle ruptures, forming a crust. New lesions develop daily for 3–7 days, and typically lesions are scattered over the body in various states of evolution at the same time. Ulcerative lesions on the buccal mucosa are common. The infection is contagious from the onset of the prodrome until the last of the lesions has crusted over.

Differential Diagnosis

Varicella usually presents as an unmistakable clinical picture, but the rash may be missed in children with mild disease.

Complications

In immunocompetent children, the most common complication is bacterial superinfection of the lesions, causing cellulitis or impetigo. Other, more serious complications are most common in children younger than 5 years or adults older than 20 years of age. Meningoencephalitis and cerebellar ataxia can occur. These normally resolve within 1–3 days without sequelae. Viral hepatitis is common but normally subclinical. Varicella pneumonia is uncommon in healthy children; it usually resolves after 1–3 days but may progress to respiratory failure in rare cases.

Treatment

Treatment is ordinarily symptomatic, including antipruritic medications if needed. Aspirin should be avoided to prevent development of Reye syndrome. Patients with signs of disseminated varicella, such as encephalitis and pneumonia, should be treated with intravenous acyclovir.

Prognosis

Varicella is normally a benign, self-limited disease. Complications in immunocompetent children are rare.

3. *Erythema Infectiosum (Fifth Disease)*

ESSENTIALS OF DIAGNOSIS

- *Prodrome of mild upper respiratory–like symptoms.*
- *Rash begins as erythema of cheeks, then becomes more generalized—macular at first, then reticular.*
- *Rash lasts 1–3 weeks.*

General Considerations

Erythema infectiosum (fifth disease) is a common childhood infection that rarely causes clinically significant disease.

Pathogenesis

The disease is caused by parvovirus B19. It appears sporadically but often in epidemics in communities. Children are infectious during the prodromal stage, which is inapparent or mild and usually indistinguishable from an upper respiratory infection. The rash is an immune-mediated phenomenon that occurs after the infection, so children with the rash are not infectious and should not be restricted from school or other activities.

Clinical Findings

Erythema infectiosum begins with a prodromal stage of upper respiratory symptoms, headache, and low-grade fever. This stage may be clinically inapparent.

The rash occurs in three phases, often transient enough to go unnoticed. The first stage is facial flushing, described as a "slapped cheek" appearance. Shortly afterward, the rash becomes generalized over the body, initially as a faint erythematous, often confluent, macular rash. In the third stage, the central regions of the macules clear, leaving a distinctive faint reticular rash. The rash comes and goes evanescently over the body and can last from 1 to 3 weeks. There are rarely any other associated findings.

Differential Diagnosis

Erythema infectiosum is usually clinically recognizable, but it may be confused with other viral exanthems.

Complications

Arthritis is rare in children but may occur in adolescents. Thrombocytopenic purpura and aseptic meningitis are rare complications.

Fetal hydrops and fetal demise may be seen in fetuses whose mothers contract the infection. It is estimated that 5% or fewer of infected fetuses will be affected by the virus.

Treatment & Prognosis

There is no known treatment for this disease. Except for rare complications in children, this is a benign infection. Fetal complications are unusual.

INFLAMMATORY DISORDERS OF THE SKIN

ATOPIC DERMATITIS

ESSENTIALS OF DIAGNOSIS

- *Pruritus is the cardinal symptom.*
- *Lesions are excoriated, scaly, and may become lichenified.*

General Considerations

Atopic dermatitis is a common skin disorder in children, affecting 10–15% of the population. It appears during the first year of life in 60% of cases and during the first 5 years in 85%.

Pathogenesis

The cause of atopic dermatitis is unclear. It has a strong association, both in the individual and in families, with allergic rhinitis and asthma, and is classified as an atopic disorder. Food allergies, primarily to cow's milk, wheat, eggs, soy, fish, and peanuts, have been implicated in 20–30% of cases.

Clinical Findings

The diagnosis is based on the presence of three of the following major criteria: pruritus, lesions with typical morphology and distribution, facial and extensor involvement in infants and children, chronic or chronically relapsing dermatitis, and personal or family history of atopic disease.

Pruritus is the hallmark of the disease, usually preceding the skin lesions, which usually develop as a reaction to scratching. The skin becomes excoriated, develops weeping and crusting, and later may become scaly or lichenified. Secondary bacterial infection is common. In infants, the lesions usually involve the face but may appear in a generalized pattern over much of the body. In young children, the extensor surfaces of the extremities are often involved. In older children and adults, the disease often moves to involve the flexion areas of the extremities instead. The disease typically is chronic, although remissions and relapses are common.

Differential Diagnosis

Atopic dermatitis may be confused with seborrheic dermatitis, especially in infants, in whom facial lesions are common. Atopic dermatitis does not usually follow the distribution of oil glands, as is typical with seborrheic dermatitis. It may also be confused with psoriasis, contact dermatitis, scabies, and cutaneous fungal infections.

Complications

The most common complication is secondary bacterial infection. Low-grade bacterial infection should be considered as a factor in lesions that do not respond well to usual therapies.

Treatment

Nonpharmacologic measures are important in the treatment of this disease. Long baths and bathing in hot water exacerbate dryness of the skin and should be avoided. Use of soaps that do not contain fragrances may be helpful, or it may be necessary to use nonsoap cleansers instead. Moisturizers that contain fragrances and other irritants will aggravate the problem. If secondary infection is suspected, systemic antibiotics effective against streptococci and staphylococci should be given.

Topical corticosteroids are the mainstay of treatment. The lowest potency preparation that is effective should be used, especially on the face and the diaper area, which are more sensitive to the skin atrophy associated with the prolonged use of higher-potency steroids. Systemic steroids are useful for severe acute flares. Antipruritic medications may be useful, but these all have significant sedative side effects. Tacrolimus and pimecrolimus, topical immune modulators, are less effective than high-potency topical steroids. Whether they are as effective or less effective than medium-potency steroids is unclear. Because these drugs do not cause skin atrophy, they may be useful for prolonged treatment of facial lesions. Doxepin, a tricyclic antidepressant with strong antihistaminic effects, is often useful in patients with severe manifestations.

Prognosis

Although it is usually fairly easily controlled, atopic dermatitis is a chronic skin disorder. It often becomes less severe as children grow into school age, but relapses and persistence of some disease into adulthood is common.

Topical pimecrolimus (Elidel) for treatment of atopic dermatitis. Med Lett 2002;44:48. [PMID: 12045753]

Topical tacrolimus for treatment of atopic dermatitis. Med Lett Drugs Ther 2001:43:33. [PMID: 11309535]

SEBORRHEIC DERMATITIS

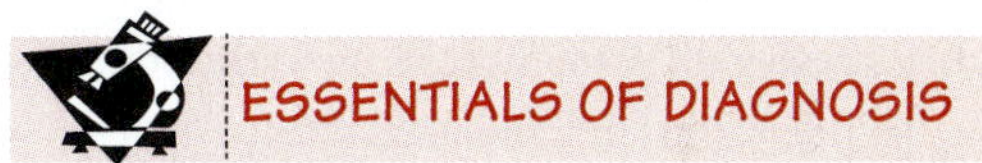

- *Inflamed lesions with yellowish or brownish crusting.*
- *Lesions may be localized or generalized.*

General Considerations

Seborrheic dermatitis is a common inflammatory disorder of the skin. It is most common in infancy and adolescence, when the sebaceous glands are more active. It generally resolves or lessens in severity after infancy, but localized lesions or mild, generalized scalp disease may be seen throughout adulthood.

Pathogenesis

The cause of seborrheic dermatitis is unknown. The fungus *Pityrosporum ovale* has been implicated, but whether it is causative in all cases is not known.

Clinical Findings

The typical lesions of seborrheic dermatitis are inflammatory macular lesions, usually with brownish or yellowish scaling. Inflammation may begin during the first month of life, and it usually becomes evident within the first year. In infants, the lesions may be generalized, but in older children, lesions are most common in areas where sebaceous glands are concentrated, such as the scalp, face, and axillae. Marginal blepharitis may be seen. Cradle cap is a common variant seen in infants, either by itself or in association with other lesions. This is seen as scaling and crusting of the scalp, often with extremely heavy buildup of scale in untreated infants.

Differential Diagnosis

Atopic dermatitis is the main element in the differential diagnosis. The disease may also be confused with psoriasis and other cutaneous fungal infections.

Complications

Secondary infection, either bacterial or fungal, is a common complication.

Treatment

Topical corticosteroids are the main treatment for inflammatory lesions. Medium and high-potency preparations are usually unnecessary. Scalp lesions usually respond to antiseborrheic shampoos, such as selenium sulfide. Topical treatment with antifungal creams or shampoo may also be helpful. Cradle cap is treated by soaking the scales with mineral oil and then gently debriding them with a toothbrush or washcloth. Following debridement, cleansing with baby shampoo is normally adequate for control; antiseborrheic or antifungal shampoos usually are not necessary.

Prognosis

Seborrheic dermatitis generally resolves or lessens in severity after infancy, but localized lesions or mild, generalized scalp disease may be seen throughout adulthood.

ACNE VULGARIS

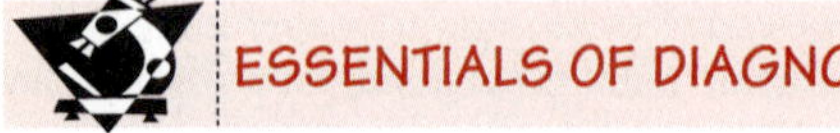

- *Comedones, open or closed.*
- *Papules, pustules, or nodules.*

General Considerations

Acne vulgaris is an extremely common skin disease in older children and adolescents. The prevalence of this disorder increases with age: 30–60% of 10- to 12-year-olds and 80–95% of 16- to 18-year-olds are affected.

Pathogenesis

Acne is caused by the interaction of several factors in the pilosebaceous unit of the skin. The basic abnormality is excessive sebum production caused by sebaceous gland hyperplasia and generally related to androgenic influences. Hyperkeratinization of the hair follicle results in obstruction of the follicle and the formation of a microcomedo. Sebum and cellular debris accumulate, forming an environment that can become colonized by *Propionibacterium acnes*. The presence of the bacteria provokes an immune response that includes the production of inflammatory mediators. Lesions are most commonly seen in areas of the body that have the highest concentration of sebaceous glands. The face is the most common site for lesions to develop, but the chest, back, neck, and upper arms may be affected as well.

Although the androgenic influences that cause the increase in sebum production are generally related to puberty, a number of factors can cause or aggravate acne. Mechanical obstruction or irritation (eg, by shirt collars) can be a factor. Cosmetics can occlude follicles and trigger eruptions. Medications, most commonly anabolic steroids, corticosteroids, lithium, and phenytoin, can cause or aggravate acne. Hyperandrogenic states, such as polycystic ovary syndrome, are often associated with acne. Emotional stress has been shown to exacerbate the problem. Finally, the role of diet has long been controversial. No specific foods have been found to aggravate acne, despite common assumptions. However, acne is almost uniformly a disease of western cultures, and some authorities are studying the role of the high-glycemic-index western diet in its development. This diet leads to higher levels of insulin-like growth factor, which has androgenic effects.

Clinical Findings

Several types of lesions characterize this disease, and they can occur in varying combinations and degrees of severity. Microcomedones can evolve into visible comedones, either open ("blackheads") or closed ("whiteheads"). Inflammatory papules and pustules may develop. Nodules are pustules larger than 5 mm in size. Hyperpigmentation and scarring may develop at the sites of more severe lesions.

Multiple classification systems have been devised to characterize this disorder. The disease may be classed as comedonal, papulopustular (inflammatory), and nodulocystic (also inflammatory, but more severe). The American Academy of Dermatology defines three levels of severity. In mild acne, there are a few to several papules and pustules, but no nodules. In moderate acne, there are several to many papules and pustules and a few to several nodules. In severe disease, there are extensive papules and pustules, along with many nodules.

Differential Diagnosis

The diagnosis is usually straightforward. The physician should consider drug-induced acne if the patient is taking any medications. Severe acne in athletes raises the possibility of anabolic steroid use. In women, severe acne, hirsutism, and other signs of virilization suggest an underlying hyperandrogenic condition.

Complications

The primary morbidity of acne is psychological. This can be a serious problem for the adolescent patient. Hyperpigmentation and scarring may result from more severe disease, especially from nodulocystic acne.

Treatment

The various treatments for acne are aimed at reducing infection and inflammation, normalizing the rate of desquamation of follicular epithelium, or correcting hormone excesses or other systemic factors. Treatments work better in combination than singly.

A. Topical Antibiotics

Antibiotics are directed at the infectious component of acne. By reducing infection, they also have a beneficial effect on the inflammatory component of the disease. *P acnes* has been developing antibiotic resistance worldwide, and this may be responsible for some treatment failures.

Available topical antibiotic preparations include erythromycin, clindamycin, benzoyl peroxide, and azelaic acid. Available evidence shows that erythromycin and clindamycin work better in combination with benzoyl peroxide than either agent alone. The different strengths of benzoyl peroxide appear to be about equally effective.

B. Oral Antibiotics

It is generally believed that oral antibiotics are more effective than topical agents and therefore more useful in severe disease. However, because few, if any, good-quality comparisons of the two modalities exist, it is impossible to be certain of this. Tetracycline is the mainstay of oral antibiotic treatment. Side effects are minimal—primarily gastrointestinal upset. Doxycycline may be taken with food to minimize gastric upset, but this agent is more photosensitizing than tetracycline. Minocycline is a more effective agent against *P acnes* than the other tetracyclines, but it is more expensive and has a higher incidence of serious side effects, such as vertigo and lupus-like syndrome. It is generally best reserved for disease that does not respond to first-line agents. All tetracyclines bond to calcium in bone and teeth and can cause staining of dental enamel. They should not be given to children younger than 10 years of age. Erythromycin is an alternative when tetracyclines cannot be used.

C. Topical Retinoids

Retinoids are derivatives of vitamin A. They prevent the formation of comedones by normalizing the desquamation of the follicular epithelium. Tretinoin has been in use much longer than the other agents, adapalene and tazarotene. All agents have the main adverse effect of excessive drying, burning, and inflammation of the skin. This can be ameliorated by changing to a lower concentration of the agent or by periodically skipping a day of application. Although tretinoin has been rated pregnancy category C, and there are no clear indications of teratogenicity, the role of topical retinoids in pregnancy is a matter of debate. Tazarotene has been designated pregnancy category X.

All agents are available in various strengths and vehicles. The choice of vehicle is determined by the patient's skin type.

D. Isotretinoin

Isotretinoin is a metabolite of vitamin A that reduces sebaceous gland size, decreases sebum production, and normalizes desquamation of follicular epithelium. It is effective for severe nodular acne and for acne unresponsive to other treatments. Adverse effects are common, including dry eyes, dry skin, headache, and mild elevation in liver enzymes and serum lipids. Benign intracranial hypertension is less common but must be considered if the patient develops headaches. Despite commonly held beliefs, evidence does not support the idea that depression is a side effect of this drug. Isotretinoin is extremely teratogenic, with major malformations occurring in 40% of infants exposed during the first trimester, so it must be used only after a negative pregnancy test—preferably after two negative tests—and with strict attention to contraception.

E. Hormonal Therapy

Because of the antiandrogenic effect of the progestin component, combined oral contraceptives are effective in reducing the severity of acne in women. Although some newer brands have been explicitly marketed for this indication, they have not been proved superior to older, less-expensive brands.

F. Combination Therapy

Agents for the treatment of acne work best in combination. The choice of agents can be tailored to the severity of the disease. Because of the time required for complete turnover of the epithelium, at least 6–8 weeks of treatment should be given before assessing the effectiveness of the regimen. If the disease is not adequately controlled, the regimen may be intensified (eg, by increasing the concentration of a retinoid, changing from a topical to an oral antibiotic, or adding another agent). Patients should be advised that total suppression of lesions may not be possible, but otherwise, the patient's assessment can be used as a guide to decide whether more intensive treatment is necessary.

For patients with comedones only, retinoids are the first line of therapy. These are applied once a day to the entire area involved.

For those with mild to moderate inflammatory acne, topical antibiotics are the treatment of choice. As mentioned previously, erythromycin and clindamycin are more effective in combination with benzoyl peroxide than alone. These are applied twice daily. Retinoids can be added if comedones are present.

For moderate to severe inflammatory acne, oral antibiotics can be substituted for topical agents.

For severe nodulocystic acne or for disease unresponsive to other regimens, isotretinoin is the treatment of choice.

For women with acne, oral contraceptives are a reasonable first-line treatment.

Prognosis

Although in general, acne diminishes at the end of adolescence, it may persist into adult life.

Haider A, Shaw J: Treatment of acne vulgaris. JAMA 2004;292: 726. [PMID: 15304471]

Liao D: Management of acne. J Fam Pract 2003;52:43. [PMID: 12540312]

Routine Childhood Vaccines

7

Richard Kent Zimmerman, MD, MPH, Donald B. Middleton, MD, & Sanford R. Kimmel, MD

Routine vaccination has had a tremendous worldwide impact on the burden of childhood diseases. The magnitude of this impact justifies the conclusion that immunizations constitute one of the major medical achievements of the 20th century.

Important topics to consider when making decisions that concern routine vaccination include disease burden, rationale for vaccination, vaccine efficacy, adverse reactions, and official recommendations. Except for trace amounts in some formulations of influenza vaccine, thimerosal has been removed from all routine childhood vaccines.

HEPATITIS B VACCINE

In the United States the number of potentially infectious persons chronically infected with hepatitis B virus (HBV) is estimated at 1.25 million. Chronic HBV infection occurs in 90% of those infected as infants, 30–60% of those infected before the age of 4 years, and only 5–10% of those infected as adults. Thirty-six percent of persons in the United States with chronic HBV infection contracted the infection during childhood. Up to 25% of individuals infected with HBV as infants will die of HBV-related chronic liver disease as adults.

Hepatitis B can be contracted from persons who are acutely or chronically infected with the virus. Transmission occurs primarily by blood exchange or by sexual contact, but in 30–40% of hepatitis B cases, the source of infection is not identified. Some of those cases may result from inapparent contamination of skin lesions or mucosal surfaces. Hepatitis B surface antigen (HBsAg) has been found in impetigo lesions and saliva of persons chronically infected with HBV. Epidemiologic studies show that HBV can be transmitted between young children.

Rationale for Routine Hepatitis B Vaccination

The duration of immunity in healthy persons is based on immunologic memory. Although antibody levels may diminish slowly over several years following vaccination, most persons remain protected by the immunologic memory in B lymphocytes. Immunologic memory and the long incubation period of HBV infection allow most immunized persons who have low titers to mount an anamnestic immune response.

Factors that affect immunogenicity include genetics, the number of doses administered, intervals between doses, prematurity, and underlying medical conditions. After the third dose of hepatitis B vaccine, more than 95% of children undergo seroconversion. The third dose is required for optimal protection; furthermore, titers improve with longer intervals between the second and third doses, supporting the concept that the vaccine series does not need to be restarted in those whose series is interrupted or delayed. Underlying medical conditions associated with a lower seroconversion rate include prematurity with low birth weight and immunosuppression. Premature infants who weigh less than 2 kg at birth have reduced seroconversion until they have gained weight and reached 30 days of age. Therefore, hepatitis B vaccination should be delayed until 1 month of age in preterm infants weighing less than 2 kg, unless the infant is born to a mother who is HBsAg-positive or whose HBsAg status is unknown, in which case the vaccine should be given within 12 hours of birth. The full three-dose series is still required as the infant ages.

Efficacy (ie, protection against HBV infection) is high for hepatitis B vaccine.

Adverse Reactions

The most common adverse event after administration of hepatitis B vaccine is pain at the injection site in 3–9% of children. Mild, transient systemic adverse events such as fatigue and headache have been reported in about 8–18% of children. Temperature higher than 37.7°C (99.8°F) has been reported in 1–6% of vaccinees.

Recommendations

The prevalence of HBV infection and its associated morbidity and mortality have led to the development of a comprehensive US hepatitis B vaccination policy that includes: (1) prevention of perinatal HBV infection, including emphasis on a birth dose, (2) routine vaccination of infants (Figure 7–1), (3) catch-up immunization of adolescents not previously vaccinated, and (4) catch-up immunization of young children at high risk for infection.

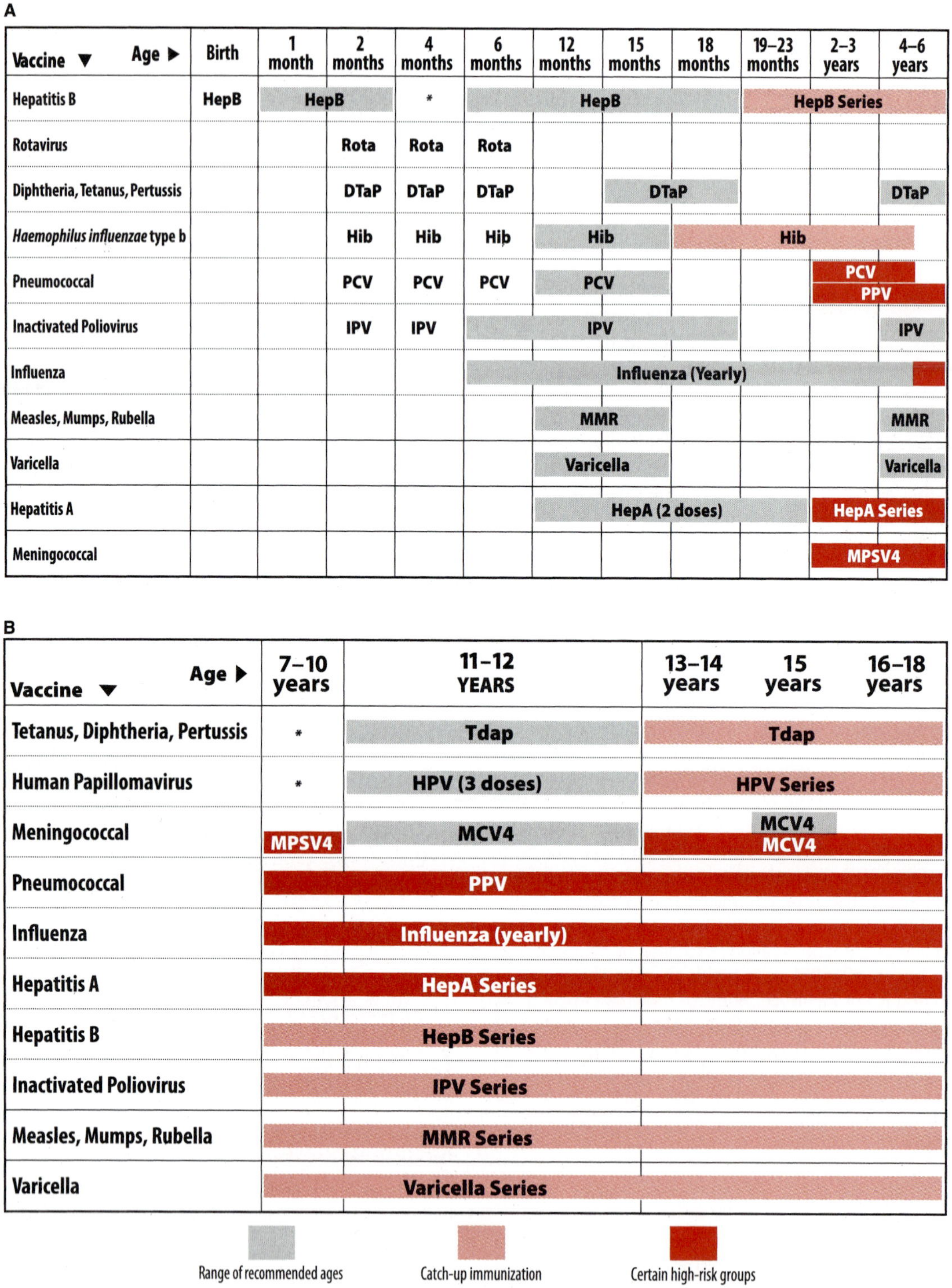

A

Vaccine ▼ Age ▶	Birth	1 month	2 months	4 months	6 months	12 months	15 months	18 months	19–23 months	2–3 years	4–6 years
Hepatitis B	HepB	HepB		*	HepB				HepB Series		
Rotavirus			Rota	Rota	Rota						
Diphtheria, Tetanus, Pertussis			DTaP	DTaP	DTaP		DTaP				DTaP
Haemophilus influenzae type b			Hib	Hib	Hib	Hib		Hib			
Pneumococcal			PCV	PCV	PCV	PCV				PCV PPV	
Inactivated Poliovirus			IPV	IPV	IPV						IPV
Influenza					Influenza (Yearly)						
Measles, Mumps, Rubella						MMR					MMR
Varicella						Varicella					Varicella
Hepatitis A						HepA (2 doses)				HepA Series	
Meningococcal										MPSV4	

B

Vaccine ▼ Age ▶	7–10 years	11–12 YEARS	13–14 years	15 years	16–18 years
Tetanus, Diphtheria, Pertussis	*	Tdap	Tdap		
Human Papillomavirus	*	HPV (3 doses)	HPV Series		
Meningococcal	MPSV4	MCV4	MCV4	MCV4	
Pneumococcal	PPV				
Influenza	Influenza (yearly)				
Hepatitis A	HepA Series				
Hepatitis B	HepB Series				
Inactivated Poliovirus	IPV Series				
Measles, Mumps, Rubella	MMR Series				
Varicella	Varicella Series				

Range of recommended ages — Catch-up immunization — Certain high-risk groups

Figure 7–1. Recommended childhood and adolescent immunization schedule, 2007 United States. **(A)** Recommended immunization schedule for persons aged 0–6 years. **(B)** Recommended immunization schedule for persons aged 7–18 years. *See footnotes on CDC Web site at http://www.cdc.gov/nip/recs/child-schedule.htm. (From Centers for Disease Control and Prevention. Recommended immunization schedule for persons 0–18 years—United States, 2007. MMWR Morb Mortal Wkly Rep 2006;55 (51 & 52):Q1–Q4.)

Postvaccination testing is not indicated after routine vaccination of infants, children, or adolescents. Postvaccination testing at 9–15 months of age for anti-HBs is recommended for infants born to HBsAg-positive mothers. A titer of 10 mIU/mL or greater indicates an adequate antibody response to vaccination.

PERTUSSIS VACCINE

More than 25,000 cases of pertussis were reported in the United States in 2004, representing an estimated total case burden of 800,000 to three million infections. Waning immunity from childhood pertussis vaccination and improved detection are the apparent reasons for this increase. Clinically, pertussis in older persons ranges from mild cough to classic paroxysms of cough truncated by inspiratory "whoop," cyanosis, apnea, and posttussive vomiting, or any of these in combination. Cough often lasts for months, creating significant morbidity and disruption of daily activities.

The majority of pertussis-related hospitalizations and serious complications occur in infants. One fifth of reported cases occur in infants younger than 6 months of age who are too young to receive three doses of vaccine, and half occur in children younger than 5 years. The case-fatality rate is 0.6% for infants younger than 12 months. Girls are somewhat more likely to exhibit clinical pertussis than boys, possibly because girls have smaller airways.

Complications of pertussis include pneumonia, seizures, encephalopathy, and permanent brain damage. Pneumonia is the leading cause of death. Encephalopathy, possibly due to hypoxia or minute cerebral hemorrhages, occurs in about 1% of cases, is fatal in approximately one third of those afflicted, and causes permanent brain damage in another third.

Pertussis is highly contagious: 70–100% of susceptible household contacts and 50–80% of susceptible school contacts become infected following exposure to someone who is contagious. Adults and adolescents are the primary source of pertussis infection for young infants. The reported incidence rate among adults and adolescents has risen recently, perhaps partly as a result of improved diagnosis with polymerase chain reaction testing and improved physician awareness.

Rationale for Vaccination

Before pertussis vaccination of children became routine, peaks in whooping cough incidence occurred approximately every 3–4 years, and virtually all children eventually were infected. Between 1925 and 1930, 36,013 persons in the United States died as a result of pertussis-related complications. More than one million cases of pertussis were reported in the United States from 1940 through 1945. After pertussis vaccination became widespread in the mid-1940s, the incidence of pertussis dropped by more than 95%, although it has been increasing in recent years, reaching 25,827 cases in the United States in 2004.

Vaccine Efficacy

Diphtheria, tetanus, acellular pertussis (DTaP) vaccines have an efficacy rate of 80–89%. The duration of protection from acellular vaccines is not yet known, although cohorts from earlier trials show no loss of protection in 2- to 6-year follow-up periods.

Adverse Reactions

The DTaP vaccines have approximately one quarter to half the number of common and uncommon adverse reactions associated with DTP. Minor adverse reactions associated with DTaP vaccination include localized edema at the injection site, fever, and fussiness.

Uncommon adverse reactions after DTaP vaccination are persistent crying for 3 or more hours, an unusually high-pitched cry, seizures, and hypotonic-hyporesponsive episodes. Most seizures that occur after DTaP vaccination are simple febrile seizures that do not have any permanent sequelae. Many experts state that on rare occasions a child might have an anaphylactic reaction to DTaP, prohibiting further doses of DTaP. Rarely, temporary swelling of the entire limb has occurred after administration of the fourth or fifth DTaP dose.

Recommendations

The DTaP vaccine is recommended for all children younger than 7 years of age. Premature infants should be vaccinated with full doses at the appropriate chronologic age, according to the recommended childhood immunization schedule. Full doses should be used because fractional doses may not be as immunogenic and might not lessen the risk for adverse reactions. Completing the recommended series is important for optimal efficacy.

To reduce the incidence of adolescent and adult pertussis and, as a secondary goal, infection of infant siblings, the Advisory Committee on Immunization Practices (ACIP) recommended that tetanus toxoid, reduced diphtheria toxoid, and reduced acellular pertussis (Tdap) vaccine replace Td vaccine in adolescents aged 11–18 years. These recommendations are available online at http://www.cdc.gov/nip/vaccine/tdap/tdap_acip_recs.pdf. If the recommended childhood DTP/DTaP vaccine series is complete and no Td or Tdap has yet been given, all adolescents should receive a single dose of Tdap, preferably at age 11–12 years. For those who previously received Td, a single dose of Tdap is encouraged after a 5-year interval. In some situations (close contact with an infant younger than 6 months of age or in a pertussis outbreak), shorter intervals (2 years) are acceptable. Similarly, all adults—including health care personnel with direct patient contact—should receive one dose of Tdap rather than Td.

PNEUMOCOCCAL CONJUGATE VACCINE

Streptococcus pneumoniae is a gram-positive diplococcus with a polysaccharide capsule that helps protect it from host-defense mechanisms. Over 90 capsular serotypes have been identified. Droplets from respiratory tract secretions spread infection. Prior to the introduction of pneumococcal conjugate vaccine (PCV), *S pneumoniae* caused about 17,000 cases of invasive disease, including 200 deaths annually, among children younger than 5 years. Invasive disease consists of bacteremia, meningitis, or infection in a normally sterile site, excluding the middle ear and sinuses. *S pneumoniae* is the most common bacterial cause of community-acquired pneumonia, sinusitis, and acute otitis media in young children. After the tremendous success of *Haemophilus influenzae* type b (Hib) vaccines in reducing meningitis, *S pneumoniae* became the leading cause of bacterial meningitis in the United States.

Risk factors that place individuals at high risk for infection include splenic dysfunction similar to that of sickle cell disease, African-American or Native-American heritage, and underlying medical disease such as diabetes mellitus.

Rationale for Vaccination

Currently, two vaccines that protect against pneumococcus are available: the 23-valent polysaccharide vaccine and the 7-valent conjugate vaccine.

PPV contains T cell–independent antigens, which stimulate mature B-lymphocytes to produce effective antibody. Thus, T cell–independent immune responses do not produce an anamnestic response and may not be long-lasting. The vaccine is effective in older children but not in children younger than 2 years of age because an infant's immune system does not respond well to such antigens. PPV does not reduce nasopharyngeal colonization of *S pneumoniae.*

A seven-valent immunogenic conjugate vaccine was licensed in the United States in 2000. PCV covers the seven serotypes (4, 6B, 9V, 14, 18C, 19F, and 23F) most common in children. These serotypes account for about 80% of invasive infections in children younger than 6 years but only 50% of infections in those aged 6 years and older. Unlike PPV, PCV elicits a T cell–dependent immune response that leads to anamnestic response on rechallenge and is effective in infants. The vaccine also reduces nasopharyngeal carriage rates of *S pneumoniae,* which might improve herd immunity.

In the primary efficacy analysis, a randomized, double-blind controlled trial conducted in 1995–1998 found that PCV efficacy against invasive disease was 100%. In the follow-up analysis done 8 months later, the vaccine's efficacy against invasive disease was 94% for serotypes included in the vaccine. In the intention-to-treat analyses, the vaccine's efficacy rates were 11% against clinical pneumonia, 33% against clinical pneumonia with radiographic evidence of infiltrate, and 73% against pneumonia with radiographic evidence of consolidation of 2.5 cm or greater. Radiographic evidence of consolidation is typical of pneumococcal pneumonia.

Adverse Reactions

No serious adverse reactions are associated with PCV. When given with DTaP vaccine but at another site, fever of 38°C (100.4°F) or less occurs in 15–24% of those vaccinated with PCV, compared with 9–17% of those receiving a control experimental meningococcal conjugate vaccine. Among PCV vaccinees, 10–14% develop redness at the injection site and 15–23% develop tenderness at the injection site.

Recommendations

PCV is recommended for routine infant immunization. Although the American Academy of Pediatrics (AAP) allows use of PCV in older children up to 13 years of age who have high-risk conditions, it should not replace PPV, which is recommended for those aged 2 years and older with certain high-risk conditions, including chronic disorders of the pulmonary system (excluding asthma), cardiovascular diseases, diabetes mellitus, chronic liver diseases, chronic renal failure or nephrotic syndrome, functional or anatomic asplenia (eg, sickle cell disease or splenectomy), immunosuppressive conditions (eg, congenital immunodeficiency), and children receiving chemotherapy with alkylating agents, antimetabolites, or long-term systemic corticosteroids. One-time revaccination after 3–5 years (age dependent) is recommended for persons with chronic renal failure or nephrotic syndrome, functional or anatomic asplenia (eg, sickle cell disease or splenectomy), immunosuppressive conditions (eg, congenital immunodeficiency, HIV infection), and in those receiving chemotherapy with alkylating agents, antimetabolites, or long-term systemic corticosteroids.

POLIOVIRUS VACCINE

More than 18,000 paralytic cases of poliomyelitis occurred in 1954 in the United States. Poliovirus is quite infectious: 73–96% of those infected will transmit the virus to susceptible household contacts, primarily by the fecal-oral route, although oral-oral transmission can occur. The incubation period ranges from 3 to 35 days.

The results of poliovirus infection, in decreasing order of likelihood, are subclinical infection (up to 95% of cases), nonspecific viral illnesses with complete recovery (~5% of cases), nonparalytic aseptic meningitis (1–2% of cases), and paralytic poliomyelitis (< 2% of cases). The ratio of inapparent to paralytic illness is about 200:1 (range, 50:1 to 1000:1). The case-fatality rate is 2–5% in children and 15–30% in adults.

Rationale for Vaccination

Poliovirus vaccination programs have dramatically decreased disease incidence. Circulation of indigenous wild polioviruses ceased in the United States in the 1960s, and the last case of wild poliomyelitis contracted in the United States was reported in 1979. The last case of poliomyelitis due to indigenous virus in the Americas occurred in 1991 in Peru, and in 1994, the Americas were declared free of indigenous poliomyelitis. Poliovirus was isolated from a few Amish children in the United States in 2005.

Recommendations

Poliovirus vaccination continues to be recommended because of outbreaks in other countries, ease of importation of wild virus, and the highly contagious nature of the virus. The all-inactivated poliovirus vaccine (IPV) schedule is recommended for the United States. Oral poliovirus vaccine (OPV), which is no longer recommended for routine use in the United States, is recommended by the World Health Organization for global eradication efforts and provides timely mucosal immunity. Prior to school entry, four doses of poliovirus vaccine generally are recommended; any combination of IPV and OPV, or either, is acceptable.

INFLUENZA VACCINE

During the influenza season, hospitalizations increase because of pneumonia and other complications. Hospitalization rates are increased among preschoolers, especially infants aged 1 year or younger. Complications of influenza include secondary bacterial pneumonia, worsening of chronic respiratory and cardiac diseases, sinusitis, otitis media, primary viral pneumonia (uncommon), and Reye syndrome, which is rare and associated with salicylate use concomitant with influenza type A or B infection in children. Recently, neurologic complications of influenza in children, including encephalopathy and death, have been recognized more widely.

Human influenza is extremely contagious and is transmitted from person to person, usually by the airborne route. Persons in crowded environments, such as students, are at high risk of exposure. Infected persons are most contagious during the period of peak symptoms. The incubation period is usually 2 days (range, 1–5 days), but young children can shed virus for up to 6 days before onset of symptoms. The illness attack rate is highest in children (14–40% yearly). Children frequently infect their families.

Vaccine Types

Two influenza vaccines are currently licensed: trivalent inactivated influenza vaccine (TIV) and live attenuated influenza vaccine (LAIV). TIV consists of subvirion or purified surface antigen preparations, which have lower rates of side effects than older inactivated vaccines.

The LAIV is a trivalent, cold-adapted, temperature-sensitive vaccine. Master donor viruses, developed by serial passage at sequentially lower temperatures in chick kidney cells, attain three genetic changes: cold-adaptation with good replication at 25°C (77°F), temperature sensitivity, and attenuation so as not to produce classic influenza symptoms. The master donor strains are cultured with the strains chosen annually for influenza vaccination; then reassortants are selected that replicate at 25°C, a temperature at which wild strains do not grow well. The LAIV replicates somewhat in the nasopharynx, where the temperatures are cooler, but inefficiently in lower airways where temperatures are warmer.

Vaccine Efficacy

The effectiveness of influenza vaccine in preventing or attenuating illness varies, depending primarily on the degree of similarity between the virus strains included in the vaccine and those that circulate during the influenza season, and on the immunocompetence of the vaccine recipient.

TIV has moderate efficacy in young children and good efficacy in older children. A study of children aged 1–15 years found TIV to be 77–91% efficacious against influenza type A respiratory illness, with efficacies defined by seroconversion of 44–49% among children between the ages of 1 and 5 years. In the first year of another study, efficacy was 66% against culture-confirmed influenza among 6- to 24-month-olds. Immunity from TIV wanes following vaccination and may not persist beyond a year. Hence, annual vaccination just prior to the influenza season is recommended. It may take up to 2 weeks after vaccination to develop protection.

In healthy children, LAIV was 87% efficacious against culture-confirmed influenza in the first year of a randomized, double-blind, placebo-controlled trial among the 60- to 71-month-old subset for which the vaccine is licensed. During the second year of the study, in which the strain was not well-matched against one serotype, the efficacy was 87% among the 60- to 84-month-old subset. As a secondary benefit, a 27% reduction in febrile otitis media occurred.

Safety of & Adverse Reactions to Influenza Vaccines

A. Trivalent Inactivated Influenza Vaccine

TIV can cause local reactions such as soreness at the injection site that lasts less than 2 days. In persons previously exposed to influenza disease or vaccination, studies comparing split-virus vaccine with placebo show similar rates of systemic reactions such as fever. However, in young children not previously exposed to influenza vaccine, fever, malaise, and myalgia can occur after TIV. A study from the Vaccine Safety Datalink found no serious reactions from TIV among 251,600 children younger than 18 years, including 8446 children aged 6–23 months who received over 438,000 doses of TIV. Persons with severe egg allergy should not receive TIV vaccination.

B. Live Attenuated Influenza Vaccine

Persons vaccinated with LAIV shed vaccine virus. In one unpublished study of children attending day care, 80% of vaccinees aged 8–36 months shed one or more temperature-sensitive strains for a mean of 7.6 days. One unvaccinated contact contracted the vaccine virus, which retained its temperature-sensitive, attenuated properties without genetic change; the transmission rate was estimated at 0.6–2.4%. Adverse events among children included nasal congestion and rhinorrhea (20–75%), headache (2–46%), fever (0–26%), vomiting (3–13%), abdominal pain (2%), and myalgia (0–21%); these were reported more commonly by vaccinees than by placebo recipients, were self-limited, and occurred more commonly after the first dose. Additional safety data are needed before LAIV can be considered for high-risk persons, such as those with asthma.

Recommendations

TIV is neither licensed nor recommended by the US Food and Drug Administration (FDA) for infants younger than 6 months of age. Until further data are available on safety and efficacy, LAIV is not recommended by the FDA for children younger than 5 years, persons with chronic cardiopulmonary conditions, or patients who require medical care for chronic metabolic disease, renal failure, or hemoglobinopathies.

Routine, annual vaccination with TIV is recommended for children aged 6–59 months. TIV also is recommended for individuals with chronic cardiopulmonary diseases; persons who require regular medical care for chronic metabolic diseases, renal failure, or hemoglobinopathies; patients with immunosuppression (including HIV); and children receiving long-term aspirin therapy. Influenza vaccine (either TIV or LIAV) is recommended for contacts of children younger than 59 months of age and for contacts of the aforementioned high-risk persons. Influenza vaccine recommendations often change every other year, with the addition of new age groups to routine annual vaccination recommendations.

Children younger than 9 years of age who receive TIV and have not had any previous doses should receive two doses, at least 1 month apart. Previously vaccinated children subsequently require only one dose each year. Dose varies by age: 0.25 mL intramuscularly for children aged 6–35 months and 0.5 mL intramuscularly for those aged 3 years and older (an inadvertent 0.25-mL dose given to children in this older age group must be repeated at any time).

Children aged 5–8 years who receive LAIV and have not had a previous dose of either TIV or LAIV should have two doses of LAIV separated by 6–10 weeks. All previously vaccinated persons or those aged 9 years and older require only one dose each year.

MEASLES, MUMPS, & RUBELLA (MMR) VACCINE

Throughout the 20th century, the burden of disease due to measles, mumps, and rubella ("German measles") dramatically declined because of widespread vaccination. In the United States, the number of cases reported in 2004 dropped from annual peaks of 503,000 to 11 indigenous cases for measles, from 152,000 to 258 for mumps, and from 50,000 to 50 for rubella.

Measles can be severe and sometimes acutely fatal. The disease may be complicated by a delayed fatal encephalopathy (called subacute sclerosing panencephalitis), the onset of which tends to occur in early adolescence. Worldwide, measles kills many people every year. Mumps produces excruciating bilateral parotitis and sometimes pancreatitis, orchitis, cerebellar ataxia, or death. Although mild rubella usually causes only posterior cervical adenopathy, arthralgia, and minimal rash, the disease can also produce a devastating fetal infection termed *congenital rubella syndrome.*

Measles cases often are imported in the United States. Outbreaks occur because the attack rate among unvaccinated household contacts is 90% or higher, and infected persons may transmit the disease from 4 days prior to 4 days after the appearance of the rash.

Rationale for Vaccination

The first dose of measles vaccine protects 95% of children. A small number fail to undergo seroconversion, usually due to the presence of higher initial titers of maternally acquired antibody. Mothers who have acquired immunity as a result of wild viral disease, rather than through vaccination, confer higher initial levels of immunity to their infants, who then have protective antibody levels until about 11 months of age. In such cases, seroconversion rates are optimal when administration of MMR vaccine is delayed until children are 15 months old. Today, because maternal immunity to measles is due primarily to vaccination, the duration of immunity transferred to infants has decreased to about 8–9 months of age, making vaccination at 12 months of age ideal. Failure to undergo seroconversion after the initial dose of measles vaccine occurs at a rate of 2–5%, necessitating a second vaccine dose. In comparison, the rate of waning immunity is less than 0.2%.

After MMR vaccination, seroconversion rates are 95% for children vaccinated at 12 months of age and 98% at 15 months of age. Immunity is probably lifelong in almost all vaccinated persons who initially seroconvert. After two doses, more than 99% of persons are immune.

Adverse Reactions

Pain, irritation, and redness at the site of injection are common but mild. Delayed reactions to measles vaccine include fever that is usually below 38.8°C (102°F), occurring between days 7 and 12, or a rash occurring between days 5 and 20. Adverse reactions to rubella vaccine include generalized lymphadenopathy in children and arthralgia in young women, but no reports of long-term arthritis. Adverse reactions to mumps vaccine include transient orchitis in young men. MMR vaccine does not cause autism. Transient thrombocytopenia due to the measles component of MMR (1 in 25,000 to two million) has been reported.

Recommendations

MMR vaccine is given routinely to all healthy children at age 12–15 months, with a second dose at age 4–6 years. A second dose is especially important for college students. MMRV (measles, mumps, rubella, varicella) combination vaccine was licensed in 2005 and may be used for both doses. It is preferable to receive the MMR or MMRV vaccine, rather than the separate vaccines for each component.

VARICELLA VACCINE

In the prevaccine era varicella-zoster virus (VZV) caused chickenpox in children, generally a self-limited and benign illness. Prior to the introduction of varicella vaccine, roughly four million cases of VZV infection occurred annually in the United States, with a hospitalization rate of 5 cases per 1000 population. Because secondary attack rates are as high as 90% and because communicability via aerosol droplets begins 1–2 days prior to the appearance of the rash, prevention of spread requires a universal vaccination. Complications of chickenpox include secondary bacterial skin infection (both impetigo and invasive group A streptococcal disease), pneumonia, Reye syndrome (now rare), encephalomeningitis, glomerulonephritis, thrombocytopenia, purpura fulminans, cerebellar ataxia, arthritis, and hepatitis. The lifetime risk for the late complication of herpes zoster (shingles) is at least 10%.

Rationale for Vaccination

In the prevaccine era, VZV hospitalization rates were 23 per 10,000 for children between the ages of 1 and 4 years. The majority of individuals hospitalized each year for VZV-related complications are in this group because VZV is so common at those ages. Although most hospitalized individuals were immunologically normal, many have developed the secondary complications mentioned earlier, sometimes with fatal outcomes. Routine vaccination is a cost-effective measure to reduce VZV morbidity and mortality and lost time from work and school; each dollar spent on universal immunization of children avoids approximately $5 in costs.

The current varicella vaccine contains live attenuated virus and is 97% effective against moderately severe and severe disease and 44–85% protective against any infection for at least 7 years. When the disease does develop in vaccinees, it is usually mild, producing fewer than 30 pox lesions. Due to break-through cases, a second dose of varicella is now recommended for all age groups.

Adverse Reactions

Local pain and erythema occur in 2–20% of children after the first dose and up to 47% develop local reactions with the second dose. From 4% to 10% develop a few (median of 5) varicella-like lesions 5–41 days after administration; these lesions last 2–8 days. A brief low-grade fever develops in 12–30% of vaccinees. In rare cases, vaccine virus can be transmitted to healthy immunocompetent siblings and parents, especially if the vaccinee has developed a varicelliform rash. No severe reactions have been associated with vaccination. Rare hypersensitivity reactions to gelatin or neomycin have been reported. Those with previously unrecognized VZV infection or prior immunization are not at increased risk. The risk for zoster is less among vaccinees than those who have been infected naturally.

Recommendations

The ACIP, AAFP, and AAP recommend that children receive two doses of VZV vaccine, unless they have a history of prior infection. To assess for immunity to varicella, the physician can start the assessment by asking if the patient has had varicella. About 80% of those without a history of chickenpox are actually immune. Although serologic tests may be cost-efficient, such tests are not required because the vaccine is well tolerated. Households with immunocompromised persons require no special precautions unless the vaccinee develops a rash, after which direct contact should be avoided.

Postexposure Prophylaxis

VZV vaccine is effective in preventing or modifying varicella if given within 3 days (and possibly up to 5 days) of exposure to wild varicella. Ideally, intravenous immune globulin (IGIV) or investigational varicella-zoster immune globulin (VariZIG) should be given within 96 hours of varicella exposure to exposed immunosuppressed patients; during early pregnancy to susceptible, exposed mothers; to newborns of mothers who develop chickenpox 5 days before to 2 days after delivery; and to exposed premature, low-birth-weight infants.

MENINGOCOCCAL CONJUGATE VACCINE

Neisseria meningitidis causes approximately 2200–3000 cases of invasive disease in the United States each year, with an annual incidence of 0.8–1.5 cases per 100,000 persons. *N meningitidis* is now the most common cause of bacterial meningitis in children and young adults in the United States. Death occurs in about 10% of cases, and sequelae such as limb loss, neurologic disabilities, and hearing loss occur in another 11–19%.

N meningitidis is transmitted from person to person via respiratory tract droplets. Disease most often occurs in children younger than 5 years of age. Fortunately, most cases of meningococcal disease are sporadic and not linked to outbreaks.

Serogroup B accounts for more than 30% of cases of meningococcal disease and tends to occur in children younger than 2 years. Serogroup Y also accounts for about 30% of sporadic cases, and serogroup C caused many of the outbreaks reported to state health departments. Although the incidence of meningococcal infection among Maryland college students was found to be similar to that among other persons of the same age, students residing in dormitories on campus had at least a threefold greater relative risk of contracting meningococcal infection than did students living off campus. A nationwide survey found that the incidence of meningococcal disease for first-year students living in dormitories was 5.1 per 100,000, compared with 0.7 per 100,000 undergraduates and 1.4 per 100,000 18- to 23-year-olds in the general population.

Vaccine Types

The quadrivalent meningococcal polysaccharide vaccine (MPSV-4, Menomune—A/C/Y/W-135, Aventis Pasteur) contains polysaccharide antigens to meningococcal groups A, C, Y, and W-135. Although it is not effective in children younger than 2 years of age, its efficacy is as high as 85% in school-aged children. Immunity probably decreases 3 years after initial administration as measured by declining levels of antibody to groups A and C, especially in children younger than 5 years. The vaccine is given subcutaneously. Pain, tenderness, and redness at the injection site are the most common local reactions. Fever, malaise, and headache also occur in a small percentage of vaccinees.

The meningococcal (groups A, C, Y, and W-135) polysaccharide diphtheria toxoid conjugate vaccine (Menactra, Aventis Pasteur), or MCV-4, is licensed for use in adolescents and adults aged 11–55 years. Conjugated vaccines stimulate immunologic memory with a longer duration of immunity than occurs from polysaccharide vaccines. The vaccine achieves seroconversion rates of serum bactericidal antibody titers similar to or higher than the unconjugated MPSV-4 for all four serogroups. A study in 2- to 10-year-old children found that the serum bactericidal antibody titers were significantly higher for all serogroups in MCV-4 recipients compared with MPSV-4 recipients at 28 days and 6 months after vaccination.

The MCV-4 vaccine is given intramuscularly, and the most commonly reported adverse events were local pain, headache, and fatigue. Local reactions were more frequent after MCV-4 than MPSV-4 vaccination, but most reactions were mild for both vaccines. Mild or moderate systemic reactions such as fever, fussiness, and drowsiness were similar in those receiving MCV-4 and MPSV-4.

The ACIP recommends that MCV-4 be given to 11- to 12-year-olds at a routine preadolescent appointment and for the next 2–3 years to teenagers who are entering high school (catch-up immunization). College freshman living in dormitories are at increased risk for meningococcal disease and should be vaccinated with either MCV-4 or MPSV-4. Other adolescents who want to decrease their risk for meningococcal disease may also be vaccinated

Vaccination is also recommended for the following high-risk groups: (1) persons with anatomic or functional asplenia, (2) persons with deficiencies in terminal complement components, and (3) travelers to, and residents of, hyperendemic areas such as sub-Saharan Africa.

NEWER VACCINES

In 2005–2006, several new vaccines were licensed or recommended for routine use, including hepatitis A vaccine, rotavirus vaccine, and human papillomavirus vaccine. Information about each vaccine is summarized below. The clinician is referred to the CDC web site for more detailed information (http://www.cdc.gov/nip).

A. Hepatitis A

Despite the progress in hepatitis A vaccination in the United States over the past decade, annually 5000–7000 hepatitis A cases are reported and an estimated 20,000–30,000 cases occur. Most cases now occur in states that did not have routine hepatitis A childhood vaccination in 1999–2004, raising the question of why vaccination policies should differ by state. The package label for hepatitis A vaccines was recently expanded by the FDA for use in 12- to 23-month-olds. In 2005, the ACIP guidelines were changed to recommend universal vaccination of children aged 12–23 months of age in all states using two doses, spaced 6 or more months apart.

B. Rotavirus

Rotavirus is the most common cause of severe gastroenteritis worldwide. In the United States, rotavirus causes 55,000–70,000 hospitalizations annually. In February 2006, a live, oral, pentavalent human-bovine reassortant rotavirus vaccine was licensed for use among infants. The CDC recommends routine vaccination of US infants with three doses administered orally at ages 2, 4, and 6 months. The first dose must be administered between the ages of 6 and 12 weeks. Subsequent doses should be administered at 4- to 10-week intervals, and all three doses must be administered by age 32 weeks. Side effects are minimal and include mostly gastrointestinal upset. Intussusception is not linked to the new vaccine. A dose of vaccine that is vomited up should not be repeated.

C. Human Papillomavirus

The American Cancer Society estimates that 10,370 new cases of cervical cancer and 3710 deaths occur annually in the United States. The cause of cervical cancer is human papillomavirus (HPV), which is the most common sexually transmitted infection in the United States. Quadrivalent HPV vaccine is licensed by the FDA for use in girls and women aged 9–26 years against the viral types that cause 70% of cervical neoplasia (types 16 and 18) and more than 95% of genital warts (types 6 and 11). The vaccine is 95–100% efficacious against cervical intraepithelial neoplasia and 99% efficacious against genital warts caused by serotypes in the vaccine. Localized pain at the injection site and swelling are the main side effects. Routine vaccination of girls at 11–12 years of age is recommended by CDC because at this age most girls have not yet become sexually active; catch-up vaccination is recommended for adolescent and young women aged 13–26 years who have not yet been vaccinated.

D. Routine Vaccine Schedules

Routine vaccine schedules for childhood, for catch-up vaccination, for adolescents, for adults, and for medical indications are available online at http://www.cdc.gov/nip. Schedules are updated at least annually for children and adolescents. Free downloads of Shots, a program for handheld computers and Palm Pilot devices is also available at that site or at http://www.immunizationEd.org. Prior to the receipt of any vaccine, parents and older patients should read the Vaccine Information Statements available in multiple languages at the CDC site. This site also discusses other nonroutine vaccines for use in appropriate situations.

Centers for Disease Control and Prevention; Atkinson W et al, eds: *Epidemiology and Prevention of Vaccine-Preventable Diseases,* 9th ed. Public Health Foundation, 2006.

Centers for Disease Control and Prevention: General recommendations on immunization: Recommendations of the Advisory Committee on Immunization Practices (ACIP) and the American Academy of Family Physicians (AAFP). MMWR Recomm Rep 2002;51:1. [PMID: 11848294]

Pickering LD: *Red Book: 2006 Report of the Committee on Infectious Diseases,* 27th ed. American Academy of Pediatrics, 2006.

Plotkin SA, Orenstein WA: *Vaccines,* 4th ed. Elsevier, 2004.

Disruptive Behavioral Disorders in Children

8

William S. Sykora, MD, COL, USAF, MC

We expect our children to be active and energetic, but when they exceed the norms for their age in their displays of activity, their lack of impulse control, or their inability to focus attention, they are likely to experience problems in social, familial, academic, and emotional interactions. Self-esteem is adversely affected, and these individuals are at greater risk of developing antisocial disorders, substance abuse disorders, academic failure, employment failure, and secondary mood and anxiety disorders. These behavioral variants, therefore, cause a significant social burden and are often brought to the attention of primary care physicians. This chapter addresses three Axis I childhood behavioral problems likely to be encountered in the primary care setting: attention-deficit/hyperactivity disorder (ADHD), oppositional defiant disorder (ODD), and conduct disorder (CD).

The controversies surrounding behavioral problems and their treatments have generated several comprehensive reviews that have improved understanding of these conditions. In 1998, the American Medical Association Council on Scientific Affairs concluded that there was little evidence of overtreatment with neurostimulants in the United States. That same year, the National Institutes of Health (NIH) conducted a Consensus Conference on the Diagnosis and Treatment of ADHD that concluded "there is validity in the diagnosis of ADHD as a disorder with broadly accepted symptoms and behavioral characteristics that define the disorder." Details are available at http://odp.od.nih.gov/consensus/cons/110/110_statement.htm. An International Consensus Letter from prominent leaders in the field in 2002 concluded decisively that "All the major medical associations and government health agencies recognize ADHD as a genuine disorder because the scientific evidence indicating it is so is overwhelming."

ATTENTION-DEFICIT/HYPERACTIVITY DISORDER

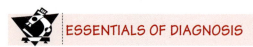

ESSENTIALS OF DIAGNOSIS

- *A persistent pattern of inattention, hyperactivity, or both; more frequent and severe displays of impulsivity.*
- *Academic underachievement and behavioral problems.*

General Considerations

Up to 20% of school-aged children in the United States have behavioral problems and at least half of these involve attention or hyperactivity difficulties. ADHD is the most common and well-studied of the childhood behavioral disorders. All family physicians have encountered the classically hyperactive child and his or her beleaguered parents and teachers in practice and in social interactions, but, likewise, may have overlooked the quiet but inattentive "daydreamer." The seeming dichotomy between the hyperactive and the inattentive types of ADHD can be confusing to both clinicians and the public. Primary care physicians should be familiar with the features of this disorder and are ideally positioned to evaluate and treat the majority of children and families dealing with this condition.

Pathogenesis

Neurophysiologic data suggest that there is no single cognitive or behavioral deficit common to all individuals with ADHD. Emerging data suggest that individuals with ADHD have abnormalities in the frontal-striatal circuits but the exact problem has not been isolated.

The current behavioral models for ADHD identify the primary defect as a lack of behavioral inhibition, which then affects four executive functions: (1) prolongation and working memory; (2) self-regulation of affect, motivation, and arousal; (3) internalization of speech; and (4) reconstitution. These executive functions then affect motor control and fluency. This model helps to give some conceptual framework to the behaviors seen in ADHD and areas where medications or cognitive and behavior modification therapy may play a role.

There is good evidence that ADHD is not caused by too much television (although patients may be attracted and distracted by it); by food allergies (although the rare child may display inattention secondary to such allergies); by excess sugar, artificial flavorings, colorings, or preservatives in food; by poor home life or parenting skills (although the behaviors of ADHD do set up the classic parent-child confrontation seen in ODD and account for some of that common comorbidity); or by poor schools or teachers. Some data suggest that maternal smoking, cocaine use, and alcohol use in pregnancy could play a role in some children with ADHD. Fetal alcohol syndrome results in similar problems with hyperactivity, inattention, and impulsivity.

Evidence now favors ADHD as a lifelong process. Preschoolers are being identified with great predictability for developing ADHD symptoms once in school. Up to 80% of ADHD children have features into adolescence and 65% into adulthood. The family physician is ideally placed to assist patients across the life span.

Epidemiology & Cultural Demographics

Analysis by the Centers for Disease Control and Prevention (CDC) of data from the 2003 National Survey of Children's Health places the national prevalence of ADHD in the United States among children aged 4–17 years at 7.8% (11% of males and 4.4% of females) and shows that 4.3% of children are currently being treated with medications (http://www.cdc.gov/mmwr/preview/mmwrhtml/mm5434a@.htm). The ratio of male to female children is estimated at 4:1 for the hyperactive type of ADHD and 2:1 for the inattentive type. For ADHD alone, without comorbid factors such as CD, there are no differences along socioeconomic classes. Among races in the United States, the CDC reports the following prevalences: 8.6% of white children, 7.7% of black children, 9.7% of multiracial children, and 4.5% of others. It would seem that ADHD arises across ethnic groups and, although cultural and ethnic factors may contribute to variations in diagnosis, there is no cultural or ethnic component to the etiology and true prevalence of ADHD.

Studies support a substantial genetic contribution to ADHD. Sibling studies show a risk of ADHD among siblings of a child with the diagnosis that is two to three times that in normal controls. The parents of children with ADHD have a higher incidence of the condition than societal norms and have a higher incidence of other psychiatric problems, and relatives have a higher incidence of mood problems, anxiety disorders, learning disabilities, CD, antisocial personality disorder, substance abuse problems, depression, and marital dysfunction.

Clinical Findings

A. Diagnostic Criteria

There is no single diagnostic test or tool for ADHD. The diagnostic criteria included in the *Diagnostic and Statistical Manual of Mental Disorders,* Fourth Edition, Text Revision (*DSM-IV-TR*) are the current basis for the identification of individuals with ADHD. Meeting these criteria (Table 8–1) does not exclude the possibility of other conditions, and the full differential diagnosis must be considered by the evaluating physician (see Table 8–2). There is rarely a need for extensive laboratory analysis, but screening for iron deficiency and thyroid dysfunction is reasonable.

The American Academy of Child and Adolescent Psychiatry and the American Academy of Pediatrics (AAP), with input from members of the American Academy of Family Physicians, have formulated evidence-based practice guidelines to aid in the improvement of current diagnostic and treatment practices. These guidelines can be accessed at the AAP's web site (http://aappolicy.aappublications.org/cgi/content/full/pediatrics;105/5/1158). The diagnosis is made by parent interview, direct observation, and use of standardized and scored behavioral checklists that are specific for ADHD and should include input from both parents and teachers. The criterion for diagnosis on the checklists is two standard deviations above the mean in the number of ADHD symptoms displayed.

Three subtypes of ADHD are recognized (see Table 8–1): predominantly inattentive (accounting for 20–30% of ADHD individuals), predominantly hyperactive-impulsive (accounting for < 15%), and the combined subtype (the most common, accounting for 50–75% of cases). Individuals with the inattentive subtype have fewer behavioral problems but are subject to mood fluctuations. Those with an inattentive component have more academic problems than those with a purely hyperactive component. Individuals with the combined subtype have the highest incidence of comorbid psychiatric problems and problems with substance abuse, and are the most impaired.

Some children may not fully meet *DSM-IV-TR* criteria. A useful reference for these children has been supplied by the AAP in its *Diagnostic and Statistical Manual for Primary Care (DSM-PC), Child and Adolescent Version.* The *DSM-PC* considers environmental and developmental influences on the more common variations in behavior to help in the diagnosis and management of children with attention, hyperactivity, and impulsivity.

B. Comorbidities

ADHD is often associated with other Axis I diagnoses, especially in patients referred to psychiatrists. From 35% to 60% of referred ADHD children have ODD, and 25–50% will develop CD. Of these, 15–25% progress to antisocial personality disorder in adulthood. Indeed, ADHD can be used as a reliable early predictor of disruptive behavior disorders. A family history of conduct problems aids this prediction. Among children with ADHD, those who are most hyperactive-impulsive are at greatest risk for development of ODD; however, it is possible to distinguish between the two disorders. ODD behaviors, such as "loses temper," "actively defies," and "swears," are less characteristic of children with ADHD.

Anxiety disorders are more common in the predominantly inattentive type of ADHD; for example, 25–40% of referred children have a concurrent anxiety disorder. As

Table 8–1. *DSM-IV-TR* diagnostic criteria for attention-deficit/hyperactivity disorder.

A. Either (1) or (2):
(1) Six (or more) of the following symptoms of **inattention** have persisted for at least 6 months to a degree that is maladaptive and inconsistent with developmental level:

Inattention
(a) often fails to give close attention to details or makes careless mistakes in schoolwork, work, or other activities
(b) often has difficulty sustaining attention in tasks or play activities
(c) often does not seem to listen when spoken to directly
(d) often does not follow through on instructions and fails to finish schoolwork, chores, or duties in the workplace (not due to oppositional behavior or failure to understand instructions)
(e) often has difficulty organizing tasks and activities
(f) often avoids, dislikes, or is reluctant to engage in tasks that require sustained mental effort (such as schoolwork or homework)
(g) often loses things necessary for tasks or activities (eg, toys, school assignments, pencils, books, or tools)
(h) is often easily distracted by extraneous stimuli
(i) is often forgetful in daily activities

(2) Six (or more) of the following symptoms of **hyperactivity-impulsivity** have persisted for at least 6 months to a degree that is maladaptive and inconsistent with developmental level:

Hyperactivity
(a) often fidgets with hands or feet or squirms in seat
(b) leaves seat in classroom or in other situations in which remaining seated is expected
(c) often runs about or climbs excessively in situations in which it is inappropriate (in adolescents or adults, may be limited to subjective feelings of restlessness)
(d) often has difficulty playing or engaging in leisure activities quietly
(e) is often "on the go" or often acts as if "driven by a motor"
(f) often talks excessively

Impulsivity
(g) often blurts out answers before questions have been completed
(h) often has difficulty awaiting turn
(i) often interrupts or intrudes on others (eg, butts into conversations or games)

B. Some hyperactive-impulsive or inattentive symptoms that caused impairment were present before age 7 years.

C. Some impairment from the symptoms is present in two or more settings (eg, at school [or work] and at home).

D. There must be clear evidence of clinically significant impairment in social, academic, or occupational functioning.

E. The symptoms do not occur exclusively during the course of a pervasive developmental disorder, schizophrenia, or other psychotic disorder and are not better accounted for by another mental disorder (eg, mood disorder, anxiety disorder, dissociative disorder, or a personality disorder).

Code Based on Type:

314.01 Attention-Deficit/Hyperactivity Disorder, Combined Type: if both Criterion A1 and A2 are met for the past 6 months
314.00 Attention-Deficit/Hyperactivity Disorder, Predominantly Inattentive Type: if Criterion A1 is met but Criterion A2 is not met for the past 6 months
314.01 Attention-Deficit/Hyperactivity Disorder, Predominantly Hyperactive-impulsive Type: if Criterion A2 is met but Criterion A1 is not met for the past 6 months

Coding Note: For individuals (especially adolescents and adults) who currently have symptoms that not longer meet full criteria, "In Partial Remission" should be specified.

314.9 Attention-Deficit/Hyperactivity Disorder: Not Otherwise Specified: this category is for disorders with prominent symptoms of inattention or hyperactivity/impulsivity that do not meet criteria for attention-deficit/hyperactivity disorder. Examples include:
1. Individuals whose symptoms and impairment meet the criteria for attention-deficit/hyperactivity disorder, predominantly inattentive type but whose age at onset is 7 years or after
2. Individuals with clinically significant impairment who present with inattention and whose symptom pattern does not meet the full criteria for the disorder but have a behavioral pattern marked by sluggishness, daydreaming, and hypoactivity

Reproduced, with permission, from American Psychiatric Association: *Diagnostic and Statistical Manual of Mental Disorders*, 4th ed, text revision. APA, 2000.

Table 8–2. Differential diagnosis of ADHD.

General Medical Conditions	Neurologic Conditions	Psychiatric Conditions	Environmental Conditions
Hearing impairment	Learning disability[1]	Conduct disorder[1]	Improper learning environment (eg, unsafe, disruptive)[1]
Visual impairment	Tic disorders (eg, Tourette syndrome)	Oppositional defiant disorder[1]	Mismatch of school curriculum with child's ability (eg, gifted, learning-disabled)
Medication effects (eg, antihistamine decongestants, β-agonists, anticonvulsants)	Seizure disorders	Substance abuse	Family dysfunction or stressful home environment[1]
Asthma	Mental retardation (eg, fetal alcohol syndrome, fragile X syndrome, phenylketonuria)	Anxiety[1]	Poor parenting (eg, inappropriate, inconsistent, punitive)[1]
Allergic rhinitis	Developmental delays	Obsessive-compulsive disorder[1]	Child neglect or abuse[1]
Eczema	Brain injury	Post-traumatic stress disorder	Parental psychopathology[1]
Enuresis[1]	Sleep disorders	Depression[1]	
Encopresis			
Malnutrition			
Hypothyroidism			
Lead toxicity			

[1]Common comorbid and associated conditions.
Reproduced, with permission, from Smocker WD, Hedayat M: Evaluation and treatment of ADHD. Am Fam Physician 2001;64:817.

many as 50% of referred children with ADHD eventually develop a mood disorder—most commonly depression, diagnosed in adolescence. The diagnosis of bipolar disease in childhood increases the risk of the concurrent label of ADHD because of the overlap of behaviors. About half the children with Tourette syndrome have ADHD, and the symptoms of ADHD usually precede the other symptoms of that syndrome. The medical treatment of Tourette syndrome and ADHD is complicated by the effects of stimulant medications on tics. Determination of the coexistence of ADHD and Tourette syndrome is vital to ensure that appropriate social and educational services are obtained for these children. (Tourette syndrome is discussed in detail in Chapter 43.)

There appears to be a strong correlation between sleep disorders and ADHD. Children who snore are almost twice as likely as their nonsnoring counterparts to meet diagnostic criteria for ADHD. This is particularly true for younger (under 8) boys, for whom the risk is three times higher in snorers. Whether this is a cause-and-effect phenomenon needs further study, but this link should be kept in mind when taking a history.

There is a definite association among ADHD, academic problems, and learning disabilities. Between 20% and 50% of children with ADHD have at least one type of learning disorder. In any child with ADHD in whom academic achievement seems to lag behind intelligence, testing for learning disabilities should be performed. The documentation of a learning disability makes it easier to obtain academic accommodations and modifications through individual educational plans as protected by the Individuals with Disabilities Education Act (IDEA). Individuals with ADHD have a higher risk of reading problems, as well as arithmetic and writing difficulties. They are often poor spellers and have poor penmanship. These problems are associated with difficulties in the executive functions of integration of working memory and motor coordination and fluency, all mediated by the lack of intact inhibitory processes.

There does not seem to be an association between intelligence and ADHD, although the verbal scores, mental arithmetic scores, and digital span scores in many intelligence quotient (IQ) tests can be lower in children with ADHD due to problems with working memory. These differences disappear when hyperactive behavior is factored out of the testing and are thought to be due to the methodology rather than true differences in intelligence. The true impact of ADHD is on the application of intelligence in everyday functioning and academic work.

Willens TE et al: Attention deficit/hyperactivity disorder across the lifespan. Annu Rev Med 2002;53:113. [PMID: 11818466]

Differential Diagnosis

Table 8–2 lists the differential diagnosis for ADHD.

Treatment

A. Pharmacotherapy

Medications commonly used in the treatment of ADHD are listed in Table 8–3.

1. Stimulants—The efficacy of this class has been proven in controlling some of the manifestations of ADHD but they are not a "cure." The fact that stimulants are controlled substances (Schedule II) with an

Table 8–3. Pharmacotherapy of ADHD.

Drug	Dosing	Cautions
Methylphenidate		
(Ritalin)—immediate release	5–20 mg twice or three times daily Initial: 0.3 mg/kg twice daily	Dependency in emotionally unstable patients
(Ritalin LA)—extended release	10–40 mg once daily Initial: 20 mg in the morning; increase every 7 d	As above
(Concerta)—extended release	18–54 mg once daily Initial: 18 mg once daily; increase every 7 d	As above
(Daytrana)—transdermal (on 9 h, off 15 h)	10–30 mg once daily Initial: 10 mg every 9 h; increase every 7 d	Local skin reactions
Mixed amphetamine salts		
(Adderall)—immediate release	5–30 mg twice daily Initial: 4 mg twice daily; increase by 5 mg every 7 d	Higher abuse potential, potential dependency
(Adderall XR)—extended release	5–30 mg once daily Initial: 5–10 mg in the morning; increase by 5–10 mg every 7 d	As above
Atomoxetine (Strattera)	10–100 mg once daily Initial: 0.5 mg/kg; increase every 28 d	Suicidality, rare hepatic problems

abuse potential justifies the close scrutiny of their use. About 65% of children with ADHD show improvement in the core symptoms of hyperactivity, inattention, and impulsivity with their first trial of a stimulant and up to 95% will respond when given appropriate trials of the various stimulants. The management of these medications can be complex, and treatment failures may more often be the result of improper treatment strategies than ineffective medication.

The pharmacokinetics of stimulants are characterized by rapid absorption, low plasma protein binding, and rapid extracellular metabolism. Up to 80% may be excreted in the urine unchanged or de-esterized. Therefore half-lives are short and frequent dosing or sustained-release preparations are necessary. Response does not seem to be weight dependent so weight-dependent dosing strategies are not as helpful as with other medications. Plasma levels of these agents have not been shown to be useful in determining optimal dosing.

Successful management of the stimulants used in ADHD treatment requires a systematic approach such as that outlined in the following model. It comprises four phrases: (1) counseling, (2) titration, (3) maintenance, and (4) potential termination.

a. Counseling Phase—The goals of this phase are to explain the rationale for the trial of the medication with both the expected positive effects and potential negative effects. Children must understand why they are being treated. They should know that the physician and not their parents or teachers is responsible for the treatment. The details of the treatment should also be discussed, including the choice of medication, dosage, and expected frequency of follow-up. Parents should be told which behaviors to monitor, what side effects to expect, and how they will be dealt with. Physicians should also explain the expected changes in dosing and timing of medications, and the anticipated eventual shift from short-acting to sustained-release preparations.

An important step is to determine the targeted symptoms, which will be unique for each child and family. This requires that the physician and parents review the child's symptoms and prioritize them based on their effect on the child's performance. Responders have shown specific effects, as outlined below.

Motor Effects

- Reduced hyperactivity.
- Decreased excessive talking and disruption.
- Improved handwriting.
- Improved fine motor control.

Social Effects

- Reduction in off-task behaviors.
- Improved ability to play and work independently.

- Decreased intensity of behavior.
- Reduced anger.
- Improved (but not normalized) peer social interaction.
- Improved parent-child interactions.
- Reduce verbal and physical aggression.

Cognitive Effects

- Greater sustained attention.
- Reduced distractibility.
- Improved short-term memory.
- Increased work completed.
- Increased accuracy of academic work.

Perhaps the most important step at this phase is the choice of medications. The current choices include methylphenidate and dexmethylphenidate, dextroamphetamine and methamphetamine, plus a combination of mixed amphetamine salts. (Pemoline [Cylert] had been used in the past, but concerns about liver toxicity have limited its role. It requires biweekly monitoring of liver enzymes and the signing of an informed consent. It is generally considered a final resort.) Most of these agents are available in short-acting (2–4 hours) and long-acting (6–8 hours) formulations. There appears to be little overall difference in the available agents as to the number of children who respond initially, and the side-effect profiles appear to be very similar. A methylphenidate transdermal system (MTS) was approved by the Food and Drug Administration (FDA) in 2006 and is marketed under the name Daytrana. The MTS is indicated for treatment of ADHD in children and adults who have difficulty swallowing oral medications. This route appears to be safe and effective but has a statistically significant higher side-effect profile, with insomnia and anorexia and the potential of reactions to the patch or adhesive. Each child will react differently to the various stimulants, and finding the optimal agent and dose is a matter of trial and error. The patient and parents must be aware of this and active in the decisions that will follow. Many times a combination of short- and long-acting medications is necessary to ensure the best coverage for the periods of peak target symptoms. A useful analogy is to insulin therapy in diabetes mellitus.

Absolute contraindications to the use of stimulants include concomitant use of monoamine oxidase (MAO) inhibitors, psychosis, glaucoma, underlying cardiac conditions, existing liver disorders, a history of stimulant drug dependence. Deaths have been associated with the use of stimulants in children with underlying heart and seizure disorders. The FDA has not yet put a "black box" warning on these agents, but physicians should be aware of the rare but serious cardiovascular risks. Most manufacturers do not recommend the use of stimulants in patients younger than 6 years of age, although several agents are approved for use in children as young as 3 years.

b. Titration Phase—Medication management requires close monitoring of behaviors and frequent dosing modifications in timing and strength to achieve optimal results. Titration usually lasts several months and entails weekly monitoring by the physician, much of which can be done by phone. Neither drug levels nor laboratory tests will determine appropriate dosing, and there is wide variation in response and side effects. Patients and families should be counseled that the initial dose may be ineffective and that the process of identifying the optimal dose will take time to do properly.

The most common side effects of stimulants are appetite suppression, which may be accompanied by nausea or stomach pain (but usually not); difficulty falling asleep; irritability; sadness; or rebound in hyperactive behaviors as the medication wears off. Side effects are the most common reason for discontinuation of these medications. Table 8–4 lists common side effects of stimulants and strategies to manage those side effects.

Most of the short-acting agents have their effect on symptoms for about 3–4 hours. The mixed amphetamine salts (Adderall) have an intermediate length of action of 4–6 hours. Dexmethylphenidate (Focalin) has an extended version that can be opened and sprinkled on food. The MTS patch (Daytrana) is designed to be worn for 9 hours and to have similar action to the release mechanics seen in the long-acting methylphenidate (Concerta). Long–acting medications are preferable to shorter acting agents because they have less rebound phenomenon and they do not require a noontime dose in school. The effects of the longer acting agents on the target symptoms must be compared with the effects established by the shorter agents. The longer acting agents have a delayed onset of action (usually about 1 hour compared with 20 minutes for the shorter acting agents.) In addition, the longer acting agents may be less potent milligram for milligram; therefore, conversion is not always straightforward.

The final step of the titration phase is an attempt to convert from the shorter acting agents to longer acting agents or even combining them to obtain the maximum benefit. It is possible to use a lower dose of the long-acting agent as a baseline and give shorter acting agents for periods where control is needed the most. Dosage modification is always an individual process and requires a great deal of communication among the patient, parents, teacher, and prescribing physician.

c. Maintenance Phase—Once the dosage of a long-acting agent is established and target symptoms are controlled, the frequency of visits between the physician and the patient can decrease. Because stimulants are Schedule II controlled substances, prescriptions with no refills are usually written monthly; however, several states allow 3-month prescriptions. In the large MTA cooperative study in 1999, the children with the best outcomes had monthly

Table 8–4. Common side effects of stimulants and their management.

Appetite Suppression
Will decrease with time (why stimulants eventually fail as "diet pills")
Try to time meals when medication effect is minimal or worn off
Make breakfast a major meal, prior to dosing
Make favorite foods for lunch
Offer substantial meal at bedtime
Delayed Sleep Onset
Determine if problem was preexisting, in which case an afternoon dose may actually help
If real, consider decreasing afternoon dosing
Usual sleep hygiene maintenance (same bedtime routine, bed just for sleep, etc)
Rarely consider second agent such as clonidine or trazadone (usually with consultation)
Rebound or "Wearing-off" Phenomenon
Check dosing, consider a 4 PM dosing of a short-acting agent
Switch to longer acting agents (pharmacokinetics decrease withdrawal)
Tics
Check child for emergence of Tourette syndrome
Simple tics are common and not necessarily associated with stimulants; they can be observed
If troublesome or irretractible, stop stimulant and consider adding or substituting another agent (such as a centrally acting α-agonist) with consultation
Depression
Check timing of symptoms; if they concur with medication timing consider a different agent
Make sure that attention problems were not really a mood problem
Consider consultation
Social Withdrawal
Uncommon effect of "zombie-like" behavior due to excessive dosing
Check timing of symptoms and dosing; decrease dose or increase intervals

30-minute medication visits. Growth and vital signs should be checked and documented, and it is vital to monitor the medication effects and the child's progress. Issues to address include (1) adequacy and timing of the dosage, (2) compliance with the regimen, (3) changes in school or out-of-school activities that may affect medical therapy, and (4) maintenance of appropriate growth. An initial drop-off in weight gain usually occurs during the titration phase, but over 2 years this reverses, resulting in no long-term sustained growth suppression from stimulant use. Drug holidays are no longer standard procedure, but parents may opt for their children to have periods off the medications to minimize potential unknown drug effects or to assess the continuing need for the medication.

d. Termination of Stimulant Medication—The decision to stop stimulant therapy is based on a clinical trial off of the medication and close monitoring of target symptoms. If there is an immediate return of targeted behaviors when medication is accidentally forgotten, the child is not yet ready for a trial off medication. In planning a trial off medication, the physician should choose a less-stressful period such as school vacations. Completion of a 2-week period without return of symptoms warrants an extended trial. The child's behavior should be monitored for about 1 year before deciding to permanently discontinue stimulant therapy.

A 14-month randomized clinical trial of treatment strategies for attention-deficit/hyperactivity disorder. The MTA Cooperative Group. Multimodal Treatment Study of Children with ADHD. Arch Gen Psychiatry 1999;56:1073. [PMID: 10591283]

Greenhill LL et al: Practice parameter for the use of stimulant medications in the treatment of children, adolescents, and adults. J Am Acad Child Adolesc Psychiatry 2002;41:26S. [PMID: 11833633]

Wender EH: Managing stimulant medication for attention-deficit/hyperactivity disorder: An update. Pediatr Rev 2002;23:234. [PMID: 12093933]

2. Nonstimulants—Many nonstimulant medications are being used for ADHD, alone and in combination with neurostimulants. Nonstimulant agents are less well-studied and are summarized here to inform the physician about their use. These medications usually are used when comorbidities are involved, and they may best be managed in partnership with a pediatric psychiatrist through close follow-up. They vary from established effective treatments such as the tricyclic antidepressants to potentially effective ones such as the highly selective catecholamine reuptake inhibitors (eg, atomoxetine [Strattera]), discussed below. Nonstimulants are often used to treat both ADHD and comorbid states, and their effectiveness alone is generally less than that of the neurostimulants. Fear and misunderstanding about the effects of neurostimulants make these nonstimulant agents attractive to parents. An excellent review of these alternative medications appears in *Child and Adolescent Psychiatric Clinics of North America* (see Popper CW, Pharmacologic alternatives to psychostimulants for ADHD, 2000;9:605).

FDA approval in 2003 of atomoxetine HCl for the treatment of ADHD in children older than 6 years of age and adults added a noncontrolled medication to the treatment arsenal for this disorder. Initially developed as a selective serotonin reuptake inhibitor (SSRI), this agent was found to have more selective norepinephrine reuptake inhibition and subsequently shown to have some effect in patients with ADHD. As with SSRIs, there appears to be an increase in suicidal thoughts in children who take atomoxetine (an increase of ~0.5% over placebo). The FDA has placed a black box warning on atomoxetine, and parents should be made aware of this risk. Atomoxetine has also been associated with rare but serious liver failure.

Atomoxetine has been found to be effective in both children and adults with both predominantly inattentive and predominantly hyperactive forms of ADHD for up to 10 weeks. Similar compounds have been shown to be less effective for the core problems of distractibility and hyperactivity than the 95% response rate seen with the neurostimulants, but the lack of addictive and abuse potential makes this class of agents attractive to many parents and physicians. Adverse effects include abdominal pain, decreased appetite, nausea, vomiting, and somnolence. As with stimulants, this medication class interacts with MAO inhibitors. Cardiovascular side effects include increases in blood pressure and heart rate, and atomoxetine has caused urinary retention problems in adults. The drug has also been shown to potentiate the cardiovascular effects of albuterol, and it should be used with great caution in patients with asthma. In adults, it appears to have similar sexual side effects as SSRIs.

Dosing of atomoxetine is by weight at an initial dose of 0.5 mg/kg/day, increasing every 3 days to a target dosage of 1.2 mg/kg/day. It is dosed once daily and is believed to have effects for 16 hours. The total daily dose should not exceed 1.4 mg/kg/day or 100 mg total, whichever is less. As with other selective neurotransmitter reuptake inhibitors, the full effects may not be seen for several weeks. For now, this agent could be considered when patients fail to respond to properly titrated stimulants, cannot tolerate stimulants, or refuse to try stimulants.

Atomoxetine (Strattera) for ADHD. Med Lett Drugs Ther 2003; 45:11. [PMID: 12571539]

B. Psychotherapeutic Interventions

1. Behavioral Modification—Behavioral modifications are designed to improve specific behaviors, social skills, and performance in specific settings. Behavioral approaches require detailed assessment of the child's responses and the conditions that elicited them. Strategies are then developed to change the environment and the behaviors while maintaining and generalizing the behavioral changes. The most prudent approach to the treatment of ADHD is multimodal, and combination therapy with psychosocial interventions and medications produces the best results.

Behavioral therapy alone is less effective than protocol-based medication alone and has shown little additional benefits when added to medications for inattention, impulsivity, and hyperactivity. The efficacy of behavioral modification comes from enhanced academic and social successes, which are hard to measure and generalize. Intensive behavioral therapy alone was shown to have equal efficacy to the usual care in the community even if medications were given to the community care group. This confirms the viability of specialized behavioral treatment in parents who prefer nonpharmacologic therapy of ADHD.

2. Educational Interventions—Teachers and schools play a huge role in the identification and subsequent management of ADHD. The education of children with ADHD is covered by three federal statutes: the Individuals with Disabilities Education Act (IDEA), Section 504 of the Rehabilitation Act of 1973, and the Americans with Disabilities Act (ADA) of 1990. The diagnosis of ADHD alone is not enough to qualify for special educational services. The ADHD must impair the child's ability to learn. A 1991 Department of Education Policy Clarification Memorandum specifies three categories by which ADHD children may be eligible for special education. They are (1) health impaired (other documented condition such as Tourette syndrome), (2) specific learning disability (could be ADHD alone if there is a significant discrepancy between a child's cognitive ability or intelligence and his or her academic performance), and (3) seriously emotionally disturbed. It is therefore vital to document all comorbid conditions in these children. For children who qualify, the accommodation strategies and specific goals should be outlined in the student's Individualized Education Plan (IEP) which is mandated under IDEA and is usually put together by teachers and parents along with school psychologists and administrators. Occasionally parents will ask for physician input into this process as they advocate for their children. Physician documentation of the diagnosis and management of ADHD is necessary to obtain accommodations for college entry examinations and other testing.

3. Parent Education and Training—Parental understanding of ADHD is vital to successful treatment. Parents must know the difference between nonadherence and inability to perform. They need to understand that ADHD is not a choice but a result of nature. Parent education can be frustrating at times because parents of children with ADHD often have features of the disorder themselves. Many parents respond well to referral to local and national support groups such as Children and Adults with Attention Deficit/Hyperactivity Disorder (CHADD) or the Attention Deficit Disorder Association (ADDA).

Formal parental behavior modification may be necessary for nonadherent, oppositional, and aggressive children. The most effective of these training programs use written materials, verbal instruction in social learning principles, modeling by the clinician (usually a psychologist), and role playing.

Some families require formal family therapy to treat the dysfunction that is caused or aggravated by raising a child with ADHD. The basic strategies focus on helping the family solve problems together. Table 8–5 outlines some of the strategies parents and families can use to manage ADHD behaviors.

4. Other Behavioral Approaches—Many other behavioral strategies have been used in the treatment of children with ADHD. These include social skills training, academic skills training, cognitive behavior modification, therapeutic recreation, and individual psychotherapy. These approaches must be individualized for each situation and require the involvement of a trained therapist who works with the physician. They require time and, in many cases, financial commitment.

Table 8–5. Advice for parents and families of children with ADHD.

Make a Schedule
- Set specific times for waking up, eating, playing, doing homework, doing chores, watching TV or video games, and going to bed.
- Post the schedule where the child will always see it.
- Explain any changes to the routine in advance.

Make Simple House Rules
- Explain what will happen when the rules are obeyed and when they are broken.
- Write down the rules and the consequences of not following them.

Make Sure Your Directions Are Understood
- Get the child's attention and look directly into his or her eyes. Then tell the child in a clear, calm voice specifically what you want.
- Keep directions short and simple. Ask the child to repeat the directions back to you.

Reward Good Behavior
- Congratulate the child when he or she completes each step of a task.

Make Sure the Child Is Supervised at All Times
- Because they are impulsive, children with ADHD need more supervision than other children their age.

Watch the Child around His or Her Friends
- It is harder for ADHD children to learn social skills. Reward good play behaviors.

Set a Homework Routine
- Pick a regular place for doing homework away from distractions such as other people, TV, and video games.
- Break homework tasks into small parts and schedule breaks.

Focus on Effort, Not Grades
- Reward the child when he or she tries to finish schoolwork, not just for good grades.
- Give extra rewards for earning better grades.

Talk with the Child's Teachers
- Find out how the child is doing at school: in class, at playtime, at lunchtime.
- Ask for daily or weekly progress notes from teachers.

Source: American Academy of Family Physicians. Available at: http://familydoctor.org.

C. Alternative and Complementary Therapies

Because ADHD does not have an easily understood etiology and no pharmacologic "magic bullet" exists to cure the disorder, and because of the stigma associated with the use of stimulant medications, there exists an eager market for alternative therapies. Caution should be used whenever a remedy claims to work for everyone with ADHD, uses only testimonials as evidence, cites only one study for support, fails to list the active ingredients, or is based on a "secret formula" and describes itself as harmless because it is "natural." Likewise, one should be careful not to alienate patients who find that a certain remedy is working for them, allowing for social and academic success. The physician's role is to advocate, educate, and protect patients in making decisions about alternative therapies.

Although some of these therapies have received good reviews from prestigious backers, they have shown little or no evidence of efficacy. Some therapies, such as elimination diets, have shown promise with a very small subset of patients (enough to allow for some outstanding testimonials) but have never been proven better than placebo in controlled studies. Sugar has often been labeled as the cause of all behavioral problems in children, but the studies have either been inconclusive or shown no correlation between sugar intake and attention and learning. Vitamin therapy has shown efficacy only in proven deficiency states, and megadoses can be potentially dangerous. There is also no evidence that caffeine is effective for ADHD in adolescents or adults. Although many "cures" for ADHD claim to have been tested in clinical trials, the NIH's National Center for Complementary and Alternative Medicine (NCCAM) has found no studies that prove efficacy. An excellent review of alternative treatments can be found at http://psychservices.psychiatryonline.org/cgi/content/full/53/9/1096.

Prognosis

Follow-up studies of children with ADHD show that adult outcomes vary greatly. There are three general outcome groups. The largest group is the 50–60% of affected children who continue to have concentration, impulsivity, and social problems in adulthood. These problems lead to workplace difficulties, troubled relationships, poor self-esteem, and emotional lability; however, success is possible if these individuals are matched to the right spouse and job. About 30% of affected children function well in adulthood and have no more difficulty than controlled normal children. The final group comprises about 10–15% who, in adulthood, have significant psychiatric or antisocial problems. Predictors for bad outcomes include comorbid CD, low IQ, and concurrent parental pathology. Treatment for all groups has been shown to be effective for the core symptoms over the short term, and the continuation of treatment may be necessary to maintain gains and improve the quality of life for patients and their families. Long-term treatment and outcome studies have yet to be performed.

The consequences of ADHD are significant. Up to 40% of children with ADHD require some form of special education by adolescence, 25–35% are retained in grade at least once, 10–25% are expelled, and 10–35% never finish high school. Individuals with ADHD are at increased risk of serious injuries, accidental poisoning, cigarette smoking, and substance use, and early death.

The exact financial impact of ADHD is unknown, but one study placed the national costs at $31.6 billion. Studies have shown that ADHD children incur twice the annual per capita health care costs of children without ADHD. They have 10 times the number of mental health visits, 3 times the number of prescriptions, and 1.6 times the number of primary care visits above and beyond their mental health visits.

WEB SITES

Attention Deficit Disorder Association (ADDA):

http://www.add.org

Children and Adults with Attention Deficit/Hyperactivity Disorder (CHADD):

http://www.chadd.org

OPPOSITIONAL DEFIANT DISORDER

ESSENTIALS OF DIAGNOSIS

- *A persistent pattern of negative, defiant, disobedient, and hostile behavior toward authority figures that is not part of a psychotic, mood, or conduct disorder.*
- *Age-inappropriate display of angry, defiant, irritable, and oppositional behaviors that have occurred for at least 6 months.*

General Considerations

ODD is defined by the age-inappropriate display of angry, defiant, irritable, and oppositional behaviors that have occurred for at least 6 months. Although many parents would categorize their teenagers as fitting this description, the object in applying this diagnosis is to define and help individuals whose behavior clearly impairs their functioning. The diagnosis is not made if an individual's behaviors are part of a psychotic or mood disorder, nor can it be made if the criteria for CD are met.

The experts who created this category hoped to provide a means of diagnosing the aggressive and antisocial behaviors exhibited in early and middle childhood that do not attain the severity seen in CD. Children with ODD do not usually have significant problems with the law and are not physically aggressive. Most do not progress to CD, but if no action were taken until the destructive behaviors of CD were manifested, valuable time could be lost. There is much overlap and comorbidity with ODD and ADHD but also clear evidence of divergence from attention deficit syndromes. In children with ODD, the problem is more an inability to inhibit moody outbursts and less an issue of executive functioning, as in ADHD. Owing to its relatively new emergence as a separate diagnostic entity, ODD has not been extensively studied and is usually linked to CD.

Psychopathology

ODD is seen as a behavioral disorder and is not associated with any known physical or biochemical abnormality. There is some evidence that children with ODD have higher androgen levels than normal controls, but this finding is not conclusive. The cause is generally related to social, parental, and child factors.

A. Social Factors

A correlation exists between ODD and living in crowded conditions such as high-rise buildings with inadequate play space. There is a correlation between social class and ODD, but no correlation to paternal employment or maternal employment. Finally, there appears to be some correlation to the quality of the day care if the mother is employed.

B. Parental Factors

It is difficult to tell whether parental behavior causes ODD or vice versa, but there are strong correlations between the way parents act and oppositional behavior. Parents of ODD children (not all, but certainly in pattern) tend to be critical, rejecting, lacking in warmth, passive, and unstimulating. Mothers, especially, demonstrate high levels of anxiety and depression. Family relationships, especially the marital relationship, tend to be strained. This sets up a vicious cycle as the child becomes more insecure and more difficult to handle, to which the parents react with more rejection.

C. Child Factors

It has been impossible to determine if the adverse temperamental factors that contribute to ODD are present from birth. ODD children are more likely to have language delay and have a higher incidence of enuresis beyond age-controlled peers.

The presentation of oppositional behaviors is highly variable. During the preschool years, transient oppositional behavior is normal. However, when these behaviors are of a persistent nature and last beyond the preschool years, the development of more disruptive behaviors is likely. On the basis of research data, two possible developmental trajectories have been suggested. In most oppositional children, especially those who are not physically aggressive, oppositional behaviors peak around age 8 years and decrease beyond that. In a second group of children, delinquent behaviors follow the onset of oppositional behaviors. Early physical aggression is a key element of this group, with physically aggressive children being more likely to progress to the violation of other property and rights that categorize CD.

Prevalence & Demographics

The reported prevalence of ODD varies from 2–16% of the school-aged population. Studies show an increasing rate of diagnosis from grade school to middle school to high school and then a decrease in college-aged individuals. Unlike CD and ADHD, gender differences are minimal in ODD, and boys are only slightly more likely to receive a diagnosis of ODD than girls. Conclusive data on racial or cultural differences do not exist, but worldwide ODD and CD are more prevalent among families of low socioeconomic status who tend to live in close quarters. Early onset of disruptive behaviors in which the rights of others rights are violated (as in CD), which has a worse prognosis and the highest social burden, seems to be concentrated in cities in the United States.

Certain familial situations are associated with the diagnosis of ODD. ODD is more common when at least one parent has a history of a mood disorder, CD, antisocial personality disorder, or a substance-related disorder, and 18% of children with ODD have alcoholic fathers. Family adversity scores in children with ODD are usually intermediate between those of children with CD and normal children. Whether this is a cause or effect is unknown, but the family physician is ideally suited to help address and untangle these complex issues.

Clinical Findings

A. Symptoms and Signs

Common manifestations of ODD include persistent stubbornness, resistance to directions, and unwillingness to negotiate and compromise with others. Defiant behaviors include persistent testing of limits, arguing, ignoring orders, and denying blame for misdeeds. Hostility usually takes the form of verbal abuse and aggression. The most common setting is the home, and behavioral problems may not be evident to teachers or others in the community. Because the symptoms of the disorder are most likely to be manifested toward individuals that the patient knows well, they are rarely apparent during clinical examination. Children with ODD do not see themselves as the problem but instead view their behavior as a reasonable response to unreasonable demands. They have problems with low self-esteem, lability of mood, and low tolerance of frustration and are more likely to be involved with substance abuse. These are difficult children to live with and difficult homes to live in, and families frequently turn to their physicians for help.

B. Diagnostic Criteria

DSM-IV-TR has specific diagnostic criteria for ODD (Table 8–6). The clinical features that bring children to family physicians' offices are based on control issues, aggression, and activity. Control issues start early, with battles over bedtime and mealtime starting at age 3 or 4 years. Children with ODD demonstrate verbal aggression toward their parents almost as soon as they can talk. This may progress to physical aggression that is usually directed at parents or caretakers and rarely at strangers. Activity levels are variable and may depend on the common comorbid condition of ADHD. Other features include anxiety and an increased incidence of temper tantrums and breath-holding attacks.

Table 8–6. *DSM-IV-TR* diagnostic criteria for oppositional defiant disorder.

A. A pattern of negativistic, hostile, and defiant behavior lasting at least 6 months, during which four (or more) of the following are present:

(1) often loses temper, (2) often argues with adults, (3) often actively defies or refuses to comply with adults' requests or rules, (4) often deliberately annoys people, (5) often blames others for his or her mistakes or misbehavior, (6) is often touchy or easily annoyed by others, (7) is often angry and resentful, (8) is often spiteful or vindictive.

Note: Consider a criterion met only if the behavior occurs more frequently than is typically observed in individuals of comparable age and developmental level.

B. The disturbance in behavior causes clinically significant impairment in social, academic, or occupational functioning.

C. The behaviors do not occur exclusively during the course of a psychotic or mood disorder.

D. Criteria are not met for conduct disorder, and, if the individual is age 18 years or older, criteria are not met for antisocial personality disorder.

Reproduced, with permission, from American Psychiatric Association: *Diagnostic and Statistical Manual of Mental Disorders*, 4th ed, text revision. APA, 2000.

DSM-IV-TR does not establish an age of onset for the diagnosis other than "younger than 18." The average onset of ODD behaviors is 6 years, and behaviors tend to peak at age 8. Diagnosis is made by parental, patient, or teacher history and direct observation.

Some behavioral checklists are available that can identify the pattern of ODD. They include the Child Behavioral Checklist and the Rochester Adaptive Behavior Inventory. A structured interview such as the Diagnostic Interview for Children and Adolescents or the Child and Adolescent Psychiatric Assessment may be helpful. It is rare that any medical testing or neuropsychiatric testing is necessary, unless comorbid states are present.

C. Comorbidities

ODD is common among children with ADHD. The disruptive behaviors of ADHD tend to bring out the parental behaviors associated with ODD. The combination of ADHD, ODD, family adversity, and low verbal IQ are predictors of progression to more serious conduct disorders and antisocial behaviors as adults. However, although up to 50% of ADHD children have ODD behaviors, only about 15% of those diagnosed with ODD have ADHD.

About 15% of ODD children have anxiety disorders and approximately 10% have depression or mood disorders. Addressing these problems can often help with the oppositional behaviors.

Differential Diagnosis

All the behaviors of ODD are present in CD; thus, ODD is not diagnosed in the presence of CD. Although comorbidity is seen with mood disorders, the diagnosis of ODD should not be made if a major mood disorder or a psychotic disorder is present. ODD should be distinguished from ADHD although both may be present in many children, in which case both diagnoses should be given. Physical causes for oppositional behavior must be considered, especially if hearing or auditory comprehension is impaired. The diagnosis of ODD in mentally retarded individuals is difficult and can only be made if the behaviors exceed those usually seen in individuals with corresponding cognitive impairment and age. Bipolar disease can be confused with ODD. Any of the social or medical conditions listed earlier in Table 8–2 could also be confused with ODD.

Treatment

Management of ODD depends on the extent of behavioral problems. Children with ODD demonstrate lower degrees of impairment and are more socially competent than children with CD. Furthermore, children with CD come from less advantaged families and, by definition, have greater conflict with school and judicial systems compared with children with ODD. These differences can be used to predict which children may need more aggressive intervention.

A. Behavioral Therapy

The vast majority of these patients and their families can be managed with behavioral therapies, especially parental training and family therapy.

Parental-controlled behavioral modification is based on social learning theory and uses naturally occurring consequences to teach social skills and self-evaluation. Parents are taught to minimize emotional reactions to oppositional behaviors, to give clear instructions and limits, to positively reinforce good behaviors, and to use punishment selectively. Parent training is usually conducted by psychologists or trained social workers and can be conducted in groups. Advice to parents includes the importance of communicating with each other to avoid situations in which the child plays one against the other. Communication with teachers and principals is also important.

Studies have shown that children who watch 4–6 hours of television a day are more violent, more likely to use drugs, and more preoccupied with sex, and the AAP recommends that television viewing be limited to 1–2 hours per day. Likewise, video games can be addictive and children who play violent video games are more physically aggressive and not as intelligent as controls.

Many families of children with ODD are characterized by low socioeconomic status, parental psychopathology, and marital conflict. These issues also need to be addressed by counseling or medication if behavioral modification techniques are to be successful with the child. Family therapy may be indicated to address family dysfunction from the oppositional behavior or from primary parental or marital problems. Behavioral intervention can be performed in which the family learns how to negotiate together. One technique for adolescents is parent-child contracting, which involves written agreements for behavioral changes in both parties based on specified contingencies.

B. Pharmacotherapy for Comorbid Conditions

There is no accepted pharmacologic treatment for oppositional behaviors, but comorbid conditions such as ADHD or depression must be properly addressed and appropriately treated. For children who do not respond to nonmedical interventions or are extremely impaired, it is best to consult a pediatric psychiatrist. Medications used for ODD include clonidine, lithium, carbamazepine, valproic acid, and risperidone; all have significant risks and their use should be monitored carefully.

Prognosis

The most serious consequence of ODD is the development of more dangerous conduct problems. Although the majority of children with ODD will not develop CD, in some cases ODD appears to represent a developmental precursor of CD. This seems to hold true for boys more than for girls. In cases in which ODD precedes CD, the onset of CD is typically before age 10 years (childhood-onset CD). For children in whom such symptoms subsequently decrease with maturity, the prognosis is good. If oppositional behaviors progress and begin to involve the violation of others' rights, then the child will probably progress to CD.

Lavigne JV et al: Oppositional defiant disorder with onset in preschool years: Longitudinal stability and pathways to other disorders. J Am Acad Child Adolesc Psychiatry 2001;40:1393. [PMID: 11765284]

CONDUCT DISORDER

ESSENTIALS OF DIAGNOSIS

- *A repetitive and persistent pattern of behavior in which the basic rights of others and major age-appropriate societal norms are violated.*
- *Behavior characterized by aggression toward people and animals, destruction of property, deceitfulness or theft, and serious violation of rules.*

General Considerations

The most serious disruptive behavioral problem of childhood seen in primary care is CD. Although many normal children have lapses in judgment and break rules or hurt others, CD represents a persistent or repetitive pattern of such behaviors. These behaviors represent a significant problem for patients, their families, and society in general, and often physicians are consulted to help. Social norms tend to be culturally specific, and significant differences may exist among cultures or societal groups in determining when (and what) behavior is deemed antisocial. Physicians and professionals must be aware that their judgments of abnormality will be affected by the values of their particular society.

CD is a condition in which the expertise of physicians has implications for society in general as well as for individual patients and their families. It is also a condition that is a referral diagnosis for most primary care physicians and may be best addressed by working in conjunction with specialized pediatric and adolescent psychiatrists and therapists. Family physicians may be called on for brief behavioral counseling and sometimes pharmacotherapy; however, their biggest role may be the determination and treatment of the many comorbid conditions found in these individuals. CD also comprises a public health concern by contributing to school and gang violence, weapon use, substance abuse, and high drop-out rates. It is therefore important to identify these behaviors and intervene as early as possible.

Psychopathology

The etiology of CD is unknown but seems to involve an interaction of genetic or constitutional factors with familial and environmental factors.

A. Constitutional Factors

The risk of CD is higher in children whose biological or adoptive parents have antisocial personality disorder, and siblings of children with CD have a higher risk for developing the condition as well. CD is also more common in children whose biological parents have ADHD, CD, alcohol dependence, mood disorders, and schizophrenia. Studies examining physiologic factors that might explain CD have centered around a decreased autonomic response to various stimuli in these individuals. Essentially, it seems to take a lot of stimulation to generate an autonomic and visceral response in individuals with CD, especially those with the early-onset form of the disorder. Hormonal factors have been studied, in particular, the influence of testosterone on aggression and cortisol on anxiety. Trends but no distinct cause-and-effect relationship have been noted. Neurotransmitters also play a role in aggression, and current research points to serotonin as an important mediator.

B. Environmental Factors

Exposure to antisocial behavior in a caregiver increases the risk of CD. Child abuse also increases the risk, especially sexual abuse in girls. Although once thought to play a role, divorce does not seem to be a contributor once one controls for parental pyschopathology. There is no doubt that the caregiver-child interaction contributes to disruptive behavior. The influence is bidirectional, with parents' behavior influencing the child's and vice versa. Factors in these relationships include (1) low levels of parental involvement in the child's activities, (2) poor supervision, and (3) harsh and inconsistent disciplinary practices. The child views behavioral problems as strategies to secure attention and become closer to the caregiver or parent. Neighborhood and peer factors also contribute to the incidence of CD. Being poor, living in crowded conditions in a high-crime neighborhood, and having a "deviant" peer group all increase the risk of CD.

Prevalence & Demographics

The prevalence of CD varies from 1% to 10% overall, depending on the studied population, with ranges of 6–

16% in boys and 2–9% in girls younger than 18 years of age. CD tends to increase from middle childhood to adolescence. Although certain behaviors (eg, physical fighting) decrease with age, the most serious aggressive behaviors (eg, robbery, rape, and murder) increase during adolescence. The differing incidence of CD in boys and girls does not occur until after age 6 years, and boys and girls with CD manifest differing behaviors. Boys exhibit more fighting, stealing, vandalism, and school discipline problems, whereas girls are more likely to lie, be truant, run away, and abuse substances.

The incidence of CD does not seem to have racial or ethnic correlations if one controls for socioeconomic group and for high-crime neighborhoods. Although some observers contend that the incidence of CD is on the rise, many authorities would argue that differences between generations in the perception of youth crime are influenced by recall bias in the older population.

Clinical Findings

The key to the diagnosis of CD is the disregard for the rights of others and the rules of society shown by affected individuals. The *DSM-IV-TR* allows for a broad range of behaviors and makes a clear distinction between early-onset and later-onset CD. This distinction is useful because the prognosis is much better if onset of these behaviors is after age 10.

A. Symptoms and Signs

Children with CD are referred to physicians by either parents or authorities. Younger children may present with behaviors that include outright refusal to cooperate with examinations or immunizations and a history of frequently running away from parents. Older children may be referred by teachers or school administrators, who request a medical evaluation prior to allowing a suspended student back into school. Adolescents may present after they have been arrested for violent or destructive behaviors. These behaviors are not only disruptive but involve blatant breaking of societal rules and violation of the rights of others.

B. Diagnostic Criteria

Because of some significant differences in CD that occurs before or after age 10, the disorder is subtyped into two groups: early onset and late onset. There are four main groupings of behaviors in CD: (1) aggression to people or animals, (2) destruction of property, (3) deceitfulness or theft, and (4) serious violation of rules. Due to the diversity of disruptive behaviors, *DSM–IV-TR* includes "specifiers" that classify behaviors into mild, moderate, and severe. These are useful in trying to predict the nature of the presenting problems, the developmental course, and the outcomes.

Behavioral disorders must be differentiated from normal reactions to abnormal circumstances. The *DSM–IV-TR* states that the diagnosis of CD should not be made when behaviors are in response to the social context. Screening questions might include asking about troubles with police, involvement in physical fights, suspensions from school, running away from home, sexual activity, and the use of tobacco, alcohol, and drugs.

Physicians must distinguish normal adolescent risk-taking and antisocial behaviors from CD. Normal experimentation usually does not harm others and does not recur persistently. According to the *DSM–IV-TR,* three specific CD behaviors should be present for at least 6 months to make the diagnosis. The full *DSM-IV-TR* criteria are listed in Table 8–7.

It has become more common to utilize standardized interviews in making the diagnosis of CD. These include the National Institute of Mental Health (NIMH) Diagnostic Interview Schedule for Children Version IV, the Child and Adolescent Psychiatric Assessment, the Schedule for Affective Disorders and Schizophrenia for School-Age Children, and the Diagnostic Interview for Children and Adolescents. These interviews are time consuming and expensive but yield more information than behavioral checklists. Pictorial instruments are available for very young children. Because parents and authorities usually do not know the full extent of the child's behaviors, it is useful to interview them as well.

Most primary care physicians refer cases of CD to pediatric psychiatrists but may be involved in the initial workup. Rarely are any special tests necessary.

C. Comorbidities

A clear majority (75%) of children with CD have at least one other psychiatric diagnosis. The relationship between ADHD and CD has been studied the most. Thirty percent to 50% of children with CD also have ADHD. ADHD can be conceptualized as a cognitive-developmental disorder, with an earlier age at onset than CD. Children with ADHD more frequently show deficits on measures of attention and cognitive function, have hyperactivity, and have greater neurodevelopmental abnormalities than children with CD. Furthermore, children with CD tend to be characterized by higher levels of aggression and greater familial dysfunction than those with ADHD.

A significant proportion of children present with symptoms of both ADHD and CD, and both conditions should be diagnosed when this occurs. Comorbid ADHD and CD is consistently reported to be more disabling than either disorder alone. These children have the problems found in both disorders and tend to show increased levels of aggressive behaviors at an early age, which remain remarkably persistent. This is in contrast to the more typical episodic course seen in children with

Table 8–7. *DSM-IV-TR* diagnostic criteria for conduct disorder.

A. A repetitive and persistent pattern of behavior in which the basic rights of others or major age-appropriate societal norms or rules are violated, as manifested by the presence of three (or more) of the following criteria in the past 12 months, with at least one criterion present in the past 6 months:

Aggression to people and animals
(1) often bullies, threatens, or intimidates others
(2) often initiates physical fights
(3) has used a weapon that can cause serious physical harm to others (eg, a bat, brick, broken bottle, knife, gun)
(4) has been physically cruel to people
(5) has been physically cruel to animals
(6) has stolen while confronting a victim (eg, mugging, purse snatching, extortion, armed robbery)
(7) has forced someone into sexual activity

Destruction of property
(8) has deliberately engaged in fire setting with the intention of causing serious damage
(9) has deliberately destroyed others' property (other than by fire setting)

Deceitfulness or theft
(10) has broken into someone else's house, building, or car
(11) often lies to obtain goods or favors or to avoid obligations (ie, "cons" others)
(12) has stolen items of nontrivial value without confronting a victim (eg, shoplifting, but without breaking and entering; forgery)

Serious violations of rules
(13) often stays out at night despite parental prohibitions, beginning before age 13 years
(14) has run away from home overnight at least twice while living in parental or parental surrogate home (or once without returning for a lengthy period)
(15) is often truant from school, beginning before age 13 years

B. The disturbance in behavior causes clinically significant impairment in social, academic, or occupational functioning.

C. If the individual is age 18 years or older, criteria are not met for antisocial personality disorder.

Code based on age at onset:

312.81 Conduct Disorder, Childhood-Onset Type: onset of at least one criterion characteristic of conduct disorder prior to age 10 years
312.82 Conduct Disorder, Adolescent-Onset Type: absence of any criteria characteristic of conduct disorder prior to age 10 years
312.89 Conduct Disorder, Unspecified Onset: age at onset is not known

Specify severity:

Mild: few if any conduct problems in excess of those required to make the diagnosis and conduct problems cause only minor harm to others
Moderate: number of conduct problems and effect on others intermediate between "mild" and "severe"
Severe: many conduct problems in excess of those required to make the diagnosis or conduct problems cause considerable harm to others

Reproduced, with permission, from American Psychiatric Association: *Diagnostic and Statistical Manual of Mental Disorders*, 4th ed, text revision. APA, 2000.

CD alone, who tend to do bad things impulsively and tend to get caught. Finally, children with comorbid ADHD and CD appear to have a much worse long-term outcome than those with either disorder alone. In children who have late-onset CD, symptoms of ODD and ADHD are usually not present during early childhood.

Other psychiatric diagnoses commonly seen in association with CD include substance abuse, mania, schizophrenia, somatoform disorder, and obsessive-compulsive disorder. This is not surprising, considering that these diagnoses are more common in the parents of children with CD. Anxiety disorders and mood disorders are also commonly diagnosed in children with CD (25%), especially in girls.

Differential Diagnosis

All of the social or medical conditions listed earlier in Table 8–2 may cause behaviors that could mimic CD. ODD is often thought of as existing on a continuum with CD, with the line being crossed when others' rights or societal rules are broken. If a child meets the criteria for both disorders, the diagnosis of CD takes precedence.

Table 8–8. Drug classes used in the treatment of conduct disorder.

Drug Class	Target Symptoms	Precautions
Neurostimulants	Depression and aggression	Abuse potential, cardiac effects
Antidepressants (eg, bupropion)	Depression and aggression	Agitation, GI side effects
Selective serotonin reuptake inhibitors	Depression, obsessive behaviors	Agitation, serotonin syndrome
Anticonvulsants	Aggression	LFTs and CBC abnormalities
Lithium	Mania, aggression	Weight gain, cholinergic effects
Antipsychotics	Aggression	Weight gain, cholinergic effects
α-Blockers (eg, clonidine)	Aggression, sleep problems	Cardiac effects, dry mouth

GI, gastrointestinal; LFTs, liver function tests; CBC, complete blood count.
Reproduced, with permission, from Searight HR et al: Conduct disorder: Diagnosis and treatment in primary care. Am Fam Physician 2001;63:1579.

Children with ADHD have disruptive and impulsive behavior but their behavior does not violate age-appropriate societal norms and rarely hurts others. If the diagnostic criteria for both disorders are met, the child is given both diagnoses.

Children with major depression may present with acting-out behaviors. Mood disorders are usually associated with affective symptoms, sleep disturbances, and appetite disruption. Having CD and depression places a child at great risk for impulsive suicidal behavior. Bipolar disease can manifest in irrational behavior and conduct problems, but the episodic nature of the behaviors and other symptoms of mania are usually apparent. It is possible to have both disorders.

Intermittent explosive disorder features sudden aggressive outbursts that are usually unprovoked. These individuals do not intend to hurt anyone but say they "snapped" and, without realizing it, attacked another person. Intermittent explosive disorder is distinguished from CD in that these episodes are the only signs of behavioral problems and these individuals do not engage in other rule violations.

Late onset of CD may be associated with substance abuse or dependence, especially in the previously normal child. There may be a large overlap of such abuse with CD. Repeated use of alcohol at an early age (10–13 years) is a marker for development of CD.

Treatment

The family physician is usually the first health professional consulted by parents of children with CD. A key element in the initial treatment of these children is to obtain parental involvement. Although many parents of children with CD have problems themselves, they do not want their children to follow their path. All parties need to be aware of the possibility of a poor prognosis without the interventions of the caregiver.

Behavioral interventions are similar to those for ODD. Parents need to establish monitoring of their child's activities and friends. They need to structure those activities and set consistent behavioral guidelines with consistent and clear consequences. Referral to family counseling can help with communication problems. For children with mild CD, this may be all that is needed, but for those with moderate to severe CD, referral to a subspecialist who can devote the time necessary to these patients is best. Individual psychotherapy seems to be more effective in CD than in ODD.

Pharmacotherapy should be considered an adjunct to behavioral therapies or can be directed at specific comorbid states. Medications target specific symptoms as there is no approved medication for CD. Table 8–8 summarizes some of the medications that are used in the treatment of CD. These should be prescribed in collaboration with a specialist unless the primary physician is very familiar and comfortable with the medication and the condition.

Prognosis

The social burden and public health concerns associated with CD make diagnosis and treatment of this condition very important. About 40% of children with early-onset CD are diagnosed in adulthood with antisocial personality disorder or psychopathology. Overall about 30% of children with CD continue to demonstrate a repetitive display of illegal behaviors. Antisocial behavior rarely begins in adulthood, and the family cycle of such behaviors is difficult to break. It is therefore critical that early onset of CD be diagnosed and appropriate interventions implemented to avoid a lifetime of criminal activity or prison and a continuation of such behaviors in subsequent generations. As with all the disruptive behaviors of childhood, family physicians can have a significant impact through screening, recognition, treatment, and referral.

Loeber R et al: Oppositional defiant and conduct disorder: A review of the past 10 years, part 1. J Am Acad Child Adolesc Psychiatry 2000;39:1468. [PMID: 11128323]

Seizures

9

Donald B. Middleton, MD

ESSENTIALS OF DIAGNOSIS

- *Occurrence of an aura.*
- *Alteration in or impaired consciousness or behavior.*
- *Abnormal movement.*
- *Interictal trauma or incontinence.*
- *Eyewitness account.*
- *Presence of fever.*
- *Postictal confusion, lethargy, or sleepiness.*
- *Diagnostic electroencephalogram.*
- *Abnormality on neuroimaging.*

General Considerations

Despite an alarming appearance, a single seizure rarely causes permanent sequelae or signals the onset of epilepsy. The lifetime risk of having a seizure is 10% but only about 3% of the population develops epilepsy, defined as spontaneous or unprovoked, recurrent seizures. The annual number of new seizures in children and adolescents is 50,000–150,000, 15,000–30,000 of which constitute epileptic seizures. The majority of seizure victims will not have a recurrence or develop epilepsy.

Epilepsy has an annual incidence of 50 per 100,000 population with a prevalence of 5–10 per 1000. The incidence is high in childhood, decreases in midlife, and then peaks in the elderly. Generally to be classified as epilepsy, seizures must be repetitive, but even a single seizure coupled with a significant abnormality on neuroimaging or a diagnostic electroencephalogram (EEG) can signify epilepsy. During childhood the incidence of partial seizures is 20 per 100,000; generalized tonic-clonic seizures, 15 per 100,000; and absence seizures, 11 per 100,000.

Of the 10% of children who experience one seizure, only about 30% seek a medical evaluation. In contradistinction, more than 80% of children with a second seizure obtain medical assistance. Persons at the lowest risk for seizure recurrence are those with recognizable, treatable seizure etiologies; negative family histories; normal physical examination findings; lack of head trauma; normal EEG findings; and normal neuroimaging results. Each year about 3% of 6-month-old to 6-year-old children suffer from a febrile seizure, the most common seizure entity. The likelihood of these children developing epilepsy is extremely low.

Chang BS, Lowenstein DH: Epilepsy. N Engl J Med 2003;349:1257. [PMID: 14507951]

Shneker BF, Fountain NB: Epilepsy. Dis Mon 2003;49:426. [PMID: 12838266]

Pathogenesis

A seizure results from an abnormal, transient outburst of involuntary neuronal activity. Anoxic degeneration, focal neuron loss, hippocampal sclerosis (the major pathologic finding in temporal lobe epilepsy), and neoplasia are examples of pathologic central nervous system (CNS) changes that can produce seizures. Why a seizure spontaneously erupts is unclear, but the fact that most antiepileptic drugs (AEDs) alter ion flow suggests that abnormal ion flow in damaged neurons is the initiating event.

Seizures are either generalized (a simultaneous discharge from the entire cortex) or partial (focal, a discharge from a focal point within the brain). Generalized seizures impair consciousness and, with the exception of some petite mal (absence) spells, cause abnormal movement, usually intense muscle contractions termed *convulsions.* Because generalized convulsions occur most commonly in the absence of a focal defect, the initiating mechanism of a generalized seizure is less well understood than that of a partial seizure secondary to a focal CNS lesion. Partial seizures may either impair consciousness (complex) or not (simple) and can start with almost any neurologic complaint or aura, including abnormal smells, visions, movements, feelings, or behaviors. Partial seizures can progress to and thus mimic generalized seizures, a fact that sometimes obscures the true nature of the problem because of the commotion of the convulsion.

During childhood the majority of seizures are reactive (ie, due to an inciting event such as head trauma, CNS

Table 9–1. Classification of seizures.

I. Generalized
  A. Convulsive: tonic, clonic, tonic-clonic
  B. Nonconvulsive: absence (petit mal), atypical absence, myoclonic, atonic
II. Partial (focal or localization related)
  A. Simple (consciousness preserved): motor, somatosensory, special sensory, autonomic, psychic
  B. Complex (consciousness impaired): at onset, progressing to loss of consciousness
  C. Evolving to secondary generalized
III. Unclassified
  A. Syndrome: West syndrome (infantile spasms), Lennox–Gastaut syndrome, neonatal seizures, others
  B. Other

infection, drug ingestion, or metabolic abnormalities such as hypoglycemia or hyponatremia), but the cause of many reactive seizures remains unknown. Nonspecific etiologies such as stress or sleep deprivation are often blamed for lowering the seizure threshold. A genetic predisposition to seize is probably distributed throughout the population.

Unprovoked seizures are more likely to be epilepsy. The majority of epileptic seizures have no known cause and so are termed *cryptogenic.* Those with identifiable causes are called *symptomatic.* If genetic inheritance is at fault, the epilepsy is *idiopathic.* Hence, possible etiologies for a partial seizure include inheritance (idiopathic), head injury (symptomatic), or unknown cause (cryptogenic). Genetic predisposition to epilepsy has been clearly defined for many entities, including juvenile myoclonic epilepsy and tuberous sclerosis, each of which is linked to a specific chromosomal defect.

Table 9–1 presents a scheme of seizure description to guide treatment and predict outcome. Some forms of epilepsy are specially categorized as epilepsy syndromes (eg, infantile spasms [West syndrome] or benign childhood epilepsy with centrotemporal spikes [rolandic epilepsy]). Table 9–2 lists a general classification of epilepsy syndromes.

National Institute for Clinical Excellence (UK): The epilepsies: The diagnosis and management of the epilepsies in adults and children in primary and secondary care. NICE Clinical Guideline 20, October 2004. Available at: http://www.nice.org.uk/page.aspx?o=229249.

Prevention

Primary prevention includes advice to pregnant mothers to avoid addictive drug use (alcohol, cocaine, benzodiazepines), trauma (automobile safety), and infection (young kittens with risk for toxoplasmosis). Modern obstetric techniques minimize birth trauma and cerebral anoxia, which can result in cerebral palsy, an unfortunately persistent disorder despite efforts to reduce its incidence. Family history may reveal significant inborn errors of metabolism (Gaucher disease) or chromosomal abnormalities, some of which are amenable to treatment. Strict attention to childhood immunization to prevent sepsis and meningitis, especially from pneumococcus and *Haemophilus influenzae* type b, and to safety during childhood activities (using car seats and wearing bicycle helmets, supervision when swimming or in the bathtub) and for adolescents (wearing seatbelts), and avoidance of addictive drugs (cocaine, phencyclidine) are examples of appropriate, primary seizure prevention strategies. Annual influenza vaccination decreases the potential for febrile illness and secondary seizures. A full night's sleep, regular exercise, and a well-rounded diet are extremely important in the primary prevention of seizures.

Secondary prevention requires attention to the triggers of seizures, such as drugs that lower seizure threshold or cause seizures *de novo* (Table 9–3). Some children seize after prolonged fasting, possibly from hypoglycemia: for example, the unfed infant who seizes on Sunday morning when the parents oversleep after a late Saturday night out, the so-called "Saturday night seizure." Stimulation from light or noise, startle responses, faints, fever, metabolic derangements, or certain video games, television shows, or computer programs can cause repetitive seizures. Avoidance of any known prior precipitant of seizure is required to reduce future likelihood of another event. Known individuals with epilepsy should not drive until seizure free for 6 months, swim or take baths alone, or engage in any potentially dangerous activity. Patient education and referral to outside sources such as the Epilepsy Foundation play important roles in keeping patients healthy and active.

Diagnosis and management of epilepsy in adults. A national clinical guideline. (2) Diagnosis and management of epilepsy in adults. Update to printed guideline. Scottish Intercollegiate Guidelines Network–National Government Agency [Non-US]. April 2003 (addendum released June 7, 2004). NGC: 003832.

Evidence based clinical guideline for medical management of first unprovoked seizure in children 2 to 18 years of age revised; July 2002. Available at: http://www.guideline.gov/summary/summary.aspx?doc_id.

Clinical Findings

A. Symptoms and Signs

The primary tool for seizure assessment is the history, including (1) age at onset; (2) family history; (3) developmental status; (4) behavior profile; (5) health at seizure onset, including fever, vomiting, diarrhea, or illness exposure; (6) precipitating events, including exposure to toxin or trauma; (7) sleep pattern; and (8) dietary pattern. Any symptom can constitute an aura. Whether an aura occurred prior to the seizure is a critical feature that commonly points to a partial seizure, although an aura can also accompany a generalized seizure. The patient who reports

Table 9–2. Classification of epilepsies and epileptic syndromes.

I. Localization-related (focal, local, partial) epilepsies and syndromes
  A. Idiopathic (genetic) with age-related onset
    1. Benign childhood epilepsy with centrotemporal spikes (rolandic)
    2. Childhood epilepsy with occipital paroxysms
    3. Primary reading epilepsy
  B. Symptomatic (remote or preexisting cause)
  C. Cryptogenic (unknown etiology)
II. Generalized epilepsies and syndromes
  A. Idiopathic with age-related onset in order of age at onset
    1. Benign neonatal familial convulsions
    2. Benign neonatal convulsions
    3. Benign myoclonic epilepsy in infancy
    4. Childhood absence epilepsy (pyknolepsy)
    5. Juvenile myoclonic epilepsy (impulsive petit mal)
    6. Epilepsy with grand mal seizures on awakening
    7. Other
  B. Cryptogenic and/or symptomatic epilepsies in order of age at onset
    1. Infantile spasms (West syndrome)
    2. Lennox–Gastaut syndrome
    3. Epilepsy with myoclonic-astatic seizures
    4. Epilepsy with myoclonic absences
  C. Symptomatic
    1. Nonspecific etiology
      a. Early myoclonic encephalopathy
    2. Specific syndromes
      a. Diseases presenting with or predominantly evidenced by seizures
III. Epilepsies and syndromes undetermined as to whether they are focal or generalized
  A. With both types
    1. Neonatal seizures
    2. Severe myoclonic epilepsy in infancy
    3. Epilepsy with continuous spike waves during slow wave sleep
    4. Acquired epileptic aphasia (Landau-Kleffner syndrome)
  B. Without unequivocal generalized or focal features
    1. Sleep-induced grand mal
IV. Special syndromes
  A. Situation-related seizures
    1. Febrile convulsions
    2. Related to other identifiable situations: stress, hormonal changes, drugs, alcohol, sleep deprivation
  B. Isolated, apparently unprovoked epileptic events
  C. Epilepsies characterized by specific modes of seizure precipitation
  D. Chronic progressive epilepsia partialis continua of childhood

Sources: Leppik IE: *Contemporary Diagnosis and Management of the Patient with Epilepsy,* 5th ed, Handbooks in Health Care, 2000; Commission on Classification and Terminology of the International League Against Epilepsy: Proposal for the classification of epilepsy and epilepsy syndromes. Epilepsia 1989;30:389; and Guberman AH, Bruni J: *Essentials of Clinical Epilepsy,* 2nd ed. Butterworth Heinemann, 1999.

an aura usually requires more extensive evaluation in a search for a focal CNS lesion. Because 20% of childhood seizures occur only at night, a description of early morning behavior, including transient neurologic dysfunction or disorientation, is especially important. Specific areas for investigation are summarized in Table 9–4. Reports of preictal, ictal, and postictal events from both the patient and witnesses help to clarify the seizure type and therapy.

Children and adolescents with seizures tend to have fewer correctable associated conditions. Impact seizures are common after head trauma, but the 5-year risk for epilepsy is only 2%. On the other hand, 15–30% of children with depressed skull fractures develop epilepsy. Syncopal episodes with diminished CNS perfusion often result in minor twitching or even major tonic-clonic seizures but do not portend epilepsy.

Table 9–3. Drugs linked to seizures.

A. Over-the-counter
  1. Antihistamines: cold remedies
  2. Ephedrine: common in diet supplements
  3. Insect repellents and insecticides: benzene hexachloride
  4. "Health" and "diet" drugs
B. Prescription
  1. Antibiotics: penicillins, imipenem, fluoroquinolones; acyclovir; metronidazole; mefloquine; isoniazid
  2. Asthma treatments: aminophylline, theophylline, high-dose steroids
  3. Chemotherapeutic agents: methotrexate, tacrolimus
  4. Mental illness agents: tricyclics, selective serotonin reuptake inhibitors, methylphenidate, lithium, antipsychotics, bupropion
  5. Anesthetics and pain relievers: meperidine, propoxyphene, tramadol; local (lidocaine) or general anesthesia
  6. Antidiabetic medications: insulin and oral agents
  7. Miscellaneous: some β-blockers, immunizations, radiocontrast
C. Drugs of abuse
  1. Alcohol
  2. Cocaine
  3. Phencyclidine
  4. Amphetamine
  5. LSD
  6. Marijuana overdose
D. Drug withdrawal
  1. Benzodiazepines: diazepam, alprazolam, chlordiazepoxide
  2. Barbiturates
  3. Meprobamate
  4. Pentazocine may precipitate withdrawal from other agents
  5. Alcohol
  6. Narcotics
  7. Antiepileptic drugs: rapid drop in levels

Sources: Leppik IE: *Contemporary Diagnosis and Management of the Patient with Epilepsy,* 5th ed. Handbooks in Health Care, 2000; Menkes JH, Sankar R: Paroxysmal disorders. In Menkes JH, Sarnat HB, eds: *Child Neurology,* 6th ed. Lippincott Williams & Wilkins, 2000; and Guberman AH, Bruni J: *Essentials of Clinical Epilepsy,* 2nd ed. Butterworth Heinemann, 1999.

The most common conditions associated with repetitive seizures are mental retardation and cerebral palsy. Other cognitive deficiencies linked to epilepsy include attention deficit, memory difficulties, and learning disorders. Associated psychological difficulties are common and often make recognition or control of seizure disorders difficult. Affective problems such as depression or personality disorders are occasionally present in all age groups. In adolescents, psychoses, anxiety disorders (including panic attacks), and eating disorders (anorexia nervosa) should be considered. In adults sleep apnea can cause recurrent seizures. Several causes of seizures are listed in Table 9–5; this myriad of etiologies requires diligence to elucidate.

Table 9–4. Historical evaluation of possible seizure.[1]

I. Behavior: mood or behavior changes before and after the seizure
II. Preictal symptoms or aura
  A. Vocal: cry or gasp, slurred or garbled speech
  B. Motor: head or eye turning, chewing, posturing, jerking, stiffening, automatisms (eg, purposeless picking at clothes or lip smacking), jacksonian march, hemiballism
  C. Respiration: change in or cessation of breathing, cyanosis
  D. Autonomic: drooling, dilated pupils, pallor, nausea, vomiting, urinary or fecal incontinence, laughter, sweating, swallowing, apnea, piloerection
  E. Sensory changes
  F. Consciousness alteration: stare, unresponsiveness, dystonic positioning
  G. Psychic phenomena: delusion, déjà vu, daydreams, fear, anger
III. Postictal symptoms
  A. Amnesia
  B. Paralysis: up to 24 h, may be focal
  C. Confusion, lethargy, or sleepiness
  D. Nausea or vomiting
  E. Headache
  F. Muscle ache
  G. Trauma: tongue, head, bruising, fracture, laceration
  H. Transient aphasia

[1]For further information, see Hirtz D et al: Practice parameters: Evaluating a first nonfebrile seizure in children. Neurology 2000;55:616.

The etiology of epilepsy in childhood is 68% idiopathic, 20% congenital, 5% traumatic, and 4% postinfectious, but only 1% each vascular, neoplastic, and degenerative. The latter three are much more common in adulthood: 16% vascular, 11% neoplastic, and 3% degenerative. Complex partial seizures, the most difficult type to control, afflict 21% of children; generalized tonic-clonic seizures, the easiest to control, 19%; absence seizures, which almost universally cease prior to adulthood, 12%; simple partial seizures 11%; other generalized seizures 11%; simultaneous multiple types, often syndrome associated, 7%; myoclonic seizures, which are often difficult to recognize because of limited motor activity, 14%; and other types 5%. In adults, 39% of epilepsy cases are complex partial seizures, 25% generalized, 21% simple partial, and 15% other types.

Table 9–5. Some causes of seizures.

Cause	Examples
Reflex	
Visual	Photic stimulation, colors, television, video games
Auditory	Music, loud noise, specific voice or sound
Olfactory	Smells
Somatosensory	Tap, touch, immersion in water, tooth brushing
Cognitive	Math, card games, drawing, reading
Motor	Movement, swallowing, exercise, eye convergence, eyelid fluttering
Other	Startle, eating, sudden position change, sleep deprivation
Genetic	Neurofibromatosis, Klinefelter syndrome, Sturge-Weber syndrome, tuberous sclerosis
Structural	Hippocampal sclerosis, neoplasia
Congenital	Hamartoma, porencephalic cyst
Cerebrovascular	Arteriovenous malformation, stroke
Infectious	Syphilis, tuberculosis, toxoplasmosis, HIV infection, meningitis, encephalitis
Metabolic	Porphyria, phenylketonuria, electrolyte disorder (eg, hypoglycemia, hypocalcemia, hypomagnesemia), hyperosmolality, hyperventilation, drugs
Trauma	Depressed skull fracture, concussion
Other	Collagen vascular disease (systemic lupus erythematosus), eclampsia, demyelinating disease (multiple sclerosis), blood dyscrasias (sickle cell disease, idiopathic thrombocytopenia), mental disease (autism)

1. Generalized Seizures—Major motor seizures with tonic-clonic movement (grand mal) are both the most common and the most readily recognized. A short cry just before the seizure, apnea, and cyanosis are usual. The majority of these seizures are reactive and nonrecurrent. Convulsions usually last less than 3 minutes but can last up to 15 minutes without major sequelae. Other generalized seizures may be more difficult to identify. Typical absence spells (petit mal) are 10–30-second losses of consciousness without collapse characterized by a blank, unresponsive stare with occasional chewing or lip smacking. Normal activity is interrupted only briefly. Common from ages 3 to 20 years, these spells can be precipitated by photic stimulation or hyperventilation. Up to 50% of petit mal seizures evolve into tonic-clonic seizures later in life, especially if the onset of absence was during adolescence. About 10% of epileptic children have atypical absence spells with some motor activity of the extremities, duration greater than 30 seconds, and postictal confusion. Many of these children are mentally handicapped. Both types of absence spells can occur up to hundreds of times per day, creating havoc with school performance and recreational activities. Affecting 1–3 per 1000 persons, juvenile myoclonic epilepsy is genetically linked to chromosome 6. When myoclonic or tonic-clonic epilepsy begins between ages 8 and 18 years in otherwise normal children, prospects for permanent remission are poor: about 90% relapse when AED treatment is stopped.

2. Partial Seizures—Benign epilepsy with centrotemporal spikes (BECTS or rolandic epilepsy) accounts for 15% of all epilepsy and has an onset between ages 2 and 14 years. BECTS presents with guttural noises, paresthesias, and tonic or clonic face or arm contractions. An aura of numbness or tingling in the mouth often precedes motor arrest of speech and excessive salivation in a conscious child. Nocturnal BECTS may generalize into grand mal convulsions, often in the early morning. BECTS is not usually dangerous. About 20% of these children have only one episode whereas 25% develop repetitive seizures unless treated. By age 16 years almost all are seizure free.

The classic, albeit rare, simple partial seizure is the jacksonian march, an orderly progression of clonic motor activity, distal to proximal, indicating a focal motor cortex defect. The arm on the side to which the head turns may be extended while the opposite arm flexes, creating the classic fencer's posture. Many of these seizures generalize into clonic-tonic convulsions. In childhood, Todd's postictal paralysis can persist for up to 24 hours following a convulsion but usually does not suggest an underlying structural lesion.

Myoclonic jerks consist of single or repetitive contractions of a muscle or muscle group and account for 7% of seizures in the first 3 years of life. Benign occipital epilepsy has an onset between ages 1 and 14 years with a peak incidence between ages 4 and 8 years. These otherwise normal children develop migraine-like headaches with vomiting, loss of vision, visual hallucinations, or illusions. These episodes usually stop during adolescence.

In normal children complex partial seizures usually begin after age 10 years and usually last 1–2 minutes. Fifty percent to 75% are accompanied by automatisms and postictal confusion. Consciousness may be lost at onset or gradually over time. Behavior alteration, including hissing, random walking or wandering, sleepwalking, and irrelevant or incoherent speech; affective change such as fearfulness, anger, daydreaming, aggression, and searching behavior; nausea, vomiting, abdominal pain, pallor, flushing, enuresis, falling, illusions, and drooling demonstrate the variety of manifestations. Especially common are changes in body or limb position, confusion during activities, and a dazed expression. The child always exhibits amnesia for these events upon recovery. Repetitive episodes warrant evaluation.

Syndromes such as Lennox–Gastaut usually present with several different types of seizures closely linked in time. Myoclonic jerks, grand mal seizures, and absence spells in the same, usually mentally deficient individual should suggest this syndrome.

B. Physical Findings

Because 3% of children have simple febrile convulsions, fever is by far the most important physical finding. A stiff neck coupled with a fever mandates a lumbar puncture. Focal infection such as pneumonia can also cause febrile seizures. Many febrile seizures are linked to herpesvirus 6, the cause of roseola.

Preexisting focal deficits, mental deficiency, abnormal neurologic findings, and postictal focal deficits point to the need for imaging studies. Common neurologic findings include cerebral palsy or stroke, which is often complicated by seizures. Failure to return to baseline alertness should trigger more intensive evaluation.

Trauma such as a fractured tooth provides definitive evidence of seizure activity. Trauma is generally absent if syncope rather than a seizure is at fault. Significant complications of seizures include oral lacerations, fractures, dislocations, bruises, cuts, burns, concussion, arrhythmias, pulmonary edema, myocardial infarction, drowning, and death. Fluid leak from the nose suggests cribriform plate fracture. Many of these problems arise from well-intentioned but misdirected bystanders whose attempts to stop the seizure or stop the tongue from "being swallowed" lead to trauma. Lacerations or fractures can also suggest child abuse. Shaken baby syndrome with CNS hemorrhage can present with a seizure.

Café-au-lait spots, adenoma sebaceum and hypopigmented spots (tuberous sclerosis), port-wine stain (Sturge–Weber), or cutaneous telangiectasia (Louis–Bar) on the skin or cherry red spots in the eyes suggest various underlying etiologies. The lungs can reveal signs of aspiration pneumonia, or the heart cardiac rhythm disturbances or murmurs. The possibility of cancer metastasis or primary tumor is a particularly important consideration in patients who smoke and in those with unexplained weight loss, HIV infection, or lymphadenopathy.

Sudden unexpected death in epilepsy occurs in 1–2 persons per 1000 per year. Tonic-clonic seizures, treatment with three or more AEDs, and an intelligence quotient (IQ) of less than 70 are risk factors for sudden death, whereas choice of AED and serum levels are not. Sudden death, which is uncommon in childhood, peaks at age 50–59 years.

Walczak TS et al: Incidence and risk factors in sudden unexpected death in epilepsy. Neurology 2001;56:519. [PMID: 11222798]

C. Laboratory Findings

The decision to perform laboratory or radiographic evaluations is based on (1) the patient's age (younger than 6 months requires action); (2) history of preceding illness, especially gastroenteritis and dehydration; (3) history of substance abuse or drug exposure; (4) type of seizure (eg, complex partial seizures generally require evaluation); (5) failure to return to a normal state following a seizure; and (6) abnormal neurologic examination upon recovery from the seizure. Table 9–6 lists the usual battery of examinations, which can be augmented with cardiac, pulmonary, or liver testing or arterial blood gases. The majority of evidence fails to support routine testing, especially for first-time, tonic-clonic seizures.

An EEG is diagnostic in only 30–50% of first-time seizure victims, but its accuracy improves to 90% with repetitive testing. A focally abnormal EEG suggests the need for neuroimaging. Among patients suspected clinically of having epilepsy, the EEG has a 95% positive predictive value. Unfortunately, up to a third of seizure victims with normal EEGs eventually are proven to have epilepsy. Many experts advise that an EEG is indicated for evaluation of all patients with first nonfebrile seizures or repetitive febrile seizures, about 5% of whom develop epilepsy. Awake, asleep, hyperventilation, and photic-stimulated EEG tracings give the best chance of uncovering an abnormality. Risk of seizure reoccurrence is about 50% with an abnormal EEG and 25% with a normal nonepileptic EEG. Because tracings within 48 hours of a seizure may be falsely abnormal, the optimal timing for an EEG is unclear. EEG patterns are particularly diagnostic in absence spells, BECTS, and juvenile myoclonic epilepsy. When doubt exists as to the veracity of a seizure diagnosis, video-EEG recording can be diagnostic, especially in detecting psychogenic seizures. Twenty-four-hour EEG monitoring often reveals a seizure frequency much greater than otherwise suspected.

However, obtaining an EEG after the first seizure may not be worthwhile, especially as treatment with an AED often causes new dilemmas. It fails to accurately predict who will have a seizure recurrence, and about 2% of normal children have abnormal EEGs. Similar criticism can be leveled at neuroimaging. In children and adolescents in the absence of other abnormalities, an underlying brain tumor is extremely rare, but seizures are not. In an international review of 3291 children with brain tumors, only 35 otherwise normal children (1%) had a seizure as the initial difficulty. The key is to perform a complete neurologic examination and provide follow-up.

The clinical presentation should serve as a guide regarding who needs an EEG or neuroimaging. Parental acquiescence with delayed evaluation until a second seizure occurs is advisable.

Table 9–6. Recommendations for evaluation of a first seizure.

Study	Recommendation	Strength of Recommendation[1]
Electroencephalogram	All patients[2]	A[3–5]
Blood tests (electrolytes, glucose, blood urea nitrogen [BUN], creatinine, calcium, magnesium)	Individual basis: especially indicated for age 6 mo or younger; continued illness; history of vomiting, diarrhea, or dehydration	A[6]
Toxicology screening	If any possibility of drug or substance of abuse exposure	C[6]
Lumbar puncture	If possibility of meningitis or central nervous system (CNS) infection; continued CNS dysfunction	B[7]
CNS imaging		
Computed tomography (CT)	Value limited largely to head trauma	A[6,8]
Magnetic resonance imaging (MRI)	Best performed for	A[6]
	Prolonged postictal paralysis or failure to return to baseline	
	Persistent significant cognitive, motor, or other unexplained neurologic abnormality	
	Age younger than 12 mo	
	Perhaps with partial seizures	
	An EEG indicative of nonbenign seizure disorder	
Prolactin level	Variable benefit; 15–30 min after a seizure	B[6]
Creatine kinase level	Variable benefit	C[6]

[1]A, supported by clinical studies and expert opinion; B, expert opinion; limited evidence for support; C, limited to specific situations; insufficient evidence for or against this evaluation.
[2]Somewhat in debate.
[3]Martinovic Z, Jovic N: Seizure recurrence after a first generalized tonic-clonic seizure, in children, adolescents and young adults. Seizures 1997;6:461.
[4]Shinnar S et al: The risk of seizure recurrence following a first unprovoked afebrile seizure in childhood: an extended follow-up. Pediatrics 1996;98:216.
[5]Stroink H et al: The first unprovoked, untreated seizure in childhood: a hospital based study of the accuracy of diagnosis, rate of recurrence, and long term outcome after recurrence. Dutch study of epilepsy in childhood. J Neurol Neurosurg Psychiatry 1998;64:595.
[6]Hirtz D et al: Practice parameters: Evaluating a first nonfebrile seizure in children. Neurology 2000;55:616.
[7]Rider LG et al: Cerebrospinal fluid analysis in children with seizures. Pediatr Emerg Care 1995;11:226.
[8]Garvey MA et al: Emergency brain computed tomography in children with seizures: Who is most likely to benefit. J Pediatr 1998;133:664.

Magnetic resonance imaging (MRI) is preferred over a computed tomography (CT) scan. Although abnormalities are detected in up to one third of MRIs, only 1–2% of these findings influence either treatment or prognosis, especially in otherwise normal children. Table 9–7 lists recommended evaluations for neuroimaging for each seizure type. Neuroimaging is primarily useful for those who have focally abnormal neurologic examinations or a history suggesting deteriorating behavior or school function, infection, or trauma; the extremely young infant; those with persistent focal seizures except for BECTS; focal EEG abnormalities; or persons older than 18 years of age. Patients presenting with status epilepticus, 27% of whom have abnormal MRI findings, deserve study. Prior to CNS surgery, MRI or cerebral angiography and positron emission tomography (PET) scans are needed to assess the extent of the surgical procedure.

Routine blood tests are more often abnormal in patients with isolated seizures than in those with epilepsy, with the caveat that those taking carbamazepine or many other medications (eg, diuretics) can develop hyponatremia. Glucose, magnesium, calcium, blood urea nitrogen (BUN), creatinine, and electrolyte levels, and complete blood counts (CBC) usually are normal. A high creatine phosphokinase or prolactin level may indicate prior seizure activity. A toxicology screen is useful if drug exposure or ingestion is elicited. Other helpful evaluations include pregnancy tests in young women and psychometric studies to detect focal mental defects or psychiatric disease. Lumbar puncture is required only if meningitis is suspected, an unusual problem in a fully immunized

Table 9–7. Imaging recommendations for childhood seizures.

Seizure Type	Imaging Study
Neonatal	Cranial ultrasound preferred CT acceptable
Partial	MRI preferred CT acceptable
Generalized	
Neurologically normal	MRI or CT but low yield
Neurologically abnormal	MRI preferred CT acceptable
Intractable or refractory	MRI preferred SPECT acceptable PET acceptable
Febrile	"No study" recommended
Post-traumatic (seizures within 1 week of trauma)	CT preferred MRI acceptable

person. Meningococcal meningitis still remains a hazard and is most likely to affect young infants, first-year college students residing in a dormitory room, or travelers returning from the Middle East.

Kim LG et al: Prediction of risk of seizure recurrence after a single seizure and early epilepsy: Further results from the MESS trial. Lancet Neurol 2006;5:317. [PMID: 16545748]

Practice parameter: Evaluating a first nonfebrile seizure in children. Report of the Quality Standards Subcommittee of the American Academy of Neurology, the Child Neurology Society, and the American Epilepsy Society. American Academy of Neurology–Medical Specialty Society; American Epilepsy Society–Disease Specific Society; Child Neurology Society–Medical Specialty Society. September 2000 (reviewed 2003). NGC: 002055.

Differential Diagnosis

Gastroesophageal reflux, brief shuddering, benign nonepileptic myoclonus, or the Moro reflex in infants can mimic seizures. Breath-holding spells, night terrors, and benign paroxysmal vertigo in toddlers can raise concern about epilepsy. Tics and behavior problems can precede true seizures or act as seizure mimics. Children and adolescents who suffer from psychogenic seizures (pseudoseizures) must be carefully evaluated for underlying psychiatric disturbances, especially depression or suicidal ideation. Psychogenic seizures, which account for 20% of referrals to epilepsy centers, often coexist with true seizures. Hysteria, panic attacks, transient global amnesia, and hyperventilation can mimic a seizure disorder. Malingering to avoid stressful situations such as school or true conversion reactions are uncommon during childhood but can occur in adolescents or adults. Malingering patients may use soap to simulate frothing at the mouth, bite their tongues, or urinate or defecate voluntarily to simulate seizures.

The differential diagnosis includes drugs of abuse, narcolepsy, migraine, cough-induced or vasovagal syncopal convulsions, shuddering attacks, hereditary tremors, and Tourette syndrome. Syncopal seizures are best treated with efforts to control syncope, not seizures. Cardiac entities such as prolonged QT interval (electrocardiogram), aortic stenosis (echocardiogram), or hypertrophic cardiomyopathy (echocardiogram) should be considered in those with a family history of fainting or appropriate physical findings. In difficult situations, neurologic consultation, video-EEG recording, 24-hour EEG recording, and watchful waiting almost always provide the correct diagnosis eventually.

Austin JK et al: Behavior problems in children before first recognized seizures. Pediatrics 2001;107:115. [PMID: 11134444]

Gudmundsson O et al: Outcome of pseudo-seizures in children and adolescents: A 6-year symptom survival analysis. Dev Med Child Neurol 2001;43:547. [PMID: 11508920]

Treatment

A. First Aid and Initial Care

Acute assistance for a seizure requires placing the patient prone, removing eyeglasses, loosening clothing and jewelry, clearing the area of harmful objects, and *not* putting any object into the patient's mouth or attempting to apply any restraint. After the seizure, the patient should be placed on one side and observed until awake. Families should call for medical assistance if a seizure lasts longer than 3 minutes, the patient requests assistance or is injured, or a second seizure occurs. After a tonic-clonic seizure, vigorous stimulation may reduce postictal apnea and perhaps sudden death. To reduce the risk of sudden death, patients with epilepsy should be encouraged to sleep in the *supine* position. Hospitalization is necessary only if the patient is at high risk, lives alone without appropriate supervision, or remains ill. Postictal confusion, sleepiness, headache, muscle soreness, and lethargy are common. Following a seizure, a patient appreciates an explanation of what transpired and information as to how to avoid further difficulties. Follow-up arrangements need to be definite. Avoidance of seizure-provoking activities, provocative drugs, or other seizure-inducing behaviors is adequate treatment for reactive seizures.

B. Pharmacotherapy

Correctable provoked seizures or unprovoked seizures that are not likely to be dangerous or frequent do not require AEDs. Most experts do not treat after a single seizure. Side effects of medication include worsening seizure severity or frequency, organ damage, or even death. AEDs do not positively affect long-term prognosis nor do they always provide seizure control. In fact, 20–30% of those on AEDs still have significant seizure activity.

Nonetheless, all primary care physicians should have a command of basic AED use and side effect profiles. Table 9–8 provides information on the most useful AEDs. Other drugs (adrenocorticotropic hormone [ACTH], nitrazepam, pyridoxine [vitamin B_6], and vigabatrin [which may damage the eyes] for infantile spasms; acetazolamide for absence spells; felbamate [highly toxic and rarely used] for Lennox–Gastaut syndrome; oxcarbazepine for partial seizures; tiagabine for complex partial epilepsy; and zonisamide for myoclonus) usually require specialist help. Lamotrigine is approved for those older than 2 years of age for treatment of generalized tonic-clonic epilepsy and partial epilepsy. Lamotrigine is started at 0.15 mg/kg/day, divided into two doses and is increased by 0.15 mg/kg every 2 weeks to a maintenance dose of 1–5 mg/kg/day (maximum of 400 mg/day). It interacts with valproic acid. Levetiracetam is approved for partial epilepsy in those older than 4 years of age and for myoclonic epilepsy in those older than 12 years. Topiramate is approved for generalized tonic-clonic and partial seizures in those older than 10 years.

The selection of AED is based on the seizure type, which unfortunately is inaccurately identified at least 25% of the time. The least toxic AED, usually carbamazepine, valproic acid, or phenytoin, is initiated. Primary generalized seizures respond best to valproic acid, which controls seizures in 80% of patients when given as monotherapy. Divalproex produces fewer side effects, especially of the gastrointestinal tract. Lamotrigine, carbamazepine, and phenytoin are also good choices to control tonic-clonic convulsions. Ethosuximide is an ideal choice for absence spells, for which lamotrigine is also effective. Juvenile myoclonic epilepsy responds well to valproic acid but is unlikely to respond to other agents so is sometimes difficult to control. Partial seizures are best treated with carbamazepine or phenytoin. Lamotrigine, gabapentin, or pregabalin can be added when control is inadequate. Side effects of some AEDs are listed in Table 9–9. These are sometimes serious and often unfamiliar to primary care physicians. Any new symptom or sign in a patient on an AED must trigger a search in a standard reference for AED side effects. Many of the newer agents are also expensive. Although costly, oxcarbazepine at 8–10 mg/kg/day (maximal starting dose 300 mg divided twice a day) offers a significant reduction in side effects compared with carbamazepine.

Use of one drug to control seizures—increased to its maximum or to just below toxicity, as necessary—is best. If one drug proves ineffective, the current AED should be withdrawn slowly over at least 7 days to several weeks at the same time as another AED is started. Polytherapy is fraught with drug side effects and often loss of seizure control. However, in 25% of patients, seizures require two drugs to achieve satisfactory control. Because newer drugs generally cause unfamiliar side effects, neurologic consultation is often a superior choice to random new drug use.

Serum AED levels should be obtained (1) as a check on compliance; (2) to detect toxicity, especially for those taking multiple agents or who are too young or mentally handicapped to communicate their symptoms; (3) when the drug regimen is changed; (4) for poor seizure control; and (5) when a problem develops that can affect drug levels. Table 9–10 provides a scheme for monitoring the effects of the three most commonly utilized AEDs: valproic acid, phenytoin, and carbamazepine. Levels of AEDs, especially ethosuximide, phenytoin, and carbamazepine, help to guide dosage. Valproic acid levels often fail to predict toxicity or seizure control. Whether seizure-free patients require periodic drug level monitoring is unclear. Unlike adults, children are rapidly growing, so levels of steady-dose AEDs lessen over time. Some experts advise allowing a child to "grow out" of the AED as a slow taper off medication to see if a seizure recurs. If this path is chosen, patients and parents must be informed about the plan. Patients on phenobarbital may "outgrow" the dose, resulting in a slow taper off the drug. If seizures do not recur, phenobarbital should not be restarted; it is no longer considered an acceptable AED for general use because of adverse effects on personality.

Whether routine checks of hematologic or liver functions can prevent organ damage is also unclear. Certainly all patients and parents should be warned to be alert for fever, jaundice, itching, bruising, bleeding, and other signs of bone marrow or liver toxicity. Many physicians choose to follow CBCs, liver and renal tests, and serum AED levels periodically, once or twice a year. In special circumstances (pregnancy, uremia, hypoalbuminemia, or concurrent drug use with agents that displace AED off protein, ie, salicylate use), serum free-AED levels may be a better guide to dosing, especially for phenytoin and valproic acid.

Because all AEDs can cause fetal malformations, during pregnancy the drug that controls seizures the best, with the possible exception of valproic acid, should be continued. A fetal sonogram can identify malformations. Folic acid (up to 4 mg daily before and throughout pregnancy) and vitamins D and K (given during the last 4 weeks) minimize problems for the fetus. Phenytoin dose must often be increased during pregnancy and slowly decreased after delivery.

Some AEDs, especially carbamazepine, felbamate, oxcarbazepine, phenobarbital, phenytoin, primidone, and topiramate, may interfere with oral contraceptives. Midcycle bleeding indicates possible oral contraceptive failure. This problem can be avoided with alternative contraceptive methods, a higher estrogen content product, or prescription of a noninteracting AED such as gabapentin or lamotrigine. Women who take AEDs can safely breast-feed.

Because of its low cost and broad effectiveness, phenytoin is a favorite AED choice, but side effects of phenytoin prohibit its use for everyone. Dose-related problems

Table 9–8. Drugs for the treatment of seizures.

Drug	Seizure Type	Pediatric Dosage (mg/kg)		Maximal Dose	Number of Daily Doses	Therapeutic Level (mcg/mL)	Dosage Forms		Notes
		Starting Dose	Usual Daily Dose				Pill (mg)	Liquid	
Phenytoin	GM, CPS, SPS	5 orally, 10–20 intravenously	5–15	700 mg daily 1000 mg loading	1–3	10–20	C: 100 EC: 30, 100 CT: 50	S: 125 mg/5 mL (use not recommended)	Gen/Tr (some forms)
Carbamazepine	GM, CPS, SPS	5–10	15–30	2000	2–4	4–12	T: 200; CT: 100; ET: 100, 200, 300, 400	S: 100 mg/5 mL	Gen/Tr (some forms)
Valproic acid	GM, PM, CPS, SPS, M	10–15	15–60	3000	2–4	50–120	C: 250 CS: 125 ET: 500 DT: 125, 250, 500	SY: 250 mg/5 mL	Gen/Tr (some forms)
Ethosuximide	PM	10–20	10–40	2000	1–2	40–100	C: 250	SY: 250 mg/5 mL	Gen/Tr (some forms)
Clonazepam	M	0.01–0.03	0.025–0.2	20	2–3	18–80	T: 0.5, 1, 2	—	Gen/Tr
Gabapentin	Additive only; GM, CPS, SPS	10–15	25–50	4800	3	> 2	C: 100, 300, 400 T: 600, 800	Sol: 50 mg/5 mL	Tr
Primidone	GM, CPS, SPS	10	10–30	1500	2–4	5–15	T: 50, 250	S: 250 mg/5 mL	Gen/Tr (some forms)

GM, grand mal; PM, petit mal; CPS, complex partial seizures; SPS, simple partial seizure; M, myoclonic; C, capsule; EC, extended release capsule; T, tablet; CT, chewable tablet; S, suspension; ET, extended release tablet; SY, syrup; CS, capsule sprinkles; DT, delayed release tablet; Sol, solution; Gen, generic; Tr, trade.

Table 9–9. Side effects of selected antiepileptic drugs.

Drug[1]	Common Side Effects
Phenytoin	Hirsutism, coarse facial appearance, gum hyperplasia, nystagmus
Carbamazepine	Hyponatremia (up to 10% of patients)
Valproic acid	Hair loss, weight gain, edema, pancreatitis, thrombocytopenia
Lamotrigine	Life-threatening rash (~1 out of 50 children)
Phenobarbital	Personality change
Topiramate	Renal stones
Zonisamide	Renal stones
Ethosuximide	Abdominal pain, abnormal behavior

include nystagmus (an excellent marker for overdose), hypotension, ataxia, blurred vision, dysarthria, and drowsiness. With prolonged use, folate deficiency–related anemia, osteomalacia, neuropathy, coarseness of facial features, gingival hyperplasia (preventable with dental flossing and regular dental cleaning), acne, hirsutism, lymphadenopathy, and mental dullness can occur. Some of these problems are idiosyncratic. Rarely, bone marrow suppression, toxic rash, or hepatic failure develops. Drugs that increase phenytoin levels include warfarin, isoniazid, disulfiram, alcohol acutely ingested, benzodiazepines, and other anticonvulsants. Decreased levels occur with chronic alcohol use, amiodarone, rifampin, folic acid, or certain chemotherapies. Phenytoin can change serum levels of warfarin, lithium, acetaminophen, oral contraceptives, thyroid hormone, quinidine, and insulin. Whenever any agent is added to or withdrawn from the drug regimen of a patient who takes phenytoin, a serum level should be obtained, usually 5–7 days later. Because phenytoin dosing does not follow first-order kinetics, a wise rule is to increase the amount less than appears necessary and decrease the amount more than appears necessary. A patient with a toxic serum level should stop the drug for several days until the serum level is satisfactory and then restart it at a reduced dose.

For home treatment of acute repetitive seizures, rectal diazepam (0.2–0.5 mg/kg) or buccal or intranasal midazolam (0.25–1 mg/kg) both appear to be safe and effective. Rectal diazepam is available as a gel and midazolam as a liquid.

No specific seizure-free time interval predicts resolution of epilepsy. A single seizure type, normal neurologic examination, normal IQ, and normal EEG all predict good outcomes if the AED is stopped. Of 1013 patients free of seizures for 2 years, 40% had a recur-

Table 9–10. Recommended monitoring parameters for antiepileptic drugs.

Drug	Monitoring
Carbamazepine	Complete blood count (CBC) with platelets at baseline, then twice monthly for first 2 mo, and annually or as clinically indicated Blood chemistries with emphasis on hepatic and renal function and electrolytes at baseline, then at 1 mo, and annually or as clinically indicated Electrocardiogram (ECG) at baseline for patients > 40 y and as clinically indicated Carbamazepine level weekly for 2 wk, then at 1 mo and annually or as clinically indicated in older patients
Phenytoin	CBC at baseline and as clinically indicated Blood chemistries with emphasis on hepatic and renal functions at baseline, annually, and as clinically indicated ECG at baseline for patients > 40 y and as clinically indicated Phenytoin level in 1 wk, then in 1 mo, and annually or as clinically indicated in older patients
Valproic acid	CBC with platelets at baseline, then twice monthly for first 2 months, and annually or as clinically indicated Blood chemistries with emphasis on hepatic function at baseline, then at 1 mo, and annually or as clinically indicated Protime, international normalized ratio (INR), partial prothrombin time (PPT) at baseline and annually Valproic acid level weekly for 2 wk, then annually or as clinically indicated in older patients

Sources: Scottish Intercollegiate Guidelines Network (SIGN): Diagnosis and management of epilepsies in children and young people. Scottish Intercollegiate Guidelines Network (SIGN), Publication no. 81, March 2005, p 53. Available at: http://www.guideline.gov/summary/summary.aspx?doc_id; Texas Tech University Management Health Care Network Pharmacy and Therapeutics Committee: Acute seizures and seizure disorder. University of Texas Medical Branch Correctional Managed Care; April 2003. Available at: http://www.guideline.gov/summary/summary.aspx?doc_id; and Cincinnati Children's Hospital Medical Center: Evidence based clinical practice guideline for first unprovoked seizure for children 2 to 18 years of age. Cincinnati Children's Hospital Medical Center, July 2002. Available at: http://www.gov/summary.aspx?dox_id.

rence following drug withdrawal compared with 12% of those who maintained AED treatments. Freedom from drug side effects and daily medication must be weighed against this 28% difference with potential loss of job or driving ability or possible injury. A recent abnormal EEG would make a decision to stop therapy more difficult. Phenytoin, carbamazepine, and valproic acid should be slowly withdrawn over at least 6–10 weeks. Once children grow into young adulthood, assuming a 2- to 5-year period without seizures, an attempt to stop AED treatment ought to be strongly considered.

Britton JW: Antiepileptic drug withdrawal: Literature review. Mayo Clin Proc 2002;77:1378. [PMID: 12479528]

Marson A et al: Immediate versus deferred antiepileptic drug treatment for early epilepsy and single seizures: A randomised controlled trial. Lancet 2005;365:2007. [PMID: 15950714]

National Institute for Clinical Excellence: Newer drugs for epilepsy in adults, full guidance. Technology Appraisal Guidance 76, March 2004. Available at: http://www.nice.org.uk/TA076guidance.

Specchio LM et al: Discontinuing antiepileptic drugs in patients who are seizure free on monotherapy. J Neurol Neurosurg Psychiatry 2002;72:22. [PMID: 11784819]

C. Referral or Hospitalization

Poorly controlled or complicated seizures or developmental delay should prompt neurologic consultation. Hospitalization is necessary for prolonged or complicated seizures, status epilepticus, inadequate family resources, or parental or physician anxiety. In general, seizures are not dangerous, but persons with repetitive seizures must be guarded from injury and other complications.

D. Surgery and Other Treatments

At least twenty percent of patients with epilepsy are inadequately controlled with AEDs alone. Surgery for epilepsy, including severing of the corpus callosum or temporal lobe resection, results in 80% seizure-free outcomes for specific epilepsy types. Candidates for surgery should have recurrent uncontrolled seizures, focal EEGs, and consistent focal abnormalities on neuroimaging. PET or single photon emission computed tomography (SPECT) imaging often reveals unsuspected abnormalities.

Vagal nerve stimulation is less invasive and controls or reduces seizures in about 40% of patients with previously refractory epilepsy. The ketogenic diet reduces episodes by about 50%. These treatments all require referral and extensive evaluation prior to institution.

Andrade DM et al: Long-term follow-up of patients with thalamic deep brain stimulation for epilepsy. Neurology 2006;66:1468. [PMID: 16540602]

Tellez-Zenteno JF et al: Long-term seizure outcomes following epilepsy surgery: A systematic review and meta-analysis. Brain 2005;128:1188. [PMID: 15758038]

Uthman BM et al: Effectiveness of vagus nerve stimulation in epilepsy patients: A 12-year observation. Neurology 2004;63:1124. [PMID: 15452317]

E. Family Counseling

Family members, other caregivers, teachers, and co-workers need instruction in proper seizure first aid. Helpful information and group support are available from the American Epilepsy Society (http://www.aesnet.org) and the Epilepsy Foundation of America (http://www.efa.org) or local epilepsy foundations. Vocational help and assistance to defray medical costs are often needed. A close physician-patient relationship serves the interests of the patient and family. Adequate sleep and exercise, stress reduction, and avoidance of alcohol or sedative drugs benefit all.

A seizure per se does not lower IQ or cause brain damage, but dealing with epilepsy is difficult. Although the negative consequences of a seizure disorder to daily life should not be underestimated, most otherwise normal patients with epilepsy lead full, productive lives. About 25% of untreated epilepsy is debilitating. In general an individual can lead a normal existence despite seizure recurrence. Scheduled activities for each day may help. Some children respond better to home schooling until seizures are controlled. For those who develop psychological dysfunction, especially depression, psychiatric consultation or medication is usually helpful.

Centers for Disease Control and Prevention (CDC): Health-related quality of life among persons with epilepsy—Texas, 1998. MMWR Morb Mortal Wkly Rep 2001;50:24. [PMID: 11215719]

Shackleton DP et al: Living with epilepsy: Long-term prognosis and psychosocial outcomes. Neurology 2003;61:64. [PMID: 12847158]

F. Alternative Therapies

Few of the commonly utilized alternative therapies have evidence-based support. Some such as pyridoxine (vitamin B_6) and magnesium have scientific grounding for use in specific seizure disorders. Many web sites present unfounded claims for acupuncture, chiropractic, or naturopathic manipulation. Food allergies are occasionally blamed for seizures, without scientific proof. Most alternative therapy sources advise avoidance of alcohol, caffeine, and aspartame, the first two of which are at least logical. Proof that taurine, folic acid, vitamin B_{12}, manganese, zinc, dimethylglycine, megavitamins, or a diet high in fat, low in protein, and low in carbohydrates reduce seizure frequency or medication requirements is absent or marginal. Herbal remedies such as passionflower, skullcap, valerian, belladonna, causticum, cicuta, or cuprum metallicum, have not been adequately studied. On the other hand, any nontoxic technique to reduce stress and bring order to a patient's life may help. Some patients have learned to control seizures with self-relaxation or special techniques such as looking at a particular piece of jewelry as an aura comes on. Hence, those families who wish to augment medical treatment with noninvasive treatments may be permitted to do so after physician review for safety and if the treatments appear to help over time.

Additional information is available at web sites such as http://home.mdconsult.com or http://healthcare.micromedex.com. The veracity of advice on these sites is left to the user to investigate.

Febrile Convulsions

The most common seizure disorder, febrile convulsions affect 3% of children between ages 6 months and 6 years. After age 14 years febrile seizures are rare. Despite a recurrence rate of 30%, only 3% of these individuals develop epilepsy. Those with a family history of epilepsy, abnormal neurologic or developmental status prior to the seizure, or a prolonged (> 15 minute) focal seizure have at least a 15% chance of later epilepsy. Commonly, the young toddler with an upper respiratory infection, nonpolio enterovirus, or roseola suddenly seizes during an afternoon nap. Usually short tonic-clonic convulsions, such seizures are multiple in one third of cases. Postictal sleepiness can last several hours. Generally laboratory tests are unnecessary unless meningitis is suggested by failure to arouse, continued focal seizures, suggestive physical findings (stiff neck, bulging fontanel, rash), or age younger than 6 months. Seizures that occur in the office or emergency department can also be more indicative of serious infection.

Treatment consists of reassurance to worried parents that the worst has passed and that these seizures leave no permanent brain damage. Controlling fever with warm baths, acetaminophen (10–15 mg/kg every 4 hours), or ibuprofen (5–10 mg/kg every 6 hours) may reduce immediate risk of recurrence. If begun at the onset of fever, buccal or intranasal midazolam, 0.25–1 mg/kg, acutely; oral or rectal valproic acid, 20 mg/kg every 8 hours for 1–3 days; or diazepam, 0.5 mg/kg every 8 hours for 1–3 days; can reduce recurrence. Intravenous lorazepam is the drug of choice for prolonged febrile seizures. Hospitalization is best if seizures are prolonged beyond 30 minutes or are recurrent or complicated, if follow-up is inadequate, or if parents or the physician want observation. Chronic treatment is advised only for the child with multiple recurrences, persistent neurologic abnormality, or worrisome EEG findings.

Baumann RJ: Prevention and management of febrile seizures. Paediatr Drugs 2001;3:585. [PMID: 11577923]

Gordon KE et al: Treatment of febrile seizures: The influence of treatment efficacy and side-effect profile on value to parents. Pediatrics 2001;108:1080. [PMID: 11694684]

Status Epilepticus

Any recurrent or prolonged seizure uninterrupted by consciousness for more than 30 minutes is termed *status epilepticus* (SE). About 5% of children with febrile convulsions and 20% of all persons with epilepsy have SE at least once. Newly diagnosed epileptic patients often develop SE. These individuals run a low risk of permanent residual brain damage or other complications, which can be minimized through rapid treatment. Although all seizure types—including simple partial seizures—can present in SE, most commonly consciousness is severely impaired. A persistent grand mal seizure is usually readily identified as SE, but myoclonic SE with preserved consciousness is more difficult to recognize. Perhaps the most difficult is the patient in SE who has no abnormal motor movement but is comatose. Confused but moving persons may be in absence or complex partial epilepsy SE. Diagnosis is based on clinical presentation with typical EEG findings. Death is usually related to a serious underlying etiology for the SE rather than the SE itself.

Management requires stabilization of vital signs. Adolescents and adults should be given 100 mg of thiamine followed by 50 mL of 50% glucose (children: 2–4 mL/kg of 25% glucose) intravenously coupled with naloxone (0.1 mg/kg up to 2 mg) repeated as necessary. Lorazepam, 0.1 mg/kg (maximum of 4 mg) intravenous push at 2 mg/min, is successful in stopping 80% of SE episodes in 2–3 minutes. A second dose in 10 minutes is frequently successful in the remaining 20%. An alternative is diazepam, 0.5 mg/kg (maximum of 20 mg) intravenous push at 5 mg/min. Poorly controlled SE responds to phenytoin, 20 mg/kg intravenous push at 50 mg/min, while monitoring the electrocardiogram and blood pressure, or its more safe prodrug, fosphenytoin, given at 30 mg/kg intravenous push at 150 mg/min. Other alternatives are phenobarbital and propofol. Immediate serum AED levels define adequacy of therapy. Some SE in children younger than 18 months of age responds to pyridoxine, 50 mg intravenously. For information about other drugs for SE, the clinician is referred to the Cochrane Database. Once the SE is controlled, a

Table 9–11. Evaluation of neonatal seizures.

I. History
  A. Pregnancy related
    1. Infection: toxoplasmosis, rubella, cytomegalovirus, herpes, syphilis (TORCHS); immunoglobulin M level
    2. Maternal addiction: smoking, alcohol, cocaine, heroin, barbiturates
    3. Maternal behavior: inadequate prenatal care, lack of folic acid
  B. Delivery related
    1. Anoxia
    2. Trauma
  C. Family history: chromosomal disorders, errors of metabolism
II. Physical findings
  A. Recognizable patterns of malformation: eyes, ears, hands, facies, head shape
  B. Neurologic evaluation: motor, sensory, cranial nerves
  C. Odor: phenylketonuria
  D. Dermatologic signs: crusted vesicles, abnormal creases, hypopigmentation, nevi
  E. Ocular: chorioretinitis, cataracts, coloboma, cherry red spot
III. Laboratory evaluation
  A. Neuroimaging: cranial ultrasound, magnetic resonance imaging (MRI), computed tomography (CT) scan
  B. Chest radiograph
  C. Cerebral spinal fluid: culture, cell count, Gram stain, India ink, VDRL, glycine, glucose, protein, xanthochromia
  D. Blood test: cultures, complete blood count, electrolytes, renal function, glucose, magnesium, calcium, karyotype, glycine, lactate, ammonia, long-chain fatty acid levels
  E. Urine: culture, glucose, protein, cells

Sources: Hill A: Neonatal seizures. Pediatr Rev 2000;21:117 and Moshe SL: Seizure early in life. Neurology 2000;54:635.

Table 9–12. Clinical practice guidelines for management of patients with seizure disorders.

Clinical Scenario	Guideline
Febrile seizure	Children with febrile seizures, even if recurrent, should rarely be treated with antiepileptic drugs (AEDs).
Provoked seizure	Long-term prophylactic AED treatment for children with head injuries or correctable causes of seizure is not indicated.
Unprovoked, tonic-clonic epileptic seizure	AED treatment should generally not be commenced routinely after a first, unprovoked tonic-clonic seizure.
Generalized epilepsy	The choice of first AED should be determined, where possible, by the syndromic diagnosis and potential adverse effects.
Focal seizure	When appropriate monotherapy fails to reduce seizure frequency, combination therapy should be considered.
Monitoring for adverse effects of AEDs	Routine AED level monitoring is generally not required.
Withdrawal of AEDs	Withdrawal of AED treatment should be considered for individuals who have been seizure free for 2 or more years.
Prolonged or serial seizure	Prolonged or serial seizures can be treated with either intranasal or buccal midazolam or rectal diazepam.

search for the underlying cause should be conducted to minimize the risk of recurrence.

Prasad K et al: Anticonvulsant therapy for status epilepticus. Cochrane Database Syst Rev 2005;(4):CD003723. [PMID: 16235337]

Neonatal Seizures

In the first month of life, clonic-tonic seizure activity is uncommon. Hence, most neonatal seizures are difficult to recognize. Focal rhythmic twitches, recurrent vomiting, unusual high-pitched crying, posturing, chewing, apnea, cyanosis, and excessive salivation should raise alarm. Diligent inquiry into family history, prenatal history, and maternal habits is warranted. Definitive diagnosis rests on neurologic consultation, CNS ultrasound to detect hemorrhage, and EEG tracings. Often difficult to control, these seizures may have a dismal outcome. Treatment for maternal drug addiction with resultant neonatal drug withdrawal seizures, which often leave no residual defects, includes paregoric, methadone, chlorpromazine, and phenobarbital. Table 9–11 lists suggested evaluations.

Booth D, Evans DJ: Anticonvulsants for neonates with seizures. Cochrane Database Syst Rev 2004;(4):CD004218. [PMID: 15495087]

Prognosis

Clinical practice guidelines for management of patients with seizure disorders are presented in Table 9–12. Overall about one third of patients have a second seizure, and about 75% of these experience a third seizure. However, no adverse outcomes are likely even with up to 10 untreated seizures. A study of 220 children indicated that 92% of those treated for idiopathic seizures remained seizure free for as long as 5 years. The same was true for 62% of those with cryptogenic epilepsy: over 25% of patients off all medicine had no seizures for 5 years, but unfortunately many of those with severe CNS damage died. This information reaffirms the need to carefully consider AED treatment before institution and before discontinuation. Eventually 60% of epileptic children become seizure free.

National statement of good practice for the treatment and care of people who have epilepsy. Joint Epilepsy Council–Disease Specific Society. March 2002. NGC: 003525.

SECTION II
Adolescence

Physical Activity in Adolescents 10

Mark B. Stephens, MD, MS, FAAFP[1]

"Do it, move it, make it happen. No one ever sat their way to success."

—*Unknown*

The United States is in the midst of a growing epidemic of physical inactivity and obesity. During the past two decades, physical inactivity has played a major role in the staggering rise of obesity among children and adolescents. Longitudinal data from the National Health and Examination Surveys show that the percentage of overweight female adolescents has increased from 5% to 10% of the population and the percentage of overweight male adolescents, from 5% to 12% (Figure 10–1). Currently, one in four adolescents in the United States is either overweight or at risk for becoming overweight. Overweight youth are much less likely to engage in physical activity and are much more likely to report chronic health problems compared with peers of normal weight.

During adolescence, levels of spontaneous physical activity drop precipitously from childhood levels. One third of US high-school students are not regularly active; one half of high school seniors are not enrolled in physical education classes, and 70% of all high school students watch at least 1 hour of television every day of the week. For those students enrolled in physical education, the actual amount of class time devoted to physical activity has dropped significantly over the past decade. Students spend a majority of time in physical education class standing around, waiting for instructions, or socializing.

[1]The opinions herein are those of the author. They do not represent official policy of the Uniformed Services University, the Department of the Navy, or the Department of Defense.

Individuals who are overweight during adolescence are far more likely to be overweight as adults. Teens spend a majority of their days engaged in sedentary activities, averaging a mere 12 min/day of vigorous physical activity. Teens who are active in school sporting activities are more likely to be active as adults. The bottom line is that behaviors that are initiated in childhood tend to consolidate during adolescence. Therefore, health-related behaviors, such as dietary habits and physical activity patterns, solidify during adolescence and persist into adulthood. Recognition of individuals who are insufficiently active, overweight, or obese during adolescence is important.

Gordon-Larsen P et al: Longitudinal physical activity and sedentary behavior trends: Adolescence to adulthood. Am J Prev Med 2004;27:277. [PMID: 15488356]

Janz KF et al: Tracking physical fitness and physical activity from childhood to adolescence: The Muscatine Study. Med Sci Sport Exer 2000;32:1250. [PMID: 10912890]

Lowry R et al: Recent trends in participation in physical education among US high school students. J Sch Health 2001;71:145. [PMID: 11357870]

Malina RM: Physical activity and fitness: Pathways from childhood to adulthood. Am J Hum Biol 2001;13:162. [PMID: 11460860]

US Department of Health and Human Services, Centers for Disease Control and Prevention: Youth risk behavior surveillance—United States, 2005. MMWR Morb Mortal Wkly Rep 2006;55(SS-5):1.

DEFINITIONS

The following definitions apply to the discussion of physical activity and obesity (Table 10–1). *Physical fitness* refers to a general state of well-being that allows an

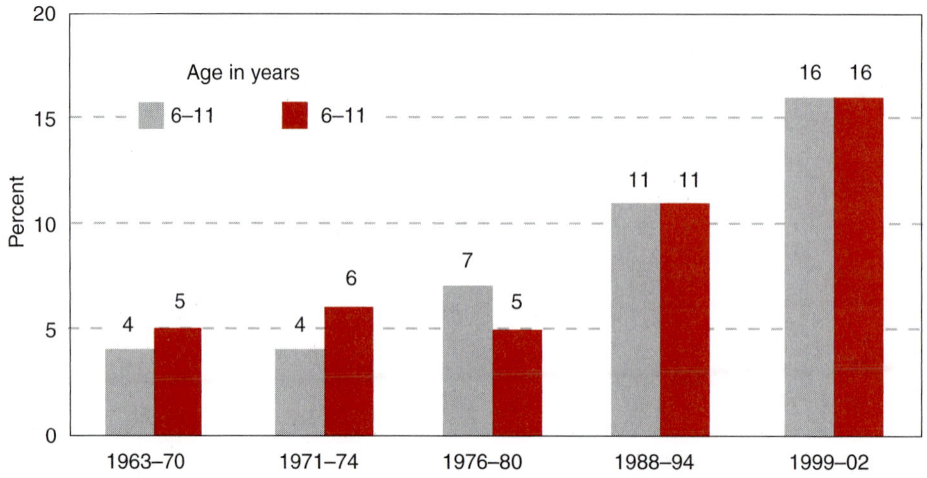

Figure 10–1. Prevalence of overweight among children and adolescents aged 6–19 years. (From Centers for Disease Control and Prevention, Atlanta, Georgia. Available at: http://www.cdc.gov/nchs/products/pubs/pubd/hestats/overfig1.gif.)

individual to perform activities of daily living in a vigorous manner. Physical fitness is further described in terms of health-related characteristics and skill-related characteristics. Health-related components of physical fitness include cardiorespiratory endurance, muscular strength, muscular endurance, flexibility, and body composition. Skill-related components of physical fitness include power, speed, agility, and balance. Historically, physical education programs have focused on skill-related activities and athletic ability. From a public health perspective, however, the health-related components of physical fitness are more important in terms of overall morbidity and mortality from chronic diseases related to physical inactivity.

Physical activity refers to any bodily movement resulting in the expenditure of energy. Physical activity occurs in a broad range of settings. Leisure-time activities, occupational activities, routine activities of daily living, and dedicated exercise sessions are all valid forms of physical activity. Physical activity varies along a continuum of intensity from light (eg, housework) to moderate (eg, jogging) to more vigorous (eg, strenuous bicycling). *Exercise* is a structured routine of physical activity specifically designed to improve or maintain one of the components of health-related physical fitness. Historically, society has placed more emphasis on formal exercise programs as the primary means of achieving physical fitness rather than promoting physical activity in a more general sense.

Body mass index (BMI) is the anthropometric measurement of choice for assessing body composition in children, adolescents, and adults. BMI is calculated by dividing an individual's weight (in kilograms) by the square of the individual's height (in meters). Charts and digital tools for the office (http://www.cdc. gov/nccdphp/dnpa/bmi/calc-bmi.htm) and for handheld computers (http://hin.nhlbi.nih.gov/bmi_palm.htm) are available for rapid calculation of BMI. Normative values for

Table 10–1. Definitions of physical activity, physical fitness, and exercise.

Physical activity	Any bodily movement that results in the expenditure of energy
Physical fitness	A general state of overall well-being that allows individuals to conduct the majority of their activities of daily living in a vigorous manner
Health-related physical fitness	Aerobic capacity (cardiorespiratory endurance) Body composition Muscular strength Muscular endurance Flexibility
Skill-related physical fitness	Power Agility Speed Balance Coordination Reaction time
Exercise	A structured routine of physical activity specifically designed to improve or maintain one of the components of health-related physical fitness

Table 10–2. Definitions of overweight and obesity for adolescents and adults.

Definition	Clinical Parameter
Obesity (adults)	BMI > 30
Overweight (adults)	BMI 25.1–29.9
Overweight (adolescents)	BMI > 95th percentile for age
At risk for overweight (adolescents)	BMI > 85th percentile for age
Underweight (adolescents)	BMI < 5th percentile for age

Source: Centers for Disease Control and Prevention (http://www.cdc.gov/nccdphp/dnpa/bmi/bmi-for-age.htm).

underweight, normal weight, overweight, and obesity for adolescents have been established, and are presented in Table 10–2. BMI-for-age charts have replaced standard weight-for-height charts as the preferred mechanism for tracking weight in children and adolescents (Figures 10–2 and 10–3).

Grunbaum JA et al: *School Health Profiles: Characteristics of Health Programs Among Secondary Schools (Profiles 2004).* Centers for Disease Control and Prevention, 2005.

Ogden CL et al: Prevalence of overweight and obesity in the United States, 1999–2004. JAMA 2006;295:1549. [PMID: 16595758]

RISKS ASSOCIATED WITH PHYSICAL INACTIVITY

Physical inactivity is a primary risk factor for cardiovascular disease and all-cause mortality. A sedentary life-style also contributes to increased rates of diabetes, hypertension, hyperlipidemia, osteoporosis, cerebrovascular disease, and colon cancer. Adolescents who are less physically active are more likely to smoke cigarettes, less likely to consume appropriate amounts of fruits and vegetables, less likely to routinely wear a seat belt, and more likely to spend increased time watching television.

Physical activity serves numerous preventive functions. In addition to preventing chronic diseases such as hypertension, diabetes, and cardiovascular disease, sufficient levels of physical activity on a regular basis are associated with lower rates of mental illness. Physically active adolescents have lower levels of stress and anxiety and have higher self-esteem than sedentary peers. Active adolescents also have fewer somatic complaints, are more confident about their own future health, have improved relationships with parents and authority figures, and have a better body image.

Lotan M et al: Physical activity in adolescence. A review with clinical suggestions. Int J Adolesc Med Health 2004;16:13. [PMID: 15900808]

Suris JC, Parera N: Don't stop, don't stop: Physical activity and adolescence. Int J Adolesc Med Health 2005;17:67. [PMID: 15900813]

US Department of Health and Human Services: The Surgeon General's call to action to prevent and decrease overweight and obesity. DHHS, Public Health Service, Office of the Surgeon General, 2001.

FACTORS INFLUENCING PHYSICAL ACTIVITY

Despite the overwhelming evidence supporting the health-related benefits of physical activity, young Americans are increasingly sedentary. A complex interaction of social, cultural, gender-based, environmental, and familial factors associated with "modern living" has contributed to decreased rates of physical activity.

Social Factors

Socioeconomic status is one of the strongest predictors of physical activity in both adolescents and adults. Lower socioeconomic status is associated with lower levels of spontaneous physical activity. Youth of higher socioeconomic status engage in more spontaneous physical activity, are more frequently enrolled in physical education classes, and are more active during physical education classes compared with peers of lower socioeconomic status. This relationship persists when controlling for age, gender, and ethnicity.

Social mobility also plays an important role in shaping levels of physical activity. Specifically, achieved levels of social positioning are more strongly associated with positive health behaviors and increased levels of physical activity than the social class of origin. Youth with active friends are more likely to be active. Youth with sedentary friends are more likely to be sedentary. There are also significant differences in patterns of spontaneous physical activity when youth attending public schools are compared with youth attending private secondary schools. In the public school system, individuals are more likely to enroll in physical education classes. In private schools, adolescents are more likely to participate in organized team sports. Participation in organized sports is associated with higher levels of physical activity in adulthood.

Unfortunately, all Americans have become increasingly reliant on automated transportation. This has had a negative impact on the simplest form of physical activity: walking. Historically, most youth walked to school. This is no longer the case. It is estimated that of all trips Americans take under 1 mile in distance, 75% are made via automobile or some other form of automated transportation. Americans rely too heavily on automated forms of transportation.

Cultural & Ethnic Factors

Cohort studies consistently suggest that there are inherent cultural differences in levels of spontaneous physical

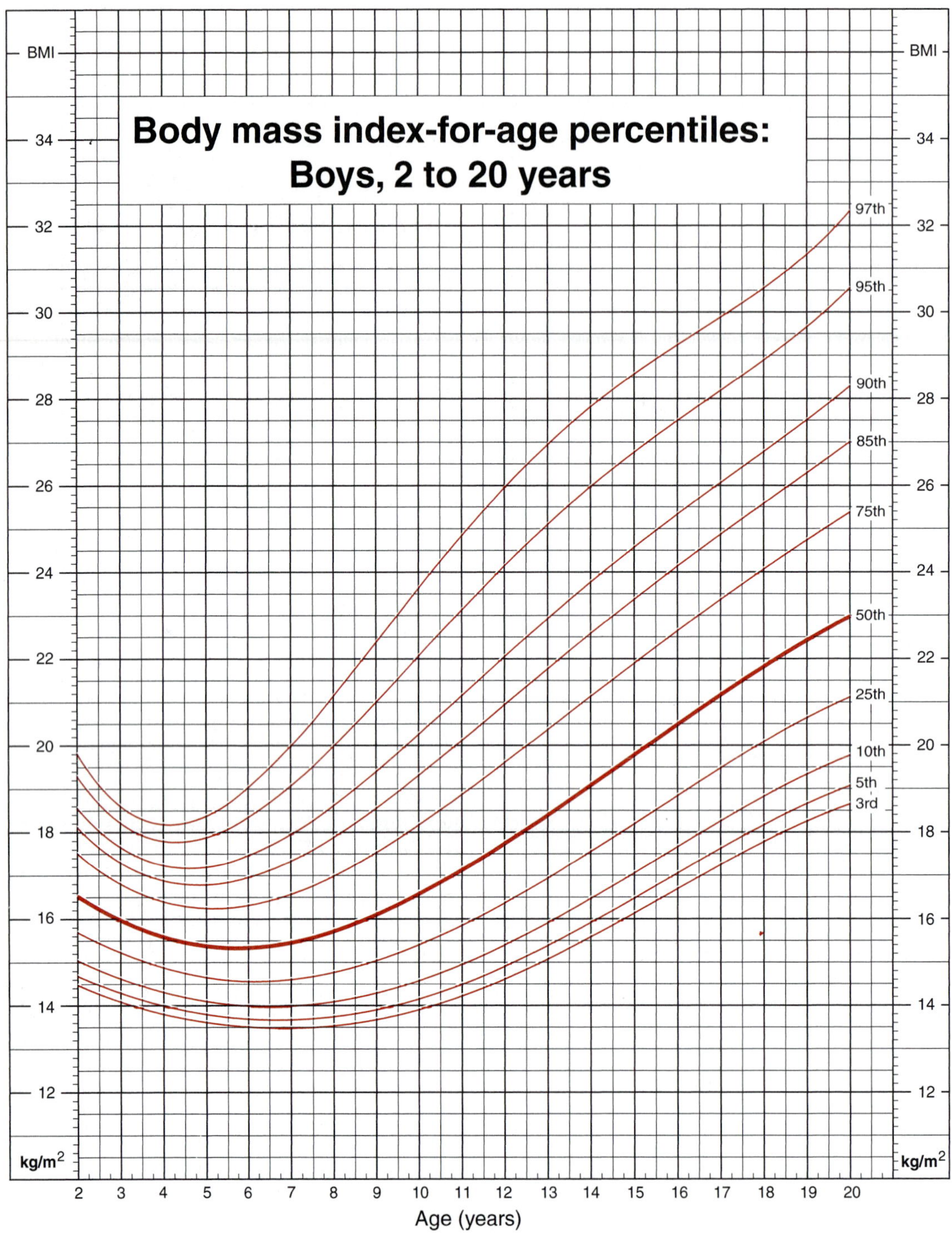

Figure 10–2. Body mass index for age—males. (From Centers for Disease Control and Prevention, Atlanta, Georgia. Available at: http://www.cdc.gov/nchs/about/major/nhanes/growthcharts/set1/chart15.pdf.)

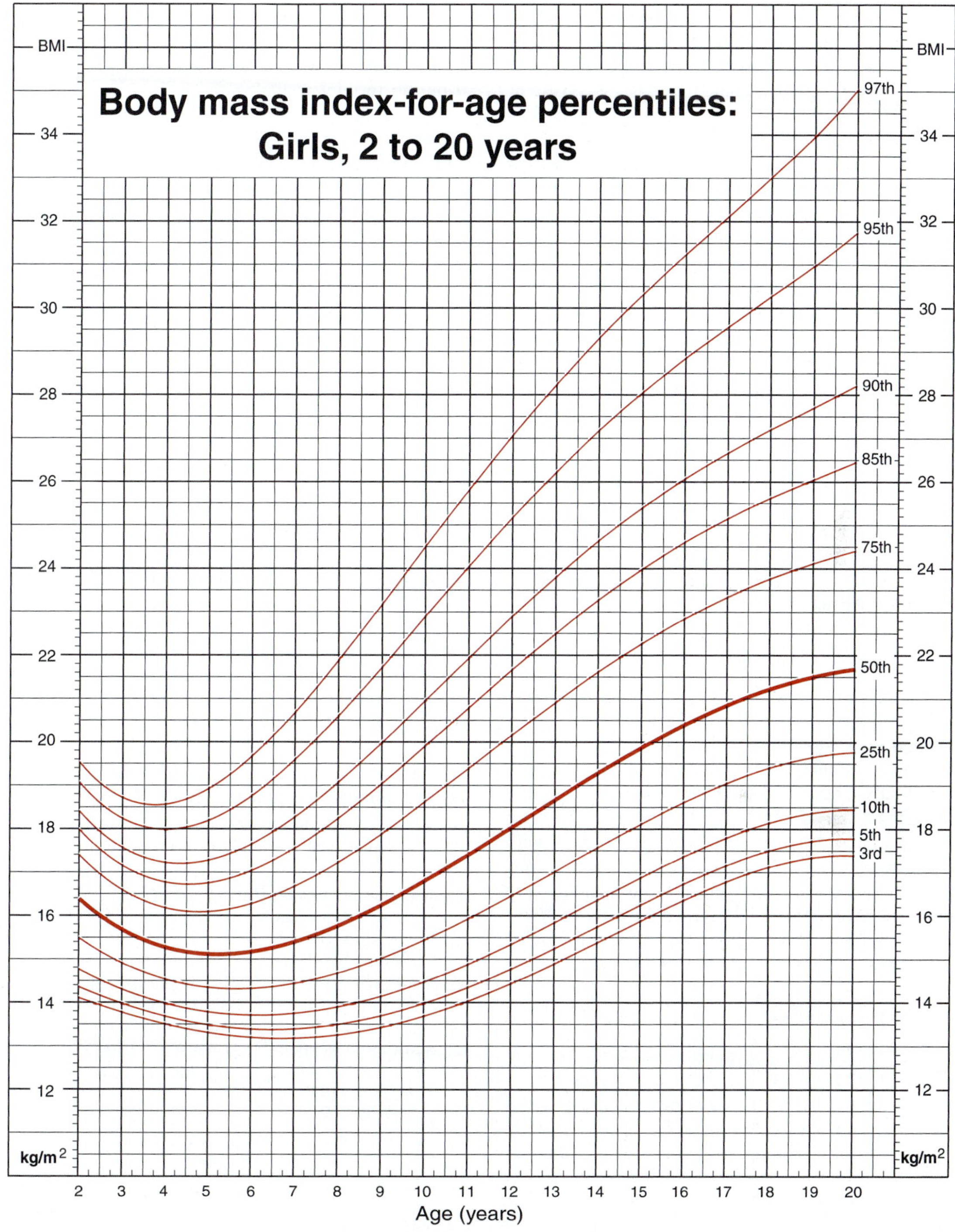

Figure 10–3. Body mass index for age—females. (From Centers for Disease Control and Prevention, Atlanta, Georgia. Available at: http://www.cdc.gov/nchs/about/major/nhanes/growthcharts/set1/chart16.pdf.)

activity. Data from the Youth Risk Behavior Survey and the National Longitudinal Study of Adolescent Health show that minority adolescents engage in the lowest levels of physical activity. These findings are consistent for both leisure-time physical activity and activity during physical education class.

Currently, 25% of adolescents consider themselves to be "too fat." Hispanic youth are more likely to view themselves as overweight when compared with African-Americans and non-Hispanic whites. Those adolescents who view themselves as overweight are significantly less physically active than their normal-weight peers and are less likely to engage in healthy behaviors. Compared with non-Hispanic whites, African-American and Hispanic youth are at significantly higher risk for being overweight and obese.

There are important cultural differences in perceptions about the inherent value of exercise. Not all cultures encourage using leisure time for fitness activities. In fact, dedicating time for exercise as an isolated activity can be viewed as either selfish or a waste of time. Cultural and ethnic differences also exist in television viewing habits. Hispanic and African-American adolescents spend significantly more time watching television than do non-Hispanic whites.

Gender-Specific Factors

There are significant differences in levels of spontaneous physical activity between male and female adolescents. Boys are more active than girls from childhood through adolescence. Levels of physical activity decline for both boys and girls during adolescence, but there is a disproportionate decline for girls. The reasons for this are unclear. Factors that are positively associated with an increased likelihood of physical activity among female adolescents include perceived competence at a particular activity, perceived value of the activity, favorable physical appearance during and after the activity, and positive social support for the activity.

Environmental Factors

Many of the barriers to physical activity are environmental. Of these, television and video games are the most important. It is estimated that between the ages of 8 and 18, youth spend an average of 4.5 h/day watching television or videotapes, playing video or computer games, or surfing the Internet. This translates to over 25% of waking hours being spent in front of a video monitor. By contrast, adolescents spend less than 1% of their time (an estimated 12–14 min/day) engaged in vigorous physical activity. The impact of television, video, personal computers, and handheld gaming devices on the activity levels of youth is so significant that the American Academy of Pediatrics has released a position statement recommending that youth watch a maximum 1–2 hours of television per day.

Television is not the only environmental issue contributing to adolescent inactivity and obesity. Adolescents are more reliant than ever on labor-saving devices. Elevators and escalators take precedence over staircases, and high-technology tools such as the Internet have further reduced the incentive to get up and get moving. Acquisition of a driver's license often represents the pinnacle of adolescence, providing an excuse for adolescents to drive everywhere. Poor community planning has resulted in a paucity of safe gymnasiums or playing fields for adolescents to use during their leisure time. In addition, there is an abundance of readily available, inexpensive, calorically dense foodstuffs. The rate of processed food consumption parallels the rise in overweight and obesity in adolescents.

Familial Factors

Finally, there are factors inherent within individual families that shape how active young individuals will be. Children and adolescents with overweight parents are more likely to be overweight themselves. Interestingly, parental levels of physical activity do not correlate with their children's levels of physical activity. Children and youth from larger families are more active than children from small families. Children whose parents are available to provide transportation to organized sporting activities are more likely to be physically active. Individuals who are forced to exercise as children are less likely to be physically active as adults. Thus, although it is important for parents to model physical activity, clearly there are external forces at work in an adolescent's life shaping individual patterns of health-related behaviors.

Forshee RA et al: The role of beverage consumption, physical activity, sedentary behavior and demographics on body mass index of adolescents. Int J Food Sci Nutr 2004;55:463. [PMID: 15762311]

Gordon-Larsen P et al: Determinants of adolescent physical activity and inactivity patterns. Pediatrics 2000;105:E83. [PMID: 10835096]

Koivusilta LK et al: Health-related lifestyle in adolescence—origin of social class differences in health? Health Educ Res 1999; 14:339. [PMID: 10539226]

Tammelin T et al: Physical activity and social status in adolescence as predictors of physical inactivity in adulthood. Prev Med 2003;37:375. [PMID: 14507496]

Yang X et al: Risk of obesity in relation to physical activity tracking from youth to adulthood. Med Sci Sports Exerc 2006;38: 919. [PMID: 16672846]

ASSESSMENT

There are three ways to assess physical activity levels in adolescents: (1) direct observation, (2) activity or heart

Table 10–3. Sixty-minute screening measure for moderate-to-vigorous physical activity in adolescents: PACE + (Patient-Centered Assessment and Counseling for Exercise Plus Nutrition).

Physical activity is any activity that increases your heart rate and makes you get out of breath some of the time

Physical activity can be done in sports, playing with friends, or walking to school

Some examples of **physical activity** include running, brisk walking, rollerblading, biking, dancing, skateboarding, swimming, soccer, basketball, football, and surfing.

Add up all the time you spend in physical activity each day (don't include your physical education or gym class).

1. Over the past 7 days, on how many days were you physically active for a total of at least 60 minutes per day?

   _1 _2 _3 _4 _5 _6 _7

2. Over a typical or usual week, on how many days are you physically active for a total of at least 60 minutes per day?

   _1 _2 _3 _4 _5 _6 _7

Scoring: Add the value from question 1 and question 2 and divide by 2 (Q1 + Q2/2). If this score is less than 5, the individual is not meeting current physical activity guidelines

Source: Reproduced, with permission, from Prochaska JJ, Sallis JF, Long B: A physical activity screening measure for use with adolescents in primary care. Arch Pediatr Adolesc Med 2001;155:554.

rate monitors, and (3) self-report questionnaires. Of these, direct observation is the gold standard. It is also the most labor intensive. Therefore, several attempts have been made to provide valid, accurate, and rapid clinical tools for assessing physical activity levels in adolescents.

The Patient-Centered Assessment and Counseling for Exercise Plus (PACE+) Nutrition program has been developed to assist clinicians in assessing physical activity levels and to counsel patients regarding appropriate levels of physical activity and proper nutrition. As part of this program, a rapid screening tool has been developed specifically to screen levels of adolescent physical activity (Table 10–3). This simple two-question survey provides clinicians with a valid assessment of whether adolescents are achieving recommended levels of physical activity on a regular basis. The combination of BMI and the PACE+ activity measure allows for a rapid clinical assessment of adolescents' physical activity status, weight status, and potential health risk.

Sirard JR, Pate RR: Physical activity assessment in children and adolescents. Sports Med 2001;31:439. [PMID: 11394563]

GUIDELINES & CLINICAL INTERVENTIONS

It is known that risk factors for chronic disease track from childhood into adolescence and from adolescence into adulthood. Overweight adolescents are more likely to become overweight adults. Because levels of obesity are rising sharply among adolescents and levels of physical activity are declining, there is an acute need for interventions to promote physical activity in children and adolescents. The following guidelines can assist clinicians in providing activity counseling for their adolescent patients (Table 10–4).

American College of Sports Medicine

The American College of Sports Medicine (ACSM) published the initial set of guidelines for physical activity in adults in 1978. Recommendations call for 15–60 minutes of exercise, 3–5 days per week at an intensity of 60–90% of an individual's maximum heart rate. These guidelines emphasize physical training as opposed to physical activity. In 1990, this position was modified to include conditioning for muscular strength and endurance.

American College of Sports Medicine position statement on the recommended quantity and quality of exercise for developing and maintaining fitness in healthy adults. Med Sci Sport Exerc 1978;10:vii. [PMID: 723501]

International Consensus Conference on Physical Activity Guidelines for Adolescents

Convened in 1993, this expert panel recommends that adolescents be physically active on most if not all days of the week. Adolescents should strive for activity 3–5 days per week for 20 minutes or more at levels requiring moderate to vigorous exertion. Activity should routinely occur as part of play, games, sporting activities, work, recreation, physical education, or planned exercise sessions. These guidelines also emphasize the importance of considering family, school, and community factors when counseling adolescents about physical activity.

Twisk JW: Physical activity guidelines for children and adolescents: A critical review. Sports Med 2001;31:617. [PMID: 1147523]

ACSM/CDC Consensus Statement

This 1995 statement serves as a consensus for several national societies, and calls for all Americans to engage in regular physical activity according to their individual abilities. Simply stated, adolescents should strive to obtain 30 minutes of moderate to vigorous physical activity on most if not all days of the week.

Table 10–4. Guidelines for physical activity in adolescence.

Guideline Source	Recommendation
American College of Sports Medicine (ACSM)	Fifteen to 60 min of exercise per day Exercise 3–5 d/wk Intensity of 60–90% of maximal heart rate
International Consensus Conference on Physical Activity Guidelines for Adolescents	Physical activity 3–5 d/wk Activity sessions of 20 min or more requiring moderate to vigorous physical exertion Emphasis on consideration of familial, social, and community factors when promoting activity
ACSM/CDC Consensus Statement	All Americans should strive to be physically active on most, preferably all days of the week according to individual abilities Goal of accumulating 30 min of moderate to vigorous physical activity each day
Surgeon General's Report	Sedentary individuals benefit from even modest levels of physical activity Sufficient levels of activity can be accumulated through independent bouts of activity throughout the day
Healthy People 2010	Increase the proportion of adolescents who engage in moderate physical activity for at least 30 min on 5 or more d/wk Increase the proportion of adolescents who engage in vigorous activity 3 or more d/wk for 20 min or more per occasion Increase the proportion of adolescents participating in daily physical education Increase the proportion of adolescents who spend at least 50% of class time during physical education engaged in physical activity Increase the proportion of adolescents who walk to school (less than 1 mile) Increase the proportion of adolescents who bicycle to school (less than 2 miles)
Dietary Guidelines for Americans	Accumulate 60 min of moderate activity per day
Surgeon General's Call to Action	Clinicians, schools, communities, and families should work together to promote physical activity and healthy life-style choices for all individuals

Pate RR et al: Physical activity and public health: A recommendation from the Centers for Disease Control and Prevention and the American College of Sports Medicine. JAMA 1995;273:402. [PMID: 7823386]

Surgeon General's Report: Physical Activity and Health

In 1996, the surgeon general released a report summarizing available medical evidence relating to the health benefits of regular physical activity. This report emphasizes that even modest amounts of physical activity have important health benefits for sedentary individuals. It also states physical activity need not be overly strenuous to be beneficial.

Healthy People 2010

In 1991, the US Department of Health and Human Services released a series of national public health goals. This initiative, *Healthy People 2000,* failed to significantly change activity patterns in children or adolescents. As a result, a follow-up initiative, *Healthy People 2010,* was announced. The number one priority in this initiative is to promote physical activity. Of the 13 adolescent health objectives outlined in *Healthy People 2010,* 6 are specifically targeted to promote physical activity. Objectives relating specifically to physical activity in adolescents are presented in Table 10–4.

US Department of Health and Human Services: *Healthy People 2010: Understanding and Improving Health.* DHHS, Government Printing Office, 2000.

Dietary Guidelines for Americans

Now in its sixth edition, these guidelines are the cornerstone for providing clinical nutritional advice. Emphasizing the inherent relationship between physical activity, dietary choices, and resultant weight issues, the current edition of the *Guidelines* is the first to specifically recommend physical activity as a part of routine dietary practice. Adolescents should aim to accumulate 60 minutes or more of moderate physical activity on a daily basis.

US Department of Health and Human Services; US Department of Agriculture: *Dietary Guidelines for Americans 2005,* 6th ed. Government Printing Office, 2005.

Surgeon General's Call to Action

Recognizing the need for further action, the surgeon general has recently released an additional report recommending that individuals, families, schools, worksites, health care providers, and communities work together to combat the increasing problem of physical inactivity, overweight, and obesity in the United States.

US Department of Health and Human Services: *The Surgeon General's Call to Action to Prevent and Decrease Overweight and Obesity.* DHHS, Public Health Service, Office of the Surgeon General, 2001.

PROMOTING PHYSICAL ACTIVITY: WHAT CAN WE DO TO IMPROVE?

Health care professionals play a central role in promoting physical activity among adolescents. Adolescents have the lowest utilization of health care services of any segment of the population. They do, however, rely on their physician as a reliable source of health care information. Clinicians must, therefore, take the opportunity to provide preventive advice at each adolescent visit in accordance with the guidelines established by the US Preventive Services Task Force. During each adolescent visit, "appropriate counseling to promote physical activity and a healthy diet should be provided."

Unfortunately, very few visits with adolescents actually document preventive counseling. In a study of counseling services during routine adolescent visits, only one of four patients received specific advice from his or her provider regarding nutrition or physical activity. When reviewing guidelines or recommending life-style changes with adolescent patients, it is important to promote the concept of physical activity as opposed to physical fitness. Adolescents should be aware that cumulative bouts of physical activity are just as effective as sustained periods of exercise in attaining health-related benefits. For changes to be effective in adolescence, physical activity must be enjoyable and there should be social support for the activity either from family or from peers. Using established guidelines within the context of social, cultural, familial, and environmental factors, clinicians must improve preventive counseling services to adolescents.

Ma J et al: U.S. adolescents receive suboptimal preventive counseling during ambulatory care. J Adol Health 2005;36:441e1. [PMID: 15841517]

US Preventive Services Task Force: The *Guide to Clinical Preventive Services, Recommendations of the U.S. Preventive Services Task Force.* DHHS, Agency for Healthcare Research and Quality, 2005.

SPECIAL CONSIDERATIONS

Performance-Enhancing Supplements

Over the past decade, the use of performance-enhancing supplements has exploded. One half of the US population consumes some form of nutritional supplement on a regular basis, resulting in over $44 billion in annual sales. Reasons cited for the use of dietary nutritional supplements include ensuring good nutrition, preventing illness, improving performance, warding off fatigue, and enhancing personal appearance.

Estimates suggest that roughly 5% of all adolescents have used some form of performance-enhancing nutritional supplements. Adolescents, in particular, are vulnerable to the allure of performance-enhancing products.

Creatine is the most commonly used performance-enhancing supplement. Creatine is reported to increase energy during short-term intense exercise, increase muscle mass, increase strength, increase lean body mass, and decrease lactate accumulation during intense exercise. Although it is clear that supplementation with exogenous creatine can raise intramuscular creatine stores, it is not clear how effective creatine is as a performance aid. In general, creatine supplementation may be useful for activities requiring short, repetitive bouts of high-intensity exercise. There is conflicting evidence, however, as to whether it is effective in increasing muscle strength or muscle mass. There are no scientific data regarding the safety or effectiveness of long-term use of creatine in adolescents.

Anabolic-androgenic steroids (AAS) are another important category of performance-enhancing substances used by adolescents. Testosterone is the prototypical androgenic steroid hormone. Many synthetic modifications have been made to the basic molecular structure of testosterone in an attempt to promote the anabolic, muscle-building effects of testosterone while minimizing androgenic side effects. Androstenedione is one of several oral performance-enhancing supplements that are precursors to testosterone. The effectiveness of androstenedione as a performance-enhancing supplement is debatable. To date, the largest controlled trial examining its effectiveness showed no significant gains in muscular strength compared with a standard program of resistance training. The Anabolic Steroid Control Act of 2004 expanded the definition of anabolic steroids to include androstenedione and tetrahydrogestrinone (THG)—a designer steroid whose use was implicated in accusations of steroid use by several famous US athletes—as controlled substances, making their use as performance-enhancing drugs illegal.

Despite this ban, it is estimated that 3–10% of adolescents have used anabolic steroids. Importantly, adolescents who use anabolic steroids have been shown to be more likely to engage in high-risk personal health behaviors such as tobacco use and excessive alcohol consumption. Users of other nutritional performance-enhancing supplement have also been shown to engage in similar predictable high-risk behaviors. The American Academy of Pediatrics has recently published a position statement strongly discouraging the use of performance-enhancing substances.

Clinicians should be aware of the prevalence of performance-enhancing supplement use in the adolescent population. They should also be aware of health-related behaviors that often accompany the use of these products and provide preventive counseling accordingly. The preparticipation physical examination represents an excellent opportunity for clinicians to provide information about performance-enhancing products to young athletes. When counseling adolescents about the use of performance-enhancing products it is helpful to ask the following questions: (1) Is the product safe to use? (2) Why does the adolescent want to use a particular product? (3) Is the product effective in helping to meet the desired goal? (4) Is the product legal? Many adolescents will either try or continue to use performance-enhancing products regardless of the information or advice they receive. Nevertheless, they should be aware of potential health risks or bans from competition that accompany use of performance-enhancing products. The use of performance-enhancing supplements in adolescents should be discouraged.

Gomez J, American Academy of Pediatrics Committee on Sports Medicine and Fitness: Use of performance-enhancing substances. Pediatrics 2005;115:1103. [PMID: 15805399]

Koch JJ: Performance-enhancing substances and their use among adolescent athletes. Pediatr Rev 2002;23:310. [PMID: 12205298]

Stephens MB, Olsen C: Ergogenic supplements and health-risk behaviors. J Fam Pract 2001;50:696. [PMID: 11509164]

Female Athlete Triad

Although many adolescents engage in too little physical activity, there is a segment of the population for whom too much exercise leads to specific physiologic side effects. The female athlete triad refers to the combination of disordered eating, amenorrhea, and osteoporosis that can accompany excessive physical training in young female athletes. Athletes particularly at risk include those who participate in gymnastics, ballet, figure skating, distance running, or any other sport that emphasizes a particularly lean physique.

The preparticipation physical examination represents an excellent opportunity for clinicians to screen for and to prevent the female athlete triad. During this examination, screening questions for female athletes should include careful menstrual, dietary (including a history of disordered eating practices), and exercise histories. When elicited, a history of amenorrhea (particularly in a previously menstruating woman) should be taken seriously. The American College of Sports Medicine recommends that these women be considered at risk for the female athlete triad and that a formal medical evaluation should be undertaken within 3 months.

Hobart JA, Smucker DR: The female athlete triad. Am Fam Physician 2000;61:3357. [PMID: 10865930]

Exercise & Sudden Death

Another small segment of the adolescent population is at risk during exercise. These individuals are predisposed to sudden cardiac death during physical activity. Highly publicized events among well-known athletes have further focused attention on this issue. Although the incidence of sudden cardiac death in young athletes is fortunately quite low, proper screening is still important. Here again, the preparticipation physical examination represents an excellent clinical opportunity for prevention.

When screening for sudden death in young athletes, the medical history should include questions about exercise-related syncope or near-syncope, shortness of breath, chest pain, or palpitations. The clinician should ask about a family history of premature death or premature cardiovascular disease. Any prior history of a cardiac murmur or specific knowledge of an underlying cardiac abnormality (either structural, valvular, or arrhythmic) in the athlete should be elicited as well. If the examining clinician has any suspicion that the athlete might have a symptomatic arrhythmia, that individual should be withheld from physical activity pending consultation with a cardiologist.

On physical examination, blood pressure should be recorded. The precordial fields should be auscultated in the supine, squatting, and standing positions. Murmurs that increase with moving from the squatting to standing position or that increase with the Valsalva maneuver are of potential concern and merit further evaluation. The equality of the femoral pulses should be noted. If any abnormalities are noted on the initial preparticipation history or physical examination, a more detailed evaluation is warranted.

O'Connor FG et al: Sudden death in young athletes: Screening for the needle in a haystack. Am Fam Physician 1998;57:2763. [PMID: 9636339]

Eating Disorders 11

Evelyn L. Lewis, MD, MA, & Tracy Sbrocco, PhD

General Considerations

More than eight million Americans suffer from eating disorders. Approximately 90% of them are young women; however, middle-aged women, children, and young men are also affected. The prevalence of eating disorders appears to vary by the population being studied. Eating disorders have been found to be more prevalent in industrialized societies (where food is abundant and attractiveness is linked to being thin) than in developing countries.

Women in western countries traditionally have exhibited greater concern for body habitus than those in developing countries, who appear to be more accepting of and comfortable with a fuller body shape. In many of the latter societies, a fuller figure has been considered the cultural stereotype of attractiveness, although this appears to change when individuals from these societies integrate into western societies.

Clinicians sometimes fail to diagnose eating disorders in women of color, perhaps because these disorders have been reported much less frequently among African Americans, Asian Americans, Hispanic Americans, and American Indians. Incorrect diagnosis may also derive from the widely accepted but false belief that eating disorders affect only middle- to upper-middle-class white adolescent girls and women. This oversight or unconscious cultural bias can undermine appropriate treatment.

Westernization has affected many countries, and individuals from other cultures should not be excluded from consideration of an eating disorder diagnosis. Although no culture appears immune to the occurrence of eating disorders, the evidence seems to support a higher incidence of eating disorders in westernized societies as well as in societies experiencing enormous changes.

Agras WS: The consequences and costs of the eating disorders. Psychiatr Clin North Am 2001;24:371. [PMID: 11416936]

Normal versus Abnormal Eating

Before detailing the clinical characteristics of various eating disorders, it is necessary to identify what is meant by "normal eating." In so doing, it becomes apparent that a great deal of dieting occurs in western culture as part of normal eating. In fact, estimates suggest that anywhere from 15% to 80% of the population may be dieting at a given time.

Despite these statistics, over 60% of the adult population and 16% of children and adolescents aged 6–19 years are considered overweight or obese (22% of African-American and Hispanic children compared with 12% of non-Hispanic white children). Women are most likely to restrict their food intake to control their weight or lose weight, but increasingly men are also engaging in dieting behavior. Most disconcerting is the prevalence of dieting among adolescents and even children. Statistics show that 40% of 9-year-old girls have dieted, and even 5-year-olds voice concern about their diet that appear to be linked to cultural standards. Although not all individuals who diet develop an eating disorder, dieting, in combination with other factors, may be an important precipitant to the development of eating disorders. In addition, dieting is a factor to consider in the prevention of eating disorders, particularly among adolescents whose parents pressure them to lose weight. Lastly, the acceptance of dieting as "normal" may stand in the way of the clinician's recognition of problem eating.

The prevalence and incidence rates for eating disorders vary significantly, depending on the disorder and the population. Generally speaking, of patients with classic signs and symptoms of anorexia nervosa (AN) or bulimia nervosa (BN), 90% are female, 95% are white, and 75% are adolescent when they develop the disorder. These data are substantiated by several cross-cultural studies that have reported few, if any, cases in rural areas of Africa, the Middle East, or Asia with the exception of Japan, the only nonwestern country that has seen a substantial and persistent increase in eating disorders.

AN has been implicated as a "culture-bound syndrome" because certain cultural mores are reflected in the signs and symptoms of the disorder. This view is backed by findings that indicate that as individuals (particularly girls and women) from cultures in which AN is unknown or extremely rare immigrate to westernized societies with higher rates of AN, they tend to develop disorders as they attempt to acculturate. In the United States, the frequency of AN among young Hispanic women appears to be about as common as that seen in non-Hispanic whites.

However, several studies have shown that other abnormal eating behaviors may be as common or more so among African-American women (eg, purging by laxatives vs vomiting). Black women are also more likely to develop BN or binge eating disorder (BED) than AN, and a recent study found a strong association between BED and obesity in this population. Given the high rates of obesity in ethnic minority populations, experts have postulated that BED is a significant problem among these groups. Contributing elements appear to be increased influence by the media (eg, television and advertising that depict thin beauty ideals), rise in the standard of living, lack of physical activity, and increased food availability that make weight gain common.

Most patients with eating disorders are of middle to upper socioeconomic status. Age-specific and sex-specific estimates suggest that about 0.5–1% of adolescent girls develop AN, whereas 5% of older adolescent and young adult women develop BN. This population also exhibits a high frequency of coexistence between AN and BN. It has been reported that as many as 50% of AN patients may exhibit bulimic behaviors while 30–80% of patients with BN have a history of AN. Although constituting a small segment of patients with eating disorders, male adolescents must not be forgotten. Most, however, tend to have a diagnosis of BN or BED.

Data suggest that approximately 4% of people surveyed in a general population have BED. Although being overweight is not a criterion for making the diagnosis of BED, it has been estimated that slightly over 11% of individuals who join Weight Watchers and 30% of individuals who present to hospital-based weight control programs meet the diagnosis of BED.

Finally, it should be noted that despite the emphasis on AN, BN, and BED in both the literature and the media, the diagnostic category of "eating disorder not otherwise specified" (EDNOS) is the most prevalent eating disorder in the United States, affecting 6–10% of young women.

Crago M et al: Eating disturbances among American minority groups: A review. Int J Eat Disord. 1996;19:239. [PMID: 8704722]

de Zwaan M: Binge eating disorder and obesity. Int J Obes Relat Metab Disord Suppl 2001;1:S51. [PMID: 11460589]

Meshreki LM, Hansen CE: African American men's female body size preferences based on racial identity and environment. J Black Psychol 2004;30(4):451.

Miller MN, Pumariega AJ: Culture and eating disorders: A historical and cross-cultural review. Psychiatry 2001;64:93. [PMID: 11495364]

Petersons M et al: Effect of ethnicity on attitudes, feelings, and behaviors toward food. Eat Disord 2000;8:207.

Pathogenesis

The origins of eating disorders (AN, BN, and BED) are extremely complex and poorly understood. However, biological, psychological, cultural, and societal factors are likely contributors to the predisposition, precipitation, and perpetuation of these disorders.

A. Women at Risk

Risk factors for developing an eating disorder include participation in activities that promote thinness (eg, ballet dancing, modeling, and athletics) and certain personality traits, such as low self-esteem, difficulty expressing negative emotions, difficulty resolving conflict, and being perfectionistic. Mounting data also support substantial biological predispositions to AN and BN. Mothers and sisters of probands who had AN were found to have eight times the risk of developing an eating disorder compared with the general population. Genetic studies also lend strong support to the underlying biological supposition regarding eating disorders. Twin studies have shown heritability estimates in the 50–90% range for AN and 35–50% for BN, with monozygotic twins having higher concordance than dizygotic twins. A strong association between AN and BN in families has also been found in the Virginia Twin Registry.

Eating disorders may also be precipitated by psychosocial factors in vulnerable individuals. These precipitating factors often relate to developmental tasks of adolescence and include maturation fears, particularly those related to sexual development, peer group involvement, independence and autonomy struggles, family conflicts, sexual abuse, and identity conflicts. Two other psychological factors that figure permanently in the pathogenesis of BN or BED are sexual trauma and depression. Patients with either of these disorders are predisposed to have a family and personal history of depression. Therefore, it is important to note the presence of depression or history of sexual trauma during the initial patient assessment.

Mehler PS: Diagnosis and care of patients with anorexia nervosa in primary care settings. Ann Intern Med 2001;134:1048. [PMID: 11388818]

Misra M et al: Effects of anorexia nervosa on clinical, hematologic, biochemical, and bone density parameters in community-dwelling adolescent girls. Pediatrics 2004;114:1574. [PMID: 15574617]

Rome ES et al: Children and adolescents with eating disorders: The state of the art. Pediatrics 2003;111:e98. [PMID: 12509603]

B. Men at Risk

Most people, including many health care providers, associate AN with upper-middle-class, overachieving, young white women. The National Association of Anorexia Nervosa and Associated Disorders estimates that as many as one million American men suffer from eating disorders, although the actual number may be much larger. Manifestations of eating disorders in men are similar to those in women and include an excessive fear of gaining weight, excessive dieting or compulsive overeating, and dissatisfaction with one's body.

In the past two decades, the number of men who openly report dissatisfaction with their physical appearance has tripled and today, nearly as many men as women say they are unhappy with how they look. Meanwhile, therapists report seeing 50% more men for evaluation and treatment for eating disorders than they did in the 1990s. The root of this trend may be an obsession with "six-pack abs" and bulging biceps that seems especially common among athletes and other fitness enthusiasts.

Exercise status and sexual orientation are two risk factors for eating disorders in men. Often men who develop eating disorders have a history of being overweight when they were younger. The following groups of men are considered to be at increased risk of developing eating disorders:

- Athletes, especially those participating in sports that work against gravity, such as gymnastics.
- Men with gender issues.
- Men with personality traits such as perfectionism and impulsive behaviors, and those who have anxiety.
- Obese boys who face teasing and have low self-esteem.

Leit RA et al: The media's representation of the ideal male body: A cause for muslce dysmorphia? Int J Eat Disord 2002;31:344. [PMID: 11920996]

Prevention & Screening

Eating disorders are serious and complex problems, and the earlier an eating disorder is identified, the better the patient's chance of recovery. This makes a compelling argument for targeted screening of at-risk groups (male and female), including gymnasts, runners, body builders, wrestlers, dancers, rowers, and swimmers. These groups warrant close monitoring because their sports or livelihood dictate weight restriction. The populations at highest risk for AN and BN are female adolescents and young adults, and screening should occur at about ages 14 and 18 years. This correlates with the transition to high school and college and the associated stressors. Almost all individuals seeking treatment for weight control should be screened for BED because of the high incidence of this disorder in this group. Although these individuals may fall short of meeting the full criteria for BED, the problematic attitudes associated with the disorder will likely be uncovered. The tools used for screening can be very sophisticated and vary with the population being assessed. However, there are some that are easily incorporated into the routine primary care office visit (Table 11–1). These questions are very helpful for the early detection of BN and BED, because individuals with these disorders can be uncovered using self-report alone. Those with AN on the other hand, are resistant to self-reporting and usually require reporting by others (ie, parents, friends). Therefore, it is imperative that parents, friends, teachers, family, dentists, and physicians become educated about the possible signs and symptoms associated with these difficult-to-manage disorders to facilitate prevention or early management of these individuals.

Table 11–1. Screening questionnaire.

1. Has there been any change in your weight?
2. What did you eat yesterday?
3. Do you ever binge?
4. Have you ever used self-induced vomiting, laxatives, diuretics, or enemas to lose weight or compensate for overeating?
5. How much do you exercise in a typical week?
6. How do you feel about how you look?
7. Are your menstrual periods regular?

Reproduced, with permission, from Powers PS: Initial assessment and early treatment options for anorexia nervosa and bulimia nervosa. Psychiatr Clin North Am 1996;19(4):639.

Clinical Findings

A. Symptoms and Signs

The multiple symptoms experienced by the patient and signs noted by the physician are related to the numerous methods used to manipulate weight. When initially screening a patient, a symptom checklist can facilitate taking a history (Table 11–2). Questions are usually answered honestly except in the case of the anorexic patient, who is usually reticent to be seen or report any problem with weight.

If the review of systems contains primarily positive results, this may be indicative of a significant problem for the patient. Most commonly, female patients with AN complain of amenorrhea, depression, fatigue, weakness, hair loss, and bone pain (which may be indicative of pathologic fracture secondary to osteopenia). Constipation or abdominal pain, or both, occur frequently but may be commonly mistaken as symptoms of endometriosis or pelvic inflammatory disease, which are disorders common to both anorexia and bulimia. Unlike AN, BN may be missed initially by the inexperienced clinician because these patients may present with normal or near-normal body weight or be slightly underweight. In addition to constipation and gastrointestinal pain, bulimic patients may present with menstrual irregularity, food and fluid restrictions, abuse of diuretics and laxatives (causing dizziness and bloody diarrhea), misuse of diet pills (leading to palpitations and anxiety), frequent vomiting (resulting in throat irritation and pharyngeal

Table 11–2. Evaluation of eating disorders: the history.

History should include questions on the following:
- Weight (minimum/maximum, as well as ideal)
- Menstrual history and pattern (if applicable: age of menarche, date of last period)
- Body image (thin, normal, heavy; satisfaction/dissatisfaction with current weight)
- Exercise regimen (amount, intensity, response to inability to exercise)
- Eating habits
- Sexual history (if applicable, a history of current sexual activity, number of partners, review of health habits and sexual practices that might place the patient at risk for sexually transmitted diseases [STD])
- Current and past medication
- Laxative/diuretic/diet pill use, ipecac, cigarettes, alcohol, drugs
- Substance abuse (eg, cigarettes, alcohol, drugs)
- Binge-eating and purging behavior (identify a binge: how much, what kinds of food; presence of triggers: foods, time of day, feelings; frequency of binge eating; identify vomiting methods: finger, toothbrush)
- Psychiatric history (substance abuse, mood/anxiety/personality disorders)
- Suicidal ideation

trauma), sexually transmitted diseases (which appears to be related to impulsive, risk-taking behaviors associated with this disorder), and bone pain. Mouth sores, weaknesses, dental caries, heartburn, muscle cramps and fainting, hair loss, easy bruising, and cold intolerance are some of the more obvious presenting complaints.

B. Diagnostic Criteria

Since the 1950s and 1960s there has been a concomitant recognition of eating disorders as clinical syndromes and a drive for thinness among individuals, particularly women, as they strive to attain a thin beauty ideal. AN and BN first appeared in 1980 in the *Diagnostic and Statistical Manual of Mental Disorders,* Third Edition (*DSM-III*) under the category of "Disorders First Evident in Childhood and Adolescence." Over the ensuing decades, the increased clinical recognition and the research focus on the problem has led to a substantial increase in the understanding of eating disorders, their treatment, and, more recently, preventative strategies. These syndromes have been further defined and now appear in a separate section in the *DSM-IV-TR* (Fourth edition, Text Revision) entitled "Eating Disorders."

The hallmark of AN is the refusal to eat anything but minimal amounts of food, resulting in low body weight, whereas the hallmark of BN is the attempt to restrict food intake that eventually leads to out-of-control eating episodes followed by inappropriate compensatory behaviors (eg, vomiting). The commonalities among the eating disorders include disturbance in body image (both body shape and body weight) and a drive for thinness. In part, these themes are present in the population as a whole.

Currently, there is an increased focus on the binge eating disorders as well as the overlap among obesity, eating disorders, and other mental disorders. As previously noted, the most prevalent eating disorder listed in *DSM-IV-TR* is "eating disorder not otherwise specified" (EDNOS); it is important that clinicians consider this possibility in the differential diagnosis of patients with eating disorders.

1. Anorexia nervosa—The diagnostic criteria for AN are defined and listed in the *DSM-IV-TR* (Table 11–3). The hallmark of AN is the refusal to maintain minimum body weight, defined as maintenance of 85% of expected weight or BMI greater than 17.5 kg/m^2 or failure to make appropriate weight gains with growth. Anorexic patients exhibit an intense fear of weight gain and body image disturbance, which may include any or all of its three components: emotional (eg, self-disgust),

Table 11–3. *DSM-IV-TR* criteria for anorexia nervosa.

A. Refusal to maintain body weight at or above a minimally normal weight for age and height (eg, weight loss leading to maintenance of body weight less than 85% of that expected, or failure to make expected weight gain during period of growth, leading to body weight less than 85% of that expected).

B. Intense fear of gaining weight or becoming fat, even though underweight.

C. Disturbance in the way in which one's body weight or shape is experienced, undue influence of body weight or shape on self-evaluation, or denial of the seriousness of the current low body weight.

D. In postmenarcheal females, amenorrhea, ie, the absence of at least three consecutive menstrual cycles. (A woman is considered to have amenorrhea if her periods occur only following hormone, eg, estrogen, administration.)

Restricting Type: During the current episode of anorexia nervosa, the person has not regularly engaged in binge eating or purging behavior (ie, self-induced vomiting or the misuse of laxatives, diuretics, or enemas).

Binge Eating/Purging Type: During the current episode of anorexia nervosa, the person has regularly engaged in binge eating or purging behavior (ie, self-induced vomiting or the misuse of laxatives, diuretics, or enemas).

perceptual (eg, "my thighs are too fat"), and cognitive (eg, "people will hate me if I'm fat"). Amenorrhea (albeit occasionally controversial) is also a defining element. In prepubertal girls menarche is delayed, and in postmenarchal women, at least three consecutive menstrual cycles are absent. The amenorrhea is attributed to low levels of follicle-stimulating hormone (FSH) and luteinizing hormone (LH) and may eventually precede weight loss in up to 20% of patients.

Two subtypes of AN are identified: a binge eating–purging type and a restricting type. The binge eating–purging subtype includes patients who engage in diuretic laxative abuse, vomiting, and overuse of enemas to eliminate calories. Patients who do not engage in either binge eating or purging behaviors are categorized as having the restrictive subtype. Patients with the AN binge eating–purging subtype differ from those with BN in weight criteria, size of the binge (usually smaller), and consistency of purging (less frequent).

2. Bulimia nervosa—BN, or "hunger of an ox," is more common than AN and largely confined to collegiate women, although the disorder usually starts in the late teenage years. The hallmark of BN is the patient's attempt to restrict food intake. This results in out-of-control eating and is followed by inappropriate compensatory behaviors. Patients with BN may be slightly more difficult to initially identify than those with AN, because 10% are within normal weight for age and height.

The *DSM-IV-TR* defined criteria for BN (Table 11–4) include recurrent episodes of binge eating in which more food than normal is consumed in a discrete period of time. The patient must also engage in recurrent inappropriate compensatory behaviors. Both criteria occur on average of two times per week for 3 months. BN is also divided into two subtypes: a purging type and a nonpurging type. The purging subtype requires regular engagement in self-induced vomiting and abuse of laxatives, diuretics, or enemas. The nonpurging subtype highlights other inappropriate behaviors, such as fasting and excessive exercise, but does not include vomiting or the abuse of laxatives, enemas, or diuretics. About two thirds of bulimic patients are purgers, and this subgroup has been found to exhibit more severe pathology, including more frequent binging and higher comorbidity of other psychological disorders, than nonpurgers.

3. Binge eating disorder—The most recent of the eating disorder diagnostic categories is BED. BED is not fully recognized by the *DSM-IV-TR.* It is listed as a disorder meriting further study and patients currently are considered to meet the diagnostic criteria for EDNOS. (Research criteria for BED are found in an appendix to the *DSM-IV-TR.*)

Evidence suggests that BED affects women and men (3:2) more evenly, affects a broader age range of individuals (aged 20—50 years), and likely affects African Americans as often as whites. Most people with BED are obese and have a history of "yo-yo" dieting. The hallmark of BED is binge eating in the absence of compensatory behaviors. Patients report feeling a "loss of control" while they consume larger amounts of food than is typical for most people in a discrete period of time. The episodes are associated with rapid eating, eating until uncomfortable, eating large amounts when they are not hungry, and eating alone. Other diagnostic markers and criteria include feeling depressed, disgusted, or guilty (regarding their binging behavior), and the presence of these behaviors 2 days per week for at least 6 months.

4. Eating disorder not otherwise specified—Persons with EDNOS include those who meet all the criteria for AN but have regular menses, normal-range weight, and less-frequent binges (Table 11–5). With this in mind, it is easy to understand the importance of identifying and treating these individuals. Nonetheless, many are frequently not treated by clinicians because they fail to meet the full diagnostic criteria for AN. Other unique features of this disorder not seen in AN, BN, or BED include regular use of compensatory behaviors after consuming small amounts of food and chewing and spitting out of food before swallowing.

Table 11–4. *DSM-IV-TR* criteria for bulimia nervosa.

A. Recurrent episodes of binge eating. An episode of binge eating is characterized by both of the following:
   (1) Eating, in a discrete period of time (eg, within any 2-h period), an amount of food that is definitely larger than most people would eat during a similar period of time and under similar circumstances.
   (2) A sense of lack of control over eating during the episode (eg, a feeling that one cannot stop eating or control how much one is eating).
B. Recurrent inappropriate compensatory behavior in order to prevent weight gain, such as self-induced vomiting, misuse of laxatives, diuretics, enemas, or other medications; fasting, or excessive exercise.
C. The binge eating and inappropriate compensatory behaviors both occur, on average, at least twice a week for 3 months.
D. Self-evaluation is unduly influenced by body shape and weight.
E. The disturbance does not occur exclusively during episodes of anorexia nervosa.

Reproduced, with permission, from American Psychiatric Association: *Diagnostic and Statistical Manual of Mental Disorders*, 4th ed, text revision. APA, 2000:326. Copyright 2000 by the American Psychiatric Association.

C. Physical Examination

Whenever suspicion of an eating disorder is raised, a detailed physical and dental examination should be con-

Table 11–5. *DSM-IV-TR* criteria for eating disorder not otherwise specified.

The eating disorder not otherwise specified category is for disorders of eating that do not meet the criteria for any specific eating disorder. Examples include:

1. For females, all of the criteria for anorexia nervosa are met except that the individual has regular menses.
2. All of the criteria for anorexia nervosa are met except that, despite significant weight loss, the individual's current weight is in the normal range.
3. All of the criteria for bulimia nervosa are met except that the binge eating and inappropriate compensatory mechanisms occur at a frequency of less than twice a week or for a duration of less than 3 months.
4. The regular use of inappropriate compensatory behaviors by an individual of normal body weight after eating small amounts of food (eg, self-induced vomiting after the consumption of two cookies).
5. Repeatedly chewing and spitting out, but not swallowing, large amounts of food.
6. Binge eating disorder: recurrent episodes of binge eating in the absence of the regular use of inappropriate behaviors characteristic of bulimia nervosa.

Reproduced, with permission, from American Psychiatric Association: *Diagnostic and Statistical Manual of Mental Disorders*, 4th ed, text revision. APA, 2000:326. Copyright 2000 by the American Psychiatric Association.

ducted (Table 11–6). Complications of AN and BN can affect most organ systems; however, early in the diagnosis the "good-looking" or "normal-weight" patient may elude diagnosis by even the most astute physician. Multilayered, baggy clothing worn by adolescents may be representative of the latest fads in fashion or a significant eating disturbance. Just as baggy clothing may be used to conceal cachexia, patients may use increased fluid consumption and the addition of undergarment weights to normalize their weight prior to weigh-ins.

A thorough physical examination addresses several issues. It may indicate the presence of another condition (eg, Crohn disease or central nervous system lesion [papilledema]) or emphasize to the patient that the body is adapting to an unhealthy state. This objective evidence can be particularly effective, because the use of "scare tactics" to motivate healthy behaviors is usually futile.

One of the most significant disturbances associated with patients undergoing evaluation for eating disorders will be detected by assessing pulse, resting, and other static measurements. These should be assessed at the initial evaluation and at each follow-up. Anorexic patients often have significant bradycardia (< 60 beats per minute in up to 91% of patients in various series). Eighty-five percent of anorexics may have hypotension with pressures lower than 90/60––90/50 secondary to a chronic volume-depleted state. Symptomatic orthostatic hypotension has been suggested as a reason for hospitalization. Cardiac arrhythmias are also common. Abuse of laxatives and diuretics causes the most serious damage for bulimic patients. The misuse of syrup of ipecac to induce vomiting is extremely dangerous in this population and often results in irreversible cardiomyopathy. Assessment of vital signs is critical and often leads to the detection of cardiac arrhythmias (resulting from hypokalemia), metabolic acidosis, hypotension, and faint pulse.

Height, weight, and BMI should also be recorded regularly and at each visit. This is helpful in establishing the patient's weight trends, because few anorexic patients are overweight prior to the onset of their disease. These weight trends also help to identify the patient's failure to gain weight during normal adolescent growth spurts. It is vitally important to obtain accurate readings. Therefore, patients should be weighed in a hospital gown, not in personal clothing, because of the various strategies they employ to disguise their weight loss.

Careful examination of the patient's body should also be performed. Signs of AN such as brittle hair and nails,

Table 11–6. Key components of the physical examination in patients with eating disorders.

Physical examination, including:
- Assessment of vital signs
  - Body temperature (hypothermia: <35.5°C [96°F])
  - Heart rate (bradycardia: <50)
  - Blood pressure (hypotension: 90/50 mm Hg)
- Weight (taken with the patient dressed in a hospital gown) and height assessment should take into account previous height and weight percentiles, anticipated growth, and average weights of healthy adolescents of the same sex, height, and sexual maturation [prepared from National Center for Health Statistics (NCHS) data]
- Evaluation of body mass index (BMI):
  - Quetelet BMI (weight-to-height relationship: defined as weight in kilograms divided by height in meters squared; this BMI is then compared with reference data; percentile tables for BMI for age and sex based on NCHS data have been developed for children and adolescents)

Gynecologic examination (if applicable):
- Pelvic evaluation (atrophic vaginitis)
- Breast evaluation (atrophy)
- Pregnancy testing (where appropriate)
- Sexually transmitted disease testing (where appropriate)

Reproduced, with permission, from Fisher M et al: Eating disorders in adolescents: A background paper. J Adolesc Health 1995;16:420.

dry scaly skin, loss of subcutaneous fat, fine facial and body hair (lanugo hair), carotene pigmentation, breast atrophy, and atrophic vaginitis may be readily observable. Physical examination findings more representative of bulimic patients include the callused finger (Russell sign) used to induce vomiting, dry skin, and dull hair. Periodontal diseases are well-recognized sequelae of BN and may present as erosion of tooth enamel, mouth sores, dental caries, gum inflammation, chipped teeth, and sialadenosis (swelling of the parotid glands).

D. Laboratory Findings

There are no confirmatory laboratory tests specific to the diagnosis of eating disorders, and reported findings may be normal. Nonetheless, screening or baseline evaluations are recommended and should include a complete blood count with differential, urinalysis, blood chemistries (electrolytes, calcium, magnesium, and phosphorus), thyroid function tests, an amenorrhea evaluation, and baseline electrocardiogram, as indicated. Generally speaking, laboratory abnormalities are due to the weight-control habits or methods used by the patient, or the resulting complications.

In the early stages of anorexia, laboratory findings may show elevated BUN, which may be secondary to dehydration; leukopenia due to increased margination of neutrophils; and pancytopenia. In addition, low circulatory levels of LH and FSH, osteopenia and osteoporosis, deficiency of gonadotropin-releasing hormone, low estradiol, elevated cortisol, low triiodothyronine(T_3) and free thyroxine (T_4), an increase in reverse T_3, and hypoglycemia with diminished circulating insulin levels may be observed.

Laboratory testing in bulimic patients is also usually normal. However, when an abnormality is present (ie, metabolic alkalosis), it is usually due to the effects of binge eating and purging. Significant hypokalemia due to purging places the patient at high risk for cardiac arrhythmias, the most common cause of death in bulimics. Hypophosphatemia, metabolic acidosis (secondary to laxative abuse), and osteopenia and osteoporosis (in BN patients with a past history of AN) are also possible findings.

Laboratory findings in male patients with AN are characterized by low testosterone and diminished LH and FSH_9 and decreased testicular volume. Likewise, libido and sexual functioning are diminished in these patients during the starved state. Also of note is the presence of osteopenia in male adolescents and young men with eating disorders. Although relatively common, this is usually an unrecognized clinical problem in these patients.

American Academy of Pediatrics, Committee on Adolescence: Identifying and treating eating disorders. Pediatrics 2003;111:204. [PMID: 12509579]

Gowers S, Bryant-Waugh R: Management of child and adolescent eating disorders: The current evidence base and future directions. J Child Psychol Psychiatry 2004;45:63. [PMID: 14959803]

Differential Diagnosis

In patients presenting with weight loss, other differential diagnoses, both medical and psychiatric, must be considered. Eating disorder symptoms may be caused by numerous medical disorders, including brain tumors, malignancy, connective tissue disease, malabsorption syndrome, hyperthyroidism and infection, gastrointestinal disease (inflammatory bowel disease [IBD], Crohn disease, ulcerative colitis), menstrual irregularities, cystic fibrosis, and substance abuse (eg, cocaine, amphetamines).

The psychiatric differential diagnosis includes affective and major depressive disorders, schizophrenia, obsessive-compulsive disorder, and somatization disorder. However, the diagnosis of an eating disorder is made by confirming, by history and mental state examination, the core psychopathology of a morbid fear for fatness and not by ruling out all conceivable medical causes of weight loss or binge-purge behavior. Because eating disorders and affective disorders have both been shown to have an increased incidence in first-degree relatives of anorexics, a through family history should also be performed.

Carney CP, Andersen AE: Eating disorders. Guide to medical evaluation and complications. Psychiatr Clin North Am 1996; 19:657. [PMID: 8933601]

Davis AJ, Grace E: *Dying to Be Thin: Patients With Anorexia and Bulimia.* Continuing Education Monograph of the North American Society for Pediatric and Adolescent Gynecology, 1999.

Complications

Complications of eating disorders are listed in Table 11–7.

Treatment

Overall, eating disorders present an unusual challenge for clinicians. Much of the denial, resistance, and anger of the patient and occasionally the family may now be directed at the physician. However, awareness that patients with these disorders are frequently ambivalent, desiring but often afraid of recovery and making the physician the target of their emotions and of the inner conflict, serves to facilitate the building of a trusting relationship, the foundation of effective therapy.

A. Early-Stage Eating Disorders

Although it is well documented that the number of girls and boys in elementary, middle, and high schools engaging in dieting and disordered eating behaviors is alarmingly high, most do not progress to classic eating

Table 11–7. Complications of eating disorders.

Cardiovascular	Constipation
Bradycardia	Delayed gastric emptying
Congestive heart failure	Esophageal or gastric rupture
Dysrythmias	Esophagitis
Electrocardiographic abnormalities	Fatty infiltration and focal necrosis of liver
Ipecac-induced cardiomyopathy	Gallstones
Mitral valve prolapse	Intestinal atony
Pericardial effusion	Mallory-Weiss tears
Orthostatic hypotension	Parotid hypertrophy
	Perforation/rupture of the stomach
Dermatologic	Perimolysis and increased incidence of dental caries
Acrocyanosis	Superior mesenteric artery syndrome
Brittle hair and nails	
Carotene pigmentation	**Hematologic**
Edema	Bone marrow suppression
Hair loss	Impaired cell-mediated immunity
Lanugo hair	Low sedimentation rate
Russell sign	
	Neurologic
Endocrine	Cortical atrophy
Amenorrhea	Myopathy
Diabetes insipidus	Peripheral neuropathy
Growth retardation	Seizures
Hypercortisolism	
Hypothermia	**Skeletal**
Low T_3 syndrome	Osteopenia
Pubertal delay	Osteoporosis
	Osteoporotic fracture
Gastrointestinal	
Acute pancreatitis	
Barrett esophagus	
Bloody diarrhea	

disorders. In fact, many of these individuals fall into the *DSM-IV-TR* category of EDNOS. This includes patients who have one or two disordered eating habits and display subthreshold attitudes, behaviors, or signs.

Management of the early or mild stages of an eating disorder diagnosis begins with the assessment of weight loss or weight control and establishment of a working relationship and rapport with the patient and family. Next, the physician focuses on the patient's methods of weight loss or weight control. This opens the door to educating the patient on the importance of maintaining good health—including a discussion of normal eating, nutrition, and exercise—and assisting the patient to establish a goal weight that will serve as a boundary for excessive weight loss.

In addition to the institution of an appropriate diet and weight goal, patients should also be instructed on beginning and maintaining a food diary. This assists the physician in identifying patterns and triggers for dysfunctional habits and gives patients a way of exerting some control over their eating behavior.

Another important component of treatment is to acknowledge the possibility of relapse and have a plan in place. Discussing some of the potential triggers of relapse—relationship problems, family issues (eg, divorce, separation), academic and peer pressure—and the strategies to cope with them can help patients avoid feelings of hopelessness when they are experienced. The patient who relapses should be reevaluated within 3–6 weeks. Information obtained on the follow-up visit is helpful in determining if weight is changing precipitously, if there are changes in physical examination findings, or, most importantly, if the dysfunctional eating habits are more entrenched. These markers help to determine if the patient will require referral.

B. Established Eating Disorders

Patients who clearly meet the criteria for an established eating disorder typically require management by a multidisciplinary team that includes a physician (family physician, pediatrician, or internist), nutritionist or dietician, nurse, mental health professional, and other support staff.

If the family physician is not an integral part of an established eating disorder treatment team, then his or her role is to coordinate and facilitate transfer. This role is critical because the trust in the primary care physician may not be readily transferred to the team of specialists. It is essential that the family physician remain involved in the patient's treatment by providing regular medical assessments, supporting the patient and family, clarifying the tasks performed by each of the team members, reinforcing the importance of the referral, and preventing premature discontinuation of treatment.

Among the various approaches to the management of eating disorders are family therapy, cognitive-behavioral therapy (CBT, a type of short-term psychotherapy), behavior modification, and psychoactive medications. Based on the condition of the patient (see Table 11–6), they may be applied in the inpatient or outpatient setting.

1. Anorexia nervosa—The primary treatment goal for patients with AN is to develop a trusting relationship and restore the patient to a healthy weight. In the female patient, this means a weight at which ovulation and menses can occur; in the male patient, it entails return to normal hormone levels and sexual drive; and in adolescents and children, return to normal physical and sexual maturation. Other goals include treating medical and physical complications, motivating patients to cooperate and participate in treatment education regarding healthy nutrition and eating patterns, treating comorbid psychiatric conditions, encouraging and supporting family participation, and, ultimately, preventing relapse. Because of the variation and severity of symptoms presented, a comprehensive approach to available services and their clinical dimensions must be considered by the multidisciplinary team.

The cornerstone of the multidisciplinary approach to treatment is inpatient or outpatient psychiatric management. Mental health professionals target treatment of the underlying psychological causes and symptoms of eating disorders, including distorted cognitions, body image issues, self-image and ego strength problems, and comorbid conditions (ie, mood and anxiety disorders). They employ various behavioral or psychological therapies, including individual dynamic therapy, family therapy, behavior modification, and CBT. Although these interventions are viewed as distinctly separate treatments, they frequently overlap. For example, the primary responsibility of the nutritional program entails reestablishing normal eating patterns and meeting nutritional requirements for normal maturation. Rehabilitation combines emotional nurturance and any one of a variety of behavioral interventions, which typically combine reinforcers that link exercise, bed rest, and privileges to target weight and desired behaviors. As the patient improves (and gains weight), other types of individual psychotherapeutic modalities may be employed.

The chronic and complex characteristics of AN are also inherent problems in the use of psychosocial modalities for treatment. Although behavior modification and family therapy are often effective during the acute refeeding program, psychodynamic therapies and CBT are not. However, psychotherapy is thought to be very helpful once malnutrition is corrected. Clinicians use the CBT approach to restructure or modify distorted beliefs and attitudes regarding strict food rituals and dichotomous thinking (viewing the world as "black or white," "all or none"). Individual psychodynamic and group therapy are also used by many therapists to address underlying personality disturbances after the acute phase of weight restoration has occurred.

The treatment services available range from intensive inpatient settings, through partial hospital and residential programs, to varying levels of outpatient care. The pretreatment patient evaluation (weight, cardiac, and metabolic status) is essential in determining where treatment will occur. For example, patients who are significantly malnourished, weighing less than 75% of their individually estimated ideal body weight, are likely to require a 24-hour hospital program. For these patients, hospitalization should occur before the onset of medical instability (ie, marked orthostatic hypotension, bradycardia of >40 beats/min, tachycardia >110 beats/min, hypothermia, seizures, cardiac dysrhythmia, or failure), which could otherwise result in greater risks when refeeding and a more problematic prognosis overall. In such patients, hospitalization is based on psychiatric and behavioral grounds such as acute food refusal, uncontrollable binge eating and purging, failure of outpatient management, and comorbid psychiatric diagnosis (Table 11–8).

For milder cases of AN, successful alternatives to intensive inpatient programs have been partial hospitalization and day treatment programs. These programs typically involve a high level of parental participation and are indicative of the patient's motivation to participate in treatment. Initially, these programs require the patient's presence and participation for 14 hours a day. However, as patients approach their target weight, they can be seen in outpatient sessions three times per week. Once the target weight is reached, follow-up is less frequent.

The least intrusive treatment arena is the outpatient setting. Patients selected for treatment in this setting are highly motivated; have brief symptom duration; cooperative, supportive families; no serious medical complications; and BMI greater than 17.5. Their management should also be orchestrated by a multidisciplinary team that includes a primary care physician (family practitioner, pediatrician), nutritionist, psychotherapist, family therapist, and support staff, because success is highly dependent on careful monitoring of weight obtained in a hospital gown and after voiding, orthostatic vital signs, temperature, urine specific gravity, and the patients' eating disorder symptoms and behaviors. As an initial step, a clearly and concisely written behavioral contract with the patient and family (if appropriate) can be established. The contract serves as an agreement to maintain an acceptable mini-

Table 11–8. Criteria for hospitalization.

Any one or more of the following would justify hospitalization:
- Severe malnutrition (weight, 75% ideal body weight)
- Dehydration
- Electrolyte disturbance
- Cardiac dysrhythmia
- Physiologic instability (eg, severe bradycardia, hypotension, hypothermia, orthostatic changes)
- Arrested growth and development
- Failure of outpatient treatment
- Acute food refusal
- Uncontrollable binge eating and purging
- Acute medical complications of malnutrition, such as syncope, seizures, cardiac failure
- Acute psychiatric emergencies, such as suicidal ideation or acute psychosis, and any comorbid diagnosis that interferes with treatment, such as severe depression, obsessive-compulsive disorder, or severe family dysfunction

Reproduced, with permission, from Fisher M et al: Eating disorders in adolescents: A background paper. J Adolesc Health 1995; 16:420.

mum weight and vital signs or be hospitalized. Criteria for treatment failure and hospitalization are also included. However, it should be noted that although behavioral contracts are encouraged, they may not be as effective in the outpatient setting because they are more difficult to monitor. Nonetheless, they are helpful in achieving the goal of outpatient management, which is to get the patient to self-monitor and assume responsibility for appropriate eating.

In the anorexic patient, daily structure is key and should include three meals and several snacks each day. Parents should ensure that healthy foods are readily available and that mealtimes are planned. Although this results in a gradual increase in caloric intake, it may still be necessary to limit physical activity to facilitate weight gain of up to a pound per week. This incremental weight increase prevents the gastric dilation, edema, and congestive heart failure experienced by patients who have restricted their eating for a prolonged period of time.

Psychotropic medications are not useful in treatment of AN when patients are in a malnourished state. However, they are frequently used after sufficient weight restoration has occurred for maintenance and the treatment of other associated psychiatric symptoms. Psychotropic medications other than selective serotonin reuptake inhibitors (SSRIs) are most often used. They include neuroleptics for obsessive-compulsive symptoms and anxiety disorders, and acute anxiety agents to reduce anticipatory anxiety associated with eating.

2. Bulimia nervosa—Most patients with uncomplicated BN do not require hospitalization. Indications for the few patients (<5%) who require inpatient care include severe disabling symptoms that have not responded to outpatient management, binge-purge behavior causing severe physiologic or cardiac disturbances (ie, dysrhythmias, dehydration, metabolic abnormalities), psychiatric disturbances (ie, suicidal ideation or attempts, substance abuse, major depression). If hospitalization is warranted, the treatment focus is on metabolic restoration, nutritional rehabilitation, and mood stabilization. These patients may also require assistance with laxative, diuretic, and illicit drug withdrawal. Hospitalization is usually brief and management then transfers to partial hospitalization programs or outpatient treatment facilities. Partial hospitalization programs usually require the patient to be present 10 hours per day, 5 days a week. Support is usually provided in a group format and family participation is often required. Many of the treatment modalities for BN resemble those for AN. However, the primary focus differs significantly. Although some bulimia patients may be slightly underweight, most are of normal weight; hence nutritional rehabilitation targets the patient's pattern of binging and purging in weight restoration. Therefore, nutritional counseling serves as an adjuvant to other treatment modalities and has been noted to enhance the effectiveness of the overall treatment program.

Interventions targeting the psychosocial aspects surrounding BN address the issues of binging and purging, food restriction, attitudes related to eating patterns, body image and developmental concerns, self-esteem and sexual difficulties, family dysfunction, and comorbid conditions (ie, depression). The most efficacious psychosocial approach is CBT, a relatively short-term approach specifically focused on the eating disorder symptoms and underlying cognitions (ie, low self-esteem, body image concerns) of bulimic patients. Patients managed with CBT demonstrate profound decrements in three very characteristic behaviors: binge eating, vomiting, and laxative abuse. However, the percentage of patients who can achieve total abstinence from binge-purge behavior is invariably small.

Other types of individual psychotherapy that are used in clinical practice are interpersonal, psychodynamic, and psychoanalytic approaches. These approaches may be helpful in treating some of the underlying causes of BN, including comorbid mood, anxiety, trauma, and abuse. BN can also be treated using group psychotherapy. Success is moderate, but improvement and alleviation of symptoms have been maintained at the 1-year follow-up. The efficacy of this approach is increased when it is combined with nutritional counseling and frequent clinic visits. Family or marital therapy should also be considered in conjunction with other treatment modalities for adolescents living at home, older patients from dysfunctional homes, and patients experiencing marital discord.

Another important aspect of eating disorder management is pharmacotherapy with antidepressants (ie, SSRIs). These agents were first used in the acute phase of treatment for BN because of its well-established comorbid association with clinical depression. It was later reported that nondepressed patients also responded to these medications. Multiple clinical studies have shown the SSRIs to have an antibulimic (reduction in binge eating and vomiting rates) effect independent of their antidepressant effect. Therapists have also noted improvement in mood and anxiety symptoms. Other antidepressant medications used in the treatment of BN include the tricyclic antidepressants (imipramine-desipramine), the monoamine oxidase inhibitors (MAOIs; phenelzine and isocarboxazid). The MAOIs should be used with great caution and only in patients with severe BN. At this time, fluoxetine is the only SSRI approved by the Food and Drug Administration for the treatment of BN. A 20 mg/day dose is used to initiate treatment, with doses of 40–60 mg/day required for maintenance.

3. Binge eating problems—Although most individuals with binge eating problems are obese, normal-weight people are also affected. Therefore, treatment usually focuses on the distress experienced by individuals rather than on their weight problem. Several treatment modalities are available, including CBT, antidepressants, behavioral and group therapy, and self-help groups. All are effective to varying degrees; however,

CBT, which teaches techniques to monitor eating habits and alternative responses to difficult situations, appears to be the most efficacious. The great majority of those affected can be treated as outpatients and hospitalization is rarely needed.

American Psychiatric Association: Clinical Guidelines for Eating Disorders. Available at: http://www.psychorg/clin_res/guide.bk_2.cfm.

Fisher M: Treatment of eating disorders in children, adolescents, and young adults. Pediatr Rev 2006;27:5. [PMID: 16387924]

Kreipe RE, Yussman SM: The role of the primary care practitioner in the treatment of eating disorders. Adolesc Med 2003; 14:133. [PMID: 12529197]

Prognosis

The prognosis for full recovery of patients with AN is modest. Many individuals demonstrate symptomatic improvement over time, but a substantial number have persistent problems with body image, disordered eating, and psychological challenges. A review of multiple carefully conducted follow-up studies of hospitalized populations (at least 4 years after onset of illness) showed that the outcomes for 44% could be rated as good (weight restored to within 15% of recommended weight for height; regular menses established), 24% were poor (weight never reached 15% of recommended weight for height; menses absent or sporadic), about 28% fell between the good and poor groups, and about 5% had died (early mortality). About two thirds of patients continued to have morbid food and weight preoccupation and psychiatric symptoms, and about 40% continued to have bulimic symptoms. Lower initial weight, previous treatment failure, vomiting, family dysfunction, and being married have all been associated with a worse prognosis. Adolescents have better outcomes than adults, and younger adolescents have better outcomes than older adolescents.

The outcomes for patients with BN are less certain. Generally speaking, the short-term success rate for patients treated with psychosocial modalities and medication is reported to be 50–70%, with relapse rates between 30% and 50% after 6 months to 6 years of follow-up. Data also suggest that slow, steady progress continues when the follow-up period is extended 10–15 years.

Characteristically, bulimic patients who have onset at an early age, milder symptoms at start of treatment, a good support system, and those more likely to be treated as outpatients, often have a better prognosis. In summary, bulimic patients typically have one or more relapses during recovery whereas anorexic patients generally have a more protracted and arduous course, requiring long-term, intensive therapy.

Agras WS et al: Outcome predictors for cognitive behavior treatment of bulimia nervosa: Data from a multisite study. Am J Psychiatry 2000;157:1302. [PMID: 10910795]

Becker AE et al: Genes and/or jeans?: Genetic and socio-cultural contributions to risk for eating disorders. J Addict Dis 2004; 23:81. [PMID: 15256346]

Adolescent Sexuality 12

Margaret R. H. Nusbaum, DO, MPH, & Peter J. Katsufrakis, MD, MBA

Although nearly 90% of parents want their children to have it, 23 states require it, 13 other states encourage its teaching, and over 90 national organizations believe that all children should have it, only 5% of children in the United States receive sex education. Adolescence is a time of tremendous physical and emotional turmoil. Family and cultural values, as well as personal experiences, including fears, lead to different sex education needs, such as understanding their bodies and body functions, exploring personal values, and setting sexual limits with partners. Unfortunately, not only parents but many clinicians are ill prepared to discuss health issues related to sex with adolescents. Additionally, teens may be uncomfortable discussing sexual issues with their peers and adults. This leaves adults with the responsibility for facilitating the discussion.

Lack of comprehensive sex education programs as well as differences in cognitive and physical maturity put adolescents at increased risk for unwanted or unhealthy consequences of sexual activity. This includes increased susceptibility for contracting sexually transmitted diseases and increased risk for morbidity associated with sexual activity.

Sexuality Information and Education Council of the United States: *Guidelines for Comprehensive Sexuality Education: Kindergarten–12th Grade,* 3rd ed. National Guidelines Task Forces, 2004.

SCOPE OF THE PROBLEM

Unwanted & Unhealthy Consequences of Sexual Activity

About 50% of US adolescents begin having sexual intercourse between the ages of 15 and 18 years, over 50% of adolescent girls and nearly 75% of adolescent boys have had sexual intercourse by the time they graduate from high school, and nearly 90% have had sexual intercourse by age 22. About 40% of all 15- to 19-year-olds have had sexual intercourse in the past 3 months. For adolescents who want to have intercourse, the primary reasons given are sexual curiosity (50% of boys; 24% of girls) and affection for their partner (25% of boys; 48% of girls). For adolescents who agree to have intercourse but do not really want to, the primary reasons given are peer pressure (about 30%), curiosity (50% of boys; 25% of girls), and affection for their partner (> 33%). With little sex education, adolescents are poorly prepared to openly discuss their need for contraception, negotiate safe sex, and negotiate the types of behavior in which they are willing to participate. Sexual behavior that contradicts personal values is associated with emotional distress and lower self-esteem. As adolescents are learning to develop appropriate interpersonal skills, damage to self-esteem can be significant when sexual activity is exchanged for attention, affection, peer approval, or reassurance about their physical appearance. Furthermore, early unsatisfactory sexual experiences can set up patterns for repeated unsatisfactory sexual experiences into adulthood.

Unintended Pregnancy

Nearly 50% of all pregnancies in the United States are not planned, with the highest rates of unintended pregnancies occurring among adolescents, lower income women, and black women. About 10% of 15- to 19-year-olds become pregnant every year and more than 40% become pregnant before age 20. Despite similar rates of adolescent sexual activity, the United States has the highest rate of adolescent pregnancy among developed nations.

Unintended pregnancy is socially and economically costly. Medical costs include lost opportunity for preconception care and counseling, increased likelihood of late or no prenatal care, increased risk for a low-birth-weight infant, and increased risk for infant mortality. The social costs include reduced educational attainment and employment opportunity, increased welfare dependency, and increased risk of child abuse and neglect. In addition to being confronted with adult problems prematurely, adolescent parents' ability to lead productive and healthy lives and to achieve academic and economic success is compromised.

Although abortion rates are higher for women in their 20s, accounting for 80% of total induced abortions, a greater proportion of adolescent pregnancies end in abortion (29%) than do pregnancies for women over 20 years of age (21%). Adolescents who terminate pregnancies are less likely to become pregnant over the next 2 years, more likely to graduate from high school, and more likely to show lower anxiety, higher self-esteem, and more internal control than adolescents who do not terminate pregnancies. For an adolescent, postponement of childbearing appears to improve social, psychological, academic, and economic outcomes of life (see Chapter 16).

Sexually Transmitted Diseases

Adolescents (10–19 years old) and young adults (20–24 years old) have the highest rate of sexually transmitted diseases, and rates of chlamydial and gonorrheal infection are highest among women aged 15–19 years. Additionally, one in five cases of AIDS in the United States is diagnosed in men and women aged 20–29 years, with the likelihood that HIV infection was acquired up to 10 years earlier. Education is key to preventing sexually transmitted diseases, and vaccination for hepatitis B and human papillomavirus—if not already done prior to adolescence—can reduce disease risk in this population (see Chapter 14).

Sexual Abuse

More than 100,000 children are victims of sexual abuse each year. Sexual abuse contributes to sexual and mental health dysfunction as well as public health problems such as substance abuse. Victims of sexual abuse may have greater difficulty with identity formation as well as problems establishing and maintaining healthy relationships with others. Additionally, they may engage in premature sexual behavior, frequently seeking immediate release of sexual tension, and have poor sexual decision-making skills, attempting to create intimacy through sex.

Although only a relatively small proportion of rapes are reported, a major national study found that 22% of women and approximately 2% of men had been victims of a forced sexual act. Unfortunately, adolescent boys are more likely to believe that sexual coercion is justifiable.

Delinquency and homelessness are associated with a history of physical, emotional, and sexual abuse, as well as negative parental reactions to sexual orientation. Homelessness is associated with exchanging sex for money, food, or drugs. Additionally, homeless adolescents are at high risk for repeated episodes of sexual assault.

Institute of Medicine; Brown SS, Eisenberg L, eds: *The Best Intentions: Unintended Pregnancy and the Well-Being of Children and Families.* National Academy Press, 1995.

Institute of Medicine; Eng TR, Butler WT, eds: *The Hidden Epidemic: Confronting Sexually Transmitted Diseases.* National Academy Press, 1997.

US Department of Health and Human Services: *Child Maltreatment 1998: Reports from the States to the National Child Abuse and Neglect Data System.* Government Printing Office, 2000.

DEVELOPMENT

Adolescence is a time of complex physical, psychosocial, sexual, and cognitive changes. With earlier onset of puberty, physical changes occur in advance of cognitive changes. Not until maturity is reached in all of these realms does the adolescent acquire mature decision-making skills and the ability to make healthy decisions regarding sexual activity. Sexuality involves more than just anatomic gender or physical sexual behavior; it incorporates how individuals view themselves as male or female, how they relate to others, and their ability to enter into and maintain an intimate relationship on a giving and trusting basis. Adolescents who are sexually active before having achieved the capacity for intimacy are at risk for unwanted or unhealthy consequences of sexual activity. Adolescent sexual development forms the basis for further adult sexuality and future intimate relationships. The child's successful achievements during each stage have major implications for both physical and psychosocial development, positive self-concept, and, ultimately, healthy sexuality.

Physical Changes

Adolescents often feel uncomfortable, clumsy, and self-conscious because of the rapid changes in their bodies. Disproportionate physical development among girls and boys contributes additionally to the awkwardness of adolescence. Adolescents must adapt to a new physical identity, which includes hormonal changes, menstruation (often irregular or unpredictable for the first 18–24 months), unpredictable spontaneous erections, nocturnal ejaculations ("wet dreams"), growth of pubic and axillary hair, and even the odors from maturing apocrine glands, necessitating deodorant use.

As adolescents are learning to adjust and grow comfortable with their changing bodies, questions concerning body image are common (eg, penis size, breast size and development, distribution of pubic hair, and changing physique in general). In addition to adapting to a new body, adolescents must develop social skills and learn to interact with peers and adults.

Psychosocial Changes

Adolescent psychosocial development necessitates that the adolescent develop a realistic and positive self-image and identity. Adolescent identity includes the development of physical, cognitive, and social skills; emotional and spiritual maturity; and sexual identity, including sexual orientation. Adolescents must develop the ability not only to view themselves realistically but also to relate to others. This necessitates successfully achieving independence from the family. Successful acquisition of a stable sense of self allows the adolescent to move on to face the task of the young adult: achieving intimacy by developing openness, mutual trust, sharing, self-abandon, and commitment to another. Core developmental tasks of adolescence include the following:

1. Developing independence: becoming emotionally and behaviorally independent rather than dependent; in particular, developing independence from the family.
2. Acquiring educational and other experiences needed for adult work roles and developing a realistic vocational goal.
3. Learning to deal with emerging sexuality and to achieve a mature level of sexuality.
4. Resolving issues of identity (essentially being reborn) and achieving a realistic and positive self-image.
5. Developing interpersonal skills, including the capacity for intimacy, and preparing for intimate partnering with others.

This development includes both internal (introspective) and external forces. Peers, parents or guardians, teachers, and coaches have an important influence on adolescent expectations, evaluations, values, feedback, and social comparison. Failure to accomplish the developmental tasks necessary for adulthood results in identity or role diffusion: an uncertain self-concept, indecisiveness, and clinging to the more secure dependencies of childhood. With physical, cognitive, and social changes, it is natural for adolescents to explore sexual relationships and sexual roles in their social interactions, which contributes to self-identity. The adolescent's task is to successfully manage the conflict between sexual drives and the recognition of the emotional, interpersonal, and biological results of sexual behavior.

Sexual Changes

Gender identity forms a foundation for sexual identity. Gender identity, the sense of maleness or femaleness, is established by age 2 years, solidifying as adolescents experience and integrate sexuality into their identity.

Sexual identity is the erotic expression of self as male or female and the awareness of self as a sexual being who can be in a sexual relationship with others. The task of adolescence is to integrate sexual orientation into sexual identity. Heterosexual orientation is taken for granted by society. For lesbian and gay individuals, this creates a clash between outside cultural expectations and their inner sense of self. Currently in US society, the primary developmental task of the gay adolescent is to adapt to a socially stigmatized sexual role. Same-sex orientation emerges during adolescence but is far more subtle and complex; it includes behavior, sexual attraction, erotic fantasy, emotional preference, social preference, and self-identification—felt to be a continuum from completely heterosexual to completely homosexual (see Chapter 62).

Sexual orientation is typically determined by adolescence, or earlier, and there is no valid scientific evidence that sexual orientation can be changed. Nonetheless, society often stigmatizes homosexual behavior, identity, and relationships. These antihomosexual attitudes are associated with significant psychological distress for gay, lesbian, and bisexual (GLB) persons and have a negative impact on mental health, including a greater incidence of depression and suicide (as many as one third have attempted suicide at least once), lower self-acceptance, and a greater likelihood of hiding sexual orientation. When GLB adolescents disclose their orientation to their families, they often experience overt rejection at home as well as social isolation. GLB adolescents often lack role models and access to support systems. They frequently run away and become homeless, which places them at higher risk for unsafe sex, drug and alcohol use, and exchanging sex for money or drugs. Although the research is limited, transgendered persons are reported to experience similar problems. Negative attitudes within society toward gay, lesbian, bisexual, and transgendered (GLBT) individuals lead to antigay violence. Media coverage of the Matthew Shepard case brought such violence to greater public awareness. Data from over two dozen studies indicate that 80% of gay men and lesbians have experienced verbal or physical harassment on the basis of their orientation, 45% have been threatened with violence, and 17% have experienced a physical attack.

Adolescents with questions or concerns about sexual orientation need the opportunity to talk about their feelings, their experiences, and their fears of exposure to family and friends. GLBT adolescents need reassurance about their value as a person, support regarding parental and societal reactions, and access to role models. Parents, Families and Friends of Lesbians and Gays (PFLAG) is a nationwide organization whose purpose is to assist parents with information and support (see Chapter 62).

Problems with sexual identity may manifest in extremes—sexually acting out or repression of sexuality. Frequent sexual activity and a variety of sexual partners, negative risk factors for physical or psychological health, suggest poor integration of sexual identity in adolescents. Sexual behavior might be used to gain a sense of security in terms of gender and sexual identity or to gain acceptance or status in a peer group.

Cognitive Changes

Cognitively, the shift from concrete thinking to abstract thinking (the cognitive development of formal operations) begins in early adolescence (11–12 years) and usually reaches full development by 15–16 years—so 10- to 14-year-olds should not be expected to function with full capacity for abstract thinking. In contrast to younger children, adolescents:

- Show an increased ability to generate and hold in mind more than one complex mental representation.
- Show an appreciation of the relativity and uncertainty of knowledge.
- Tend to think in terms of abstract rather than only concrete representations; they think of consequences and the future (abstract) versus a sense of being omnipotent, invincible, infallible, and immune to mishaps (concrete).
- Show a far greater use of strategies for obtaining knowledge, such as active planning and evaluation of alternatives.
- Are self-aware in their thinking, being able to reflect on their own thought processes and evaluate the credibility of the knowledge source.
- Understand that fantasies are not acted out.
- Have the capacity to develop intimate, meaningful relationships.

Adolescents have the task of figuring out what should and should not be done sexually. In concrete thinking risks of sexual behavior are not completely understood or thought out. Abstract thinking allows the capacity for responsible sexual decision making. The concept of relationship is abstract. Sexual intimacy includes not only eroticism but also a sense of commitment: emotional closeness, mutual caring, vulnerability, and trust. The level of intimacy and cognitive development influences sexual decision making. It is estimated that one third of the adult population may never have fully achieved operational thinking.

American Psychiatric Association: *Position Statement on Therapies Focused on Attempts to Change Sexual Orientation (Reparative or Conversion Therapies)*. APA, 2000.

Auslander BA et al: Sexual development and behaviors of adolescents. Pediatr Ann 2005;34:785. [PMID: 16285632]

Ponton LE, Judice S: Typical adolescent sexual development. Child Adolesc Psychiatr Clin N Am 2004;13:497. [PMID: 1518337]

SEXUAL BEHAVIOR & INITIATION OF SEXUAL ACTIVITY

Adolescents often learn about sexuality from a wide range of sources outside of school (family, friends, television, movies, advertising, magazines, the Internet, partners, church, and youth organizations). In addition to physical changes, early to middle-stage adolescents begin to experience sexual urges that may be satisfied by masturbation. Masturbation is the exploration of the sexual self and provides a sense of control over one's body and sexual needs. Masturbation starts in infancy, providing children with enjoyment of their bodies. Parents are typically uncomfortable observing this behavior. In contrast to this activity in younger children, masturbation in adolescents is accompanied by fantasies. In early adolescence, masturbation is an important developmental task, allowing the adolescent to learn what forms of self-stimulation are pleasurable and integrating this with fantasies of interacting with another. Sexual curiosity intensifies. Typical reasons for sexual activity in early to mid-adolescence are curiosity, peer pressure, seeking approval, physical urges, and rebellion. Sexual activity can be misinterpreted by the adolescent as evidence of independence from the family or individuation. With older adolescents, the autoeroticism of masturbation develops into experimentation with others, including intercourse.

Adolescent girls may misinterpret sexual activity as a measure of a meaningful relationship. When sexual activity is used to meet needs such as self-esteem, popularity, and dependency, it delays or prevents developing a capacity for intimacy and is associated with casual and less responsible sexual activity. The adolescent must emerge from the transitional stage of sexual development into relational sexual intimacy by participating in sexual activities in a mature and responsible manner. Sexual activity then becomes an expression of the depth and meaningfulness of the relationship. Mature and responsible sexual activity is not used to satisfy social or personal needs, is neither coercive nor exploitive, and occurs in an atmosphere of trust and respect in which each individual feels free to engage or refuse to engage. Sexual intimacy typically includes identity as a "couple."

Appropriate education, parental support, and a positive sexual self-concept are associated with a later age of first intercourse, a higher consistent use of contraceptives, and a lower pregnancy rate. Sexual self-concept seems to improve with age.

Parental supervision and limit setting, living with both parents in a stable environment, high self-esteem, higher family income, and orientation toward achievement are associated with delayed initiation of sexual activity.

Commitment to a religion or affiliation with certain religious denominations appears to have an effect on sexual behavior. For example, an adolescent's frequent attendance at religious services is associated with a greater likelihood of abstinence. On the other hand, for adolescents who are sexually active, frequency of attendance is associated with decreased contraceptive use by girls and increased use by boys.

Evidence suggests that school attendance reduces adolescent sexual risk-taking behavior. Worldwide, as the percentage of girls completing elementary school has increased, adolescent birth rates have decreased. In the United States, adolescents who have dropped out of school are more likely to initiate sexual activity earlier, fail to use contraception, become pregnant, and give birth. Among those who remain in school, greater involvement with school, including athletics for girls, is related to less sexual risk taking, including later age of initiation of sex and lower frequency of sex, pregnancy, and childbearing.

Schools structure students' time, creating an environment that discourages unhealthy risk taking, particularly by increasing interactions between children and adults. They also affect selection of friends and larger peer groups. Schools can increase belief in the future and help adolescents plan for higher education and careers, and they can increase students' sense of competence, as well as their communication and refusal skills. Parents vary widely in their own knowledge about sexuality, as well as their emotional capacity to explain essential health issues related to sex to their children. Schools often have access to training and communications technology and also provide an opportunity for the kind of positive peer learning that can influence social norms.

Evaluation of school-based sex education programs that typically emphasize abstinence, but also discuss condoms and other methods of contraception, indicates that the programs either have no effect on, or, in some cases, result in a delay in the initiation of sexual activity. There is strong evidence that providing information about contraception does not increase adolescent sexual activity by hastening the onset of sexual intercourse, increasing the frequency of sexual intercourse, or increasing the number of sexual partners. More importantly, providing this information results in increased use of condoms or contraceptives among adolescents who were already sexually active.

Early age of first intercourse and lack of contraceptive use are associated with early pubertal development, a history of sexual abuse, lower socioeconomic status, poverty, lack of attentive and nurturing parents, single-parent homes, cultural and familial patterns of early sexual experience, lack of school or career goals, and dropping out of school. Additional factors include low self-esteem, concern for physical appearance, peer group pressure, and pressure to please partners.

Compared with those not sexually active, sexually active male adolescents used more alcohol, engaged in more fights, and were more likely to know about HIV and AIDS. Similarly sexually active female adolescents used more alcohol and cigarettes. Both sexually active male and female adolescents had higher levels of stress. Alcohol and drug use is associated with greater risk taking, including unprotected sexual activity.

Coyle K et al: Short-term impact of Safer Choices: A multi-component school-based HIV, other STD and pregnancy prevention program. J Sch Health 1999;69:181. [PMID: 10363221]

Kirby D: Effective approaches to reducing adolescent unprotected sex, pregnancy, and childbearing. J Sex Res 2002;39:51. [PMID: 12476257]

Kirby DB et al: The "Safer Choices" intervention: Its impact on the sexual behaviors of different subgroups of high school students. J Adolesc Health 2004;35:442. [PMID: 15581523]

SOURCES OF INFORMATION

The Family

Although not the most important source of information about sexuality, parents exert more influence on sexual attitudes. Furthermore, parent-adolescent communication mediates the strength of peer influence on sexual activity. Adolescents need stable environments, parenting that promotes healthy social and emotional development, and protection from abuse. They also need education, the development of skills, experiences that promote self-esteem, and access to sex health information and services, along with positive expectations and sound preparation for their future roles as partners in committed relationships and as parents.

Several family factors are known to be associated with increased adolescent sexual behavior and the risk of pregnancy. These include living with a single parent; having older siblings who have had sexual intercourse, have become pregnant, or have given birth; and, for girls, the experience of sexual abuse in the family. Family factors associated with decreased sexual activity and increased use of contraception include parents with higher education and income; close, warm parent-child relationships; and parental supervision and monitoring of children. However, parental control can be associated with negative effects if it is excessive or coercive.

The developmental tasks of adolescence include the transition from dependence on family to establishing an independent identity. The stresses of families tend to peak during adolescence, which is attributed to the desire among adolescents for an independent identity, the parents' own unresolved parent-child conflicts, and possible changing gender role identities. Additionally, adolescent sexuality can be very threatening to adults, who may not have resolved their own issues concerning sexuality. With escalating stresses, the self-esteem of parents may decline, making them either highly impulsive or overly controlling or rigid. Heightening levels of anxiety contribute to blocked communication.

Both parental lack of rules and discipline as well as very strict discipline have been strongly associated with adolescent sexual activity, whereas parents who supervised their children's dating and insisted on reasonable curfews were least likely to have adolescents who exhibited irresponsible sexual behaviors.

Because many parents are uncomfortable discussing sexuality with their children, family physicians must be

Table 12–1. How to talk to your child about sex.

1. **Be available.** Watch for clues that show they want to talk. Remember that your comfort with the subject is important. They need to get a feeling of trust from you. If your child doesn't ask, look for ways to bring up the subject. For example, you may know a pregnant woman, watch the birth of a pet, or see a baby getting a bath. Use a TV program or film to start a discussion. Libraries and schools have good books about sex for all ages.
2. **Answer their questions** honestly and without showing embarrassment, even if the time and place do not seem appropriate. A short answer may be best for the moment. Then return to the subject later. It's OK to say, "I don't know." Not being able to answer a question can be an opportunity to learn with your child. Tell your child that you'll get the information and continue the discussion later, or do the research together. Be sure to do this soon. Answer the question that is asked. Respect your child's desire for information. But don't overload the child with too much information at once. Try to give enough information to answer the question clearly, yet encourage further discussion.
3. **Use correct names** for body parts and their functions to show that they are normal and OK to talk about.
4. **Practice talking about sex** with your partner, another family member, or a friend. This will help you feel more comfortable when you do talk with your child.
5. **Talk about sex more than once.** Children need to hear things again and again over the years to really understand, because their level of understanding changes as they grow older. Make certain that you talk about feelings and not just actions. It is important not to think of sex only in terms of intercourse, pregnancy, and birth. Talk about feeling oneself as man or woman, relating to others' feelings, thoughts, and attitudes, and feelings of self-esteem.
6. **Respect their privacy.** Privacy is important, for both you and your child. If your child doesn't want to talk, say, "OK, let's talk about it later," and do. Don't forget about it. Never search a child's room, drawers, or purse for "evidence." Never listen in on a telephone or private conversation.
7. **Listen to your children.** They want to know that their questions and concerns are important. The world they're growing up in is different from what yours was. Laughing at or ignoring a child's question may stop them from asking again. They will get information, accurate or inaccurate, from other sources. When the problem belongs to your child, listen, watch their body language to know when they are ready for you to talk, repeat back to them what you think you heard, listen, respond, and guide them through solving their problem. Talk to your children, trust them, have confidence in them, and respect their feelings.
8. **Share your values.** If your jokes, behaviors, or attitudes don't show respect for sexuality, then you cannot expect your child to be sexually healthy. They learn attitudes about love, caring, and responsibility from you, whether you talk about it or not. Tell your child what your values are about sex and about life. Find out what they value in their lives. Talk about your concern for their health and their future.
9. **Make it easier for your children to talk with you.** Choose words wisely to keep communication open. Use "I" statements because "you" statements can sound accusatory or like a put-down. Instead of telling them what to do, share your values but don't try to control your children. If you act in a controlling manner by telling them what to do, your reaction is likely to lead to their being resentful, insecure, or even rebellious. But you don't want to give them freedom without responsibility for their actions as they are likely to become self-centered, demanding, or even anxious. Teach your child how to make decisions: (a) have your child identify the problem, (b) analyze the situation, (c) search for options or solutions, (d) think about possible consequences to these options, (e) choose the best option, (f) take action, and then (g) watch for the results.

Sources: Facts of Life Netline: Planned Parenthood of Toronto; and Adolescent Sexuality: A Guide for Parents. Tape #5. Adolescent Wellness Series by Health Learning Systems, Inc., Lyndhurst, NJ, 1990.

proactive in initiating and facilitating conversations about the topic.

The Family Physician

Adolescents, in a developmental phase between childhood and adulthood, are often uncomfortable with body changes. Encouraging open communication at home is crucial. Making a handout (Table 12–1) available to parents might help facilitate discussions about sexuality. The quality of discussions at home about sexual matters is the most important factor of family life affecting the risk of teenage pregnancy. If information is not available at home, the family physician, uniquely positioned to serve as a resource, should take a proactive approach by creating the proper environment for discussion, initiating the topic of sexuality, and providing anticipatory guidance for both adolescents and their families (Table 12–2).

A. Creating the Environment

The physician should provide a confidential place that fosters open and nonjudgmental communication, which augments or fulfills the parental role. The individuation of the adolescent should be supported by having a separate discussion with parents or guardians and adolescent. Ensuring confidentiality for the preadolescent or adolescent helps create a trusting environment. An office letter

Table 12–2. Office approach to adolescent health care.

1. Establish comfortable, friendly relationships that permit discussion in an atmosphere of mutual trust well before sensitive issues arise. Ensure confidentiality before the need arises. Establish separate discussions with parents and adolescents as a matter of routine.
2. Take a firm, proactive role to initiate developmentally appropriate discussions of sexuality. Recognize and use teachable moments regarding sexuality.
3. Provide anticipatory guidance and resources to facilitate family discussions about sexuality and cue families and preteens about upcoming physical and psychosocial developmental changes.
4. Enhance communication skills. Use reflective listening. With a nonjudgmental manner, accept what adolescents have to say without agreeing or disagreeing.
5. Use a positive approach when discussing developmental changes and needed interventions, complementing pubertal changes.
6. Increase knowledge of family systems and the impact physicians can have on the family.
7. Discuss topics about sexuality incrementally over time to improve assimilation and decrease embarrassment. Avoid scientific terms. Keep answers to questions thorough yet simple. Be cautious about questions that might erode trust.
8. Know your limitations. Use other professional staff and referrals when necessary.

Reproduced, with permission, from Croft CA, Asmussen L: A developmental approach to sexuality education: Implications for medical practice. J Adolesc Health 1993;14:109.

to the parent can outline policies regarding confidentiality and clearly communicate the desire to work with parents in making the office as accessible to adolescents as possible. Many states have particular laws regarding the ability of adolescents to seek health care for specific issues—such as contraception, mental health, substance abuse, and pregnancy—without parental presence or approval. Family physicians need to be familiar with the nuances of these laws in their practicing state.

B. Proactive Approach

Physicians should recognize opportunities to provide anticipatory guidance, such as to adults who are seeing them for their health needs and mention having a preteen or teen at home. They should cue the preteen positively about upcoming physical changes and cue the parent or family by recommending that issues concerning sex be discussed with the adolescent at home. In the office and at home, sexuality should be discussed incrementally over time. Parents are more influential in early adolescence whereas peer groups are more influential in later adolescence; the extent to which adolescents can balance these two factors influences their risk-taking behavior.

C. Asking the Question

Family physicians should initiate the topic of sexuality with adolescents during health maintenance or perhaps even acute care visits. Questions might include the following: Are you dating? Whom are you attracted to? Conversations about sexuality should be tailored to the adolescent's stage of physical, social, and emotional development (Table 12–3). Because abstract thinking is still undergoing development, adolescents need explicit examples to understand ideas. History taking must be specific and directive. Instructions should be concrete. Answers to questions should be simple and thorough.

Concerns in early adolescence typically relate to body image and what is "normal," both physically and socially. Information and reassurance about pubertal changes are critical parts of physical examinations. Conversations may include addressing concerns about obesity, acne, and body image that affect self-perception of acceptability and attractiveness. Discussions about how to handle peer pressure may always be helpful. The adolescent's understanding of safer sexual practices as well as the ability to negotiate the behavior in which they are willing or not willing to participate should be explored. Giving the adolescent the opportunity to role-play the discussion regarding these issues may contribute to confidence in successfully negotiating with a current or future partner.

Although it is important not to make assumptions about sexual orientation, an adolescent who presents with depression and suicidal ideation should be questioned about this. Hiding one's orientation increases stress. It is important to be aware of community resources for GLBT adolescents such as psychologists and counselors, GLBT community support groups, and organizations such as PFLAG.

Caring for adolescents can be exciting and challenging. Physicians should recognize that their own projections of unfinished sexual issues from their adolescence may surface in caring for adolescent patients. This can make discussions, particularly about sensitive subjects such as drugs, alcohol, nicotine, and sex, difficult. Recognizing and addressing these issues or referring adolescents to colleagues with greater experience and comfort with these matters would be appropriate.

The role of family physicians is to provide a supportive, sensitive, and instructive environment in which they neither ignore nor judge adolescent sexual activity but reassure, listen, clarify, and provide correct information about this important aspect of adolescent development. Consultation or referral is appropriate when it is in the best interest of the patient. Open and frank communication, ensuring confidentiality, nonjudg-

Table 12–3. Adolescent sexual development.

	8–12 Years	13 Years and Older
Sexual knowledge	Knows correct terms for sexual parts, commonly uses slang. Understands sexual aspects of pregnancy. Increasing knowledge of sexual behavior: masturbation, intercourse. Knowledge of physical aspects of puberty by age 10.	Understands sexual intercourse, contraception, and sexually transmitted diseases (STDs).
Body parts and function	Should have complete understanding of sexual, reproductive, and elimination functions of body parts. All need anticipatory guidance on upcoming pubertal changes for both sexes, including menstruation and nocturnal emissions.	Important to discuss health and hygiene, as well as provide more information about contraceptives, STDs/HIV, and responsible sexual behaviors. Access to health care, especially gynecologic care, is important.
Gender identity	Gender identity is fixed. Encouragement to pursue individual interests and talents regardless of gender stereotypes is important.	Discuss men and women in social perception. Males tend to perceive social situations more sexually than females and may interpret neutral cues (eg, clothing, friendliness, etc) as sexual invitations.
Sexual abuse prevention	Assess their understanding of an abuser and correct misconceptions. Explain how abusers, including friends, relatives, and strangers, may manipulate children. Help them to identify abusive situations, including sexual harassment. Practice assertiveness and problem solving skills. Teach them to trust their body's internal cues and to act assertively in problematic situations.	Teach them to avoid risky situations (eg, walking alone at night, unsafe parts of town). Discuss dating relationships and, in particular, date/acquaintance rape and its association with alcohol and drug use, including date rape drugs. Encourage parents to make themselves available for a ride home anytime their teenager finds himself or herself in a difficult or potentially dangerous situation. Consider a self-defense class for children.
Sexual behavior	Sex games with peers and siblings: role-play and sex fantasy, kissing, mutual masturbation, and simulated intercourse. Masturbation in private. Shows modesty, embarrassment: hides sex games and masturbation from adults. May fantasize or dream about sex. Interested in media sex. Uses sexual language with peers. Talk about making decisions in the context of relationships. Provide information about contraceptives, STDs/HIV, and responsible sexual behaviors.	Pubertal changes continue: most girls menstruate by 16, boys capable of ejaculation by 15. Dating begins. Sexual contacts are common: mutual masturbation, kissing, petting. Sexual fantasy and dreams. Sexual intercourse may occur in up to 75% by age 18. Encourage parents to share attitudes and values. Provide access to contraceptives. Respect need and desire for privacy. Set clear rules about dating and curfews.
Developmental issues:[1] most sexual concerns are related to the developmental tasks.	Early adolescence (Tanner I and II): Physical changes, including menstruation and nocturnal emissions. Often ambivalent over issues of independence and protection and family relationships. Egocentric. Beginning struggles of separation and emerging individual identity. Seemingly trivial concerns to adults can reach crisis proportions in young adolescents. Common concerns include fears of too slow or too rapid physical development, especially breasts and genitalia; concern and curiosity about their bodies; sexual feelings; and sexual behavior of their peer group as well as adults around them. Although masturbation is very healthy and normal, reassurance may be needed given persistence of myths and mixed messages.	Middle adolescence (Tanner III and IV): Peer approval. Experimentation and risk-taking behavior arise out of the developmental task of defining oneself socially. Sexual intercourse may be viewed as requisite for peer acceptance. Curiosity, need for peer approval, self-esteem, and struggle for independence from parents can lead to intercourse at this stage. Feelings of invincibility lead to sexual activity that is impulsive and lacking discussion about sexual decision making, such as contraception, preferences for behavior, relationship commitment, or safe sex. Increasing insistence on control over decisions. Increasing conflict with parents.

(continued)

Table 12–3. Adolescent sexual development. (Continued)

	8–12 Years	13 Years and Older
	Developmental tasks: 1. Independence and separation from the family. 2. Development of individual identity. 3. Beginning to shift from concrete to abstract thinking.	Developmental tasks: 1. Development of adult social relationships with both sexes. 2. Continued struggle for independence. 3. Continued development of individual identity. 4. Continued shifting from cognitive to abstract thinking. Late adolescence (Tanner V): With cognitive maturation, issues regarding peer acceptance and conflicts with parents regarding independence lessen. Intimacy, commitment, and life planning, including thoughts of future parenthood. Self-identity continues to solidify, moral and ethical values, exploration of sexual identity. Crises over sexual orientation may surface at this stage. Increasing ability to recognize consequences of own behavior. Developmental tasks: 1. Abstract (futuristic) thinking. 2. Vocational plans. 3. Development of moral and ethical values. 4. Maturation toward autonomous decision making.

[1]These are general categories; adolescents vary in their physical, psychosocial, and cognitive development.
Sources: Gordon BN, Schroeder CS: *Sexuality: A Developmental Approach to Problems.* Plenum Press, 1995; and Alexander B, et al: Adolescent sexuality issues in office practice. Am Fam Physician 1991;44:1273.

mental listening, and the provision of clear, accurate information help develop a successful physician-patient relationship. Ideally the goal should be to delay sexual activity until adolescents have the knowledge and tools needed to make healthy decisions about sex. However, identifying adolescents at risk, educating about safer sex, establishing sexual limits, and providing information about support and educational resources for adolescents who are currently sexually active are critical activities for the family physician.

Catallozzi M et al: Lesbian, gay, bisexual, transgendered, and questioning youth: The importance of a sensitive and confidential sexual history in identifying the risk and implementing treatment for sexually transmitted infections. Adolesc Med Clin 2004;15:353. [PMID: 15449849]

Miller BC: *Families Matter: A Research Synthesis of Family Influences on Adolescent Pregnancy.* National Campaign to Prevent Teen Pregnancy, 1998.

Ryan C, Futterman D: Caring for gay and lesbian youth. Contemp Pediatr 1998;15:107.

Web Sites

American Association of Family Physicians: *Information from Your Family Doctor: Sex: Take Time to Make the Right Decision,* 2000. Available from:

http://www.familydoctor.org/handouts/276.html.

Gay and Lesbian Medical Association (GLMA):

http://www.glma.org

Parents, Families and Friends of Lesbians and Gays (PFLAG):

http://www.pflag.org

Menstrual Disorders 13

Mary V. Krueger, DO, MPH, MAJ, MC, USA

Menstrual disorders are a heterogeneous group of conditions that are both physically and psychologically debilitating. Although once considered nuisance problems, menstrual disorders are now recognized to take a significant toll on society, both in days lost from work, as well as the pain and suffering experienced by individual women. Many women consider the occurrence of their monthly cycle evidence that their body is functioning properly and are disturbed when irregularities in this cycle occur. These disorders may arise from physiologic (ie, pregnancy), pathologic (ie, endocrine abnormalities), or iatrogenic (ie, secondary to contraceptive use) conditions.

Irregularities in menstruation may manifest as complete absence of menses, dysfunctional uterine bleeding, dysmenorrhea, or premenstrual syndrome. Establishing an accurate diagnosis is essential for appropriate treatment and avoidance of potential complications. Because it is essential to know what is normal in order to define that which is abnormal, normal menstrual parameters are listed in Table 13–1. This chapter discusses the evaluation, diagnosis, and treatment of patients whose menses fall outside these norms.

The menstrual cycle relies on the action and interaction of hormones released from the hypothalamus, pituitary, and ovaries and their effect on the endometrium through feedback mechanisms. Any disease state that affects one or more of these organs, or that interferes with the timing of hormone release, may result in a menstrual disorder. A solid understanding of this cycle and its complex interactions will serve the clinician well in evaluation and diagnosis of menstrual disorders.

AMENORRHEA

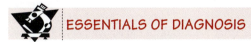

ESSENTIALS OF DIAGNOSIS

- *Primary amenorrhea—absence of menses by 16 years of age in a patient with secondary sex characteristics, or absence of menses by 14 years of age in a patient without secondary sex characteristics.*
- *Secondary amenorrhea—absence of a period for at least 6 months in a woman with previously normal menses, or at least 12 months or six cycles without a period in a woman with previously irregular menses.*

General Considerations

Amenorrhea is the natural result of menopause, pregnancy, and lactation, but can be very distressing when it occurs outside of these conditions. Amenorrhea is a symptom, not a diagnosis, and may occur secondary to a number of endocrine and anatomic abnormalities. Classifying amenorrhea into primary and secondary amenorrhea can aid in evaluation and simplify diagnosis.

1. Primary Amenorrhea

Primary amenorrhea is defined as absence of menses by 16 years of age in a patient with secondary sex characteristics, or the absence of menses by 14 years of age in a patient without secondary sex characteristics. The most common causes are gonadal dysgenesis and physiologic delay of puberty.

Clinical Findings

A. Symptoms and Signs

The patient with primary amenorrhea is often brought to the physician by her mother, who is concerned about the patient's delay in reaching developmental milestones of adolescence. The clinician should be aware that the patient may be uncomfortable discussing her sexuality, especially in the presence of a parent. The adolescent's rights as a patient must be respected. Important elements of the history are listed in Table 13–2. This targeted history will help to narrow the differential and eliminate unnecessary laboratory and radiologic testing.

B. Physical Examination

Assessment should focus on appearance of secondary sexual characteristics (axillary and pubic hair), breast development, external genitalia, height percentile, female body shape, and pelvic examination findings—specifically the presence or absence of a uterus. The clinician should be careful to acknowledge and allay patient fears, as this will

Table 13–1. Normal menstrual parameters.

Age of menarche	< 16 years old
Age of menopause	> 40 years old; mean age 52
Length of menstrual cycle	22–45 days
Length of menstrual flow	3–7 days
Amount of menstrual flow	≤ 80 mL

often be her first pelvic examination. Body mass index (BMI) should be calculated and compared with prior visits to assess for anorexia, rapid weight loss, or significant weight gain. Presence or absence of breast development and presence or absence of the uterus and cervix are decision points for further testing and diagnostic categories. Table 13–3 lists causes of primary amenorrhea.

1. Absent Breast Development with Normal Pelvic Examination Findings

a. Hypothalamic Failure—This is the common pathway for amenorrhea resulting from constitutional delay, anorexia nervosa, excessive exercise, severe stress (ie, due to abuse or psychosocial deprivation), chronic infection, malignancy, or systemic illness. All these conditions are believed to suppress hypothalamic gonadotropin-releasing hormone (GnRH) secretion through neuronal pathways in the arcuate nucleus. Those patients with with constitutional delay will display delayed but otherwise normal secondary sexual characteristics and there may be a history of the mother or sisters also being "late bloomers."

Table 13–2. Evaluation of primary amenorrhea: the history.

Recent History
- History of head trauma (damage to hypothalamic-pituitary axis)
- History of weight loss and amount of regular physical activity (female athlete triad)
- Timeline of development of secondary sexual characteristics (if present)

Past History
- Diabetes mellitus
- Juvenile rheumatoid arthritis
- Inflammatory bowel disease
- Malignancy
- Chronic infection

Family History
- Onset of menarche in patient's mother and sisters
- Family history of gonadal dysgenesis

Medications
- Medication or supplement use (particularly hormonal)

Social History
- Sexual activity
- History of psychosocial deprivation or abuse

Symptoms
- Anosmia (Kallman syndrome)
- Monthly abdominal pain (imperforate hymen)

Table 13–3. Etiologies of primary amenorrhea.

Physiologic
- Constitutional delay
- Pregnancy

Pathologic
- Absent breast development, normal pelvic examination findings
  - Hypothalamic failure
    - Anorexia nervosa, excessive weight loss, excessive exercise, stress
    - Chronic illness (juvenile rheumatoid arthritis, diabetes, irritable bowel syndrome)
  - Gonadotropin deficiency
    - Kallman syndrome (associated with anosmia)
    - Pituitary dysfunction after head trauma or shock
    - Infiltrative or inflammatory processes
    - Pituitary adenoma
    - Craniopharyngioma
  - Gonadal failure
    - Gonadal dysgenesis (ie, Turner syndrome)
- Normal breast development, normal pelvic examination findings
  - Hypothyroidism
  - Hyperprolactinemia
- Normal breast development, abnormal pelvic examination findings
  - Testicular feminization
  - Anatomic abnormalities (uterovaginal septum, imperforate hymen)

b. Pituitary Failure—Pituitary failure results in hypogonadotropic hypogonadism. This may occur as a result of inadequate GnRH stimulation secondary to Kallman syndrome (in which the GnRH neurons fail to migrate from the olfactory bulb) and can be identified by its association with anosmia. Head trauma, severe hypotension (shock), infiltrative or inflammatory processes, pituitary adenoma, or craniopharyngioma may damage the pituitary gland, resulting in decreased or absent gonadotropin (luteinizing hormone [LH] and follicle-stimulating hormone [FSH]) release. These patients often display symptoms relating to deficiency of other pituitary hormones as well.

c. Gonadal Dysgenesis—This condition, which results from chromosomal anomalies, is the most common cause of primary amenorrhea, responsible for 45% of cases. Turner syndrome (45,XO) is the most familiar type and is associated with short stature, widely spaced nipples, a webbed neck, and sexual infantilism. Ovaries are vestigial "streak gonads" and produce little to no estradiol. Mosaic variants may also occur, which can result in both subtle abnormalities and more striking ambiguous genitalia.

2. Normal Breast Development and Normal Pelvic Examination Findings

a. Hypothyroidism and Hyperprolactinemia—Both conditions can suppress the secretion of GnRH, FSH, and LH, resulting in suppression of the menstrual cycle. Pubarche and thelarche should progress normally in this setting. Conversely, profound hypothyroidism can result in precocious puberty due to the FSH-like effect of high levels of circulating thyroid-stimulating hormone (TSH).

b. Polycystic Ovarian Syndrome—This syndrome may cause primary amenorrhea, although it is more commonly thought of as a cause of secondary amenorrhea. Acne, hirsutism, and obesity are commonly seen in patients with this disorder.

3. Normal Breast Development with Abnormal Pelvic Examination Findings

a. Testicular Feminization—Androgen resistance prevents the influence of testicular androgens on a chromosomally male (XY) fetus, resulting in female external genitalia. The testes secrete a müllerian duct inhibitory hormone to which the fetus does respond, thus preventing development of the upper vagina and uterus.

b. Anatomic Abnormalities—Failures of uterovaginal communication due to either uterovaginal septum or imperforate hymen are anatomic causes of primary amenorrhea. They are often accompanied by cyclic pelvic pain and hematocolpos. Rokitansky–Kuster–Hauser syndrome, failure of uterine development, is associated with renal anomalies.

C. Laboratory Findings

Laboratory examination should be guided by the history and physical findings, and the tests discussed here are based on etiology. A pregnancy test should be performed on all individuals presenting for primary amenorrhea who have secondary sexual characteristics and functional anatomy. Although the initial cycles after menarche are often anovulatory, pregnancy can occur before the first recognized menstrual cycle. A sensitive discussion of this subject is necessary to facilitate understanding and avoid conflict with the patient, her mother, or both.

Patients with normal findings on pelvic examination, but absent breast development, should have serum FSH measured to distinguish peripheral (gonadal) from central (pituitary or hypothalamic) causes of amenorrhea. A high FSH level suggests gonadal dysgenesis. A karyotype should be performed to identify patients who are 46,XY, because these individuals have a high peripubertal risk for gonadoblastoma and dysgerminoma.

If the uterus is absent, serum testosterone should be measured and a karyotype obtained. Elevated testosterone in the presence of a Y chromosome indicates functional testicular tissue that should be excised to prevent later neoplastic transformation.

In patients with both normal breast development and a normal pelvic examination, serum prolactin and TSH should be measured to rule out hyperprolactinemia and hypothyroidism. If these values are in the normal range, investigation should proceed according to the secondary amenorrhea algorithm.

D. Imaging Studies

Radiographic studies are targeted toward the diagnosis suggested by history, and by the physical and laboratory findings. Magnetic resonance imaging (MRI) is indicated in patients in whom pituitary pathology is suspected. Computerized visual field testing may be added if the examination or MRI indicates compression of the optic chiasm. Pelvic ultrasound should be performed in patients with suspected pelvic anomalies.

Treatment

Successful treatmentof primary amenorrhea is based on correct diagnosis of the underlying etiology. The goals of treatment are to establish a firm diagnosis, to restore ovulatory cycles and treat infertility, to treat hypoestrogenemia and hyperandrogenism, and to assess and address risks associated with a persistent hypoestrogenemic state.

A. Medical Therapy

Patients with anorexia can manifest amenorrhea as a result of hypothalamic failure due to rapid weight loss, excessive exercise, abuse, or stress. (See the discussion of eating disorders in Chapter 11.)

Pituitary adenomas, resulting in hyperprolactinemia, can be treated with either bromocriptine or cabergoline. Bromocriptine may be used in pregnancy and has the best-established safety record of all the dopamine agonists. Cabergoline is longer acting and may have fewer side effects in some patients but is very expensive. Tumors that are large enough to affect vision or produce a mass effect should be surgically removed through trans-sphenoidal excision. Initial success rates are high, but late recurrence rates may approach 20%.

Patients with gonadal dysgenesis should be given hormone replacement therapy to prevent the negative effects of a hypoestrogenic state. Patients with an intact uterus may undergo induction of menstruation with cyclic progesterone and estrogen therapy. If testing reveals a 46,XY karyotype, surgical removal of the gonads is necessary, because gonadal dysgenesis with this karyotype is associated with a high peripubertal risk of dysgerminoma or gonadoblastoma.

Only providers experienced in this field should perform induction of puberty in patients with constitutional delay. Estrogen is responsible for epiphyseal closure as well as the adolescent growth spurt; mistimed administration could have significant effects on the final achieved height in these patients.

B. Surgical Intervention

Structural anomalies should be addressed surgically. In patients with congenital absence of a uterus, investigation should be undertaken for associated renal anomalies.

2. Secondary Amenorrhea

The most common type of amenorrhea, secondary amenorrhea, is diagnosed when a woman with previously normal menses goes at least 6 months without a period, or when a woman with previously irregular menses goes at least 12 months or at least six cycles without a period. It can have either physiologic or pathologic etiologies and can be a topic of great concern for the patient. The causes of secondary amenorrhea can be broken down into those with and those without evidence of hyperandrogenism.

Clinical Findings

A. Symptoms and Signs

Pertinent history in the evaluation of secondary amenorrhea includes previous menstrual history (timing and quality of menses), pregnancies (including terminations and complicated deliveries), symptoms of endocrine disease, medication history, weight loss or gain, exercise level, and masculinizing characteristics noticed by the patient or family.

B. Physical Examination

General examination should assess pubertal development and secondary sexual characteristics while looking for evidence of hyperandrogenism. These latter findings may include oily skin, acne, and hirsutism. Pelvic examination should note clitoral size, with clitorimegaly defined as length × width product of greater than 40 mm^2. Evidence of hyperandrogenism assists in classifying etiologies of secondary amenorrhea.

1. Evidence of Hyperandrogenism on Examination

a. Polycystic Ovarian Syndrome (PCOS)—Responsible for 30% of secondary amenorrhea, PCOS is the most common reproductive female endocrine disorder, occurring in 5–7% of women. Its clinical manifestations may include menstrual irregularities, signs of androgen excess, and obesity. Insulin resistance, impaired glucose tolerance, and elevated serum LH levels are also common features in PCOS. PCOS is associated with an increased risk of type 2 diabetes, abdominal obesity, hypertension, hypertriglyceridemia, and cardiovascular events. Dysfunctional uterine bleeding and endometrial carcinoma may also occur secondary to endometrial hyperstimulation by the continuous presence of estrogen and progesterone. There is no cyclical decrease of these hormones due to anovulation and the failure of a dominant ovarian follicle to develop.

b. Autonomous Hyperandrogenism—Tumors of adrenal or ovarian origin may secrete androgens. Virilization is more pronounced than in PCOS and may manifest as frontal balding, increased muscle bulk, deep voice, clitorimegaly, and severe hirsutism.

c. Late-Onset or Mild Congenital Adrenal Hyperplasia—This rare condition may be diagnosed with the finding of an increased 17-hydroxyprogesterone level in the setting of secondary amenorrhea and hyperandrogenism.

2. No Evidence of Hyperandrogenism on Examination

a. Medication Use—History should be reviewed for use of contraceptives, particularly progesterone-only preparations. These may take the form of oral contraceptives (OCPs), implants, injectables, or intrauterine devices. Amenorrhea secondary to OCP use is an important side effect to address, because it may lead to patient concern and discontinuation. It is important to educate women that 20% of patients who take progestin-only pills become amenorrheic within the first year of use. Rates are even higher for those using injectable progesterone, with 55% of women at 1 year and 68% of women at 2 years reporting amenorrhea.

b. Functional Hypothalamic Amenorrhea—Patients who are significantly underweight; who have experienced recent, rapid weight loss; who exercise rigorously; or who are under emotional stress may experience amenorrhea due to a functional suppression of GnRH. Careful history taking will aid in detection of these factors. Amenorrhea in this setting may be part of the female athlete triad of amenorrhea, disordered eating, and osteoporosis addressed in Chapter 10.

c. Hypergonadotropic Hypogonadism—Premature ovarian failure (cessation of ovarian function before 40 years of age) may be autoimmune, idiopathic, or occur secondarily due to radiotherapy or chemotherapy (cyclophosphamide is associated with destruction of oocytes). A history of Addison disease, autoimmune thyroid disease, or diabetes mellitus type 1 should raise suspicion of an autoimmune cause, whereas a history of treatment for Hodgkin lymphoma, breast cancer, or Wilms tumor points to cytotoxic drugs as a primary etiology.

d. Hyperprolactinemia—Pituatary adenomas may present with amenorrhea and galactorrhea, and are responsible for 20% of cases of secondary amenorrhea. Prolactin secreted by these tumors acts directly on the hypothalamus to suppress GnRH secretion. Dopamine receptor–blocking agents, hypothalamic masses, and hypothyroidism are less common causes of hyperprolactinemia.

e. Thyroid Disease—Profound hypothyroidism or hyperthyroidism affects the feedback control of LH, FSH, and estradiol on the hypothalamus, causing menstrual irregularities.

f. Hypogonadotropic Hypogonadism—Head trauma, severe hypotension (shock), infiltrative or inflammatory processes, pituitary adenoma, or craniopharyngioma may damage the pituitary, resulting in decreased or absent gonadotropin (LH and FSH) release. These patients often display symptoms relating to deficiency of other pituitary hormones as well.

C. Laboratory Findings

Initial studies should include a pregnancy test, fasting glucose, TSH, and prolactin levels. In the absence of significant abnormalities in these values, a progestin challenge test should be performed to assess the patient's estrogen status. The patient is given medroxyprogesterone, 5–10 mg orally, daily for 5–7 days. Women with adequate levels of circulating estrogen should experience withdrawal bleeding within 2 weeks of administration. Some patients who do not respond to oral administration will respond to intramuscular injection. FSH should be measured in women who do not experience withdrawal bleeding within the designated time period. A high FSH value (> 30 IU/L) is indicative of ovarian failure, whereas normal or low values indicate either an acquired uterine anomaly (Asherman syndrome) or hypothalamic-pituitary failure. Ovarian failure is confirmed with a low serum estradiol level, less than 30 pg/mL. Serum LH and FSH should be drawn on women who do not experience withdrawal bleeding after the progesterone challenge and have a normal estrogen level. An elevated LH value is highly suggestive of PCOS, especially in a woman with clinical features of virilization. If the LH level is normal, an LH to FSH ratio should be determined. This ratio is elevated (> 2.5) in women with PCOS even when FSH and LH values are within normal limits. This diagnosis can be confirmed by measurement of serum testosterone and dehydroepiandrosterone sulfate (DHEA-S), which should be normal or just mildly elevated in PCOS. An increased testosterone to DHEA-S ratio is suggestive of an adrenal source. This finding warrants further study with determination of 17-hydroxyprogesterone. This level is elevated in late-onset congenital adrenal hyperplasia and Cushing syndrome. Cushing syndrome may be excluded with a 24-hour urinary free cortisol and dexamethasone suppression testing.

D. Imaging Studies

Computed tomographic (CT) scanning of the adrenal glands and ultrasound of the ovaries should be performed in women with clinical features of virilization and increased testosterone (> 200 ng/dL) or DHEAS-S (> 7 mcg/mL). Even though these are the most sensitive imaging modalities, normal ovarian ultrasound does not exclude neoplasm. Surgical exploration may be necessary in situations where this is still a concern. A CT or MRI scan of the pituitary should be performed if pituitary pathology is suspected.

Treatment

Treatment depends on correct diagnosis of the underlying etiology. As in primary amenorrhea, the goals of treatment are to establish a firm diagnosis, to restore ovulatory cycles and treat infertility (when possible), to treat hypoestrogenemia and hyperandrogenism, and to assess and address risks associated with a persistent hypoestrogenemic state.

A. Medical Therapy

Patients with identified hypothyroidism should be treated with thyroxine replacement. Patients with hyperprolactinemia secondary to prolactinoma may be treated with either surgical resection or dopamine agonist therapy. Although there are strong proponents for each therapy, many authorities currently favor medical therapy. Treatment with a dopamine agonist can suppress prolactin secretion, induce ovulation, and decrease tumor size while maintaining the pituitary reserve. Bromocriptine is often used in women who desire to conceive, because there is no increased incidence of congenital malformations. The main side effects are nausea, vomiting, and postural hypotension. Patients experiencing these side effects may be treated with cabergoline, also a dopamine agonist. Given weekly in a depot formulation, it has a much lower incidence of nausea.

Patients found to have empty sella or Sheehan syndrome should be treated with replacement of pituitary hormones.

Women younger than 40 years of age whose amenorrhea is secondary to absent ovarian function have premature ovarian failure. Those who experience ovarian failure before 30 years of age should undergo karyotype testing to screen for y-chromosome elements, which are associated with malignancies. These patients are at a high risk of osteoporosis and cardiovascular disease due to their hypoestrogenemic state. Estrogen replacement should be undertaken, with progesterone for those patients with an intact uterus, to prevent these sequelae. Assisted reproduction technology with a donor oocyte can make it possible for women desiring pregnancy to give birth.

Patients with PCOS may achieve resumption of menses with weight loss. The assistance of a registered dietician should be sought to improve success rates in this daunting task. Metformin, a biguanide insulin sensitizer, has been used to treat PCOS, with reports of success in both inducing ovulation and improving laboratory markers for cardiovascular risk. Metformin is effective in achieving ovulation in women with PCOS with odds ratios of 3.88 (CI 2.25–6.69) for metformin versus placebo. It also lowers fasting insulin levels, blood pressure, and low-density lipoprotein cholesterol (LDL). A recent review showed no evidence of effect on BMI or waist to hip ratio. Based on this evidence of intermediate outcomes and the side effects of nausea, bloating, and diarrhea, metformin should be used as an adjuvant to general life-style improvements, and not as a replacement for adequate physical activity and healthy diet.

B. Surgical Intervention

Women with adrenal or ovarian androgen-secreting tumors should undergo appropriate surgical intervention. Likewise, women found to have Asherman syndrome as a cause for their amenorrhea should undergo lysis of adhesions followed by endometrial stimulation with estrogen. These patients are at increased risk of placenta accreta in subsequent pregnancies.

Lord JM et al: Insulin-sensitising drugs (metformin, troglitazone, rosiglitazone, pioglitazone, D-chiro-inositol) for polycystic ovary syndrome. Cochrane Database Syst Rev 2003;(3):CD003053. [PMID: 12917943]

Nestler JE: Role of hyperinsulinemia in the pathogenesis of the polycystic ovary syndrome, and its clinical implications. Semin Reprod Endocrinol 1997;15:111. [PMID: 9165656]

Verhelst J et al: Cabergoline in the treatment of hyperprolactinemia: A study in 455 patients. J Clin Endocrinol Metab 1999;84:2518. [PMID: 10404830]

DYSFUNCTIONAL UTERINE BLEEDING

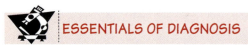

- *Menses that are too heavy (> 80 mL per cycle), too frequent (occurring every 22 days or less), or too long (> 7 days of flow).*

General Considerations

Vaginal bleeding caused by hormonal abnormalities, in the absence of pregnancy, tumor, infection, or coagulopathy is termed *dysfunctional uterine bleeding.* Vaginal bleeding attributed to causes other than menstrual dysfunction is addressed in Chapter 32. The most frequent cause of dysfunctional uterine bleeding is continuous estrogen production associated with anovulation, a common condition in adolescents. This condition carries significant physical, psychological, cultural, and societal morbidity. Women losing more than 60 mL of blood per month are at risk of developing iron deficiency anemia with the attendant lethargy, decreased immune function, and restriction in activities of daily living. Some cultures view menstruating women as "unclean," unable to prepare food, participate in daily activities, or have sexual intercourse. For all these reasons, it is important for the family physician to be familiar with assessment, diagnosis, and treatment of dysfunctional uterine bleeding.

Clinical Findings

A. Symptoms and Signs

The initial history should include a detailed description of menstrual bleeding, including age of onset of menses, length of cycles, length of menses, presence of clots, number of pads or tampons used per day, and change in character or timing of menses. A symptom diary is helpful in obtaining this information. A sexual history, including number of partners, form of contraception, number and timing of pregnancies, number and timing of elective terminations, and history of sexually transmitted diseases, should also be documented. Patients using an intrauterine device (IUD) for contraception should be questioned about the onset of dysfunctional uterine bleeding in relation to the insertion of the IUD. Symptoms of anemia (eg, fatigue, lethargy, and lightheadedness) may be present. The patient should also be asked about both personal and family history of bleeding disorders.

B. Physical Examination

The physical examination should include initial evaluation of hemodynamic stability followed by a pelvic examination with cervical smear and cultures. IUD placement should be confirmed in patients using this method of contraception. Special note should be made of pallor, tachycardia, hypotension, or excessive bruising. Uterine size should be noted, as enlargement may indicate fibroids, a common cause of heavy menstrual bleeding.

C. Laboratory Findings

A pregnancy test should be performed on all patients with dysfunctional uterine bleeding, especially if onset is recent, as this may represent an ectopic pregnancy. A complete blood count (CBC) should also be undertaken in all women, as hemoglobin is a surrogate assessment for excessive menstrual loss, white blood cell count may indicate chronic infection, and indices can provide an assessment of the whole body iron stores. Coagulation screens, thyroid function tests, endometrial sampling, and other endocrine investigations should be performed only as indicated by the history and physical examination.

D. Imaging Studies

Pelvic ultrasound should be performed only in the evaluation of pelvic disorders discovered during clinical examination, in women who weigh 90 kg or more, or in women who are 45 years of age or older.

Treatment

A. Medical Therapy

The treatment strategy described in this section assumes that the clinician has ruled out infection, neoplasm, pregnancy, trauma, or coagulopathy as the cause of abnormal vaginal bleeding. Adolescents with irregular menstrual bleeding that does not involve excessive blood loss should be counseled on the possible etiologies and all available treatment options. If the patient is within 2 years of menarche, anovulatory cycles are the most likely cause for dysfunctional uterine bleeding, and OCPs may be used to regulate cycles. This may not be an acceptable option to all patients because of the stigma associated with OCP use. Expectant management may be a preferable choice in these situations.

In patients with dysfunctional uterine bleeding due to underlying endocrine disorders, the underlying disorder should be addressed.

If menorrhagia is the primary complaint, and no underlying pathology is suspected, OCPs, nonsteroidal anti-inflammatory drugs (NSAIDs), levonorgestrel IUDs, luteal phase progesterone, and danazol are all medical therapies that have shown efficacy in reducing regular heavy menstrual bleeding. Clinicians must be aware of contraindications to these treatments and tailor therapy to the individual patient. NSAIDs, OCPs, progesterone IUDs, and luteal phase progesterone are equally effective at reducing heavy menstrual bleeding, although none are as effective as danazol. Use of danazol is limited by adverse androgenic side effects that include weight gain, acne, deepened voice, and hirsutism. NSAIDs have the added benefit of decreasing accompanying dysmenorrhea.

B. Surgical Intervention

Surgical therapy should be limited to patients in whom a structural cause for dysfunctional uterine bleeding exists (eg, fibroids, polyps, or neoplasm). Although endometrial ablation and hysterectomy are common surgical treatments for menorrhagia unresponsive to medical therapy, their use should be balanced against the associated morbidity and mortality, as well as the patient's wishes for fertility. Dilation and curettage (D&C) is generally not therapeutic in cases of heavy menstrual bleeding.

Working Party for Guidelines for the Management of Heavy Menstrual Bleeding: An evidence-based guideline for the management of heavy menstrual bleeding. N Z Med J 1999; 112:174. [PMID: 10391640]

Lethaby A et al: Nonsteroidal anti-inflammatory drugs for heavy menstrual bleeding. Cochrane Database Syst Rev 2001(4):20. [PMID: 11869575]

Royal College of Obstetrics and Gynaecology Menorrhagia Guideline Development Group: *The Management of Menorrhagia in Secondary Care,* vol 5. Evidence-based Clinical Guidelines. RCOG Press, 1999:77.

Stabinsky SA et al: Modern treatments of menorrhagia attributable to dysfunctional uterine bleeding. Obstet Gynecol Surv 1999;54:251. [PMID: 9891301]

DYSMENORRHEA

General Considerations

Dysmenorrhea—painful menstruation—is one of the most common gynecologic problems seen by the family physician. It affects 50% of all women and between 20% and 90% of all adolescent women. Approximately 1% of all adult and 15% of adolescent women describe their dysmenorrhea as severe. It is a leading cause of morbidity in female high school students, resulting in absence from school and nonparticipation in sports. For diagnostic purposes, dysmenorrhea is classified as either primary or secondary, with primary dysmenorrhea being defined as the presence of painful menses in the absence of pelvic disease and secondary dysmenorrhea being the occurrence of painful menstruation caused by pelvic disease.

Pathogenesis

Primary dysmenorrhea is thought to be caused by the release of prostaglandin $F_2\alpha$ from the endometrium at the time of menstruation. The endometrium, stimulated by estrogen and progesterone released from the dominant follicle, releases large amounts of prostaglandins as the cells lyse with menstruation. This explains why younger adolescents who are often anovulatory, and who do not development a dominant follicle, experience less dysmenorrhea. Prostaglandins induce smooth muscle contraction in the uterus, as well as in the intestine, bronchi, and vasculature, which may account for the systemic symptoms of diarrhea, asthma exacerbation, hypertension, and headache experienced by women with primary dysmenorrhea. As contractions cause the pressure within the uterus to exceed that of the systemic circulation, ischemia ensues, causing an anginal equivalent in the uterus.

The causes of **secondary dysmenorrhea** vary with the underlying disease and include adenomyosis, myomas, polyps, infection, endometriosis, tumors, adhesions, leiomyomas, intrauterine devices, blind uterine horn (rare), obstructed outflow of menstrual blood secondary to anatomic causes, bladder pathology, and gastrointestinal pathology.

Clinical Findings

A. Symptoms and Signs

Patients with a history of primary dysmenorrhea often report pain beginning with the onset of menstruation and lasting 12–72 hours. The pain is characterized as crampy and intermittent in nature, is often most intense in the lower abdomen, and may radiate to the low back or upper thighs. Headache, nausea, vomiting, diarrhea, and fatigue may accompany the pain. Symptoms are often worst on the first day of menses and then gradually resolve. The patient may report that her dysmenorrhea began gradually, with the first year of menses, and then became worse as her periods became regular. Conversely, patients with secondary amenorrhea report symptoms beginning after age 20, lasting for 5–7 days, and progressive worsening of pain with time. These patients may also report pelvic pain that is not associated with menstruation.

B. Physical Examination

A pelvic examination with cervical smear and cultures should be performed in all patients presenting with a chief complaint of dysmenorrhea. Findings of cul-de-sac induration and uterosacral ligament nodularity on pelvic examination are indicative of endometriosis. Adnexal masses could indicate endometriosis, neoplasm, hydrosalpinx, or scarring from chronic pelvic inflammatory disease (PID). Likewise, uterine abnormalities or tenderness should raise the examiner's index of suspicion for underlying pathology as the cause of dysmenorrhea.

C. Laboratory Findings

Any woman with acute onset of pelvic pain should have a pregnancy test. Women with a history consistent with primary dysmenorrhea do not require initial laboratory tests. In those who fail to respond to therapy for primary dysmenorrhea or in whom a diagnosis of secondary dysmenorrhea is suspected, a CBC and an erythrocyte sedimentation rate (ESR) may help in detection of underlying infection or inflammation.

D. Imaging Studies

Patients with abnormal findings on pelvic examination who do not respond to therapy for primary dysmenorrhea or who have a history suggestive of pelvic pathology should undergo pelvic ultrasound. In those patients in whom endometriosis is suggested, diagnostic laparoscopy may be indicated. Because high rates of treatment and diagnostic failure are associated with laparoscopy, empirical treatment of patients with a presumptive diagnosis of endometriosis, consisting of GnRH analogues for 3 months, has been recommended. Proponents argue this provides both diagnostic and therapeutic functions, while forgoing surgical complications.

Treatment

A. Medical Therapy

Treatment of primary dysmenorrhea focuses on reducing endometrial prostaglandin production. This can be accomplished with medications that inhibit prostaglandin synthesis; with contraceptives that suppress ovulation, administered orally or intravaginally, by injection, by IUD; or by other hormonal means (Table 13–4).

Ibuprofen, 400 mg orally four times daily, is the first-line therapy based on its favorable risk-benefit ratio. In women who can predict the onset of their menses, treatment should begin the day before menstruation and be continued for 3–4 days. Patients who do not respond to this therapy can be tried on second-line agents. Patients are most satisfied with medications that have a rapid onset of action. Patients unable to tolerate the gastrointestinal side effects of traditional NSAIDs may alternatively consider cyclooxygenase-2 (COX-2) inhibitors, but the question of risk of myocardial infarction with use must be weighed against the benefit and availability of alternative therapies.

For patients who do not desire fertility, combination oral contraceptives (those containing both estrogen and progesterone) are an effective treatment for primary dysmenorrhea, although most studies evaluated older formulations containing more than 35 mcg of estrogen. These combination products suppress ovulation, inhibiting endogenous progesterone production, and prevent normal endometrial growth—actions that dramatically reduce prostaglandin release. An adequate trial of OCPs for 3–6 months should be undertaken to evaluate their efficacy. Hormonal delivery by injection (depo-medroxyprogesterone acetate) and hormonal IUD (levonorgestrel IUD) are also effective at reducing severity of pain with dysmenorrhea, whereas the contraceptive patch is less effective.

B. Physical Modalities

Physical modalities utilizing heat, acupuncture or acupressure, and spinal manipulation have been proposed for inclusion in the treatment of dysmenorrhea. A heated abdominal patch was demonstrated to have efficacy similar to ibuprofen (400 mg) in the treatment of dysmenorrhea, and quicker, but not greater, relief was observed with the combination of ibuprofen and heat. Acupuncture has been shown to relieve pain in 91% of patients with dysmenorrhea compared with 36% of control patients who received sham acupuncture. Finally, a systematic review of spinal manipulation in the treatment of dysmenorrhea showed no evidence of efficacy with this approach.

C. Alternative and Complementary Therapies

Numerous supplements and herbal formulations are touted as relieving the symptoms of dysmenorrhea, but few of these claims are backed by solid evidence. One randomized, double-blind, placebo-controlled study evaluated vitamin E in the treatment of dysmenorrhea in adolescent girls. Use of vitamin E, 200 units twice daily, beginning 2 days before menses and continuing through the first 3 days

Table 13–4. Medications used in the treatment of primary dysmenorrhea.

Medication	Mechanism of Action	Primary Side Effects/ Complications	Efficacy (Strength of Recommendation)[1]	Comments
NSAIDs[2] (diclofenac, ibuprofen, mefenamic acid, naproxen, ASA)	Inhibits prostaglandin synthesis	Gastrointestinal upset and bleeding	Effective (A)	Most effective when started before onset of pain
Danazol	Suppresses menses	Amenorrhea, vaginal dryness, jaundice, eosinophilia	Probably effective (B)	Significant side effects, primarily severe endometriosis
Leuprolide	Suppresses menses	Weight gain, hirsutism, elevation of blood pressure	Probably effective (B)	Very expensive with significant side effects; not first-line treatment
Depo-medroxyprogesterone acetate	Suppresses menses	Amenorrhea, hypermenorrhea	Probably effective (B)	Weight gain may be significant
Contraceptives: oral and intravaginal	Reduces prostaglandin release during menstruation	Irregular menses, mood swings, acne, deep venous thrombosis	Possibly effective (B)	Use with caution in patients older than 35 y and in those who smoke cigarettes
COX-2 inhibitors	Inhibits prostaglandin synthesis	Cardiovascular risk, acute renal failure	Possibly effective (B)	Contains sulfa moiety; consider safer NSAIDs first
Levonorgestrel IUD[3]	Thins uterine lining through inhibition	Hypertension, acne, weight gain	Possibly effective (B)	Effective for 5 y
Nifedipine[4]	Induces uterine relaxation	Hypotension, peripheral edema	Uncertain efficacy (C)	Provides moderate to good pain reduction but has high rate of side effects
Transdermal contraceptive patch[5]	Reduces prostaglandin release during menstruation	Local irritation, irregular menses	Uncertain efficacy (B)	Less effective than OCPs; efficacy varies with patient weight

NSAID, nonsteroidal anti-inflammatory drug; ASA, acetylsalicylic acid; COX-2, cyclo-oxygenase-2; IUD, intrauterine device; OCP, oral contraceptive pill.

[1]A indicates consistent, good quality, patient-oriented evidence; B, inconsistent or limited-quality patient-oriented evidence; C, consensus, disease-oriented evidence, usual practice, opinion, or case series.

[2]Procter M, Farquhar C: Dysmenorrhea. Clin Evid 2002;(7):1639.

[3]Baldaszti E, Wimmer-Puchinger B: Acceptability of the long-term contraceptive levonorgestrel-releasing intrauterine system (Mirena): A 3-year follow-up study. Contraception 2003;67:87.

[4]Ulmsten U: Calcium blockade as a rapid pharmacological test to evaluate primary dysmenorrhea. Gynecol Obstet Invest 1985;20:78.

[5]Audet MC, Moreau M: Evaluation of contraceptive efficacy and cycle control of a transdermal contraceptive patch vs an oral contraceptive; a randomized trial. JAMA 2001;285:2347.

of bleeding, resulted in a shorter duration and lower intensity of pain than placebo. This confirmed results of a similar trial using 500 units of vitamin E to treat dysmenorrhea in adolescent girls. Treatment with a fish oil supplement (1080 mg of eicosapentaenoic acid, 720 mg of docosahexaenoic acid) has also been shown to significantly decrease symptoms of dysmenorrhea; however, the supplement was given with 1.5 mg of vitamin E, which may have influenced the findings.

D. Behavioral Modification

Strenuous exercise and caffeine intake are both life-style factors that can modulate prostaglandin-induced uterine contractions. Strenuous exercise can increase uterine tone, resulting in increased periods of uterine "angina" and accompanying increases in prostaglandins. Decreasing strenuous exercise in the first few days of a woman's menses may reduce her dysmenorrhea. Conversely, caffeine decreases uterine tone by increasing uterine cyclic adenosine monophosphate levels.

E. Surgical Intervention

If a patient continues to have significant dysmenorrhea with the preceding treatment modalities, further testing for causes of secondary dysmenorrhea should be considered. Women with chronic pelvic pain that does not respond to supportive therapy often have adhesions, endometriosis, or chronic PID discovered on diagnostic laparoscopy. For those with refractory primary amenorrhea, hysterectomy is an option. Disruption of the nerve pathways through presacral neurectomy or laparoscopic uterine nerve ablation (LUNA) can be used in patients with severe dysmenorrhea; however, there is insufficient evidence to recommend this treatment for patients with less severe cases.

Akin MD et al: Continuous low-level topical heat in the treatment of dysmenorrhea. Obstet Gynecol 2001;97:343. [PMID: 11239634]

Audet MC, Moreau M: Evaluation of contraceptive efficacy and cycle control of a transdermal contraceptive patch vs an oral contraceptive: A randomized trial. JAMA 2001;285:2347. [PMID: 11343482]

Baldaszti E et al: Acceptability of the long-term contraceptive levonorgestrel-releasing intrauterine system (Mirena): A 3-year follow-up study. Contraception 2003;67:87. [PMID: 12586318]

Barbieri RL: Primary gonadotropin-releasing hormone agonist therapy for suspected endometriosis: A nonsurgical approach to the diagnosis and treatment of chronic pelvic pain. Am J Manag Care 1997;3:285. [PMID: 10169263]

Davis AR, Westhoff CL: Primary dysmenorrhea in adolescent girls and treatment with oral contraceptives. J Pediatr Adolesc Gynecol 2001;14:3. [PMID: 11358700]

Harel Z, Biro FM: Supplementation with omega-3 polyunsaturated fatty acids in the management of dysmenorrhea in adolescents. Am J Obstet Gynecol 1996;174:1335. [PMID: 8623866]

Proctor M, Farquhar C: Dysmenorrhoea. Clin Evid 2002;(7):1639. [PMID: 16973091]

Proctor ML, Smith CA: Surgical interruption of pelvic nerve pathways for primary and secondary dysmenorrhoea. Cocharane Database Syst Rev 2004;(3):CD001896.

Proctor ML et al: Combined oral contraceptive pill (OCP) as treatment for primary dysmenorrhea. Cochrane Database Syst Rev 2001;(4):CD002120. [PMID: 11687142]

Proctor M et al: Spinal manipulation for primary and secondary dysmenorrhea. Cochrane Database Syst Rev 2004(3):CD002119. [PMID: 16855988]

Ziaei S et al: A randomised controlled trial of vitamin E in the treatment of primary dysmenorrhoea. BJOG 2005;112: 466.

PREMENSTRUAL SYNDROME

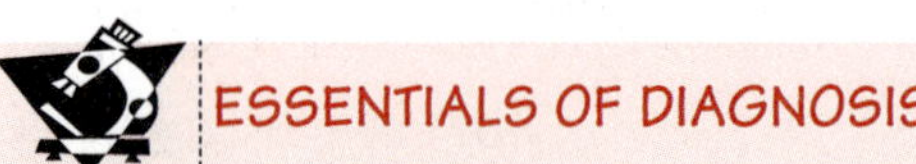

- *Any of the following disorders or symptoms occurring during the luteal phase of the menstrual cycle:*
  - *Premenstrual dysphoric disorder.*
  - *Affective or cognitive disturbances.*
  - *Alterations in appetite.*
  - *Fluid retention*
  - *Pain.*

General Considerations

Premenstrual syndrome (PMS) is a group of disorders and symptoms occurring during the luteal phase of the menstrual cycle that include: premenstrual dysphoric disorder (PMDD), affective disturbances, alterations in appetite, cognitive disturbances, fluid retention, and pain. In 40% of women with PMS, symptoms are significant enough to interfere with daily life and relationships, and 5% of women experience severe impairment. Onset may occur at any time during the reproductive

Table 13–5. Abraham's classification of symptoms of premenstrual syndrome.

A: Anxiety
Nervous tension
Mood swings
Irritability
Anxiety
C: Cravings
Headache
Craving for sweets
Increased appetite
Heart pounding
Fatigue
Dizziness or faintness
D: Depression
Depression
Forgetfulness
Crying
Confusion
Insomnia
H: Water-related symptoms
Weight gain
Swelling of extremities
Breast tenderness
Abnormal bloating

years, but once established, PMS tends to persist until menopause. Evaluation, diagnosis, and treatment of PMS should be undertaken prudently, as it is often mistaken for other disorders and sometimes treated with counterproductive and even harmful approaches. The clinician must be sensitive in addressing issues of reduced self-worth, frustration, and depression that may be present in women suffering from this condition.

Clinical Findings

A. Symptoms and Signs

PMS is a cluster of affective, cognitive, and physical symptoms that occurs before the onset of menses, and not at other times during the month. Symptoms may include irritability, bloating, depression, food cravings, aggressiveness, and mood swings. Abraham's classification of PMS (Table 13–5) helps the clinician to organize history taking for affected patients.

Factors associated with an increased risk of PMS include stress, alcohol use, exercise, smoking, and the use of certain medications. It is not clear whether some of these factors are causative or are forms of self-medication used by sufferers. A prospective symptom diary kept for at least 2 months is helpful in assessing the relationship of symptoms to the luteal phase of menses. The absence of a symptom-free week early in the follicular phase, the time period just after menses, suggests that a chronic psychiatric disorder may be present. A record of symptoms that are temporally clustered before menses and that decline or diminish 2–3 days after the start of menses is highly suggestive of PMS.

B. Physical Examination

Patients with PMS experience fluid retention and fluctuating weight gain in relation to their menses. Mild edema may or may not be evident on physical examination.

C. Laboratory and Imaging Studies

No laboratory or radiologic tests are useful in the diagnosis of PMS. Nutrient deficiency tests are not recommended, as they do not adequately assess the patient's physiologic state.

Treatment

The treatment goals for PMS are to minimize symptoms and functional impairment while optimizing the patient's overall health and sense of well-being. Therapy should take an integrative approach, including education, psychological support, exercise, diet, and pharmacologic intervention, if necessary. The clinician should begin by reassuring the patient and displaying genuine empathy. By providing education about the prevalence

Table 13–6. Selected pharmacologic and supplemental therapies for PMS.

Medication	Indication(s) for Use in PMS	Dosing	Primary Side Effects/ Complications	Evidence Supporting Use
Mefenamic acid	Pain relief	500 mg loading dose then 250 g orally four times a day for up to 7 days	Diarrhea, nausea, vomiting, drowsiness; with prolonged use decreased renal blood flow and renal papillary necrosis	RCCT[1]
GnRH agonists (nafrelin, leuprolide)	Severe PMS; relief of all symptoms in 50% of patients	Nafrelin; 200 mg intranasal twice a day Leuprolide: 3.75 mg depot intramuscularly every 4 weeks or 0.5 mg subcutaneously every day	Vaginal dryness, accelerated bone loss, hot flashes	Controlled clinical trial[2]
Danazol	Severe PMS	200 mg orally every day in the luteal phase	Acne, weight gain, hirsutism, virilization	RCCTs[3,4]
Alprazolam[5]	Anxiety caused by PMS	0.25 mg orally three times a day during the late luteal phase of the cycle	Drowsiness, increased appetite; discontinue if patient exhibits withdrawal symptoms	RCCT[6]

(continued)

Table 13–6. Selected pharmacologic and supplemental therapies for PMS. *(Continued)*

Medication	Indication(s) for Use in PMS	Dosing	Primary Side Effects/ Complications	Evidence Supporting Use
SSRIs (fluoxetine, sertraline, paroxetine, venlafaxine, citalopram)	Depression, anger, and anxiety caused by PMS	20 mg/day orally all month or just during the luteal phase	Nervousness, insomnia, drowsiness, nausea, anorexia	EBM review[7]
Diuretics (metolazone, spironolactone)	Bloating, edema, breast tenderness (especially in women with >1.5 kg premenstrual weight gain)	Metolazone: 2.4 mg/day orally Spironolactone: 25 mg orally four times a day	Electrolyte imbalance	EBM review[8]
Bromocriptine	Breast tenderness and fullness	2.5 mg orally twice a day or three times a day	Postural hypotension, nausea	Use not supported by RCCTs
Oral contraceptives	General symptoms	Varies by formulation	Varies by formulation	Use not supported by RCCTs for treatment of PMS
Vitamin B_6	Depression and general symptoms	50 mg orally every day or twice a day	Ataxia, sensory neuropathy	EBM review[9]
γ-Linoleic acid	Breast tenderness, bloating, weight gain, edema	3 g/day in the late luteal phase of menstrual cycle	Headache, nausea	Efficacy not supported[10]
Calcium	Depression, anxiety and dysphoric states	800–1600 mg/day in divided doses	Bloating, nausea	RCCT[11]

GnRH, gonadotropin-releasing hormone; SSRI, selective serotonin reuptake inhibitor.

[1]Gunston KD: Premenstrual syndrome in Cape Town. Part II. A double-blind placebo-controlled study of the efficacy of mefenamic acid. South African Med J 1986;70:159.

[2]Brown CS, et al: Efficacy of depot leuprolide in premenstrual syndrome: effect of symptom severity and type in a controlled trial. Obstet Gynecol 1994;84:779.

[3]Sarno AP Jr et al: Premenstrual syndrome: beneficial effects of periodic, low-dose danazol. Obstet Gynecol 1987;70:33.

[4]O'Brien PM, Abukhalil IE: Randomized controlled trial of the management of premenstrual syndrome and premenstrual mastalgia using luteal phase-only danazol. Am J Obstet Gynecol 1999;180(1, Pt 1):18.

[5]Second-line treatment; primarily treats depressive symptoms; highly addictive potential.

[6]Freeman EW et al: A double-blind trial of oral progesterone, alprazolam, and placebo in treatment of severe premenstrual syndrome. JAMA 1995;274:51.

[7]EBM Reviews—ACP Journal Club: Review: selective serotonin reuptake inhibitors reduce symptoms in the premenstrual syndrome. ACP J Club 2001;134:83.

[8]Vellacott ID, O'Brien PM: Effect of spironolactone on premenstrual syndrome symptoms. J Reprod Med 1987;32:429.

[9]EBM Reviews— ACP Journal Club: Review: vitamin B6 is beneficial in the premenstrual syndrome. ACP J Club 1999;131.

[10]Budeiri D et al: Is evening primrose oil of value in the treatment of premenstrual syndrome? Control Clin Trials 1996;17:60.

[11]Thys-Jacobs S et al: Calcium carbonate and the premenstrual syndrome: effects on premenstrual and menstrual symptoms. Premenstrual Syndrome Study Group. Am J Obstet Gynecol 1998;179:444.

and treatability of PMS, the clinician can destigmatize the disease and encourage the patient to take responsibility for the treatment plan. Providers should be familiar with alternative therapies so they can adequately advise patients who are interested in pursuing these treatments.

Many first-line treatments for PMS, although not based on well-designed prospective trials, have general health benefits, are inexpensive, and have few side effects. These include dietary modifications, as recommended by the American Heart Association, and moderate exercise at least three times a week. Patients should begin to see the results of these life-style changes 2–3 months after initiation. Patients should be counseled to expect improvement in their symptoms, rather than cure. They should know that multiple approaches may be required before finding the optimal treatment.

For patients with continued symptoms, secondary treatment strategies may be employed. Dietary supplements, specifically vitamin B_6, calcium, and magnesium have been suggested to correct possible deficiencies. Current therapies are listed in Table 13–6, along with their levels of supporting evidence, primary benefits, and potential side effects. Pharmacotherapy, if utilized, should be tailored to the patient's symptoms.

Numerous alternative therapies exist for premenstrual symptoms. These include herbal medicine, dietary supplements, relaxation, massage, reflexology, manipulative therapy, and biofeedback. Although some small trials have shown promising results, there is no compelling evidence from well-designed studies that supports the use of any of these therapies in the treatment of PMS.

Abraham GE: Nutritional factors in the etiology of the premenstrual tension syndromes. J Reprod Med 1983;28:446. [PMID: 6684167]

Barbieri R, Ryan K: The menstrual cycle. In Ryan K et al, eds: *Kistner's Gynecology & Women's Health,* 7th ed. Mosby, 1999:23.

Deuster PA et al: Biological, social, and behavioral factors associated with premenstrual syndrome. Arch Fam Med 1999;8:122. [PMID: 10101982]

Stevinson C, Ernst E: Complementary/alternative therapies for premenstrual syndrome: A systematic review of randomized controlled trials. Am J Obstet Gynecol 2001;185:227. [PMID: 11483933]

Stubblefield P: The role of hormonal contraceptives; menstrual impact of contraception. Am J Obstet Gynecol 1994;170:1513. [PMID: 8178900]

Sexually Transmitted Diseases 14

Peter J. Katsufrakis, MD, MBA, & Kimberly A. Workowski, MD, FACP

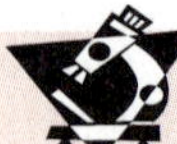

ESSENTIALS OF DIAGNOSIS

- *Privacy, confidentiality, and legal disease reporting concerns affect detection and treatment.*
- *Suspicion or diagnosis of one sexually transmitted disease (STD) should prompt screening tests for others.*
- *Diagnosis of an STD should always include identification and treatment of partners, and education to reduce risk of future infection.*

General Considerations

STDs include sexually transmitted infections and the clinical syndromes they cause. Based on estimates there are up to 19 million new STDs in the United States annually, of which 9.1 million (48%) are among persons aged 15–24 years. Rates in the United States are among the highest in the developed world.

Although all sexually active individuals are susceptible to infection, adolescents and young adults are most commonly affected. Reasons for this include (1) adolescents' biological susceptibility to increased morbidity (eg, cervical cancer in women exposed to human papillomavirus [HPV] as adolescent girls), (2) an attitude of invincibility, (3) lack of knowledge about the risks and consequences of STDs, and (4) barriers to health care access. International travelers may be another population at increased risk for STDs and may benefit from pretravel counseling.

This chapter emphasizes the clinical presentation, diagnostic evaluation, and treatment of STDs commonly found in the United States. Readers of this chapter should be able to:

- Differentiate common STDs on the basis of clinical information and laboratory testing.
- Treat STDs according to current guidelines.
- Intervene in patients' lives to reduce risk of future STD acquisition.

The discussion draws greatly from the most recent Centers for Disease Control and Prevention (CDC) guidelines for treatment of STDs. We are indebted to the individuals who worked to develop these recommendations.

Federal and state laws create disease-reporting requirements for many STDs. Gonorrhea, chlamydial infection, syphilis, and AIDS are reportable in every state. HIV and chancroid are reportable in many states. Because reporting requirements for other diseases vary by state, clinicians should contact their local health department for pertinent information.

Privacy and confidentiality concerns are different for STDs than for general medical information. Patients generally experience greater anxiety about information pertaining to a possible diagnosis of an STD, and this may limit their willingness to disclose clinically pertinent information. Conversely, legal requirements for disease reporting and health department partner notification programs can inadvertently compromise patient confidentiality if not handled with the utmost professionalism. Furthermore, although minors generally require parental consent for nonemergent medical care in all states, minors can be diagnosed and treated for STDs without parental consent. Additionally, in some states legislation may permit physicians to prescribe treatment for partners of patients with chlamydial infection without examining the partner. Thus, laws in different jurisdictions create additional options and complexity in treating STDs. Practitioners need to be familiar with local requirements.

Centers for Disease Control and Prevention; Workowski KA, Berman SM: Sexually transmitted disease treatment guidelines, 2006. MMWR Recomm Rep 2006;55(RR-11):1. [PMID: 16888612]

Weinstock H et al: Sexually transmitted diseases among American youth: Incidence and prevalence estimates, 2000. Perspect Sex Reprod Health 2004;36:6. [PMID: 14982671]

Prevention

Intervening in patients' lives to reduce their risk of disease due to STDs is no less important than reducing risk due to smoking, inadequate exercise, poor nutrition, and other health risks. STD risk assessment should prompt providers to undertake risk reduction, and thus disease prevention. Physicians' effectiveness depends on their ability to obtain an accurate sexual history employing effective counseling skills. Specific techniques include creating a trusting, confidential environment; obtaining permission to ask questions about STDs; demonstrating a nonjudgmental, optimistic attitude; and combining information collection with patient education, using clear, mutually understandable language (see Chapter 17). Prevention is facilitated by an environment of open, honest communication about sexuality.

A. Counseling

Recommendations for changes in behavior should be tailored to the patient's specific risks and needs. Brief counseling using personalized risk reduction plans and culturally appropriate videos can significantly increase condom use and prevent new STDs, and can be conducted even in busy public clinics with minimal disruption to clinic operations. Effective interventions to reduce STDs in adolescents can extend beyond the examination room and include school-based and community-based education programs. Although abstinence has been advocated by some, research suggests that this may not be the most effective intervention to prevent STD transmission. Individuals with chronic infections (eg, herpes simplex virus [HSV] and HPV) will need counseling tailored to help them accurately understand their infection and effectively manage symptoms and transmission risk.

B. Condoms

For sexually active patients, male condoms are effective in reducing transmission of many STDs and HIV. When used correctly and consistently, male latex condoms are effective in preventing sexual transmission of *Chlamydia,* gonorrhea, and trichomonas. Condoms may afford some protection against transmission of HSV, and may mitigate some adverse consequences of infection with HPV, as their use has been associated with higher rates of regression of cervical intraepithelial neoplasia and clearance of HPV in women.

Effectiveness depends on correct, consistent use. Patients should be instructed to use only water-based lubricants, and providers should consider demonstrating how to place a condom on the penis via a suitable model, especially for persons who may be inexperienced with condom use. Condoms substantially reduce STD risk, but are not foolproof, in part because of the biology of STD transmission and because of the difficulty in maintaining correct and consistent condom use.

Nonoxonyl-9 spermicide has not been shown to increase condom effectiveness for reducing *Chlamydia,* gonorrhea, or HIV transmission. Some patients confuse contraception with disease prevention; they need to understand that nonbarrier methods of contraception such as hormonal contraceptives or surgical sterilization do not protect against STDs. Women employing these methods should be counseled about the role of condoms in prevention of STDs.

C. Vaccination

Vaccination for hepatitis B virus (HBV) is indicated for all nonimmune patients undergoing evaluation for an STD, as well as for persons with multiple sex partners, men who have sex with men, sex partners of individuals with chronic HBV infection, persons with hepatitis C infection, and illicit drug users. Prevaccination testing of adolescents is not cost effective and may reduce compliance. The prevalence of past exposure to HBV in homosexual men and injection drug users may render prevaccination testing cost effective, although it may lower compliance. For this reason, if prevaccination testing is employed, patients should receive their first vaccination dose when tested. If employed, HBV core antibody testing is an effective screen for immunity.

Vaccination for hepatitis A virus (HAV) is indicated for homosexual or bisexual men, persons with chronic liver disease (including hepatitis B and C), and persons who use illicit drugs. In cases of sexual or household contact with someone with HAV, immune globulin given within 2 weeks of exposure is effective in preventing HAV infection in more than 85% of people. (For additional information on hepatitis A and B, see Chapter 31.) A vaccine for HPV was licensed by the Food and Drug Administration (FDA) in 2006, and vaccines are also being explored for other STDs, including gonorrhea, HSV, and HIV.

D. Partner Treatment

Following treatment of an individual patient, "epidemiologic treatment" of asymptomatic partners of a diagnosed patient is commonly employed in STD treatment. For patients with multiple partners, it may be difficult to identify the source of infection. Partner treatment should be recommended for sexual contacts occurring prior to diagnosis within the time intervals indicated for each disease:

- Chancroid, 10 days.
- Granuloma inguinale, 60 days.
- Lymphogranuloma venereum, 30 days.
- Syphilis, up to 90 days, even if the partner tests seronegative.
- Chlamydial infection, 60 days.
- Gonorrhea, 60 days.
- Epididymitis, 60 days.
- Pelvic inflammatory disease, 60 days.
- Pediculosis pubis, 30 days.
- Scabies, 30 days.

These are "best guess" estimates of incubation periods, and depending on the organism, infection may persist for even longer periods.

Table 14–1. US Preventive Services Task Force (USPSTF) recommendations for STD screening.[1]

Infection	Recommendation
Chlamydia	Screen *all* sexually active women aged 25 y and younger, and other asymptomatic women at increased risk for infection (eg, unmarried, African-American race, having a prior history of STD, having new or multiple sex partners, having cervical ectopy)
Gonorrhea	Screen all sexually active women, including those who are pregnant, for gonorrhea infection if they are at increased risk for infection (eg, age < 25 y, previous gonorrhea or other STD, new or multiple sex partners, inconsistent condom use, sex work, and drug use)
Hepatitis B	Screen all pregnant women at their first prenatal visit
HIV	Screen all pregnant women Screen all adolescents and adults at increased risk for HIV infection (eg, men who have had sex with men after 1975; men and women having unprotected sex with multiple partners; past or present injection drug users; men and women who exchange sex for money or drugs or have sex partners who do; individuals whose past or present sex partners were HIV-infected, bisexual, or injection drug users; persons being treated for STDs; persons with a history of blood transfusion between 1978 and 1985; persons seen in high-risk or high-prevalence clinical settings; and persons who request an HIV test)
Syphilis	Screen all pregnant women Screen persons at increased risk for syphilis infection (eg, men who have sex with men and engage in high-risk sexual behavior, commercial sex workers, persons who exchange sex for drugs, and those in adult correctional facilities)

[1]The USPSTF does not presently recommend routine screening for hepatitis C, human papillomavirus, or herpes simplex.
Source: Agency for Healthcare Research and Quality (AHRQ) of the United States Department of Health and Human Services (HHS). Available at: http://www.ahrq.gov/clinic/.

Although in general physicians must examine a patient directly before prescribing treatment, when prior medical evaluation and counseling is not feasible, or resource limitations constrain evaluation and diagnosis, other partner management options may be considered. One of these is partner-delivered therapy, in which the diagnosed patient delivers the prescribed treatment to his or her partner; this option is affected by state laws and regulations.

Repeat diagnostic testing as a "test of cure" following treatment is generally not indicated. If test of cure is employed using nucleic acid–based tests, up to 1 month may need to elapse to eliminate false-positive results due to the presence of dead organisms.

Patients should also be instructed to avoid sexual contact for the duration of therapy to prevent further transmission. Patients taking single-dose azithromycin should be instructed to avoid sexual contact for 7 days, as the medication's long half-life makes actual duration of effect much longer than the duration of medication ingestion. Patients must also be instructed to avoid contact with their previous partner(s) until they are treated.

E. Screening

Some form of STD screening, such as questions asked during the history interview or included in routine history forms, should be a universal practice for *all* patients, with periodic and regular updating. Content, frequency, and additional screening should be determined by individual patient circumstances, local disease prevalence, and research documenting effectiveness and cost–benefit. Barriers exist to talking about sexuality and STDs with most patients, especially adolescents. Table 14–1 summarizes current recommendations for STD screening from the US Preventive Services Task Force (USPSTF).

1. *Chlamydia* and gonorrhea—Annual laboratory screening for *Chlamydia* may be indicated for all sexually active adolescent women, and has been recommended in areas in which the prevalence of infection is 2% or higher. Both the CDC and the USPSTF recommend screening all sexually active women aged 25 years and younger and other asymptomatic women at increased risk for infection (defined as women with more than one sex partner who have had an STD in the past or who do not use condoms consistently and correctly). The argument and data supporting screening in girls and young women are convincing. Screening women has been shown to reduce pelvic inflammatory disease, and screening sexually active women up to age 25 has been shown to be cost effective. To date there are less compelling cost–benefit data supporting screening in boys and young men, although clearly men infect most women with *Chlamydia.*

The USPSTF believes there is insufficient evidence to support screening asymptomatic sexually active men, although it does support screening women 25 years and younger for gonorrhea, as well as older women at increased risk.

2. Pregnancy—Recommendations for screening pregnant women vary somewhat depending on the source. According to the CDC, pregnant women should receive a serologic test for syphilis at the onset of prenatal care, again early in the third trimester, and at delivery for high-risk women. Hepatitis B surface antigen (HBsAg) testing should be performed at the onset of prenatal care and repeated late in pregnancy for unvaccinated HBsAg-negative women at high risk (ie, those who have had more than one sex partner in the previous 6 months; have been evaluated for an STD; are current injection drug users; or have an HBsAg-positive partner). Furthermore, women at risk for HBV infection should be vaccinated for hepatitis B.

Providers of obstetric care should test for *Neisseria gonorrhoeae* at the onset of care if local prevalence of gonorrhea is high or if the woman is at increased risk, and testing should be repeated in the third trimester if the woman is at continued risk. Providers should test for *Chlamydia* at the first prenatal visit. Women younger than 25 years and those at increased risk for chlamydial infection (ie, those who have multiple partners or who have a partner with multiple partners) should also be tested in the third trimester. Evaluation for bacterial vaginosis may be conducted at the first prenatal visit for asymptomatic women who are at high risk for preterm labor (ie, those with a past history of preterm delivery).

3. HIV—HIV screening is recommended for patients aged 13–64 years in all health care settings after the patient is notified that testing will be performed unless the patient declines. Repeat annual testing for HIV is indicated for any high-risk patient, including patients with a diagnosed STD or with a history of behaviors that could expose her or him to HIV. Testing is also indicated for patients who present with a history and findings consistent with the acute retroviral syndrome (ARS), symptoms and frequency of which appear in Table 14–2. Appropriate testing regimens include an HIV-1 screening antibody test such as enzyme immunoassay, with a confirmatory test such as the Western immunoblot. HIV-2 prevalence in the United States is very low, so routine testing is not indicated; it should be considered for persons coming from areas of high HIV-2 prevalence (eg, parts of West Africa, particularly Cape Verde, Ivory Coast, Gambia, Guinea-Bissau, Mali, Mauritania, Nigeria, and Sierra Leone).

Early diagnosis of ARS may present a very narrow window of opportunity to alter the course of HIV infection in the recently infected patient, and to block the source of most presumed new HIV transmission. Symptoms are common and nonspecific, making diagnosis difficult without a high index of suspicion; they include fever, malaise, lymphadenopathy, pharyngitis, and skin rash. Appropriate testing should include a nucleic acid test for HIV such as HIV-RNA polymerase chain reaction (PCR) or b-DNA; routine HIV antibody tests are not sufficient, because they generally will not have become positive during ARS. Individuals with positive HIV tests should be referred immediately to an expert in HIV care.

HIV-infected individuals pose particular challenges for STD risk reduction. Reducing high-risk behaviors of known HIV-infected patients is a top priority, both to decrease the further spread of HIV and to limit the exposure of HIV patients to additional STDs. Persons with

Table 14–2. Acute retroviral syndrome: associated signs and symptoms and expected frequency.

Symptoms and Signs	Frequency (%)
Fever	96
Lymphadenopathy	74
Pharyngitis	70
Rash	70
Erythematous maculopapular with lesions on face and trunk and sometimes extremities, including palms and soles	
Mucocutaneous ulceration involving mouth, esophagus, or genitals	
Myalgia or arthralgia	54
Diarrhea	32
Headache	32
Nausea and vomiting	27
Hepatosplenomegaly	14
Weight loss	13
Thrush	12
Neurologic symptoms	12
Meningoencephalitis or aseptic meningitis	
Peripheral neuropathy or radiculopathy	
Facial palsy	
Guillain-Barré syndrome	
Brachial neuritis	
Cognitive impairment or psychosis	

Source: AIDSinfo project, sponsored by the National Institute of Health: Office of AIDS Research, National Institute of Allergy and Infectious Diseases, National Library of Medicine; Centers for Disease Control and Prevention; Health Resources and Service Administration; and Centers for Medicaid & Medicare Services. Available at: http://www.ncbi.nlm.nih.gov/books/bv.fcgi?rid=hstat2.table.10610.

HIV also have substantial medical, psychological, and legal needs that are beyond the scope of this chapter.

4. Other STDs—Accepted national guidelines directing screening for syphilis and other STDs do not exist. If undertaken, additional screening should be guided by local disease prevalence and an individual patient's risk behaviors.

Centers for Disease Control and Prevention. *Expedited Partner Therapy in the Management of Sexually Transmitted Diseases.* US Department of Health and Human Services, 2006. Available at: http://www.cdc.gov/std/treatment/eptfinalreport2006.pdf.

Hollier LM, Workowski K: Treatment of sexually transmitted infections in pregnancy. Clin Perinatol 2005;32:629. [PMID: 16085024]

Leung DT, Sacks SL: Current recommendations for the treatment of genital herpes. Drugs 2000;60:1329. [PMID: 11152015]

McCree DH et al: Status of and pharmacists' role in patient-delivered partner therapy for sexually transmitted diseases. Am J Health Syst Pharm 2005;62:643. [PMID: 15757888]

Stammers T: Abstinence, monogamy, and sex. Lancet 2002;360:1792. [PMID: 12480469]

Stanberry LR, Rosenthal SL: Progress in vaccines for sexually transmitted diseases. Infect Dis Clin North Am 2005;19:477. [PMID: 15963884]

Warren T, Ebel C: Counseling the patient who has genital herpes or genital human papillomavirus infection. Infect Dis Clin North Am 2005;19:459. {PMID: 15963883]

Zenilman JM: Behavioral interventions—rationale, measurement, and effectiveness. Infect Dis Clin North Am 2005;19:541. [PMID: 15963887]

Web Sites

HIV InSite Knowledge Base:

http://hivinsite.ucsf.edu/InSite.jsp? page=KB

US Public Health Service: Guidelines for the Use of Antiretroviral Agents in HIV-Infected Adults and Adolescents:

http://www.hivatis.org/trtgdlns.html

SEXUALLY TRANSMITTED INFECTIONS & SYNDROMES

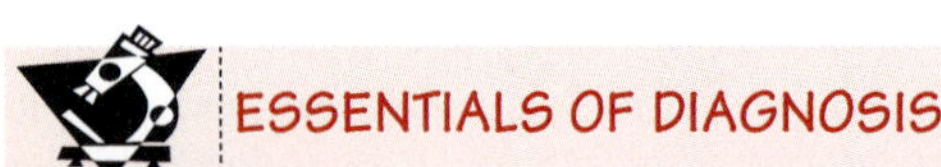

- *Presenting clinical syndromes often guide diagnosis and treatment.*
- *History and findings can justify presumptive treatment while awaiting laboratory confirmation of a diagnosis.*

Patients who are infected with STDs rarely present with accurate knowledge of their microbiological diagnosis. More commonly, patients present with clinical syndromes consistent with one or more diagnoses, so that providers frequently employ syndromic evaluation and treatment. This approach is useful for several reasons, including the fact that more than one disease may be present, and has been employed most commonly in resource-poor settings with limited access to advanced diagnostic technology.

The following recommendations for testing strategies and use of empiric treatment pending laboratory results should be adapted to take into consideration local availability of specific tests, the probability of the diagnosis based on the history and examination, the risk of further transmission while awaiting diagnosis, and the likelihood that an untreated patient will return for laboratory test results and treatment. Treatment information is summarized in Table 14–3 and additional treatment information appears within the text description of specific diseases where applicable.

GENITAL ULCER DISEASES

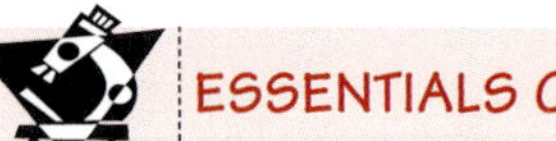

- *Herpes is the most common cause of genital ulcers in the United States.*
- *Most persons infected with herpes simplex virus type 2 (HSV-2) have not been diagnosed with genital herpes.*
- *All genital ulcer patients need syphilis testing via serologic tests (rapid plasma reagin [RPR] or Venereal Disease Research Laboratories [VDRL]), darkfield microscopy, or direct immunofluorescence testing for* Treponema pallidum.

General Considerations

In the United States, herpes simplex is the most common cause of genital ulcer diseases (GUD). Other causes such as syphilis, chancroid, lymphogranuloma venereum, and granuloma inguinale are much less common. Because this is not true throughout the world, physicians treating international travelers or recent arrivals to the United States may need to consider a broad spectrum of potential etiologies. The approach to diagnosis needs to include consideration of the likelihood of the different etiologies based on the patient's history, physical examination, and local epidemiology. Furthermore, all types of GUD are associated with increased risk of HIV transmission, making HIV testing a necessary part of GUD evaluation.

Table 14–3. STD treatment guidelines for adults and adolescents.

Disease	Recommended Regimens	Dose/Route	Alternative Regimens
Chlamydia Uncomplicated infections in adults/adolescents[1]	Azithromycin **or** Doxycycline[2]	1 g po 100 mg po bid × 7 d	Erythromycin base 500 mg po qid × 7 d **or** Erythromycin ethylsuccinate 800 mg po qid × 7 d **or** Ofloxacin[3] 300 mg po bid × 7 d
Pregnant women[4]	Amoxicillin **or** Azithromycin **or** Erythromycin base	500 mg po tid × 7 d 1 g po 500 mg po qid × 7 d	Erythromycin base 250 mg po qid × 14 d **or** Erythromycin ethylsuccinate 800 mg p qid × 7 d **or** Erythromycin ethylsuccinate 400 mg po qid × 14 d
Gonorrhea[5] Uncomplicated infections in adults/adolescents	Ceftriaxone **or** Cefixime[6] **plus** a *Chlamydia* recommended regimen listed above	125 mg IM 400 mg po	Ceftizoxime 500 mg IM **or** Cefotaxime 500 mg IM **or** Cefoxitin 2 g IM **plus** probenecid 1 g po **or** Spectinomycin 2 g IM **plus**[5] a *Chlamydia* recommended regimen
Pregnant women	Ceftriaxone **or** Cefixime[6] **plus**[5] a *Chlamydia* recommended regimen listed above	125 mg IM 400 mg po	Spectinomycin[8] 2 g IM **plus**[5] a *Chlamydia* recommended regimen
Pelvic inflammatory disease	**Parenteral**[9] Cefotetan **or** Cefoxitin **plus** Doxycycline[2] **or** Clindamycin **plus** Gentamicin **Oral treatment** Ceftriaxone **or** Cefoxitin **with** Probenecid **plus** Doxycycline[2] ± Metronidazole	 2 g IV q 12 h 2 g IV q 6 h 100 mg po or IM q 12 h 900 mg IV q 8 h 2 mg/kg IV or IM followed by 1.5 mg/kg IV or IM q 8 h 250 mg IM 2 g IM 1 g po 100 mg po bid × 14 d 500 mg bid × 14 d	**Parenteral** Ampicillin/sulbactam 3 g IV q 6 h **plus** Doxycycline[2] 100 mg po or IV q 12 h If parenteral cephalosporin therapy is not feasible, use of fluoroquinolones (levofloxacin 500 mg orally once daily or ofloxacin 400 mg twice daily for 14 days) with or without metronidazole (500 mg orally twice daily for 14 days) may be considered **if** the community prevalence and individual risk of gonorrhea is low. Tests for gonorrhea must be performed prior to instuting therapy and the patient managed as follows: If NAAT test is positive, parenteral cephalosporin is recommended. If culture for gonorrhea is positive, treatment should be based on results of antimicrobial susceptibility. If isolate is quinolone-resistant or antimicrobial susceptibility cannot be assessed, parenteral cephalosporin is recommended.

(continued)

Table 14–3. STD treatment guidelines for adults and adolescents. (*Continued*)

Disease	Recommended Regimens	Dose/Route	Alternative Regimens
Cervicitis[10]	Azithromycin **or** Doxycycline[2]	1 g po 100 mg po bid × 7 d	Erythromycin base 500 mg po qid × 7 d **or** Erythromycin ethylsuccinate 800 mg po qid × 7 d **or** Ofloxacin[3] 300 mg po bid × 7 d **or** Levofloxacin[3] 500 mg po qd × 7 d
Nongonococcal urethritis[10]	Azithromycin **or** Doxycycline[2]	1 g po 100 mg po bid × 7 d	Erythromycin base 500 mg po qid × 7 d **or** Erythromycin ethylsuccinate 800 mg po qid × 7 d **or** Ofloxacin[3] 300 mg po bid × 7 d **or** Levofloxacin[3] 500 mg po qd × 7 d
Epididymitis	Ceftriaxone **plus** Doxycycline For acute epididymitis most likely caused by enteric organisms or with negative gonococcal culture or nucleic acid amplification test Ofloxacin[3] **or** Levofloxacin	250 mg IM 100 mg po bid × 10 d 300 mg orally twice a day for 10 days 500 mg orally once daily for 10 days	Levofloxacin[3] 500 mg po pd × 10 d
Trichomoniasis	Metronidazole **or** Tinidazole	2 g po 2 g po	Metronidazole 500 mg po bid × 7 d **or** For failure, Tinidazole or Metronidazole 2 g po × 5 d
Vulvovaginal candidiasis	Butoconazole cream[11] Butoconazole 2% cream (SR)[11] Clotrimazole cream[11] Clotrimazole vaginal tablet[11] Miconazole cream[11] Miconazole vaginal suppository[11] Nystatin Tioconazole cream[11] Terconazole cream[11] Terconazole vaginal suppository[11]	2%, 5 g intravaginally × 3 d Single application 1% 5 g intravaginally × 7d 100 mg intravaginally × 7 d 200 mg intravaginally × 3 d 2% 5 g intravaginally × 7 d 100 mg intravaginally × 7 d 200 mg intravaginally × 3 d 1200 mg intravaginally × 1 100,000 units intravaginal tablet × 14 d 6.5% 5 g intravaginally once 0.4% 5 g intravaginally × 7 d 0.8% 5 g intravaginally × 3 d 80 mg intravaginally × 3 d	Fluconazole 150 mg po once
Bacterial vaginosis Adults/adolescents	 Metronidazole **or**	 500 mg po bid × 7 d	 Clindamycin 300 mg po bid × 7 d **or**

	Clindamycin cream[11] **or** Metronidazole gel	2%, one full applicator (5 g) intravaginally at bedtime × 7 d 0.75%, one full applicator (5 g) intravaginally, bid × 5 d	Clindamycin ovules 100 g intravaginally qhs × 3 d
Pregnant women	Metronidazole Clindamycin	250 mg po tid × 7 d **or** 500 mg bid × 7 d 300 mg po bid × 7 d	
Chancroid	Azithromycin **or** Ceftriaxone **or** Ciprofloxacin[3]	1 g po 250 mg IM 500 mg po bid × 3 d	Erythromycin base 500 mg po tid × 7 d
Lymphogranuloma venereum	Doxycycline[2]	100 mg po bid × 21 d	Erythromycin base 500 mg po qid × 21 d Azithromycin 1 g po q week × 3 weeks
Human papillomavirus External genital/perianal warts	**Patient applied** Podofilox[12] 0.5% solution or gel **or** Imiquimod[13] 5% cream **Provider administered** Cryotherapy **or** Podophyllin[12] resin 10–25% in tincture of benzoin **or** Trichloroacetic acid (TCA) **or** Bichloroacetic acid (BCA) 80–90% **or** Surgical removal		Intralesional interferon or laser surgery
Vaginal warts	Cryotherapy **or** TCA or BCA 80–90% **or** Surgical removal		
Urethral meatus warts	Cryotherapy **or** Podophyllin[12] 10–25% in tincture of benzoin		
Anal warts	Cryotherapy **or** TCA or BCA 80–90% **or** Surgical removal		
Herpes simplex virus[13] First clinical episode of herpes	Acyclovir[14] **or** Acyclovir[14] **or** Famciclovir[14] **or** Valacyclovir[14]	400 mg po tid × 7–10 d 200 mg po 5 × q d × 7–10 d 250 mg po tid × 7–10 d 1 g po bid × 7–10 d	

(continued)

Table 14–3. STD treatment guidelines for adults and adolescents. (*Continued*)

Disease	Recommended Regimens	Dose/Route	Alternative Regimens
Herpes simplex virus[13] Episodic therapy for recurrent episodes	Acyclovir[13] **or** Acyclovir[13] **or** Acyclovir[13] **or** Famciclovir[13, 14] **or** Famciclovir[13, 14] **or** Valacyclovir[13, 14] **or** Valacyclovir[13, 14]	400 mg po tid × 5 days 800 mg po bid × 5 d 800 mg po tid × 2 d 125 mg po bid × 5 d 1000 mg po bid × 1 d 500 mg po bid × 3 d 1 g po qd × 5 d	
Herpes simplex virus[13] Suppressive therapy	Acyclovir[13] **or** Famciclovir[14] **or** Valacyclovir[14] **or** Valacyclovir[14]	400 mg po bid 250 mg po bid 500 mg po qd 1 g po qd	
Syphilis Primary, secondary, and early latent	Benzathine penicillin G	2.4 million units IM	Doxycycline[2] 100 mg po bid × 2 weeks **or** Tetracycline[2] 500 mg po qid × 2 weeks
Late latent and unknown duration	Benzathine penicillin G	7.2 million units, administered as 3 doses of 2.4 million units IM, at 1 week intervals	Doxycycline[2] 100 mg po bid × 4 weeks **or** Tetracycline[2] 500 mg po qid × 4 weeks
Neurosyphilis[15]	Aqueous crystalline penicillin G	18–24 million units daily, administered as 3–4 million units IV q 4 h × 10–14 d	Procaine penicillin G, 2.4 million units IM qd × 10–14 d **plus** Probenecid 500 mg po qid × 10–14 d Ceftriaxone 2 g IM or IV qd × 10–14 d (penicillin-allergic patient)
Pregnant women[15] Primary, secondary, and early latent[16]	Benzathine penicillin G	2.4 million units IM	None
Late latent and unknown duration	Benzathine penicillin G	7.2 million units, administered as 3 doses of 2.4 million units IM, at 1 week intervals	None
Neurosyphilis[15]	Aqueous crystalline penicillin G	18–24 million units daily, administered as 3–4 million units IV q 4 h × 10–14 d	Procaine penicillin G, 2.4 million units IM qd × 10–14 d **plus** Probenecid 500 mg po qid × 10–14 d **or** Desensitization if penicillin allergic
Congenital syphilis	Procaine penicillin G	50,000 U/kg IM daily for 10–14 d	Aqueous crystalline penicillin G 100,000–150,000 U/kg/day in doses of 50,000 U/kg IV q 12 h for 7 days then q 8 h for 3–7 days

Children: early (primary)	Benzathine penicillin G	50,000 U/kg IM once (max. 2.4 million units)	
Children: late latent or >1 y late	Benzathine penicillin G	50,000 U/kg IM for 3 doses at 1 week intervals, to max. total dose of 7.2 million units	
HIV infection			
Primary, secondary, and early latent	Benzathine penicillin G	2.4 million units IM	The efficacy of nonpenicillin regimens in HIV-infected persons has not been well studied
Late latent and unknown duration[15] with normal CSF examination	Benzathine penicillin G	7.2 million units, administered as 3 doses of 2.4 million units IM, at 1 week intervals	None
Neurosyphilis[15]	Aqueous crystalline penicillin G	18–24 million units daily, administered as 3–4 million units IV q 4 h × 10–14 d	Procaine penicillin G, 2.4 million units IM qd × 10–14 d **plus** Probenecid 500 mg po qid × 10–14 d
Pediculosis pubis[17] "crab lice"	Permethrin creme rinse	1% applied to affected areas, rinsed after 10 min	Malathion 0.5% lotion applied for 8–12 h and washed off **or** Ivermectin 0.25 mg/kg po repeated in 2 weeks
	Pyrethrins with piperonyl butoxide	Apply to affected area, wash after 10 min	
Scabies[17]	Permethrin cream	5% applied to entire body below neck, washed off after 8–14 h	Lindane 1% 1 oz lotion or 30 g cream applied thinly to entire body below neck, washed off after 8 h[2,18]
	Ivermectin	0.2 mg/kg po repeated in 2 weeks	

po, orally; bid, twice a day; tid, three times a day; qid, four times a day; IM, intramuscularly; IV, intravenously; SR, sustained release; q, every; qd, every day; d, day; h, hours.

[1]Screen adolescents and women younger than 24 y annually, especially if new or multiple partners.

[2]Contraindicated for pregnant and nursing women.

[3]Contraindicated for pregnant and nursing women, and children younger than 18 y.

[4]Test-of-cure follow-up recommended because the regimens are not highly efficacious (amoxicillin and erythromycin) or the data on safety and efficacy are limited (azithromycin).

[5]Cotreatment for *Chlamydia* infection is indicated if coinfection rates are high (>20%), no nucleic acid amplification test for *Chlamydia* was done, or follow-up is uncertain.

[6]Not recommended for pharyngeal gonococcal infection.

[7]If risk of gonorrhea is low and pre-treatment gonorrhea testing is available; if nucleic acid amplification test is positive, treat with cephalosporin, or if culture is positive, treat according to suceptibility.

[8]For patients who cannot tolerate cephalosporins or quinolones; not recommended for pharyngeal gonococcal infection.

[9]Discontinue 24 h after patient improves clinically and continue with oral therapy for a total course of 14 d.

[10]Testing for gonorrhea and *Chlamydia* is recommended because a specific diagnosis may improve compliance and partner management and these infections are reportable.

[11]Might weaken latex condoms and diaphragms because oil based.

[12]Contraindicated during pregnancy.

[13]Counseling especially about natural history, asymptomatic shedding, and sexual transmission is an essential component of herpes management.

[14]Safety in pregnancy has not been established.

[15]Patients allergic to penicillin should be treated with penicillin after desensitization.

[16]Some experts recommend a second dose of 2.4 million units of benzathine penicillin G administered 1 week after the initial dose.

[17]Because efficacy of these therapies has not been established and compliance with some of these regimens is difficult, close follow-up is essential. If compliance or follow-up cannot be ensured, the patient should be desensitized and treated with benzathine penicillin.

[18]Bedding and clothing should be decontaminated (machine washed, machine dried, or dry cleaned) or removed from body contact for >72 h.

[19]Contraindicated for children younger that 2 y.

Sources: CDC STD treatment guidelines (2006), Region IX infertility clinical guidelines, and California STD treatment guidelines for adults and adolescents.

1. Herpes Simplex

Serologic studies suggest that 50 million people in the United States are infected with HSV-2. Data on genital HSV-2 seroprevalence from the National Health and Nutrition Examination Survey (NHANES) III conducted in 1988–1994 reveal HSV-2 seroprevalence among persons at least 12 years of age was 21.9%, 30% higher than the age-adjusted HSV-2 seroprevalence from NHANES II conducted a decade earlier. Increases in seroprevalence occurred primarily in persons aged 12–39 years.

Clinical Findings

A. Symptoms and Signs

A first episode of genital herpes classically presents with blisters and sores, with local tingling and discomfort. Visible lesions may be preceded by a prodrome of tingling or burning. Some patients also report dysesthesia or neuralgic-type pain in the buttocks or legs and malaise with fever. The clinical spectrum of disease can include atypical rashes, fissuring, excoriation and discomfort of the anogenital area, cervical lesions, urinary symptoms, and extragenital lesions. Recent data suggest that only 37% of patients who acquire HSV-2 have symptoms, although overt disease may follow. Atypical genital herpes can present as large, chronic, hyperkeratotic ulcers. It is seen in immunocompromised patients and is sometimes due to acyclovir-resistant HSV.

Both HSV-1 and HSV-2 cause genital disease, although HSV-1 produces fewer clinical recurrences and may be less severe. Symptoms during recurrences are generally less intense and shorter in duration. Infectious virus is shed intermittently and unpredictably in some asymptomatic patients. Latex condoms, when used correctly and consistently, may reduce the risk of genital HSV transmission.

B. Laboratory Findings

Diagnosis of HSV is based on either culture of the vesicle base or ulcer, or PCR test for HSV DNA. PCR assays for HSV DNA are more sensitive and have been used instead of viral culture; however, PCR tests are not FDA-approved for testing of genital specimens. Cytologic detection of cellular changes of herpes virus infection is insensitive and nonspecific, both in genital lesions (Tzanck smear) and cervical Papanicolaou (Pap) smears, and so should not be relied on. Type-specific serologic assays may be useful in patients with recurrent symptoms and negative HSV cultures, those with a clinical diagnosis of genital herpes without laboratory confirmation, or in patients who have a partner with genital herpes.

Treatment

Treatment of HSV is either episodic (ie, in response to an episode of disease) or suppressive, with daily medication continuing for months or years. Treatment for an initial outbreak consists of 7–10 days of oral medication (see Table 14–3). Episodic treatment is effective when medication is started during the prodrome or on the first symptomatic day. No benefit will be seen if treatment of recurrences is delayed until lesions are vesicular; thus, patients should be given a prescription to have available for use when needed.

Suppressive therapy is traditionally indicated for patients with frequent recurrences (> 5 per year) although this may be individualized based on the stress and disability caused by recurrences. Available experience suggests that long-term suppression is safe and is not associated with development of antiviral resistance. Suppressive therapy seems to reduce but not eliminate asymptomatic shedding. Daily treatment with valacyclovir, 500 mg, has been shown to decrease the rate of HSV-2 transmission in discordant heterosexual couples in which the source partner has a history of genital HSV-2 infection. Suppression does not change the natural history of a patient's infection; however, because the frequency of recurrences diminishes with time, suppression may be particularly useful during the time period immediately following initial infection. Suppressive therapy may reduce risk of HIV transmission or acquisition. Available therapies appear to be safe in pregnant women, although data for valacyclovir and famciclovir are limited.

2. Syphilis

General Considerations

Syphilis cases reported to the CDC had declined since the early 1950s until a resurgence was noted in the 1990s. In 1999, the CDC launched "The National Plan to Eliminate Syphilis from the United States." In 2004, 7980 cases of primary and secondary syphilis were reported, an 11% increase over the previous year. Of concern, national numbers have increased every year since 2000, and recent resurgences of syphilis in some populations and geographic areas indicate the need for continued vigilance.

Clinical Findings

A. Symptoms and Signs

Syphilis infection is characterized by stages, and accurate staging is vital to determine appropriate therapy. **Primary syphilis** is characterized by the appearance of a painless, indurated ulcer—the chancre—occurring 10 days to 3 months after infection with *T pallidum.* The chancre usually heals by 4–6 weeks, although associated painless bilateral lymphadenopathy may persist for months.

Secondary syphilis has variable manifestations, but usually includes symmetric mucocutaneous macular, papular, papulosquamous, or pustular lesions with generalized nontender lymphadenopathy. In moist skin areas such as the perianal or vulvar regions, papules may become superficially eroded to form pink or whitish condylomata lata. Constitutional symptoms such as fever, malaise, and weight loss occur commonly. Less common complications include meningitis, hepatitis, arthritis, nephropathy, and iridocyclitis.

Latent syphilis is diagnosed in persons with serologic evidence of syphilis infection *without* other current evidence of disease. "Early" latent syphilis is defined as infection for less than 1 year. A diagnosis of early latent syphilis is demonstrated by seroconversion, a definitive history of primary or secondary syphilis findings within the past year, or documented exposure to primary or secondary syphilis in the past year. Asymptomatic patients with known infection of more than 1 year or in whom infection of less than 1 year cannot be conclusively demonstrated are classified as having late latent syphilis or latent syphilis of unknown duration, respectively. These two categories of syphilis are treated equivalently. The magnitude of serologic test titers cannot reliably differentiate early from late latent syphilis.

Neurosyphilis is diagnosed by positive cerebrospinal fluid (CSF) VDRL test. It is suggested by positive CSF fluorescent treponemal antibody absorption (FTA-ABS), although false-positive results occur in the absence of neurosyphilis, and is suggested by CSF pleocytosis (> 5 white blood cells [WBCs]/mm^3), although HIV infection and other conditions may also cause increased WBCs in the CSF.

Tertiary syphilis is diagnosed in patients with syphilitic aortitis, and in patients with one or more gummas, a syphilitic granuloma. Patients are infectious during primary, secondary, and early latent stages of syphilis.

B. Laboratory Findings

Positive darkfield examination or direct fluorescent antibody tests of lesion exudates definitively diagnose primary syphilis. More typically, syphilis is diagnosed by positive results of both a nontreponemal test (VDRL or RPR) and a treponemal test (*T pallidum* particle agglutination [TP-PA] or FTA-ABS).

Nontreponemal tests are sometimes falsely positive due to other medical conditions (eg, some collagen vascular diseases). When positive due to syphilis, their titers generally rise and fall in response to *T pallidum* infection and treatment, respectively, and usually return to normal (negative) following treatment, although some individuals remain "serofast" and have persistent low positive titers. Treponemal tests usually yield persistent positive results throughout the patient's life following infection with *T pallidum*. Treponemal test titers do not correlate with disease activity or treatment.

Lumbar puncture is indicated for (1) neurologic or ophthalmologic signs or symptoms, (2) active aortitis or gumma, (3) treatment failure (a fourfold increase in titer or a failure to decline fourfold or more within 12–24 months), or (4) patients with late or unknown duration latent syphilis and coexisting HIV infection.

Treatment

Treatment for syphilis as described in Table 14–3 is based on current CDC guidelines. Follow-up testing of patients diagnosed with syphilis is a vital part of care, as it determines the effectiveness of therapy and provides useful information to differentiate potential future serofast patients from those with recurrent infection.

The 6-month post-treatment, nontreponemal test titer should have fallen fourfold or more (eg, from 1:32 to 1:8 or less) for persons with primary or secondary syphilis. If it does not, consider this a treatment failure or an indication of reinfection. In evaluating such a potential treatment failure, the patient should, at minimum, receive continued serologic follow-up, and repeat HIV serology if previously negative. Lumbar puncture should also be considered, and if the results are normal, the patient should be treated with 2.4 million units of benzathine penicillin weekly for 3 weeks and followed as described above.

3. Chancroid

Although very common in other parts of the world, in 2004 a total of 31 cases of chancroid were reported in the United States. These data should be interpreted with caution, however, in view of the fact that *Haemophilus ducreyi* is difficult to culture, and thus this condition may be substantially underdiagnosed.

Definitive diagnosis is difficult, requiring identification of *H ducreyi* on special culture medium that is generally not readily available. Presumptive diagnosis rests on the presence of painful genital ulcer(s) with a negative HSV test and negative syphilis serology, with or without regional lymphadenopathy.

Treatment consists of oral antibiotics as listed in Table 14–3. Healing of large ulcers may require more than 2 weeks. If patients do not show clinical improvement after 7 days, consider the accuracy of the diagnosis, medication nonadherence, antibacterial resistance, or a combination of these. Fluctuant lymphadenopathy may require drainage via aspiration or incision.

Although definitive diagnosis generally rests on laboratory testing, history and examination often lead to a presumptive diagnosis. Table 14–4 summarizes findings for different causes of GUD.

Table 14–4. Differentiation of common causes of genital ulcers.[1]

	Herpes	Syphilis	Chancroid	Lymphogranuloma Venereum	Granuloma Inguinale
Ulcer(s) Appearance	Often purulent	"Clean"	Purulent	May be purulent	"Beefy," hemorrhagic
Number	Usually multiple	Single[2]	Often multiple	Single or multiple	Multiple
Pain	Yes	No	Yes	Ulcer: no Nodes: yes	No
Preceded by	Papule, then vesicle	Papule	Papule	Papule; ulcer often unnoticed	Nodule(s)
Adenopathy	Painful with primary outbreak	Painless	Painful; may suppurate	Painful; may suppurate	No, unless secondary bacterial infection
Systemic symptoms	Often with primary outbreak	Usually not	Occasionally	Usually not	No

[1]A diagnosis based solely on medical history and physical examination is often inaccurate.
[2]Up to 40% of patients with primary syphilis have more than one chancre.

4. Other Causes of GUD

Granuloma inguinale or donovanosis is caused by *Calymmatobacterium granulomatis,* which is endemic in some tropical nonindustrialized parts of the world and is rarely reported in the United States. The bacterium does not grow on standard culture media; diagnosis rests on demonstration of so-called Donovan bodies in a tissue specimen. Infection causes painless, progressive, beefy red, highly vascular lesions without lymphadenopathy. Treatment is often prolonged, and relapse can occur months after initial treatment and apparent cure.

Lymphogranuloma venereum is caused by serovars L1, L2, and L3 of *C trachomatis.* The small ulcer arising at the site of infection is often unnoticed or unreported. The most common clinical presentation is painful unilateral lymphadenopathy. Rectal exposure in women and in men who have sex with men may result in proctocolitis (mucus or hemorrhagic rectal discharge, anal pain, constipation, fever, or tenesmus). Diagnosis rests on clinical suspicion, epidemiologic information, exclusion of other etiologies, and *C trachomatis* tests. In addition to antibiotics, treatment may require aspiration or incision and drainage of buboes, and despite this patients may still experience scarring.

Beauman JG: Genital herpes: A review. Am Fam Physician 2005;72:1527. [PMID: 16273819]

Centers for Disease Control and Prevention (CDC): Lymphogranuloma venereum among men who have sex with men–Netherlands, 2003–2004. MMWR Morb Mortal Wkly Rep 2004;53:985. [PMID: 15514580]

Peterman TA et al: The changing epidemiology of syphilis. Sex Transm Dis 2005;32:S4. [PMID: 16205291]

Trager JD: Sexually transmitted diseases causing genital lesions in adolescents. Adolesc Med Clin 2004;15:323. [PMID: 15449848]

URETHRITIS

ESSENTIALS OF DIAGNOSIS

- *Coinfection with* C trachomatis *is common in those with* N gonorrhoeae, *justifying treatment for both.*
- *Nucleic acid amplification tests (PCR and others) of urine have largely supplanted older culture tests for diagnosis.*

The best estimates from population studies of adolescents and young adults suggest 3–5% have chlamydial infection and 0.4% have gonorrhea, although prevalence for each of these infections in some populations may exceed 10%.

STDs causing urethritis are typically diagnosed in men, although women may also experience urethritis as a consequence of an STD. For clinical management, urethritis can be divided into "nongonococcal urethritis" (NGU) and urethritis due to *N gonorrhoeae* infection.

1. Nongonococcal Urethritis

One frequent cause of NGU is *C trachomatis.* In 2004, 210,396 *Chlamydia* cases were reported in males; female cases were more than threefold greater at 716,675, and, although significant, these numbers likely dramatically underestimate actual cases of *C trachomatis* infection. The spectrum of *C trachomatis*–caused disease includes extragenital manifestations, among them ophthalmic infection and a reactive arthritis.

Causes of nonchlamydial NGU cases may include *Mycoplasma genitalium, Ureaplasma urealyticum, Trichomonas vaginalis,* herpes simplex, and adenovirus. Diagnosis of NGU can be based on (1) purulent urethral discharge, (2) urethral secretions with 5 or more WBCs per high-power field (HPF) and no gram-negative intracellular diplococci (which if present would indicate gonorrhea), (3) first-void urine with positive leukocyte esterase, or more than 10 WBCs/HPF, or (4) a positive nucleic acid amplification–based test performed on a urine specimen. Nucleic acid amplification tests offer greater convenience and better sensitivity than culture and represent the best tests currently available to diagnose *C trachomatis* infection or gonorrhea.

2. Gonorrhea

General Considerations

In 2004, gonorrhea was reported in 157,303 men and 172,142 women in the United States.

Clinical Findings

A. Symptoms and Signs

If symptomatic, gonorrhea typically causes dysuria and a purulent urethral discharge; however, it may also cause asymptomatic infection or disseminated systemic disease, including skin lesions, septic arthritis, tenosynovitis, arthralgias, perihepatitis, endocarditis, and meningitis. In these cases, there is usually minimal genital inflammation.

Clinical differentiation between *C trachomatis* and gonorrhea may be difficult. Characteristically, urethral exudate in gonorrhea is thicker, more profuse, and more purulent in appearance than the exudate caused by *C trachomatis,* which is often watery with mucus strands. However, differentiation of etiology based on clinical appearance is notoriously unreliable.

B. Laboratory Findings

Nucleic acid amplification technology has largely supplanted culture for diagnosis due to enhanced sensitivity, excellent specificity, and greater patient acceptance. Tests can be performed on a urine specimen, eliminating more invasive specimen collection.

Diagnostic evaluation identifies disease etiology and may facilitate the public health missions of contact tracing and disease eradication. For an individual patient, however, the physician may treat empirically if follow-up cannot be assured and an insensitive diagnostic test was used. Decisions about diagnostic testing should consider both public health goals and how information obtained will influence patient (and partner) treatment.

In patients presenting with recurrent urethritis, diagnostic evaluation may be necessary to identify the etiology. In evaluating recurrent urethritis, the physician should assess medication compliance and potential reexposure; perform wet mount, culture, or both, for *T vaginalis;* and treat as indicated by findings, or empirically as per Table 14–3.

Treatment

Treatment of NGU generally employs azithromycin or doxycycline, with alternatives as listed in Table 14–3. If findings of urethritis are present, treatment is generally indicated pending results of diagnostic tests. Because diagnostic testing typically does not look for all potential causes of urethritis, patients with negative tests for gonorrhea and *C trachomatis* may also benefit from treatment. Empiric treatment of symptoms without documentation of urethritis is recommended only for patients at high risk for infection who are unlikely to return for a follow-up evaluation. Such patients should be treated for gonorrhea and *Chlamydia.* Partners of patients treated empirically should be evaluated and treated. If treatment is not offered at the initial visit, diagnostic testing should use the most sensitive test available, with additional treatment as indicated by test results and symptom persistence.

When treating for gonorrhea, practitioners should treat also for *C trachomatis,* as coinfection is common and treatments for the former are generally inadequate for the latter. Quinolone-resistant gonorrhea exists and is spreading worldwide and throughout the United States, and quinolones are no longer recommended for treatment of gonorrhea.

Treatment failures should be followed by repeat culture and sensitivity testing, and any resistance should be reported to the public health department.

Bradshaw CS et al: Etiologies of nongonococcal urethritis: Bacteria, viruses, and the association with orogenital exposure. J Infect Dis 2006;193:336. [PMID: 16388480]

Centers for Disease Control and Prevention. Update to CDC's Sexually Transmitted Disease Treatment Guidelines, 2006: Fluoroquinolones No Longer Recommended for Treatement of Gonococcal Infections. MMWR 2007;56:332–6.

Miller WC et al: Prevalence of chlamydial and gonococcal infections among young adults in the United States. JAMA 2004;291:2229. [PMID: 15138245]

EPIDIDYMITIS

The cause of epididymitis varies with age. It is most commonly due to gonorrhea or *C trachomatis* in men 35 years of age or younger, or to gram-negative enteric organisms in men 35 years of age or older who engage in unprotected insertive anal intercourse, who have undergone recent urologic surgery, or who have anatomic abnormalities. Patients usually present with unilateral testicular pain and inflammation with onset over several days. The clinician must differentiate epididymitis from testicular torsion, a surgical emergency requiring immediate correction. The laboratory evaluation of suspected epididymitis is essentially the same as for urethritis, and includes Gram stain, culture or antigen test, and serologic testing for HIV and syphilis.

PROCTITIS, PROCTOCOLITIS, & ENTERITIS

Proctitis, proctocolitis, and enteritis may arise from anal intercourse or oral-anal contact. Depending on organism and anatomic location of infection and inflammation, symptoms can include pain, tenesmus, rectal discharge, and diarrhea. Etiologic agents include *C trachomatis* (lymphogranuloma venereum), *N gonorrhea, T pallidum,* HSV, *Giardia lamblia, Campylobacter, Shigella,* and *Entamoeba histolytica.* In HIV-infected patients, additional etiologic agents include cytomegalovirus, *Mycobacterium avium intracellulare, Salmonella, Cryptosporidium, Microsporidium,* and *Isospora.* Symptoms may also arise as a primary effect of HIV infection.

Diagnosis involves examination of stool for ova, parasites, occult blood, and WBCs; stool culture; and anoscopy or sigmoidoscopy. If the patient's clinical situation permits, diagnostic evaluation may proceed in a stepwise fashion, delaying endoscopy until other tests prove nondiagnostic.

Treatment should generally be based on results of diagnostic studies. However, if the onset of symptoms occurs within 1–2 weeks of receptive anal intercourse, and there is evidence of purulent exudates or polymorphonuclear neutrophils on Gram stain of anorectal smear, the patient can be treated presumptively for gonorrhea and chlamydial infection, reserving additional evaluation and treatment for patients who fail to respond to this therapy.

VAGINITIS

ESSENTIALS OF DIAGNOSIS

- *Pelvic examination.*
- *Examination of vaginal discharge by wet mount, potassium hydroxide (KOH) preparation, pH, and odor.*
- *Disease-specific point-of-care test or vaginal fluid culture if indicated.*

Patients with vaginitis may present with vaginal discharge, vulvar itching, irritation, or all of these, and sometimes with complaints of abnormal vaginal odor. Common etiologies include *C albicans, T vaginalis,* and bacterial vaginosis. Diagnostic evaluation typically includes physical examination and evaluation of a saline wet mount and potassium hydroxide (KOH) preparation. Differences between common causes of vaginitis are summarized in Table 14–5 and described below.

1. Vulvovaginal Candidiasis

Vulvovaginal candidiasis (VVC) is typically caused by *C albicans,* although occasionally other species are identified. More than 75% of all women will have at least one episode of VVC during their lifetime. The diagnosis is presumed if the patient has vulvovaginal pruritus and erythema with or without a white discharge, and is confirmed by wet mount or KOH preparation showing yeast or pseudohyphae, or culture showing a yeast species.

VVC can be classified as uncomplicated, complicated, or recurrent. Uncomplicated VVC encompasses sporadic, nonrecurrent, mild to moderate symptoms due to *C albicans* that, in an otherwise healthy patient, are sensitive to routine therapy. Complicated VVC implies recur-

Table 14–5. Common causes of vaginitis.

	Findings Characteristic of		
Diagnostic Test	**Candida albicans**	**Trichomonas vaginalis**	***Bacterial Vaginosis***
pH	<4.5		>4.5
KOH to slide	Yeast or pseudohyphae		Amine or "fishy" odor
Saline to slide	Yeast or pseudohyphae	Motile *T vaginalis* organisms	"Clue" cells
Culture	Yeast species	*T vaginalis*	Nonspecific (not recommended)

rent or severe local disease in a patient with impaired immune function (eg, diabetes or HIV), or infection with resistant yeast species. Recurrent VVC is defined as four or more symptomatic episodes annually.

Treatment is summarized in Table 14–3. Uncomplicated candidiasis should respond to short-term or single-dose therapies as listed. Complicated VVC may require prolonged treatment. Treatment of women with recurrent vulvovaginal candidiasis should begin with an intensive regimen (7–14 days of topical therapy or a three-dose fluconazole regimen) followed by 6 months of maintenance therapy to reduce the likelihood of subsequent recurrence. Symptomatic candidal vaginitis is more frequent in HIV-infected women and correlates with severity of immunodeficiency.

VVC is not usually acquired through sexual intercourse; treatment of sex partners is not recommended but may be considered in women who have recurrent infection. Some male sex partners have balanitis and may benefit from topical antifungal agents.

2. Trichomoniasis

Vaginitis due to *T vaginalis* presents with a thin, yellow or yellow-green frothy malodorous discharge and vulvar irritation that may worsen following menstruation. Diagnosis can often be made via prompt examination of a freshly obtained wet mount, which reveals the motile trichomonads. Although culture is more sensitive, it may not be as readily available, and results are delayed. Point-of-care tests (eg, Osom Trichomonas Rapid Test and Affirm VPIII) are also available. Partners of women with trichomonas infection require treatment; although men are usually asymptomatic, they will reinfect female partners if untreated.

3. Bacterial Vaginosis

Bacterial vaginosis arises when normal vaginal bacteria are replaced with an overgrowth of anaerobic bacteria. Although not thought to be an STD, it is associated with having multiple sex partners or a new sex partner. The cause of microbiological change is uncertain.

Diagnosis can be based on the presence of three of four clinical criteria: (1) a thin, homogeneous vaginal discharge, (2) a vaginal pH value of more than 4.5, (3) a positive KOH test, and (4) the presence of clue cells in a wet mount preparation.

Culture is generally not indicated. Treatment relieves symptoms and may also reduce the incidence of preterm delivery in pregnant women (who have a history of previous preterm birth) and who have asymptomatic bacterial vaginosis. If treated, consider test of cure 1 month later, as recurrence in both pregnant and nonpregnant women is common. Treatment of the male partner does not affect symptoms in the female patient.

4. Cervicitis

Cervicitis is characterized by purulent discharge from the endocervix, which may or may not be associated with vaginal discharge or cervical bleeding. The diagnostic evaluation should include testing for *Chlamydia,* gonorrhea, bacterial vaginosis, and trichomonas. Absence of symptoms should not preclude additional evaluation and treatment, as approximately 70% of chlamydial infections and 50% of gonococcal infections in women are asymptomatic.

Any positive test results require treatment. Urine nucleic acid tests for *Chlamydia* demonstrate sensitivity and specificity comparable to cervical or urethral specimens, although reduced sensitivity for gonorrhea makes urine specimens inferior to a cervical specimen. Empiric treatment should be considered in areas with high prevalence of *C trachomatis* or gonorrhea, or if follow-up is unlikely.

Cook RL et al: Systematic review: Noninvasive testing for *Chlamydia trachomatis* and *Neisseria gonorrhoeae.* Ann Intern Med 2005;142:914. [PMID: 15941699]

French L et al: Abnormal vaginal discharge: What does and does not work in treating underlying causes. J Fam Pract 2004;53:890. [PMID: 15527726]

Marrazzo JM et al: Predicting chlamydial and gonococcal cervical infection: Implications for management of cervicitis. Obstet Gynecol 2002;100:579. [PMID: 12220782]

PELVIC INFLAMMATORY DISEASE

ESSENTIALS OF DIAGNOSIS

- *Diagnosis is challenging, requiring the clinician to balance underdiagnosis with overtreatment.*
- *Consequences of untreated pelvic inflammatory disease (PID) can include chronic pain, sterility, and death.*

PID is defined as inflammation of the upper genital tract, including pelvic peritonitis, endometritis, salpingitis, and tuboovarian abscess due to infection with gonorrhea, *C trachomatis,* or vaginal or bowel flora. Diagnosis is challenging due to often vague symptoms, lack of a single diagnostic test, and the invasive nature of technologies needed to make a definitive diagnosis. Lower abdominal tenderness and uterine, adnexal, or cervical motion tenderness without other explanation of illness is sufficient to diagnose PID. Other criteria enhance the specificity of the diagnosis (but reduce diagnostic sensitivity):

- Fever higher than 38.3 °C (101 °F).
- Abnormal cervical or vaginal discharge.

- Abundant WBCs in saline microscopy of vaginal secretions.
- Elevated sedimentation rate.
- Elevated C-reactive protein.
- Cervical infection with gonorrhea or *C trachomatis*.

Definitive diagnosis rests on techniques that are not always readily available and that are not generally used to make the diagnosis. These include laparoscopic findings consistent with PID, evidence of endometritis on endometrial biopsy, and ultrasonographic findings showing thickened fluid-filled tubes with or without free pelvic fluid or tuboovarian complex.

Determination of appropriate therapy should consider pregnancy status, severity of illness, and patient compliance. Less severe disease can generally be treated with oral antibiotics in an ambulatory setting, whereas pregnant patients and those with severe disease may need hospitalization. Options are listed in Table 14–3.

Ness RB et al: Effectiveness of inpatient and outpatient treatment strategies for women with pelvic inflammatory disease: Results from the Pelvic Inflammatory Disease Evaluation and Clinical Health (PEACH) Randomized Trial. Am J Obstet Gynecol 2002;186:929. [PMID: 120165517]

EXTERNAL GENITAL WARTS

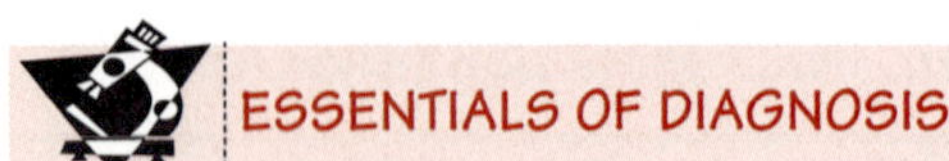

- *Diagnosis typically rests on appearance, and biopsy is rarely indicated for diagnosis.*
- *Treatment does not eradicate HPV infection, but treatment may reduce risk of neoplastic change.*

General Considerations

It is estimated that over 20 million Americans are infected with HPV, with one million new infections and 250,000 initial visits to physicians for genital warts occurring annually. Over 100 types of HPV have been identified, and over 30 types cause genital lesions. Types 6, 11, and others typically produce benign exophytic warts, whereas types 16, 18, 31, 33, 35, and others are associated with dysplasia and neoplasia. Thus, cervical and anogenital squamous cancer can be considered STDs, and other cancers may also be sexually transmitted.

Clinical Findings

Diagnosis is almost always based on physical examination with bright light and magnification, and rarely requires biopsy. If the diagnosis is uncertain, consider referral to a physician with extensive experience in external genital warts. Biopsy should be considered for warts that are larger than 1 cm; indurated, ulcerated, or fixed to underlying structures; atypical in appearance; pigmented; or resistant to therapy. Application of 3–5% acetic acid as an aid to visualization is generally not useful, and the resulting nonspecific acetowhite reaction may lead to overdiagnosis of genital warts.

Cancer screening via cervical Pap smear, if not done in the past 12 months, is indicated, and may be collected after other specimens (eg, cervical culture swabs). Regular cervical Pap smears are also indicated for women who have sex with women, a population sometimes erroneously felt to have limited risk for cervical cancer. Genital warts are not an indication for screening more frequently than every 12 months.

Type-specific HPV DNA tests may be useful in the triage of women with atypical squamous cells of undetermined significance (ASCUS) or in screening women 30 years of age or older in conjunction with the Pap test. Abnormal Pap results should be managed according to current recommendations.

Because of the increased incidence of anal cancer in HIV-infected homosexual and bisexual men and high-risk women, screening for anal cytologic abnormalities is recommended by some specialists. However, there are limited data on the natural history of anal intraepithelial neoplasias, the reliability of screening methods, the safety of and response to treatments, and the programmatic considerations that would support this screening approach.

Treatment

The therapeutic goal in treatment of external genital warts is elimination of warts, *not* elimination of HPV infection. Treatment strives to eliminate symptoms, and a potential theoretical benefit is reduced likelihood of transmission. Clinicians should be certain of the diagnosis prior to instituting therapy, and should not apply treatments to skin tags, pearly penile papules, sebaceous glands, or other benign findings that do not require (and will not respond to) genital wart treatment.

No evidence suggests any treatment is superior to others. The possibility of spontaneous resolution may justify no treatment, if that is the patient's wish.

Treatments can be categorized as provider applied or patient applied. Physicians should familiarize themselves with at least one or two treatments in each category, as described in Table 14–3. Most treatments work via tissue destruction. Imiquimod uses a different mechanism; by inducing production of interferon, it may be more effective than other therapies in treating some genital warts or other skin conditions, including molluscum contagiosum. Patients unresponsive to an initial course of treatment may require another round of treatment, more aggressive treatment, or referral to a specialist.

Patients with HPV need to understand the chronic nature of this infection, its natural history, and treatment options, and should receive adequate education and counseling to achieve optimal treatment outcomes. The chronic nature of HPV infection combined with the serious, albeit relatively infrequent, complication of cancer creates significant challenges to patient coping and provider counseling.

Beutner KR et al: External genital warts: Report of the American Medical Association Consensus Conference. Clin Infect Dis 1998;27:796. [PMID: 9798036]

Kodner CM, Nasraty S: Management of genital warts. Am Fam Physician 2004;70:2335. [PMID: 15617297]

MOLLUSCUM CONTAGIOSUM

Molluscum contagiosum appears in individuals of all ages and from all races, but has been reported more commonly in the white population and in males. Lesions are due to infection with poxvirus, which is transmitted through direct skin contact, as occurs among children in a nursery school and among adults during sexual activity. Diagnosis is typically based on inspection, which reveals dimpled or umbilicated flesh-colored or pearly papules several millimeters in diameter; if needed, a smear of the core stained with Giemsa reveals cytoplasmic inclusion bodies. Lesions usually number less than 10–30, but may exceed 100, especially in HIV-infected patients who may have verrucous, warty papules, as well as mollusca greater than 1 cm in diameter. Lesions usually resolve spontaneously within months of appearance, but can be treated with cryotherapy, cautery, curettage, or removal of the lesion's core, with or without local anesthesia.

Trager JDK: Sexually transmitted diseases causing genital lesions in adolescents. Adolesc Med 2004;15:323. [PMID: 15449848]

HEPATITIS

Vaccines for prevention of viral hepatitis and indications have been previously described. Diagnostic and treatment considerations of viral hepatitis are reviewed in Chapter 31.

ECTOPARASITES

Pediculosis pubis results from infestation with "crab lice" or *Phthirus pubis.* Affected patients usually present with pubic or anogenital pruritus, and may have identified lice or nits. The physician should be able to identify lice or nits with careful examination, and their absence calls into question the diagnosis despite compatible history.

Scabies, resulting from infestation with *Sarcoptes scabiei,* usually presents with pruritus not necessarily limited to the genital region. The intensity of pruritus may be increased at bedtime, and may be out of proportion to modest physical findings of erythematous papules, burrows, or excoriation from scratching. A classic finding on physical examination is the serpiginous burrow present in the web space between fingers, although this finding is frequently absent in individuals with scabies.

Scabies can be sexually transmitted in adults, although sexual contact is not the usual route of transmission in children. Pruritus may persist for weeks after treatment. Retreatment should be deferred if intensity of symptoms is diminishing and no new findings appear. In HIV-infected patients with uncomplicated scabies, treatment is the same as for HIV-uninfected patients. However, HIV-infected patients are at risk for a more severe infestation with Norwegian scabies, which should be managed with expert consultation.

Ambroise-Thomas P: Parasitic diseases and immunodeficiencies. Parasitology 2001;122:S65. [PMID: 11442198]

GENERAL PRINCIPLES OF THERAPY FOR STDS

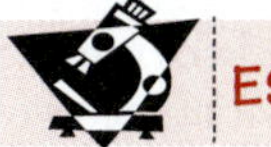

ESSENTIAL FEATURES

- *Presumptive treatment while awaiting laboratory test results is common practice.*
- *Coexisting HIV infection may modify STD treatment regimens.*
- *Patient education and partner treatment are essential to reduce disease spread.*

Treatments may be empirically targeted to agents most likely causing the presenting clinical syndrome, or targeted to a specific infection diagnosed definitively. Regardless, there are overarching concerns affecting STD treatment that pertain to adherence and treatment success, HIV status, partner treatment, test of cure, and pregnancy.

Adherence considerations may favor shorter or single-dose regimens. For example, although single-dose azithromycin is more expensive than 7-day doxycycline therapy, reduced medication compliance and attendant costs of follow-up evaluation for patients treated with doxycycline may favor the use of azithromycin.

With HIV coinfection, treatments are generally the same as for uninfected patients unless stated otherwise. One potential difference is that HSV often causes more significant and prolonged symptoms in HIV-infected than in uninfected patients, so that HIV-infected patients may require longer treatment or higher medication dosages, or both. Syphilis treatment is the same as for HIV-uninfected patients, although some experts recommend extending benzathine penicillin therapy weekly for primary, secondary, and early latent syphilis. Careful follow-up is even more important, as treatment failure or progression to neurosyphilis may be more common in the presence of HIV.

STD treatment can reduce HIV transmission, although the benefit of STD treatment with respect to HIV transmission may diminish as HIV prevalence increases. Ulcerative and nonulcerative STDs increase the risk of HIV transmission approximately three- to fivefold.

Pregnancy imposes constraints and special considerations for therapy. Where applicable, these are noted in the treatment recommendations in Table 14–3.

As previously described, patients often present with a clinical syndrome potentially attributable to more than one infectious agent, and optimally focused therapy depends on microbiological identification. However, delaying therapy may allow symptoms to continue, resulting in untreated infection or continued spread (if the patient fails to return for follow-up or heed advice to avoid sexual contact until cured), and contribute to increased long-term morbidity. Consequently, it may be desirable to "overtreat" upon initial presentation to avoid the risk of these undesirable sequelae, or at least discuss with patients the risks and benefits of immediate presumptive treatment versus delayed targeted treatment. This syndromic management has been employed in other countries as a strategy to reduce HIV transmission with variable success. However, even where successful, generalization from studies performed elsewhere may not be appropriate. It appears that for several STDs, prevalence and patient presentation in African cohorts may be different than in studies of patients in industrialized countries.

Web Sites

American Social Health Association (ASHA):
http://www.ashastd.org/
CDC STD Treatment Guidelines:
http://www.cdc.gov/nchstp/dstd/
Infectious Diseases Society of America (IDSA):
http://www.idsociety.org/

SEXUAL ASSAULT

Management of victims of sexual assault encompasses much more than treatment or prevention of STDs. Providers must heed legal requirements and effectively manage the psychological trauma, while not compromising the best course of medical care.

Proper medical management of sexual assault victims includes collection of evidence, diagnostic evaluation, counseling, and medical therapies to treat infection and unintended pregnancy. The diagnostic evaluation should include the following:

- Culture or FDA-approved nucleic acid amplification tests for *N gonorrhoeae* and *C trachomatis* from specimens collected from any sites of penetration or attempted penetration.
- Vaginal wet mount and culture for *T vaginalis.*
- Serum tests for syphilis, hepatitis B, and HIV.

Repeat wet mount and cultures should be obtained 2 weeks after initial evaluation to detect organisms that may have been present initially in small numbers and thus were undetected, unless the patient was treated prophylactically. Providers should also consider a late screen for hepatitis C virus, transmission of which has been documented following sexual assault.

Prophylactic treatment for STDs may be offered or recommended. Hepatitis B vaccine should be administered according to the routine schedule; hepatitis B immune globulin is not necessary. Azithromycin, 1 g orally, plus ceftriaxone 125 mg intramuscularly, plus metronidazole, 2 g orally, may be offered to treat *C trachomatis, N gonorrhea,* and *Trichomonas.* Gastrointestinal side effects, especially when combined with postcoital oral contraceptive pills, may make this regimen intolerable, and alternative therapies or watchful waiting may be preferable.

Need for and benefit from HIV postexposure prophylaxis is difficult to predict. If instituted, the greatest benefit results from initiation of therapy as soon after exposure as possible. For guidance in deciding whether to begin postexposure HIV prophylaxis and in selecting appropriate treatment and monitoring, providers may contact the National Clinician's Post-Exposure Prophylaxis Hotline (PEPline) at 888-HIV-4911 (888-448-4911).

After the neonatal period, STDs in children most commonly result from sexual abuse. In addition to vaginal gonococcal infection, pharyngeal and anorectal infection are common and often asymptomatic. Diagnostic techniques should rely only on FDA-approved tests due to the legal ramifications of the results, and ideally will include confirmatory tests using different methodologies, with specimen preservation for future testing when needed.

Centers for Disease Control and Prevention; Workowski KA, Berman SM: Sexually transmitted diseases treatment guidelines, 2006. MMWR Recomm Rep 2006;55(RR-11):1. [PMID: 16888612].

Smith DK et al; US Department of Health and Human Services: Antiretroviral postexposure prophylaxis after sexual, injection-drug use, or other nonoccupational exposure to HIV in the United States: Recommendations from the US Department of Health and Human Services. MMWR Recomm Rep 2005;54(RR-2):1. [PMID: 15660015]

SECTION III
Adults

Preconception Care 15

Essam Demian, MD, MRCOG

There were 4,089,950 births in the United States in 2003, 2% more than the previous year. Although most infants are born healthy, of critical importance is that the infant mortality rate in the United States ranks 28th among developed nations. Preconception care has been advocated as a measure to improve pregnancy outcomes. Its components parallel those of prenatal care: risk assessment, health promotion, and medical and psychosocial interventions. Preconception care can be provided most effectively as part of ongoing primary care. It can be initiated during visits for routine health maintenance, during examinations for school or work, at premarital or family planning visits, after a negative pregnancy test, or during well-child care for another family member.

Jack BW, Culpepper L: Preconception care. Risk reduction and health promotion in preparation for pregnancy. JAMA 1990;264:1147. [PMID: 2002323]

Martin JA et al: Births: final data for 2003. Natl Vital Stat Rep 2005;54:1. [PMID: 1617606]

NUTRITION

A woman's nutritional status before pregnancy may have a profound effect on reproductive outcome. Obesity is the most common nutritional disorder in developed countries. Obese women are at increased risk for prenatal complications such as hypertensive disorders of pregnancy, gestational diabetes, and urinary tract infections. They are also more likely to deliver large-for-gestational age infants and, as a result, have a higher incidence of intrapartum complications. Because dieting is not recommended during pregnancy, obese women should be encouraged to lose weight prior to conception.

On the other hand, underweight women are more likely than women of normal weight to give birth to low-birth-weight infants. Low birth weight may be associated with an increased risk of developing cardiovascular disease and diabetes in adult life (the "fetal origin hypothesis").

At the preconception visit, the patient's weight and height should be assessed and inquiries should be made regarding anorexia, bulimia, pica, vegetarian eating habits, and use of megavitamin supplements.

Vitamin A is a known teratogen at high doses. Supplemental doses exceeding 5000 IU/day should be avoided by women who are, or who may become, pregnant. The form of vitamin A that is teratogenic is retinol, not β-carotene, so large consumption of fruits and vegetables rich in β-carotene is not a concern.

Folic acid supplementation: Neural tube defects (NTDs), including spina bifida, anencephaly, and encephalocele, affect approximately 4000 pregnancies each year in the United States. Although anencephaly is almost always lethal, spina bifida is associated with serious disabilities including paraplegia, bowel and bladder incontinence, hydrocephalus, and intellectual impairment.

Over the past 30 years, multiple studies conducted in various countries have shown a reduced risk of NTDs in infants whose mothers used folic acid supplements. The strongest evidence was provided by the Medical Research Council Vitamin Study in the United Kingdom, which showed a 72% reduction of recurrence of NTDs with a daily dose of 4 mg of folic acid started 4 weeks prior to conception and continued through the first trimester of pregnancy. Additionally, other studies showed a reduction in the incidence of first occurrence NTD with lower doses of folic acid (0.36–0.8 mg). Since 1992, the Centers for Disease Control and Prevention (CDC) has recommended that all women of childbearing age who are capable of becoming pregnant take 0.4 mg of folic acid daily to reduce the risk of NTDs in pregnancy. It is also recommended that patients who had a previous pregnancy affected by an NTD take 4 mg of folic acid daily starting 1–3 months prior to planned conception and continuing through the first 3 months of pregnancy.

Despite the recommendations, compliance has been poor. As of 1998 and in an effort to ensure an increased intake of folic acid, the US Food and Drug Administration (FDA) mandated the fortification of cereals and grains with folic acid at doses of 0.14 mg per 100 g of grain, an amount estimated to increase folic acid consumption by an average of 0.1 mg/day. By reducing plasma homocysteine levels, folic acid fortification could also have a beneficial effect on the rates of cerebrovascular and coronary heart disease in the general population.

The American College of Preventive Medicine advocates fortification at the higher level of 0.35 mg folic acid per 100 g product. It could be argued that this level of food fortification may mask the megaloblastic anemia associated with vitamin B_{12} deficiency and allow the progression of neurologic symptoms. This is unlikely to occur in women of childbearing age, but can develop in the elderly who are at high risk for vitamin B_{12} deficiency.

Centers for Disease Control and Prevention (CDC): Knowledge and use of folic acid by women of childbearing age—United States, 1997. MMWR Morb Mortal Wkly Rep 1997;46(31):721. [PMID: 9498295]

Prevention of neural tube defects: Results of the Medical Research Council Vitamin Study. MRC Vitamin Study Research Group. Lancet 1991;338:131. [PMID: 1677062]

Recommendations for the use of folic acid to reduce the number of cases of spina bifida and other neural tube defects. MMWR Recomm Rep 1992;41(RR-14):1. [PMID: 1522835]

EXERCISE

More and more women wish to continue with their exercise programs during pregnancy. Among a representative sample of US women, 42% reported exercising during pregnancy. Walking was the leading activity (43% of all activities reported), followed by swimming and aerobics (12% each).

Available data suggest that moderate exercise is safe for pregnant women who have no medical or obstetric complications. A meta-analysis review of the literature on the effects of exercise on pregnancy outcomes found no significant difference between active and sedentary women in terms of maternal weight gain, infant birth weight, length of gestation, length of labor, or Apgar scores.

Exercise may actually reduce pregnancy-related discomforts and improve maternal fitness and sense of self-esteem. The American College of Obstetricians and Gynecologists recommends that exercise in the supine position and any activity that increases the risk of falling (gymnastics, horseback riding, downhill skiing, and vigorous racquet sports) be avoided during pregnancy. Contact sports (such as hockey, soccer, and basketball) should also be avoided as they can result in trauma to both the mother and the fetus. Scuba diving is contraindicated during pregnancy because the fetus is at risk for decompression sickness. Absolute contraindications to exercise during pregnancy are significant heart or lung disease, incompetent cervix, premature labor or ruptured membranes, placenta previa or persistent second- or third-trimester bleeding, and preeclampsia or pregnancy-induced hypertension.

ACOG Committee on Obstetric Practice: ACOG Committee opinion, Number 267, January 2002: Exercise during pregnancy and the postpartum period. Obstet Gynecol 2002;99:171. [PMID: 11777528]

MEDICAL CONDITIONS

Diabetes

Congenital anomalies occur two to six times more often in the offspring of women with diabetes mellitus and have been associated with poor glycemic control during early pregnancy. Preconceptional care with good diabetic control during early embryogenesis has been shown to reduce the rate of congenital anomalies to essentially that of a control population. In a recent meta-analysis of 18 published studies, the rate of major anomalies was lower among preconception care recipients (2.1%) than nonrecipients (6.5%).

According to the American Diabetes Association recommendations, the goal for blood glucose management in the preconception period and in the first trimester is to reach the lowest A_{1c} level possible without undue risk of hypoglycemia to the mother. A_{1c} levels that are less than 1% above the normal range are desirable. Suggested pre- and postprandial goals are as follows: before meals, capillary plasma glucose 80–110 mg/dL; 2 hours after meals, capillary plasma glucose less than 155 mg/dL.

Prior to conception, a baseline dilated eye examination is recommended, because diabetic retinopathy can worsen during pregnancy. Hypertension, frequently present in diabetic patients, needs to be controlled. Angiotensin-converting enzyme inhibitors and diuretics should be avoided as they have been associated with adverse effects on the fetus. Oral hypoglycemic agents should be discontinued because they may cause fetal anomalies and neonatal hypoglycemia, and insulin should be prescribed for patients with either type 1 or type 2 diabetes.

Epilepsy

Epilepsy occurs in 1% of the population and is the most common serious neurologic problem seen in pregnancy. There are approximately one million women of childbearing age with epilepsy in the United States, of whom around 20,000 deliver infants every year. Much can be done to achieve a favorable outcome of pregnancy in women with epilepsy. Ideally, this should start before conception. Menstrual disorders, ovulatory dysfunction, and infertility are relatively common problems in women with epilepsy and should be addressed.

Women with epilepsy must make choices about contraceptive methods. Certain antiepileptic drugs (AEDs), such as phenytoin, carbamazepine, phenobarbital, primidone, and topiramate, induce hepatic cytochrome P450 enzymes, leading to an increase in the metabolism of the estrogen and progestin present in the oral contraceptive pills. This increases the risk of breakthrough pregnancy. The American Academy of Neurology recommends the use of oral contraceptive formulations with at least 50 mcg of ethinyl estradiol or mestranol for women with epilepsy who take enzyme-inducing AEDs.

Both levonorgestrel implants (Norplant) and the progestin-only pill have reduced efficacy in women taking enzyme-inducing AEDs. Other AEDs that do not induce liver enzymes (eg, valproic acid, lamotrigine, vigabatrin, gabapentin, and felbamate) do not cause contraceptive failure.

Because many AEDs interfere with the metabolism of folic acid, all women with epilepsy who are planning a pregnancy should receive folic acid supplementation at a dose of 4–5 mg/day. Withdrawal of AEDs can be considered in any woman who has been seizure free for at least 2 years and has a single type of seizure, normal neurologic examination and intelligence quotient, and an electroencephalogram that has normalized with treatment. Because the risk of seizure relapse is greatest in the first 6 months after discontinuing AEDs, withdrawal should be accomplished before conception. If withdrawal is not possible, monotherapy should be attempted to reduce the risk of fetal malformations. Offspring of women with epilepsy are at increased risk for intrauterine growth restriction, congenital malformations that include craniofacial and digital anomalies, and cognitive dysfunction. The term *fetal anticonvulsant syndrome* encompasses various combinations of these findings and has been associated with use of virtually all AEDs. Some recent studies have indicated a higher risk for birth defects as well as for lower verbal intelligence in association with valproic acid compared with other AEDs, mainly carbamazepine.

Phenylketonuria

Phenylketonuria (PKU) is one of the most common inborn errors of metabolism. It is associated with deficient activity of the liver enzyme phenylalanine hydroxylase, leading to an accumulation of phenylalanine in the blood and other tissues. If untreated, PKU can result in mental retardation, seizures, microcephaly, delayed speech, eczema, and autistic-like behaviors. All states have screening programs for PKU at birth. When diagnosed early in the newborn period and when treated with a phenylalanine-restricted diet, affected infants have normal development and can expect a normal life span.

Dietary control is recommended for life in individuals with PKU and especially in women planning conception. Studies have shown a strong relationship between high maternal phenylalanine levels and mental retardation, microcephaly, and congenital heart disease in the offspring.

The Maternal Phenylketonuria 12-year Collaborative Study has demonstrated that the institution of a phenylalanine-restricted diet before conception or by 8–10 weeks' gestation can significantly reduce the incidence of congenital heart disease. Their preliminary data, however, suggest that optimum intellectual status in the offspring is achieved only when dietary treatment is started prior to conception.

American Diabetes Association: Preconception care of women with diabetes. Diabetes Care 2004;27(suppl 1):s76. [PMID: 14693933]

Platt LD et al: The international study of pregnancy outcome in women with maternal phenylketonuria: Report of a 12-year study. Am J Obstet Gynecol 2000;182:326. [PMID: 10694332]

GENETIC COUNSELING

The ideal time for genetic counseling is before a couple attempts to conceive, especially if the history reveals advanced maternal age, previously affected pregnancy, consanguinity, or family history of genetic disease.

Certain ethnic groups have a relatively high carrier incidence for certain genetic disorders. For example, Ashkenazi Jews have a 1:25 chance of being a carrier for Tay–Sachs disease, a severe degenerative neurologic disease that leads to death in early childhood. Carrier status can easily be determined by a serum assay for the level of the enzyme hexosaminidase A. Screening for Tay–Sachs disease is recommended prior to conception, because testing on serum is not reliable in pregnancy and the enzyme assay on white blood cells that is used in pregnancy is more expensive and labor intensive. Ashkenazi Jews are at risk not only for Tay–Sachs disease, but also for Canavan disease, Gaucher disease, and cystic fibrosis, all of which can be screened for by DNA analysis.

Cystic fibrosis is the most common autosomal-recessive genetic disorder among whites in the United States, with a carrier rate of 1:22–25. It is characterized by the production of thickened secretions throughout the body, but particularly in the lungs and the gastrointestinal tract. In 1997, the National Institutes of Health recommended that cystic fibrosis carrier screening be offered to all couples planning a pregnancy or seeking prenatal testing. However, this recommendation has not yet been implemented. The complete text of the consensus statement can be found online at http://consensus.nih.gov/cons/106/106_statement.pdf.

Other common genetic disorders for which there is a reliable screening test for carriers are sickle cell disease in African Americans, β-thalassemia in individuals of Mediterranean descent, and α-thalassemia in Southeast Asians. Sickle cell carriers can be detected with solubility testing (Sickledex) for the presence of hemoglobin S. However, the American College of Obstetricians and Gynecologists recommends hemoglobin electrophoresis screening in all patients considered at risk for having a child affected with a sickling disorder. Solubility testing is described as inadequate because it does not identify carriers of abnormal hemoglobins such as the β-thalassemia trait or the HbB, HbC, HbD, or HbE traits. A complete blood count with indices is a simple screening test for the thalassemias and will show a mild anemia with a low mean corpuscular volume.

Fragile X syndrome is the most common cause of mental retardation after Down syndrome and is the most common inherited cause of mental retardation. It affects approximately 1 in 4000 men and 1 in 8000 women and results from a mutation in a gene on the long arm of the X chromosome. The X-linked inheritance is atypical in that unaffected males can transmit the disorder and up to 30% of female carriers are affected.

In addition to mental retardation, fragile X syndrome is characterized by physical features such as macroorchidism, large ears, a prominent jaw, and behavioral problems such as hyperactivity and avoidance of eye contact. Preconception screening should be offered to women with a known family history of fragile X syndrome or a family history of unexplained mental retardation, and to women who have learning disabilities or mental retardation.

American College of Obstetrics and Gynecology, Committee on Genetics: ACOG Committee opinion. Genetic screening for hemoglobinopathies, number 238, July 2000. Committee on Genetics Int J Gynaecol Obstet 2001;74:309. [PMID: 11579910]

Genetic testing for cystic fibrosis. National Institutes of Health Development Conference Consensus Statement on genetic testing for cystic fibrosis. Arch Intern Med 1999;159:1529. [PMID: 10421275]

IMMUNIZATIONS

The preconception visit is an ideal time to screen for rubella immunity, because rubella infection in pregnancy can result in miscarriage, stillbirth, or an infant with congenital rubella syndrome (CRS). The risk of developing CRS abnormalities (hearing impairment, eye defects, congenital heart defects, and developmental delay) is greatest if the mother is infected in the first trimester of pregnancy. From 2001 through 2004, only four cases of CRS were reported to the CDC; the mothers of three of the children were born outside the United States.

Immunization should be offered to any woman with a negative rubella titer and advice given to avoid conception for 1 month due to the theoretical risk to the fetus. Inadvertent immunization of a pregnant woman with rubella vaccine should not be a reason to consider termination of pregnancy as there is no evidence that the vaccine causes any malformations or CRS.

If a pregnant woman acquires varicella before 20 weeks' gestation, the fetus has a 1–2% risk of developing fetal varicella syndrome, which is characterized by skin scarring, hypoplasia of the limbs, eye defects, and neurologic abnormalities. Infants born to mothers who manifest varicella 5 days before to 2 days after delivery may experience a severe infection and have a mortality rate as high as 30%.

At the preconception visit, patients who do not have a prior history of chickenpox and who are seronegative should be offered vaccination. In 1995, the live attenuated varicella vaccine was introduced and the recommended regimen for patients older than 13 years is two doses 4 weeks apart. Patients should avoid becoming pregnant for at least 4 weeks after the second dose.

Since 1988, the CDC has recommended universal screening of pregnant women for hepatitis B. Although hepatitis B vaccine can be given during pregnancy, women with social or occupational risks for exposure to hepatitis B virus should ideally be identified and offered immunization prior to conception.

Centers for Disease Control and Prevention (CDC): Elimination of rubella and congenital rubella syndrome—United States, 1969–2004. MMWR Morb Mortal Wkly Rep 2005;54(11):279. [PMID: 15788995]

LIFE-STYLE CHANGES

Caffeine

Caffeine is present in many beverages, in chocolate, and in over-the-counter medications such as cold and headache medicines. One cup of coffee contains approximately 120 mg of caffeine, a cup of tea has 40 mg of caffeine, and soft drinks such as cola contain 45 mg of caffeine per 12-oz serving. Consumption of caffeine during pregnancy is quite common, but its metabolism is slowed. Cigarette smoking increases caffeine metabolism, leading to increased caffeine intake.

Several epidemiologic studies have suggested that caffeine intake may be associated with decreased fertility, increased spontaneous abortions, and decreased birth weight. As a result in 1980 the FDA advised pregnant women to avoid caffeine during pregnancy. However, a recent extensive literature review of the effects of caffeine concluded that pregnant women who consume moderate amounts of caffeine (≤ 5–6 mg/kg/day) spread throughout the day and do not smoke or drink alcohol have no increase in reproductive risks.

Tobacco

Between 12% and 22% of pregnant women smoke during pregnancy, subjecting themselves and their infants to a number of adverse health effects. Smoking during pregnancy has been associated with spontaneous abortion, prematurity, low birth weight, intrauterine growth restriction, placental abruption, placenta previa, as well as an increased risk for sudden infant death syndrome. Accumulating evidence also indicates that maternal tobacco use is associated with birth defects such as oral clefts and foot deformities. Paradoxically, smoking during pregnancy has reportedly been associated with a reduced risk of preeclampsia. However, the smoking-related adverse outcomes of pregnancy outweigh this benefit.

The use of nicotine replacement products to help with smoking cessation has not been sufficiently evaluated during pregnancy to determine its safety. Nicotine gum was contraindicated during pregnancy when it was initially approved (ie, category X). In 1992, the FDA downgraded the contraindication to pregnancy category C (risk cannot be ruled out). Transdermal nicotine systems are graded as pregnancy category D (positive evidence of risk).

Women who are contemplating pregnancy should be advised to quit smoking prior to conception, and nicotine replacement could then be prescribed. Smoking cessation either before pregnancy or in early pregnancy is associated with improvement in maternal airway function and an infant birth weight comparable to that observed among nonsmoking pregnant women.

Alcohol

In 1981, the surgeon general of the United States recommended that women abstain from drinking alcohol during pregnancy and when planning a pregnancy, because such drinking may harm the fetus. Despite that, approximately 15% of pregnant women report drinking alcohol.

The most severe consequence of exposure to alcohol during pregnancy is fetal alcohol syndrome (FAS), characterized by a triad of prenatal or postnatal growth retardation, central nervous system neurodevelopmental abnormalities, and facial anomalies (short palpebral fissures, smooth philtrum, thin upper lip, and midfacial hypoplasia). FAS is the largest preventable cause of birth defects and mental retardation in the western world. The most recent prevalence rate of FAS in the United States is 0.97 per 1000 births.

Some ethnic groups are disproportionately affected by FAS. American Indians and Alaska Native populations have a prevalence of FAS 30 times higher than white populations. It also appears that binge drinking produces more severe outcomes in offspring than more chronic exposure, possibly because of *in utero* withdrawal and its concomitant effects.

At the preconception visit, physicians should counsel their patients that there is no safe level of alcohol consumption during pregnancy and that the harmful effects on the developing fetal brain can occur at any time during pregnancy. High alcohol consumption in women has also been associated with infertility, spontaneous abortion, increased menstrual symptoms, hypertension, and stroke. Mortality and breast cancer are also increased in women who report drinking more than two drinks daily.

Illicit Drugs

Illicit drug use during pregnancy remains a major health problem in the United States. The National Institute on Drug Abuse estimates that about 5.5% of women use an illicit drug while pregnant. Marijuana is used by 2.9%, cocaine by 1.1%, and heroin by 0.1%. At the preconception visit, all patients should be questioned about drug use and offered counseling, referral, and access to recovery programs.

Marijuana is the most frequently used illicit drug in pregnancy. It does not appear to be teratogenic in humans and there is no significant association between marijuana usage and preterm birth or congenital malformations. A recent study, however, reported that prenatal exposure to marijuana was associated with increased hyperactivity, impulsivity, and inattention symptoms in children at age 10 years.

Cocaine use during pregnancy has been associated with spontaneous abortion, premature labor, intrauterine growth restriction, placental abruption, microcephaly, limb reduction defects, and urogenital malformations. Initial reports that suggested "devastating" outcomes for prenatal exposure to cocaine, have not been substantiated. A recent meta-analysis concluded that cocaine exposure *in utero* has not been demonstrated to affect physical growth and that it does not appear to independently affect developmental scores from infancy to age 6 years.

Maternal use of heroin and other opiates is associated with low birth weight due to both premature delivery and intrauterine growth restriction, preeclampsia, placental abruption, fetal distress, and sudden infant death syndrome.

Infants born to heroin-dependent mothers often develop a syndrome of withdrawal known as neonatal abstinence syndrome within 48 hours of delivery. Neonatal withdrawal is characterized by central nervous system hyperirritability, respiratory distress, gastrointestinal dysfunction, poor feeding, high-pitched cry, yawning, and sneezing. Methadone has long been used to treat opioid dependence in pregnancy because of its long half-life. It has been associated with increases in birth weight. However, the use of methadone is controversial because more than 60% of neonates born to methadone-maintained mothers require treatment for withdrawal. Also, a substantial number of patients on methadone maintenance continue to use street narcotics and other illicit drugs. Buprenorphine, a recently developed partial opiate agonist, may have important advantages over methadone, including fewer withdrawal symptoms and a lower risk of overdose.

Bradley KA et al: Medical risks for women who drink alcohol. J Gen Intern Med 1998;13:627. [PMID: 9754520]

Christian MS, Brent RL: Teratogen update: Evaluation of the reproductive and developmental risks of caffeine. Teratology 2001;64:51. [PMID: 11410911]

Frank DA et al: Growth, development, and behavior in early childhood following prenatal cocaine exposure: A systematic review. JAMA 2001;285:1613. [PMID: 11268270]

Goldschmidt L et al: Effects of prenatal marijuana exposure on child behavior problems at age 10. Neurotoxicol Teratol 2000;22:325. [PMID: 10840176]

National Institute on Drug Abuse: Pregnancy and drug use trends. Available at: http://nida.nih.gov/Infofax/pregnancytrends.html.

US Department of Health and Human Services, Public Health Services Office of the Surgeon General: *Women and Smoking: A Report of the Surgeon General.* DHHS, 2001.

SEXUALLY TRANSMITTED DISEASES

The latest estimates suggest that there are up to 19 million new cases of sexually transmitted diseases (STDs) in the United States each year (see Chapter 14). The preconception visit is a good opportunity to screen for genital infections such as *Chlamydia,* gonorrhea, syphilis, and HIV.

Chlamydia and gonorrhea are two of the most prevalent STDs and both are often asymptomatic in women. In pregnancy, both *Chlamydia* and gonorrhea have been associated with premature rupture of membranes, preterm labor, postabortion and postpartum endometritis, and congenital infection.

Infants whose mothers have untreated *Chlamydia* infection have a 30–50% chance of developing inclusion conjunctivitis and a 10–20% chance of developing pneumonia. Inclusion conjunctivitis typically develops 5–14 days after delivery and is usually mild and self-limiting. Pneumonia due to *Chlamydia* usually has a slow onset without fever and can have a protracted course if untreated. Long-term complications may be significant. Ophthalmia neonatorum is the most common manifestation of neonatal gonococcal infection. It occurs 2–5 days after birth in up to 50% of exposed infants who did not receive ocular prophylaxis. Corneal ulceration may occur, and unless treatment is initiated promptly, the cornea may perforate, leading to blindness.

Congenital syphilis occurs when the spirochete *Treponema pallidum* is transmitted from a pregnant woman with syphilis to her fetus. Untreated syphilis during pregnancy may lead to spontaneous abortion, nonimmune hydrops, stillbirth, neonatal death, and serious sequelae in liveborn infected children. In 1999, the CDC launched the National Plan to Eliminate Syphilis in the United States, and CDC officials believe syphilis can be almost completely eradicated before the end of this decade. During 2000–2002, the rate of congenital syphilis decreased 21.1%, from 14.2 to 11.2 cases per 100,000 live births.

Women are increasingly affected by HIV. In untreated HIV-infected pregnant women, the risk of mother-to-child transmission varies from 16% to 40%. However, it is possible to dramatically reduce the transmission rates by using highly active antiretroviral therapy (HAART) during pregnancy, by offering elective cesarean delivery at 38 weeks if the viral load at term is higher than 1000 copies/mL, and by discouraging breast-feeding. In developed countries, transmission rates as low as 1–2% have been achieved.

Centers for Disease Control and Prevention (CDC): Congenital syphilis—United States, 2002. MMWR Morb Mortal Wkly Rep 2004;53:716. [PMID: 15306757]

MEDICATIONS

Therapeutic regimens for chronic illnesses are best modified, when possible, in the preconception period to include those drugs that have been used the longest and have been determined to pose the lowest risk.

Antihypertensives

Women with chronic hypertension who are receiving angiotensin-converting enzyme inhibitors should be advised to discontinue them before becoming pregnant or as soon as they know they are pregnant because of the possible hazards to the fetus. This class of drugs can result in fetal renal impairment, anuria leading to oligohydramnios, intrauterine growth restriction, hypocalvaria, persistent patent ductus arteriosus, and stillbirth. In the absence of congestive heart failure or pulmonary edema, diuretics are best avoided during pregnancy because they reduce maternal plasma volume, which may diminish uteroplacental perfusion. Methyldopa is the drug of choice for treatment of hypertension during pregnancy, with proven maternal and fetal safety.

Anticoagulants

Warfarin (Coumadin) readily crosses the placenta and is a known human teratogen. The critical period for fetal warfarin syndrome is exposure during weeks 6–9 of gestation. This syndrome primarily involves nasal hypoplasia and stippling of the epiphyses. Later drug exposure may also be associated with intracerebral hemorrhage, microcephaly, and mental retardation. In patients who require prolonged anticoagulation therapy, discontinuing warfarin in early pregnancy and substituting heparin will reduce the incidence of congenital anomalies, because heparin does not cross the placenta.

Antithyroid Drugs

Both propylthiouracil and methimazole are effective in the management of hyperthyroidism in pregnancy. Propylthiouracil is generally the preferred agent because in addition to inhibition of tetraiodothyronine (T_4) synthesis, it also inhibits the peripheral conversion of T_4 to triiodothyronine (T_3). Methimazole crosses the placenta in larger amounts and has been associated with aplasia cutis, a congenital defect of the scalp. If the patient is taking methimazole, it is reasonable to switch to propylthiouracil prior to conception.

Oral Hypoglycemics

As discussed earlier, patients with diabetes who take oral hypoglycemic agents should be switched to insulin before pregnancy.

Risk Categories

The FDA has defined five risk categories (A, B, C, D, and X) that are used by manufacturers to rate their products for use during pregnancy.

A. Category A

Controlled studies in women fail to demonstrate a risk to the fetus in the first trimester (and there is no evidence of risk in later trimesters), and the possibility of fetal harm appears remote (eg, folic acid and thyroxine).

B. Category B

Either animal reproduction studies have not demonstrated fetal risk but no controlled studies in pregnant women have been conducted, or animal reproduction studies have shown an adverse effect (other than a decrease in fertility) that was not confirmed in controlled studies in women in the first trimester and there is no evidence of risk in later trimesters (eg, acetaminophen, penicillins, and cephalosporins).

C. Category C

Either studies in animals have revealed adverse effects on the fetus (teratogenic, embryocidal, or other) but no controlled studies in women have been reported, or studies in women and animals are not available. Drugs should be given only if the potential benefit justifies the potential risk to the fetus (eg, acyclovir and zidovudine).

D. Category D

Positive evidence of human fetal risk exists, but the benefits from use in pregnant women may be acceptable despite the risk, especially if the drug is used in a life-threatening situation or for a severe disease for which safer drugs cannot be used or are ineffective (eg, tetracycline and phenytoin).

E. Category X

Studies in animals or humans have demonstrated fetal abnormalities, or evidence of fetal risk exists based on human experience, or both, and the risk of using the drug in pregnant women clearly outweighs any possible benefit. The drug is contraindicated in women who are or may be pregnant (eg, isotretinoin, misoprostol, warfarin, and statins).

OCCUPATIONAL EXPOSURES

Increasing numbers of women are entering the workforce worldwide, and most are in their reproductive years. This has raised concerns for the safety of pregnant women and their fetuses in the workplace. The preconception visit is the best time to identify and control exposures that may affect parental health or pregnancy outcome. The three most common occupational exposures reported to affect pregnancy are video display terminals, organic solvents, and lead.

Video Display Terminals

In 1980, a cluster of four infants with severe congenital malformations was reported in Canada. The cluster was linked to the fact that the mothers had all worked with video display terminals (VDTs) during their pregnancy, at a newspaper department in Toronto. Many epidemiologic studies have since investigated the effects of electromagnetic fields emitted from VDTs on pregnancy outcome. Most studies found only equivocal or no associations of VDTs with birth defects, preterm labor, and low birth weight. Thus, it is reasonable to advise women that there is no evidence that using VDTs will jeopardize pregnancy.

Organic Solvents

Organic solvents comprise a large group of chemically heterogeneous compounds that are widely used in industry and common household products. Occupational exposure to organic solvents can result from many industrial applications, including dry cleaning, painting, varnishing, degreasing, printing, and production of plastics and pharmaceuticals. Smelling the odor of organic solvents is not indicative of a significant exposure, because the olfactory nerve can detect levels as low as several parts per million, which are not necessarily associated with toxicity. A recent meta-analysis of epidemiologic studies demonstrated a statistically significant relationship between exposure to organic solvents in the first trimester of pregnancy and fetal malformations. There was also a tendency toward an increased risk for spontaneous abortion. Women who plan to become pregnant should minimize their exposure to organic solvents by routinely using ventilation systems and protective equipment.

Lead

Despite a steady decline in average blood levels of lead in the US population in recent years, approximately 0.5% of women of childbearing age may have blood levels of lead higher than 10 mcg/dL. The vast majority of exposures to lead occur in artists using glass staining and in workers involved in paint manufacturing for the automotive and aircraft industries. Other occupational sources of exposure to lead include smeltering, printing, and battery manufacturing. The most worrisome consequence of low to moderate lead toxicity is neurotoxicity. A review of the literature suggested that low-dose exposure to lead *in utero* may cause developmental deficits in the infant. However, these effects seem to be reversible if further exposure to lead is avoided. It is crucial to detect and treat lead toxicity prior to conception because the chelating agents used (dimercaprol, ethylenediaminetetraacetate, and penicillamine) can adversely affect the fetus if used during pregnancy.

Bentur Y, Koren G: The three most common occupational exposures reported by pregnant women: an update. Am J Obstet Gynecol 1991;165:429. [PMID: 1872354]

DOMESTIC VIOLENCE

Domestic violence is increasingly recognized as a major public health issue. Findings from the 1998 National Violence Against Women Survey showed that in the United States 1.5 million women are raped or physically assaulted by an intimate partner every year. Domestic violence crosses all socioeconomic, racial, religious, and educational boundaries. Even physicians are not immune: in a survey, 17% of female medical students and faculty had experienced abuse by a partner in their adult life, an estimate comparable to that of the general population. Victims of domestic violence should be identified preconceptionally, because the pattern of violence may escalate during pregnancy. The prevalence of domestic violence during pregnancy ranges from 0.9% to 20.1%, with most studies identifying rates between 3.9% and 8.3%. Whereas violence in nonpregnant women is directed at the head, neck, and chest, the breasts and the abdomen are frequent targets during pregnancy. Physical abuse during pregnancy is a significant risk factor for low birth weight and maternal complications of low weight gain, infections, anemia, smoking, and alcohol or drug usage. If it is identified that a patient is the victim of domestic violence, the physician should assess her immediate safety and make timely referrals to local community resources and shelters.

Tjaden P, Thoennes N: *Prevelance, Incidence and Consequence of Violence Against Women: Findings from the National Violence Against WomenSurvey.* US Department of Justice: National Institue of Justice and Centers for Disease Control and Prevention, 1998.

Contraception

16

Susan C. Brunsell, MD

In the United States, 49% of pregnancies are unintended and 54% of these end in abortion. These rates remain higher than rates of many other industrialized countries. Addressing family planning and contraception is an important issue for providers of care to women of reproductive age. An increasing number of contraceptive options are becoming available on the US market. It is dependent on physicians and other health care providers to maintain currency with the recent advances in information concerning counseling, efficacy, safety, and side effects.

COMBINED ORAL CONTRACEPTIVES

Hormonal contraception is used by over 100 million women worldwide and by over 12 million women in the United States. The year 2000 marked the fourth decade of oral contraceptive use. The introduction of lower-dose combination oral contraceptives (COCs), containing less than 50 mcg of ethinyl estradiol, has provided many women a highly effective, safe, and tolerable method of contraception.

COCs suppress ovulation by diminishing the frequency of gonadotropin-releasing hormone pulses and halting the luteinizing hormone surge. They also alter the consistency of cervical mucous, affect the endometrial lining, and alter tubal transport. Most of the antiovulatory effects of COCs derive from the action of the progestin component. The estrogen doses are not sufficient to produce a consistent antiovulatory effect. The estrogenic component of COCs potentiates the action of the progestin and stabilizes the endometrium so that breakthrough bleeding is minimized. When administered correctly and consistently, they are more than 99% effective at preventing pregnancy. However, the 1995 National Survey of Family Growth estimated that the failure rates of COCs were as high as 8.3% during the first year of typical use. Noncompliance is the primary reason cited for the difference between these rates, frequently secondary to side effects such as abnormal bleeding and nausea.

Hormonal Content

The estrogenic agent most commonly used in COCs is ethinyl estradiol, in doses ranging from 20 to 35 mcg. Mestranol, which is infrequently used, is less potent than ethinyl estradiol, such that a 50-mcg dose of mestranol is equivalent to 30–35 mcg of ethinyl estradiol. It appears that decreasing the dose of estrogen to 20 mcg reduces the frequency of estrogen-related side effects but increases the rate of breakthrough bleeding. In addition, there may be a lower margin of error with low-dose preparations; thus, missing pills may be more likely to result in breakthrough ovulation.

Multiple progestins are used in COC formulations. Biphasic and triphasic oral contraceptives, which vary the dose of progestin over a 28-day cycle, were developed to decrease the incidence of progestin-related side effects and breakthrough bleeding, although there is no convincing evidence that multiphasics indeed cause fewer adverse effects. The most commonly used progestins include norgestrel, levonorgestrel, and norethindrone. As with estrogens, some progestins (norethindrone and levonorgestrel) are biologically active, whereas others are prodrugs that are activated by metabolism. Norethindrone acetate is converted to norethindrone and norgestimate is metabolized into several active steroids, including levonorgestrel. Progestins that do not require hepatic transformation tend to have better bioavailability and a longer serum half-life. For example, levonorgestrel has a longer half-life than norethindrone. In the 1990s COCs with different progestins—norgestimate and desogestrel—were introduced to decrease the incidence of androgenic side effects.

Drospirenone, a derivative of spironolactone, is available combined with ethinyl estradiol under the trade name Yasmin. Drospirenone differs from other progestins because it has mild antimineralocorticoid activity. Contraceptive efficacy, metabolic profile, and cycle control are comparable to other COCs. The clinical implications of the diuretic-like potential of drospirenone are not yet clear. Because of its antimineralocorticoid effects and the potential for hyperkalemia, drospirenone should not be used in women with severe renal disease or hepatic dysfunction.

Most COCs are designed to provide 21 days of hormone therapy and 7 days of placebo tablets, during which withdrawal bleeding occurs. An exception is Mircette (Organon), which is formulated to provide 21 days of 150 mcg of desogestrel and 20 mcg of ethinyl estradiol, 2 days of placebo, and 5 days of 10 mcg of ethinyl estradiol in a 28-day pack. This formulation is meant to decrease breakthrough ovulation and decrease early cycle bleeding.

The belief that a monthly period is normal and healthy for women is being challenged. The "tri-cycle" regimen in which women take 42–84 active pills in a row was first described more than 20 years ago. Monophasic COCs are usually used. Skipping the pill-free week has been prescribed to treat menstrual headache, estrogen withdrawal symptoms, and to suppress endometriosis. This regimen has been shown to be safe, effective, and acceptable to women. Approved in 2003, Seasonale is a monophasic combination of ethinyl estradiol and levonorgestrel that extends the duration of hormonally active tablets to 12 weeks followed by 1 week off. Initial breakthrough spotting is considerably more common than with conventional COCs; however, this side effect decreases with time.

Side Effects

Side effects may be due to the estrogen component, the progestin component, or both. Side effects attributable to progestin include androgenic effects, such as hair growth, male-pattern baldness, and nausea. Switching to an agent with lower androgenic potential may decrease or resolve these problems. Estrogenic effects include nausea, breast tenderness, and fluid retention. Weight gain is commonly thought to be a side effect of COCs; however, multiple studies have failed to confirm a significant effect. Weight gain can be managed by switching to a different formulation; however, appropriate diet and exercise should be emphasized.

Bleeding irregularity is the side effect most frequently cited as the reason for discontinuing COCs. Patients should be counseled that irregular bleeding or spotting is common in the first 3 months of COC use and will diminish with time. Spotting is also related to missed pills. Patients should be counseled regarding the importance of taking the pill daily. If the bleeding does not appear to be related to missed pills, the patient should be evaluated for other pathology such as infection, cervical disease, or pregnancy. If this evaluation is negative, the patient may be reassured. Another approach would be to change the pill formulation to increase the estrogen or progestin component. The doses can be tailored to the time in the cycle when the bleeding occurs. If bleeding precedes the menses, the patients can be switched to a triphasic pill that increases the dose of estrogen (Estrostep) or progestin (eg, Ortho-Novum 7/7/7) sequentially through the cycle. If bleeding follows the menses, Mircette, which incorporates only 2 hormone-free days, may be tried. The estrogen or progestin component, or both, should be increased midcycle for patients with midcycle bleeding (eg, Triphasil).

COCs may cause a small increase in blood pressure in some patients. The risk increases with age. The hypertension usually resolves within 3 months if the COC is discontinued. Both estrogens and progestins are known to affect blood pressure. Therefore, switching to a lower estrogen formulation or a progestin-only pill may not resolve the problem.

Major Sequelae

Use of most oral contraceptive products containing less than 50 mcg of estrogen approximately triples a woman's risk of venous thromboembolism. Before 1995, the progestin component of COCs was not generally thought to contribute to the risk of thrombosis. However, more recent studies with formulations containing gestodene (not available in the United States) or desogestrel have shown a nearly sevenfold increased risk of thrombosis compared with nonusers of COCs. Bias and confounding in these studies do not explain the consistent epidemiologic findings of an increased risk. Obesity and increasing age are contributing risk factors. The identification of the factor V Leiden mutation in 1993 introduced another risk factor. In women who carry the mutation and also use COCs, the risk of venous thromboembolism is increased by a factor of 35 over the baseline risk for women who do not carry the mutation and do not use COCs. The best approach to identify women at higher risk of venous thromboembolism before taking COCs is controversial. Universal screening for the factor V Leiden mutation is not cost effective. Furthermore, family history of venous thromboembolism has unsatisfactory sensitivity and positive predictive value for identifying carriers of other common defects.

The risk of thrombotic or ischemic stroke among users of COCs appears to be relatively low. There is no evidence that the type of progestin influences risk or mortality associated with ischemic stroke. The risk of ischemic stoke appears to be directly proportional to estrogen dose, but even the newer low-estrogen preparations convey a slightly increased risk for users compared with nonusers. Hypertension, cigarette smoking, and migraine headaches interact with COC use to substantially increase the risk of ischemic stroke. The risk of hemorrhagic stroke in young women is low and is not increased by the use of COCs in the absence of risk factors. The major risk factors are hypertension and cigarette smoking. History of migraine without focal neurologic signs is not a contraindication to hormonal contraception.

Current use of COCs is associated with an increased risk of acute myocardial infarction among women with known cardiovascular risk factors (diabetes, cigarette smoking, hypertension) and among those who have not been effectively screened for risk factors, particularly for hypertension. There is no increased risk for acute myocardial infarction with increasing duration of use or with past use of COCs.

In 1990, more than 20 studies that evaluated changes in carbohydrate metabolism associated with 6 or more months of low-dose COC use were reviewed. It was concluded that most studies demonstrated a low degree of alterations in carbohydrate metabolism, that most changes observed were not statistically significant, and that clinical relevance of those minimal statistically significant differences was unlikely.

Many epidemiologic studies have reported an increased risk of breast cancer among COC users. For current users of COCs, the relative risk of breast cancer compared with never-users is 1.24. This small risk persists for 10 years but essentially disappears after this time period. Although the risk of breast cancer is increased modestly in COC users, the disease tends to be localized. The pattern of disappearance of risk after 10 years coupled with the tendency toward localized disease suggests that the overall effect may represent detection bias or perhaps a promotional effect. A population-based, case-control study that enrolled over 8000 women evaluated risk of breast cancer in COC users later in life when the risk of cancer is higher. The results of this study, reported in 2002, showed that among women aged 35–64 years, current or previous contraceptive use was not associated with a significantly increased risk of breast cancer.

Noncontraceptive Health Benefits

Most studies evaluating the relationship between COCs and ovarian cancer have shown a protective effect for oral contraceptives. There appears to be an overall decrease in risk of 40–80% among users, with protection beginning 1 year after starting use, and a 10–12% decrease in risk annually for each year of use. Protection persists for 15–20 years after discontinuation. The mechanisms by which COCs may produce these protective effects include suppression of ovulation and the suppression of gonadotropins.

The use of COCs conveys protection against endometrial cancer as well. The reduction in risk of up to 50% begins 1 year after initiation, and persists for up to 20 years after COCs are discontinued. The mechanism of action is likely reduction in the mitotic activity of endometrial cells because of progestational effects.

Several epidemiologic studies demonstrate that the use of COCs will reduce the risk of salpingitis by 50–80% compared with the risk to women not using contraception or who use a barrier method. There is no protective effect against the acquisition of sexually transmitted diseases (STDs) of the lower genital tract. The purported mechanisms for protection include progestin-induced thickening of the cervical mucus, so that ascent of bacteria is inhibited, and a decrease in menstrual flow, resulting in less retrograde flow to the fallopian tubes. Other noncontraceptive benefits of COCs include decreased incidence of benign breast disease, relief from menstrual disorders (dysmenorrhea and menorrhagia), reduced risk of uterine leiomyomata, protection against ovarian cysts, reduction of acne, improvement in bone mineral density, and reduced risk of colorectal cancer.

Burkman RT: Oral contraceptives: Current status. Clin Obstet Gynecol 2001;44:62. [PMID: 11219247]

Hatcher RA et al: *Contraceptive Technology,* 18th ed. Ardent Media, 2004.

TRANSDERMAL CONTRACEPTIVE SYSTEM

A transdermal contraceptive patch containing norelgestromin, the active metabolite of norgestimate, and ethinyl estradiol is marketed by Ortho-McNeil under the trade name Ortho Evra. The system is designed to deliver 150 mcg of norelgestromin and 20 mcg of ethinyl estradiol daily directly to the peripheral circulation. The treatment regimen for each cycle is three consecutive 7-day patches (21 days) followed by one patch-free week so that withdrawal bleeding can occur. The patch can be applied to one of four sites on a woman's body: abdomen, buttocks, upper outer arm, or torso (excluding the breast).

The efficacy of Ortho Evra is comparable to that of COCs. Compliance with the patch is much higher than with COCs, which may result in fewer pregnancies overall. However, pregnancy is more likely to occur in women weighing more than 198 pounds (89.8 kg). Breakthrough bleeding, spotting, and breast tenderness are slightly higher for Ortho Evra than for COCs in the first two cycles, but there is no difference in later cycles. Amenorrhea occurs in only 0.1% of patch users. Patch-site reactions occur in 2–3% of women.

Initiation of patch use is similar to initiation of COC use. Women apply the first patch on day 1 of their menstrual cycle. Another option is to apply the first patch on the Sunday after their menses begins. This becomes their patch change day. Subsequently, they change patches on the same day of the week. After three cycles they have a patch-free week during which they can expect their menses. A backup contraceptive should be used for the first 7 days of use.

In November 2005, the US Food and Drug Administration (FDA) approved updated labeling for the Ortho Evra patch to warn health care providers and patients that this product exposes women to higher levels of estrogen than most birth control pills. Average concentration at steady state for ethinyl estradiol is approximately 60% higher in women using Ortho Evra compared with women using an oral contraceptive containing 35 mcg of ethinyl estradiol. In contrast, peak concentrations for ethinyl estradiol are approximately 25% lower in women using Ortho Evra. In general, increased estrogen exposure may increase the risk of blood clots. The potential risks related to increased estrogen exposure with the patch should be balanced against the risk of pregnancy if patients have difficulty following the daily regimen associated with typical birth control pills.

Burkman RT: The transdermal contraceptive system. Am J Obstet Gynecol 2004;190:S49. [PMID: 15105798]

INTRAVAGINAL RING SYSTEM

The vaginal contraceptive ring (NuvaRing; Organon, Inc) was approved by the FDA in October 2001. It is a flexible, transparent ring made of ethylene vinylacetate copolymers, delivering an average of 120 mcg of etonogestrel and 15 mcg of ethinyl estradiol per day. A woman inserts the NuvaRing herself, wears it for 3 weeks, then removes and discards the device. After one ring-free week, during which withdrawal bleeding occurs, a new ring is inserted. Small studies have shown that the ring can be used for extended periods (6 or 12 weeks of continuous use) without an increase in the pregnancy rates. However, there is an increase in irregular bleeding with extended-use regimens. Rarely, the vaginal ring can slip out of the vagina if it has not been inserted properly or while removing a tampon, moving the bowels, straining, or with severe constipation. If the ring has been out of the vagina for more than 3 hours, breakthrough ovulation may occur. Patients may be counseled to check the position of the NuvaRing before and after intercourse.

Peak serum concentrations of etonogestrel and ethinyl estradiol occur about 1 week after insertion and are 60–70% lower than peak concentrations produced by standard COCs. The manufacturer recommends using backup birth control for the first 7 days of use if not switching from another hormonal contraceptive. The vaginal ring prevents pregnancy by the same mechanism as COCs. Pregnancy rates for users of the ring are between one and two per 100 women-years of use.

The side effects of the ring are similar to those of COC pills with the main adverse effect being disrupted bleeding. Breakthrough bleeding or spotting occurs in 2.6–11.7% of cycles and absence of withdrawal bleeding occurs in 0.6–3.8% of cycles. Fewer than 1–2% of women experience discomfort or reported discomfort from their partners with the ring. Its use is associated with increased vaginal secretions, which is a result of both hormonal and mechanical effects. Twenty-three percent of users reported vaginal discharge; however, the normal vaginal flora appears to be maintained. The ring is not associated with either adverse cytologic effects or bacteriologic colonization of the vaginal canal. The contraindications to use of the vaginal ring are similar to those of COCs. In addition, the ring may not be an appropriate choice for women with conditions that make the vagina more susceptible to irritation or that make expulsion of the ring more likely to occur, such as vaginal stenosis, cervical prolapse, cystocele, or rectocele.

Johansson ED, Sitruk-Ware R: New delivery systems in contraception: Vaginal rings. Am J Obstet Gynecol 2004;190:S54. [PMID: 15105799]

Miller L et al: Extended regimens of the contraceptive vaginal ring: A randomized trial. Obstet Gynecol 2005;106:473. [PMID: 16135576]

PROGESTIN-ONLY PILL

Progestin-only oral contraceptives (POPs), sometimes called the "minipill," are not widely used in the United States. Their use tends to be concentrated in select populations, notably breast-feeding women and those with contraindications to estrogen. Two formulations of POPs are available, one containing norgestrel, the other with norethindrone. POPs appear to prevent conception through several mechanisms, including suppression of ovulation, thickening of cervical mucus, alteration of the endometrium, and inhibition of tubal transport. Efficacy of POPs requires consistent administration. The pills should be taken at the same time every day without interruption (ie, no hormone-free week). If a pill is taken more than 3 hours late, a backup method of contraception should be used for the next 48 hours. No increase in the risk for thromboembolic events has been reported for POPs. The World Health Organization has deemed this contraceptive method to be acceptable for use in women with a history of venous thrombosis, pulmonary embolism, diabetes, obesity, or hypertension. Vascular disease is no longer considered a contraindication to use. The most common side effects of POPs are menstrual cycle disruption and breakthrough bleeding. Other common side effects include headache, breast tenderness, nausea, and dizziness. In general, POP use protects against ectopic pregnancy by lowering the chance of conception. If POP users do become pregnant, an average of 6–10% of pregnancies are extrauterine—a higher rate than in women not using contraception. Therefore POP users should be aware of the symptoms of ectopic pregnancy.

INJECTABLE CONTRACEPTIVES

Injectable long-acting contraception offers users convenient, safe, and reversible birth control as effective as surgical sterilization. Depo-Provera (depot medroxyprogesterone acetate; DMPA), a 3-month progestin-only formulation, contains 150 mg medroxyprogesterone acetate per injection. It is administered by deep intramuscular injection into the gluteus or deltoid muscle. Depo-SubQ Provera 104 is a new formulation of medroxyprogesterone acetate that patients can be taught to self-administer subcutaneously four times a year. Self-administration facilitates access to injectable contraception for many women, eliminating the need for an office visit. In addition to contraception, Depo-SubQ Provera is also indicated for the treatment of pain associated with endometriosis. Lunelle, a monthly injectable estrogen-progestin contraceptive, was introduced in 2000. Its use was associated with regular withdrawal bleeding and rapid return to fertility, but in 2003 the manufacturer elected to discontinue availability.

Depo-Provera acts primarily by inhibiting ovulation. With typical use, the failure rate of DMPA is 0.3 per 100 woman-years, which is comparable to that of levonorgestrel implants, copper intrauterine devices (IUDs), or surgical sterilization. Neither variations in weight nor use of concurrent medications has been noted to alter efficacy, apparently because of high circulating levels of progestin.

The first injection of DMPA should be administered within 5 days of the onset of menses or within 5 days of a first-trimester abortion. If a woman is postpartum and breast-feeding, the drug should not be administered until at least 6 weeks postdelivery. When switching from COCs, the first injection may be given any time while the active pills are being taken or within 7 days of taking the last active pill. Repeat injections of DMPA should be administered every 12 weeks. If a patient presents at 13 weeks or later, the manufacturer recommends excluding pregnancy before administering a repeat injection.

Use of DMPA has no permanent impact on fertility; however, return of fertility may be delayed after cessation of use. Fifty percent of women who discontinue DMPA to become pregnant will have conceived within 10 months of the last injection. In a small proportion of women fertility is not reestablished until 18 months after the last injection.

Menstrual changes are the most common side effects reported by users of DMPA. After 1 year of use, approximately 75% of women receiving DMPA report amenorrhea, with the remainder reporting irregular bleeding or spotting. Some women, especially adolescents, view amenorrhea as a potential benefit of use. Women who voice concern over this side effect can be reassured that the amenorrhea is not harmful. Patients with persistent bleeding or spotting should be evaluated for genital tract neoplasia and infection as appropriate. If these conditions are excluded and the symptoms are bothersome to the patient, a 1–3 month trial of low-dose estrogen can be considered. Options include conjugated equine estrogen (0.625, 1.25, or 2.5 mg), ethinyl estradiol (20 mcg), or a COC. Early reinjection (eg, every 8–10 weeks) does not seem to decrease bleeding.

Other side effects attributed to DMPA include weight changes, mood swings, reduced libido, and headaches. Due to concerns regarding decreased bone mineral density after prolonged use, the manufacturer no longer recommends use for longer than 2 years. Reassuringly, results from several studies indicate almost complete recovery of bone mineral density 2 years after discontinuation. Many clinicians recommend that users take supplemental calcium and vitamin D. DMPA may be used safely by smokers 35 years or older, and by other women at increased risk for arterial or venous events. Use of DMPA has not been associated with clinically significant alterations in hepatic function.

Kaunitz AM: Injectable long-acting contraceptives. Clin Obstet Gynecol 2001;44:73. [PMID: 11219248]

INTRAUTERINE DEVICES

Throughout the world, the most common form of reversible contraception is the IUD, used by almost 100 million women. Relatively few women in the United States use IUDs, although those who do express a high degree of satisfaction. Currently two IUDs are marketed for use in the United States. The most common IUD used is the copper-T 380A (ParaGard), made of polyethylene with fine wire copper wrapped around the stem and copper in the sleeves of each horizontal arm. It is approved for 10 years of use. The levonorgestrel IUD (Mirena) has a polyethylene frame that releases 20 mcg of levonorgestrel per day for as long as 5 years. Both IUDs are visible on radiographs.

The contraceptive action of IUDs is probably a result of a combination of factors. The IUD induces an inflammatory foreign body reaction within the uterus that causes prostaglandin release. This release results in altered uterine activity, inhibited tubal motility, and a direct toxic effect on sperm. The copper present in the ParaGard enhances the contraceptive effects by inhibiting transport of ovum and sperm. IUDs containing a progestin produce a similar effect and, in addition, thicken cervical mucus and suppress ovulation. IUDs are not abortifacients; they prevent conception. The IUD is one of the most effective methods of reversible contraception available. Among women who use the IUD perfectly (checking strings regularly to detect expulsion), the probability of pregnancy in the first year of use is 0.6% for ParaGard and 0.1% for Mirena. The progestational activity of the levonorgestrel IUD results in noncontraceptive benefits. It improves menorrhagia, and early investigations indicate it will likely benefit women with endometriosis, adenomyosis, and fibroids.

Screening is critical for identifying women at risk for IUD-associated complications. The main goal of patient selection is to prevent insertion of an IUD in a patient who has an STD or is at high risk for exposure to one. Women who have more than one sex partner or whose partner has other sex partners are at high risk for acquiring an STD and are more likely to develop pelvic inflammatory disease (PID) if they use an IUD instead of other barrier or hormonal methods of birth control. The risk of developing PID associated with IUD use is related to insertion of the IUD and subsequent exposure to STDs. The greatest risk of PID occurs during the first few weeks following insertion, possibly because of contamination of the endometrial cavity at the time of insertion. The use of prophylactic antibiotics at the time of IUD insertion has not been shown to decrease the risk of PID. Concern about the potential risk of PID and subsequent tubal infertility has led to the recommendation that they not be placed in women who have never been pregnant. However, a case control study of over 1800 women showed that the IUD can be used safely in appropriately selected nulligravid women with no increased risk of tubal infertility.

The most common side effects reported by IUD users are cramping and bleeding. These symptoms can be minimized with the use of a nonsteroidal anti-inflammatory drug. However, if symptoms are persistent or severe the patient should be evaluated for infection or perforation. Patients can be reassured that the amount of bleeding and cramping usually decreases with time.

Expulsion occurs in 2–10% of women in the first year of use, with most expulsions occurring in the first 3 months. Nulliparity, abnormal amount of menstrual flow, and severe dysmenorrhea are risk factors for expulsion. In addition, the expulsion rate may be higher when the IUD is inserted at the time of the menses. Pregnancy may be the first sign of expulsion. Therefore, patients should be taught to check for the IUD strings after each menstrual cycle. If a pregnancy does occur with an IUD in place, the IUD should be removed as soon as possible. In the presence of an IUD 50–60% of pregnancies spontaneously abort. The risk drops to 20% when the IUD is removed. Septic abortion is 26 times more common in women with an IUD. The copper-T IUD protects against ectopic pregnancy, whereas the progesterone IUD increases the risk of ectopic pregnancy almost twofold.

The management of actinomyces discovered on routine Papanicolaou (Pap) smear is one of the most controversial areas in the IUD literature. This finding on cervical cytology is more common in IUD users than in other women. There was concern that actinomyces was associated with IUD-related PID. However, this relationship has been questioned. If actinomyces is detected on Pap smear and the patient has signs or symptoms of PID, the IUD should be removed immediately and the patient treated with doxycycline. If the patient is asymptomatic, antibiotic treatment is not recommended and the Pap smear is repeated in 1 year.

Kaunitz AM: Beyond the pill: New data and options in hormonal and intrauterine contraception. Am J Obstet Gynecol 2005;192:998. [PMID: 15846172]

BARRIER CONTRACEPTION

Condom use, both at first intercourse and currently, has increased markedly since the 1970s, with over nine million women in the United States reportedly using condoms for contraception or protection from STDs. Condoms are inexpensive, easy to use, and available without a prescription. Until the late 1990s, most commercially available condoms were manufactured from latex. Now, polyurethane condoms are also available for latex-sensitive individuals. Although polyurethane and latex condoms offer similar protection against pregnancy, breakage and slippage rates appear to be higher with the polyurethane condom. Natural membrane condoms (made from sheep intestine) are also available; however, they do not offer the same degree of protection from STDs. Because couples vary widely in their ability to use condoms consistently and correctly, the failure rate also varies. The percentage of women experiencing an unintended pregnancy within the first year of use ranges from 3% with perfect use to 14% with typical use. Women relying on condoms for contraception and protection from STDs should be reminded that oil-based lubricants reduce the integrity of a latex condom and facilitate breakage. Because vaginal medications (eg, for yeast infections) often contain oil-based ingredients, they can damage latex condoms as well.

Several vaginal barrier contraceptives are available that are both easy to use and effective. The contraceptive efficacy of all barrier methods depends on their consistent and correct use. The percentage of women experiencing an unintended pregnancy within the first year of typical use ranges from 15% to 32%.

The female condom is a soft, loose-fitting polyurethane sheath with two flexible polyurethane rings at either end. One ring is inserted into the vagina and lies adjacent to the cervix. The other ring remains outside of the vagina, against the perineum. Sperm are captured within the condom. The sheath is coated on the inside with a silicone-based lubricant. The female condom is available without a prescription and is intended for one-time use. Female and male condoms should not be used together because the two condoms can adhere to one another, causing slippage and displacement. With correct and consistent use, the female condom can decrease the transmission of STDs, including HIV/AIDS.

The diaphragm is a dome-shaped rubber cup with a flexible rim. It is inserted, with a spermicide, into the vagina before intercourse. Once in position, the diaphragm provides contraceptive protection for 6 hours. If a longer interval has elapsed, insertion of additional spermicide is required. After intercourse the diaphragm must be left in place for 6 hours, but no longer than 24 hours. Use of the diaphragm has been associated with an increased risk of urinary tract infections (UTIs). Spermicide exposure is an important risk factor for UTI (due to alterations in vaginal flora), although it is possible mechanical factors in diaphragm use also may contribute to the risk of UTI. Use of the diaphragm requires an appointment with a health care provider for education, fitting, and a prescription. Oil-based vaginal products should not be used with the latex diaphragm.

The contraceptive sponge is a small, pillow-shaped polyurethane sponge containing a spermicide. The sponge protects for up 12–24 hours, no matter how many times intercourse occurs. After intercourse, the sponge must be left in place for at least 6 hours before it is removed and discarded. The sponge comes in one universal size and does not require a prescription.

The newest barrier device on the market is Lea's Shield. It is a reusable elliptical bowl made of medical-grade silicone rubber that is used with spermicide. It has an anterior loop to assist with removal and a centrally located valve that allows passage of cervical secretions. Lea's Shield offers several advantages over other vaginal barriers. Because the device is made of silicone, latex allergy and reaction with vaginal medications are not a concern. The device comes in only one size, simplifying the fitting process, and can be worn for up to 48 hours. Unlike the diaphragm, Lea's Shield does not require application of additional spermicide for repeated acts of intercourse. It is available by prescription only.

Spermicides are an integral component of several of the barrier contraceptives. Nonoxynol-9, the active chemical agent in spermicides available in the United States, is a surfactant that destroys the sperm cell membrane. It comes in a variety of formulations, including gel, foam, cream, film, suppository, and tablet. Spermicide use may lower the chance of becoming infected with a bacterial STD by as much as 25%. Women at high risk for acquiring HIV should not use products containing nonoxynol-9 because some studies have shown it causes vaginal lesions, which could then be entry points for HIV.

McNaught J, Jamieson MA: Barrier and spermicidal contraceptives in adolescence. Adolesc Med Clin 2005;16:495. [PMID: 16183536]

EMERGENCY CONTRACEPTION

There are three million unintended and unwanted pregnancies in the United States each year, 80% of which occur in women older than 19 years. As many as half of these pregnancies result from condom failure, missed birth control pills, or incorrect or inconsistent use of barrier contraception. Optimal use of emergency contraception could reduce unintended pregnancy in the United States by as much as 50%. Emergency contraception, available as COC pills, progestin-only pills, and the copper-T IUD, are safe and effective. When taken as directed, emergency contraceptive pills (ECPs) can reduce the risk of pregnancy by 75–89% after a single act of unprotected intercourse, and a copper-containing IUD inserted within 5 days of intercourse can reduce the risk by 99%.

Emergency contraception is appropriate when no contraception was used or when intercourse was unprotected due to contraceptive accidents. Because pill regimens involve only limited exposure to hormones, ECPs are safe. They have not been shown to increase the risk of venous thromboembolism, stroke, myocardial infarction, or any other cardiovascular event. In addition, ECPs will not disrupt an implanted pregnancy and will not cause birth defects. The mechanism of action of ECPs is not fully understood, but it is thought to involve inhibition of ovulation and prevention of fertilization, implantation, or both. ECPs do not protect against STDs.

The use of COCs for emergency contraception is frequently referred to as the Yuzpe method. Commercially available COCs containing ethinyl estradiol and levonorgestrel or norgestrel can be used as emergency contraception. Each of two doses separated by 12 hours must contain at least 100 mcg of ethinyl estradiol plus 0.5 mg of levonorgestrel or 1.0 mg of norgestrel (eg, Lo/Ovral: 4 white pills per dose). When used correctly, the Yuzpe method decreases expected pregnancies by 75%. More specifically, 8 out of every 100 women who have unprotected intercourse once during the second or third week of their cycles will become pregnant; 2 out of 100 will become pregnant if the Yuzpe method is used. The most common adverse effects are nausea (50%) and vomiting (20%). Antiemetics taken 30–60 minutes before each dose help to minimize these symptoms. Other side effects include delayed or early menstrual bleeding. Some women also experience heavier menses.

When used for emergency contraception, the initial dose of progestin-only ECP is 0.75 mg of levonorgestrel taken no more than 72 hours after unprotected intercourse and repeated in 12 hours. This regimen is marketed under the trade name Plan B. If Plan B is not available the dosage can be formulated from commercially available POPs. The initial dose of Ovrette, for example, is 20 pills, which is repeated 12 hours later. The progestin-only regimen may be somewhat more effective than the Yuzpe method, preventing 85% of expected pregnancies in one study. In addition, nausea occurs in fewer than 25% of patients and vomiting is reduced to about 5% in women taking the progestin-only regimen. Recent trials have found that treatment is effective when initiated up to 5 days after unprotected intercourse and that a single dose of 1.5 mg is as effective as two 0.75-mg doses administered 12 hours apart.

To prevent pregnancy, a copper-containing IUD can be inserted up to 5 days after unprotected intercourse. The IUD is highly effective and can be used for long-term contraception. An IUD is not recommended for anyone at risk for STDs or ectopic pregnancy, or if long-term contraception is not desired. The IUD is the most effective method of emergency contraception, with failure rates of less than 1%.

Screening of patients for emergency contraception focuses on identifying the time of unprotected intercourse and the date of the last normal menstrual period. There are no preexisting disease contraindications, and inadvertent use in pregnancy has not been linked to birth defects. Neither a pregnancy test nor a pelvic examination is required, although the latter may be done for other reasons (eg, screening for STDs). In contrast, IUD insertion for emergency contraception is an office-based procedure that requires appropriate counseling and screening as for any patient desiring an IUD for contraception.

Counseling regarding the availability of emergency contraception can occur anytime that contraception or family planning issues are discussed. It is especially appropriate if the patient is relying on barrier methods or does not have a regular form of contraception. The counseling can be reinforced when patients present with contraceptive "mishaps." Information that should be discussed includes the definition of emergency contraception, indications for use, mechanism of action, lack of protection against STDs, instructions on use, and follow-up plans, including ongoing contraception.

American Academy of Pediatrics, Committee on Adolescence: Emergency contraception. Pediatrics 2005;116:1026. [PMID: 16147972]

Trussell J et al: The role of emergency contraception. Am J Obstet Gynecol 2004;190:S30. [PMID: 15105796]

IMPLANTS

Progestin-releasing contraceptive implants provide highly effective, convenient birth control. Difficulty with insertion and removal of the Norplant system, in conjunction with complaints of irregular bleeding, prompted the manufacturer to cease marketing the product. A single rod implant (Implanon), which releases etonogestrel, is easier to insert and remove than Norplant and is associated with less bleeding. Implanon was approved by the FDA in July 2006 and is effective for up to 3 years. The manufacturer, Organon, will be conducting a national clinical training program to train health care providers on the insertion and removal procedures associated with the device. Only health care professionals trained through the company-sponsored programs will be able to prescribe the medication for their patients.

Funk S et al: Safety and efficacy of Implanon, a single-rod implantable contraceptive containing etonogestrel. Contraception 2005;71:319. [PMID: 15854630]

SPECIAL POPULATIONS

Adolescents

Adolescent pregnancy continues to be a serious public health problem in the United States. Nearly 1 in 10 female adolescents becomes pregnant each year, with half of those pregnancies ending in abortion. The general approach to adolescent contraception should focus on keeping the clinician-patient encounter interactive. Suggestions include avoiding "yes/no" questions, keeping clinician speaking time short and focused, and avoiding the word "should."

Abstinence deserves emphasis, especially in young teenagers. The focus of counseling should be "know how to say no" rather than "just say no." Oral contraceptives (COCs) and condoms are the most common contraceptive methods chosen by teens. Many clinicians promote using both methods simultaneously as an approach to pregnancy and STD prevention. COC use is associated with health benefits that are especially important during adolescence, including treatment for acne and menstrual cycle irregularity, decreased risk of PID and functional ovarian cysts, and decreased dysmenorrhea. The main concern adolescents have regarding COCs is the development of side effects, especially weight gain. They can be reassured that many studies have proven that COCs do not cause weight gain. Another issue that may contribute to the reluctance of adolescents to seek contraception is fear of a pelvic examination. Contrary to popular belief, a pelvic examination is not necessary when contraception is prescribed, especially if it will delay the sexually active teen's access to needed pregnancy prevention. Adolescents should be counseled regarding missed pills and given anticipatory guidance about breakthrough bleeding and amenorrhea. The contraceptive patch may be an attractive alternative to some teens who find it difficult to take a daily pill.

DMPA (Depo-Provera) is in some ways an ideal contraceptive for adolescents. The dosing schedule allows flexibility and minimal maintenance, and the failure rate is extremely low. However, concerns regarding bone loss in long-term users have prompted the recommendation that use not extend beyond 2 years. Although available data on adolescents are scant, they indicate that this group may be especially vulnerable to bone mineral density loss. It is not known whether bone loss before achieving peak bone density is recoverable, or to what extent the loss influences future risk of fracture. In addition, adolescents are likely to demonstrate other risk behaviors for bone loss, including early sexual activity, smoking, alcohol use, and poor diet choices. Until the results of larger studies are available definitive recommendations in teenagers cannot be made.

Vaginal barrier contraceptives are not ideal choices for several reasons. Many adolescents are not prepared to deal so intimately with their own bodies and do not wish to prepare so carefully for each episode of intercourse. However, these methods can be effective for highly motivated, educated adolescents. The IUD is normally not appropriate for adolescents because of the risk of PID in this population.

A discussion of emergency contraception should be part of contraceptive counseling for all adolescents. To increase the availability of emergency contraception, teens may be given a replaceable supply of ECPs to keep at home. Several studies in adolescents have shown that direct access to emergency contraception increases its rate of use but does not result in repetitive use. Although concern for improper use persists, women who are provided education on this method use it correctly, and incorrect use does not pose a health risk beyond unintended pregnancy.

Breast-feeding Women

Lactational amenorrhea is a highly effective, temporary method of contraception. However, to maintain effective protection against pregnancy, another method must be used as soon as menstruation resumes, the frequency or duration of breast-feeding is reduced, bottle-feeding or regular food supplements are introduced, or the infant reaches 6 months of age. Other contraceptive options for lactating women include barrier methods, progestin-only methods, or an IUD. Some experts recommend that breast-feeding women delay using progestin-only contraception until 6 weeks postpartum. This recommendation is based on a theoretical concern that early neonatal exposure to exogenous steroids should be avoided if possible. The combined pill is not a good option for lactating women because estrogen decreases the supply of breast milk.

Perimenopausal Women

Women older than 40 years of age have the second highest proportion of unintended pregnancies, exceeded only by girls 13–14 years old. Although women still need effective contraception during perimenopause, issues such as bone loss, menstrual irregularity, and vasomotor instability also need to be addressed. Oral contraceptives offer many benefits for healthy, nonsmoking perimenopausal women. They have been found to decrease the risk of postmenopausal hip fracture, regularize menses in women with dysfunctional uterine bleeding, and decrease vasomotor symptoms.

POPs can be used by women who have contraindications to estrogen. However, irregular bleeding patterns can create problems for perimenopausal women. Abnormal bleeding that is persistent, even if contraceptive hormone exposure is the most likely cause, will need to be evaluated. Other contraceptive options include condoms, vaginal barriers, and IUDs.

Physiologically, menopause is the permanent cessation of menstruation as a consequence of termination of ovarian follicular activity. Determining the exact onset of menopause in a woman who is using hormonal contraception can be tricky. Many clinicians measure the level of follicle-stimulating hormone (FSH) during the pill-free interval to diagnose menopause. However, because suppression of ovulation can vary from month to month, a single FSH value is unreliable. In addition, in women who use COCs, FSH levels can be suppressed even on the seventh pill-free day. Given that many women do not become menopausal until their mid-50s, and considering the limited utility of FSH testing, one approach to managing this transition avoids FSH testing entirely: women continue to use their COCs until age 55, at which time they can discontinue use.

Brown RT, Braverman PK, eds: Adolesc Med Clin 2005;16(3). [Entire issue devoted to contraception and adolescents.]

Davis AR, Teal SB: Controversies in adolescent hormonal contraception. Obstet Gynecol Clin North Am 2003;30:391. [PMID: 12836727]

Kaunitz AM: Oral contraceptive use in perimenopause. Am J Obstet Gynecol 2001;185:S32. [PMID: 11521120]

Adult Sexual Dysfunction 17

Charles W. Mackett III, MD, Margaret R. H. Nusbaum, DO, MPH, & T. A. Miller, MD

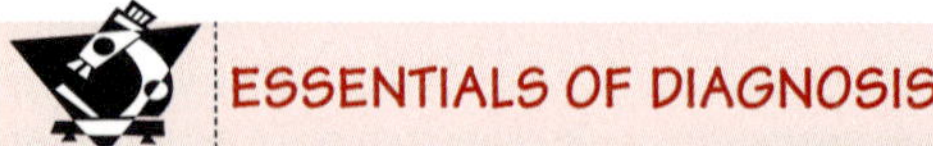

ESSENTIALS OF DIAGNOSIS

- *Disturbance in one or more aspects of the sexual response cycle.*
- *Cause is often multifactorial, associated with medical conditions, therapies, and life-style.*

General Considerations

Sexual dysfunction is a disturbance in one or more of the aspects of the sexual response cycle. It is a common problem that can result from communication difficulties, misunderstandings, and side effects of medical or surgical treatment, as well as underlying health problems. Because sexual difficulties often occur as a response to stress, fatigue, or interpersonal difficulties, addressing sexual health requires an expanded view of sexuality that emphasizes the importance of understanding individuals within the context of their lives and defining sexual health across physical, intellectual, emotional, interpersonal, environmental, cultural, and spiritual aspects of their lives and their sexual orientation. Family physicians are ideally situated to address the sexual health needs of both men and women, and it is likely that the therapeutic options for addressing these needs will continue to expand over the next decade.

Sexual dysfunction is extremely common. A survey of young to middle-aged adults found that 31% of men and 43% of women in the general population reported some type and degree of sexual dysfunction. The prevalence of sexual concerns and difficulties is even higher in clinical populations.

Recognition of sexual dysfunction is important whether specific treatment is available or desired. Sexual dysfunction may be the initial manifestation of significant underlying disease or provide a marker for disease progression and severity. It should be a consideration when managing a number of chronic medical conditions.

Sexual dysfunction is positively correlated with low physical and emotional relationship satisfaction, as well as low general happiness. Despite this, only 10% of men and 20% of women with sexual dysfunction seek medical care for their sexual difficulties. The key to the identification of sexual function disorders is for the provider to inquire about their presence. A discussion of sexual health can be initiated in a variety of ways. Educational material or self-administered screening forms, placed in the waiting area or the examination rooms, send the message that sexual health is an important topic that is discussed in the clinician's office. Table 17–1 lists several questionnaires that can be incorporated into self-administered patient surveys for office practices.

Sexual history can be included as part of the social history, as part of the review of systems under genitourinary systems, or in whatever manner seems most appropriate to the clinician. There are many other opportunities to bring a discussion of sexual health into the clinical encounter, as outlined in Table 17–2. Clinician anxiety may be reduced by asking the patient for permission prior to taking the sexual history.

Once the history confirms the existence of sexual difficulties, obtain as clear a description as possible of the following elements: the aspect of the sexual response cycle most involved, the onset, the progression, and any associated medical problems. Asking the patient what he or she believes to be the cause can help the clinician identify possible relationship, health, and iatrogenic etiologies. Asking the patient what he or she has tried to do to resolve the problems and clarifying the patient's expectations for resolution can help facilitate an appropriate therapeutic approach. Involving the partner in both identification and subsequent management can be very valuable.

Sexual dysfunction is associated with many factors, including medical conditions and therapies and lifestyle choices (Table 17–3). In some instances the underlying medical condition may be the cause of the sexual dysfunction (eg, arterial vascular disease causing erectile dysfunction). In other instances the sexual dysfunction contributes to the associated condition (eg, erectile dysfunction leads to loss of self-esteem and depression). Sexual difficulties can begin with one aspect of the sexual response cycle and subsequently affect other aspects; for example, arousal difficulties can lead to depression, which can then negatively affect sexual interest.

Table 17–1. Sexual health screening questionnaires.

Sexual Health Inventory for Men (SHIM)
International Index of Erectile Function (IIEF)
World Health Organization (WHO) Intensity Score
Androgen Deficiency in the Aging Male (ADAM)
Female Sexual Function Index (FSFI)
Sexual Energy Scale
Brief Index of Sexual Function Inventory (BISF-W)
Changes in Sexual Functioning Questionnaire (CSFQ)

Nusbaum MR, Hamilton CD: The proactive sexual health inquiry. Am Fam Physician 2002;66:1705. [PMID: 12449269]

DISORDERS OF DESIRE

General Considerations

Difficulties with sexual desire are the most common sexual concern. Over 33% of women and 16% of men in the general population report experiencing an extended period of lack of sexual interest. Other investigators have reported prevalence rates as high as 87% in specific populations. Women who were younger, separated, black, less educated, and of lower socioeconomic status reported the highest rates. Among men, the same demographics as well as increasing age were associated with the highest rates.

Table 17–2. Sexual health inquiry.

Review of systems or social history
What sexual concerns do you have?
Has there been any change in your (or partner's) sexual desire or frequency of sexual activity?
Are you satisfied with your (or partner's) present sexual functioning?
Is there anything about your sexual activity (as individuals or as a couple) that you (or your partner) would like to change?
Counseling about healthy life-style (smoking or alcohol cessation, exercise program, weight reduction)
Discussing effectiveness and side effects of medications
Inquire before and after medical event or procedures likely to impact sexual function (myocardial infarction, prostate surgery)
Inquire when there is about to be or has been a life cycle change such as pregnancy, new baby, teenager, children leaving the home, retirement, menopause, "discovery" of past abuse

Sources: Nusbaum MRH: *Sexual Health*. American Academy of Family Physicians, 2001; Nusbaum MR, Hamilton C: The proactive sexual health inquiry: Key to effective sexual health care. Am Fam Physician 2002;66:1705; and Nusbaum M, Rosenfeld J: *Sexual Health Across the Lifecycle: A Practical Guide for Clinicians.* Cambridge University Press, 2004:20.

Table 17–3. Factors associated with sexual dysfunction.

Aging
Chronic disease
Diabetes mellitus
Heart disease
Hypertension
Lipid disorders
Renal failure
Vascular disease
Endocrine abnormalities
Hypogonadism
Hyperprolactinemia
Hypo/hyperthyroidism
Life-style
Cigarette smoking
Chronic alcohol abuse
Neurogenic causes
Spinal cord injury
Multiple sclerosis
Herniated disc
Penile injury/disease
Peyronie plaques
Priapism
Pharmacologic agents
Psychological issues
Depression
Anxiety
Social stresses
Trauma/injury
Pelvic trauma/surgery
Pelvic radiation

Classification

Decrease in sexual desire can be related to decrease or loss of interest in or an aversion to sexual interaction with self or others, or both. It can be lifelong (primary) or acquired (secondary), generalized or situational in occurrence. Sexual aversion is characterized by persistent or extreme aversion to, and avoidance of, sexual activity. Separating these difficulties can be difficult or impossible. For example, a patient who has experienced sexual trauma may have difficulties with subsequent partners and ultimately develop an aversion to sexual activity.

A common situation in clinical practice is discrepancy in sexual desire within a partnership, in which partners differ in their level of sexual desire. Although most couples negotiate a workable solution, in some instances it may be significant enough to cause relation-

Table 17–4. Common medical conditions that may affect sexual desire.

Pituitary/hypothalamic
Infiltrative diseases/tumors
Endocrine
Testosterone deficiency
Castration, adrenal disease, age-related bilateral salpingo-oophorectomy, adrenal disease
Thyroid deficiency
Endocrine-secreting tumors
Cushing syndrome
Adrenal insufficiency
Psychiatric
Depression and stress
Substance abuse
Neurologic
Degenerative diseases/trauma of the central nervous system
Urologic/gynecologic (indirect cause)
Peyronie plaques, phimosis
Gynecologic pain syndromes
Renal
End-stage renal disease, renal dialysis
Conditions that cause chronic pain, fatigue, malaise
Arthritis, cancer, chronic pulmonary or hepatic disease

Table 17–5. Drugs most commonly associated with sexual dysfunction.

Drug Class	Negative Effect on Sexual Response Cycle
Antihypertensives	Arousal difficulties
Diuretics	Arousal and desire
Thiazides	
Spironolactone	
Sympatholytics	
Central agents (methyldopa, clonidine)	Arousal and desire
Peripheral agents (reserpine)	Arousal and desire
α-Blockers	Arousal and orgasm
β-Blockers (particularly nonselective agents)	Arousal and desire
Psychiatric medications	
Antipsychotics	Multiple phases of sexual function
Antidepressants	
Tricyclic antidepressants	Arousal and desire
MAO inhibitors	Multiple phases of sexual function
SSRIs	Arousal and orgasm
Anxiolytics	
Benzodiazepines	Arousal difficulties
Antiandrogenic Agents	
Digoxin	Arousal and desire
H_2 receptor blockers	Arousal and desire
Others	
Alcohol (long-term, heavy use)	Arousal and desire
Ketoconazole	Arousal and desire
Niacin	Arousal and desire
Phenobarbital	Arousal and desire
Phenytoin	Arousal and desire

MAO, monoamine oxidase; SSRI, selective serotonin reuptake inhibitor.

ship dissatisfaction. It can also be a marker for extrarelationship affairs or domestic violence.

Pathogenesis

Changes in or a loss of sexual desire can be the result of biological, psychological, or social and interpersonal factors. Numerous medical conditions directly or indirectly affect sexual desire (Table 17–4). Illnesses and medications that decrease relative androgen levels, increase the level of sex hormone–binding globulin, or interfere with endocrine and neurotransmitter functioning can negatively affect desire. Examples include exogenous hormones (eg, estrogens and progesterones), diabetes, and depression, as well as erectile difficulties due to arterial vascular disease or dyspareunia due to estrogen deficiency–induced atrophic vaginitis. In both men and women, sexual desire is linked to levels of androgens, testosterone, and dehydroepiandrosterone (DHEA). In men, testosterone levels begin to decline in the fifth decade and continue to do so steadily throughout later life. For both genders, DHEA levels begin to decline in the 30s, decrease steadily thereafter, and are quite low by age 60.

Decreased sexual desire is a common manifestation of some psychiatric conditions, particularly affective disorders. Several medications can negatively affect desire and the sexual response cycle (Table 17–5). The agents most commonly associated with these changes are psychoactive drugs, particularly antidepressants, and medications with antiandrogen effects. Many psychosocial issues affect sexual desire. Factors as widely varied as religious beliefs, primary sexual interest in individuals outside of the main relationship, specific sexual phobias or aversions, fear of pregnancy, lack of attraction to partner, and poor sexual skills in the partner can all diminish sexual desire.

Clinical Findings

A. Symptoms and Signs

The evaluation of decreased sexual desire should include a detailed sexual problem history, which may clarify difficulties with sexual desire, identify predisposing conditions, and help establish a therapeutic plan. In addition to loss of desire, a diminished sense of well being, depression, lethargy, osteoporosis, loss of muscle mass, and erectile dysfunction are other manifestations of androgen deficiency.

The physical examination in patients with an acquired generalized loss of desire should be directed toward the identification of unrecognized conditions such as endocrine abnormalities (eg, hypogonadism, hypothyroidism).

B. Laboratory Findings

An assessment of hormone status may be helpful. In men, an assessment of androgen status is indicated. In women, an assessment of both androgens and estrogens is indicated.

Assessment of the total plasma testosterone level, obtained in the morning, is the most readily available study. In most men, levels below 300 ng/dL are symptomatic of hypogonadism; however, 200 ng/dL might be a more appropriate cutoff for diagnosis in older men. Free testosterone more accurately reflects bioavailable androgens. Levels less than 50 pg/mL suggest hypogonadism.

Measurement of other androgenic agents formed earlier in the steroid hormone synthesis pathway are advocated by some authorities. If low testosterone is confirmed, further endocrine assessment and imaging is indicated to determine the specific underlying etiology.

Treatment

Treatment is directed at the underlying etiology and consists of both nonspecific and specific therapy. Asking sex partners about each other's sexual function can be useful.

Educating couples about the impact of extraneous influences—fatigue, preoccupation with child rearing, work stress, and interpersonal conflict—can improve awareness of these issues. Encouraging couples to set time aside for themselves, to schedule "dates," can be very effective. Educating partners about gender generalities and encouraging communication about sexual needs and desires can be helpful. The quality of the relationship appears to be a critical component in women's sexual response cycle.

Although largely unstudied, the quality of the relationship is likely of equal import in men's sexual interaction. An emotionally and physically satisfying relationship enhances sexual desire and arousal and has a positive feedback on the quality of the relationship. The importance of allowing time for sexual relations, incorporating the senses, understanding what is pleasing to one's partner, and incorporating seduction cannot be overemphasized.

The impact of potentially reversible medical conditions or medications on sexual desire should be addressed. Treating organic etiologies such as depression, hypothyroidism, hyperprolactinemia, and androgen deficiency can often restore sexual interest.

Options available when decreased sexual desire is attributed to medical therapy can be challenging. Treatment approaches can include lowering the dosage, suggesting drug holidays, discontinuing potentially offensive medications, or switching to a different agent. Where continuation of therapy is indicated, adding specific agents to address the sexual manifestations can be useful.

In men and women with acquired decreased sexual interest, hormone supplementation may be considered.

A. Androgen Replacement

The goal of replacement therapy is to raise the level to the lowest physiologic range that promotes satisfactory response (Table 17–6). For both genders, oral testosterone is not recommended due to the prominent first-pass phenomenon and the potential for significant liver toxicity. Intramuscular injections result in dramatic fluctuations in blood levels. Topical preparations offer the advantage of consistent levels in the normal range. Local skin reactions are common with patches. Topical gels tend to have fewer skin side effects.

A diagnosis of androgen insufficiency should only be made in women who are adequately estrogenized, whose free testosterone is at or below the lowest quartile of the normal range for the reproductive age (20–40 years), and who present with clinical symptoms.

Androgen supplementation can be helpful for desire and arousal difficulties in both men and women. Dehydroepiandrosterone sulfate (DHEAS) is available over the counter and is dosed 25–75 mg/day based on response. Transdermal testosterone can be compounded as 1–2% cream, gel, or lotion that can be applied to the labial and clitoral area. Oral methyltestosterone, available as Estratest for women, has been used safely for years. Oral administration of methyltestosterone is a less preferred route given erratic absorption and concerns about liver effects.

Exogenous estrogens and progestins, in the form of hormone replacement therapy, lower physiologically available androgens and can contribute to decreased sexual interest. Addition of androgens, methyltestosterone, or DHEAS can offset this negative impact. If no benefit occurs from this change, the physician should reassess the quality of the sexual relationship and also consider discontinuing the exogenous hormones. All oral contraceptive agents lower bioavailable androgen levels as a result of high sex hormone–binding globulin levels. Changing to oral contraceptive pills with greater androgen activity, such as those containing norgestrel, levonorgestrel, and norethindrone acetate, may be an effective change (Table 17–7).

Table 17–6. Androgen therapy: agents, routes, and dosages.

Route/Agent	Dosage for Women	Dosage for Men
Oral[1]		
Methyltestosterone	10 mg: 1/4 to 1/2 tablet daily or 10 mg Monday, Wednesday, Friday	10–50 mg/day
Fluoxymesterone	2 mg: 1/2 tablet daily or 1 tablet every other day	5–20 mg/day
Estratest and Estratest HS	Either 1.25 or 0.625 mg	
Dehydroepiandrosterone	25–75 mg 3 times weekly to daily[1]	
Buccal		
Methyltestosterone[3]	5–25 mg daily USP tablet, 0.25 mg[2]	5–25 mg/day
Sublingual		
Methyltestosterone Testosterone micronized USP tablet	0.25 mg[2]	
Transdermal		
Testosterone patch	2.5–5.0 mg applied every day or every other day	4–6 mg/day
Topical testosterone	1% vaginal cream daily to clitoris and labia	5–10 mg/day (Androderm)
Testosterone micronized	1–2% gel daily to clitoris and labia[2]	
Intramuscular		
Testosterone enanthate	200 mg/mL: 0.25–0.5 ml every 3–5 wk	50–400 mg every 2–4 wk
Testosterone propionate	100 mg/mL: 1/4–1/2 mL every 3–4 weeks	25–50 mg 2–3 times weekly

[1]Oral methyltestosterone, aside from the combination estratest, should be used only short term due to the risk of hepatotoxicity.
[2]Must be compounded by a pharmacist.
[3]Guay A: Advances in the management of androgen deficiency in women. Med Aspects Hum Sexuality, 2001.
Adapted from Nusbaum M, Rosenfeld J: *Sexual Health Across the Lifecycle: A Practical Guide for Clinicians.* Cambridge University Press, Chaps 6 and 7.

B. Contraindications and Risk of Testosterone Therapy

Because testosterone treatment may stimulate tumor growth in androgen-, estrogen-, or progesterone-dependent cancers, it is contraindicated in men with prostate cancer and in men and women with a history of breast cancer. Although it is known that testosterone accelerates the clinical course of prostate cancer and may stimulate the growth of previously undiagnosed prostate tumors, there is no conclusive evidence in short-term studies that testosterone therapy increases the incidence of prostate cancer.

Certain patient populations such as the elderly and patients who have a first-degree relative with prostate cancer may be at increased risk. Preexisting sleep apnea and hyperviscosity, including deep venous thrombosis or pulmonary embolism, are relative contraindications to testosterone use. Serious hepatic and lipid changes have been associated with the use of oral preparations available in the United States. Benign prostatic hypertrophy, lipid changes, gynecomastia, sleep apnea, and increased oiliness of skin or acne are other reported side effects.

If androgen therapy is initiated for both men and women, close follow-up is recommended to assess androgen levels, lipid profile, hematocrit levels, and liver function. Periodic assessment of the prostate-spe-

Table 17–7. Relative androgenicity of progestational components of oral contraceptive agents.

Relative androgenicity
Least
Norethindrone (0.4–0.5 mg)[1]
Norgestimate (0.18–0.25 mg)
Desogestrel (0.15 mg)
Ethynodiol diacetate (1.0 mg)
Medium/neutral
Norethindrone (0.5–1.0 mg)[1]
Greatest
Levonorgestrel (0.1–0.15 mg)
Norgestrel (0.075–0.5 mg)
Norethindrone acetate (1.0–1.5 mg)

[1]Norethindrone (0.35 mg) without estrogen, in progestin-only oral contraceptive pills, has medium relative androgenicity.
Sources: Nusbaum MRH: *Sexual Health.* American Academy of Family physicians, 2001; and Burham T, Short R (eds): *Drug Facts and Comparisons.* Mosby, 2001.

cific antigen level may be considered. Until more data regarding long-term use are available, it is probably most prudent to check androgen, hematocrit, liver, and lipid levels every 3–6 months.

Basson R et al: Report of the international consensus development conference on female sexual dysfunction: Definitions and classifications. J Urol 2000;163:888. [PMID: 10688001]

Snyder PJ: Hypogonadism in elderly men—what to do until the evidence comes. N Eng J Med 2004;350:440. [PMID: 14749451]

DISORDERS OF EXCITEMENT & AROUSAL

General Considerations

Arousal disorders appear to affect 18.8% of women and 5% of men in the general population. The prevalence of arousal difficulties for both men and women is much higher in patient populations with coexisting illnesses such as depression, diabetes, and heart disease. Abuse also has a negative effect on arousal and sexual health.

Pathogenesis

Arousal difficulties most likely result from a mix of organic and psychogenic etiologies. Organic causes include vascular, neurogenic, and hormonal etiologies. Vascular arterial or inflow problems are by far the most common. Regardless of the primary etiology, a psychological component frequently coexists. Although influenced by other systems, arousal is primarily a neurovascular process. Optimal function requires an intact nervous system and responsive arterial vasculature. Sexual stimulation results in nitric oxide release, which initiates a cascade of events leading to a dramatic increase in blood flow to the penis in men and the vagina and clitoris in women. Nitric oxide enters into vascular smooth muscle cells causing an increase in the production of cyclic guanosine monophosphate (cGMP). As cGMP concentrations rise, vascular smooth muscle relaxes, allowing increased arterial blood flow. The cGMP buildup is countered by the enzyme phosphodiesterase type 5 (PDE-5).

Inhibiting the action of PDE-5 results in higher levels of cGMP, causing increased and sustained vasodilation. Arousal disorders appear to increase with age, but it is more likely that increase in chronic illnesses and their therapeutic intervention are the root cause. Life-style factors such as tobacco, alcohol, exercise, and diet also contribute.

Clinical Findings

A. Symptoms and Signs

The first step in assessment is to ensure that arousal problems are the primary problem. Some men may complain of erectile difficulties but on detailed questioning may not be experiencing erections due to lack of desire or may not be able to sustain the erection due to premature ejaculation. Detailed information about onset, duration, progression, severity, and association with medical conditions, medications, and psychosocial factors will enable the provider to identify if the patient's problem has a primarily organic or psychogenic etiology.

Physical examination should be focused and directed by the history. The clinician should assess overall health, including life-style topics such as exercise, tobacco use, and alcohol use. Additionally, screening for manifestations of affective, cardiovascular, neurologic, or hormonal etiology should be performed.

B. Laboratory Findings

If not previously done, basic laboratory studies such as lipid profile and fasting blood glucose should be considered to identify unrecognized systemic disease that may predispose to vascular disease. Measurement of androgen levels (including DHEA) should be performed if androgen supplementation is being considered.

Treatment

Chronic medical conditions should be treated or controlled to reverse or slow the progression of associated conditions. Medications contributing to arousal problems (eg, antihypertensive agents) should be replaced with other agents, if possible, or reduced in dosage. Potentially reversible causes should be addressed.

Maximizing glucose control in diabetic patients, moderating alcohol consumption, encouraging exercise, and smoking cessation are important life-style changes necessary to maintain healthy sexual response. Nitric oxide appears to be androgen sensitive, so correction of androgen levels may be necessary before PDE-5 inhibitors will be successful. Sexual lubricants such as Astroglide, Replens, and K-Y jelly can add lubrication and enhance sensuality.

A. Oral Agents

Sildenafil, vardenafil, and tadalafil are PDE-5 inhibitors approved for the treatment of male erectile dysfunction. Inhibitors do not result in spontaneous erection and require erotic or physical stimulation, or both, to be effective. PDE-5 inhibitors are contraindicated in patients who take organic nitrates of any type. Nitrates are nitric oxide donors. The concomitant use of a PDE-5 inhibitor and a nitrate can result in profound hypotension. PDE-5 inhibitors are also contraindicated in patients with recent cardiovascular events or who are clinically hypotensive.

The side effects of PDE-5 inhibitors are related to the presence of PDE-5 in other parts of the body and cross-reactivity with other PDE enzyme subtypes. A transient disturbance in color vision, characterized typically by a greenish-blue hue, is due to a slight cross-reactivity with PDE-5 isoenzyme in the retina. Because of this cross-reactivity, PDE-5 inhibitors should not be used in patients with retinitis pigmentosa. Side effects tend to be mild and transient, and include headache, flushing, dyspepsia, and rhinitis.

Although PDE-5 inhibitors are not approved by the Food and Drug Administration for use in women, it is likely that these agents will have a role in treating female arousal difficulties. One study reported significant effectiveness in improving arousal and orgasm in a group of young premenopausal women with arousal difficulties. Additionally, the frequency of sexual fantasies, sexual intercourse, and enjoyment improved. Studies of genital stimulation devices and topical warming gels have shown these adjuncts to be beneficial to sexual functioning.

B. Vacuum Constriction Devices

These devices are effective for most causes of erectile dysfunction, are noninvasive, and are a relatively inexpensive treatment option. The device consists of a cylinder, vacuum pump, and constriction band. The flaccid penis is placed in the cylinder. Pressing the cylinder against the skin of the perineum forms an airtight seal. Negative pressure from the pump draws blood into the penis, resulting in increased firmness. When sufficient blood has entered the erectile bodies, a constriction band is placed around the base of the penis preventing the escape of blood. Following intercourse the band is removed. Side effects include penile pain, bruising, numbness, and impaired ejaculation.

C. Intracavernosal Injection

With this method, synthetic formulations of prostaglandin E_1 (alprostadil alone or in combination with other vasoactive agents) is injected directly into the corpus cavernosum. This results in spontaneous erection. Intracavernosal injection is effective in producing erection in most patients with erectile dysfunction, including some who failed to respond to oral therapy.

D. Penile Prosthesis

In patients not responding to other therapies, a permanent penile prosthesis has proven to be safe and effective in many patients. Current models have a 7- to 10-year life expectancy or longer. Overall patient satisfaction is excellent.

Caruso S et al: Premenopausal women affected by sexual arousal disorder treated with sildenafil: A double-blind, cross-over, placebo-controlled study. BJOG 2001;108:623. [PMID: 11426898]

SEXUAL PAIN SYNDROMES

Sexual pain syndromes can negatively affect arousal for both men and women. Sexual pain syndromes occur in 14% of women and 3% of men in the general population, and over 70% of samples of female patients. Peyronie plaques or other penile deformity, priapism, and lower urinary tract symptoms can be etiologic in male sexual pain syndrome. For women, vaginitis, vestibulitis, pelvic pathology, vaginismus, and inadequate vaginal lubrication are among the etiologies of sexual pain syndromes for women. Sexual pain syndromes negatively affect desire, arousal, and thus orgasm.

Nusbaum MR, Gamble G: The prevalence and importance of sexuality concerns among female military beneficiaries. Mil Med 2001;166:208. [PMID: 11263020]

Nusbaum MRH et al: The high prevalence of sexual concerns among women seeking routine gynecological care. J Fam Pract 2000;49:229 [PMID: 1073548]

DISORDERS OF EJACULATION & ORGASM

Premature ejaculation affects 29% of men in the general population, and orgasm difficulties affect 8% of men and 24% of women. Over 80% of women in patient populations report difficulties with orgasm.

Premature ejaculation results from a shortened plateau phase. In addition to heightened sensitivity to erotic stimulation and, often, learned behavior from rushed sexual encounters, organic etiology is also likely. The ejaculatory reflex involves a complex interplay between central serotonergic and other neurons. From studies of rodents, premature ejaculation is speculated to be a dysfunction of serotonergic receptors.

Although premature ejaculation tends to improve with age by the natural lengthening of the plateau phase, it persists well into aging for many men. Like erectile dysfunction, premature ejaculation is often associated with shame and depression. Orgasmic difficulties can feed back negatively on arousal and then desire. A man with premature ejaculation can develop erectile dysfunction and ultimately have decreased sexual desire because of the emotional effects.

Difficulty or inability to achieve orgasm affects a greater number of women than men and typically results from a prolonged arousal phase caused by inadequate stimulation. Medications can also interfere. Selective serotonin reuptake inhibitors (SSRIs) raise the threshold for orgasm, which makes them highly effective treatment options for men with premature ejaculation, but highly problematic for both genders who have difficulty achieving orgasm. Medications that lower the threshold for orgasm can be very problematic for men with premature ejaculation but can be very effective for treating problems with orgasm. These include cyproheptadine, bupropion, and possibly PDE-5 inhibitors. These agents can be helpful for men with delayed ejaculation. Psychotropic agents and alcohol often cause

Table 17–8. Antidotes for psychotropic-induced sexual dysfunction.

Drug	Dosage
Yohimbine	5.4–16.2 mg, 2–4 h prior to sexual activity
Bupropion	100 mg as needed or 75 mg three times daily
Amantadine	100–400 mg as needed or daily
Cyproheptadine	2–16 mg a few hours before sexual activity
Methylphenidate	5–25 mg as needed
Dextroamphetamine	5 mg sublingually 1 h prior to sex
Nefazodone	150 mg 1 h prior to sex
Sildenafil	50–100 mg as needed

Sources: Nusbaum MRH: *Sexual Health.* American Academy of Family Physicians, 2001; and Maurice W: Ejaculation/orgasm disorders. In: *Sexual Medicine in Primary Care.* Mosby, 1999: 192.

delayed ejaculation. Medications used as rescue agents for treating sexual side effects of psychotropic agents or to lower the threshold for orgasm for women having difficulty with orgasm are also useful for treating delayed ejaculation (Table 17–8).

Retrograde ejaculation occurs when the seminal fluid is ejaculated from the posterior urethra into the bladder. This is caused by abnormal function of the internal sphincter of the urethra and can result from anatomic disruption (eg, transurethral prostatectomy), sympathetic nervous system disruptions (eg, damage from surgery), lymph node invasion, or diabetes. Retrograde ejaculation can result from interference with the sphincter function from medications such as antipsychotics, antidepressants, and antihypertensive agents as well as alcohol use. Dextroamphetamine, ephedrine, phenylpropanolamine, and pseudoephedrine are potentially effective in treating retrograde ejaculation.

Evaluation should include a history of sexual problems, medications, and quality of the relationship. Treatment approaches include discontinuing, decreasing the dosage of, or drug holidays from offending medications. Small studies have shown a benefit from rescue agents that can be added as standing (or as needed) medications (see Table 17–8). SSRIs are the treatment of choice for premature ejaculation. It is helpful if women become familiar with the type of stimulation they require for orgasm and communicate that to their partners. An excellent reference for patients is the book *Becoming Orgasmic.*

The resolution phase is typically not problematic for either gender, but misunderstandings of age-related changes can occur. Men, and their partners, need to understand that with increasing age the refractory period to sexual stimulation lengthens, sometimes up to 24 hours. Men may require more direct penile stimulation for sexual response as they age.

Heiman JR, LoPicolo J: *Becoming Orgasmic: A Sexual & Personal Growth Program for Women.* Prentice Hall, 1988.

Waldinger MD: The neurobiological approach to early ejaculation. J Urol 2002:168;2359. [PMID: 12441918]

SEXUAL ACTIVITY & CARDIOVASCULAR RISK

Sexual activity and intercourse are associated with physiologic changes in heart rate and blood pressure. A patient's ability to meet the physiologic demands related to sexual activity should be assessed, particularly if the patient is not accustomed to the level of activity associated with sex or may be at increased risk of a cardiovascular event. Typical sexual intercourse is associated with an oxygen expenditure of 3–4 metabolic equivalents (METS), whereas vigorous sexual intercourse can expend 5–6 METS. Patients unaccustomed to the level of exercise associated with sexual activity and who have risk factors for cardiovascular events present a clinical challenge. An algorithm based on expert opinion can assist clinicians in determining which patients can be safely advised that sexual activity and treatment can be undertaken without further risk stratification and which should have further evaluation. In this algorithm patients are classified as low risk if they have fewer than three risk factors (age, hypertension, diabetes, obesity, cigarette smoking, dyslipidemias, and sedentary life-style). Patients in the intermediate risk group should undergo risk stratification into either the low-risk or high-risk group. This assessment may include cardiac stress testing.

Debusk R et al: Management of sexual dysfunction in patients with cardiovascular disease: Recommendations of the Princeton Consensus Panel. Am J Cardiol 2000;86:175. [PMID: 10913479]

Acute Coronary Syndrome 18

Stephen A. Wilson, MD, & Jacqueline S. Weaver-Agostoni, DO, MPH

ESSENTIALS OF DIAGNOSIS

- *At least two of the following findings: ischemic symptoms, diagnostic electrocardiogram (ECG) changes, and an elevated serum marker of cardiac injury.*
- *Chest pain, often accompanied by diaphoresis, is common; pain often radiates to the left arm, shoulder, jaw, or neck.*
- *Shortness of breath is more common in patients who are elderly, black, or female.*

General Considerations

Acute coronary syndrome (ACS) is an umbrella term that encompasses unstable angina, ST-elevation myocardial infarction (STEMI), and non–ST-elevation myocardial infarction (NSTEMI). It is the symptomatic cardiac end product of cardiovascular disease, resulting in reversible or irreversible cardiac injury, and even death.

Cultural issues can affect the diagnosis, treatment, and outcome of ACS. Some clinical symptoms are more common in certain patient populations (see Symptoms and Signs, later). Other notable differences exist between patient populations that relate to diagnosis and treatment of cardiac disease. Both men and women with ACS respond to early invasive treatment. Women tend to have more severe first ACS, are less likely to receive thrombolysis, and are at greater risk for death and hospital readmission at 6 months. Patients experiencing ACS are less often hospitalized, thus increasing their mortality, if they are women younger than 55 years of age, are nonwhite, have shortness of breath as their chief complaint, or have a normal or indeterminate ECG.

Patients are more likely to adhere to treatment plans they can afford, and this should be taken into account when deciding which medication to prescribe and which diet and exercise plans to recommend. In addition to promoting healthy habits, family physicians provide continuity of care for patients with ACS and can help monitor adherence and response to treatment.

Glaser R et al: Benefit of an early invasive management strategy in women with acute coronary syndromes. JAMA 2002;288:3124. [PMID: 12495392]

Link N, Tanner M: Coronary artery disease: Part I. Epidemiology and diagnosis. WJM 2001;174:257. [PMID: 11290684]

Pathogenesis

Cardiovascular disease includes all diseases of the heart and vasculature (eg, stroke and hypertension). Coronary artery disease (CAD), synonymous with coronary heart disease (CHD), affects the coronary arteries, diminishing their ability to supply oxygenated blood to the heart.

A. Progression of Atherosclerosis

Atherosclerotic disease is the thickening and hardening (loss of elasticity) of the arterial wall due to the accumulations of lipids, macrophages, T lymphocytes, smooth muscle cells, extracellular matrix, calcium, and necrotic debris. Figures 18–1 through 18–3 grossly depict the multifactorial and complex depository, inflammatory, and reactive processes that collaborate to occlude coronary arteries.

B. Genetic Predisposition

The best indicator of CAD risk is family history of CAD. Some inherited risk factors (eg, dyslipidemia and propensity for diabetes mellitus) are modifiable; others (eg, age and sex) are not. Genes affect the development and progression of disease and its response to risk factor modification and life-style decisions: nature (genetics) meets nurture (environment) and they responsively interrelate (Table 18–1).

Grech ED: Pathophysiology and investigation of coronary artery disease. BMJ 2003;306:1027. [PMID: 12742929]

Scheuner MT: Genetic predisposition to coronary artery disease. Curr Opin Cardiol 2001;16:251. [PMID: 11574787]

Worthley SG et al. Coronary artery disease: Pathogenesis and acute coronary syndromes. Mt Sinai J Med 2001;68:167. [PMID: 11373689]

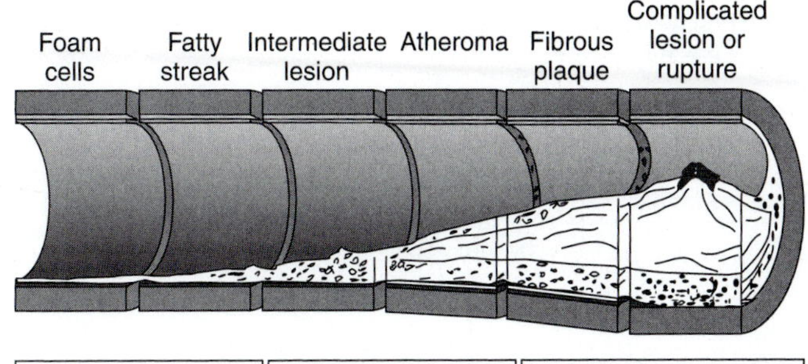

Figure 18–1. **Atheromatous plaque progression.** (Reproduced, with permission, from Grech ED: Pathophysiology and investigation of coronary artery disease. BMJ 2003;326:1027.)

Prevention

The cascade of events that leads to ACS can be interrupted, delayed, or treated. *Primary prevention* tries to prevent disease before it develops (ie, prevent or delay development of risk factors). *Secondary prevention* attempts to prevent disease progression by identifying and treating risk factors or preclinical, asymptomatic disease. *Tertiary prevention* involves treatment of established disease to restore and maintain highest function, minimize negative disease effects, and prevent complications (ie, help recovery from and prevent recurrence of ACS).

A. Primary Prevention

Primary prevention of ACS should begin in childhood by avoiding tobacco use, eating a diet rich in fruits and vegetables and low in saturated fats, engaging in regular exercise of 20–30 minutes five times a week, and maintaining a body mass index (BMI) between 18 and 25 (calculated by dividing weight in kilograms by height in meters squared).

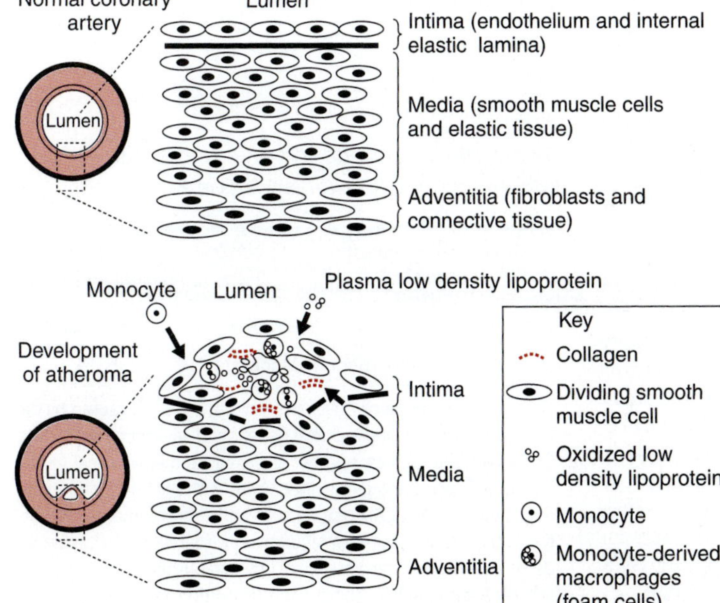

Figure 18–2. **Mechanism of plaque development.** (Reproduced, with permission, from Grech ED: Pathophysiology and investigation of coronary artery disease. BMJ 2003;326:1027.)

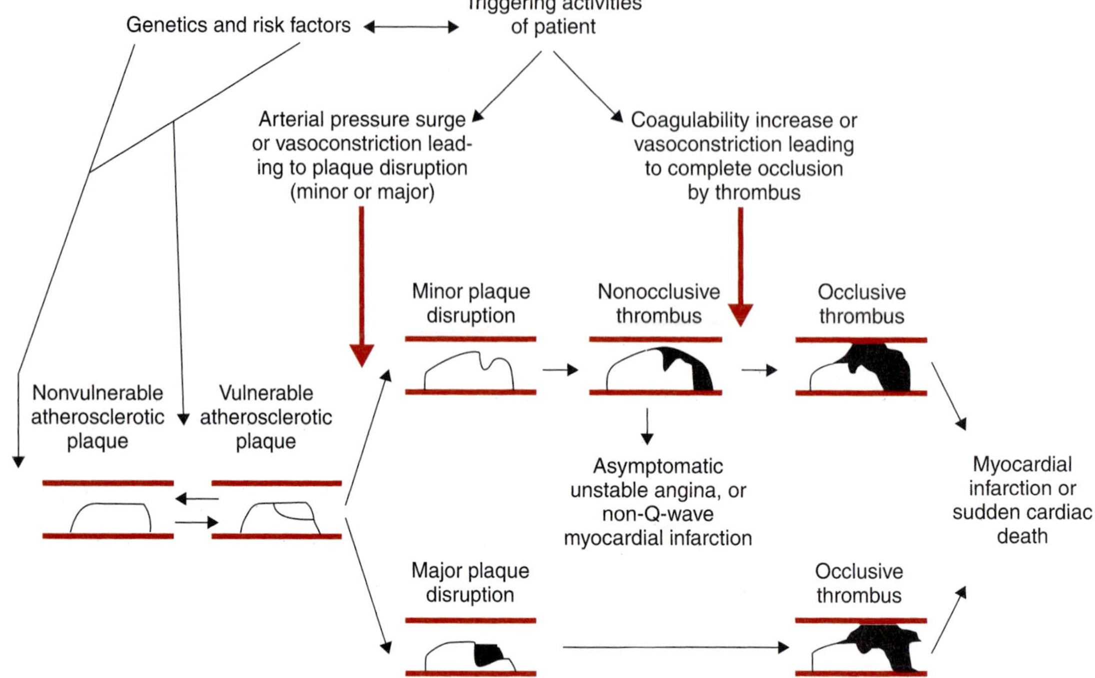

Figure 18–3. Mechanism of coronary artery thrombosis. Hypothetical methods of possible trigger for coronary thrombosis: (1) physical or mental stress leads to hemodynamic changes leads to plaque rupture; (2) activities causing an increase in coagulability; and (3) stimuli leading to vasoconstriction. The role of coronary thrombosis in unstable angina, myocardial infarction, and sudden cardiac death has been well described. (From Muller JE et al: Triggers, acute risk factors and vulnerable plaques: The lexicon of a new frontier. J Am Coll Cardiol 1994;23:809. Reprinted, with permission, from the American College of Cardiology. Chasen CA, Muller JE: Triggers of myocardial infarction. Cardiol Special Ed 1997;3:57.)

B. Secondary and Tertiary Prevention

Secondary and tertiary prevention involves progressively more aggressive management of patients who have known risk factors for or have experienced ACS (Figure 18–4 and Table 18–2). Although the association between cholesterol and ACS death is weaker in those older than 65 years, statin drugs can still have a positive impact on morbidity and mortality in this age group.

Research into preventive measures is ongoing, and some once-touted therapies have been shown to be ineffective. In particular, estrogen/progestin hormone replacement therapy should not be used as primary, secondary, or tertiary prevention of CAD due to lack of positive effect and the potential for harm. Antibiotics and the antioxidants vitamins C and E likewise do not improve ACS morbidity and mortality and are not recommended as preventive measures.

Table 18–1. Genetic and environmental influences on CAD predisposition.[1]

Gene–Environment Interaction	Favorable Genes	Unfavorable Genes
Favorable environment	Low risk	Moderate risk
Unfavorable environment	Moderate risk	High risk

[1]The manifestation of coronary artery disease (CAD) is caused by the interaction of several unfavorable genetic and environmental factors. Those with the greatest number of genetic and environmental risk factors will face the highest risks. Those with favorable genotypes might not develop CAD despite substantial environmental risk factors. Conversely, those with favorable environmental factors might develop CAD given the presence of unfavorable genetic factors.

Source: Scheuner MT: Genetic predisposition to coronary artery disease. Curr Opin Cardiol 2001;16:251.

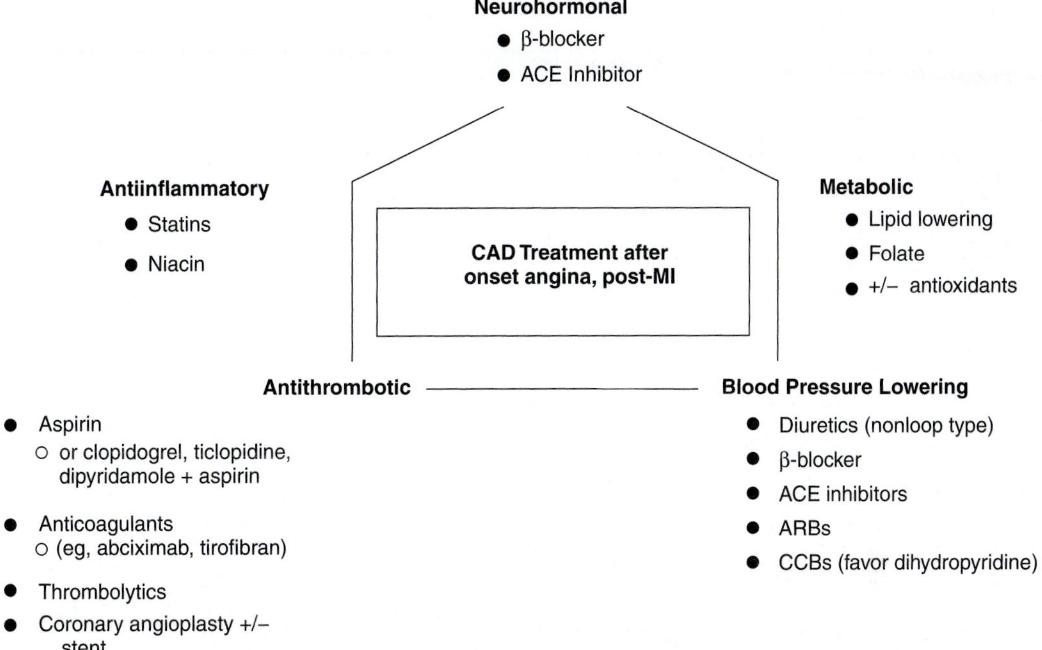

Figure 18–4. Tertiary prevention for coronary artery disease (CAD). ACD, angiotensin-converting enzyme; ARB, angiotensin receptor blocker; CCB, calcium channel blocker.

C. Cardiac Rehabilitation

Cardiac rehabilitation attempts to prevent disease progression in patients who have experienced an ACS episode or who have established CAD, by focusing on three areas: exercise, risk factor modification, and psychosocial intervention. Exercise-based rehabilitation programs reduce both all-cause and cardiac mortality in patients with a prior history of myocardial infarction or surgical intervention (ie, percutaneous coronary intervention [PCI] or coronary artery bypass grafting [CABG]) and in those who have stable CAD.

Risk factor modification addresses the measures outlined in Table 18–2 and includes dietician-led nutritional training and emphasis on smoking cessation via counseling, bupropion therapy, nicotine replacement, and formal cessation programs.

Psychosocial intervention emphasizes the identification and management of the psychological and social effects associated with ACS. These effects can include depression, anxiety, family issues, and job-related problems. Depression has been linked to increased mortality in patients with CAD. Although psychosocial intervention alone does not decrease total or cardiac mortality, it reduces depression and anxiety in these patients.

Andraws R et al: Effects of antibiotic therapy on outcomes of patients with coronary artery disease. A meta-analysis of randomized controlled trials. JAMA 2005;293:2641. [PMID: 15928286]

Barth J et al: Depression as a risk factor for mortality in patients with coronary heart disease: A meta-analysis. Psychosom Med 2004;66:802. [PMID: 15564343]

McGrath PD: Review: Exercise-based cardiac rehabilitation reduces all-cause and cardiac mortality in coronary heart disease. ACP J Club 2004;141:62. [PMID: 15518446]

Rees K et al: Psychological interventions for coronary heart disease. Cochrane Database System Rev 2004;(2):CD002902. [PMID: 15106183]

Clinical Findings

The diagnosis of ACS requires the presence of at least two of the following findings: ischemic symptoms, diagnostic ECG changes, and an elevated serum marker of cardiac injury (ie, troponin I or T).

A. Symptoms and Signs

Having known risk factors for CAD (Table 18–3) increases the likelihood of ACS. Up to one third of people with CAD progress to an ACS episode accompanied by chest pain. Chest pain is the predominant symptom of ACS but is not always present. Patients may report a range of symptoms, including:

Table 18–2. Guide to comprehensive risk reduction for patients with coronary artery disease.

<table>
<tr><th>Risk Intervention</th><th colspan="5">Recommendation</th></tr>
<tr><td>Smoking
Goal: complete cessation</td><td colspan="5">Strongly encourage patient and family to stop smoking.
Provide counseling, nicotine replacement, and formal cessation programs as appropriate.</td></tr>
<tr><td>Lipids
Primary goal:
LDL <100 mg/dL
Secondary goals:
HDL >35 mg/dL
TG <200 mg/dL</td><td colspan="5">Start AHA Step II diet in all patients (30% fat, <200 mg/day cholesterol).
Assess fasting lipid profile. In post-MI patients, lipid profile may take 4–6 weeks to stabilize. Add drug therapy according to the following:</td></tr>
<tr><td rowspan="6"></td><td>LDL <100 mg/dL</td><td colspan="2">LDL 100–130 mg/dL</td><td>LDL >130 mg/dL</td><td>HDL <35 mg/dL</td></tr>
<tr><td>No drug therapy</td><td colspan="2">Consider adding drug therapy to diet, as follows:</td><td>Add drug therapy to diet, as follows:</td><td rowspan="4">Emphasize weight management and physical activity. Advise smoking cessation. If needed to achieve LDL goals, consider niacin, statin, fibrates.</td></tr>
<tr><td></td><td colspan="3">Statins as first-line suggestion drug therapy</td></tr>
<tr><td></td><td>TG <200 mg/dL</td><td>TG 200–400 mg/dL</td><td>TG >400 mg/dL</td></tr>
<tr><td></td><td>Statin
Resin
Niacin</td><td>Statin
Niacin</td><td>Consider combined drug therapy (niacin, fibrates, statin)</td></tr>
<tr><td></td><td colspan="3">If LDL goal not achieved, consider combination therapy.</td><td></td></tr>
<tr><td>Physical activity
Minimum goal: 30 min 3–4 times per week</td><td colspan="5">Assess risk, preferably with exercise test, to guide prescription. Encourage minimum of 30–60 min of moderate-intensity activity three to four times weekly (walking, jogging, cycling, or other aerobic activity) supplemented by an increase in daily life-style activities (eg, walking breaks at work, using stairs, gardening, household work). Maximum benefit 5–6 h a week. Advise medically supervised programs for moderate- to high-risk patients.</td></tr>
<tr><td>Weight management</td><td colspan="5">Start intensive diet and appropriate physical activity intervention, as outlined above, in patients >120% of ideal weight for height. Particularly emphasize need for weight loss in patients with hypertension, elevated TG, or elevated glucose levels; ideal BMI: 18.5–25 kg/m².</td></tr>
<tr><td>Antiplatelet agents/ anticoagulants</td><td colspan="5">Start aspirin 80–325 mg/day if not contraindicated.
Manage warfarin to INR = 2–3.5 for post-MI patients not able to take or fails aspirin, then consider ticlopidine, clopidogrel, or dipyridamole + aspirin.</td></tr>
<tr><td>ACE inhibitors
Post-MI</td><td colspan="5">Start early post-MI in stable patients, especially those with anterior MI, CHF, renal insufficiency, EF <40% (LV dysfunction). Maximize dose as tolerated indefinitely.
Use as needed to manage blood pressure or symptoms in all other patients.</td></tr>
<tr><td>β-Blockers</td><td colspan="5">For all patients, especially post-MI, as tolerated.</td></tr>
<tr><td>Estrogens</td><td colspan="5">Limited, if any, role. More evidence of harm than help.</td></tr>
<tr><td>Blood pressure
Goal: ≤140/90 mm Hg
Optimal: 115/75</td><td colspan="5">Initiate life-style modification: weight control, physical activity, alcohol moderation, and moderate sodium restriction in all patients with blood pressure >140 mm Hg systolic or 90 mm Hg diastolic.
Add blood pressure medication, individualize to other patient requirements and characteristics (ie, age, race, need for drugs with specific benefits) if blood pressure is not less than 140 mm Hg systolic or 90 mm Hg diastolic in 3 months or if initial blood pressure is >160 mm Hg systolic or 100 mm Hg diastolic.</td></tr>
</table>

LDL, low-density lipoprotein; HDL, high-density lipoprotein; TG, triglycerides; AHA, American Heart Association; BMI, body mass index; ACE, angiotensin-converting enzyme; MI, myocardial infarction; CHF, congestive heart failure; EF, ejection fraction; LV, left ventricular.

Adapted, with permission, from Smith SC Jr et al: AHA consensus panel statement. Preventing heart attack and death in patients with coronary disease. In: Dedwania PC, Gheorghiade M, eds. *Therapeutic Options for Effective Management of Coronary Artery Disease*. American Heart Association, 1999.

Table 18–3. Risk factors for coronary artery disease.

Nonmodifiable/Uncontrollable
Male sex
Age
Men ≥ 45 years old
Women ≥ 55 years old or postmenopausal
Positive family history of CAD
Modifiable with Demonstrated Morbidity and Mortality Benefits
Hypertension
Left ventricular hypertrophy
Dyslipidemia
HDL < 35 mg/dL
LDL > 130 mg/dL
Diabetes mellitus
Overweight and obesity
Physical inactivity
Smoking (risk abates 3 years after cessation)
Low fruit and vegetable intake
Excessive alcohol intake[1]
Potentially Modifiable but No Demonstrated Morbidity and Mortality Effects of Treatment
Stress
Depression
Hypertriglyceridemia
Hyperhomocysteinemia
Hyperreninemia
Uric acid
Lp(a) lipoprotein
Fibrinogen
High-sensitivity C-reactive protein

[1]More than 2 drinks per day in men or more than 1 drink per day in women and lighter weight persons. 1 drink = 0.5 oz (15 mL) of ethanol (eg, 12 oz beer, 5 oz wine, or 1.5 oz 80-proof whiskey).

- Typical or stable angina—substernal pain that occurs with exertion and alleviates with rest.
- Chest pain lasting more than 20 minutes.
- Dull, heavy pressure in or on the chest.
- Sensation of a heavy object on the chest.
- Pain radiating to the back, neck, jaw, left arm, or shoulder.
- Pain unaffected by inspiration and not reproducible with chest palpation.
- Accompanying diaphoresis.
- Pain initiated by stress, exercise, large meals, or anything that increases the body's demand on the heart.
- Extreme fatigue or edema after exercise.
- Shortness of breath. This may be the only sign in elderly patients, is more common in black than in white patients, and is more common in women than in men.
- Left-sided chest pain (more common in black patients).
- Levine sign—discomfort described as a clenched fist over the sternum.
- Angor anami—great fear of impending doom or death.
- Pain high in the abdomen or chest, nausea, extreme fatigue after exercise, back pain, and edema can occur in anyone, but these symptoms are more common in women.
- Nausea, lightheadedness, or dizziness.

Less commonly, patients experience mild, burning chest discomfort; sharp chest pain; pain that radiates to the right arm or back; or an urge (especially sudden) to defecate in conjunction with chest pain.

Chest pain that is present for days, pleuritic, or positional, or that radiates to the lower extremities or above the mandible is less likely to be cardiac in origin.

B. Physical Examination

Examination findings that increase the probability that symptoms are the result of ACS include hypotension, diaphoresis, systolic heart failure (new S_3 gallop), new or worsening mitral valve regurgitation, pulmonary edema, and jugular venous distention. Chest pain reproducible with palpation is unlikely to be caused by ACS.

C. Diagnostic Studies

Anyone suspected of having ACS should be evaluated with a 12-lead ECG and assessment of serum cardiac biomarkers. When initial ECG and cardiac markers are normal, repeat testing should be performed within 6–12 hours of symptom onset. If the results of repeat testing are also normal, exercise or pharmacologic cardiac stress testing should be performed to evaluate for inducible ischemia. Exercise testing is preferred, but chemical agents (dobutamine, dipyridamole, adenosine) can be used to simulate the cardiac effects of exercise in those unable to exercise enough to produce a test adequate for interpretation. When the diagnosis of ACS is unclear, other testing is performed to investigate alternative etiologies in the differential diagnosis. Similarly, more invasive testing is reserved for patients with findings or clinical indicators that warrant further investigation.

1. Electrocardiogram—Notable ECG findings include the following:

- ST-T segment and T-wave changes (ischemia).
- Q-wave (accomplished infarction).
- ST-elevation (absent in patients with unstable angina and NSTEMI).
- New bundle branch block or sustained ventricular tachycardia (higher risk of progression to infarction).

Accurate ECG interpretation is essential for both diagnosis and risk stratification, and also guides the treatment plan. Many findings are nonspecific, and the presence of bundle branch block, interventricular conduction delay, or Wolff–Parkinson–White syndrome reduces the diagnostic reliability.

Normal findings on ECG do not exclude ACS. Up to 25–50% of people with angina or silent ischemia have a normal ECG, and 10% of patients with ACS are subsequently diagnosed with a myocardial infarction after an initial normal ECG.

2. Cardiac biomarkers—Cardiac biomarkers are chemicals whose presence in blood indicates myocardial damage. Testing for troponins T and I is preferred because of their high sensitivity and specificity for myocardial injury. Because troponin T can also be elevated in patients with renal disease, polymyositis, and dermatomyositis, tropinin I is considered a more accurate indicator of cardiac disease. Troponin level is not as sensitive (ie, can be falsely negative) during the first 4–6 hours after an ACS episode. Hence, the need to recheck the troponin level if the first is negative. Levels can remain elevated for 7–10 days and can therefore help identify prior recent infarctions.

3. Exercise electrocardiography—An exercise ECG, also called an exercise stress test, is the main test for evaluating patients with suspected angina or heart disease (Table 18–4). Interpretation of the test is based on signs of stress-induced impairment of myocardial contraction, including ECG changes (Table 18–5) and symptoms and signs of angina. The false-positive rate is 10%.

Table 18–4. Exercise electrocardiography: indications and contraindications.

Indications	Contraindications
Confirmation of suspected angina	Cardiac failure
	Any febrile illness
Evaluation of extent of myocardial ischemia and prognosis	Left ventricular outflow obstruction or hypertrophic cardiomyopathy
Risk stratification after MI	Severe aortic or mitral stenosis
Detection of exercise-induced symptoms (eg, arrhythmias or syncope)	Uncontrolled hypertension
	Pulmonary hypertension
	Recent MI
Evaluation of outcome of interventions (eg, PCI or CABG)	Severe tachyarrhythmias
	Dissecting aortic aneurysm
	Left mainstem stenosis or equivalent
Assessment of cardiac transplantation	Complete heart block
Rehabilitation and patient motivation	

MI, myocardial infarction; CABG, coronary artery bypass surgery; PCI, percutaneous coronary intervention.

Source: Grech ED: Pathophysiology and investigation of coronary artery disease. BMJ 2003;326:1027.

Table 18–5. Exercise electrocardiography: findings and interpretation.

Main End Points for Abnormal Exercise Test
Target heart rate achieved (> 85% of maximum predicted heart rate)
ST-segment depression > 1 mm (downsloping or planar depression of greater predictive value than upsloping depression)
Slow ST recovery to normal (> 5 min)
Decrease in systolic blood pressure > 20 mm Hg
Increase in diastolic blood pressure > 15 mm Hg
Progressive ST segment elevation or depression
ST-segment depression > 3 mm without pain
Arrhythmias (atrial fibrillation, ventricular tachycardia)
Features Indicative of Strongly Positive Exercise Test
Exercise limited by angina to < 6 min of Bruce protocol
Failure of systolic blood pressure to increase > 10 mm Hg, or fall with evidence of ischemia
Widespread marked ST-segment depression > 3 mm
Prolonged recovery time of ST changes (> 6 min)
Development of ventricular tachycardia
ST elevation in absence of prior myocardial infarction

Source: Grech ED: Pathophysiology and investigation of coronary artery disease. BMJ 2003;326:1027.

4. Chest radiography—Chest radiography is used to assess for non-ACS causes of chest pain (eg, aortic dissection, pneumothorax, pulmonary embolus, pneumonia, rib fracture).

5. Echocardiography—Echocardiography can be used to determine left ventricle ejection fraction and valve function and to detect regional wall motion abnormalities that correspond to areas of myocardial damage. This test has high sensitivity but low specificity, which makes it most useful as a means of excluding ACS in patients whose results are normal. It can also be used as an adjunct to stress testing. Because stress-induced impairment of myocardial contraction precedes ECG changes and angina, stress echocardiography, when performed and interpreted by experienced clinicians, can be superior to exercise stress testing.

6. Myocardial perfusion imaging—Adding radionuclide myocardial perfusion imaging to exercise stress testing can improve sensitivity, specificity, and accuracy, especially in patients with a nondiagnostic exercise test or limited exercise ability (Table 18–6). Acute rest myocardial perfusion imaging is very similar, but is performed during or shortly after resolution of anginal symptoms that were not induced by a stress test. Radionuclide exercise stress testing can be advantageous in women because exercise testing alone is less accurate in women than in men.

Table 18–6. Indications for use of radionuclide perfusion imaging rather than exercise electrocardiography.[1]

Complete left bundle branch block
Electronically paced ventricular rhythm
Preexcitation (Wolff–Parkinson–White) syndrome or other, similar electrocardiographic conduction abnormalities
More than 1 mm of ST-segment depression at rest
Inability to exercise to a level high enough to give meaningful results on routine stress electrocardiography[2]
Angina and a history of revascularization[3]

[1]Guidelines were developed by the American College of Cardiology, American Heart Association, American College of Physicians, and American Society of Internal Medicine.
[2]Patients with this factor should be considered for pharmacologic stress tests.
[3]In patients with angina and a history of revascularization, characterizing the ischemia, establishing the functional effect of lesions, and determining myocardial viability are important considerations.
Source: Lee TH, Boucher CA: Clinical practice: Noninvasive tests in patients with stable coronary artery disease. N Engl J Med 2001;344:1840.

7. MRI and CT scanning—Cardiac magnetic resonance imaging does not yet have a clinical role in diagnosis of ACS because its sensitivity and specificity for detecting significant CAD plaque do not eclipse angiography, the gold standard. Electron-beam computer tomography lacks utility because a positive test does not correlate well with an ACS episode.

8. Coronary angiography—Coronary angiography remains the gold standard in evaluation of ACS. The main indications for angiography are listed in Table 18–7. Risks include death (1 in 1400), stroke (1 in 1000), coronary artery dissection (1 in 1000), arterial access complications (1 in 500), and minor risks such as arrhythmia. Ten to 30% of angiography studies are normal.

Achar S et al: Diagnosis of acute coronary syndrome. Am Fam Physician 2005;72:119. [PMID: 16035692]

Fletcher GF et al: Exercise standards for testing and training: A statement for healthcare professionals from the American Heart Association. Circulation 2001;104:1694. [PMID: 11581152]

Pope JH, Selker HP: Acute coronary syndromes in the emergency department: Diagnostic characteristics, tests, and challenges. Cardiol Clin 2005;23:423. [PMID: 16278116]

Saadeddin SM et al: Markers of inflammation and coronary artery disease. Med Sci Monit 2002;8:RA5. [PMID: 11782689]

Differential Diagnosis

The differential diagnosis for ACS is included in Table 18–8.

Complications

The leading complications of ACS are myocardial infarction and cardiac disability. Life-style and activity options are diminished in patients with ACS because of the inability of the coronary arteries to supply the heart muscle, which in turn leaves the heart unable to supply the body with sufficient oxygenated blood to fulfill demand.

Treatment

A. Management of Acute Infarction

The key to ACS treatment can be summarized as follows: time = tissue. ACS causes myocardial infarction in three ways: (1) Plaque buildup increases until the artery is totally occluded. (2) An atheromatous plaque ruptures or tears, leading to occlusions via inflammatory response and thrombus formation as platelets adhere to the site to seal off the plaque. (3) A thrombus becomes superimposed upon a disrupted atherosclerotic plaque. The goal of treatment is to save cardiac muscle by reducing myocardial oxygen demand, increasing oxygen supply, or both.

Patients with ACS should be hospitalized, medically stabilized, and given appropriate further cardiac evaluation and treatment. The acronym HOBANAS summarizes the initial steps in medical management:

Heparin (use of low molecular weight heparin results in fewer myocardial infarctions and deaths)
Oxygen
Beta-blocker (if patient is hemodynamically stable)

Table 18–7. Main indications for coronary angiography.

Uncertain diagnosis of angina (coronary artery disease cannot be excluded by noninvasive testing)
Assessment of feasibility and appropriateness of various forms of treatment (percutaneous intervention, bypass surgery, medical)
Class I or U stable angina with positive stress test or class III or W angina without positive stress test
Unstable angina or non–Q-wave myocardial infarction (medium- and high-risk patients)
Angina not controlled by drug treatment
Acute myocardial infarction—especially cardiogenic shock, ineligibility for thrombolytic treatment, failed thrombolytic reperfusion, reinfarction, or positive stress test
Life-threatening ventricular arrhythmia
Angina after bypass surgery or percutaneous intervention
Before valve surgery or corrective heart surgery to assess occult coronary artery disease

Source: Grech ED: Pathophysiology and investigation of coronary artery disease. BMJ 2003;326:1027.

Table 18–8. Differential diagnosis of CAD.

Prinzmetal angina (coronary vasospasm)—more common in women
Esophagitis
Esophageal spasm
Gastritis
Hiatal hernia
Gastroesophageal reflux disease (GERD)
Peptic ulcer disease (PUD)
Duodenal ulcer
Cholecystitis
Costochondritis
Pleurisy/pleuritis
Pulmonary hypertension
Pulmonary embolus
Pneumothorax
Aortic aneurysm
Aortic dissection
Cardiomyopathy
Supraventricular tachycardia
Diaphragmatic irritation/inflammation due to
Mass effect from nearby cancer
Infection
Pancreatitis
Hepatitis
Pulmonary edema/effusion
Pericardial effusion
Cardiac tamponade
Shoulder arthropathy
Radiculopathy
Generalized anxiety disorder (GAD)
Panic attack
Stress reaction/anxiety
Anemia
Hyperthyroidism
High-altitude exposure
Vasculitis

Aspirin (325 mg)

Nitroglycerin (for pain; should be discontinued if hypotension develops)

ACE inhibitor (at 24 hours)

Statins (HMG-CoA-reductase inhibitors)

Clopidogrel should be added in patients with STEMI if PCI is unlikely to be performed. If PCI is likely, the drug should be added to the medical regimen after the procedure. In either case, duration of treatment is 9 months. Platelet glycoprotein IIb/IIIa receptor inhibitors (GP IIb/IIIa) should be used judiciously if there is no plan for revascularization: the clinician should keep in mind that 100 episodes of STEMI need to be treated with GP IIb/IIIa to prevent one myocardial infarction or death; however, for every one case that is prevented there is one major bleeding complication. Morphine may be added for pain and anxiety relief. It also provides some reduction of afterload.

If cardiac tissue is to survive, blood flow must be restored. Some situations (active infarctions) require medical thrombolysis or emergent angioplasty to achieve this goal. When necessary (and possible), thrombolytic agents should be started within 30–60 minutes, and PCI or CABG should be initiated within 60–90 minutes. If blood flow is not restored with thrombolytic therapy, then PCI or CABG should be performed within 2–3 hours. A "cooling off" period increases mortality without decreasing bleeding complications.

The 2-year risk of death or recurrent myocardial infarction is the same for patients undergoing PCI or CABG. In that time, an extra 5% of patients who have CABG report fewer episodes of angina.

B. Postinfarction Care

Postinfarction care centers around the tertiary prevention measures outlined earlier under Cardiac Rehabilitation (see also Figure 18–4 and Table 18–2). Because each incremental increase of 20 mm Hg in systolic pressure or 10 mm Hg in diastolic pressure across the entire range from 115/75 to 185/115 mm Hg doubles the risk of CAD, in patients aged 40–70 years with CAD, blood pressure is optimally maintained at or near 115/75 mm Hg. Cyclooxygenase-2 (COX-2) nonsteroidal anti-inflammatory drugs and naproxen should be avoided, because these agents increase the risk of ACS. In some patients, warfarin (goal INR 2.0–2.5) taken together with aspirin, or warfarin alone (goal INR 3.0–4.0), results in a better all-cause mortality than aspirin alone.

C. Referral

Once ACS is suspected, the diagnostic evaluation and management often requires the involvement of specialists (eg, cardiologist, cardiothoracic surgeon, nutritionist, rehabilitation therapist). Family physicians coordinate this collaborative effort while continuing to manage the rest of the patient's conditions, within the context of each patient's psychosocial and environmental realities.

Boersma E et al: Platelet glycoprotein IIb/IIIa inhibitors in acute coronary syndromes. Lancet 2002;360:342. [PMID: 12147403]

Braunwald E et al: ACC/AHA 2002 guideline update for the management of patients with unstable angina and non-ST-segment elevation myocardial infarction. A report of the American College of Cardiology/American Heart Association Task Force on Practice Guidelines. J Am Coll Cardiol 2002;40:1366. [PMID: 12383588]

Cannon CP et al: Intensive versus moderate lipid lowering with statins after acute coronary syndromes. N Engl J Med 2004;350:1495. [PMID: 15007110]

Eikelboom JW et al: Unfractionated heparin and low-molecular-weight heparin in acute coronary syndrome without ST elevation: A meta-analysis. Lancet 2000;355:1936. [PMID: 10859038]

Fox KA et al: Interventional versus conservative treatment for patients with unstable angina or non-ST-elevation myocardial infarction: The British Heart Foundation RITA 3 randomised trial. Randomized Intervention Trail of unstable Angina. Lancet 2002;360:743. [PMID: 12241831]

Goodman SG et al: Randomized evaluation of the safety and efficacy of enoxaparin versus unfractionated heparin in high-risk patients with non-ST-segment elevation acute coronary syndromes receiving the glycoprotein IIb/IIIa inhibitor eptifibatide. Circulation 2003;107:238. [PMID: 12538422]

Neumann FJ et al: Evaluation of prolonged antithrombotic pretreatment ("cooling-off" strategy) before intervention in patients with unstable coronary syndromes: A randomized controlled trial. JAMA 2003;2909:1593. [PMID: 14506118]

van Es RF et al: Aspirin and Coumadin after acute coronary syndromes (the ASPECT-2 study): A randomised controlled trial. Lancet 2002;360:109. [PMID: 12126819]

PROGNOSIS

An estimated 60% of deaths from myocardial infarction occur within the first hour of symptom onset. Prognosis following a survived infarction without subsequent intervention carries a mortality rate of 10% during the first year and 5% in each additional year. Sudden death following ACS, more common in patients with a lower ejection fraction, occurs in 1.4% of patients during the first month and decreases to 0.14% per month after 2 years.

When troponin T or I level is normal at 2, 4, and 6 hours after the onset of chest pain in patients with a normal ECG result, the 30-day risk of cardiac death and nonfatal acute myocardial infarction is nearly zero.

Normal troponin T level 10–12 hours after symptom onset in patients who have chest pain and a normal ECG indicates a low-risk of adverse events for the next 12 months. Elevated cardiac troponin levels, even if slight, in patients with unstable angina and NSTEMI help identify high-risk patients who may benefit the most from early invasive treatment.

Web-site–accessible scoring systems can help in risk stratification of patients with chest pain and in determining prognosis given a range of different circumstances by analyzing various patient characteristics and test results. Prognostic tools are valuable aids for the clinician when educating patients about possible outcomes, and when discussing and deciding upon treatment options.

deFilippi CR et al: Cardiac troponin T in chest pain unit patients without ischemic electrocardiographic changes: Angiographic correlates and long-term outcomes. J Am Coll Cardiol 2000;35:1827. [PMID: 10841231]

Law MR et al. The underlying risk of death after myocardial infarction in the absence of treatment. Arch Intern Med 2002;162:2405. [PMID: 12327397]

Mahaffey KW et al, for the SYNERGY Trial Investigators: High-risk patients with acute coronary syndromes treated with low-molecular-weight or unfractionated heparin. Outcomes at 6 months and 1 year in the SYNERGY trial. JAMA 2005;294:2594. [PMID: 16304073]

Morrow DA et al: Ability of minor elevations of troponins I and T to predict benefit from an early invasive strategy in patients with unstable angina and non-ST elevation myocardial infarction. Results from a randomized trial. JAMA 2001;286:2405. [PMID: 11712935]

Solomon SD et al; Valsartan in Acute Myocardial Infarction Trial (VALIANT) Investigators: Sudden death in patients with myocardial infarction and left ventricular dysfunction, heart failure, or both. N Engl J Med 2005;352:2581. [PMID: 15972864]

WEB SITES

American Academy of Family Physicians:
http://www.aafp.org and http://familydoctor.org
American College of Cardiology:
http://www.acc.org
American Heart Association:
http://www.americanheart.org
Centers for Disease Control:
http://www.cdc.gov
Facts about Coronary Artery Disease:
http://home.mdconsult.com/das/patient/body/0/10041/5558.htm
National Heart, Lung, and Blood Institute:
http://www.nhlbi.nih/health/public/heart/other/chdfacts.htm
Medtronic:
http://www.medtronic.corn/cad
National Institutes of Health—health topics:
http://health.nih.gov/
National Women's Health Information Center:
http://www.4woman.gov/faq/coronary.htm
Family Practice Notebook:
http://fpnotebook.com/CV.htm
UPMC Patient Information:
http://patienteducation.upmc.com/C.htm#Cardiology

Heart Failure

19

Richard E. Rodenberg, Jr., MD, & Michael King, MD, MPH

ESSENTIALS OF DIAGNOSIS

- *Left ventricular failure:*
- *Paroxysmal nocturnal dyspnea, orthopnea, dyspnea on exertion, fatigue, and peripheral edema.*
- *Third or fourth heart sound, increased jugular venous pressure, hepatojugular reflux, displaced cardiac apex, rales, wheezing, murmur, or peripheral edema.*
- *Any electrocardiographic (ECG) abnormality, radiographic evidence of pulmonary venous congestion, cardiomegaly, or pleural effusion; elevated B-type natriuretic peptide; echocardiographic evidence of left ventricular dysfunction.*
- *Right ventricular failure: increased jugular venous pressure, hepatomegaly, peripheral edema.*

General Considerations

Increased survivorship after acute myocardial infarction (MI) and improved treatment of hypertension, valvular heart disease, and coronary artery disease (CAD) have led to a significant increase in the prevalence of heart failure in the United States. Overall prevalence of any congestive heart failure (CHF) diagnosis is estimated at 2.6% (2.7% in men; 1.7% in women). In addition, 5.6% of the population may have isolated moderate to severe diastolic dysfunction, with age greater than 65 years and female gender being consistent predictors of preserved left ventricular systolic function. Diastolic dysfunction is rarely associated with acute MI. Based on this apparent bias, the possibility of biological changes associated with increasing age and female gender have been proposed as underlying reasons for the increased likelihood of diastolic heart failure in these populations.

The prevalence of any type of heart failure increases with age. Asymptomatic left ventricular systolic dysfunction (LVSD) has been found to be as prevalent as symptomatic LVSD: 1.4% and 1.5%, respectively. Moderate or severe isolated diastolic dysfunction appears to be as common as systolic dysfunction, and systolic dysfunction appears to increase with the severity of diastolic dysfunction.

Pathogenesis

Heart failure results from a complex interplay of compensatory mechanisms used by the body to adjust for decreased cardiac output in response to stresses placed on the myocardium (Table 19–1). These compensatory mechanisms are rooted in the activation of the sodium-retaining renin-angiotensin-aldosterone and sympathetic nervous systems (neurohormonal adaptations). The purpose is to maintain blood pressure and tissue perfusion. However, these compensatory mechanisms, which increase afterload, lead to myocardial deterioration and worsening myocardial contractility. The heart then enters into a vicious cycle of increasing release of neurohormones (norepinephrine, angiotensin II, aldosterone, endothelin, vasopressin, and cytokines) that further increases afterload, allowing the heart to spiral into failure in a progressive fashion through cardiac remodeling. These neurohormones act both in an indirect and in a directly toxic fashion to affect hemodynamic stressors and myocardial cell performance and phenotype.

Causes of Cardiac Failure

With the advent of improved hypertension treatment, earlier identification of valvular heart disease, and improved survival following MI, CAD and diabetes mellitus are now the leading causes of heart failure in the United States. CAD is a substantial predictor of developing clinically evident heart failure or symptomatic versus asymptomatic LVSD. CHF has also been found to be twofold higher in all diabetic patients. Diabetes mellitus is one of the most significant factors for developing heart failure in women. Even in women with increased hyperglycemia but no diagnosis of diabetes mellitus, the risk of heart failure is increased compared with normoglycemic women. Evidence points to a diabetic cardiomyopathy independent of CAD that is more prominent in diabetic women. This raises the question of the direct effect of

Table 19–1. Possible causes of heart failure.

Coronary artery disease, including myocardial infarction
Diabetes mellitus
Hypertension
Increased BMI (overweight)
Increased age
Smoking
Primary valvular heart disease
Congenital heart disease
Cardiomyopathies (dilated [idiopathic], hypertrophic, and restrictive)
Viral myocarditis (including HIV)
Pericardial disease
Infiltrative disease (hemochromatosis, sarcoidosis, amyloidosis)
Recent pregnancy
Connective tissue disease
Hyperthyroid or hypothyroid disease
Toxin (chemotherapy, substance abuse [especially alcohol or cocaine], heavy metal)
High-output failure secondary to anemia or thiamine deficiency (beriberi)
Cor pulmonale and pulmonary hypertension (in right-sided failure)

BMI, body mass index.

diabetes on the myocardium and endothelium. This association could also be related to the overt effect of diabetes on progression of CAD. It is also unknown whether treatment of long-standing diabetes mellitus decreases the risk of developing heart failure.

Poorly controlled hypertension and valvular heart disease remain major precipitants of heart failure. Often-overlooked risk factors in the development of heart failure are smoking, physical inactivity or obesity, and lower socioeconomic status. Tobacco is estimated to cause approximately 17% of CHF cases in the United States. The effect of cigarettes may be direct or indirect in relation to promoting CAD risk. Lower socioeconomic status may limit access to higher quality health care, resulting in decreased adherence to treatment of modifiable risk factors such as hypertension, diabetes mellitus, and CAD.

Aurigemma GP et al: Predictive value of systolic and diastolic function for incident congestive heart failure in the elderly: The Cardiovascular Health Study. J Am Coll Cardiol 2001;37:1042. [PMID: 11263606]

Bibbins-Domingo K et al: Predictors of heart failure among women with coronary disease. Circulation 2004:110:1424. [PMID: 15353499]

He J et al: Risk factors for congestive heart failure in US men and women: NHANES I epidemiologic follow-up study. Arch Intern Med 2001;161:996. [PMID: 11295963]

Masoudi FA et al: Gender, age, and heart failure with preserved left ventricular systolic function. J Am Coll Cardiol 2003;41:217. [PMID: 12535812]

Rogers VL et al: Trends in heart failure incidence and survival in a community-based population. JAMA 2004;292:344. [PMID: 15265849]

Stratton IM et al: Association of glycaemia with macrovascular and microvascular complications type 2 diabetes (UKPDS 35): Prospective observational study. BMJ 2000;321:405. [PMID: 10938048]

Classification & Prevention

The American College of Cardiology (ACC)/American Heart Association (AHA) classification of heart failure emphasizes the progressive nature of the syndrome. This classification replaced the New York Heart Association (NYHA) classification with four stages that help define appropriate therapy at each level. The new classification recognizes that there are risk factors and structural prerequisites for the development of heart failure and that therapeutic interventions initiated early in the disease process can reduce morbidity and mortality and delay the onset of clinically evident disease (Table 19–2).

Patients in ACC/AHA stages A and B do not have clinical heart failure but are at risk for developing heart failure. Stage A includes those at risk but not manifesting structural heart disease. Early identification and aggressive treatment of modifiable risk factors remain the best prevention for heart failure. Life-style modification, pharmacologic therapy, and counseling can improve or correct conditions such as CAD, hypertension, diabetes mellitus, hyperlipidemia, obesity, tobacco abuse, and alcohol or illicit substance abuse. Stage B represents persons who are asymptomatic but have structural heart disease or impaired left ventricular function. Stage C comprises the bulk of persons with heart failure who have past or current symptoms and associated underlying structural heart disease. Stage D includes refractory patients with heart failure who may need advanced and specialized treatment strategies.

The NYHA classification gauges the severity of symptoms for patients with stage C and D heart failure. This is a subjective assessment that can change frequently, secondary to treatment response.

Clinical Findings

A high index of suspicion is necessary to diagnose the syndrome of heart failure early in its clinical presentation, because it is frequently manifested by nonspecific signs and symptoms. Patients are often elderly with comorbidity, symptoms may be mild, and routine clinical assessment lacks specificity. A prompt diagnosis allows for early treatment with therapies proven to delay the progression of heart failure and improve quality of life.

Table 19–2. Progression of heart failure and recommended evidence-based therapies.

	Progression of Heart Failure				
	At Risk for Heart Failure		Heart Failure		
ACC/AHA stage	Stage A: high risk	Stage B: asymptomatic, cardiac structural abnormalities or remodeling	Stage C: symptomatic or history of heart failure		Stage D: refractory end-stage heart failure
NYHA classification	Not applicable	Class I: asymptomatic	Class II: symptoms with significant exertion	Class III: symptoms on minor exertion	Class IV: symptoms at rest
Therapy Beneficial and effective; recommended	*Goals:* Disease management: • Hypertension[1] • Lipid disorders[1] • Diabetes mellitus[3] • Thyroid disease[3] • Secondary prevention of atherosclerotic vascular disease[3] Behavior change[3]: • Smoking cessation • Regular exercise • Avoidance of alcohol and illicit drug use	*Goals:* Stage A measures *Drugs* (in appropriate patients): ACEI[1] or ARB[2] β-Blockers (history of MI[1]; no MI[3])	*Goals:* Stage A and B measures Dietary sodium restriction[3] *Drugs/Devices:* Routine use: Diuretics[3] (fluid retention) ACEI[1] β-Blockers[1] In selected patients: ARB[1] Aldosterone antagonists[2] Implantable cardioverter-defibrillator[2] Cardiac resynchronization therapy[1]		*Goals:* Stage A, B, and C measures Meticulous fluid retention control[2] Decision regarding appropriate level of care and referral to heart failure program[1] *Options:* End-of-life care or hospice[3] Extraordinary measures: heart transplantation[2]
Reasonably beneficial and probably recommended	*Drugs* (in appropriate patients): ACEI[1] or ARB[3] (in patients with vascular disease or diabetes mellitus)	—	*Drugs/Devices* (in selected patients): Digitalis[2] Hydralazine or nitrates[1]		*Options* (extraordinary measures): permanent mechanical support[2]

ACC/AHA, American College of Cardiology/American Heart Association; NYHA, New York Heart Association; ACEI, angiotensin-converting enzyme inhibitor; ARB, angiotensin receptor blocker.

[1]Level of evidence A (evidence from multiple randomized trials, meta-analysis).

[2]Level of evidence B (evidence from single randomized or nonrandomized trials).

[3]Level of evidence C (expert opinion, case studies, standard of care).

Data, in part, from Hunt SA et al: ACC/AHA 2005 guideline update for the diagnosis and management of chronic heart failure in the adult. Circulation 2005;112:e154.

Evaluation is directed at confirming the presence of heart failure, determining cause, identifying comorbid illness, establishing severity, and guiding response to therapy. Heart failure is a clinical diagnosis for which no single examination or test can establish the presence or absence with 100% certainty.

Hunt SA et al; American College of Cardiology; American Heart Association Task Force on Practice Guidelines; American College of Chest Physicians; International Society for Heart and Lung Transplantation; Heart Rhythm Society: ACC/AHA 2005 guideline update for the diagnosis and management of chronic heart failure in the adult. Circulation 2005;112:e154. [PMID: 16160202]

A. Symptoms and Signs

The primary manifestations of symptomatic heart failure are dyspnea and fatigue. Limited exercise tolerance and fluid retention may eventually lead to pulmonary congestion and peripheral edema. Neither of these symptoms necessarily dominates the clinical picture at the same time. Dyspnea, whether at rest or with exertion, is present in nearly all patients with heart failure and indicates left ventricular dysfunction. Its absence makes heart failure highly unlikely. The absence of dyspnea on exertion essentially rules out the presence of heart failure due to left ventricular dysfunction in a predominantly symptomatic population with a reported 100% sensitivity.

Other symptoms that are helpful in diagnosing heart failure include orthopnea, paroxysmal nocturnal dyspnea (PND), and peripheral edema. PND has the highest specificity of any symptom for heart failure. Likewise, if PND, orthopnea, or edema are not present the likelihood of heart failure decreases. Nonspecific symptoms include chronic nonproductive cough, wheezing, and nocturia. Patients with right ventricular failure may present with right upper quadrant pain secondary to hepatic congestion and peripheral edema.

No single clinical symptom has been shown to be both sensitive and specific. A substantial portion of the population has asymptomatic left ventricular dysfunction and the history, alone, is insufficient to make the diagnosis of heart failure. However, a detailed history and review of symptoms remain the best approach in identifying the cause of heart failure and assessing response to therapy.

B. Physical Examination

The clinical examination can provide important information concerning the degree to which cardiac output is reduced and the degree of volume overload and ventricular enlargement. It can also provide clues to noncardiac causes of dyspnea. The presence of a third heart sound, S_3 (ventricular filling gallop), increases the likelihood of heart failure with the most specificity of any physical examination finding. An S_3 or a fourth heart sound, S_4 (atrial gallop), are specific for increased left ventricular end-diastolic pressure and decreased left ventricular ejection fraction. The presence of an S_3 has been found to be superior to S_4 in identifying patients with abnormal left ventricular function. Gallop rhythm (S_3 and S_4) and displacement of cardiac apex have also been found to be specific predictors of left ventricular dysfunction.

The presence of jugular venous distention, pulmonary rales, pitting peripheral edema, and hepatojugular reflux also helps to make the diagnosis, and the absence of the first three of these findings is useful for lowering the likelihood of heart failure. Cardiac murmurs may be an indication of primary valvular disease. Asymmetric rales or rhonchi on the pulmonary examination may indicate primary pulmonary pathology such as pneumonia or chronic obstructive pulmonary disease (COPD). Examination of the thyroid can exclude thyromegaly or goiter—causes of abnormal thyroid function that can precipitate heart failure. Dullness to percussion or auscultation of the lungs could indicate pleural effusion. Hepatomegaly can indicate passive hepatic congestion. The absence of any of these findings alone does little to help rule out heart failure.

C. Laboratory Findings

A complete blood count is necessary to rule out anemia as a cause of high-output failure. Electrolyte analysis may reveal deficiencies, commonplace with treatment, that can make the patient prone to arrhythmias. Hyponatremia is a poor prognostic sign indicating significant activation of the renin-aldosterone-angiotensin system. Abnormalities on liver tests can indicate hepatic congestion. Thyroid function tests can detect hyper- or hypothyroidism. Fasting lipid profile, fasting glucose, and hemoglobin A_{1c} level can reveal comorbid conditions that may need to be better controlled. Iron studies can detect iron deficiency or overload. If the patient is malnourished or an alcoholic and presents with high-output failure, thiamine testing is indicated to rule out deficiency related to beriberi. Further testing to determine etiologic factors of heart failure must be based on historical findings.

1. B-type natriuretic peptide—More specific laboratory testing includes evaluation of B-type natriuretic peptide (BNP) levels. BNP is a cardiac neurohormone secreted from the ventricles and, to some extent, the atrial myocardium in response to volume and pressure overload. Circulating BNP levels are increased in patients with heart failure and have rapid turnover, indicating that BNP responds in proportion to the size of the exacerbation and in turn increases and decreases with each individual exacerbation. Although no BNP threshold indicates the presence or absence of heart failure with 100% certainty, the BNP level is the most accurate predictor of heart failure and, in conjunction with the history and physical examination, helps

Table 19–3. Factors influencing B-type natriuretic peptide (BNP) levels.

Factors That Cause Elevated BNP (> 100 pg/mL)	Factors That Lower BNP in the Setting of Heart Failure
Heart failure	Acute pulmonary edema
Advanced age	Stable NYHA class I disease with low ejection fraction
Renal failure[1]	Acute mitral regurgitation
Acute coronary syndromes	Mitral stenosis
Lung disease with cor pulmonale	Atrial myxoma
Acute large pulmonary embolism	
High-output cardiac states	

NYHA, New York Heart Association.
[1]Adjusted levels are based on glomerular filtration rate (GFR). GFR 60–89 mL/min: no adjustment in the 100 pg/mL threshold (see text). GFR 30–59 mL/min: BNP > 201. GFR 15–29 mL/min: BNP > 225. GFR < 15 mL/min: unknown utility of BNP levels.
Source: Wang CS et al: Does this dyspneic patient in the emergency department have congestive heart failure? JAMA 2005;294:1944.

differentiate between pulmonary and cardiac causes of dyspnea (Table 19–3).

The likelihood of heart failure increases with BNP levels above 100 pg/mL, as follows:

- Less than 100 pg/mL: diagnosis of heart failure is unlikely; consider alternate diagnoses.
- 100–400 pg/mL: increased likelihood of heart failure; history, physical examination, and other tests are required to improve the probability of the diagnosis.
- Greater than 400 pg/mL: diagnosis of heart failure is highly likely.

2. Electrocardiography—LVSD is unlikely to be present if the ECG is normal (sensitivity of 94%). Left bundle branch block, left ventricular hypertrophy, and evidence of MI all significantly increase the likelihood of left ventricular dysfunction. Atrial fibrillation is the most important predictor of heart failure in a dyspneic patient, followed by new T-wave changes and any abnormal ECG finding. An abnormal ECG does not mean the patient has chronic heart failure but is an indication for echocardiography to determine whether a structural abnormality is present. The ECG also identifies possible causes of heart failure, including signs of ischemic heart disease or possible infiltrative processes, and can detect arrhythmias once heart failure is confirmed. The finding of left bundle branch block is an unfavorable prognostic indicator in patients with heart failure, among whom there is an increased 1-year mortality rate from any cause, including sudden death.

Knudsen CW et al: Diagnostic value of B-type natriuretic peptide and chest radiographic findings in patients with acute dyspnea. Am J Med 2004;116:363. [PMID: 15006584]

Krishnaswamy P et al: Utility of B-natriuretic peptide levels in identifying patients with left ventricular systolic or diastolic dysfunction. Am J Med 2001;111:274. [PMID: 11566457]

Maisel A: B-type natriuretic peptide levels: Diagnostic and prognostic in congestive heart failure: What's next? Circulation 2002;105:2328. [PMID: 12021215]

Maisel AS et al: Rapid measurement of B-type natriuretic peptide in the emergency diagnosis of heart failure. N Engl J Med 2002;347:161. [PMID: 12124404]

Mueller C et al: Use of B-type natriuretic peptide in the evaluation and management of acute dyspnea. N Engl J Med 2004;350:647. [PMID: 14960741]

Tang WH et al: Plasma B-type natriuretic peptide levels in ambulatory patients with established chronic symptomatic systolic heart failure. Circulation 2003;108:2964. [PMID: 14662703]

D. Imaging Studies

1. Chest radiography—The chest radiograph can provide valuable clues in patients presenting with acute dyspnea. The presence of venous congestion, interstitial edema, alveolar edema, cardiomegaly, or pleural effusion increases the likelihood of heart failure in dyspneic patients. Cardiomegaly (cardiac-to-thoracic width ratio > 50%) was the best predictor of decreased ejection fraction, whereas redistribution (upper lobe pulmonary vein dilation and lower lobe pulmonary vein constriction in response to a rise in pulmonary venous pressure secondary to increased left ventricular preload) and hilar haze were the best predictors of increased preload. The absence of cardiomegaly and pulmonary venous congestion were the most useful findings on chest radiography for lowering the likelihood of heart failure.

2. Cardiac Doppler echocardiography—Echocardiography is of undeniable utility in the evaluation of suspected and newly diagnosed heart failure (Table 19–4). An echocardiography study is recommended for all patients diagnosed with heart failure. It provides important information concerning cardiac systolic (ejection fraction or fractional shortening) and diastolic function.

Echocardiographic findings can help differentiate among the various causes of heart failure, including ischemic heart disease, idiopathic cardiomyopathy, hypertensive heart disease, and valvular heart disease. Echocardiography helps to distinguish segmental wall motion abnormalities, which can correlate with ischemia. An increase in cardiac mass (left ventricular hypertrophy) can be associated with hypertensive cardiomyopathy ver-

Table 19–4. Echocardiographic parameters useful in the diagnosis of heart failure.

Parameter	Information Provided
Left ventricular function (ejection fraction)	Normal value: ≥ 55–60% Abnormal value: < 50% Significant systolic dysfunction value: ≤ 35–40%
Diastolic function	Alteration of left ventricular compliance Estimation of left ventricular filling pressure
Pulmonary artery pressure	Normal value: ≤ 30–35 mm Hg

Source: Vitarelli A et al: The role of echocardiography in the diagnosis and management of heart failure. Heart Fail Rev 2003;8:181.

sus cardiac remodeling, which is an adaptive phenomenon associated with myocardial injury. The echocardiogram also helps to elucidate differences between dilated (idiopathic), hypertrophic, and restrictive cardiomyopathies. Diastolic changes can be elucidated by Doppler imaging. Left ventricular hypertrophy and a dilated left atrium are clues to the possible presence of left ventricular diastolic dysfunction. Dobutamine stress echocardiography is an important tool to assess for myocardial ischemia and viability in the form of ischemic, stunned, or hibernating myocardium. In addition to ischemia and valvular abnormalities, potential reversible etiologies of heart failure that echocardiography can help to uncover include pericardial disorders such as effusion or tamponade. It can help determine appropriate timing of therapy by uncovering asymptomatic LVSD in high-risk populations. The degree of left ventricular dysfunction, ventricular size, and shape add important prognostic information.

The routine reevaluation with echocardiography of clinically stable patients in whom no change in management is contemplated is not recommended. If the body habitus of the patient makes echocardiography impractical, radionuclide ventriculography can be performed to assess left ventricular ejection fraction and volumes.

3. Cardiac catheterization—Coronary angiography is recommended for patients with new-onset heart failure of uncertain etiology, despite the absence of anginal symptoms or negative findings on exercise stress testing. Coronary angiography should be strongly considered for patients with LVSD and a strong suspicion of ischemic myocardium based on noninvasive testing (echocardiography or nuclear imaging). Wall motion abnormalities seen on echocardiography or hibernating myocardium detected by dobutamine stress echocardiography are particularly useful indicators because they appear shortly after ischemia or infarction. The extent and severity of wall motion abnormalities have been shown to correlate with the size of the myocardium at risk. A strong association has been demonstrated between decreased mortality and revascularization (80% relative reduction in risk of death) only in patients found to have myocardial viability by thallium perfusion imaging, dobutamine echocardiography, or positron emission tomography scanning; with no apparent benefit in the absence of demonstrated viability. Therefore, evaluation of these abnormalities may have significant implications for urgency of treatment, resultant pump function, and subsequent morbidity and mortality.

Using clusters of clinical findings from the history, physical examination, and diagnostic tests is a better diagnostic strategy than using isolated findings. The clinical examination enables the clinician to categorize patients as having low, intermediate, and high pretest probabilities for the diagnosis of heart failure. More specialized testing, such as BNP results, helps clarify the diagnosis in patients determined to have an intermediate probability of heart failure.

Allman KC et al: Myocardial viability testing and impact of revascularization on prognosis in patients with coronary artery disease and left ventricular dysfunction: A meta-analysis. J Am Coll Cardiol 2002;39:1151. [PMID: 11923039]

Marcus GM et al: Association between phonocardiographic third and fourth heart sounds and objective measures of left ventricular function. JAMA 2005;293:2238. [PMID: 15886379]

Vitarelli A et al: The role of echocardiography in the diagnosis and management of heart failure. Heart Fail Rev 2003;8:181. [PMID: 12766498]

Wang CS et al: Does this dyspneic patient in the emergency department have congestive heart failure? JAMA 2005;294:1944. [PMID: 16234501]

Differential Diagnosis

Because heart failure is estimated to be present in only about 30% of patients with dyspnea in the primary care setting, clinicians need to consider differential diagnoses for dyspnea such as asthma, COPD, infection, interstitial lung disease, pulmonary embolism, anemia, thyrotoxicosis, carbon monoxide poisoning, arrhythmia, anginal equivalent (CAD), valvular heart disease, cardiac shunt, obstructive sleep apnea, and severe obesity causing hypoventilation syndrome.

Treatment

Most evidence-based treatment strategies have focused on patients with systolic rather than diastolic heart failure; hence, stage-specific outpatient management of patients with chronic systolic heart failure is the focus of the discussion that follows. Although stages A through D of the ACC/AHA heart failure classification represent progressive cardiac risk and dysfunction, the treatment strategies recommended at earlier stages are applicable to and recommended for later stages (see Table 19–2).

A. Systolic Heart Failure

1. High risk for systolic heart failure (stage A)—Individuals with conditions and behaviors that place them at high risk for heart failure but who do not have structurally abnormal hearts are classified as ACC/AHA stage A and should be treated with therapies that can delay progression of cardiac dysfunction and development of heart failure. Optimizing hypertension treatment based on the current guidelines from the Seventh Report of the Joint National Committee on Detection, Evaluation, and Treatment of High Blood Pressure (JNC VII) can reduce new-onset heart failure by 50%. Therapies such as diuretics, β-blockers, angiotensin-converting enzyme inhibitors (ACEIs), and angiotensin II receptor blockers (ARBs) are proven to be more effective than calcium channel blockers and doxazosin in preventing heart failure. Use of hydroxymethylglutaryl coenzyme A (HMG CoA) reductase inhibitors or statin therapy in CAD patients based on current hyperlipidemia guidelines (the updated Adult Treatment Panel III [ATP III]) can also reduce the incidence of heart failure by 20%.

Evidence-based disease management strategies for diabetes mellitus, atherosclerotic vascular disease, and thyroid disease, as well as patient avoidance of tobacco, alcohol, cocaine, amphetamines, and other illicit drugs that can be cardiotoxic, are also important components of early risk modification for prevention of heart failure. In diabetic patients, both ACEIs and ARBs (specifically losartan and irbesartan) have been shown to reduce new-onset heart failure compared with placebo. In CAD or atherosclerotic vascular disease patients without heart failure, reviews of the EUROPA (European Trial on Reduction of Cardiac Events with Perindopril in Stable Coronary Artery Disease) and HOPE (Heart Outcomes Prevention Trial) results show a 23% reduction in heart failure with ACEI therapy as well as reduced mortality, MIs, and cardiac arrest.

ALLHAT Officers and Coordinators for the ALLHAT Collaborative Research Group: Major outcomes in high-risk hypertensive patients randomized to angiotensin-converting enzyme inhibitor or calcium channel blocker vs. diuretic: The Antihypertensive and Lipid-Lowering Treatment to Prevent Heart Attack Trial (ALLHAT). JAMA 2002;288:2981. [PMID: 12479763]

Baker DW: Prevention of heart failure. J Card Fail 2002;8:333. [PMID: 12411985]

Brenner BM et al: Effects of losartan on renal and cardiovascular outcomes in patients with type 2 diabetes and nephropathy. N Engl J Med 2001;345:861. [PMID: 11565518]

Fox KM: Efficacy of perindopril in reduction of cardiovascular events among patients with stable coronary artery disease: Randomized, double-blind, placebo-controlled, multicentre trial (the EUROPA study). Lancet 2003;362:782. [PMID: 13678572]

Yusuf S et al: Effects of an angiotensin-converting-enzyme inhibitor, ramipril, on cardiovascular events in high-risk patients. The Heart Outcomes Prevention Evaluation Study Investigators. N Engl J Med 2000;342:145. [PMID: 10639539]

2. Asymptomatic with cardiac structural abnormalities or remodeling (stage B)—Patients who do not have clinical symptoms of heart failure but who have a structurally abnormal heart, such as a previous MI, evidence of left ventricular remodeling (left ventricular hypertrophy or low ejection fraction), or valvular disease, are at a substantial risk of developing symptomatic heart failure. Prevention of further progression in these at-risk patients is the goal, and appropriate therapies are dependent on the patient's cardiac condition.

In all patients with a recent or remote history of MI, regardless of ejection fraction, ACEIs and β-blockers are the mainstay of therapy. Both therapies have been demonstrated in randomized control trials to cause a significant reduction in cardiovascular death and heart failure. These therapies are vital in post-MI patients, as is evidence-based management of an ST-elevation MI and chronic stable angina, to help further achieve reduction in heart failure morbidity and mortality.

In asymptomatic patients who have not had an MI but have a reduced left ventricular ejection fraction (nonischemic cardiomyopathy), clinical trials reported an overall 37% reduction in heart failure when treated with ACEI therapy. The SOLVD (Studies of Left Ventricular Dysfunction) trial and a 12-year follow-up study confirmed the long-term benefit of ACEIs regarding onset of symptomatic heart failure and mortality. A substudy of the SOLVD trial showed how enalapril attenuates progressive increases in left ventricular dilation and hypertrophy, thus inhibiting left ventricular remodeling. Despite a lack of evidence from randomized controlled trials, the ACC/AHA guidelines recommend β-blockers in patients with stage B heart failure given the significant survival benefit these agents provide in worsening stages of heart failure. The RACE (Ramipril Cardioprotective Evaluation) trial provided a clue to why ACEIs are advantageous over β-blockers for nonischemic cardiomyopathy by demonstrating that ramipril is more effective than the β-blocker atenolol in reversing left ventricular hypertrophy in hypertensive patients.

There is no clear evidence for use of ARBs in asymptomatic patients with reduced left ventricular ejection fraction; however, ARB therapy is a reasonable alternative in ACEI-intolerant patients. The VALIANT (Valsartan in Acute Myocardial Infarction) trial showed that the ARB valsartan was as effective as but not superior to captopril, an ACEI, in reducing cardiovascular morbidity and mortality in post-MI patients with heart failure or a reduced left ventricular ejection fraction. The combination of both therapies was no better than captopril alone.

Agabiti-Rosei E et al: ACE inhibitor ramipril is more effective than the beta-blocker atenolol in reducing left ventricular mass in hypertension. Results of the RACE (ramipril cardioprotective evaluation) study on behalf of the RACE study group. J Hypertens 1995;13:1325. [PMID: 8984131]

Flather MD et al: Long-term ACE-inhibitor therapy in patients with heart failure or left-ventricular dysfunction: A systematic overview of data from individual patients. ACE-Inhibitor Myocardial Infarction Collaborative Group. Lancet 2000;355:1575. [PMID: 10821360]

Greenberg B et al: Effects of long-term enalapril therapy on cardiac structure and function in patients with left ventricular dysfunction. Results of the SOLVD echocardiography substudy. Circulation 1995;91:2573. [PMID: 7743619]

Maggioni AP, Fabbri G: VALIANT (VALsartan In Acute myocardial iNfarcTion) trial. Expert Opin Pharmacother 2005;6:507. [PMID: 15794740]

3. Symptomatic systolic heart failure (stage C)—Patients with a clinical diagnosis of heart failure have current or prior symptoms of heart failure and comprise ACC/AHA stage C. This stage encompasses NYHA classes II, III, and IV, excluding patients who develop refractory end-stage heart failure (see Table 19–2). In symptomatic patients with heart failure, neurohormonal activation creates deleterious effects on the heart, leading to pulmonary and peripheral edema, persistent increased afterload, pathologic cardiac remodeling, and a progressive decline in cardiac function. The overall goals in this stage are to improve the patient's symptoms, slow or reverse the deterioration of cardiac functioning, and reduce the patient's long-term morbidity and mortality.

Accurate assessment of the cause and severity of heart failure, the incorporation of previous stage A and B treatment recommendations, and correction of any cardiovascular, systemic, and behavioral factors (Table 19–5) are important to achieve control in patients with symptomatic heart failure. Moderate dietary sodium restriction (3–4 g daily) with daily weight measurement further enhance volume control and allow for lower and safer doses of diuretic therapies. Exercise training is beneficial and should be encouraged to prevent physical deconditioning, which can contribute to exercise intolerance in patients with heart failure.

Patients with symptomatic heart failure should be routinely managed with a standard therapy of a diuretic, an ACEI (or ARB if intolerant), and a β-blocker (see Table 19–2). The addition of other pharmacologic therapies should be guided by the need for further symptom control versus the desire to enhance survival and long-term prognosis. A stepwise approach to therapy is presented in Table 19–6 and expanded upon below.

Table 19–5. Factors contributing to worsening heart failure.

Cardiovascular Factors
Superimposed ischemia or infarction
Uncontrolled hypertension
Unrecognized primary valvular disease
Worsening secondary mitral regurgitation
New-onset or uncontrolled atrial fibrillation
Excessive tachycardia
Pulmonary embolism
Systemic Factors
Inappropriate medications
Superimposed infection
Anemia
Uncontrolled diabetes mellitus
Thyroid dysfunction
Electrolyte disorders
Pregnancy
Patient-related Factors
Medication noncompliance
Dietary indiscretion
Alcohol consumption
Substance abuse

Source: Colucci WS: Overview of the therapy of heart failure due to systolic dysfunction. In Rose BD, ed: *UpToDate Version 13.3.* UpToDate, 2005.

a. Diuretics—Patients with heart failure who present with common congestive symptoms (pulmonary and peripheral edema) are given a diuretic to manage fluid retention and achieve and maintain a euvolemic state. Diuretic therapy is specifically aimed at treating the compensatory volume expansion driven by renal tubular sodium retention and activation of the renin-angiotensin-aldosterone system.

Loop diuretics are the treatment of choice because they increase sodium excretion 20–25% and substantially enhance free water clearance. Furosemide is most commonly used, but patients may respond better to bumetanide or torsemide because of superior, more predictable absorptions and longer durations of action. To minimize the risk of over- and underdiuresis, the diuretic response should guide the dosage of loop diuretics (Table 19–7), with dose increases until a response is achieved. Frequency of dosing is guided by the time needed to maintain active diuresis and sustained volume and weight control.

Thiazide diuretics also have a role in heart failure, principally as antihypertensive therapy, but they can be

Table 19–6. Pharmacologic steps in symptomatic heart failure.[1]

Pharmacotherapy	Indications and Considerations
Standard Therapy	
Loop diuretic	Titrate accordingly for fluid control and symptom relief (dyspnea, edema)
Angiotensin-converting enzyme inhibitor (ACEI)	Initiate at low dose, titrating to target, during or after optimization of diuretic therapy for survival benefit[2]
β-Blocker	Initiate at low dose once stable on ADEI (or ARB) for survival benefit May initiate before achieving ACEI (or ARB) target doses and should be titrated to target doses unless symptoms become limiting
Additional Therapies[3]	
Angiotensin II receptor blocker (ARB)	Used in ACEI-intolerant patients, as above, for survival benefit May be effective for persistent symptoms and survival (NYHA class II–IV)
Aldosterone antagonist	For worsening symptoms and survival in moderately severe to severe heart failure (NYHA class III with decompensations)
Digoxin	For persistent symptoms and to reduce hospitalizations Should be maintained at preferred serum digoxin concentration
Hydralazine plus isosorbide dinitrate	Effective for persistent symptoms and survival, particularly in blacks

NYHA, New York Heart Association.
[1]Assessment of clinical response and tolerability should guide decision making and allow for variations.
[2]ARBs are recommended in patients who are intolerant to ACEIs.
[3]Decisions about whether or not to use additional therapy are guided by the need for symptom control versus mortality benefit.
Sources: Overview of the therapy of heart failure due to systolic dysfunction. In Rose BD, ed: *UpToDate Version 13.3.* UpToDate, 2005; Hunt SA et al: ACC/AHA 2005 guideline update for the diagnosis and management of chronic heart failure in the adult. Circulation 2005;112:e154.

used in combination with loop diuretics to provide a potentiated or synergistic diuresis. As a lone treatment, however, they increase sodium excretion only 5–10% and tend to decrease free water clearance overall.

Symptom improvement with diuretics occurs within hours to days as compared with weeks to months for other heart failure therapies. For long-term clinical stability, diuretics are not sufficient and exacerbations can be greatly reduced when they are combined with ACEI and β-blocker therapies.

b. ACE inhibitors—ACEIs are prescribed to all patients with symptomatic heart failure unless contraindicated and have proven benefit in alleviating heart failure symptoms, reducing hospitalization, and improving survival. Current ACC/AHA guidelines recommend that all patients with left ventricular dysfunction be started on low-dose ACEI therapy to avoid side effects and raised to a maintenance or target dose (see Table 19–7). There is, however, some uncertainty regarding target doses achieved in clinical trials, and whether these are more beneficial than lower doses. For ACEIs as a class, there does not appear to be any difference in agents in terms of effectiveness at improving heart failure outcomes.

c. β-Blockers—In patients with NYHA class II or III heart failure, the β-blockers bisoprolol, metoprolol succinate (sustained release), and carvedilol have been shown to improve mortality and event-free survival. These benefits are in addition to ACEI therapy and support the use of β-blockers as part of standard therapy in these patients. A similar survival benefit has been shown for patients with stable NYHA class IV heart failure.

β-Blocker therapy should be initiated near the onset of a diagnosis of left ventricular dysfunction and mild heart failure symptoms, given the added benefit on survival and disease progression. Titrating ACEI therapy to a target dose should not preclude the initiation of β-blocker therapy. Starting doses should be very low (see Table 19–7) but doubled at regular intervals, every 2–3 weeks as tolerated, to achieve target doses. There is no proven value to achieving a specific resting heart rate, but low doses are beneficial and there appears to be a dose-dependent improvement.

Traditionally the negative inotropic effects of β-blockers were thought to be harmful in heart failure, but this impact is outweighed by the beneficial effect of inhibiting sympathetic nervous system activation. Current evidence suggests that these beneficial effects are not necessarily equivalent among proven β-blockers. The COMET (Carvedilol or Metoprolol European Trial) findings showed that carvedilol (an α_1-, β_1-, and β_2-receptor inhibitor) is more effective than twice-daily dosed immediate-release metoprolol tartrate (a highly specific β_1-receptor inhibitor) in reducing heart failure mortality (40% vs 34%, respectively). Previous trials had investigated metoprolol succinate (sustained-release, once-daily dosing), but the COMET trial showed a mortality reduction even with metoprolol tartrate, a very cost-effective alternative.

Table 19–7. Medications used in the treatment of symptomatic heart failure in patients with reduced left ventricular ejection fraction.

Drug Therapy	Initial Daily Dose	Target or Maximum Daily Dose
Loop Diuretics		
Bumetanide	1.0 mg/dose	4–8 mg/dose
Furosemide	40 mg/dose	160–200 mg/dose
Torsemide	10 mg/dose	100–200 mg/dose
ACE Inhibitors		
Captopril	6.25 mg three times daily	50–100 mg three times daily
Enalapril	2.5 mg twice daily	10–20 mg twice daily
Fosinopril	5–10 mg once daily	20–40 mg once daily
Lisinopril	2.5–5 mg once daily	20–40 mg once daily
Perindopril	2 mg once daily	8–16 mg once daily
Quinapril	5 mg twice daily	20 mg twice daily
Ramipril	1.25–2.5 mg once daily	5 mg twice daily
Trandolapril	1 mg once daily	4 mg once daily
Angiotensin II Receptor Blockers		
Candesartan	4–8 mg once daily	32 mg once daily
Losartan	25–50 mg once daily	50–100 mg once daily
Valsartan	20–40 mg twice daily	160 mg twice daily
β-Blockers		
Bisoprolol	1.25 mg once daily	10 mg once daily
Carvedilol	3.125 mg twice daily	25 mg twice daily (50 mg twice daily, if > 85 kg [187 lb])
Metoprolol succinate, extended release (CR/XL)	12.5–25 mg once daily	200 mg once daily
Metoprolol tartrate, immediate release	12.5–25 mg once daily	100 mg once daily
Aldosterone Antagonists		
Eplerenone	25 mg once daily	50 mg once daily
Spironolactone	12.5–25 mg once daily	25 mg once or twice daily
Other Medication		
Digoxin	0.125–0.25 mg once daily	Serum concentration 0.5–1.1 ng/mL
Hydralazine plus isosorbide dinitrate	37.5 mg/20 mg three times daily	75 mg/40 mg three times daily

Source: ACC/AHA 2005 guideline update for the diagnosis and management of chronic heart failure in the adult. Circulation 2005;112:e154.

Because β-blockers may cause a 4- to 10-week increase in symptoms before improvement is noted, therapy should be initiated when patients have no or minimal evidence of fluid retention. Relative contraindications include bradycardia, hypotension, hypoperfusion, severe peripheral vascular disease, a P-R interval greater than 0.24 seconds, second- or third-degree atrioventricular block, severe COPD, or a history of asthma. Race or gender differences in efficacy of β-blocker therapy have not been noted.

d. Angiotensin II receptor blockers—ARBs have been shown in clinical trials to be nearly as effective as, but not superior to, ACEIs as first-line therapy for symptomatic heart failure. ARBs should be utilized in ACEI-intolerant patients but not preferentially over ACEIs given the volume of evidence validating ACEIs. Despite unclear evidence, the ACC/AHA guidelines recommend that ARB therapy be considered in addition to ACEI and standard therapy for patients who have persistent symptoms of heart failure.

e. Aldosterone antagonists—For selected patients with moderately severe to severe symptoms who are difficult to control (NYHA class III with decompensations or class IV), additional treatment options include the aldosterone antagonists spironolactone and eplerenone (see Table 19–7). There is no clear evidence to support the use of these therapies in patients with mild to moderate heart failure.

The addition of aldosterone antagonist therapy can cause life-threatening hyperkalemia in patients with heart failure, who are often already at risk because of reduced left ventricular function and associated renal insufficiency. Current guidelines recommend careful monitoring to ensure that creatinine is less than 2.5 mg/dL in men or less than 2.0 mg/dL in women and that potassium is maintained below 5.0 mEq/L (levels > 5.5 mEq/L should trigger discontinuation or dose reduction). Higher doses of aldosterone antagonists and ACEI therapy should also raise concern for possible hyperkalemia, and the use of nonsteroidal anti-inflammatory drugs (NSAIDs), cyclooxygenase-2 (COX-2) inhibitors, and potassium supplements should be avoided if possible. If the clinical situation does not allow for proper monitoring, the risk of hyperkalemia may outweigh the benefit of aldosterone antagonist therapy.

f. Digoxin—Digoxin therapy is only indicated to reduce hospitalizations in patients with uncontrolled symptomatic heart failure or as a ventricular rate control agent if a patient has a known arrhythmia. The DIG (Digitalis Investigation Group) trial proved the benefit of digoxin added to diuretic and ACEI therapy in improving heart failure symptom control and decreasing the rate of hospitalization by 6%, but there was no overall mortality benefit. Subsequent retrospective subgroup analysis of the trial discovered some survival improvement at a serum digoxin concentration of 0.5–0.8 ng/mL in men. A similar but nonsignificant survival trend was also noted in women. Because survival is clearly worse when the serum digoxin concentration is greater than 1.2 ng/mL, patients are best managed within the range noted to avoid potential adverse outcomes given the narrow risk/benefit ratio. Digoxin should be used cautiously in elderly patients, who may have impaired renal function that adversely affects drug levels.

g. Hydralazine and nitrates—The combination of hydralazine and isosorbide dinitrate (H-I) is a reasonable treatment in patients, particularly blacks, who have persistent heart failure symptoms with standard therapy. In V-HeFT I (Vasodilator Heart-Failure Trial), the mortality of black patients receiving H-I combination therapy was reduced, but mortality of white patients was not different than that of the placebo group. In V-HeFT II, a reduction in mortality with the H-I combination was seen only in white patients who had been receiving enalapril therapy. No effect on hospitalization was found in either trial.

The A-HeFT (African-American Heart Failure Trial) findings further supported the benefit of a fixed dose H-I combination (see Table 19–7) by showing a reduction in mortality and heart failure hospitalization rates as well as improved quality of life scores in patients with moderate to severe heart failure (NYHA class III or IV) who self-identified as black. The H-I combination was in addition to standard therapies that included ACEIs or ARBs, β-blockers, and spironolactone.

h. Anticoagulation—It is well established that patients with heart failure are at an increased risk of thrombosis from blood stasis in dilated hypokinetic cardiac chambers and peripheral blood vessels. Despite this known risk the yearly incidence of thromboembolic events in patients with stable heart failure is between 1% and 3%, even in those with lower left ventricular ejection fractions and evidence of intracardiac thrombi. Such low rates limit the detectable benefit of warfarin therapy, and retrospective data analysis of warfarin with heart failure show conflicting results, especially given the major risk of bleeding. Warfarin therapy is only indicated in heart failure patients with a history of a thromboembolic event or those with paroxysmal or chronic atrial fibrillation or flutter. Likewise, the benefit of antiplatelet therapies, such as aspirin, has not been clearly proven, and these therapies could possibly be detrimental because of their known interaction with ACEIs. Aspirin can decrease ACEI effectiveness and potentially increase hospitalizations from heart failure decompensation.

i. Adverse therapies—Therapies that adversely affect the clinical status of patients with symptomatic heart failure should be avoided. Other than for control of hypertension, calcium channel blockers offer no morbidity or mortality benefit in heart failure. Nondihydropyridine calcium channel blockers (eg, diltiazem and verapamil) and older, short-acting dihydropyridines (eg, nicardipine and nisoldipine) can worsen symptoms of heart failure, especially in patients with moderate to severe heart failure. The newer long-acting dihydropyridine calcium channel blockers amlodipine and felodipine appear to be safe when used in the treatment of hypertension but do not improve heart failure outcomes. NSAIDs can also exacerbate heart failure through peripheral vasoconstriction and by interfering with the renal effects of diuretics and the unloading effects of ACEIs. Most antiarrhythmic drugs (except amiodarone and dofetilide) have an adverse impact on heart failure and survival because of their negative inotropic activity and proarrhythmic effects. Phosphodiesterase inhibitors (cilostazol, sildenafil, vardenafil, and tadalafil) can cause hypotension and are potentially hazardous in patients with heart failure. Thiazolidinediones and metformin, both used in treatment of diabetes, can be detrimental in patients with heart failure because they increase the risk of excessive fluid retention and lactic acidosis, respectively.

j. Implantable devices—Nearly one third of all heart failure deaths occur as a result of sudden cardiac death. The ACC/AHA recommendations include use of implantable cardioverter-defibrillators (ICDs) for secondary prevention of sudden cardiac death in patients with symptomatic heart failure, a reduced left ventricular ejection fraction, and a history of cardiac arrest, ventricular fibrillation, or hemodynamically destabilizing ventricular tachycardia. ICDs are recommended for patients with NYHA class II or III heart failure, a left ventricular ejection fraction less than 35%, and a reasonable 1-year survival with no recent MI (within 40 days).

As heart failure progresses, ventricular dyssynchrony can also occur. This is defined by a QRS duration greater than 0.12 msec in patients with a low left ventricular ejection fraction (usually < 35%) and NYHA class III or IV heart failure. Clinical trials have shown that cardiac resynchronization therapy with biventricular pacing can improve quality of life, functional class, exercise capacity, exercise distance, left ventricular ejection fraction, and survival in these patients. Patients who meet criteria for cardiac resynchronization therapy and an ICD and should receive a combined device, unless contraindicated.

Brophy JM et al: Beta-blockers in congestive heart failure. A Bayesian meta-analysis. Ann Intern Med 2001;134:550. [PMID: 11281737]

de Vries RJ et al: Efficacy and safety of calcium channel blockers in heart failure: Focus on recent trials with second-generation dihydropyridines. Am Heart J 2000;139(2 Pt 1):185. [PMID: 10650289]

Goldstein S et al: Metoprolol controlled release/extended release in patients with severe heart failure: Analysis of the experience in the MERIT-HF study. J Am Coll Cardiol 2001;38:932. [PMID: 11583861]

Jong P et al: Angiotensin receptor blockers in heart failure: Meta-analysis of randomized controlled trials. J Am Coll Cardiol 2002;39:463. [PMID: 11823085]

Jong P et al: Effect of enalapril on 12-year survival and life expectancy in patients with left ventricular systolic dysfunction: A follow-up study. Lancet 2003;361:1843. [PMID: 12788569]

Juurlink DN et al: Drug-drug interactions among elderly patients hospitalized for drug toxicity. JAMA 2003;289:1652. [PMID: 12672733]

McMurray JJ et al: Effects of candesartan in patients with chronic heart failure and reduced left-ventricular systolic function taking angiotensin-converting-enzyme inhibitors: the CHARM-Added trial. Lancet 2003;362:767. [PMID: 13678869]

Pitt B et al: The EPHESUS trial: Eplerenone in patients with heart failure due to systolic dysfunction complicating acute myocardial infarction. Eplerenone Post-AMI Heart Failure Efficacy and Survival Study. Cardiovasc Drugs Ther 2001;15:79. [PMID: 11504167]

Poole-Wilson PA et al: Comparison of carvedilol and metoprolol on clinical outcomes in patients with chronic heart failure in the Carvedilol Or Metoprolol European Trial (COMET): Randomised controlled trial. Lancet 2003;362:7. [PMID: 12853193]

Rochon PA et al: Use of angiotensin-converting enzyme inhibitor therapy and dose-related outcomes in older adults with new heart failure in the community. J Gen Intern Med 2004;19:676. [PMID: 15209607]

Taylor AL et al: Combination of isosorbide dinitrate and hydralazine in blacks with heart failure. N Engl J Med 2004;351:2049. [PMID: 15533851]

4. Refractory end-stage heart failure (stage D)—Despite optimal medical therapy some patients deteriorate or do not improve and experience symptoms at rest (NYHA class IV). These patients can have rapid recurrence of symptoms, leading to frequent hospitalizations and a significant or permanent reduction in their activities of daily living. Before classifying patients as being refractory or having end-stage heart failure, providers should verify an accurate diagnosis, identify and treat contributing conditions that could be hindering improvement, and maximize medical therapy.

Control of fluid retention to improve symptoms is paramount in this stage, and referral to a program with expertise in refractory heart failure or referral for cardiac transplantation should be considered. Other specialized treatment strategies, such as mechanical circulatory support, continuous intravenous positive inotropic therapy, and other surgical management can be considered, but there is limited evidence in terms of morbidity and mortality to support the value of these therapies. Careful discussion of the prognosis and options for end-of-life care should also be initiated with patients and their families. In this scenario, patients with ICDs should receive information about the option to inactivate defibrillation.

B. Diastolic Heart Failure

Clinically, diastolic heart failure is as prevalent as LVSD, and the presentation of clinically evident diastolic heart failure is indistinguishable from clinically apparent LVSD. Elderly women, usually with a heavy prevalence of hypertension and diabetes mellitus, appear to be most at risk. When considering the diagnosis of diastolic heart failure, conditions that mimic heart failure—including obesity, lung disease, poorly controlled atrial fibrillation, and occult coronary ischemia—have to be ruled out. Management focuses on controlling systolic and diastolic blood pressure, ventricular rate, and volume status, and reducing myocardial ischemia, because these entities are known to exert effects on ventricular relaxation. Diuretics are used to control symptoms of pulmonary congestion and peripheral edema, but care must be taken to avoid overdiuresis, which can cause decreased volume status and preload, manifesting as worsening heart failure.

Dosh SA: Diagnosis of heart failure in adults. Am Fam Physician 2004;70:2145. [PMID: 15606063]

Prognosis

Despite favorable trends in survival and advances in treatment of heart failure and associated comorbidities, 50% of patients die within 5 years of diagnosis. Mortality increases in patients both with and without CHF as systolic function declines. Even patients with diastolic heart failure have significantly higher mortality rates compared with persons who have normal left ventricular systolic function and no CHF.

WEB SITES

American College of Cardiology clinical guidelines:

http://www.acc.org/clinical/statements.htm

American Heart Association (AHA):

http://www.americanheart.org

AHA heart disease and stroke statistics update:

http://www.americanheart.org/presenter.jhtml?identifier=3036355

AHA patient information:

http://www.americanheart.org/presenter.jhtml?identifier=1486

Dyslipidemias

20

Brian V. Reamy, MD, COL, USAF, MC[1]

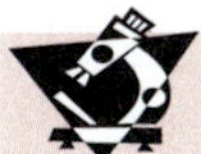

ESSENTIALS OF DIAGNOSIS

- *Serum cholesterol values greater than ideal for the prevention of atherosclerotic cardiovascular disease (ASCVD).*
- *Ideal values vary based on the risk status of the individual patient.*

General Considerations

The Framingham Heart Study firmly established an epidemiologic link between elevated serum cholesterol and an increased risk of morbidity and mortality from ASCVD. Although the benefits of lowering cholesterol were assumed for many years, not until the past decades has enough evidence accumulated to show unequivocal benefits from using dietary and pharmacologic therapy to lower serum cholesterol. Evidence in support of using statin agents is very strong and has revolutionized the treatment of dyslipidemias.

The efficacy of lipid reduction for both the secondary prevention of ASCVD (reducing further disease-related morbidity in those with manifest disease) as well as primary prevention (reducing the risk of disease occurrence in those without overt cardiovascular disease) led to the release in 2001 of treatment guidelines from the National Cholesterol Education Program (NCEP), Adult Treatment Panel (ATP) III. Subsequent research was incorporated in a revision to these guidelines in July 2004. The guidelines emphasize aggressive treatment of dyslipidemias, with the intensity of treatment titrated to those patients at the highest risk.

Pathogenesis

Serum cholesterol is carried by three major lipoproteins: high-density lipoprotein (HDL), low-density lipoprotein (LDL), and very low-density lipoprotein (VLDL). Most clinical laboratories measure the total cholesterol, total triglycerides, and the HDL fraction. The LDL level is estimated, not directly measured, using the formula:

$$\text{LDL cholesterol} = \text{Total cholesterol} - \text{HDL cholesterol} - \text{Triglycerides}/5$$

Total serum cholesterol is relatively stable over time and does not depend on whether the patient is fasting. However, the triglyceride fraction (and to a lesser extent the HDL level) varies considerably depending on the fasting status of the patient. The NCEP/ATP III guidelines recommend that only fasting measurements, including total cholesterol, triglycerides, HDL cholesterol, and LDL cholesterol, be used to guide management decisions.

Different populations have different median cholesterol values. For example, Asian populations tend to have total cholesterol values 20–30% lower than populations living in Europe or the United States. It is important to recognize that unlike a serum sodium electrolyte value, there is no normal cholesterol value. Instead, there are cholesterol values that predict higher morbidity and mortality from ASCVD if left untreated, and cholesterol values that correlate with less likelihood of cardiovascular disease if they are below certain levels.

Prevention & Clinical Trials

Basic science studies have established that atherosclerosis is an inflammatory disease. Inflammatory cells and mediators participate at every stage of atherogenesis from the earliest fatty streak to the most advanced fibrous lesion. Elevated glucose, increased blood pressure, and inhaled cigarette byproducts can trigger inflammation. One of the key factors triggering this inflammation is oxidized LDL. When LDL is taken up by macrophages it triggers the release of inflammatory mediators that can lead to thickening or rupture of plaque lining the arterial walls. Ruptured or unstable plaques are responsible for clinical events such as myocardial infarction and stroke. Lipid lowering, whether by diet or medication, can therefore be thought of as an anti-inflammatory and plaque-stabilizing therapy.

[1]The opinions contained herein are those of the author. They do not represent the opinions or official policy of the Department of the Air Force, the Department of Defense, or the Uniformed Services University.

Older trials, done in the 1980s prior to the advent of statin drugs, provided several insights into the benefits of cholesterol reduction. Several large, prospective, randomized double-blind trials of statin agents for both the primary and secondary prevention of ASCVD were completed in the 1990s. Five of these trials were especially significant (Tables 20–1 and 20–2).

Two of the trials were primary prevention trials. The West of Scotland Coronary Prevention Study (WOSCOPS; 1995) treated 6596 men with markedly elevated cholesterol levels with 40 mg/day of pravastatin. After just 5 years, coronary events were reduced by 31%, coronary artery disease (CAD) deaths by 28%, coronary revascularizations by 37%, and all-cause mortality was reduced by 22%.

The second primary prevention trial was the Air Force/Texas Coronary Atherosclerosis Prevention Study (AFCAPS/TEXCAPS; 1998). This trial treated 6605 patients (15% women) whose cholesterol values were in the average range for the United States population. All were treated with either 20 or 40 mg of lovastatin. Remarkably, even in this low risk group of patients, after 5 years of therapy there was a 25% risk reduction in nonfatal myocardial infarction and CAD deaths, a 40% risk reduction in fatal and nonfatal myocardial infarctions, and a 33% reduction in revascularizations.

Three remaining trials established the use of statins in secondary prevention. The Scandinavian Simvastatin Survival Study (4S; 1994) studied 4444 patients (19% women) for 5.4 years. Treated patients received either 20 or 40 mg of simvastatin. The patients were high risk in terms of both the presence of preexisting disease and markedly unfavorable cholesterol profiles. In this study CAD deaths were reduced by 34%, all myocardial infarcts by 42%, revascularizations by 37%, and all-cause mortality by 30%. The Long Term Intervention with Pravastatin in Ischemic Disease Study Group (LIPID; 1998) and Cholesterol and Recurrent Events (CARE; 1996) trials also showed reductions in all clinical end points.

Since the publication of ATP III in 2001, many other clinical trials of statin therapy have been completed, further reinforcing the evidence base for the treatment of hyperlipidemia. In addition, the safety and clinical utility of reducing LDL cholesterol levels to even lower values (< 70 mg/dL) was demonstrated by the 2004 Pravastatin or Atorvastatin Evaluation and Infection–Thrombolysis in Myocardial Infarction 22 (PROVE IT-TIMI 22) and the 2005 Treat to New Targets (TNT) trials.

Clinical Findings

A. Symptoms and Signs

The majority of patients with dyslipidemias have no signs or symptoms of disease. Rarely, patients with familial forms of hyperlipidemia may present with yellow xanthomas on the skin or in tendon bodies, especially the patellar tendon, Achilles tendon, and the extensor tendons of the hands. Dyslipidemia is usually detected by routine laboratory screening in an asymptomatic individual.

A few associated conditions can cause secondary hyperlipidemia (Table 20–3). These conditions should

Table 20–1. Major trials of statin treatment for coronary heart disease (CHD) primary prevention.

Trial	Number of Patients	% Men/ % Women	Treatment	Baseline Labs (mg/dL)	Post-treatment	% Risk Reduction
WOSCOPS	6596	100/0	Pravastatin, 40 mg/day	TC = 272	−20%	Nonfatal MI/CHD death −31%
				LDL = 192	−26%	CHD mortality −28%
				HDL = 44	+5%	Total mortality −22%
				TG = 164	−12%	Revascularizations −37%
AFCAPS/ TEXCAPS	6605	85/15	Lovastatin, 20–40 mg/day	TC = 221	−19%	Nonfatal MI/CHD death −25%
				LDL = 150	−26%	Fatal/nonfatal MI −40%
				HDL = 37	+5%	Total mortality no change
				TG = 158	−13%	Revascularizations −33%

WOSCOPS, West of Scotland Coronary Prevention Study (1998); TC, total cholesterol; MI, myocardial infarction; CHD, coronary heart disease; LDL, low-density lipoprotein; HDL, high-density lipoprotein; TG, triglycerides; AFCAPS/TEXCAPS, Air Force/Texas Coronary Atherosclerosis Prevention Study (1998).

Table 20–2. Major trials of statin treatment for coronary heart disease (CHD) secondary prevention.

Trial	No. Pts.	% Men/ % Women	Treatment	Baseline Labs (mg/dL)	Post-treatment	% Risk Reduction
4S	4444	81/19	Simvastatin, 20–40 mg/day	TC = 261	−26%	Nonfatal MI/CHD death −34%
				LDL = 188	−36%	Fatal/nonfatal MI −42%
				HDL = 46	+7%	Total mortality −30%
				TG = 134	−17%	CHD mortality −42%
LIPID	9014	83/17	Pravastatin, 40 mg/day	TC = 218	−18%	Nonfatal MI/CHD death −24%
				LDL = 150	−25%	Fatal/nonfatal MI −29%
				HDL = 36	+5%	Total mortality −22%
				TG = 138	−11%	CHD mortality −24%
CARE	4159	86/14	Pravastatin, 40 mg/day	TC = 209	−20%	Nonfatal MI/CHD death −24%
				LDL = 139	−28%	Fatal/nonfatal MI −29%
				HDL = 39	+5%	Total mortality −22%
				TG = 155	−14%	CHD mortality −20%

4S, Scandinavian Simvastatin Survival Study (1994); TC, total cholesterol; MI, myocardial infarction; CHD, coronary heart disease; LDL, low-density lipoprotein; HDL, high-density lipoprotein; TG, triglycerides; LIPID, Long Term Intervention with Pravastatin in Ischemic Disease Study Group (1998); CARE, Cholesterol and Recurrent Events (1996).

be considered before lipid-lowering therapy is begun or when the response to therapy is much less than predicted. In particular, poorly controlled diabetes and untreated hypothyroidism can lead to a significant elevation of serum lipids.

B. Screening

The US Preventive Services Task Force (USPSTF) bases its screening recommendations on the age of the patient. It strongly recommends (rating: A) routinely screening men 35 years of age and older and women 45 years and older for lipid disorders.

The USPSTF recommends (rating: B) screening younger adults (men 20–35 years of age and women 20–45 years of age) if they have other risk factors for CAD. They make no recommendation for or against screening in younger adults in the absence of known risk factors.

In contrast, the NCEP guidelines advise that screening should occur in adults aged 20 years or older with a fasting lipid profile once every 5 years.

Screening of children and adolescents is controversial because of scant studies proving the benefits of reducing elevated serum cholesterol and the paucity of medications indicated for treatment in children. Some expert opinion recommends screening only those children older than 2 years of age with significant family histories of hypercholesterolemia or premature ASCVD.

Treatment

The NCEP/ATP III treatment guidelines released in May 2001, and the July 2004 revision, are as rooted in evidence as possible. These guidelines are available

Table 20–3. Secondary causes of lipid abnormalities.

Hypercholesterolemia
- Hypothyroidism
- Nephrotic syndrome
- Obstructive liver disease
- Acute intermittent porphyria
- Diabetes mellitus
- Chronic renal insufficiency
- Cushing disease
- Drugs (oral contraceptives, diuretics)

Hypertriglyceridemia
- Diabetes mellitus
- Alcohol use
- Obesity
- Chronic renal insufficiency
- Drugs (estrogens, isotretinoin)

Hypocholesterolemia
- Cancer
- Hyperthyroidism
- Cirrhosis

Table 20–4. Summary of nine steps in NCEP/ATP III guidelines.

Step 1	Determine lipoprotein levels after a 9–12 h fast.
Step 2	Identify the presence of coronary heart disease or equivalents (coronary artery disease, peripheral arterial disease, abdominal aortic aneurysm, diabetes mellitus).
Step 3	Determine the presence of major risk factors, other than LDL (smoking, hypertension, HDL <40 mg/dL, family history of premature coronary disease, men ≥45 years and women ≥55 years).
Step 4	Assess level of risk [use Framingham risk tables if two or more risk factors and no coronary heart disease (or equivalent) is present].
Step 5	Determine risk category, LDL goal, and the threshold for drug treatment.
Step 6	Initiate therapeutic life-style changes (TLC) if LDL is above goal.
Step 7	Initiate drug therapy if LDL remains above goal.
Step 8	Identify the presence of the metabolic syndrome and treat. Determine the triglyceride and HDL goals of therapy.
Step 9	Treat elevated triglycerides and reduced HDL with TLC and drug therapy to achieve goals.

online (http://www.nhlbi.nih.gov), and the Framingham risk calculators can be downloaded for use in a personal data assistant (PDA).

The NCEP/ATP III clinical practice guidelines follow a nine-step process (Table 20–4). **Step 1** begins after obtaining fasting lipoprotein levels. The profile is categorized based on the LDL, HDL, and total cholesterol values:

LDL Cholesterol (mg/dL)

< 100	Optimal
100–129	Near optimal
130–159	Borderline high
160–189	High
≥ 190	Very high

HDL Cholesterol (mg/dL)

< 40	Low
≥ 60	High

Total Cholesterol (mg/dL)

< 200	Desirable
200–239	Borderline high
≥ 240	High

Step 2 focuses on determining the presence of clinical atherosclerotic disease such as CAD, carotid artery disease, peripheral arterial disease, or diabetes mellitus.

In **Step 3** the clinician should determine the presence of other major CAD risk factors, including smoking, age greater than 45 years in men (55 years in women), hypertension, HDL cholesterol less than 40 mg/dL, and a family history of premature CAD in a male first-degree relative younger than 55 years or a female first-degree relative younger than 65 years of age. An HDL cholesterol level greater than 60 mg/dL negates one risk factor.

Step 4 uses the Framingham coronary risk calculator to classify the patient into one of four risk categories: *high risk*, having coronary artery disease or a 10-year risk greater than 20%; *moderately high risk,* having a 10-year risk of 10–20%; *moderate risk*, having more than two risk factors, but a 10-year risk of less than 10%; or *low risk*, having zero to one risk factors. As previously noted, the Framingham risk tables can be downloaded to a personal computer or handheld PDA (see http://www.nhlbi.nih.gov).

Step 5 is the key step that determines the patient's suggested LDL cholesterol treatment goals and the methods to reach these goals. Table 20–5 summarizes risk category determination and treatment goals.

A. Behavior Modification

Step 6 reviews the contents of Therapeutic Lifestyle Changes (TLC). Saturated fat is limited to less than 7% of total calories, cholesterol intake to less than 200 mg/day. In addition, weight management and increased physical activity are encouraged. TLC also includes advice to increase the consumption of soluble fiber (10–25 g/day) and the intake of plant sterols (sitostanol, approximately 2 g/day). Several margarines (Benecol, Take Control) contain these plant sterols, and evidence exists that they work in conjunction with cholesterol-lowering drugs.

The cultural background of the patient will influence the choice of dietary recommendations. A skilled nutritional medicine consultant can easily adapt the fat and cholesterol intake recommendations to a variety of culturally normative diets. Indeed, components of some cultures' diets that encourage the consumption of soluble fiber, plant sterols, soy protein, or fish oils can be encouraged to enhance the cholesterol-lowering effect. Dietary advice given without regard to a patient's culturally accepted diet is counterproductive to effective cholesterol reduction.

B. Pharmacotherapy

Step 7 reviews the options for drug therapy if required (Table 20–6). Of note, NCEP/ATP III now recommends the simultaneous use of TLC and drugs in

Table 20–5. Risk category determination and LDL cholesterol goals.[1]

Risk Category	LDL Goal	LDL Level at Which to Begin Therapeutic Life-style Changes (TLC)	LDL Level at Which to Consider Drug Treatment
High-risk: Coronary heart disease or equivalent (10-y risk ≥ 20%)	<100 mg/dL (<70 mg/dL optimal)	≥100 mg/dL	≥100 mg/dL or <100 mg/dL
Moderately high risk: 10-y risk 10–20%)	<130 mg/dL (<100 mg/dL optimal)	≥130 mg/dL	≥130 mg/dL or consider if 100–129 mg/dL
Moderate risk: 2+ risk factors (10-y risk ≤ 10%)	<130 mg/dL	≥130 mg/dL	≥160 mg/dL
Low-risk: 0–1 risk factor	<160 mg/dL	≥160 mg/dL	≥190 mg/dL (160–189 mg/dL: drug use optional)

[1]Adapted from 2001 NCEP/ATP III treatment guidelines and 2004 update.

patients at the highest risk. Medications should be added to TLC after 3 months if goal LDL levels are not reached in lower risk patients. Given their proven efficacy, ease of administration, and enhanced patient compliance over other classes of medications, statin agents are the drugs of first choice for most patients. In particular, patients with diabetes or those in the highest risk category derive special benefits from their use due

Table 20–6. Pharmacologic therapy of elevated cholesterol.

Drug Class	Drugs	Typical Effects[1]	Side Effects
Statins	Lovastatin Pravastatin Simvastatin Fluvastatin Rosuvastatin Atorvastatin	LDL −20–50% HDL +5–15% TG −10–25%	Myopathy Increased liver enzymes
Bile acid sequestrants	Cholestyramine Colestipol Colesevelam	LDL −15% HDL Minimal TG May increase 10%	Gastrointestinal (GI) distress Constipation Decreased absorption of other drugs
Nicotinic acid	Immediate release Extended release Sustained release	LDL −20% HDL +20–35% TG −20–50%	Flushing GI distress Hyperglycemia Hyperuricemia Hepatotoxicity
Fibrates	Gemfibrozil Fenofibrate	LDL −5–15% HDL +15% TG −20–50%	GI distress Gallstones Myopathy
Absorption blocker	Ezetimibe	LDL −17% HDL +1.3% TG −6%	Gallstones

LDL, low-density lipoprotein; HDL, high-density lipoprotein; TG, triglycerides.

[1]Lipid effects represent the average seen in most patients. Individual patients may display markedly different effects. This reinforces the need for dosage titration and close monitoring of lipid effects during drug initiation.

to their innate anti-inflammatory effects. Myopathy and elevated liver enzymes are the main potential side effects from statin agents. An increase of serum aminotransferase levels to more than three times normal occurs in 1% of patients taking high doses of statins. Monitoring of liver function tests at 6 weeks, 12 weeks, 6 months, and annually thereafter can help identify patients with hepatic side effects and facilitate prompt discontinuation of the agents. Rhabdomyolysis occurs in less than 0.1% of cases. It can be prevented by the prompt discontinuation of the agent when muscle pain and elevated muscle enzymes occur. Unexplained pain in large muscle groups should prompt investigation for myopathy; however, routine monitoring of muscle enzymes is not supported by any evidence. Side effects from statins may not be class specific. Therefore, a side effect with one agent should not prevent a trial with another statin agent. Prior concerns about statins causing cataracts or cancer have been alleviated by the release of two large meta-analyses in 2001.

Statin agents can be combined with fibrates and nicotinic acid, but the potential for side effects is increased. A good rule-of-thumb is to halve the dose of the statin agent when adding a fibrate and then titrate the dosage of the statin upward to reach the therapeutic goal. Fibrate agents have special efficacy in patients with primarily low HDL and elevated triglycerides.

Nicotinic acid is the most potent HDL-elevating agent and the agent that affects all cholesterol subfractions in a positive fashion. Yet long-term patient compliance is difficult to achieve due to flushing, nausea, and abdominal discomfort. Additionally, nicotinic acid can cause an increase in blood glucose, which can limit its use in diabetic patients.

The bile acid sequestrants cause significant gastrointestinal side effects and can lead to decreased absorption of other medications. Given their relative decreased potency they are mainly useful as adjuncts. Ezetimibe, a cholesterol absorption inhibitor that lowers LDL and is ideally used in combination with a statin agent, has fewer side effects than the bile acid sequestrants.

C. Complementary and Alternative Therapies

Many complementary or alternative therapies are employed for cholesterol reduction, but the evidence supporting their use is variable. Several are harmless; others could lead to significant side effects. Oat bran ($^1/_2$ cup/day) is a soluble fiber that can reduce total cholesterol by 5 mg/dL and triglycerides by 5%. Fish oil (1 g daily of unsaturated omega-3 fatty acids) can reduce triglycerides by up to 30% and raise HDL slightly with long-term use.

Garlic has minimal side effects but several trials have shown that it changes lipids minimally. Soy can reduce LDL by up to 15% with an intake of 25 g/day. This amount is unlikely to be achieved in a western-style diet. Went yeast is the natural source for statin agents. As such, it is effective at lowering lipid values but carries the same side effect profile as statins. Of concern is that most patients do not undergo monitoring for potential hepatic or muscle side effects. Red wine can raise HDL; however, in amounts greater than two glasses per day, red wine will raise triglycerides and potentially cause hepatic damage and other deleterious health effects. Several other supplements, such as ginseng, chromium, and myrrh, all have putative cholesterol-lowering effects but little patient-oriented clinical outcome evidence supporting their use.

Step 8 of the NCEP/ATP III guidelines encourages clinicians to look for the "metabolic syndrome." The components of this syndrome are abdominal obesity, hypertriglyceridemia, low HDL, hypertension, and glucose intolerance. Aggressive treatment of inactivity, obesity, and hypertension, and the use of low-dose aspirin are encouraged in these patients.

Step 9 is the final step of the algorithm. This step focuses on treating elevated triglycerides and low HDL as secondary end points of cholesterol therapy. Triglycerides are classified as follows:

< 150 mg/dL Normal
150–199 mg/dL Borderline high
200–499 mg/dL High
≥ 500 mg/dL Very high

The initial steps are to employ TLC (weight reduction, increased physical activity, dietary change) and then to add a fibrate or nicotinic acid to reach goal levels. Combination therapy with a statin is frequently needed, and caution should be exercised due to the increased potential for side effects.

D. Treatment of Special Groups

The treatment of dyslipidemias in special groups presents additional problems because data on women, children, the elderly, and young adults are incomplete.

1. Women—Several statin trials included women, although they accounted for only about 15–20% of the total enrolled patient population. Subset analysis and meta-analysis reveal that statins reduced coronary events by a similar proportion in women as in men. The reduction of coronary events involved fewer nonfatal events in women.

2. Elderly—Given that ASCVD is more common in the elderly it is expected that the benefits of cholesterol-lowering would extend to this subgroup. Due to the increased frequency of ASCVD events in this population, the number needed to treat (NNT) is reduced from approximately 35:1 in patients aged 40–55 years to just 4:1 in patients aged 65–75 years. The 2002 Prospective Study of Pravastatin in the Elderly at Risk (PROSPER) study, 2003 Anglo-Scandinavian Cardiac Outcomes Trial (ASCOT), and 2002 Heart Protection Study (HPS) confirmed the benefits of lipid-lowering with statins for the primary and secondary prevention of ASCVD in patients 65–84 years of age.

3. Children—None of the large clinical trials included children. There are accumulating small reports on the safety of cholesterol lowering with statins in adolescents. However, given the theoretical concerns of interrupting cholesterol synthesis in the growing body, therapy will most likely be confined to patients deemed at very high risk. Therapeutic life-style interventions are safe and can have a profound impact on the long-term health of the child if they are followed. Cholesterol levels should not be checked in children younger than 2 years of age, because marked elevations are normal in this age group.

4. Patients younger than 35 years—Numerous studies have shown pathoanatomic evidence of ASCVD at all ages. The Pathobiological Determinants of Atherosclerosis in Youth (PDAY) study has demonstrated the ability to correlate degrees of arterial intimal narrowing with the risk factors present in a patient at the time of autopsy across all age groups.

Cholesterol treatment studies have not enrolled patients younger than 35 years of age because the frequency of clinical end points would be reduced and the duration of the studies would need to increase. The elevation of the NNT in young patients also makes treatment less economically attractive. The NCEP/ATP III guidelines specifically address this issue for patients aged 20–35 years. They state that even though clinical CAD is rare in young adults, coronary atherosclerosis may progress rapidly, and young men who smoke and have an LDL of 160–189 mg/dL may be candidates for drug therapy. In addition, for young men and women with an LDL greater than 190 mg/dL, drug therapy should be considered as in adults of other ages.

E. Patient Education

Patient education is the key portion of the behavioral modification involved in TLC. The American Heart Association web site listed at the end of this chapter is an excellent source of patient education materials, including video web casts, handouts, and dietary information.

F. Referral

Patients who do not respond to combination therapy or have untoward side effects of therapy should be considered for specialty consultation. Combinations of multiple agents or lipid plasmapheresis may sometimes be required.

Choice of lipid-regulating drugs. Med Lett Drugs Ther 2001; 43:43; also available online at: http://www.medletter.com. [PMID: 11378632]

Grundy SM et al: Implications of recent clinical trials for the National Cholesterol Education Program Adult Treatment Panel III Guidelines. Circulation 2004;110;227. [PMID: 15249516]

Third Report of the National Cholesterol Education Program (NCEP) Expert Panel on the Detection, Evaluation, and Treatment of High Blood Cholesterol in Adults (Adult Treatment Panel III). National Institutes of Health/National Heart, Lung, and Blood Institute, May 2001. Available at: http://www.nhlbi.nih.gov.

Three new drugs for hyperlipidemia. Med Lett Drugs Ther 2003; 45:17. [PMID: 12612501]

Web Sites

American Heart Association (the best peer-reviewed source for diet, exercise, and life-style information for physicians and patients):

http://www.americanheart.org

Urinary Tract Infections

21

Shersten Killip, MD, MPH

Urinary tract infections (UTIs) are the most common bacterial infection encountered in medicine. Accurately estimating incidence is difficult because UTIs are not reportable, but estimates range from 650,000 to seven million office visits per year. For a condition involving so many patients, pathophysiology and knowledge are not as well-defined as they could be.

A UTI is defined by urologists as any infection involving the urothelium, which includes urethral, bladder, prostate, and kidney infections. Some of these are diseases that have been clearly characterized (eg, cystitis and pyelonephritis), whereas others (eg, urethral and prostate infections) are not as well understood or described.

The terms *simple UTI* and *uncomplicated UTI* are often used to refer to cystitis. In this chapter *UTI* is used to refer to any infection of the urinary tract, and *cystitis* is used to specify a bladder infection. The generic term *complicated UTI* is often used to refer to cystitis occurring in a person with pre-existing metabolic, immunologic, or urologic abnormalities, including kidney stones, diabetes, and AIDS, or caused by multiply-resistant organisms.

Asymptomatic bacteriuria, two urethral syndromes, four prostatitis syndromes, uncomplicated cystitis, complicated cystitis, and pyelonephritis are discussed in this chapter. Because some of these syndromes, such as the four prostatitis syndromes, have only recently been defined, little research is available to answer basic clinical questions related to diagnosis, prevention, treatment, and prognosis. Differentiating among syndromes and deciding treatment(s) is therefore left very much to the clinician's discretion.

Antibiotic resistance is a topic that has been left mostly to the reader. General recommendations about specific antibiotics are inappropriate, given that antibiotic resistance changes from location to location. It is the responsibility of the individual physician to be familiar with local antibiotic resistances, and to determine the best first-line therapies for his or her practice. Always keep in mind that antibiotic use breeds resistance, and try to keep first-line drugs as simple and narrow-spectrum as possible.

Foxman B, Brown P: Epidemiology of urinary tract infections: Transmission and risk factors, incidence and costs. Infect Dis Clin North Am 2003;17:227. [PMID: 12848468]

ASYMPTOMATIC BACTERIURIA

ESSENTIALS OF DIAGNOSIS

- *Asymptomatic patient.*
- *Urine culture with more than 10^5 colony-forming units (CFU); bacteria in spun urine; or urine dipstick analysis positive for leukocytes, nitrites, or both.*

General Considerations

Asymptomatic bacteriuria is defined separately for men, women, and the type of specimen. For women, clean-catch voided specimens on two separate occasions must contain more than 10^5 CFU/mL of the same bacterial strain or one catheterized specimen must contain more than 10^2 CFU/mL of bacteria. For men, a single clean-catch specimen with more than 10^5 CFU/mL of bacteria or one catheterized specimen with more than 10^2 CFU/mL of bacteria suffices for the diagnosis. The patient must be asymptomatic; that is, he or she should not be experiencing dysuria, suprapubic pain, fever, urgency, frequency, or incontinence. Screening does not need to be done in young, healthy, nonpregnant women; elderly healthy or institutionalized men or women; diabetic women; persons with spinal cord injury; or catheterized patients while the catheter remains in place.

Pregnant women are now the only group that should be routinely screened and treated for asymptomatic bacteriuria. Asymptomatic bacteriuria, defined in pregnant women as one clean-catch sample at 12–16 weeks' gestation with more than 10^5 organisms on culture, is present in 2–10% of pregnant women and has been associated with premature birth. Multiple guidelines recommend screening pregnant women for asymptomatic bacteriuria. In the United States, this is usually done by urine culture because dipstick screening can miss patients without pyuria or with unusual organisms.

Treatment

Treatment should be guided by local rates of resistance. The usual first-line treatment in the absence of significant resistance or penicillin allergy is a 7-day course of amoxicillin. Nitrofurantoin or a cephalosporin is suggested for penicillin-allergic pregnant patients, again for 7 days.

Cram LF et al: Genitourinary infections and their association with preterm labor. Am Fam Physician 2002;65:241. [PMID: 11820488]

Harding GK et al: Antimicrobial treatment in diabetic women with asymptomatic bacteriuria. N Engl J Med 2002;347:1576. [PMID: 12432044]

Nicolle LE et al: Infectious Diseases Society of America guidelines for the diagnosis and treatment of asymptomatic bacteriuria in adults. Clin Infect Dis 2005;40:643. [PMID: 15714408]

ACUTE URETHRAL SYNDROME

ESSENTIALS OF DIAGNOSIS

- *Dysuria.*
- *Frequency and urgency.*
- *No vaginal discharge.*
- *Urine dipstick analysis may be negative or positive.*
- *Negative culture.*

General Considerations

Acute urethral syndrome is a term used by some to describe a young, healthy, sexually active woman who complains of recent-onset symptoms of cystitis but does not meet older, strict guidelines for diagnosis (growth of $\geq 10^4$ or 10^5 organisms on culture). Some authors now feel that even 100 CFU found on culture of a dysuric woman represent a true UTI. Because most laboratories are equipped to detect only 10^4 organisms or more, these are patients in usual practice found to have "negative" cultures. They may have positive or negative urine dipstick analysis and positive or negative spun urine for bacteria, although bacteria and white blood cells (WBCs) in the urine are more convincing for cystitis than a completely negative workup.

Clinical Findings

Testing depends on the physician's assessment of the patient. In a patient at low risk of a sexually transmitted disease (STD), no testing might be appropriate, or testing only after failure of empirical treatment for cystitis. In patients at higher risk of acquiring an STD, *Chlamydia* testing, either by cervical swab or urine polymerase chain reaction (PCR) or ligase chain reaction (LCR) might be appropriate.

Differential Diagnosis

This syndrome clearly is not well defined. It is usually taken to represent an early cystitis, but it can also be an STD (*C trachomatis* has been noted in women with the previously described symptoms).

Treatment

There is some evidence that the acute urethral syndrome will respond to antibiotics commonly used in the treatment of UTIs. Because the prevalence of *C trachomatis* was found to be high in a least one study of women with these symptoms, use of antibiotics effective against STDs or *Chlamydia* testing for patients who do not respond completely to a course of antibiotics is highly recommended.

Richards D et al: Response to antibiotics of women with symptoms of urinary tract infection but negative dipstick urine test results: Double blind randomized controlled trial. BMJ 2005; 331:143. [PMID: 15972728]

URETHRITIS

ESSENTIALS OF DIAGNOSIS

- *Pain or irritation on urination.*
- *No frequency or urgency.*
- *Discharge from the urethra (predominantly males).*
- *Vaginal discharge possible.*

General Considerations

Isolated urethritis in men or women is almost always an STD, most often caused by *C trachomatis.* This syndrome is differentiated from acute urethral syndrome by the time course of symptoms: symptoms that have a gradual onset or persist without evolution into classic cystitis symptoms, including suprapubic symptoms such as pain, urgency, or frequency, are more indicative of urethritis than of acute urethral syndrome.

Clinical Findings

It can be very difficult to differentiate a symptomatic chlamydial infection from bacterial cystitis with coliform organisms, and testing for both may be required. The advent of *Chlamydia* urine PCR or LCR tests makes ruling out *Chlamydia* much easier than in the past, as the same urine sample can be sent for both tests.

Treatment

See Chapter 14 for current diagnosis and treatment of STDs such as *Chlamydia*.

ACUTE BACTERIAL PROSTATITIS

ESSENTIALS OF DIAGNOSIS

- *Dysuria, frequency, urgency.*
- *Tender prostate.*
- *Systemic symptoms such as fever, nausea, vomiting.*
- *Leukocyte esterase or nitrite on urine dipstick analysis.*
- *Positive urine culture.*

General Considerations

Prostatitis is a very common disease among men, with a prevalence and incidence among men ranging between 5% and 8%. Some two million office visits a year are made for prostatitis (1% of all primary care office visits), so it is useful for the primary care practitioner to be able to evaluate men for symptoms of prostatitis.

Until recently, prostatitis could be described as "acute," "chronic," or "nonbacterial." The National Institutes of Health (NIH) revised the categorization of prostatitis in 1995, and the disease is now differentiated into four categories, as follows:

- Category I: acute bacterial prostatitis.
- Category II: chronic bacterial prostatitis.
- Category IIIA: inflammatory chronic pelvic pain syndrome.
- Category IIIB: noninflammatory chronic pelvic pain syndrome.
- Category IV: asymptomatic inflammatory prostatitis.

The last category is a diagnosis made incidentally, while working up other symptoms, and is not felt to require treatment. Discussion of category I, or acute bacterial prostatitis, follows. The other categories are discussed separately, later in this chapter.

Acute bacterial prostatitis is different from other types of prostatitis in that it is a well-defined entity with a relatively clear-cut etiology, diagnosis, and treatment. Acute bacterial prostatitis is caused by typical uropathogens and responds well to antibiotic treatment.

Prevention

There is no evidence for interventions that will prevent spontaneous prostatitis.

Clinical Findings

Symptoms and signs include dysuria, frequency, and urgency; low back, perineal, penile, or rectal pain; or tense or "boggy" tender prostate. Fever and chills may be present.

Laboratory findings include a urine dipstick analysis that is positive for leukocyte esterase or nitrites, or both, and urine culture that is positive for a single uropathogen. Imaging studies usually are not performed for acute uncomplicated prostatitis.

Prostatic massage is not generally performed in patients with acute bacterial prostatitis because it may lead to acute bacteremia. It can be done carefully if postmassage urine is required but should be avoided if abscess is suspected.

Differential Diagnosis

Abnormal anatomy may include urethral strictures, polyps, diverticula, redundancies, or valves anywhere in the system from the penis to the kidneys (Table 21–1).

Complications

Complications of acute bacterial prostatitis may include ascending infection, infection-related stones, abscess, fistula, cysts, and acute urinary retention. In the case of acute urinary retention precipitated by prostatitis, a suprapubic catheter rather than a Foley catheter should be placed to avoid damage to the prostate.

Treatment

The usual treatment is quinolone antibiotics for 28 days. Trimethoprim-sulfamethoxazole or trimethoprim alone is also acceptable, depending on local resistance rates for uropathogens.

Prognosis

The prognosis is very good for patients with acute uncomplicated bacterial prostatitis.

Anderson RU: Management of chronic prostatitis–chronic pelvic pain syndrome. Urol Clin North Am 2002;29:235. [PMID: 12109351]

Lummus WE, Thompson I: Prostatitis. Emerg Med Clin North Am 2001;19:691. [PMID: 11554282]

Turner JA et al: Primary care and urology patients with the male pelvic pain syndrome: Symptoms and quality of life. J Urol 2002;167:1768. [PMID: 11912406]

Table 21–1. Differential diagnosis of dysuria in men.

If Patient Has	Consider
Acute, colicky flank pain or history of kidney stones	Kidney stone; complicated cystitis
Costovertebral angle tenderness, fevers	Pyelonephritis
Urethral discharge	Sexually transmitted disease
Diabetes/immunosuppression	Complicated cystitis, unusual pathogens
Testicular pain	Torsion; epididymoorchitis
Joint pains	Spondyloarthropathy (ie, Reiter or Behçet syndrome)
History of childhood UTI or urologic surgery	Abnormal anatomy; complicated cystitis
Recurrent symptoms after treatment	Abnormal anatomy; abscess; stone; chronic prostatitis; resistant organism; inadequate length of treatment; Munchausen syndrome; somatization disorder

CHRONIC BACTERIAL PROSTATITIS

ESSENTIALS OF DIAGNOSIS

- *Dysuria, frequency, urgency.*
- *Symptoms lasting more than 3 months.*
- *Urine dipstick analysis positive for leukocyte esterase or nitrites, or both.*
- *Pyuria on microscopy.*
- *Positive four-glass or two-glass test for prostatic origin.*

General Considerations

Chronic bacterial prostatitis, or NIH category II prostatitis, is quite rare, and consequently very few studies have examined it. Bacterial disease comprises only a small percentage of the cases of chronic prostatitis. It has been estimated that the percentage of both acute and chronic bacterial prostatitis is only 5–10% of all prostatitis diagnoses, and of the bacterial cases the vast majority are acute.

Prevention

Early and sufficient treatment of acute bacterial prostatitis is felt by some authors to prevent chronic prostatitis.

Clinical Findings

A. Symptoms and Signs

Symptoms and signs include dysuria, frequency, and urgency; prostatic tenderness on examination; low back pain; and perineal, penile, or rectal pain. Symptoms are usually present for more than 3 months.

B. Laboratory and Imaging Findings

A urine dipstick analysis will be positive for leukocyte esterase or nitrites, or both. Additionally, a four-glass or two-glass test (discussed below) will be positive for prostatic origin. A transrectal prostatic ultrasound should be performed if an abscess or a stone is suspected.

C. Special Tests

1. Four-glass test—Not used by the majority of practitioners, this is a localization test for chronic prostatitis. The patient should not have been on antibiotics for a month, should not have ejaculated for 2 days, and needs a reasonably full bladder. Signs and symptoms of urethritis or cystitis should have been worked up previously and treated. To perform the test, the patient first cleans himself and carefully retracts the foreskin, then urinates the first 5–10 mL into a sterile container (VB_1). He then urinates 100–200 mL into the toilet, and a second 10–20 mL sample into a sterile container (VB_2). Prostatic massage is then done, milking secretions from the periphery to the center, and any expressed prostatic secretions are caught in a third sterile container (EPS). The patient then cleans himself again, and urinates a final 10–20 mL sample into a fourth container (VB_3).

All urine samples are examined microscopically and cultured. Expressed prostatic secretions are wet-mounted, examined, and cultured. The test is positive for prostatic localization if WBCs per high-power field (HPF) and colony counts in VB_3 are at least 10 times greater than in VB_1 or VB_2, or if there are 10 polymorphonuclear leukocytes (PMNL)/HPF in the wet mount. If there is a significant colony count in both VB_2 and VB_3, the patient should be treated for 3 days with nitrofurantoin, which does not penetrate the prostate, and the test should be repeated.

2. Two-glass test—An experimentally verified modification of the four-glass test, this test requires an initial clean-catch urine sample, prostatic massage, and a post-massage urine sample. It is functionally equivalent to the VB_2 and VB_3 portions of the four-glass test.

Differential Diagnosis

See Table 21–1.

Complications

Complications of chronic bacterial prostatitis may include ascending infection, infection-related stones, abscess, fistula, cysts, and acute urinary retention.

Treatment

Treatment with antibiotics used for prostatitis, such as trimethoprim, trimethoprim-sulfamethoxazole, or quinolones, has been suggested for up to 12 weeks in this rare population of patients.

Prognosis

The prognosis for treatment of chronic bacterial prostatitis is not known. A clear differentiation of which patients will respond to antibiotics and which will not has not been made.

CHRONIC ABACTERIAL PROSTATITIS/ CHRONIC PELVIC PAIN SYNDROME

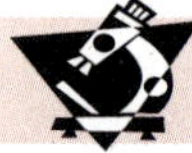

ESSENTIALS OF DIAGNOSIS

- *Not very well characterized; most suggestive symptoms include:*
- *Perineal pain.*
- *Lower abdominal pain.*
- *Penile, especially penile tip, pain.*
- *Testicular pain.*
- *Ejaculatory discomfort or pain.*
- *STDs and UTI ruled out.*

General Considerations

Chronic abacterial prostatitis was renamed by the NIH in 1995. It is now called *chronic pelvic pain syndrome* and can be further subclassified into inflammatory, meaning with inflammatory cells isolated in tests, or noninflammatory. This change was made in an attempt to recognize that the pain syndrome physicians have been referring to as "chronic abacterial prostatitis" or even "prostatodynia" in the absence of inflammatory cells on examination has never been proven to originate in the prostate.

This NIH categorization is still quite new, and, unfortunately, the literature has just begun to separate studies of chronic abacterial prostatitis into "inflammatory" and "noninflammatory" categories. In the "inflammatory" case, leukocytes are found in semen, in expressed prostatic secretions, or in a post-prostatic massage urine sample. In "noninflammatory" prostatitis, no leukocytes are found in secretions. Recent evidence suggests cytokines may play a role in diagnosis in the future. Current research efforts include the Chronic Prostatitis Clinical Research Network, funded in 1997 by the NIH to investigate the chronic pelvic pain syndrome. Their work is ongoing and not definitive at this time.

The etiology of chronic prostatitis remains unknown. Current theories include infection with unusual or fastidious organisms, lower urinary tract obstruction or dysfunctional voiding, intraprostatic ductal reflux and subsequent chemical irritation with urea from urine forced into the gland, immunologic or autoimmune processes, or neuromuscular causes, such as reflex sympathetic dystrophy. Although none of these theories has been proven, continued research, it is hoped, will increase our understanding of this problem.

Prevention

Trials of preventive measures for chronic prostatitis or chronic pelvic pain syndrome are lacking, and risk factors for prostatitis or chronic pelvic pain have not been investigated.

Clinical Findings

A. Symptoms and Signs

Symptoms include dysuria, frequency, urgency, other irritative voiding symptoms, and pain in the perineal area for more than 3 of the last 6 months.

B. Laboratory Findings

Laboratory testing shows no evidence of current cystitis or demonstrable bacterial infection. Patients with inflammatory-type chronic pelvic pain syndrome have leukocytes in expressed prostatic secretions or post-prostatic massage urine.

C. Special Tests

If the patient has hematuria, urine cytology should be performed. The two-glass test (first part of a clean-catch urine sample in one bottle; prostatic massage milking from periphery to center; second urine sample into a sterile container) has been shown to be as reliable as the more complicated four-glass test (discussed earlier) at distinguishing inflammatory or chronic bacterial prostatitis from noninflammatory prostatitis.

Differential Diagnosis

See Table 21–1.

Treatment

There is no clear-cut prescription for the treatment of chronic prostatitis of either the inflammatory or noninflammatory type. This treatment discussion therefore groups inflammatory and noninflammatory prostatitis into one entity for discussion. Type-specific information should be published soon.

Trials performed to date have investigated α-blockers (prostatitis from benign prostatic hypertrophy [BPH] or obstructive symptoms), antibiotics (prostatitis from unusual or fastidious organisms), nonsteroidal anti-inflammatory drugs (NSAIDs; prostatitis from inflammation), pentosan polysulfate (prostatitis as a form of interstitial cystitis), allopurinol (irritation from urea in prostate after reflux), Quercitin (a bioflavonoid/herbal treatment), twice-weekly ejaculation (prostatitis from "congestion" in the gland), balloon dilation (see α-blockers), transurethral and transrectal thermal treatment, transurethral needle ablation of the prostate, transurethral resection of the prostate, and radical prostatectomy.

The Cochrane Review, looking at treatments for chronic prostatitis, reported that antibiotics and α-blockers are not supported by the current literature, and that thermotherapy shows promising results but requires further investigation. Allopurinol was shown in one well-designed trial to be of benefit, but the mechanism of action is unclear, and a change in practice is not strongly recommended. Table 21–2 reviews controlled trials that have shown possible efficacy of treatments.

Despite the lack of evidence for efficacy, 28- to 42-day courses of antibiotics suitable for bacterial prostati-

Table 21–2. Effective therapies for chronic bacterial prostatitis.

Therapy	Dose	Comments
Finasteride	5 mg every day	Symptom score but not pain score dropped in one small, pilot study; placebo group had less pain to start, results may therefore be spurious[1]
Terazosin	1 mg every day for 4 days 2 mg every day for 10 days 5 mg every day for 12 wk	1.5-fold greater reduction in NIH symptom scores with terazosin than without; responders had lower pain scores to start; moderate benefit only[2]
Tamsulosin	0.4 mg every day	One small trial showed an 8-point reduction in NIH symptom scores overall; drug is well tolerated but needs to be taken for > 2 wk[3]
Quercitin	500 mg twice a day	Small pilot study with good preliminary results; decrease in symptoms from 21 (NIH) to 13 in active drug; 67% of patients on quercitin responded (with a 25% improvement in symptoms) versus 20% of placebo patients. The addition of bromelain and papain (Prosta-Q) in an open-label trial increased the response rate to 82%[4]
Allopurinol		Per the Cochrane Review, one small trial provided some evidence of benefit[5]
Pentosan polysulfate	100 mg three times a day for 6 months	Minimal improvement, with borderline statistical signficance[6]
Thermotherapy		Not enough data at this time to be considered anything but experimental[7]

[1]Leskinen M et al: Effects of finasteride in patients with inflammatory chronic pelvic pain syndrome: A double-blind, placebo-controlled, pilot study. Urology 1999;53:502.
[2]Cheah PY et al: Terazosin therapy for chronic prostatitis/chronic pelvic pain syndrome: A randomized, placebo controlled trial. J Urol 2003;169:592.
[3]Nickel JC et al: Treatment of chronic prostatitis/chronic pelvic pain syndrome with tamsulosin: A randomized double blind trial. J Urol 2004;171:1594.
[4]Shoskes DA et al: Quercetin in men with category III chronic prostatitis: a preliminary prospective, double-blind, placebo-controlled trial. Urology 1999;54:960.
[5]McNaughton CO, Wilt T: Allopurinol for chronic prostatitis. Cochrane Database Syst Rev 2002(4):CD001041.
[6]Nickel JC et al: Pentosan polysulfate sodium therapy for men with chronic pelvic pain syndrome: A multicenter, randomized, placebo controlled study. J Urol 2005;173:1252.
[7]Zeitlin SI: Heat therapy in the treatment of prostatitis. Urology 2002;60(suppl):38.

tis continue to be used by practitioners and suggested by panels of experts.

Prognosis

The prognosis for chronic prostatitis and chronic pelvic pain syndrome category III is not good. Prognosis appears to be worse for patients with previous episodes or more severe pain.

McNaughton CM et al: Diagnosis and treatment of chronic abacterial prostatitis: A systematic review. Ann Intern Med 2000; 133:367. [PMID: 10979882]

McNaughton C et al: Interventions for chronic abacterial prostatitis. Cochrane Database Syst Rev 2001;(1):CD002080. [PMID: 11279750]

McNaughton CO, Wilt T: Allopurinol for chronic prostatitis. Cochrane Database Syst Rev 2002;(4):CD001041. [PMID: 125194549]

Schaeffer AJ et al: Demographic and clinical characteristics of men with chronic prostatitis: The National Institutes of Health chronic prostatitis cohort study. J Urol 2002;168:593. [PMID: 12131316]

Schaeffer AJ et al: Overview summary statement. Diagnosis and management of chronic prostatitis/chronic pelvic pain syndrome (CP/CPPS). Urology 2002;60:1. [PMID: 12521576]

Turner JA et al: Prognosis of patients with new prostatitis/pelvic pain syndrome episodes. J Urol 2004;172:538. [PMID: 15247724]

UNCOMPLICATED BACTERIAL CYSTITIS

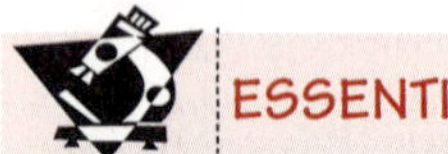

ESSENTIALS OF DIAGNOSIS

- *Dysuria.*
- *Frequency, urgency, or both.*
- *Urine dipstick analysis positive for nitrites or leukocyte esterase.*
- *Positive urine culture (> 10^4 organisms).*
- *No vaginal discharge, fever, or flank pain.*

General Considerations

Acute, uncomplicated cystitis is most common in women. Approximately one third of all women have experienced at least one episode of cystitis by the age of 24 years, and nearly half will experience at least one episode during their lifetime. Studies have established the pretest probability (the probability for disease before any tests are applied) of UTI for any young woman is 5%. However, once the young woman presents to a health care provider with one or more symptoms, her probability of UTI increases to approximately 50%. Young women's risk factors include sexual activity, use of spermicidal condoms or diaphragm, and genetic factors such as blood type or maternal history of recurrent cystitis. Healthy, noninstitutionalized older women can also experience recurrent cystitis. Risk factors among these women include changes in the perineal epithelium and vaginal microflora after the menopause, incontinence, diabetes, and history of cystitis before the menopause.

Although men can also suffer from cystitis, it is rare (annual incidence: < 0.01% of men aged 21–50 years) in men with normal urinary anatomy who are younger than 35 years. Urethritis from sexually transmitted pathogens should always be considered in this age group, and prostatitis should always be ruled out in the older age group by a rectal examination. Any cystitis in a man is complicated, due to the presence of the prostate gland, and should be treated for 10–14 days to prevent a persistent prostatic infection.

Prevention

A. Young Women

Considering the frequency and morbidity of cystitis among young women, it is hardly surprising that the lay press and medical literature contain a host of ideas about how to prevent recurrent cystitis. These range from the suggestion that cotton underwear is "healthier" to wiping habits, voiding habits, and choice of beverage. Unfortunately, the vast majority of these preventive measures do not hold up to scientific study (Table 21–3).

Recent studies have shown no effect of back-to-front wiping, pre- or postcoital voiding, tampon use, underwear fabric choice, or use of noncotton hose or tights. Behaviors that do appear to have an impact on frequency of cystitis in young women include sexual activ-

Table 21–3. UTI risk in young women.

Factors with No Evidence of Effect on Cystitis	Factors with Evidence for Effect on Cystitis	
	Promote	Prevent
Precoital voiding	Spermicide[1]	Cranberry juice
Postcoital voiding	Diaphragm[1]	Prophylactic
Underwear fabric	Cervical cap[1]	Antibiotics
Wiping pattern	Sexual activity	
Douching	Genetic predisposition	
Hot tub use		

[1]Spermicide on condoms, as contraceptive foam [Hooton TM et al: *Escherichia coli* bacteriuria and contraceptive method. JAMA 1991;265:64.], in diaphragms, and in cervical caps has been shown to adversely affect the vaginal flora, predisposing to *E coli* colonization and UTI.

ity (four or more episodes per month in one study), use of spermicidal condoms (several studies), use of unlubricated condoms (one study), use of diaphragms or cervical caps, and intake of cranberry juice.

It can be concluded from Table 21–3 that there are few behaviorally oriented strategies that can be offered to young women who suffer from recurrent cystitis. Recommending a change in contraception to oral contraceptive pills, intrauterine devices, or nonspermicidal, lubricated condoms may be helpful.

The cranberry juice question is a bit more complicated. Only one study investigated the effects of cranberry juice cocktail; it showed efficacy in preventing adhesion of trimethoprim-sulfamethoxazole resistant bacteria. Other published studies used pure cranberry juice or cranberry tablets, the optimal dose of which has not been determined. Doses ranged from 200 mL once a day to 250 mL three times a day. Although studies have shown that the cost of daily ingestion of cranberry juice far outweighs that of prophylactic antibiotics, for patients who prefer not to use medications or practitioners concerned about antibiotic resistance, suggesting a trial of cranberry juice, one to three glasses daily, or cranberry tablets twice a day (1:30 concentration minimum) is reasonable.

Prophylactic antibiotics, either low-dose daily antibiotics or postcoital antibiotics, remain the mainstay of prevention for young women and can reduce recurrence rates up to 95%.

B. Postmenopausal Women

Risk factors for cystitis in older women include urologic factors such as incontinence, cystocele, and postvoid residual; hormonal factors resulting in a lack of protective lactobacillus colonization; and a prior history of cystitis. For the above-metioned risk factors, the most easily administered effective prevention is estrogen.

There are many possible ways to administer estrogen. These include traditional oral hormone replacement therapy, which is still considered indicated (after thorough discussion with the patient of risks and benefits) for menopausal symptoms; vaginal estrogen rings; or creams.

Estriol is an end-product, low-potency estrogen that preferentially binds to urogenital binding sites, not endometrial sites. It is therefore safe to administer on its own, either as a cream or an oral pill, without adding progesterone. Overall levels of estrogen are lower when administered in pill form rather than as a cream, because of the first-pass effect of the liver on estriol, but endometrial response may be greater to the pill than the cream. Contraindications to estriol (as with all estrogens) include a history of endometrial carcinoma, breast carcinoma, thromboembolic disorders, and liver disease. Consideration should be made of patients' functional and cultural abilities before prescribing vaginal applications.

Only one study to date has investigated use of cranberry juice to prevent UTIs in hospitalized older women. Unfortunately, the study group had fewer UTIs than expected and was thus underpowered. It is likely that cranberry juice could help older women as well as younger; however, this has not been proven.

C. Young Men

The only studies focusing on prevention of UTI in young men have investigated infant circumcision, because the risk of UTI is so low in normal men these studies are prohibitively expensive. The risk of UTI in normal boys hovers around 1% in the first 10 years of life; given that, the number needed to treat (NNT) for circumcision is 111. In boys with recurrent UTI or high-grade ureteral reflux, the NNTs are 11 and 4, respectively. The complication rate of circumcision is 2–10%, with adverse sequelae ranging from minor transient bleeding (common) to amputation of the penis (extremely rare).

D. Future Trends in Prevention

Several investigators are currently evaluating the use of probiotics and vaccines for the prevention of UTI. Probiotics are benign living organisms, which in this case are used to bolster the vaginal flora. They then defend against pathologic bacteria by competing for adhesion receptors and nutrients. Some species, such as *Lactobacillus,* even produce antimicrobial substances. Vaginal vaccines are working their way through clinical trials and are not yet commercially available; whether they will prove to be more efficacious than prophylactic antibiotics is yet to be determined. One study explored intentional colonization of the urothelium with *Escherichia coli* 83972 in spinal patients; there was colonization in 13 of 21 participants, which lasted for a mean of 12.3 years. During that time no colonized patient had a symptomatic UTI.

Clinical Findings

A. Symptoms and Signs

Symptoms include dysuria, ideally felt more internally than externally, and of sudden onset; suprapubic pain; cloudy, smelly urine; frequency; and urgency.

Physical examination in the afebrile, otherwise healthy patient with a classic history is done essentially to rule out other diagnoses and to ensure that "red flags" are not present. The examination might range from checking a temperature and percussing the costovertebral angles to a full pelvic examination, depending on where the history leads. There are no pathognomonic signs on physical examination for cystitis (Table 21–4).

B. Laboratory Findings

Laboratory studies include dipstick test of urine, urinalysis, and urine culture. In some cases laboratory tests

Table 21–4. Likelihood ratios (LRs) of signs and symptoms of uncomplicated UTI in healthy, nonpregnant women.

Symptom or Sign	+LR	–LR
Dysuria and frequency *without* vaginal discharge or irritation	**24.6**[1]	—
Self-diagnosis of UTI	**4.0**	**0.0**
Hematuria	**2.0**	0.9
Frequency	**1.8**	0.6
Costovertebral angle tenderness on physical examination	**1.7**	0.9
Back pain	**1.6**	**0.8**
Dysuria	**1.5**	**0.5**
Vaginal discharge on physical examination	**0.7**	1.1
Dysuria or frequency *with* vaginal irritation or discharge	**0.7**	—
Vaginal discharge or irritation *without* dysuria	**0.3**	—
Vaginal irritation	**0.2**	2.7

[1]Bold values are significant.

Reproduced, with permission, from Bent S et al: Does this woman have an acute uncomplicated urinary tract infection? JAMA 2002;287:2701.

are not required to diagnose cystitis with high accuracy; however, they should probably only be omitted in settings where follow-up can be easily arranged in case of failure of treatment, which would of course indicate further workup. Figure 21–1 provides a diagnostic algorithm for cystitis.

1. Urine dipstick testing—Dipstick findings are positive for leukocyte esterase or nitrite, or both. Several references now support treatment of simple, uncomplicated UTI in the young, nonpregnant woman on the grounds of clinical history alone, if that history leads to high suspicion for cystitis (and low suspicion of STD). For women with an equivocal clinical history, urine dipstick analysis may be enough to reassign the women to high or low suspicion and treat or not treat accordingly. One study, using 10^4 organisms on culture as its gold standard, had a false-positive rate of 11% and a false-negative rate of 31% by sequencing clinical impression and dipstick results for diagnosis. These numbers seem high, but they are in fact comparable to other studies using rapid diagnostic methods.

2. Urinalysis—Urinalysis will be positive for WBCs, with no epithelial cells. It should be noted, however, that urinalysis is more expensive than dipstick analysis and only minimally more accurate.

3. Urine culture—One of the reasons a diagnostic algorithm is difficult to define for cystitis is that there is no agreement on what constitutes the gold standard. Some clinicians are pushing for symptoms of cystitis with as few as 100 (10^2) organisms on culture, whereas others stick to the traditional gold standard of 100,000 (10^5). Most laboratories are not equipped to detect anything fewer than 10^4 organisms. Culture is strongly suggested if a relapsing UTI or pyelonephritis is suspected to be sure of sensitivities and eradication (see Figure 21–1).

C. Imaging Studies

Imaging studies generally are not required for patients with simple uncomplicated UTIs.

D. Special Tests

These tests are generally required only for failures of treatment, symptoms suggesting a diagnosis other than cystitis, or complicated cystitis (see Complicated Cystitis, later).

Differential Diagnosis

See Table 21–5.

Complications

There are virtually no complications from repeated uncomplicated cystitis if it is recognized and treated. Delay in treatment may lead to ascending infection and pyelonephritis, but this has not been confirmed. In the case of infection with urea-splitting bacteria, "infection stones" of struvite with bacteria trapped in the interstices may be formed. These stones lead to persistent bacteriuria and must be completely removed to clear the infection. *Proteus mirabilis, S saprophyticus,* and *Klebsiella* bacteria can all split urea and lead to stones.

Treatment

A. Acute Cystitis

Current evidence-based guidelines are available from the Infectious Diseases Society of America for the treatment of uncomplicated acute bacterial cystitis in women (http://www.journals.uchicago.edu/IDSA/guidelines/p745.pdf). The guidelines note that there is evidence from randomized clinical trials to support 3-day antibiotic therapy as superior to 1-day treatment and equivalent to therapy for longer periods of time. This is true for treatment of older, noninstitutionalized women as well. Trimethoprim-sulfamethoxazole, in the absence of allergies to sulfa and local resistance rates greater than 10–20%, should be considered first-line therapy. Risk factors for trimethoprim-sulfamethoxazole resistance include recent antibiotic exposure, recent hospitalization, diabetes mellitus, three or more UTIs in the past year, and possibly use of oral contraceptive pills or estrogen

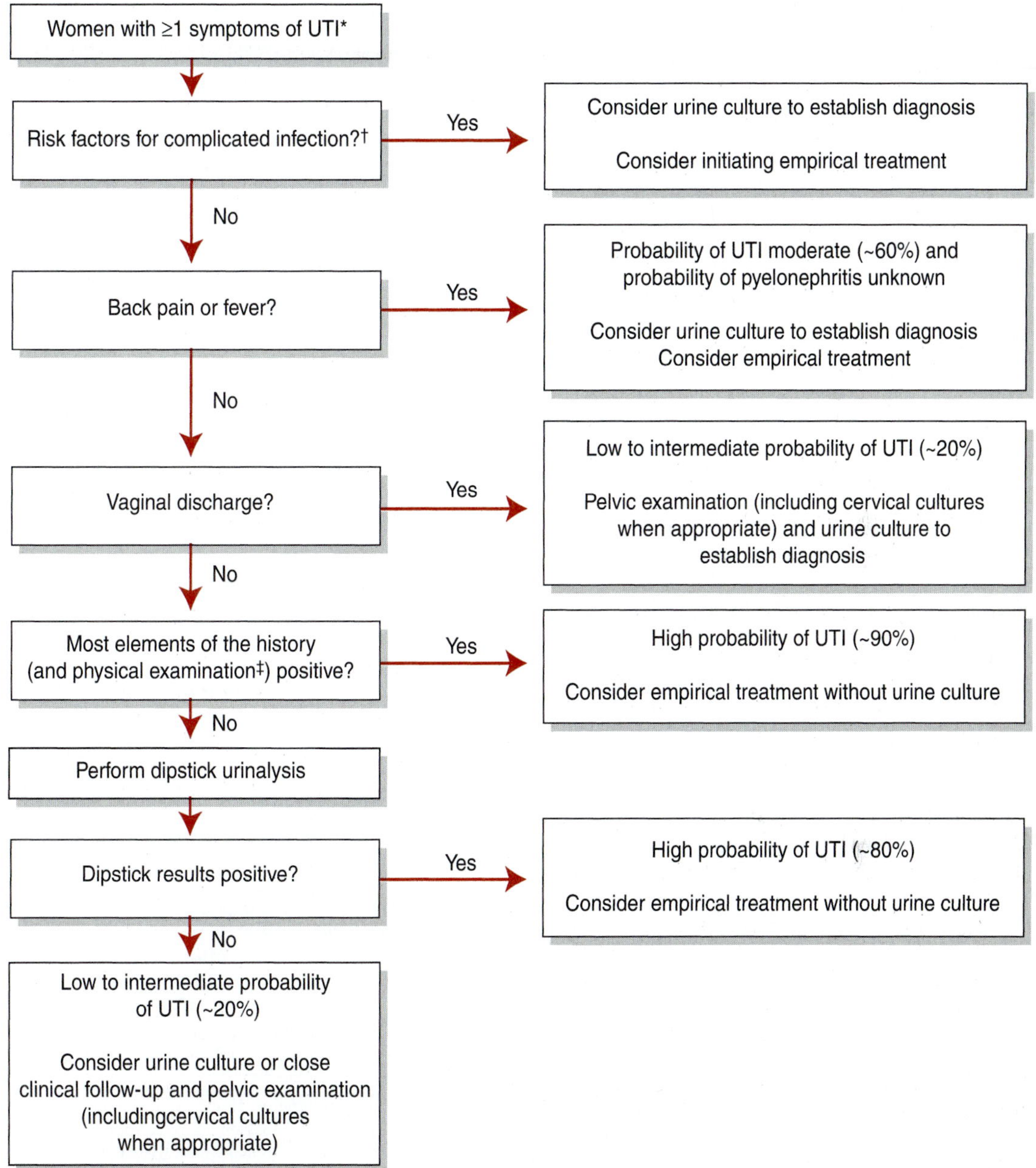

Figure 21–1. Diagnostic algorithm for cystitis. STD, sexually transmitted disease; UTI, urinary tract infection. (Reproduced, with permission, from Bent S et al: Does this woman have an acute uncomplicated urinary tract infection? JAMA 2002; 287:2701.)

*In women who have risk factors for sexually transmitted dieases (STDs), consider testing for chlamydia. The US Preventative Services Task Force recommends screnning for chlamydia for all women 25 years or younger and women of any age with more than 1 sex partner, a history of STD, or inconsistent use of condoms.

†For a definition of complicated UTI, see text.

‡The only physical examination finding that increases the likelihood of UTI is costovertebral angle tenderness, and clinicians may consider not performing this test in patient with typical symptoms of acute uncomplicated UTI (as in telephone management).

Table 21–5. Red flag symptoms and differential diagnoses.

If Patient Has	Consider
Fever	Urosepsis, pyelonephritis, pelvic inflammatory disease (PID)
Vaginal discharge	Sexually transmitted disease (STD), PID
External burning pain	Vulvovaginitis, especially candidal vaginitis
Costovertebral angle tenderness	Pyelonephritis
Nausea/vomiting	Pyelonephritis, urosepsis, inability to tolerate oral medications
Recent UTI (<2 wk)	Incompletely treated, resistant pathogen; urologic abnormality, including stones and unusual anatomy; interstitial cystitis
Dyspareunia	STD, PID, psychogenic causes
Recent trauma or instrumentation	Complicated UTI
Pregnancy	Antibiotic choice, treatment duration
Severe, colicky flank pain	UTI complicated by stones; preexisting or struvite stone caused by urea-splitting bacteria
Joint pains, sterile urine	Spondyloarthropathy, eg, Reiter or Behçet syndrome
History of childhood infections, urologic surgery	Abnormal anatomy
History of kidney stones	Complicated UTI; bacterial persistence in stones
Diabetes	Complicated UTI
Immunosuppression	Complicated UTI

replacement therapy. Use of fluoroquinolones as first-line therapy should be discouraged, considering the frequency of cystitis and the consequent potential for antibiotic resistance. β-Lactam antibiotics are not as effective as other classes of drugs against urinary pathogens and should not be used as first-line agents except in pregnant patients.

B. Acute Cystitis in the Pregnant Woman

Treatment with amoxicillin, nitrofurantoin, or another pregnancy-safe antibiotic for 7 days remains the standard, with follow-up cultures to demonstrate bacterial eradication. Asymptomatic bacteriuria, if found on cultures, is treated in pregnant women with the same antibiotics (see Asymptomatic Bacteriuria, earlier).

C. Prophylaxis for Recurrent Cystitis

Low-dose, prophylactic antibiotics have been shown to decrease recurrences by up to 95%. Most recommendations suggest starting prophylaxis after a patient has had more than three documented UTIs in 1 year. Prophylactic antibiotics are usually administered for 6 months to 1 year but can be given for longer periods of time. Antibiotics can be taken daily at bedtime or used postcoitally by women whose infections are associated with intercourse (Table 21–6). Unfortunately, prophylaxis does not change the propensity of these women for recurrent UTIs; when prophylaxis is stopped, approximately 60% of women develop a UTI within 3–4 months. Prophylaxis should not start until cultures have shown no growth after treatment, to rule out bacterial persistence.

Prognosis

Long-term prognosis in terms of kidney function is excellent; prognosis of arresting recurrent cystitis without permanent prophylaxis is not as good. New preventative treatments are currently being explored and it is hoped these will prove beneficial.

Bent S et al: Does this woman have an acute uncomplicated urinary tract infection? JAMA 2002;287:2701. [PMID: 12020306]

Hu KK et al: Risk factors for urinary tract infections in postmenopausal women. Arch Intern Med 2004;164:989. [PMID: 15136308]

Hull R et al: Urinary tract infection prophylaxis using *Escherichia coli* 83972 in spinal cord injured patients. J Urol 2000;163:872. [PMID: 10687996]

Kiel RJ et al: Clinical inquiries. Does cranberry juice prevent or treat urinary tract infection? J Fam Pract 2003;52:154. [PMID: 12585995]

Naber KG: Treatment options for acute uncomplicated cystitis in adults. J Antimicrob Chemother 2000;46(suppl 1):23; discussion 63. [PMID: 11051620]

Raz R: Hormone replacement therapy or prophylaxis in postmenopausal women with recurrent urinary tract infection. J Infect Dis 2001;183(suppl 1):S74. [PMID: 1171020]

Raz R et al: Recurrent urinary tract infections in postmenopausal women. Clin Infect Dis 2000;30:152. [PMID: 10619744]

Uehling DT et al: Phase 2 clinical trial of a vaginal mucosal vaccine for urinary tract infections. J Urol 2003;170:867. [PMID: 12913718]

Vogel T et al: Optimal duration of antibiotic therapy for uncomplicated urinary tract infection in older women: A double-blind randomized controlled trial. CMAJ 2004;170:469. [PMID: 14970093]

COMPLICATED CYSTITIS & SPECIAL POPULATIONS

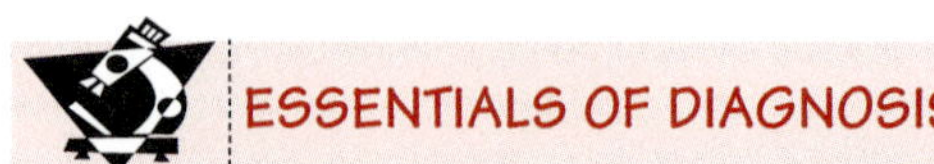

- *Any cystitis not resolved after 3 days of appropriate antibiotic treatment.*

- *Any cystitis in a special population, such as:*
  - *A diabetic patient.*
  - *A man.*
  - *A patient with an abnormal urinary tract.*
  - *A patient with stones.*
  - *A pregnant woman.*
- *Any cystitis involving multiply resistant bacteria.*

General Considerations

These are the infections for which a physician should consider further workup or referral to a urologist. These infections should all be cultured to be sure the antibiotics used are appropriate and that the organisms are sensitive to the chosen antibiotic.

Clinical Findings

Special tests should include x-ray or computed tomography (CT) to evaluate for stones, intravenous pyelogram (IVP) to evaluate anatomy and stones, and cystoscopy and biopsy to rule out interstitial cystitis, cancer, or unusual pathogens.

Treatment

Patients with complicated UTIs should be treated with long-course (10- to 14-day or more), appropriate antibiotics. Single-dose or 3-day regimens are not appropriate for this group of patients.

PYELONEPHRITIS

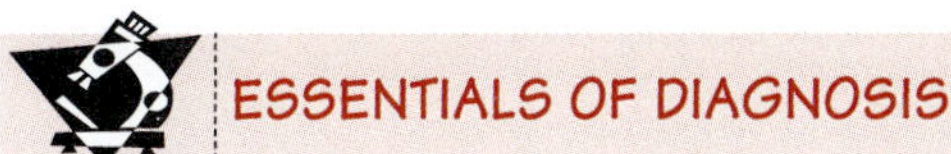

ESSENTIALS OF DIAGNOSIS

- *Fever.*
- *Chills.*
- *Flank pain.*
- *More than 100,000 CFU on urine culture.*

General Considerations

Pyelonephritis is an infection of the kidney parenchyma. It has been estimated to result in more than 100,000 hospitalizations per year. Information on outpatient visits is not easily available, but because many cases are now managed on an outpatient basis, it is likely to be seen by most primary care providers. Pyelonephritis usually results from upward spread of cystitis but can also result from hematogenous seeding of the kidney from another infectious source. The infection can be complicated by stones or renal scarring if untreated but usually resolves without sequelae in young healthy people if treated promptly.

The most common bacteria involved are the same organisms that cause uncomplicated cystitis: *E coli, S saprophyticus, Klebsiella* species, and occasionally *Enterobacter*. As with simple cystitis, women with genetic predispositions are more commonly affected than other women.

Table 21–6. Prophylactic antibiotics for recurrent UTI in women.

Regimen	Drug and Dose
Daily	Trimethoprim ,100 mg every day
	Nitrofurantoin, 50 mg every day[1]
	Nitro. macrocrystals, 100 mg every day
	Co-Trimoxazole, 240 mg every day
	Cranberry juice, 250 mL three times a day
	Cranberry tablets, 1:30 twice a day
Postcoital	One dose of any of the above antibiotics after coitus

[1]Preferred if patient could become pregnant. Trimethoprim should be avoided in the first trimester.

Prevention

There are no recent studies on prevention of pyelonephritis. Prompt treatment of cystitis may prevent some cases of pyelonephritis, but this has not been demonstrated.

Clinical Findings

Symptoms and signs include fever, chills, and malaise; dysuria; and flank pain. Nausea and vomiting may also occur.

Laboratory findings include a urine dipstick analysis that is positive for leukocyte esterase or nitrites and urine culture showing more than 100,000 CFU.

Imaging studies generally are not required unless the patient is diabetic or there is suspicion that stones are complicating the infection, in which case a CT scan is the test of choice.

Differential Diagnosis

SeeTable 21–7.

Complications

Diabetic patients can experience emphysematous pyelonephritis. This is diagnosed by an x-ray or other imag-

Table 21–7. Differential diagnosis of pyelonephritis.

If Patient Has	Consider
Negative urine dipstick or culture	Pelvic inflammatory disease; stone obstructing ureter; lower-lobe pneumonia; herpes zoster
Guarding/rebound	Acute cholecystitis; acute appendicitis; perforated viscus
Recurrent infection	Kidney stone, spontaneous or infection related; anatomic abnormality; resistant organism; inadequate treatment
Diabetes	Emphysematous pyelonephritis
History of childhood infections, urologic surgery	Abnormal anatomy
History of kidney stones	Pyelonephritis complicated by stones

ing study showing gas in the renal collecting system or around the kidney. In a diabetic patient, the treatment of choice is emergency nephrectomy, as the mortality rate in diabetics approaches 75%. This condition may rarely occur in nondiabetic patients and is often related to obstruction. In some of these cases relief of the obstruction and antibiotics may suffice.

Stones can complicate pyelonephritis by causing a partial or complete obstruction. These stones can be spontaneous or "infection" stones of struvite, caused by urea-splitting organisms. Stones complicating pyelonephritis must be removed before the infection will completely resolve.

People with a history of childhood pyelonephritis can have renal scarring and recurrent infections. These scars are unusual in healthy adults with pyelonephritis. Young men with pyelonephritis should be investigated for a cause.

Patients who do not respond to 48 hours of appropriate antibiotics should be worked up for occult complicating factors or other diagnoses.

Treatment

The best drugs for treatment of pyelonephritis are bactericidal, with a broad spectrum to cover gram-positive and gram-negative bacteria, and concentrate well in urine and renal tissues. Aminoglycosides; aminopenicillins such as amoxicillin with or without clavulanic acid, ticarcillin, or piperacillin; cephalosporins; fluoroquinolones; or, in extreme cases, imipenem, are all appropriate. First-line outpatient treatment is usually a fluoroquinolone. There are no recent studies, but cure rates have been reported to approach 90% with a 10- to 14-day course of antibiotics.

Patients experiencing severe nausea and vomiting who are unable to tolerate oral agents may need to be hospitalized for parenteral therapy. Patients with severe illness, suspected bacteremia, or sepsis should also be admitted.

Prognosis

Prognosis after an acute episode of uncomplicated pyelonephritis in a previously healthy adult is excellent.

Ramakrishnan K, Scheid DC: Diagnosis and management of acute pyelonephritis in adults. Am Fam Physician 2005;71:933. [PMID: 15768623]

Arthritis: Osteoarthritis, Gout, & Rheumatoid Arthritis

22

Bruce E. Johnson, MD

Arthritis is a complaint and a disease afflicting many patients and accounting for upwards of 10% of appointments to a generalist practice. Arthritis is multifaceted and can be categorized in several different fashions. For simplicity, this chapter focuses on conditions affecting the anatomic joint composed of cartilage, synovium, and bone. Other discussions would include localized disorders of the periarticular region (eg, tendonitis and bursitis) and systemic disorders that have arthritic manifestations (eg, vasculitides, polymyalgia rheumatica, and fibromyalgia). The chapter discusses three prototypical types of arthritis: osteoarthritis, as an example of a cartilage disorder; gout, as an example of both a crystal-induced arthritis and an acute arthritis; and rheumatoid arthritis, as an example of an immune-mediated, systemic disease and a chronic deforming arthritis.

OSTEOARTHRITIS

ESSENTIALS OF DIAGNOSIS

- *Degenerative changes in the knee, hip, thumb, ankle, foot, or spine.*
- *Pain with movement that improves with rest.*
- *Synovitis.*
- *Sclerosis, thickening, spurs formation, warmth, and effusion in the joints.*

General Considerations

Arthritis is among the oldest identified conditions in humans. Anthropologists examining skeletal remains from antiquity deduce levels of physical activity and work by searching for the presence of osteoarthritis (OA). Similarly, OA is more prevalent among people in occupations characterized by steady, physically demanding activity such as farming, construction, and production-line work. Obesity is a significant risk factor for OA, especially of the knee, Heredity and gender play a role in a person's likelihood of developing OA, regardless of work or recreational activity.

Pathogenesis

Part of the pathophysiology of OA involves microfracture of cartilage with incomplete healing. Disruption of the otherwise smooth cartilage surface allows differential pressure on the underlying bone. The debris resulting from cartilage breakdown causes a low-level inflammation within the synovial fluid.

Prevention

It is difficult to advise patients on measures to prevent arthritis. Obese persons should lose weight, but few occupational or recreational precautions can be expected to alter the natural history of OA. Arthritis has multiple etiologies and no consistent preventive steps are available to patients.

Clinical Findings

A. Symptoms and Signs

Symptomatic OA represents the culmination of damage to cartilage, usually over many years. OA progresses from symptomatic pain to physical findings to loss of function. OA can occur at any joint, but the most commonly involved joints are the knee, hip, thumb (carpometacarpal), ankle, foot, and spine. The strongly inherited spur formation at the distal interphalangeal joint (Heberden nodes) and proximal interphalangeal joint (Bouchard nodes) is often classified as OA, yet, although deforming, only infrequently causes pain or disability (Figure 22–1).

Cartilage has no pain fibers, so the pain of OA arises from secondary effects. Osteoarthritic pain is typically associated with movement, meaning that at rest the patient may be relatively asymptomatic. Recognition that at rest the joint is less painful can be maladaptive. Patients learn to "favor" the involved joint, leading to

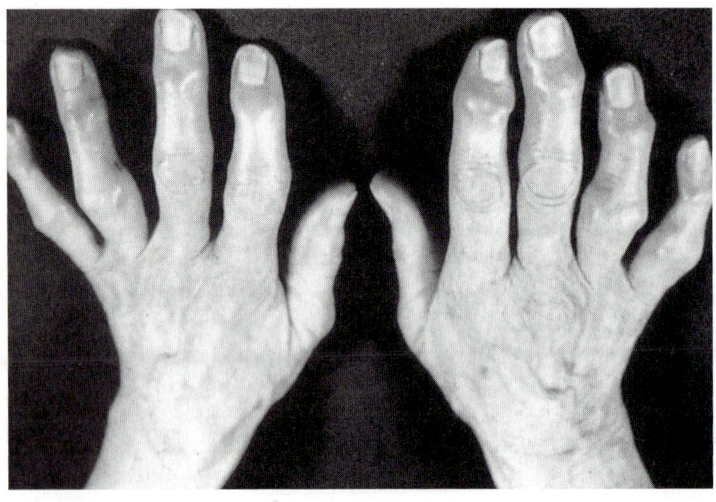

Figure 22–1. Heberden nodes (distal interphalangeal joint) noted on all fingers and Bouchard nodes (proximal interphalangeal joint) noted on most fingers.

disuse of supporting muscle groups and muscle weakness. Such weakness accounts for the complaint that a joint "gives way," resulting in dropped items (if at the wrist) or falls (if at the knee). In joints with mild OA, pain may counterintuitively improve with exercise or activity. At such joints, well-maintained muscle probably functions as a shock-absorber.

Advanced OA is characterized by bony destruction and alteration of joint architecture. Secondary spur formation with deformity, instability, or restricted motion is a common finding. Fingers, wrist, knees, and ankles appear abnormal and asymmetric. Warmth and effusion is seen in joints with advanced OA. At this stage, pain may be frequent and exacerbated by any movement, weight bearing or otherwise.

B. Laboratory Findings

There are few laboratory studies of relevance to the diagnosis of OA. Rarely, the erythrocyte sedimentation rate (ESR) will be raised, but only if an inflammatory effusion is present (and even then an elevated ESR or C-reactive protein is more likely to be misleading than helpful). If an effusion is present, arthrocentesis can be helpful in ruling out other conditions (see laboratory findings in gout, later).

OA can be secondary to other conditions, and these diseases have their own laboratory evaluation. Examples include OA secondary to hemochromatosis (elevated iron and ferritin, liver enzyme abnormalities), Wilson disease (elevated copper), acromegaly (elevated growth hormone), and Paget disease (elevated alkaline phosphatase).

C. Imaging Studies

Radiographs are usually not needed for the early diagnosis of OA. Indeed, radiographs may be misleading by suggesting more advanced disease than is consistent with the patient's symptoms. Plain films of joints afflicted with OA show changes of sclerosis, thickening, spur formation, loss of cartilage with narrowing of the joint space, and malalignment (Figure 22–2). Such radiographic changes occur relatively late in the disease process and do not always correlate with symptoms. Patients may complain of significant pain despite a relatively normal appearance of the joint and, conversely, considerable radiographic damage to a joint may exist with only modest symptoms. In addition, plain film radiography does not provide good information about cartilage, tendons, ligaments, or any soft tissue. Such findings may be crucial to explaining a patient complaint, especially if there is loss of function.

To see cartilage, ligaments, and tendon, magnetic resonance imaging (MRI) is important and, in many instances, essential. MRI can detect abnormalities of the meniscus or ligaments of the knee, cartilage or femoral head deterioration at the hip, misalignment at the elbow, rupture of muscle and fascia at the shoulder, and a host of other abnormalities. Any of these findings may be incorrectly diagnosed as "OA" before MRI scanning.

Computed tomography (CT) and ultrasonography have lesser, more specialized uses. CT, especially with contrast, can detect structural abnormalities of large joints such as the knee or shoulder. Ultrasonography is an inexpensive means of detecting joint or periarticular fluid, or unusual collections of fluid such as a popliteal (Baker) cyst at the knee.

Differential Diagnosis

In practice, it should not be difficult to differentiate among the three prototypical arthritides discussed in this chapter. Nonetheless, Table 22–1 suggests some key differential findings.

A common source of confusion and misdiagnosis occurs when a bursitis-tendinitis syndrome mimics the

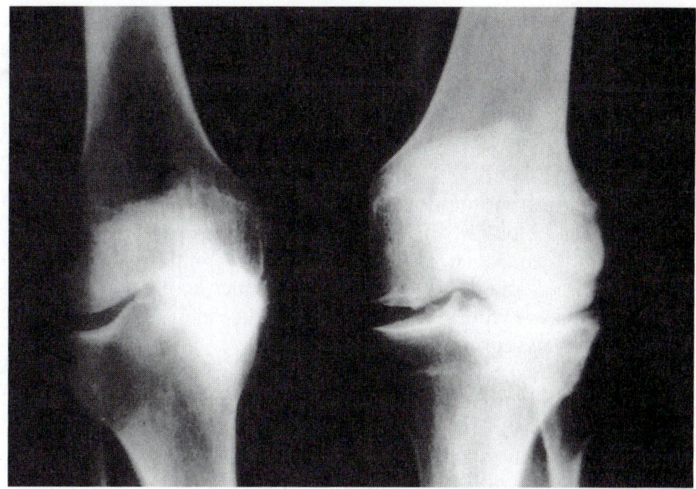

Figure 22–2. Osteoarthritis of the knees showing loss of joint space with marked reactive sclerosis and probable malalignment.

pain of OA. A common example is anserine bursitis. This bursitis, located medially at the tibial plateau, presents in a fashion similar to OA of the knee, but can be differentiated by a few simple questions and directed physical findings.

Treatment

With few exceptions, the early development of OA is silent. When pain occurs, and pain is almost always the presenting complaint, the osteoarthritic process has already likely progressed to joint destruction. Cartilage is damaged, bone reaction occurs, and debris mixes with synovial fluid. Consequently, when a diagnosis of OA is established, goals of therapy become control of pain, restoration of function, and reduction of disease progression. Although control of the patient's complaints is possible, and long periods of few or no symptoms may ensue, the patient permanently carries a diagnosis of OA.

Treatment of OA involves multiple modalities and is inadequate if only a prescription for antiinflammatory drugs is written. Patient education, assessment for physical therapy and devices, and consideration of intra-articular injections are additional measures in the total management of the patient.

Recommendations for the medical management of osteoarthritis of the hip and knee: 2000 update. American College of Rheumatology Subcommittee on Osteoarthritis Guidelines. Arthritis Rheum 2000;43:1905. [PMID: 11014340]

Table 22–1. Essentials of diagnosis.

	Osteoarthritis	Gout	Rheumatoid Arthritis
Key presenting symptoms	Pauciarticular. Pain with movement, improving with rest. Site of old injury (sport, trauma). Obesity. Occupation.	Monoarticular. Abrupt onset. Pain at rest and movement. Precipitating event (meal, physical stress). Family history.	Polyarticular. Gradual, symmetric involvement. Morning stiffness. Hands and feet initially involved more than large joints. Fatigue, poorly restorative sleep.
Key physical findings	Infrequent warmth, effusion. Crepitus. Enlargement/spur formation. Malalignment.	Podagra. Swelling, warmth. Exquisite pain with movement. Single joint (exceptions—plantar fascia, lumbar spine). Tophi.	Symmetric swelling, tenderness. MCP, MTP, wrist, ankle usually before larger, proximal joints. Rheumatoid nodules.
Key laboratory, x-ray findings	Few characteristic (early). Loss of joint space, spur formation, malalignment (late).	Synovial fluid with uric acid crystals. Elevated serum uric acid. 24 h urine uric acid.	Elevated ESR/CRP. Rheumatoid factor. Anemia of chronic disease. Early erosions on x-ray, osteopenia at involved joints.

MCP, metacarpophalangeal; MTP, metatarsophalangeal; ESR, erythrocyte sedimentation rate; CRP, C-reactive protein.

A. Patient Education

Patient education is a crucial step. The patient must be made aware of the role he or she plays in successful therapy. Many resources are available to assist the provider in patient education. Patient education pamphlets are widely available from government organizations, physician organizations (eg, American Academy of Family Physicians or American College of Physicians), insurance companies, pharmaceutical companies, or patient advocacy groups (eg, the Arthritis Foundation). Many communities have self-help or support groups that are rich sources of information, advice, and encouragement.

One of the most effective long-term measures to both improve symptoms and slow progression of disease is weight loss. Less weight carried by the hip, knee, ankle, or foot reduces stress on the involved arthritic joint, decreases the destructive processes, and probably slows progression of disease. Unfortunately, in many instances, OA makes weight loss more difficult as pain in the lower extremity joints limits exercise.

On the other hand, exercise is a crucial modality that should not be overlooked. Evaluation for appropriate exercise focuses on two issues: overall fitness and correction of any joint-specific disuse atrophy. One must be flexible in the choice of exercise. Swimming is an excellent exercise that limits stress on the lower extremities. Although many older persons are reluctant to learn to swim anew, they may be amenable to water aerobic exercises. These exercises encourage calorie expenditure, flexibility, and both upper and lower muscle strengthening in a supportive atmosphere. Stationary bicycle exercise is also accessible to most people, is easy to learn, and may be acceptable to those with arthritis of the hip, ankle or foot. Advice from a recreational therapist can be most helpful.

Thomas KS et al: Home based exercise programme for knee pain and knee osteoarthritis: Randomized controlled trial. BMJ 2002;325:752. [PMID: 12364304]

B. Physical Therapy and Assistive Devices

The pain of OA can result in muscular disuse. The best example is quadriceps weakness resulting from OA of the knee. The patient who "favors" the involved joint loses quadriceps strength. This has two repercussions: both cushioning (shock-absorption) and stabilization are lost. The latter is usually the cause of the knee "giving way." Sudden buckling at the knee, often when descending stairs, is not due to destruction of cartilage or bone but rather to inadequate strength in the quadriceps to handle the load required at the joint. Physical therapy with quadriceps strengthening is highly efficacious, resulting in improved mobility, increased patient confidence, and reduction in pain.

The physical therapist or physiatrist should also be consulted for advice regarding assistive devices. Advanced OA of lower extremity joints may cause instability and fear of falls that can be addressed by canes of various types. Altered posture or joint malalignment can be corrected by orthotics, which has the advantage, when used early, of slowing progression of OA. Braces can protect the truly unstable joint and permit continued ambulation.

C. Pharmacotherapy

The patient wants relief of pain. Despite the widespread promotion of nonsteroidal anti-inflammatory drugs (NSAIDs) for OA, there is no evidence that NSAIDs alter the course of the disease. That being the case, NSAIDs are used for their analgesic, rather than anti-inflammatory, effects. Although effective as analgesics, NSAIDs have significant side effects and are not necessarily first-line drugs.

Begin with adequate doses of acetaminophen. Acetaminophen should be prescribed in large doses, 3–4 g/day, and continued at this level until pain control is attained. Once pain is controlled, dosage can be reduced if possible. Maintenance of adequate blood levels is essential and because acetaminophen has a relatively short half-life, frequent dosing is necessary (three or four times a day). High doses of acetaminophen are generally well tolerated, although caution is important in patients with liver disease or in whom alcohol ingestion is heavy.

NSAIDs mixed as a cream and rubbed onto joints have long been advocated for small and even large joint arthritis. There undoubtedly is less GI upset when delivered in this manner but well-designed studies demonstrating prolonged effectiveness are lacking. There are two FDA-approved products on the US market, although some compounding pharmacies have these products available.

NSAIDs come in two main classes largely based on half-life. NSAIDs with shorter half-lives (eg, diclofenac, etodolac, ibuprofen, and indomethacin) need more frequent dosing than longer acting agents. Several NSAIDs are available in generic or over-the-counter form, which reduces cost. Despite differing pharmacology, there is little difference in efficacy, so choice of medication should be based on individual patient issues such as dosing intervals, tolerance, toxicity, and cost. As with acetaminophen, adequate doses must be used for maximal effectiveness. For example, ibuprofen at doses up to 800 mg three or four times a day should be maintained (if tolerated) before concluding that a different agent is necessary. Examples of NSAID dosing are given in Table 22–2.

D. Intra-articular Injections

Hyaluronic acid is a constituent of both cartilage and synovial fluid. Injection of hyaluronic acid, usually in a series of three to five weekly intra-articular insertions, is purported to provide improvement in symptomatic OA for up to 6 months. It is unknown why hyaluronic acid

Table 22–2. Selected nonsteroidal anti-inflammatory drugs with usual and maximal doses.

Drug	Frequency of Administration	Usual Daily Dose (mg/day)	Maximal Dose (mg/day)
Oxaprozin (eg, Daypro)	Every day	1200	1800
Piroxicam (eg, Feldene)	Every day	10–20	20
Nabumetone (eg, Relafen)	One to two times a day	1000–2000	2000
Sulindac (eg, Clinoril)	Twice a day	300–400	400
Naproxen (eg, Naprosyn)	Twice a day	500–1000	1500
Diclofenac (eg, Voltaren)	Two to four times a day	100–150	200
Ibuprofen (eg, Motrin)	Three to four times a day	600–1800	2400
Etodolac (eg, Lodine)	Three to four times a day	600–1200	1200
Ketoprofen (eg, Orudis)	Three to four times a day	150–300	300

helps; there is no evidence hyaluronic acid is incorporated into cartilage, and it does not slow the progression of OA. It is expensive and the injection process is painful. Use of this agent is limited to patients who have failed other forms of OA therapy.

Intra-articular injection of corticosteroids has been both under- and over utilized in the past. There is little question that steroid injection rapidly reduces inflammation and eases symptoms. The best case is one in which the patient has an exacerbation of pain accompanied by signs of inflammation (warmth, effusion). The knee is most commonly implicated and is most easily approached. Most authorities recommend no more than two injections during one episode and limiting injections to no more than two or three episodes per year. Benefits of injection are often shorter in duration than similar injection for tendinitis or bursitis, but the symptomatic improvement buys time to reestablish therapy with oral agents.

Arrich J: Intra-articular hyaluronic acid for the treatment of osteoarthritis of the knee: Systematic review and meta-analysis. CMAJ 2005;172:1039. [PMID: 15824412]

Arroll B: Corticosteroid injections for osteoarthritis of the knee: Meta-analysis. BMJ 2004;328:869. [PMID: 15039276]

E. Surgery

Until recently, orthopedic surgeons have performed arthroscopic surgery on osteoarthritic knees in an effort to remove accumulated debris and to polish or debride frayed cartilage. However, a clinical trial demonstrated that any purported benefit of this practice could be explained by the placebo effect. It remains to be seen if the numbers of these procedures will decline.

Joint replacement is a rapidly expanding option for treatment of OA, especially of the knee and hip. Pain is reduced or eliminated altogether. Mobility is improved, although infrequently to premorbid levels. Expenditures for total joint replacement are likely to increase dramatically as the baby-boomer generation reaches the age at which OA of large joints is more common. Indications for joint replacement (which also applies to other joints, including shoulder, elbow, and fingers) include pain poorly controlled with maximal therapy, malalignment, and decreased mobility. Improvement in pain relief and quality of life should be realized in about 90% of patients undergoing the procedure. Because complications of both the surgery and rehabilitation are increased by obesity, many orthopedic surgeons will not consider hip or knee replacement without at least an attempt by the patient to lose weight. Patients need to be in adequate medical condition to undergo the operation and even more so to endure the often lengthy rehabilitation process. Some surgeons refer patients for "prehabilitation" or physical training prior to the operation. Counseling of patients should include the fact that there often is a 4- to 6-month recovery period involving intensive rehabilitation.

Moseley JB et al: A controlled trial of arthroscopic surgery for osteoarthritis of the knee. New Engl J Med 2002;347:81. [PMID: 12110735]

F. Complementary and Alternative Therapies

Glucosamine, capsaicin, bee venom, and acupuncture have been promoted as alternative therapies for OA. Glucosamine and chondroitin sulfate are components of glycosaminoglycans, which make up cartilage, although there is no evidence that orally ingested glucosamine or chondroitin sulfate are actually incorporated into cartilage. Studies suggest these agents are superior to placebo in symptomatic relief of mild OA. The onset of action is delayed, sometimes by weeks, but the effect may be prolonged after treatment is stopped. Glucosamine-chondroitin sulfate combinations are available over the counter and are generally well tolerated by patients.

Capsaicin, a topically applied extract of the chili pepper relieves pain by depletion of substance P, a neuropeptide involved in pain sensation. Capsaicin is suggested for tendinitis or bursitis, but may be tried for OA of superficial joints such as the fingers. The cream should be applied three or four times a day for 2 weeks or more before making any conclusion regarding benefit.

Bee venom is prominently promoted in complementary medicine circles. A mechanism for action in OA is unclear. Although anecdotal reports are available, comparison studies to other established treatments are difficult to find.

Acupuncture can be useful in managing pain and improving function. There are more comparisons between acupuncture and conventional treatment for OA of the back and knee than for other joints. Generally, acupuncture is equivalent to oral treatments for mild symptoms at these two sites.

McAlindron TE et al: Glucosamine and chondroitin for treatment of osteoarthritis: A systemic quality assessment and meta-analysis. JAMA 2000;283:1469. [PMID: 10732937]

Prognosis

Restoring and rebuilding damaged cartilage is not possible at this time; hence, reversal of the pathophysiologic process in OA cannot be achieved. With adequate pain control, weight loss, appropriate exercise, orthotics and devices, and surgery, the successful management of osteoarthritis should be realized in most patients.

GOUT

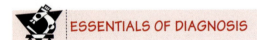

ESSENTIALS OF DIAGNOSIS

- *Podagra (intense inflammation of the first metatarsophalangeal joint).*
- *Inflammation of the overlying skin.*
- *Pain at rest and intense pain with movement.*
- *Swelling, warmth, redness, and effusion.*
- *Tophi.*
- *Elevated serum uric acid level.*

General Considerations

Gout, first described by Hippocrates in the fourth century BCE, has a colorful history, characterized as a disease of excesses, primarily gluttony. An association with diet is germane, as gout has a lower incidence in countries in which obesity is uncommon and the diet is relatively devoid of alcohol and reliance on meat and abdominal organs (liver, spleen). Gout is strongly hereditary as well, affecting as many as 25% of the men in some families.

Prevention

Despite the previously noted associations, it is difficult with any assurance to advise patients on measures to prevent gout. Even thin vegetarians develop gout, although at a markedly lower rate than obese, alcohol-drinking men. Gout has multiple etiologies and no consistent preventive steps are available to patients.

Clinical Findings

A. Symptoms and Signs

Gout classically presents as an acute monoarthritis. Podagra—abrupt, intense inflammation of the first metatarsophalangeal joint—remains the most common presentation (Figure 22–3). The first attack often occurs overnight, with intense pain awakening the patient. Any pressure, even a bed sheet on the toe, increases the agony. Walking is difficult. The overlying skin can be intensely inflamed. On questioning, an exacerbating event may be elicited. Common stories include an excess of alcohol, a heavy meal of abdominal organs, or a recent physiologic stress such as surgery or serious medical disease. Alcohol alters renal excretion of uric acid, allowing rapid buildup of serum uric acid levels. Foods such as liver, anchovies, sardines, asparagus, salmon, and legumes contain relatively large quantities of purines that, when broken down, become uric acid.

Acute gout is not limited to the great toe; any joint may be affected, although lower extremity joints are more common. The abruptness of many gouty attacks and the single joint presentation (acute monoarthritis) at any joint other than the great toe may lead to diagnostic confusion (Table 22–3).

Gout in joints other than the great toe is often misdiagnosed. Atypical gout is not uncommon in older women and in men who have already experienced multiple previous episodes of podagra. Foot pain simulating plantar fasciitis is seen in older women. Gout of the ankle (with a positive Homan sign) can be mistaken for phlebitis.

The intense inflammation at some joints, especially smaller joints such as the ankle, can be impressive. The inflammation may appear to be spreading, encompassing an area greater than that thought to be the joint. Such cases can be mistaken for cellulitis (see Figure 22–3) or superficial phlebitis. The subsequent lack of response to outpatient treatment of cellulitis can cascade to hospital admission and treatment with increasingly strong and expensive antibiotics.

Untreated, attacks of gout slowly resolve with the involved joint becoming progressively less symptomatic over 8–10 days. Long-standing gout is distinguished by the development of extra-articular manifestations. Tophi are deposits of urate crystals and are found in the ear helix or as nodules elsewhere; atypically placed tophi serve as the source of colorful medical anecdotes. Chronic, untreated

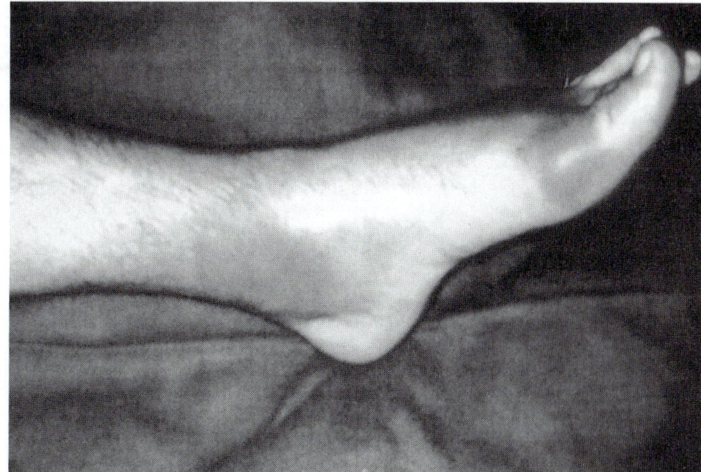

Figure 22–3. Classic podagra involving the first metatarsophalangeal joint. In this photo, the ankle is also involved and the intense erythema could be mistaken for cellulitis.

gout is a contributor to renal insufficiency (especially in association with heavy metal lead exposure).

Physiologic stress is a common precipitating factor for an acute attack. Monoarthritis within days of a surgical procedure raises concern of infection (which it should!) but is just as often due to crystal-induced gout or pseudogout. In some circumstances, prophylaxis in a person with known gout can prevent these attacks.

About 10% of kidney stones include uric acid. A person with nephrolithiasis due to uric acid stones need not have attacks of gout, but patients with gout are at increased risk of developing uric acid stones. A prior history of nephrolithiasis is an important factor in defining therapy in the patient with gout.

Gout is largely a disease of men, with a male-to-female ratio of 9:1. The first attack of podagra typically occurs in men in their 30s or 40s. One attack need not necessarily predict future attacks. In fact, in up to 20% of men who have one attack of gout a second attack never follows. Even after a second attack, a sizable percentage (as many as 5%) do not progress to chronic, recurrent gout.

Premenopausal women rarely have gout. Diagnosis of gout in postmenopausal women is infrequent, less because it does not occur than because it is uncommonly suspected.

B. Laboratory Findings

The fundamental abnormality in gout is excess uric acid. In most first attacks of gout, serum uric acid is elevated. In long-standing disease, the uric acid value may be normal yet symptoms still occur. It is important to note, however, that mild hyperuricemia has a rather high prevalence in the general population. Indeed, fewer than 25% of persons with elevated uric acid will ever have gout.

During acute attacks of gout, the white blood cell count may be slightly elevated and ESR increased, reflecting acute inflammation. Gout is not uncommon in chronic kidney disease and measurement of blood urea nitrogen and creatinine is recommended.

Gout usually results from either inappropriately low renal excretion of uric acid (implicated in 90% of patients) or abnormally high endogenous production of uric acid.

Table 22–3. Inflammatory and noninflammatory causes of monoarthritis.

Inflammatory	Noninflammatory
Crystal-induced	Fracture or meniscal tear
Gout	Other trauma
Pseudogout (calcium pyrophosphate deposition disease)	Osteoarthritis
Apatite (and others)	Tumors
Infectious	Osteochondroma
Bacteria	Osteoid osteoma
Fungi	Pigmented villonodular synovitis
Lyme disease or other spirochetes	Cancerous
Tuberculosis and other mycobacteria	Osteonecrosis
Viruses (eg, HIV, hepatitis B)	Hemarthrosis
Systemic diseases	Cancers
Psoriatic or other spondyloarthopathies	
Reactive (eg, inflammatory bowel, Reiter syndrome)	
Systemic lupus erythematosus	

Adapted from Schumacher HR: Signs and symptoms of musculoskeletal disorders. A. Monoarticular joint disease. In Klipper JH (editor). *Primer on the Rheumatic Diseases,* ed 11. Arthritis Foundation, 1997;116.

Table 22–4. Synovial fluid analysis in selected rheumatic diseases.

	Fluid	White Blood Cell Count	Differential	Glucose	Crystals
Gout	Clear/cloudy	10–100,000	>50% PMNs	Normal	Needle-shaped, negative birefringement
Pseudogout	Clear/cloudy	10–100,000	>50% PMNs	Normal	Rhomboid-shaped, positive birefringement
Infectious	Cloudy	>50,000	Often >95% PMNs	Decreased	None[1]
Osteoarthritis	Clear	2–10,000	<50% PMNs	Normal	None[1]
Rheumatoid arthritis	Clear	10–50,000	>50% PMNs	Normal or decreased	None[1]

PMNs, polymorphonuclear leukocytes.
[1]Debris in synovial fluid may be misleading on plain microscopy but only crystals respond to polarizing light.

Collecting a 24-hour urine sample for evaluation of uric acid and creatinine clearance can be useful in therapy.

For several reasons, a strong recommendation must be made to attempt arthrocentesis of the joint in suspected acute gout. First episodes of gout present as an acute monoarthritis, for which the differential diagnosis is noted in Table 22–3. Infectious arthritis is a medical emergency—the correct diagnosis must be made rapidly and appropriate antibiotic therapy begun to avoid destructive changes. Pseudogout is rarely distinguished from gout on the basis of symptoms alone. The settings of both pseudogout and gout can be similar (eg, immediately after surgery). Clinical features of many of the monoarthritides are not characteristic enough to ensure a correct diagnosis. However, finding negatively birefringent needle-shaped crystals in synovial fluid is diagnostic of gout. Characteristics of synovial fluid in selected disease settings are highlighted in Table 22–4.

C. Imaging Studies

Radiographs are not needed for the diagnosis of gout. Other means of diagnosing gout (eg, arthrocentesis) are more useful.

Differential Diagnosis

The first attack of gout must be distinguished from an acute monoarthritis. A review of Tables 22–1 and 22–3 is relevant.

Treatment

The inflammation of acute gout is effectively managed with anti-inflammatory medications. Once recognized, most cases of gout can be controlled within days, occasionally within hours. Remaining as a challenge is the decision regarding long-term treatment.

Standard therapy for acute gout is a short course of NSAIDs at adequate levels. As one of the first NSAIDs developed, indomethacin (50 mg three or four times a day) is occasionally thought to be somehow unique in the treatment of gout. In fact, all NSAIDs are probably equally effective, although many practitioners feel response is faster with short-acting agents such as naproxen (375–500 mg three times a day) or ibuprofen (800 mg three or four times a day). Pain often decreases on the first day, with treatment indicated for not much more than 3–5 days.

The classic medication for acute gout is colchicine. Typically given orally, the instructions to the patient can sound bizarre. The drug is prescribed as a 0.6-mg tablet every 1—2 hours "until relief of pain or uncontrollable diarrhea." Most attacks actually respond to the first two or three pills, with a maximum of six pills in 24 hours a prudent suggestion. Most patients develop diarrhea well before the sixth pill. Colchicine is dosed three times daily and, as with NSAIDs, is not often needed after 3–5 days.

On occasion, corticosteroids are used in acute gout. Oral prednisone (eg, up to 60 mg), methylprednisolone or triamcinolone (eg, 40–80 mg) intramuscularly, or intra-articular agents can be used. Indications include intense overlying skin involvement (mimicking cellulitis), polyarticular presentation of gout, and contraindication to NSAID or colchicine therapy. Intra-articular steroid use should be considered for ankle or knee gout, if infection is ruled out.

Decisions regarding long-term treatment of gout must take into account the natural history of attacks. The first attack, especially in young men with a clear precipitating event (such as an alcohol binge), may not be followed by a second attack for years, even decades. As stated earlier, as many as 20% of men will never have a second gouty attack. Data from the Framingham longitudinal study suggest that intervals of up to 12 years are common between first and second attacks. This is not always the case for young women with gout (who tend to have a uric acid metabolic abnormality) or for either men or women who have polyarticular gout. But for many young men, a reasonable recommendation after a first episode is not to treat prophylactically.

The physician and patient may even decide to withhold prophylactic medication after a second attack, but when episodes of gout become more frequent than one or two a year, both parties are usually ready to consider long-term medication. The primary medications used at this point are probenecid and allopurinol. Probenecid is a uric acid tubular reuptake inhibitor, which results in increased excretion of uric acid in the urine. Allopurinol inhibits the uric acid synthesis pathway, blocking the step at which xanthine is converted to uric acid. Xanthine is much more soluble than uric acid and is not implicated in acute arthritis, nephrolithiasis, or renal insufficiency. Assessing 24-hour uric acid excretion can be helpful at this time. The patient with low excretion of uric acid (< 600 mg/day) should respond to probenecid. A typical dose is 500 mg/day, with infrequent rash the only side effect. Probenecid loses effectiveness when the creatinine clearance falls below 50 mL/min, so alternative therapy is necessary in patients with chronic kidney disease. If the patient has uric acid nephrolithiasis, probenecid is contraindicated to avoid increased delivery of uric acid to the stone-forming region.

Some "underexcretors" and virtually all "overproducers" of uric acid will require allopurinol. Typically dosed at 300 mg/day, allopurinol predictably lowers serum uric acid levels and is highly effective at preventing gouty attacks. It is a well-tolerated drug with only infrequent side effects of nausea, diarrhea, or headache. The side effect of concern is rash. Although rare, allopurinol-induced rash can progress to a toxic hypersensitivity with fever, leukocytosis, epidermal necrolysis, and renal failure. Patients should be cautioned, but not alarmed, about this complication. A new xanthine oxidase inhibitor, febuxostat, has been submitted for Food and Drug Administration (FDA) approval; it is unclear whether side effects will be much different from allopurinol.

Allopurinol is especially indicated for treatment of tophaceous gout and for uric acid nephrolithiasis. Allopurinol is also the drug of choice for those with uric acid metabolic abnormalities (often young women) and polyarticular gout. Caution must be used, however, when starting allopurinol (and probenecid) for the first time. Rapid lowering of the serum uric acid causes instability of uric acid crystals within the synovial fluid and can actually precipitate an attack of gout. Consequently, prior establishment of either NSAID or colchicine therapy is necessary to prevent this complication.

Patients are occasionally seen who have been prescribed long-term therapy with colchicine. There is a conceptual attraction to this choice. Between attacks of gout, the so-called "intercritical period," examination of synovial fluid continues to show uric acid crystals. Using colchicine to prevent the spiral to inflammation seems appealing. But this choice is deceptive. Colchicine does nothing to lower uric acid levels. Long-term use allows deposition of uric acid into destructive tophi or contributes to renal disease and kidney stones. Colchicine can be an effective prophylactic agent, however, if started prior to a surgical procedure in a patient with known gout who is not using allopurinol or probenecid. But use of this drug as a solo agent courts other, significant complications.

Prognosis

Gouty attacks can be both effectively treated and prevented. A clear diagnosis is important and arthrocentesis essential. Management is relatively straightforward and no patient should have to endure tophi or repeated acute attacks.

Terkeltaub RA: Clinical practice. Gout. N Engl J Med 2003;349:1647. [PMID: 14573737]

Wise CM: Crystal-associated arthritis in the elderly. Clin Geriatr Med 2005;21:491. [PMID: 15911203]

Wortmann RL: Recent advances in the management of gout and hyperuricemia. Curr Opin Rheumatol 2005;17:319. [PMID: 15835244]

RHEUMATOID ARTHRITIS

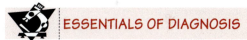

- *Arthritis of three or more joint areas.*
- *Arthritis in hands, feet, or both (bilateral joint involvement).*
- *Morning stiffness.*
- *Fatigue.*
- *Swelling, tenderness, warmth, and loss of function.*
- *Rheumatoid nodules.*
- *Elevated ESR and C-reactive protein.*
- *Positive test for rheumatoid factor.*

General Considerations

Bony changes consistent with rheumatoid arthritis (RA) have been found in the body of a Native American who lived 3000 years ago. Differentiation of RA from other types of arthritis is more recent, delineated only in the late 19th century. RA is more frequently seen in women, with the ratio of premenopausal women to age-matched men approximately 4:1; after the age of menopause, the ratio is closer to 1:1.

Pathogenesis

Although the etiology of RA is not known, the pathophysiology has been elucidated to a remarkable degree in recent decades. Important knowledge of all inflammatory processes has come from studies in RA. Early in the disease process, the synovium of joints is targeted by T cells (this is the feature that leads to the "autoimmune" moniker applied to RA). Release of interleukins, lymphokines, cytokines, tissue necrosis factor, and other messengers attracts additional inflammatory cells to the synovium. Intense inflammation ensues, experienced by the patient as pain, warmth, swelling, and loss of function. Reactive cells move to the inflammatory synovium, attempting to repair damaged tissue. Without treatment, this intense reaction develops into the pathologic tissue called *pannus,* an exuberant growth of tissue engulfing the joint space and causing destruction itself. Cartilage becomes swept into the pathologic process, resulting in breakdown, deterioration, and eventual destruction. Periarticular bone responds to inflammation with resorption, seen as erosions on radiographs. All these changes clearly are maladaptive and responsible for deformity and disability.

Prevention

It is difficult with any assurance to advise patients on measures to prevent arthritis. RA has multiple etiologies and no consistent preventive steps are available to patients.

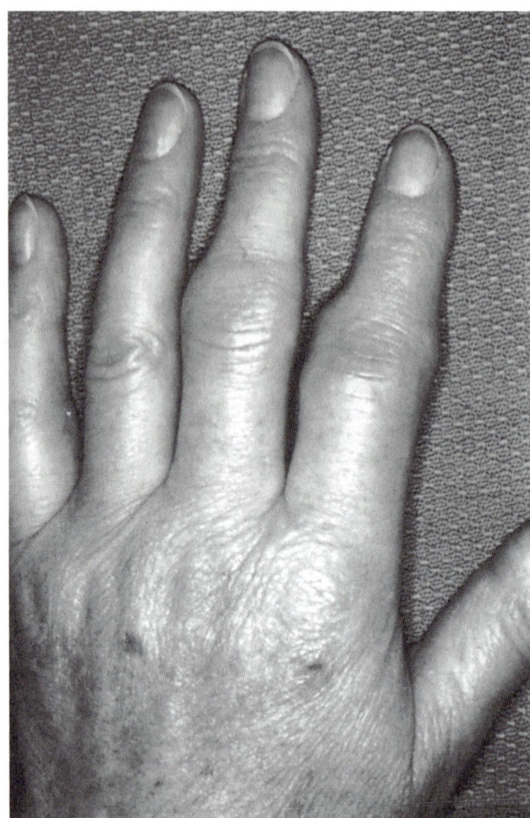

Figure 22–4. Swelling of the proximal interphalangeal joints of the second and third fingers in rheumatoid arthritis. Symmetric swelling might be expected on the other hand.

Clinical Findings

A. Symptoms and Signs

RA is a systemic disease, causing fatigue, rash, nodules, and even clinical depression as joints become progressively more stiff and inflamed. Most, but by no means all, of the initial symptoms are in the joints. There is inflammation, so the presence of swelling, warmth, and loss of function is imperative to the diagnosis. Joints of the hands (Figure 22–4) and feet are typically affected first, although larger joints can be involved at any time. The disease is classically symmetric with symptoms present bilaterally in hands or feet, or both. This mirroring is almost unique to RA; systemic lupus erythematosus, which is often confused with RA in its early stages, is not so consistently symmetric.

Fingers and wrists are stiff and sore in the mornings, requiring heat, rubbing, and movement to be functional ("morning stiffness"). Stiffness after prolonged lack of movement ("gelling") is not uncommon in many joint disorders, but the morning stiffness of RA is so prolonged and characteristic that queries regarding this symptom are one of the essentials of diagnosis.

The patient reports fatigue out of proportion to lack of sleep. Daytime naps are almost unavoidable, yet are not fully restorative. Anorexia, weight loss, even low-grade fever can be present. Along with musculoskeletal complaints, these somatic concerns may lead to mistaken diagnoses of fibromyalgia or even depression.

RA can eventually involve almost any joint in the body. Selected important manifestations of RA in specific joints are listed in Table 22–5. The cause of any one manifestation may be unique to a particular joint and the surrounding periarticular structure. Common features include inflammation-induced stretching of tendons and ligaments resulting in joint laxity, subconscious restriction of movement resulting in "frozen" joints, and consequences of inflammatory synovitis with cartilage destruction and periarticular bone erosion. An objective sign of destruction includes the high-pitched, "crunchy" sound of crepitus.

Extra-articular manifestations of RA can be seen at any stage of disease. Most common are rheumatoid nodules, found at some point in up to 50% of all patients with RA.

Table 22–5. Manifestations of rheumatoid arthritis in specific joints.

Joint	Complication
Hand	Ulnar deviation (hand points toward ulnar side) Swan-neck deformity (extension of PIP joint) Boutonniere deformity (flexion at DIP)
Wrist	Swelling causing carpal tunnel syndrome
Elbow	Swelling causing compressive neuropathy Deformity preventing complete extension, loss of power
Shoulder	"Frozen shoulder" (loss of abduction, nighttime pain)
Neck	Subluxation of C1–C2 joint with danger of dislocation and spinal cord compression ("hangman's injury")
Foot	"Cock-up" deformity and/or subluxation at MTP
Knee	Effusion leading to Baker cyst (evagination of synovial lining and fluid into popliteal space)

PIP, proximal interphalangeal; DIP, distal interphalangeal; MTP, metatarsophalangeal.

These occur almost anywhere in the body especially along pressure points (the typical olecranon site), along tendons, or in bursae. Vasculitis is an uncommon initial presentation of RA. Dry eyes and mouth are seen in the RA-associated sicca syndrome. Dyspnea, cough, or even chest pain may signal respiratory interstitial disease. Cardiac, gastrointestinal, and renal involvement in RA is not common. Peripheral nervous system symptoms are seen as compression neuropathies (eg, carpal or tarsal tunnel syndrome) and reflect not so much direct attack on nerves as consequences of squeezing compression as nerves are forced into passages narrowed by nearby inflammation.

B. Laboratory Findings

In contrast to OA, the laboratory findings in RA can be significant and helpful. A normocytic anemia is common in active RA. This anemia is almost always the so-called anemia of chronic disease. The white blood cell count is normal or even slightly elevated; an exception is the rare Felty syndrome (leukopenia and splenomegaly in a patient with known RA).

RA does not typically affect electrolytes and renal function. There is no pathophysiologic reason why transaminases, bilirubin, alkaline phosphatase, or other liver, pancreatic, or bone enzymes should be altered. Similarly, calcium, magnesium, and phosphate values should be unchanged. Most hormone measurements are normal, particularly thyroid and the adrenal axis. Any chronic inflammatory disease may alter the menstrual cycle, but measurement of luteinizing hormone and follicle-stimulating hormone is of little help.

Elevations of ESR and C-reactive protein are frequent. An elevated ESR is ubiquitous in RA. C-reactive protein is considered by many rheumatologists to be a more sensitive indicator of inflammation and might be increased in settings in which the ESR is either "normal" or minimally elevated. Although ESR is quite reliable, in some circumstances a false value may be reported (Table 22–6). For this reason, evaluation of C-reactive protein, although more expensive, is increasingly used by specialists.

The test most associated with RA is the rheumatoid factor (RF) blood test. RF is actually a family of antibodies, the most common of which is an immunoglobulin M (IgM) antibody directed against the Fc portion of immunoglobulin G (IgG). There is no question this antibody is frequently present in RA, with RF-negative RA accounting for only about 5% of all patients with RA. The problem lies with the low specificity of the test. Surveys demonstrate that in a young population, 3–5% of "normal" individuals have a high RF titer (positive test) whereas in an older cohort the prevalence of positive RF reaches 25%. With the national prevalence of RA only 1%, it is clear that many people with an elevated RF titer do not have RA. In fact, a false-positive RF titer is a com-

Table 22–6. Nondisease factors that influence the ESR.

Increase ESR	Decrease ESR	No Effect on ESR
Aging	Leukocytosis (>25,000)	Obesity
Female	Polycythemia (Hgb >18)	Body temperature
Pregnancy	Red blood cell changes	Recent meal
Anemia	Sickle cell	Aspirin
Macrocytosis	Anisocytosis	NSAID
Congenital hyperfibrinogenemia	Microcytosis	
	Acanthocytosis	
Technical factors	Protein abnormalities	
Dilutional	Dysproteinemia with hyperviscosity	
Elevated specimen temperature	Hypofibrinogenemia	
	Hypogammaglobulin	
	Technical factors	
	Dilutional	
	Inadequate mixing	
	Vibration during test	
	Clotting of specimen	

ESR, erythrocyte sedimentation rate; Hgb, hemoglobin; NSAID, nonsteroidal anti-inflammatory drug.

Modified from Brigden ML: Clinical utility of the erythrocyte sedimentation rate. Am Fam Physician 1999;60:1443.

Table 22–7. Conditions associated with a positive rheumatoid factor test.

Normal aging
Chronic bacterial infections
Subacute bacterial endocarditis
Tuberculosis
Lyme disease
Others
Viral disease
Cytomegalovirus
Epstein–Barr virus
Hepatitis B
Chronic inflammatory diseases
Sarcoidosis
Periodontal disease
Chronic liver disease (especially viral)
Sjögren syndrome
Systemic lupus erythematosus
Mixed cryoglobulinemia

mon reason for incorrect referral of patients to rheumatologists. Some of the conditions that are associated with a positive RF test are listed in Table 22–7.

Suarez-Almazor ME et al: Utilization and predictive value of laboratory tests in patients referred to rheumatologists by primary care physicians. J Rheumatol 1998;25:1980. [PMID: 9779854]

C. Imaging Studies

Radiographs are no longer needed for the initial diagnosis of rheumatoid arthritis. Other means of diagnosing RA are more useful. Nonetheless, RA is a disease of synovial tissue and, because the synovium lies on and attaches to bone, inflammation can cause changes on plain film radiography. Small erosions, or lucencies, on the lateral portions of phalanges are early indications of significant inflammation and should prompt immediate suppressive treatment.

CT, MRI, or both, have limited but useful supporting roles. An undesired complication of treatment of RA, aseptic necrosis (eg, of the femoral head) has a characteristic appearance on MRI. Scintigraphy is useful in detecting aseptic necrosis but, along with MRI, is better employed to differentiate the intense synovitis of RA from infection such as septic arthritis, overlying cellulitis, or adjacent osteomyelitis.

Differential Diagnosis

In practice, it is should not be difficult to differentiate among the three prototypical arthritides discussed in this chapter (see Table 22–1). Criteria developed by subspecialty organizations give valuable guidelines to making an accurate diagnosis of RA (Table 22–8). Because treatment started early is so generally successful, rheumatologists promote early referral—treating a new diagnosis of RA almost as a "medical emergency."

Moreland LW, Bridges SL Jr: Early rheumatoid arthritis: A medical emergency? Am J Med 2001;111:498. [PMID: 11690579]

Complications

Serious extra-articular manifestations of RA are not infrequent. Some of these are life-threatening and require sophisticated management by physicians experienced in dealing with these crises. The responsibility often remains with the primary care physician to recognize these conditions and refer appropriately. Table 22–9 lists several of these complications with a brief description of the clinical presentation.

Treatment

Therapy of RA has changed from managing inflammation to specific measures directed against the fundamental sources of the inflammation. In the past decades, treatment of RA has undergone perhaps the most wholesale shift of any of the rheumatologic conditions. Therapy is now directed at fundamental processes and begins with aggressive, potentially toxic disease-modifying drugs. The outlook can be hopeful, with preservation of joints, activity, and lifestyle a realistic goal. RA need no longer be the "deforming arthritis" by which it was known just a short time ago.

Table 22–8. 1987 American College of Rheumatology diagnostic criteria for rheumatoid arthritis.

The diagnosis of rheumatoid arthritis is confirmed if the patient has had at least four of the seven following criteria, with criteria 1–6 having been present for at least 6 weeks:

1. Morning stiffness (at least 1 h)
2. Arthritis of three or more joint areas (areas are right or left of proximal interphalangeal joints, metacarpophalangeal, wrist, elbow, knee, ankle, and metatarsophalangeal)
3. Arthritis of hand joints (proximal interphalangeal joints or metacarpophalangeal joints)
4. Symmetric arthritis, by area
5. Subcutaneous rheumatoid nodules
6. Positive test for rheumatoid factor
7. Radiographic changes (hand and wrist radiography that show erosion of joints or unequivocal demineralization around joints)

Arnett FC et al: The American Rheumatism Association 1987 revised criteria for the classification of rheumatoid arthritis. Arthritis Rheum 1988;31:315.

Table 22–9. Extraarticular manifestations of rheumatoid arthritis (RA).

Complication	Brief Comments
Rheumatoid nodules	Found over pressure points, classically olecranon. Typically fade with disease-modifying antirheumatic drug (DMARD) therapy. Also may be found in internal organs. If causing disability, may attempt intralesional steroids, or surgery.
Popliteal cyst	Usually asymptomatic unless ruptures; then mimics calf thrombophlebitis. Ultrasonography (and high index of suspicion) useful.
Anemia	Usually "chronic disease" and, despite low measured iron, does not respond to oral iron therapy. Improves with control of inflammatory disease.
Scleritis/episcleritis	Inflammatory lesion of conjunctiva. More prolonged, intense, and uncomfortable than "simple" conjunctivitis. Requires ophthalmologic management.
Pulmonary disease	Ranges from simple pleuritis and pleural effusion (noted for low glucose) to severe bronchiolitis, interstitial fibrosis, nodulosis, and pulmonary vasculitis. May require high-dose steroid therapy once diagnosis established by bronchoscopy or even open lung biopsy.
Sjögren syndrome	Often occurring with RA, includes sicca syndrome with thickened respiratory secretions, dysphagia, vaginal atrophy, hyperglobulinemia, and distal renal tubule defects. Treatment of sicca syndrome possible with muscarinic-receptor agonists; other manifestations more difficult.
Felty syndrome	Constellation of RA, leukopenia, splenomegaly, and often anemia, thrombocytopenia. Control underlying RA with DMARDs; may need granulocyte colony-stimulating factor, especially if infectious complications are frequent.
Rheumatoid vasculitis	Spectrum from digital arteritis (with hemorrhage) to cutaneous ulceration to mononeuritis multiplex to severe, life-threatening multisystem arteritis involving heart, gastrointestinal tract, and other organs. Resembles polyarteritis nodosum.

Kremers HM et al: Therapeutic strategies in rheumatoid arthritis over a 40-year period. J Rheumatol 2004;31:2366. [PMID: 15570636]

A. Assessment of Prognostic Factors

One of the early steps in treating RA is to assess prognostic factors in the individual patient. Poor prognosis leads to the decision to start aggressive treatment earlier. Some prognostic features are demographic, such as female sex, age older than 50 years, low socioeconomic status, and a first-degree relative with RA. Clinical features associated with poor prognosis include a large number of affected joints, especially involvement of the flexor tendons of the wrist, with persistence of swelling at the fingers; rheumatoid nodules; high ESR or C-reactive protein and high titers of RF; presence of erosions on radiographs; and evidence of functional disability. Formal functional testing and disease activity questionnaires are frequently employed, not only in establishing stage of disease but also at interval visits.

B. Patient Education

Therapy begins with patient education and again there are multiple sources of information from support and advocacy groups, professional organizations, government sources, and pharmaceutical companies. Patients should learn about the natural history of RA and the therapies available to interrupt the course. They should learn about joint protection and the likelihood that at least some activities need to be modified or discontinued. RA, especially before disease modification is established, is a fatiguing disorder. Patients should realize that rest is as important as appropriate types of activity. Of vital importance is the patient's acknowledgment that drug regimens about to be started are complex but that compliance is critical to successful outcomes. The patient should frankly be told that the drugs are toxic and may have adverse effects.

C. Pharmacotherapy

1. Pain relief—Pain is caused by inflammation, and establishment of effective anti-inflammatory drugs is the first goal of medication. NSAIDs, at doses recommended earlier (see Table 22–2), give the patient early relief. NSAIDs are used throughout the course of treatment; it is not uncommon to switch from one to another as effectiveness falters.

2. Alternative and complementary therapies—If the patient is reluctant to start drugs, fish oil supplementation may provide symptomatic relief. Both omega-3 and omega-6 fatty acids in fish oil modulate synthesis of highly inflammatory prostaglandin E_2 and leukotriene E_4. The fish oil chosen must contain high concentrations of the relevant fatty acids. A large number of capsules need to be taken, and palatability, diarrhea, and halitosis are frequent adverse effects. γ-Linolenic acid interrupts the pathway of arachidonic acid, another component of the inflammatory cascades. Extracted from the oils of plant seeds such as linseed, sunflower seed, and flaxseed, γ-linolenic acid demonstrates some efficacy in short-term studies using large doses of the extract.

3. Disease-modifying antirheumatic drugs—Neither NSAIDs nor "natural" products are disease modifying. Disease-modifying antirheumatic drugs (DMARDs) are drugs that suppress the underlying factors that result in synovitis, tissue reactivity (eg, pannus), erosions, ligament and tendon laxity, subluxations, and all the other complications of RA. DMARDs are almost always used in combination, both to enhance efficacy and to decrease dosage and potential toxicity. Toxicity is a major concern with DMARDs and, in fact, the monitoring for adverse effects may account for almost as much cost and inconvenience as the drugs themselves.

a. Sulfasalazine and hydroxychloroquine—Both of these drugs were initially developed for other diseases (inflammatory bowel disease and malaria, respectively) and coincidentally noted to be effective in RA. They are weak DMARDs. Hydroxychloroquine, a common first choice, requires ophthalmologic examinations every 6–12 months to detect color change or deposition of drug in the retina. The eye complications of hydroxychloroquine are rare and typically are seen with doses higher than the recommended 200 mg twice a day. Sulfasalazine is remarkably well tolerated and safe when prescribed at doses up to 2–3 g/day. A few patients experience gastric intolerance; the unlikely occurrence of leukopenia requires hematologic monitoring with some regularity (as often as every 2 months). Some patients with mild RA experience control of symptoms and delay or even suppression of disease progression with a combination of NSAID and hydroxychloroquine or sulfasalazine.

b. Gold and penicillamine—Gold preparations, either oral (auranofin) or parenteral (thiomalate, aurothioglucose), had been a standard therapy with disease-modifying properties in both short-term and intermediate use. These drugs are not easy to use and have gastrointestinal, renal, and bone marrow complications.

Penicillamine is another drug that had been widely, although cautiously, employed. It has DMARD properties and is effective enough at low doses (eg, 250 mg/day) that adverse effects are not common. But it now is prescribed only in refractory cases of RA because the adverse effects, when they do occur, are complex and difficult to treat.

c. Antibiotics—Minocycline is included in many combination therapies. This antibiotic is not used for its antibacterial effects. Rather, minocycline is an inhibitor of metalloproteinase, an enzyme involved in the production of pannus within joints. Several well-designed studies support the use of minocycline at a dose of 100 mg twice a day in moderate to even severe RA, typically in combination regimens.

d. Methotrexate—The drug that has become standard in treatment of RA is methotrexate. Especially when used in combination with an antimalarial or sulfasalazine, methotrexate truly modifies the natural course of RA. Response is common and relatively rapid, providing symptom control within weeks. Early fears of liver toxicity and cirrhosis have largely been allayed, but frequent measurement of liver enzymes is required. At recommended doses, gastrointestinal, mucocutaneous, and hematologic adverse effects are infrequent. Methotrexate affects T cells. The pathologic process in RA is complex, but enhanced activity of T cells is central to the development of destructive pannus. The ability of methotrexate to alter this activity is the key to disease modification.

Although methotrexate is the most commonly used DMARD, it is not an easy drug to take. Patients who imbibe large quantities of alcohol must alter this habit as adverse liver effects with methotrexate are considerably heightened. Folic acid is usually prescribed with methotrexate and, in addition to preventing macrocytic anemia, seems to diminish gastrointestinal side effects. Dosing starts low, as little as 5–7.5 mg/week, and is increased gradually to avoid mucositis or other gastrointestinal side effects. An early fear that long-term use of methotrexate would result in an increased incidence of infections or cancer has not been borne out. Nonetheless, awareness of infectious complications, including those from organisms such as *Pneumocystis carinii,* is necessary. Perhaps of even more concern is the development of a diffuse pulmonary alveolitis. Usually responsive to discontinuation of methotrexate and use of corticosteroids, this complication appears more likely to occur in patients with preexisting pulmonary disease.

Finally, an ironic side effect of methotrexate use is that disease flare is common (> 75%) should methotrexate have to be stopped. The flare, which develops within 2–3 months, is occasionally resistant to reinduction therapy, either with methotrexate or other DMARDs. Even so, methotrexate is almost universally used in RA, has efficacy in most patients, and ranks as one of the most significant advances in disease treatment in the past decades.

e. Azathioprine and cyclophosphamide—Azathioprine and cyclophosphamide are two other chemotherapy drugs considered for RA drug regimens. These agents have neither the efficacy nor relatively benign side effect profile of methotrexate but are chosen in circumstances in which an additional agent is needed to control symptoms or halt disease progression. Azathioprine use is limited to patients with moderate or severe RA unresponsive to other DMARDs. Gastrointestinal and hematologic adverse effects are most commonly experienced. Azathioprine has been used with success in treatment of serious extra-articular manifestations. Cyclophosphamide causes such frequent problems with bone marrow suppression, cystitis, bladder hemorrhage, and risk of cancer that its use is rare. However, used in combination with high-dose corticosteroids, cyclophosphamide is indicated in life-threatening rheumatoid vasculitis.

f. Leflunomide—Leflunomide is a pyrimidine synthesis inhibitor with efficacy equivalent to methotrexate. Even when used in low doses (10–20 mg/day after a loading dose), it causes considerable liver toxicity, and surveillance with blood tests for liver enzyme abnormalities is required. Leflunomide is not cleared from the body as rapidly as methotrexate, which is sometimes seen as an advantage (prompting the concept of a "drug holiday"). But similar to other chemotherapy agents, leflunomide is a teratogen, making the prolonged presence in body tissues a deceptive problem. Women of childbearing age must remain on effective contraception for as much as a year after stopping leflunomide. This drug is being investigated for use in moderate to severe RA, occasionally in combination with methotrexate.

g. Cyclosporine—Cyclosporine was once promoted for RA treatment as a DMARD with unique properties. It suppresses immunologic processes at steps different than chemotherapy agents. It is effective, as demonstrated in several studies. But the toxicity of cyclosporine is considerable, including the development of a particularly resistant type of hypertension and reduction in renal clearance. Cyclosporine is currently limited to combinations with methotrexate in severe RA poorly responsive to other therapies. Generally replacing these latter drugs are newer, potent, but also potentially toxic agents.

h. Tumor necrosis factor inhibitors—A different approach to management of RA has followed the development of tumor necrosis factor (TNF) inhibitors. TNF is a messenger attracting other inflammatory cells to a site. TNF is also involved in production of interferon and interleukins. Blockade of these effects diminishes the inflammatory response, both decreasing patient symptoms and slowing disease progression. Etanercept, infliximab, and adalimumab are current examples of TNF inhibitors. These drugs require subcutaneous or intravenous injection, as often as every other week. Despite that, they are relatively well tolerated and any hematologic toxicity responds to discontinuation. Although TNF inhibitors carry FDA indication for moderate to severe RA, they are increasingly given as single agents and even as first-line drugs. Following the same physiologic idea, an interleukin-1 receptor antagonist, anakinra, has also been introduced. This drug has modest benefit as both a single agent (for which it really is not recommended) and in combination with an agent such as methotrexate. Side effects are relatively common, with leukopenia and sepsis of most concern.

i. Abatacept—Abatacept (Orencia) inhibits T-cell activation. It may be used if methotrexate or TNF inhibitors fail, although some protocols use this drug in combination with methotrexate. Infectious complications and worsening of chronic obstructive pulmonary disease occurs more often than during treatment with TNF inhibitors.

j. Rituximab—Already marketed for B-cell lymphoma, rituximab (Rituxan) now carries an indication for use with methotrexate in RA patients who have not responded to treatment with TNF inhibitors. Acute infusion reactions are unfortunately common. Serious infections seem to occur at twice the rate of methotrexate alone.

k. Corticosteroids—Corticosteroid use in RA goes back to the earliest days of steroid development. It was the dramatic demonstration of symptom reduction in RA that propelled the use of corticosteroids in rheumatic diseases, resulting in a Nobel Prize in Medicine in 1950. But it was the use of high-dose steroids in RA that also led to the recognition of serious complications and the cautions physicians employ every day in decisions regarding use of steroids. Current recommendations suggest use of steroids in limited, but not infrequent, settings.

Corticosteroids suppress activity of RA while other DMARDs are being established. As initial therapy for a patient with moderate, active disease, steroids (eg, prednisone, 40–60 mg/day) can rapidly control symptoms, decrease inflammation, and provide time for DMARDs to have an effect. Similarly, if a patient has a disease flare and the decision is made to change DMARD therapy, steroids can provide "bridging" to the new therapy. If the patient has one or two joints that persist in inflammation and symptoms despite adequate overall control, intra-articular steroids provide an excellent intervention.

More controversial is the long-term use of corticosteroids at relatively low dose (eg, prednisone 5–10 mg/day). Most studies acknowledge symptom control, and a few recent studies even suggest slowing of joint destruction. Concern about progressive long-term complications to bone, skin, and other connective tissues has not been allayed with these recent reports.

Cush JJ: Safety overview of new disease-modifying antirheumatic drugs. Rheum Dis Clin North Am 2004;30:237. [PMID: 15172038]

Ranganath VK, Furst DE: Disease-modifying antirheumatic drug use in the elderly rheumatoid arthritis patient. Clin Geriatr Med 2005;21:649. [PMID: 15911212]

D. Surgery

Joint instability and resultant disability are often due to a combination of joint destruction, a primary effect of synovial inflammation, and tendon or ligament laxity, a secondary effect or "innocent bystander." The innocent bystander effect asserts that these connective tissues are stretched, weakened, or malaligned due to inflammation of the joints over which they cross but not due to a direct attack on the tendon or ligament itself. Nonetheless, at some point joint destruction and connective tissue laxity combine to produce useless, and frequently painful, joints. At this point, the surgeon has much to offer. Joint stabilization, connective tissue reinsertion, and joint replacement of both small (interphalangeal) and large (hip, knee) joints provide return of function and reduction of pain. The timing of surgery is still an art and is most effective when close collaboration exists between the primary physician and surgeon.

Prognosis

Morbidity and mortality are increased in patients with RA over age-matched persons without RA. Correlated with active disease, there is a well-described increase in stroke and myocardial infarction. These manifestations may be due to a hypercoagulable state induced by the autoimmune process and circulating antibodies. Otherwise, with long-standing RA, even under conscientious treatment, complications from infection, pulmonary and renal disease, and gastrointestinal bleeding occur at rates higher than those in the general population. Many of the latter complications are related as much to the drugs used to control the disease as to the disease itself.

Wallberg-Honsson S et al: Extent of inflammation predicts cardiovascular disease and overall mortality in seropositive rheumatoid arthritis. A retrospective cohort study from disease onset. J Rheumatol 1999;26:2562. [PMID: 10606363]

Web Sites

American Academy of Family Physicians:

http://www.aafp.org and http://www.familydoctor.org

American College of Physicians:

http://www.acponline.org

American College of Rheumatology:

http://www.rheumatology.org

Arthritis Foundation (user-friendly information for patients, written without medical jargon):

http://www.arthritis.org

National Guideline Clearinghouse:

http://www.guideline.gov

National Institute for Arthritis and Musculoskeletal and Skin Diseases (NIH):

http://www.niams.nih.gov

Low Back Pain 23

Charles W. Webb, DO, FAAFP, CAQ Sports Medicine, & Francis G. O'Connor, MD, MPH, COL, MC, USA

General Considerations

Low back pain (LBP), discomfort, tension, or stiffness below the costal margin and above the inferior gluteal folds, is one of the most common conditions encountered in primary care, second only to the common cold. LBP has an annual incidence of 15% and a lifetime prevalence of 60–90%. It is the leading cause of disability in the United States for adults younger than 45 years of age. LBP is also responsible for one third of workers' compensation costs, and accounts for direct medical costs in excess of $38 billion per year. At any given time 1% of the US population is chronically disabled and another 1% temporarily disabled as a result of back pain. Numerous studies report a favorable natural history for acute LBP, with up to 90% of patients regaining function within 6–12 weeks with or without physician intervention. Recent studies, however, suggest that back pain is often recurrent and chronically disabling. Approximately 90% of back pain has no readily identifiable cause. This chapter reviews the biomechanics of mechanical LBP, and then details an evidence-based approach to the assessment, diagnosis, and management of the adult patient with acute LBP.

LBP, as a common clinical problem with high morbidity, has been the focus of a number of evidence-based reviews and clinical practice guidelines. The evidence-based assessment and management discussed in this chapter is based on the Agency for Health Care Policy and Research (AHCPR) Clinical Practice Guideline, utilizing the Veteran's Administration/Department of Defense (VA/DoD) Clinical Practice Guideline. This guideline uses an algorithmic approach, which is divided into three phases: assessment, initial management of acute LBP, and management of chronic LBP (Figure 23–1).

Bigos S et al: *Acute Low Back Problems in Adults.* Clinical Practice Guideline, No. 14. AHCPR Publication No. 95-0642.

Drezner JA, Herring SA: Managing low-back pain: Steps to optimize function and hasten return to activity. Phys Sportsmed 2001;29:37.

Kovacs FM et al: Correlation between pain, disability, and quality of life in patients with common low back pain. Spine 2004;29:206. [PMID: 14630439]

Veterans Health Administration and Department of Defense: *Clinical Practice Guideline: Low Back Pain or Sciatica in the Primary Care Setting.* The Low Back Pain Workgroup, Contract No. V101(93) P-1633; 1999.

Prevention

LBP is a heavy medical and financial burden not only to the patients who are experiencing the ailment, but also to society. The US Preventive Services Task Force recently produced a recommendation statement on primary care interventions to prevent low back pain in adults. Currently there is insufficient evidence to support or rebuke routine use of exercise as a preventive measure for low back pain. However, regular physical activity has been shown to be beneficial in the treatment and the limitation of recurrent episodes of chronic low back pain. Lumbar supports (back belts) have not been found effective in the prevention of low back pain. Worksite interventions, including education on lifting techniques, have been shown to have some short-term effects on decreasing lost time from work for patients with back pain.

Risk factor modification may be the only way to truly prevent LBP. These risk factors can be classified as individual, psychosocial, occupational, and anatomic. Table 23–1 lists the prominent risk factors for LBP.

Manek NJ, MacGregor AJ: Epidemiology of back disorders: Prevalence, risk factors, and prognosis. Curr Opin Rheumatol 2005;17:134. [PMID: 15711224]

US Preventive Services Task Force: Primary care interventions to prevent low back pain in adults: Recommendation statement. Am Fam Physician 2005;71:2237. [PMID: 15999872]

Clinical Findings

The key elements in the correct diagnosis and treatment of problems that cause LBP include an evaluation for serious health problems, symptom control for acute LBP, and follow-up evaluation of patients whose conditions worsen. The first step is the accurate and timely identification of clinical conditions for which LBP is a symptom.

A. Symptoms and Signs

A careful medical history and physical examination is essential in determining the presence of a more serious condition in the patient presenting with acute LBP (see Figure 23–1A, Box 2). While obtaining the history and

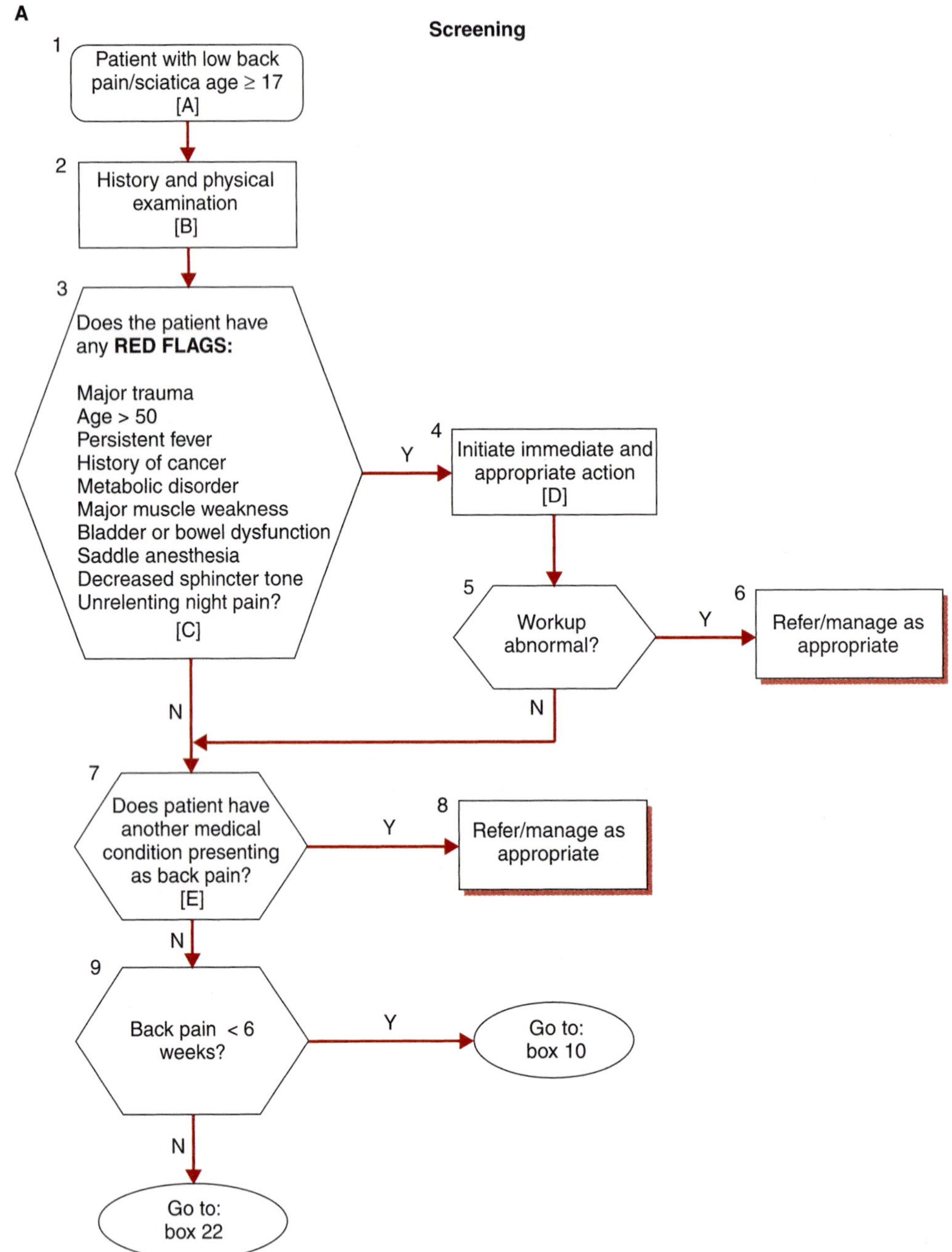

Figure 23–1. **A:** Acute LBP screening algorithm. **B:** Acute phase treatment algorithm. **C:** Chronic phase treatment algorithm. ROM, range of motion; AP, anteroposterior; Lat, lateral; LS; lumbosacral; MRI, magnetic resonance imaging; CBC, complete blood count; ESR, erythrocyte sedimentation rate; UA, urinalysis; CHEM, chemistry panel; SPEP, serum protein electrophoresis; IPEP, immunoprotein electrophoresis; UPEP, urine protein electrophoresis.

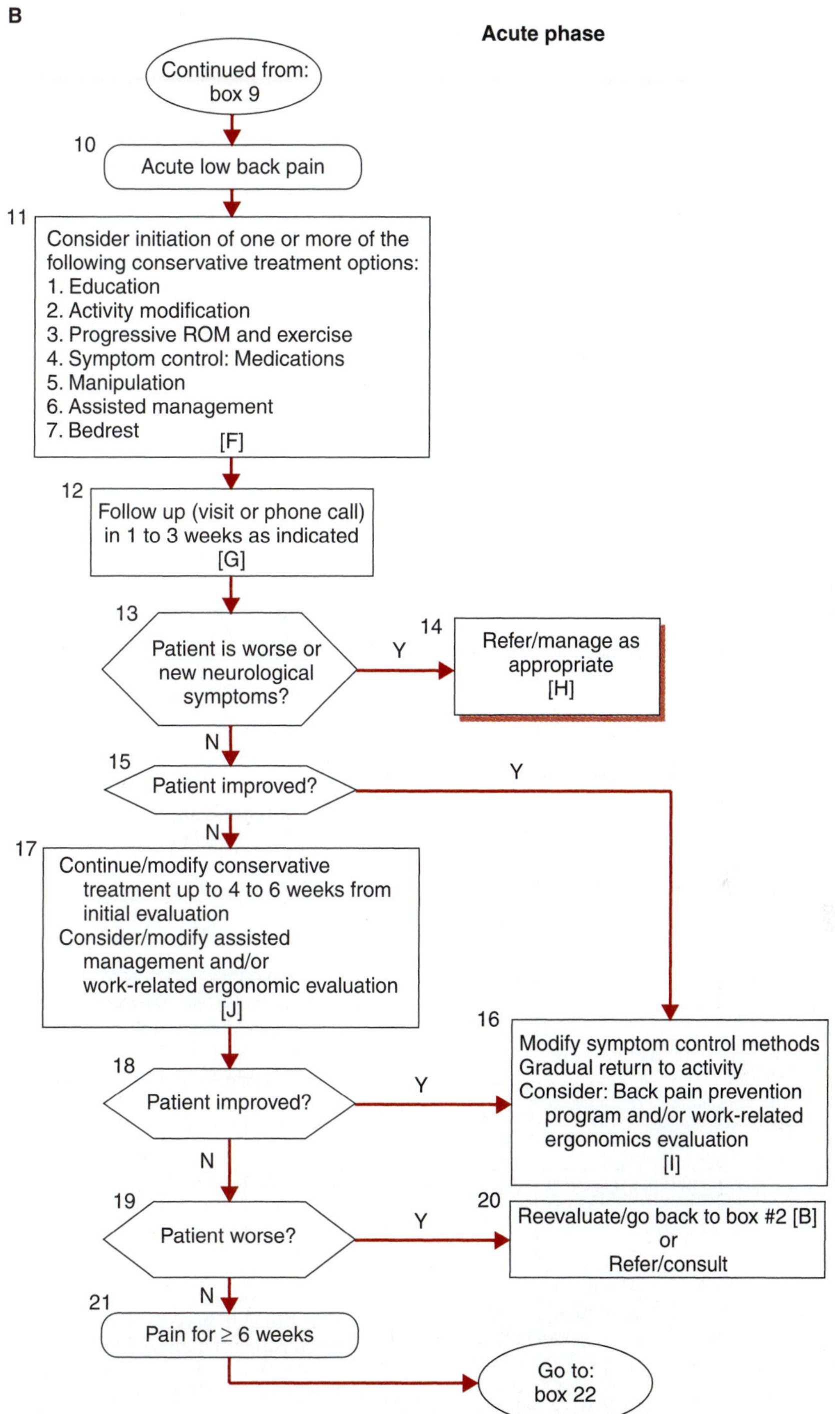

Figure 23–1. *(Continued)*

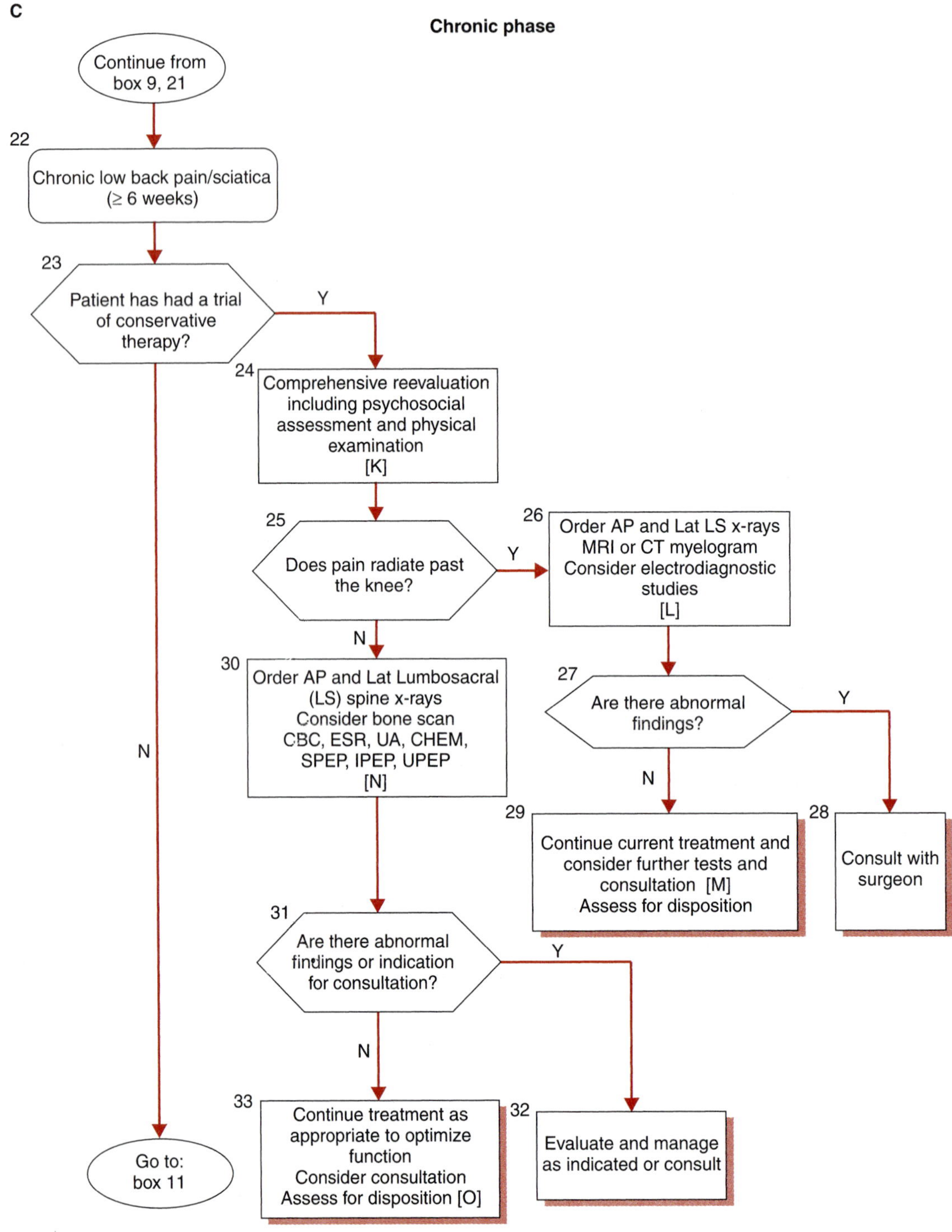

Figure 23–1. *(Continued)*

Table 23–1. Risk factors associated with LBP.

Individual
Increasing age
Smoking history
Obesity
Education level
Unemployment
High birth weight
High levels of pain
Psychosocial
Stress
Depressed mood
Decreased cognition
Somatization
Long duration of pain
Fear avoidance behavior
Occupational
Monotonous tasks
Low-control job
Manual handling of materials
Job dissatisfaction
Night-shift work
Bending, twisting, pulling, pushing
Whole-body vibration
Lifting for more than 75% of each day
Unavailability of light duty
High pressure on time
Co-worker socialization
Anatomic
Disc space narrowing
Facet joint arthritis
Synovial cysts
Lumbosacral transitional vertebra
Schmorl nodes
Annular disruption
Spondylolysis

Source: Adapted, with permission, from Manek NJ, MacGregor AJ: Epidemiology of back disorders: Prevalence, risk factors, and prognosis. Curr Opin Rheumatol 2005;17:134.

examining the patient, the primary care provider must look for "red flags" that indicate the presence of one of these conditions (see Figure 23–1A, Box 3). If any red flags are identified, patients requiring emergent or urgent care should be given immediate consultation or referral to the appropriate specialist (see Figure 23–1A, Box 4). Nonemergent patients with red flags should be scheduled for the appropriate diagnostic tests to determine if they have a condition that requires referral.

1. History—The history should focus on the location of the pain, the mechanism of injury (what the patient was doing when he or she first noticed the pain; whether it was insidious or the result of a specific trauma or activity), the character (mechanical, radicular, claudicant, or nonspecific), and duration of the pain (acute, i.e. < 6 weeks; or chronic, > 6 weeks). The provider must identify neurologic symptoms (bowel or bladder symptoms, weakness in the extremities, saddle anesthesia) suggestive of cauda equina syndrome, a true neurosurgical emergency. The functional status of the patient should be noted as should any exacerbating or ameliorating factors. The presence of fever, weight loss, and night pain is of particular concern as these could indicate a more serious disease, such as an underlying cancer. The social history should include information about drug use or abuse, intravenous drug use, tobacco use, and the presence of physical demands at work. Past medical and surgical history should also be obtained, particularly a history of previous spinal surgery or immunosuppression (history of cancer, steroid use, HIV infection). A thorough history enables the primary care provider to identify any red flags that require a more extensive medical workup to rule out potentially serious disease processes (see Figure 23–1A, Box 3).

2. Physical examination—The physical examination supplements the information obtained in the history by helping to identify underlying serious medical conditions or possible serious neurologic compromise. The primary elements of the physical examination are inspection, palpation, observation (including range-of-motion testing), and a specialized neuromuscular evaluation. The examination should start with an evaluation of the spinal curvature, lumbar range of motion, and amount of pain-free movement. Palpation should include the paraspinal muscles, the spinous processes, the sacroiliac joints, the piriformis muscles and the position of the pelvic bones (anterior and posterior superior iliac spine [ASIS and PSIS]). Because the lumbar spine is kinetically linked to the pelvis (particularly the sacroiliac area), pain from the pelvis is often referred to the lumbar spine. To address the pelvis the provider must be aware of the location of the ASIS and the PSIS in evaluating any rotational dysfunction of the pelvis as a cause for the LBP. Hip flexors and hamstring flexibility should also be assessed as a potential cause for the pain.

3. Neurologic evaluation—The neurologic evaluation should include Achilles (S1) and patellar (L2–L4) reflex testing, ankle and great toe dorsiflexion (L4–L5) and plantarflexion (S1) strength, as well as the location of sensory complaints (dermatomes involved). Light touch testing for sensation in the medial (L4), dorsal (L5), and lateral (S1) aspects of the foot should also be performed. In patients presenting with acute LBP and no specific limb complaints, a more elaborate neurologic examination is not usually necessary. The straight leg raise test (SLR) should be done in both the seated and supine positions to evaluate for nerve root impingement. This abbreviated neurologic evaluation of the lower extremity allows detection of clinically significant nerve root compromise at the L4–L5 or L5–S1 levels. These two sites make up over 90% of all significant

Table 23–2. Red flags and appropriate actions.

Condition	Red Flag	Action
Cancer	History of cancer Unexplained weight loss Age ≥50 y Failure to improve with therapy Pain ≥4–6 wk Night/rest pain	If malignant disease of the spine is suspected, imaging is indicated and CBC and ESR should be considered; identification of possible primary malignancy should be investigated, eg, PSA, mammogram, UPEP/SPEP/IPEP
Infection	Fever History of intravenous drug use Recent bacterial infection: UTI, skin, pneumonia Immunocompromised states (steroid, organ transplants, diabetes, HIV) Rest pain	If infection in the spine is suspected, MRI, CBC, ESR, and/or UA are indicated
Cauda equina syndrome	Urinary retention or incontinence Saddle anesthesia Anal sphincter tone decrease/fecal incontinence Bilateral lower extremity weakness/numbness or progressive neurologic deficit	Request immediate surgical consultation
Fracture	Use of corticosteroids Age ≥70 y or history of osteoporosis Recent significant trauma	Appropriate imaging and surgical consultation
Acute abdominal aneurysm	Abdominal pulsating mass Other atherosclerotic vascular disease Rest/night pain Age ≥60 y	Appropriate imaging (ultrasound) and surgical consultation
Significant herniated nucleus pulposus (HNP)	Major muscle weakness	Appropriate imaging and surgical consultation

CBC, complete blood count; ESR, erythrocyte sedimentation rate; PSA, prostate-specific antigen; UPEP, urine protein electrophoresis; SPEP, serum protein electrophoresis; IPEP, immunoprotein electrophoresis; UTI, urinary tract infection; HIV, human immunodeficiency virus; MRI, magnetic resonance imaging; UA, urinalysis.

radiculopathy secondary to lumbar disc herniation. Because this abbreviated examination may fail to diagnose some of the less common causes of LBP, any patient who has not improved in 4–6 weeks should return for further evaluation.

4. Risk stratification—All patients with acute LBP should be risk stratified with an initial assessment attempting to identify red flags—responses or findings in the history and physical examination that indicate a potentially serious underlying condition (eg, fracture, tumor, infections, abdominal aneurysm, or cauda equina syndrome) that can lead to considerable patient morbidity or mortality. These clinical clues include a history of major trauma, minor trauma in patients older than 50 years of age, persistent fever, history of cancer, metabolic disorder, major muscle weakness, bladder or bowel dysfunction, saddle anesthesia, decreased sphincter tone, and unrelenting night pain. The presence of red flags should prompt an earlier clinical action, such as imaging or laboratory workup (see Figure 23–1A, Box 4). Table 23–2 lists red flags and their related conditions.

B. Laboratory Findings

Laboratory testing should be reserved for patients suspected of having a condition that may masquerade as simple LBP, such as cancer or infection (Tables 23–2 and 23–3). Laboratory tests recommended in the evaluation of these patients include a complete blood count with differential and an erythrocyte sedimentation rate (ESR). An ESR over 50 mm/h is suggestive of malignancy, infection, or inflammatory disease. Blood urea nitrogen, creatinine, and urinalysis are helpful in identifying underlying renal or urinary tract disease. Serum calcium, phosphorus, and alkaline phosphatase should be checked in patients with osteopenia,

Table 23–3. Masqueraders of LBP.

System	Conditions
Vascular	Expanding aortic aneurysm
Gastrointestinal	Pancreatitis Peptic ulcers Cholecystitis Colonic cancer
Genitourinary	Endometriosis Tubal pregnancy Kidney stones Prostatitis Chronic pelvic inflammatory disease Perinephric abscess Pyelonephritis
Endocrinologic/metabolic	Osteoporosis Osteomalacia Hyperparathyroidism Paget disease Acromegaly Cushing disease Ochronosis
Hematologic	Hemoglobinopathy Myelofibrosis Mastocytosis
Rheumatologic	Spondyloathropathies Ankylosing spondylitis Reiter syndrome Psoriatic arthritis Enteropathic arthritis Behçet syndrome Familial Mediterranean fever Whipple disease Diffuse idiopathic skeletal hyperostosis
Psychogenic	Affective disorder Conversion disorder Somatization disorder Malingering
Infection	Osteomyelitis Epidural/paraspinal abscess Disc space infection Pyogenic sacroiliitis
Neoplastic	Skeletal metastases Spinal cord tumors Leukemia Lymphoma Retroperitoneal tumors Primary lumbosacral tumors Benign Malignant
Miscellaneous	Sarcoidosis Subacute endocarditis Retroperitoneal fibrosis Herpes zoster Fat herniation of lumbar space

Sources: Branch CL et al: LBP Monograph, Edition No. 185. *Home Study Self-Assessment Program.* American Academy of Family Physicians, 1994; and Bagduk N: The innervation of the lumbar spine. Spine 1983;8:286.

osteolytic vertebral lesions, or vertebral body collapse. If prostate carcinoma is suspected, prostate-specific antigen and acid phosphatase levels should be checked. If multiple myeloma is suspected, a serum immunoelectrophoresis can help guide treatment.

Historical red flags such as fever, intravenous drug abuse, and immunocompromise should raise concern for an underlying infection. An elevated white blood cell count is a clue to an underlying infection but can be within normal limits even in acute infection. The ESR and C-reactive protein can be used to monitor the efficacy of treatment of spinal infections. Urinalysis and urine culture should be obtained because urinary tract infection often precedes spinal infection. Blood cultures should be obtained as well. Although they are usually negative, positive cultures identify the infecting organism and provide antibiotic sensitivity to guide treatment.

C. Imaging Studies

Diagnostic imaging (Table 23–4) is rarely indicated in the acute setting of LBP. After the first 4–6 weeks of symptoms, the majority of patients will have regained function. However, if the patient is still limited by back symptoms, diagnostic imaging should be considered to look for other

Table 23–4. Special tests and indications/recommendations.

Special Test	Indication/Recommendation
Plain x-ray	Not recommended for routine evaluation of acute LBP unless red flags present Recommended for ruling out fractures Obliques are recommended only when findings are suggestive of spondylolisthesis or spondylolysis
Electrophysiologic tests (EMG and SEP)	Questionable nerve root dysfunction with leg symptoms ≥6 wk Not recommended if radiculopathy is obvious
MRI or CT myelography	Back-related leg symptoms and clinically detectable nerve root compromise History of neurogenic claudication suspicious for spinal stenosis Findings suggesting CES, fracture, infection, tumor
ESR	Suspected tumors, infection, inflammatory conditions, metabolic disorders
CBC	Suspected tumors, myelogenous conditions, infections
Urinalysis	Suspected UTI, pyelonephritis, myeloma
IPEP	Suspected multiple myeloma
Chemistry profile to include TSH, calcium, and alkaline phosphatase	Suspected electrolyte disorders, thyroid dysfunction, metabolic dysfunction
Bone scan	Suspected occult pars interarticularis fracture or metastatic disease Contraindicated in pregnant patients

LBP, low back pain; EMG, electromyelogram; SEP, serum electrophoresis; MRI, magnetic resonance imaging; CT, computed tomography; CES, cauda equina syndrome; ESR, erythrocyte sedimentation rate; CBC, complete blood count; UA, urinalysis; UTI, urinary tract infection; IPEP, immunoprotein electrophoresis; TSH, thyroid-stimulating hormone.

conditions that present as LBP (see Figure 23–1C, Boxes 24, 26, and 30). Patients for whom diagnostic imaging should be considered include children, patients older than 50 years of age, trauma patients, or patients for whom back pain fails to improve despite appropriate conservative treatment. Imaging studies must always be interpreted carefully, because disc degeneration and protrusion have been noted in 20–25% of asymptomatic individuals. Therefore, abnormal findings on diagnostic imaging may or may not represent the reason for the patient's pain.

Plain films remain the most widely available modality for imaging the lumbar spine. Plain radiographs are rarely useful in evaluating or guiding treatment of adults with acute LBP in the absence of red flags. Anteroposterior and lateral views allow assessment of lumbar alignment, the intervertebral disc space, bone density, and a limited evaluation of the soft tissue. Oblique views should only be used when spondylolysis is suspected as they double the radiation exposure and add only minimal information. Sacroiliac views are used to evaluate ankylosing spondylitis and, again, should only be used when this is suspected. Plain lumbar radiographs are helpful in detecting spinal fractures and evaluating tumor or infection.

Plain radiographs of the lumbar spine are recommended for ruling out fractures in patients with acute LBP when the following red flags are present: recent major trauma (any age), age greater than 50 years with history of mild trauma, history of corticosteroid use, osteoporosis, and age greater than 70 years. Plain radiographs in combination with a complete blood count and ESR may be useful for ruling out tumor or infection in patients with acute LBP when the following red flags are present: prior cancer or recent infection, fever higher than 37.7°C (100°F), intravenous drug abuse, prolonged steroid use, LBP that is worse with rest, and unexplained weight loss.

When the history or physical examination suggests an anatomic abnormality as a cause for the back pain with neurologic deficits, four imaging studies are commonly used: plain myelography, computed tomography (CT) scan, magnetic resonance imaging (MRI) scan, and CT myelography. These four tests are used in similar clinical situations and provide similar information. The objective of these studies is to define a medically or surgically remediable anatomic condition. These tests are not done routinely and should only be used for patients who present with certain clinical findings, such as radicular symptoms and clinically detectable nerve root compressive symptoms severe enough to consider surgical intervention (major muscle weakness, progressive motor deficit, intractable pain, and persistent radicular pain beyond 6 weeks). Other indications include a history of neurogenic claudication suggestive of spinal stenosis or examination findings suggesting cauda equina syndrome, spinal fracture, infection, or tumor. For a patient with a neurologic deficit and a positive tension sign (SLR with pain radiating below the knee) and a correlative imaging study, the clinical accuracy is 95%. MRI is usually the most accurate imaging modality followed by CT myelography for finding nerve root impingement.

Diagnostic imaging plays a central role in diagnosing spinal infections. Plain films should be obtained but are often only helpful in the advanced stages of the infection. MRI is the imaging modality of choice in evaluating spinal infection. When infection is identified or suspected, a spinal surgeon should be consulted immediately.

Bone scans are recommended to evaluate acute LBP only when spinal tumor, infection, or occult fracture is suspected from the medical history or physical examination. Thermography and discography are not recommended for assessing patients with acute LBP. Thermography has shown to be abnormal in a substantial proportion of asymptomatic patients as well as those with myofascial pain syndromes.

Atlas SJ, Deyo RA: Evaluating and managing acute low back pain in the primary care setting. J Gen Intern Med 2001;16:120. [PMID: 11251764]

Differential Diagnosis

After potential red flags have been ruled out, the differential diagnosis for LBP remains extensive. Table 23–3 presents a list of conditions that can present as simple LBP.

Treatment

If the patient has no red flags and the history and physical examination do not suggest an underlying cause, the diagnosis of mechanical LBP can be made, and treatment may be initiated (see Figure 23–1B, Box 11). Methods of symptom control should focus on providing comfort and keeping the patient as active as possible while awaiting spontaneous recovery. Evidence for the most common treatments currently used in the primary care setting follows. Depending on the patient, this treatment may include activity modification, bed rest (short duration), conservative medications, progressive range of motion and exercise, manipulative treatment, and patient education. This line of treatment should be used for 4–6 weeks before ordering additional diagnostic tests, unless the patient's symptoms worsen. Follow-up with patients is crucial to monitor progress and adjust treatment as tolerated (see Figure 23–1B and C, Boxes 15 and 22].

A. Patient Education

Patient education is the cornerstone of effective treatment of LBP. Patients who present to the primary care clinic with acute LBP should be educated about expectations for recovery and the potential recurrence of symptoms. Patients should be informed of safe and reasonable activity modifications, and be given information on how to limit the recurrence of low back problems through proper lifting techniques, treatment of obesity, and tobacco cessation. If medications are used, patients should be given information on their use and the potential side effects. Patients should be instructed to follow up in 1–3 weeks if they fail to improve with conservative treatment, or develop bowel or bladder dysfunction, or worsening neurologic function.

B. Activity Modification

Patients with acute LBP may be more comfortable if they are able to temporarily limit or avoid specific activities that are known to increase mechanical stress on the spine. Prolonged unsupported sitting and heavy lifting, especially while bending or twisting should be avoided. Activity recommendations for the employed patient with acute LBP should consider the patient's age, general health, and the physical demands of the job.

C. Bed Rest

A gradual return to normal activities is more effective than prolonged bed rest in the treatment of LBP. Bed rest for longer than 4 days may lead to debilitating muscle atrophy and increased stiffness and therefore is not recommended. Most patients with acute LBP do not require bed rest. For patients with severe initial symptoms, however, limited bed rest for 2–4 days remains an option.

D. Medications

Oral medications (acetaminophen, nonsteroidal anti-inflammatory drugs [NSAIDs], muscle relaxants, and opioids) and injection treatments are available for the treatment of LBP. A recent review of clinical trials found that NSAIDs are more effective for short-term symptomatic relief in patients with acute LBP. One NSAID has not been shown to be more effective than another in the treatment of LBP. Muscle relaxants are not as effective as NSAIDs in treating LBP, and no additional benefit has been noted when muscle relaxants are used in combination with NSAIDs. Muscle relaxants have more potential side effects than NSAIDs, a factor that should be considered when deciding on treatment. Because opioids are no more effective in relieving low back symptoms than other analgesics (aspirin, acetaminophen) and because of their potential for other complications (dependency), opioid analgesics, if used, should be administered over a time-limited course. Oral corticosteroids are not recommended in the treatment of acute LBP.

Injection therapy for the treatment of low back symptoms includes trigger point, ligamentous, sclerosant, facet joint, and epidural injections. Injections are an invasive treatment option that exposes patients to potentially serious complications. No conclusive studies have proven the efficacy of trigger point, sclerosant, ligamentous, or facet joint injections in the treatment of acute LBP. However, epidural and facet joint injections may benefit patients who fail conservative treatment as a means of avoiding surgery.

Curatolo M, Bogduk N: Pharmacologic pain treatment of musculoskeletal disorders: Current perspectives and future prospects. Clin J Pain 2001;17:25. [PMID: 11289086]

Nelemans PJ et al: Injection therapy for subacute and chronic benign low back pain. Spine 2001;26:501. [PMID: 11242378]

Van Tulder MW et al: Non-steroidal anti-inflammatory drugs for low back pain. Cochrane Database Syst Rev 2000. [PMID: 11013503]

E. Spinal Manipulation

There is some evidence supporting the use of manipulative therapy in the treatment of acute LBP. Spinal manipulation techniques attempt to restore joint and soft tissue range of motion. Impaired motion of synovial joints has a detrimental effect on joint cartilage, leading to degenerative spinal changes. Decreased motion in the spine also has a degenerative effect on vertebral disc metabolism. Manipulation is useful early after symptom onset for patients who have acute LBP without radiculopathy. If the patient's physical findings suggest progressive or severe neurologic deficit, manipulation should be postponed pending an appropriate diagnostic assessment. Patients who have symptoms for longer than 4–6 weeks despite manipulation should be reevaluated.

Several recent studies have investigated the use of spinal manipulation in the treatment of LBP. One study found no difference between the effects of combined manipulative and interferential (i.e., electrical tissue stimulation) therapy and manipulation alone in the treatment of acute LBP. Patients who received either spinal manipulation or interferential therapy alone demonstrated improvements in functional disability, pain, quality of life, exercise participation, and analgesic use at 12 months.

A recent randomized, controlled trial evaluated four methods of LBP treatment: medical care only, medical care with physical therapy, chiropractic care only, and chiropractic care with physical modalities. Although there was a higher patient expense for spinal manipulation than for medical care alone, medical care with physical therapy was the most costly of the interventions studied. Of note, the study did not consider the added costs of medications and their potential side effects or adverse outcomes versus spinal manipulation of the lumbosacral spine, for which there are virtually no adverse outcomes.

Childs JD et al: A clinical prediction rule to identify patients with low back pain most likely to benefit from spinal manipulation: A validation study. Ann Intern Med 2004;141:920. [PMID: 15611489]

Hurley DA et al: A randomized clinical trial of manipulative therapy and interferential therapy for acute low back pain. Spine 2004;29:2207. [PMID: 15480130]

F. Physical Agents and Modalities

There are no well-designed controlled trials to support or discourage the use of physical agents or modalities for acute LBP. Physical agents include moist heat and cold treatments. Self-administrated home programs using moist heat and ice are often used; these can be applied to the area for 20 minutes two or three times per day, although moist heat should not be used in the first 72 hours after injury.

Transcutaneous electrical nerve stimulation (TENS) is a modality that uses a small battery-operated device worn by the patient and provides a pulse of electricity to the injured area through surface electrodes. TENS is thought to modify pain perception by counterstimulation of the nervous system. Currently there is insufficient evidence on the efficacy of the TENS to recommend its routine use.

Shoe insoles (or inserts) can vary from over-the-counter foam rubber inserts to custom orthotics. These devices aim to reduce back pain due to leg length discrepancies or abnormal foot mechanics during gait. There is limited evidence that shoe orthotics (either over the counter or custom) may provide short-term benefit for patients with mild back pain, although there is no evidence supporting their long-term use. The role of leg length discrepancies in LBP has not been established, and differences of less than 2 cm are unlikely to produce symptoms.

Lumbar support devices for low back problems include corsets, support belts, various types of braces, molded jackets, and back rests for chairs and car seats. Lumbar corsets and support belts may be beneficial in preventing LBP and in reducing time lost from work for individuals whose jobs require frequent lifting; however, the evidence is lacking. Lumbar corsets have not been proven to be beneficial in the treatment of LBP. A randomized controlled trial found that mattresses of medium firmness are beneficial in reducing pain symptoms and disability in patients with chronic LBP.

Acupuncture and other dry-needling techniques have not been found to be beneficial for treating patients with acute LBP. However, recent evidence suggests that traditional Chinese acupuncture and therapeutic massage is beneficial in the treatment of chronic LBP. Acupuncture, when added to conventional therapies, improves function and pain better than conventional therapy alone. Dry-needling appears to be useful only as an adjunct to other therapies for chronic LBP and has not been found useful in the treatment of acute LBP.

Furlan AD et al: Acupuncture and dry-needling for low back pain. Cochrane Database Syst Rev 2005;(1):CD001351. [PMID: 10795434]

Hay EM et al: Comparison of physical treatments versus a brief pain-management programme for back pain in primary care: A randomized clinical trial in physiotherapy practice. Lancet 2005;365:2040. [PMID: 15950716]

Kovacs FM et al: Effect of firmness of mattress on chronic non-specific low back pain: Randomized, double-blind, controlled, multicenter trial. Lancet 2003;362:1599. [PMID: 14630439]

G. Exercise

Therapeutic exercises should be started early to control pain, avoid deconditioning, and restore function. No single treatment or exercise program has proven effective for all patients with LBP. The muscles in the hip play a major role in transferring forces from the lower extremities to the spine during upright activities. Poor endurance and abnormal firing of the hip muscles have been noted in patients with both acute and chronic LBP. Various studies have shown that the occurrence of LBP may be reduced by strengthening the back, legs, and abdomen (core muscle groups), improving muscular stabilization. Initial exercises should focus on strengthening and stabilizing the spine and stretching the hip flexors. Lower extremity muscle tightness is common with LBP and must be corrected to allow normal range of motion of the lumbar spine. Tight hip flexors (iliopsoas and rectus femoris) cause excessive anterior pelvic rotation and increased lumbar lordosis. Stretching the hip flexors and strengthening the hip extensors will potentially rotate the pelvis back to a neutral position, resulting in a decrease in LBP.

In a similar fashion tight hamstrings place excessive posterior tilt on the pelvis decreasing lumbar lordosis. This places the erector spinae at a mechanical disadvantage, making the spine less resilient to axial loads and increasing the likelihood of injury. Stretching the hamstrings and strengthening the back extensors restore the neutral pelvis positioning and reduce patient pain.

Hayden JA et al: Systematic review: Strategies for using exercise therapy to improve outcomes in chronic low back pain. Ann Intern Med 2005;142:776. [PMID: 15867410]

Nadler SF et al: Hip muscle imbalance and low back pain in athletes: Influence of core strengthening. Med Sci Sports Exerc 2002;34:9. [PMID: 11782641]

H. Behavioral Therapy

A multitude of factors play a role in decreasing pain and enabling a return to function in patients with LBP. Psychological stress (depression) has emerged as the strongest single baseline predictor of 4-year outcomes, exceeding pain intensity. Fear avoidance beliefs also have a strong influence on recovery. These factors highlight the importance of exercise as a management tool for LBP. Exercise reduces fear avoidance behavior and facilitates function despite ongoing pain. Graded behavior intervention reinforces that pain does not necessarily mean harm. Patients may still have pain but be able to function, thereby improving their prognosis over time. The results of cognitive intervention and exercise programs are similar to those for lumbar fusion in improving disability in patients with chronic back pain and disc degeneration.

Ostelo RW et al: Behavioural treatment for chronic low-back pain. Cochrane Database Syst Rev 2005;(1):CD002014. [PMID: 15674889]

I. Reevaluation

For those LBP patients whose condition worsens during the time of symptom control, reevaluation and consultation or referral to specialty care is recommended. Patients with LBP should always be reevaluated as indicated after 1–3 weeks to assess progress (see Figure 23–1C, Box 12). This can be accomplished with either a follow-up phone call or office visit. This empowers patients to take the initiative in their disease course. Patients must be advised to follow up sooner if their condition worsens. Any worsening of neurologic symptoms warrants a complete reevaluation.

Conservative treatment is warranted for 4–6 weeks from the initial evaluation. The follow-up visit is the appropriate time to consider a work-related ergonomic evaluation. As the patient improves there should be a gradual return to normal activity and a weaning of the medications. So-called "back schools" and work-related ergonomic programs might contribute to the prevention of injuries and reinjuries; however, the long-term benefits are inconclusive.

J. Referral

If a patient has LBP for more than 6 weeks despite an adequate course of conservative therapy, the patient should be reexamined in the office. A comprehensive reevaluation, including a psychosocial assessment and physical examination, should be performed (see Figure 23–1C, Box 24). During follow-up visits, questions should be directed at identifying any detriments in the patient's condition, including new neurologic symptoms, increase in pain, or new radiation of the pain. If such problems are found, the patient should be reevaluated for other health problems and consultation or referral scheduled, if necessary.

Table 23–5. Nonsurgical back specialists.

Specialist	Indications
Physiatrist/physical medicine and rehabilitation	Chronic back pain for more than 6 wk Chronic sciatica for more than 6 wk Chronic pain syndrome Recurrent back pain
Neurology	Chronic sciatica for more than 6 wk Atypical chronic leg pain (negative straight leg raising) New or progressive neuromotor deficit
Occupational medicine	Difficult workers' compensation situations Disability/impairment ratings Return to work issues
Rheumatology	Rule out inflammatory arthropathy Rule out fibrositis/fibromyalgia Rule out metabolic bone disease (eg, osteoporosis)
Primary care sports medicine specialist	Chronic back pain for more than 6 wk Chronic sciatica for more than 6 wk Recurrent back pain

For patients with pain that radiates below the knee, especially with a positive tension sign, the anatomy must be evaluated with an imaging study (see Figure 23–1C, Box 25). If there are abnormal findings then consultation with a neurosurgeon or back surgeon is appropriate (see Figure 23–1C, Box 27). If, however, the imaging study does not reveal anatomic pathology, then a nonsurgical back specialist may be necessary to help manage the patient (see Figure 23–1C, Box 29). Table 23–5 lists these specialists and indications for their referral.

If there are no abnormal findings on a comprehensive reassessment, including selected diagnostic tests, it is crucial to start patients on a program that will enable them to resume their usual activities. The management of the patient without structural pathology should be directed toward a physical conditioning program designed with exercise to progressively build activity tolerance and overcome individual limitations. This may include referral to behavior modification specialists, activity specific educators, or an organized multidisciplinary back rehabilitation program.

Kominski GF et al: Economic evaluation of four treatments for low back pain: Results from a randomized controlled trial. Med Care 2005;43:428. [PMID: 15838406]

Prognosis

The long-term course of LBP is variable. One recent review discovered that a majority of patients continue to report pain 12 months after initial onset of symptoms. However, 90% of patients will regain function with decreasing pain after 6 weeks, despite physician intervention.

Harwood MI: What is the most effective treatment for acute low back pain? J Fam Pract 2002;51:118. [PMID: 11978208]

Hestbaek L et al: Low back pain: What is the long-term course? A review of studies of general patient populations. Eur Spine J 2003;12:149. [PMID: 12709853]

Weiner DK et al: How does low back pain impact physical function in independent, well functioning older adults? Evidence from the Health ABC cohort and implications for the future. Pain Med 2003;4:311. [PMID: 14750907]

Web Sites

Agency for Healthcare Research and Quality:

http://www.achcpr.gov/consumer

American Academy of Orthopedic Surgeons information page:

http://orthoinfo.asos.org

American College of Rheumatology patient education on back pain:

http://www.rheumatology.org/public/factsheets/backpain_new.asp?aud=pat

European clinical practice guideline on the treatment of LBP, including the pediatric population:

http://medinfo.co.uk/conditions/lowbackpain/html

Institute for Clinical Systems Improvement, LBP guideline:

http://www.icsi.org/knowledge/detail.ask?catID=29&itemID=149

Intelihealth back pain page:

http://www.intelihelth.com?IH/ihtIH/WSAUSOOO/331/9519.html

Patient education handouts:

http://familydoctor.org

Quick reference to the US Agency for Health Care Policy and Research (1994) practice guideline:

http://www.chilrobase.org/07Strategy/AHCPR/ahcprclinician.html

Therapeutic Assessment Group, prescribing guidelines for LBP:

http://www.ciap.health.nsw.gov.au/nswtag/publications/guildelines/LowBackPain4=12=02.pdf

US Preventive Services Task Force:

http://preventiveservices.ahrq.gov

US Preventive Services Task Force recommendation statement on LBP, June 2005:

http://www.guideline.gov/summary/summary.aspx?doc_id=4772&nbr+003451&string+LOW+AND+BACK+AND+PAIN

Neck Pain

24

Garry W. K. Ho, MD, & Thomas M. Howard, MD

General Considerations

Neck pain is a common clinical problem experienced at some point in life by nearly two thirds of people. In addition to being a common problem, neck pain is quite disabling, in some countries accounting for nearly as much disability as low back pain. The economic impact of whiplash injuries alone is estimated to be nearly $4 billion.

Neck pain is also quite similar to low back pain in that the etiology is poorly understood and the clinical diagnoses are quite vague. Unlike low back pain, however, which has been the subject of numerous clinical practice guidelines, neck pain has received limited study. The few randomized controlled studies available lack consistency in study design. A review of the National Guidelines Clearinghouse (http://www.ngc.gov) demonstrates four published guidelines on neck pain, pertaining to the use of facet neurotomy, imaging, and selected rehabilitation interventions in neck pain. This chapter reviews the epidemiology and anatomy of neck pain and provides an evidenced-based assessment of the evaluation, diagnosis, and management of this challenging disorder.

Neck pain is most prevalent in middle-aged adults; however, prevalence tends to vary with different definitions of neck pain and with differing methodologies of neck pain surveys. One study, for example, found that 1-year prevalence in adults ranged from 16.7% to 75.1% and rose with longer time periods. Almost 85% of neck pain may be attributed to chronic stress and strains or acute or repetitive injuries associated with poor posture, anxiety, depression, and occupational or sporting risks. The acceleration and deceleration of a whiplash injury may result in sprains or strains of cervical soft tissue structures, which, in turn, are common causes of neck pain. Radicular neck pain occurs later in life, with an estimated incidence of 10% among 25- to 29-year-olds, rising to 25–40% in those older than 45 years.

Occupational neck pain is ubiquitous and not limited to any particular work setting. Predictors for occupational neck pain include little influence on the work situation, work-related psychosocial factors, and perceived general tension. Predictors of occupational neck pain include prolonged sitting at work (> 95% of the workday), especially with the neck forward flexed 20 degrees or more for more than 70% of the work time.

Ariens GA et al: Are neck flexion, neck rotation, and sitting at work risk factors for neck pain? Results of a prospective cohort study. Occup Environ Med 2001;58:200. [PMID: 1171934]

Ariens GA et al: High quantitative job demands and low coworker support as risk factors for neck pain: Results of a prospective cohort study. Spine 2001;26:1896. [PMID: 11568702]

Fejer R et al: The prevalence of neck pain in the world population: A systematic critical review of the literature. Eur Spine J 2006;15:834. [PMID: 15999284]

Narayan P, Haid RW: Treatment of degenerative cervical disc disease. Neurol Clin 2001;19:217. [PMID: 11471766]

Vasseljen O et al: Shoulder and neck complaints in customer relations: Individual risk factors and perceived exposures at work. Ergonomics 2001;44:355. [PMID: 11291820]

Functional Anatomy

The cervical spine is a highly mobile column that supports the 6- to 8-pound (2.7–3.6 kg) head and functions as a protection for the cervical spinal cord. The cervical spine consists of 7 vertebrae, 5 intervertebral discs, 14 facet joints (zygapophyseal joints or Z-joints), 12 joints of Luschka (uncovertebral joints), and 14 paired anterior, lateral, and posterior muscles. The vertebrae can be grouped into three major groups: the atlas (C1), the axis (C2), and the others (C3–C7). The atlas is a ring-shaped vertebra with two lateral masses, each with superior and inferior facets to articulate with the occiput and C2 respectively, as well as an anterior portion of the ring to articulate with the odontoid process (dens) of C2. The axis consists of a large vertebral body (the largest in the cervical spine) with the anterior odontoid process articulating with C1 and inferior and superior facet joints. This odontoid process has a precarious blood supply, placing it a risk for nonunion and malunion with fractures. The atlantooccipital articulation accounts for 50% of the flexion and extension range of motion (ROM) of the neck and the alantoaxial joint accounts for 50% of the rotational ROM of the neck.

Each of the remaining cervical vertebrae consists of an anterior body with a posterior projecting ring of the transverse and spinous processes that form the vertebral

Table 24–1. Upper extremity motor and sensory innervations.

Spinal Level	Motor	Reflex	Sensory	Peripheral Nerve
C5	Deltoid (shoulder abduction) Biceps	Biceps	Lateral shoulder	Axillary
C6	Biceps (elbow flexion) Wrist extensors	Brachioradialis	Lateral forearm Dorsal first web space	Musculocutaneous Radial
C7	Triceps (elbow extension) Wrist flexion Finger extension	Triceps	Dorsal middle finger	Median
C8	Finger flexors Thumb flexion/opposition	None	Ring finger Small finger Medial forearm	Ulnar Medial antebrachial cutaneous
T1	Hand intrinsics (finger abduction/adduction)	None	Medial arm Axilla	Medial brachial cutaneous

foramen for the spinal cord. The most prominent spinous processes that can be palpated are C2 and C7 (vertebral prominens). The spinous and transverse processes are the origin and insertion of the multiple interspinous and intervertebral ligaments and muscles. Between each vertebral body are intervertebral discs, each consisting of a gelatinous center (nucleus pulposus) with a tougher, multilayered (onion skin–like) surrounding annulus fibrosis. Each vertebral body from C3 to C7 articulates with the others through a bony lip (uncus) off the lateral margins called the joints of Luschka. These are not considered true diarthrodial joints (because they have no synovium); however, they may develop degenerative spurs, limiting motion. The facet joints are part of the transverse process and are paired superiorly and inferiorly. The facet joints have articular cartilage and a synovium that can be involved in degenerative and inflammatory processes. Among the multiple interspinous and intervertebral ligaments, the most important are the anterior and posterior longitudinal ligaments along the vertebral bodies, the ligamentum nuchae along the spinous process, and the ligamentum flavum along the anterior surfaces of the laminae. The weaker posterior longitudinal ligaments help stabilize the intervertebral discs posteriorly and are often damaged in disc herniation. Hypertrophy of the ligamentum flavum may contribute to nerve root impingement. Eight cervical nerve roots exit posterolaterally through the neuroforamina. Given that there are seven vertebrae, each cervical root emerges through a neuroforamen above the vertebra of its number (ie, the C6 root arises between C5 and C6), with C8 exiting between C7 and T1. The cervical cord gives rise to the nerves that innervate the neck, upper extremity, and diaphragm. In the evaluation of problems related to the cervical spine, the physician should have a basic understanding of the motor and sensory innervations of the upper extremity (Table 24–1).

The musculature of the cervical spine includes flexors, extensors, lateral flexors, and rotators. Major flexors include the sternocleidomastoid, scalenes, and prevertebrals. Extensors include the posterior paravertebral muscles (splenius, semispinalis, capitis) and trapezius. Lateral flexors include the sternocleidomastoid, scalenes, and interspinous (between the transverse processes) muscles, and the rotators include the sternocleidomastoid and the interspinous muscles. The ability of the cervical spine to absorb the energy from acute injuries is related to its lordotic curvature and the energy absorption of the paraspinal muscles and intervertebral discs.

The combined motion of all the preceding joints gives a significant ROM of the neck, allowing the head to scan the environment with the eyes and ears. Normal ROM includes extension of 70 degrees (chin straight up to the ceiling), flexion of 60 degrees (chin on chest, or within 3 cm of chest), lateral flexion of approximately 45 degrees (ear to shoulder), and rotation of approximately 80 degrees (looking right and left). The center of motion for flexion is C5–C6 and for extension, C6–C7; hence, degeneration and injury often occurs at these levels. ROM can be reduced by injury to muscles, vertebrae, or discs, or by the degenerative process causing spondylosis.

Prevention

Prevention strategies for high-risk groups have been employed for both neck and lower back pain. A recent review of 27 investigations into educational efforts, exercises, ergonomics, and risk factor modification found sufficient evidence for only strengthening exercises as an effective prevention strategy.

Linton SJ, van Tulder MW: Prevention interventions for back and neck pain problems. Spine 2001;26:778. [PMID: 11295900]

Clinical Findings

A. Symptoms and Signs

The mechanism of injury of the cervical spine, like that of other injuries can be classified in multiple ways: acute injuries, including a fall, blow to the head, or the whiplash injury or chronic-repetitive injury associated with recreational or occupational activities. Other classifications can include the direction of the stress or force generating an injury: flexion, extension-hyperextension, axial load, lateral flexion, or rotation. At 30 degrees of forward flexion, the cervical spine is straight and most vulnerable to axial load-type injuries. Most chronic neck pain is associated with poor posture, anxiety or depression, neck strain, or occupational and sport-related injuries.

In the evaluation of cervical spine problems the most important first step is to obtain a thorough history, ascertaining the mechanism of injury. In many cases, the mechanism of injury may identify the injury or guide the physical examination. The examiner should identify any history of prior injuries or problems with the cervical spine (eg, a history of prior disc surgery or degenerative arthritis). Radicular or radiating symptoms in the upper extremity should be identified. This includes radiating pain, motor weakness, or paresthesias of the upper or lower extremities. Additionally, the examiner should ask about any symptoms related to upper motor neuron pathology. This includes bowel or bladder dysfunction or gait disturbance.

Additional information gathered should include the duration and course of symptoms, aggravating and alleviating motions or activities, and attempted prior treatments initiated by patients on their own or by other providers. Comorbid diseases such as inflammatory spondyloarthropathies, cardiac disease, or gastrointestinal problems should be identified, as well as a history of tobacco or alcohol abuse. Current occupational and recreational activities and requirements should be identified, as they may contribute to the underlying problem and identify the desired end point for recovery and return to activity.

B. Cervical Spine Examination

The cervical spine is examined in an organized and systematic way that includes adequate exposure of the neck, upper back, and shoulders for observation; palpation of bony and soft tissues; evaluation of ROM; a Spurling test for nerve root irritation; assessment of Lhermitte sign for cervical radiculopathy; upper extremity motor and sensory examination; and evaluation for upper motor neuron symptoms.

1. Observation—Observation should begin as the patient walks into the examination room, looking for the presence or absence of normal fluid motion of the neck and arm swing with walking. After exposure, the examiner may note the posture (many patients have a poor head-forward with rounded-shoulder posture that contributes to chronic cervical muscular strain), shoulder position (looking for elevation from muscle spasm), and evidence of atrophy. The examiner should also observe for head tilt or rotation.

2. Palpation—Palpation of major bony prominences and the soft tissues should be performed. The spinous processes and the facet joints (about 1 cm lateral and deep to the spinous process) should be gently palpated, noting pain. (Caveat: If enough pressure is applied to the spinous process, pain can be produce in virtually any patient.) Palpation of the prevertebral and paravertebral muscles should be performed, noting hypertonicity, pain, or the presence of tender or trigger points. Common sites for trigger points include the levator scapulae (off the superior, medial margin of the scapula), upper trapezius, rhomboids, and upper paraspinals near the insertion into the occiput.

3. Range of motion—Active ROM should be tested first with judicious use of passive motion as pain permits. Motion should be tested in the six prime directions: forward flexion, extension, left and right lateral flexion, and left and right rotation. ROM can be recorded in degrees from the erect (neutral) position or as a percentage of the expected norm of chin on chest, chin to sky, ear to each shoulder, and rotation to each shoulder.

4. Spurling test—This test assesses for evidence of nerve root irritation, which can be related to spondylotic compression, discogenic compression, or the Stinger or Burner syndrome (a compression or stretch injury commonly seen in football). To perform the Spurling test, the physician extends, side bends, and partially rotates the patient's head toward the side being tested. An axial load is then gently applied to the top of the head. A positive test is indicated by radiation of pain, generally into the posterior shoulder or arm on the ipsilateral side. Although generally considered to be a reliable test of root irritation, one study of both normal and symptomatic patients, confirmed by electromyography (EMG), found a sensitivity of 30% and a specificity of 93% for the Spurling test. It is therefore not a definitive screening test, but is useful in helping confirm cervical radiculopathy.

5. Lhermitte sign—The Lhermitte sign may also be used to test for cervical radiculopathy. Forward flexion

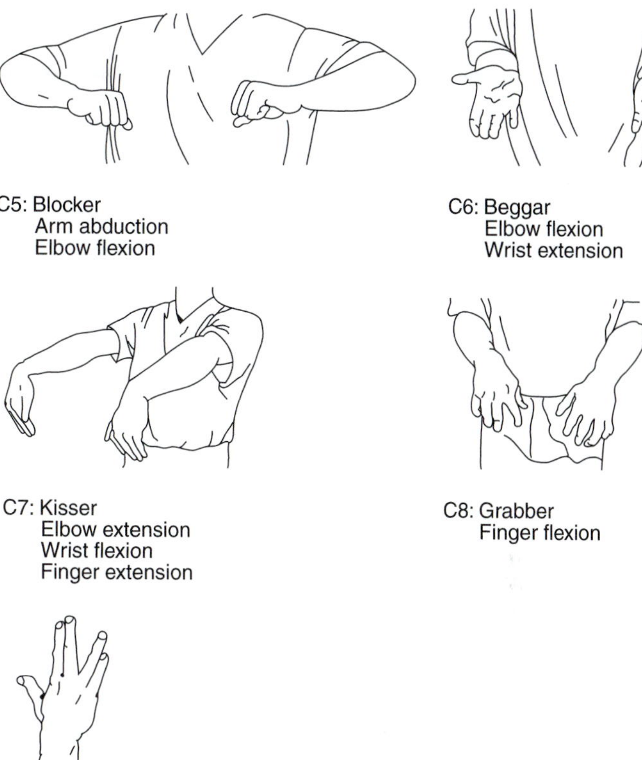

Figure 24–1. Upper extremity motor evaluation.

of the neck that causes paraesthesias down the spine or extremities suggests cervical radiculopathy, spondylosis, myelopathy, or multiple sclerosis. Manual cervical distraction may reduce neck and limb symptoms in cervical radiculopathy.

6. Upper extremity motor examination—This examination includes muscle testing and deep tendon reflexes (DTRs; see Table 24–1). A quick mnemonic to keep the upper extremity motor findings in order is *blocker, beggar, kisser, grabber, spock* (Figure 24–1). By assuming these positions, the examiner can remember the motor innervation of the cervical roots in the upper extremity. The examiner can quickly check arm abduction (blocking position) for deltoid function, then resisted elbow flexion and extension (biceps and triceps), wrist extension and flexion, grip, and finger abduction (spread fingers). DTRs should be checked for the biceps (C5), triceps (C7), and brachioradialis (C6). Sensory testing should focus on the dermatomes for the cervical roots, with focus on the lateral deltoid area (C5), dorsal first web space (C6), dorsal middle finger (C7), small finger (C8), and inner arm (T1). Upper extremity testing for upper motor neuron findings can be accomplished by looking for a Hoffman sign: With the third proximal interphalangeal joint immobilized, the patient extends the third distal interphalangeal joint with a quick flexion-flick; an abnormal flexion reflex in the thumb or other fingers is a positive test.

Testing for thoracic outlet syndrome can be accomplished with the Adson test and Roo test. In the Adson test, the patient's neck is extended, with the head rotated toward the affected side and lungs in deep inspiration, while the examiner palpates the ipsilateral radial pulse. Decrease in the amplitude of the radial pulse is a positive test. The Roo test (also called the *elevated arm stress test*) is performed with both the patient's arms (shoulders) in an abducted and externally rotated position (90 degrees each), and the elbow flexed to 90 degrees. The patient then opens and closes both hands for 3 minutes. Inability to continue this maneuver for 3 minutes due to reproduction of symptoms suggests thoracic outlet syndrome. Reasonably low false-positive rates make the Roo test the preferred test.

7. Upper motor neuron symptoms—Lower extremity testing for upper motor neuron findings should be performed, including DTRs (looking for hyperreflexia), assessment for clonus in the ankle, and testing for the Babinski reflex. The Babinski reflex may be elicited by firmly stroking the sole (plantar surface) of the foot. The reflex is present if the great toe dorsiflexes and the other toes fan out (abduct). This is normal in younger children, but abnormal after the age of 2 years. If the examiner has not queried about bowel and bladder function, it can be done at this time.

C. Laboratory Findings

In patients whose upper extremity weakness is not improving with therapy, electromyography (EMG) should be considered. EMG is useful to evaluate for upper extremity neurologic disorders and helps to distinguish between peripheral (including brachial plexus) and nerve root injuries. EMG also distinguishes between stable and active denervating or recovery processes. EMG may not be diagnostic until 3–4 weeks after an acute nerve injury, so this study should not be ordered in the acute setting. In general, however, follow-up EMG in patients with whiplash injuries may not contribute useful information to clinical and imaging findings.

Other laboratory studies, including complete blood count, sedimentation rate, rheumatoid factor, and others, should be reserved for the evaluation of spondyloarthropathies and play little role in the evaluation of most neck pain.

D. Imaging Studies

Potential imaging studies of the cervical spine can include plain radiographs, magnetic resonance imaging (MRI), computed tomography (CT), bone scan, and myelography. Bone scan does not significantly contribute to the evaluation of neck pain in acute or chronic settings. Plain films include the basic three-view series (anteroposterior, lateral, open mouth), oblique, and lateral flexion-extension views. Recommendations about the use of imaging studies in the evaluation of neck pain can be divided into recommendations for acute (traumatic) or chronic neck pain.

In the acute trauma situation the three-view radiograph is the basic study of choice. In one study of 34,000 blunt trauma patients, the three-view radiograph was abnormal and diagnostic in 498 of 818 patients, nondiagnostic in 320, and failed to note abnormality in 23. CT or lateral flexion and extension views can be used to further evaluate nondiagnostic radiographs or cases of high clinical suspicion for injury.

Cervical fractures may be ruled out on a clinical basis if the patient does not complain of neck pain when asked; does not have a history of loss of consciousness; does not have mental status change from trauma, drugs, or alcohol; does not have symptoms referable to the neck (paralysis or sensory change—present or resolved); and does not have other distracting painful injuries.

The American College of Radiology (ACR) published the ACR appropriateness criteria for imaging of suspected cervical spine trauma in 1995 and updated the criteria in 1999, and again in 2002 (http://acr.org). It concluded that cervical imaging is not required in patients who are alert; asymptomatic; without cervical tenderness, neurologic findings, or distracting injury; with or without a cervical collar; and with or without a history of unconsciousness. Those with cervical tenderness should have, at a minimum, the basic three-view series. In certain instances, a CT scan of the cervical spine may be performed along with a scan of the head while the patient is still in the CT suite, if the patient was already determined to need CT scan of the head. Patients with upper or lower extremity paraesthesias (or other neurologic findings) should also have a CT scan of the cervical spine; MRI of the cervical spine may be considered, depending on the CT findings. Patients with femur fractures should be evaluated for imaging (eg, three-view series), as previously discussed. Those who are unconscious at the time of evaluation or are in an altered mental state (due to alcohol or drugs) should receive both the three-view series and a CT scan of the cervical spine. Patients with neck pain and clinical findings suggestive of ligamentous injury, with normal radiographic and CT findings, may be considered for MRI of the cervical spine and flexion-extension radiographs.

The ACR appropriateness criteria for imaging of chronic neck pain were published in 1998 and updated in 2005. It was concluded that there are no existing guidelines for the evaluation of the patient with chronic neck pain. The initial imaging study should be the three-view series. The most common findings include a loss of lordosis (straight cervical spine) or disc space narrowing with degenerative change at the C5–C6 and C4–C5 levels. Oblique and flexion-extension views should be ordered at the discretion of the attending physician. When patients have chronic neck pain after hyperextension or flexion injury with normal radiographs and persistent pain or evidence of neurologic injury, lateral flexion-extension views should be considered to rule out instability. Abnormal findings include more than 3.5 mm horizontal displacement or more than 11 degrees of rotational difference to that of the adjacent vertebrae on resting or flexion-extension lateral radiographs. Oblique radiographs may be helpful to look for bony encroachment of the neuroforamina in the evaluation of radicular neck pain. MRI should be performed on all patients who have chronic neck pain with neurologic signs or symptoms, or both. If there is a contraindication to MRI (ie, pacemaker, nonavailability, claustrophobia, or interfering hardware in the neck), CT myelography is recommended.

American College of Radiology (ACR), Expert Panel on Musculoskeletal Imaging: *Chronic Neck Pain in ACR Appropriateness Criteria.* ACR, 2005:1–7.

American College of Radiology (ACR), Expert Panel on Musculoskeletal Imaging. *Suspected Cervical Spine Trauma in ACR Appropriateness Criteria.* ACR, 2002:1–8.

Binder A: Neck pain. Clin Evid 2006;15:1654. [PMID: 16973064]

Kimberly S: A nerve exam pantomime. Phys Sportsmed 1996;24:15.

Mower WR et al: Use of plain radiography to screen for cervical spine injuries. Ann Emerg Med 2001;38:1. [PMID: 11423803]

Steinberg FL et al: Whiplash injury: Is there a role for electromyographic studies? Arch Orthop Trauma Surg 2005;125:46. [PMID: 15611865]

Tong HC et al: The Spurling test and cervical radiculopathy. Spine 2002;27:156. [PMID: 11805661]

Differential Diagnosis

See Table 24–2.

Treatment

Multiple treatment options are available for the patient and practitioner, although there is limited evidence-based support for the efficacy of most treatment options used for such patients. Early management focuses on proper initial evaluation, use of over-the-counter analgesics, early return to motion, and judicious use of physical modalities. Acupuncture and manual therapy may help reduce pain early after injury or presentation. Chronic neck pain can be related to psychosocial factors at home and in the workplace and may be tied to litigation in whiplash-type injuries. Specialty consultation beyond physical therapy is rarely needed.

A. Initial Care

Initial management should include avoidance of aggravating factors at work or with recreational activities, as well as pain management, recognizing that most pain is self-limiting. Subsequent management should focus on early return to motion, isometric strengthening, and modification of occupational or recreational aggravating factors with return to activity (eg, observing good ergonomics).

Absolute rest should be limited to a very short period of time (ie, 1–2 days). This includes the use of cervical collars. Early motion should be encouraged as soon as severe pain allows. Early mobilization after whiplash-type injury is associated with better pain relief and return of motion. Patients should focus on proper posture (neck centered and back over the shoulders) and gentle motion of the neck in the six major motions mentioned earlier under testing for ROM. Each position should be held for 15–20 seconds. Proprioceptive neuromuscular facilitation may be employed in a structured program with physical therapy or in a home program with the goal to improve motion. This is done by having patients move the head in a direction to the point of pain. Next, they attempt to move in the opposite direction against the resistance of their own hand on the chin for a count of 5, contracting the rehabilitating

Table 24–2. Differential diagnosis of neck pain.

Acute Injury	Noninflammatory Disease	Inflammatory Disease	Infectious Causes	Neoplasm	Referred Pain
Cervical sprain, strain, spasm, whiplash Cervical tendonitis Cervical instability Fractures Vertebral body Tear drop Burst Chance Compression Spinous process Transverse process Facet Odontoid (C2) Hangman's (C2) Jefferson (C1) Stinger or Burner	Cervical osteoarthritis (spondylosis) Discogenic neck pain Cervical spinal stenosis Cervical myelopathy Myofascial pain Fibromyalgia Reflex sympathetic dystrophy/complex regional pain syndrome Migraines (or variants) Torticollis	Rheumatoid arthritis Spondyloarthropathies Juvenile rheumatoid arthritis Ankylosing spondylitis	Meningitis Osteomyelitis Infectious discitis	Primary Myeloma Cord tumor Metastatic	Temporomandibular joint Cardiac Diaphragmatic irritation Gastrointestinal Gastric ulcer Gall bladder Pancreas Thoracic outlet syndrome Shoulder disorders Brachial plexus injuries Peripheral nerve injury

muscle throughout the entire maneuver. Then they attempt to further move in the original direction, usually with improved motion. This should be done in the six major directions.

B. Pain Management

Pain management may take the form of ice, medications, or physical modalities. Application of ice (15 minutes every 2 hours) is effective for acute pain after injury or for post-activity pain during the recovery process. Medications used in the management of acute and chronic neck pain include salicylates (aspirin, 500 mg four times daily, or salsalate, 500 mg three times daily), nonsteroidal anti-inflammatory drugs (NSAIDs; ibuprofen, 600 mg four times daily or 800 mg three times daily; naproxen, 500 mg twice daily; indomethacin, 25–50 mg three times daily; piroxicam, 20 mg/d; or cyclooxygenase-2 inhibitors, eg, celecoxib, 200 mg/d), acetaminophen (500–1000 mg four times daily), muscle relaxants (diazepam, 5 mg three times daily; methocarbamol, 1000–1500 mg four times daily; and cyclobenzaprine, 10 mg three times daily), narcotic medications (acetaminophen with codeine, acetaminophen with oxycodone, acetaminophen with hydrocodone, meperidine), and corticosteroids. For acute radicular symptoms, a short course of corticosteroids may be considered (prednisone, 40–60 mg/day for 5–7 days) to reduce inflammation associated with a herniated nucleus pulposus. Although there is no literature to support use of ice or systemic steroids, anecdotal evidence suggests that they may be helpful in the acute setting.

For pain that is becoming more chronic (eg, > 30 days), tricyclic antidepressants (TCAs; nortriptyline, 25–50 mg, or amitriptyline, 10–50 mg) or selective serotonin reuptake inhibitors (SSRIs; fluoxetine, 10–60 mg, or sertraline, 25–100 mg at bedtime) may be used at night for chronic pain management and management of sleep disturbance that often accompanies chronic pain of any source. Side effects of TCAs include excessive drowsiness, dry mouth, urinary retention, and potential cardiac conduction problems. Side effects of SSRIs include insomnia, drowsiness, dry mouth, nausea, headache, and anorexia. The combination of SSRIs and TCAs may result in increased serum levels of the TCA and toxicity. Randomized controlled studies support the use of simple analgesics and NSAIDs in the management of acute pain but do not support the other treatment options.

C. Physical Modalities

Multiple physical modalities are available for the management of pain and to improve motion, although there is little clinical evidence of their effectiveness and no well-designed randomized controlled studies that support their use in management of acute or chronic neck pain. These modalities include application of heat, ultrasound, cervical traction, acupuncture, and electric stimulation (including transcutaneous electrical nerve stimulation [TENS]). Cervical traction can be effective for relief of spasm or in the management of radicular pain from a herniated nucleus pulposus or spondylosis. Traction may be performed in a controlled setting at physical therapy or with the use of home traction units. Typical sessions in physical therapy are 2–3 days per week for 30 minutes per session. A typical home cervical traction regimen would start at 10 pounds of longitudinal traction and titrate up by 5 pounds every 1–2 days until a goal of 20–30 pounds is reached. Home traction is used on a daily or every-other-day basis. Heat, ultrasound, and electric stimulation may be effective in local pain management, allowing early return to normal motion.

D. Acupuncture

Acupuncture has been shown to be effective in the treatment of acute pain, although its effectiveness beyond five treatments is limited. A home program of ischemic pressure (acupressure) with stretching has also been shown to be effective in the management of myofascial neck pain.

E. Manual Therapy

Manual therapy (osteopathic and chiropractic manipulation) is commonly used in the management of chronic neck and lower back pain, although there is limited evidence (three nonrandomized controlled studies) supporting its use. A study on the use of manual therapy in the treatment of neck and low back pain showed an average improvement of 53.8% in acute pain and 48.4% in chronic pain with 12 treatments over a 4-week period of time. A recent case report of a patient with persistent neck and arm pain after failed cervical disc surgery with resolution after a program of manual therapy and rehabilitative exercises further supports the use of manual therapy in the management of both myofascial and radicular neck pain.

F. Isometric Exercise

As patients recover, a program of strengthening should be instituted. Simple isometric exercises focusing on resisted forward flexion, extension, and right and left lateral flexion will improve pain and strength, contributing to recovery and long-term resistance to further injury.

G. Referral

Specialty referral may be considered at multiple points in the recovery process to aid in diagnosis or treatment of acute or chronic neck pain. Physical therapy may be used early in the process to incorporate physical modalities and initiate a strengthening program. However, evidence supporting the use of electrotherapy in neck disorders is lacking, limited, or conflicting. Typical consultations involve two to three sessions per week for 4–6 weeks, with follow-up evaluation by the primary provider. Physical Medicine and Rehabilitation (PM&R) involvement may be considered for comanagement of chronic pain of any source and to obtain EMGs. The input of a neurologist may be considered to obtain EMGs or for consultation in patients with confusing neurologic conditions. Neurosurgery or orthopedic-spinal surgery should be considered for patients requiring operative management. Early referral should be considered for severe muscle weakness, fractures, and evidence of myelopathy (long-track signs). Success rates for surgery have been reported to be as high as 80–90% for radicular pain and 60–70% for myelopathy. There is insignificant evidence to compare conservative treatment with surgical management of patients who have neck pain and radiculopathy. Referral for chronic pain management should be considered for patients who have chronic radiating pain after 9–12 weeks of conservative management. Referral for anesthesia or to a pain clinic should be considered for comanagement of patients with chronic pain or consideration of epidural steroid (ESI) or facet injections. Two randomized controlled studies provided limited evidence to support the use of ESI in chronic neck pain. Intramuscular injections of lidocaine, similar to those used in trigger-point injections, may be effective in patients with chronic mechanical neck pain. Intramuscular injections of botulinum toxin type A have been found to be no more efficacious than saline.

Alcantara J et al: Chiropractic care of a patient with vertebral subluxations and unsuccessful surgery of the cervical spine. J Manipulative Physiol Ther 2001;24:477. [PMID: 11562657]

Conlin A et al: Treatment of whiplash-associated disorders—Part I: Non-invasive interventions. Pain Res Manag 2005;10:21. [PMID: 15782244]

Hanten WP et al: Effectiveness of a home program of ischemic pressure followed by sustained stretch for treatment of myofascial trigger points. Phys Ther 2001;81:1059. [PMID: 11002435]

Irnich D et al: Randomized trial of acupuncture compared with conventional massage and "sham" laser acupuncture for treatment of chronic neck pain. BMJ 2001;322:1574. [PMID: 11431299]

Kroeling P et al: Electrotherapy for neck disorders. Cochrane Database Syst Rev 2005;(2):CD004251. [PMID: 15846703]

Lu DP et al: Acupuncture and clinical hypnosis for facial and head and neck pain: A single crossover comparison. Am J Clin Hypn 2001;44:141. [PMID: 11591081]

McMorland G, Suter E: Chiropractic management of mechanical neck and low-back pain: A retrospective, outcome-based analysis. J Manipulative Physiol Ther 2000;23:307. [PMID: 10863249]

Peloso P et al: Medicinal and injection therapies for mechanical neck disorders. Cochrane Database Syst Rev 2005;(2):CD000319. [PMID: 15846603]

Prognosis

Neck pain usually resolves in days to weeks, but like low back pain can become recurrent. The incidence of chronic neck pain is about 10%, and about 5% of people will experience severe disability. Patients who experience symptoms for at least 6 months have a less than 50% percent chance of recovering even with aggressive therapy. Predictors of chronic neck pain include a prior history of neck pain or injury, female gender, number of children, poor self-assessed health, poor psychological status (eg, excessive concerns about symptoms, unrealistic expectations of treatment, and psychosocial concerns), and history of low back pain.

Up to 40% of patients with whiplash injuries report symptoms for up to 15 years post injury. These patients have a three times higher risk of neck pain in the next 7 years. A Swedish study showed that 55% of an exposed group and 29% of a control group had residual symptoms up to 17 years post injury. Initial signs and symptoms that are predictive of slower recovery from whiplash-type injuries include mode of motor vehicle collision, age older than 60 years, female gender, neck pain on palpation, muscle pain, headache, and pain or numbness radiating to the arms, hands, or shoulders. High initial pain intensity is an important predictor of delayed functional recovery. The single best estimation of handicap due to whiplash injury was return of normal cervical ROM.

Albert E et al: Whiplash: Still a pain in the neck. Aust Fam Physician 2003;32:152. [PMID: 12666355]

Berglund A et al: The association between exposure to rear-end collision and future neck or shoulder pain: A cohort study. J Clin Epidemiol 2000;53:1089. [PMID: 11106881]

Bunketorp L et al: Neck pain and disability following motor vehicle accidents—a cohort study. Eur Spine J 2005;14:84. [PMID: 15241671]

Croft PR et al: Risk factors for neck pain: A longitudinal study in the general population. Pain 2001;93:317. [PMID: 11514090]

Eck JC et al: Whiplash: A review of a commonly misunderstood injury. Am J Med 2001;110:651. [PMID: 11382374]

Hoving JL et al: A critical appraisal of review articles on the effectiveness of conservative treatment for neck pain. Spine 2001;26:196. [PMID: 11154541]

Kasch H et al: Handicap after acute whiplash injury: A 1 year prospective study of risk factors. Neurology 2001;56:1637. [PMID: 11425927]

Scholten-Peeters GG et al: Prognostic factors of whiplash-associated disorders: A systematic review of prospective cohort studies. Pain 2003;104:303. [PMID: 12855341]

Suissa S: Risk factors of poor prognosis after whiplash injury. Pain Res Manag 2003;8:69. [PMID: 12879136]

Suissa S et al: The relation between initial symptoms and signs and the prognosis of whiplash. Eur Spine J 2001;10:44. [PMID: 11276835]

Web Sites

Useful sites for patient education on topics such as home rehabilitation, correction of occupational and postural risk factors:

http://www.nismat.org/orthocor/programs/neck/neckex.html

http://www.nismat.org/ptcor/neck

http://familydoctor.org/x2557.xml

Evaluation of Breast Lumps

25

Jo Ann Rosenfeld, MD

General Considerations

A woman's discovery of a breast lump always brings the specter of breast cancer, disfigurement, and death, even when it is judged benign. The physician who finds a lump or who helps a woman who has discovered a lump must realize that rapid and accurate diagnosis and appropriate treatment are essential. For this reason, so-called triple assessment—comprising clinical examination, imaging, and pathology—is now the standard approach to all breast lumps.

There are many causes of breast lumps, many of them normal or benign (Table 25–1). Most benign disorders are related to normal processes of a woman's reproductive life (ie, hormonal cycles and pregnancy). Cysts are the most common mass found in patients in a breast clinic.

The number of lumps found and the risk that the lump is malignant correlates with patient age. The percentage of lumps that are cancerous increases with age from less than 1% of all breast lumps in women younger than age 30 years to 70% of breast lumps in women older than 70 years (Figure 25–1). In women younger than 20 years, cancer is uncommon and premenarchal breast buds and fibroadenomas are much more common. Localized benign breast masses, cysts, and fibroadenomas are the most common causes of breast lumps in women younger than 50 years. In women aged 30–35 years, cancer is still uncommon, at a rate of 25 per 100,000 women. Conversely, a new breast lump in a postmenopausal woman is very worrisome. During pregnancy, mastitis or breast abscesses are the most common cause of a breast mass. Galactoceles are also found.

Prominent or asymmetric ribs; inflammatory lymph nodes in the axilla; sebaceous cysts, often in the axillae; scars; and accessory breasts may be causes of breast lumps in women at any age.

Fibrocystic breast disease, a cause of multiple or recurrent breast cysts and lumps, occurs in approximately 19% of women. The cysts usually manifest in women during their 20s and 30s and increase with age. The lumps are usually multiple and bilateral and cause cyclic pain, which is often reduced with use of oral contraceptives. However, there may be just one "lump" at any one time. Fibrocystic disease and its symptoms should decrease with menopause.

Breast lumps may be an incidental finding on a mammogram or may be found by the woman in self-breast examinations or by the physician in a clinical breast examination. Associated symptoms may be pain, discharge, or skin changes.

Hughes LE et al: *Benign Disorders and Diseases of the Breast: Concepts and Clinical Management,* 2nd ed. Saunders, 1999.

Clinical Filndings

A. Symptoms and Signs

The duration and relation of the lump in size to the menstrual period and whether the lump is tender or painful may help determine the etiology. New breast pain is the presenting complaint for cancer in fewer than 6% of women with breast cancer. Figure 25–2 outlines the evaluation of breast lumps.

Because lumps or cysts may be related to the menstrual cycle, evaluating the woman twice—once immediately and once 2 weeks later—may be advisable, especially in a young woman who is nearing her menses. If any associated symptoms are more worrisome or the woman is postmenopausal, waiting 2 weeks before proceeding to radiologic studies and pathology may not be sensible.

Although radiologic tests may be definitive, the clinical breast examination can contribute to the diagnosis and delineation of the cause of a lump. Both breasts should be examined in detail, from the axillae to the areolae, visually and by palpation.

Skin changes are important; dimpling, thickening of the skin of the breast (peau d'orange—"orange skin"), or nipple inversion is worrisome for cancer. Nipple retraction is often, but not always, a sign of cancer. Two benign lumps, skin fixation, or a chronic abscess can cause nipple retraction or skin attachment.

Noting whether the lump is soft, cystlike, hard, or firm and noting its size and mobility (whether it is attached to the chest wall, other breast tissue, or freely moving) are important. Fibroadenomas are usually rubbery, smooth, and mobile. Cysts can be soft or hard, depending on the pressure of the contents, and are usually less mobile than fibroadenomas. Abscesses are often tender, fluctuant, and warm, and the surrounding tissue is often erythematous.

Table 25–1. Causes of breast lumps.

Normal nodularity
Fat lobules, prominent ribs, etc
Inflammatory
Abscess; fat necrosis
Common benign changes
Fibroadenomas, cysts, galactoceles
Benign tumors
Duct papillomas, lipomas
Malignant
Carcinoma *in situ*, primary or secondary cancers
Skin lesions
Sebaceous cysts, hidroadenitis, malignant or benign skin tumors

Data from Hughes LE, et al: *Benign Disorders and Diseases of the Breast*, 2nd ed. Saunders, 1999: 94–121.

Lymph node enlargement, tenderness, or thickening should be noted. The presence and placement of other lumps or breast tissue should be observed. Drawing pictures of the breast with placement and sizing of the lump(s) in the medical record is also useful.

The woman whose lump is not felt by the physician should nonetheless be subject to the same complete evaluation.

B. Laboratory Findings

No laboratory tests will help define the breast lump. A white blood count and other tests may be useful if an abscess, cellulitis, or cancer is suspected, but the information only adds to the data.

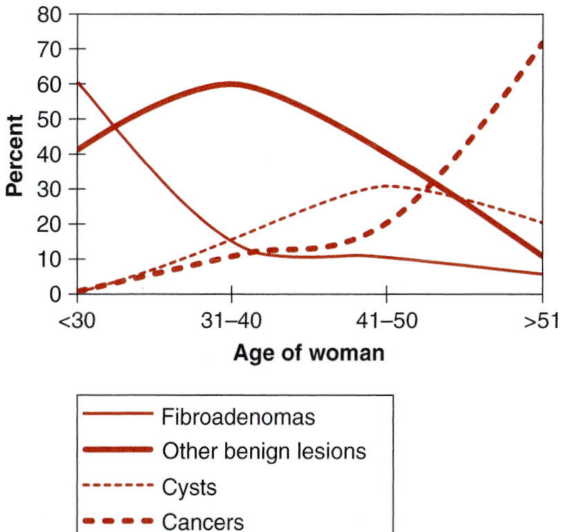

Figure 25–1. Types of breast lumps by age. (Data from Dixon JM, Mansel RE: ABC of breast diseases: Symptoms assessment and guidelines for referral. Br Med J 1994;309:722.)

C. Imaging Studies

The primary way to image the breast is with mammography. Despite current controversy over the relative benefits of prevention or detection of cancer by mass screening, every woman older than 25 years of age who has a lump needs a mammogram, even if a screening mammogram has recently been done. Mammography is the imaging technique of first choice in women 35 years of age or older. In women younger than age 35 years, breasts are usually denser and more glandular, cancer occurs less often, and, thus, ultrasonography becomes the primary radiologic study.

1. Mammography—Mammography is safe, reliable, and often sufficient to make the diagnosis of a breast lump. Benign breast lesions are usually rounded or ovoid with smooth margins. Benign lesions, such as cysts or fibroadenomas, may show "halos" of compressed fat that suggest there has been no infiltration. Cysts may also show eggshell-like rims of calcifications whereas fibroadenomas often show popcorn-like calcifications. Calcifications in benign lesions are often smooth or follow the ducts.

Additional specific mammographic views and ultrasonography often are needed to delineate the cause of a breast lump.

2. Ultrasonography—Ultrasound is used, often in conjunction with mammography, to determine whether a lump is cystic solid, discrete or associated with other nodularity, and to assist in localization and targeting for needle and other biopsy.

3. Fine-needle aspiration—Use of fine-needle aspiration (FNA) has become almost mandatory in the diagnosis of breast lumps. FNA will assess the consistency of a mass, aspirate fluid, "cure" the lump if it is a cyst, and even provide a specimen for cytology, if possible. Usually it is performed under mammographic or ultrasound direction.

Cytologic evaluation of a specimen obtained with FNA has an accuracy of up to 99%, with as few as 0.4% false positives. In patients with normal ultrasound, physical examination, and cytologic findings, a negative FNA has an almost 100% negative predictive value. Ultrasound-guided FNA is more accurate than freehand biopsy. Even FNA with scant cellularity can be reassuring in the presence of normal breast imaging studies and clinical breast examination.

Geller BM et al: Use of the American College of Radiology BI-RADS to report on the mammographic evaluation of women with signs and symptoms of breast disease. Radiology 2002;222:536. [PMID: 11818625]

Houssami N et al: Florence-Sydney Breast Biopsy Study: Sensitivity of ultrasound-guided versus freehand fine needle biopsy of

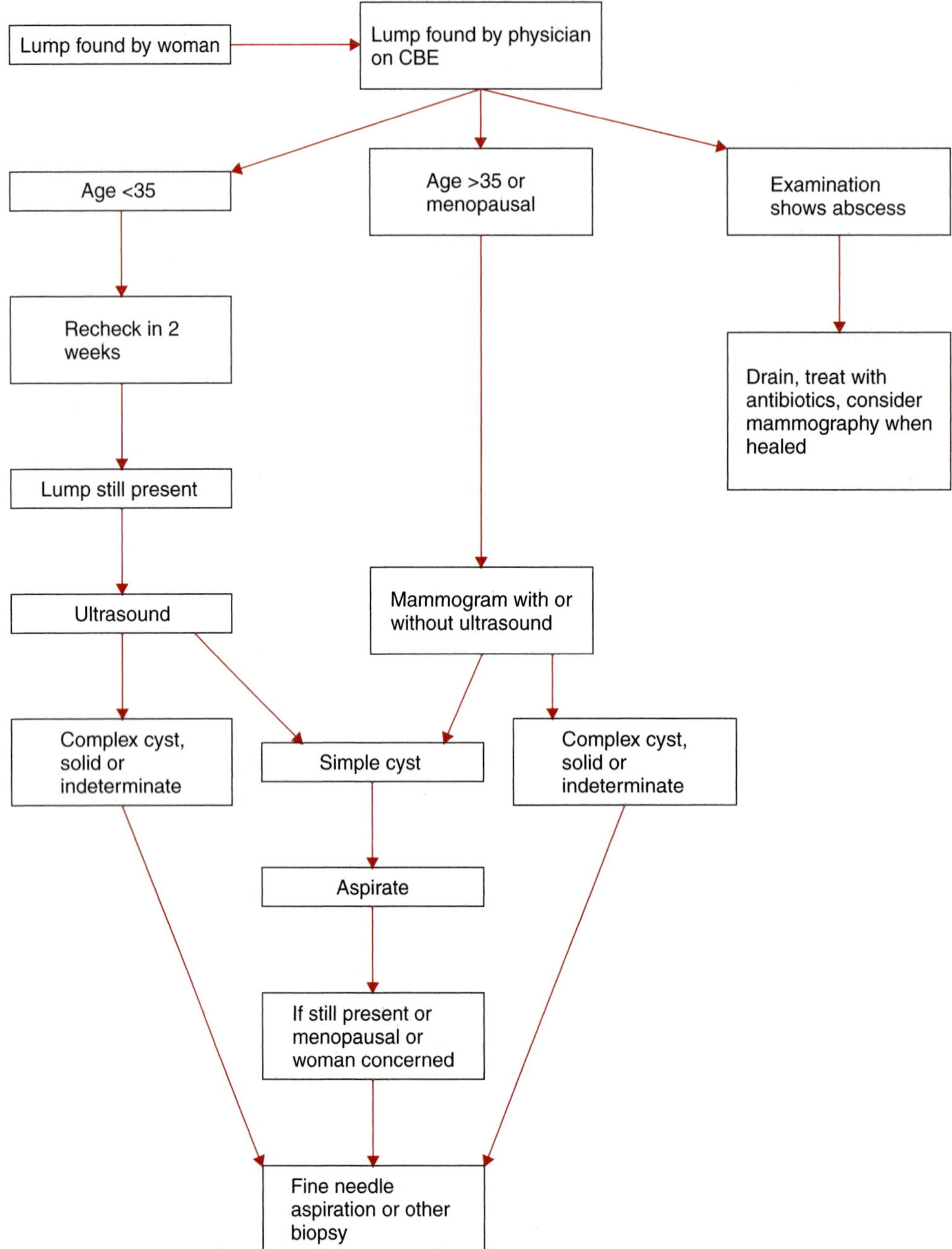

Figure 25–2. Evaluation of breast lumps. CBE, clinical breast examination.

palpable breast cancer. Breast Cancer Res Treat 2005;89:55. [PMID: 15666297]

Lau SK et al: The negative predictive value of breast fine needle aspiration biopsy: The Massachusetts General Hospital experience. Breast J 2004;10:487. [PMID: 15569203]

Vetto JT et al: Breast fine needle aspirates with scant cellularity are clinically useful. Am J Surg 2005;189:621. [PMID: 15862508]

Treatment

Treatment depends on diagnosis. If there is uncertainty after FNA, a wide needle or open biopsy is indicated. Abscesses should be drained; consultation with a surgeon may be necessary, especially if the abscesses are large, deep, or involved.

Skin abscesses such as those from sebaceous cysts and those in the axillae can often be drained in the office. Antibiotics, oral or parenteral, are indicated. If the woman is not breast-feeding and surgical drainage is performed, the excised tissue should be sent for cytologic evaluation or the woman should have another mammogram after the abscess heals to evaluate for inflammatory cancers.

Physicians comfortable with the procedure can drain cysts. If the examination, mammogram, and ultrasound show the lump is a cyst, an aspiration can be diagnostic and therapeutic. If after anesthesia, the needle encounters fluid, and when aspirated, the lump disappears, the lump was definitely a cyst and further evaluation may not be needed. The fluid can be sent for cytologic study. Larger cysts may need to be aspirated or drained surgically. However, women with breast cysts have a moderately higher risk of breast cancer.

Lumps definitely diagnosed by mammography as fibroadenomas can be watched or excised. Recent research suggests that for younger women conservative watching may be acceptable psychologically and a reasonable risk. Repeat mammography in 6 months may be an adequate evaluation and no other treatment is necessary.

The treatment of fibrocystic breast disease has not been extensively studied. Dietary additions and avoidance of caffeine, chocolate, and alcohol have been suggested by observational studies without proof of efficacy in case-controlled studies. Diuretics have not beenshown to be useful. Use of oral contraceptives for 12–24 months has resulted in some reduction in cysts and pain. In severe cases, danazol and gonadotropin-releasing hormone analogs have been used, but they are not approved for use in fibrocystic disease.

Women whose lumps show pathologic changes indicative of cancer or *in situ* cancer should be immediately referred to an oncologist, preferably one specializing in breast cancers.

Greenberg R et al: Management of breast fibroadenomas. J Gen Intern Med 1998;13:640. [PMID: 9754521]

Marchant DJ: Controversies in benign breast disease. Surg Oncol Clin North Am 1998;7:285. [PMID: 9537977]

Respiratory Problems 26

William J. Hueston, MD

Respiratory infections and chronic lung diseases are among the most common reasons that patients consult primary care physicians. Most of the respiratory problems encountered by primary care physicians are acute, with the majority comprising respiratory infections, exacerbations of asthma, chronic obstructive pulmonary diseases, and pulmonary embolism.

UPPER RESPIRATORY TRACT INFECTIONS

COMMON COLDS/UPPER RESPIRATORY TRACT INFECTIONS

ESSENTIALS OF DIAGNOSIS

- *Sore throat, congestion, low-grade fever, mild myalgias, and fatigue.*
- *Symptoms lasting for 12–14 days.*

General Considerations

Although colds are mild, tend to get better on their own, and are of short duration, they are a leading cause of sickness and of industrial and school absenteeism. Each year, colds account for 170 million days of restricted activity, 23 million days of school absence, and 18 million days of work absence.

Most colds are caused by viruses. Rhinoviruses are the most common type of virus and are found in slightly more than half of all patients. Coronaviruses are the second most common cause. In rare instances (0.05% of all cases), bacteria can be cultured from individuals with cold symptoms. It is not clear if these bacteria cause the cold, are secondary infectious agents, or are simply colonizers. Bacterial pathogens that have been identified include *Chlamydia pneumoniae, Haemophilus influenzae, Streptococcus pneumoniae,* and *Mycoplasma pneumoniae.*

Prevention

The mechanisms of transmission suggest that colds can be spread through contact with inanimate surfaces, but the primary transmission appears to be via hand-to-hand contact. The beneficial effects of removing viruses from the hands are supported by observations that absences due to colds among children in day-care or school settings have been reduced through the use of antiseptic hand wipes throughout the day.

Clinical Findings

Colds generally last 12–14 days. Telling patients that colds last no longer than a week underestimates the actual natural history of an uncomplicated viral respiratory tract infection and leads patients to believe that symptoms that persist beyond a week are not normal. When the symptoms of congestion persist longer than 2 weeks, consideration should be given to other causes of chronic congestion (Table 26–1).

Symptoms of colds include sore throat, congestion, low-grade fever, and mild myalgias and fatigue. In general, early in the development of a cold the discharge is clear. As more inflammation develops, the discharge takes on some coloration. A yellow, green, or brown-tinted nasal discharge is an indicator of inflammation, not secondary bacterial infection. Discolored nasal discharge raises the likelihood of sinusitis, but only if other predictors of sinusitis are present. In addition, several studies have shown that patients with discolored discharge respond to antibiotics no better than they respond to placebos.

Complications

Primary complications from upper respiratory tract infection are otitis media and sinusitis. These complications develop from obstruction of the eustachian tube or sinus ostia from nasal passage edema. Although treatment of these infections with antibiotics is common, the vast majority of infections clear without antibiotic therapy.

Table 26–1. Differential diagnosis for congestion and rhinorrhea.

Common cold
Sinusitis
Viral
Allergic
Bacterial
Fungal
Seasonal allergic rhinitis
Vasomotor rhinitis
Rhinitis secondary to α-agonist withdrawl
Drug-induced rhinitis (eg, cocaine)
Nasal foreign body

One misconception is that using antibiotics during the acute phase of a cold can prevent these complications. Evidence shows that taking antibiotics during a cold does not reduce the incidence of sinusitis or otitis media.

Differential Diagnosis

The differential diagnosis of colds includes complications of the cold such as sinusitis or otitis media, acute bronchitis, and noninfectious rhinitis. Influenza shares many of the symptoms of a common cold, but generally patients have a much higher fever, myalgias, and more intense fatigue.

Treatment

Despite the widespread recognition that viruses cause common colds, several studies have shown that patients with the common cold who are seen in physicians' offices are often treated with antibiotics. The prescribing of antibiotics for colds occurs more often in adults than children. Although this practice appears to have declined in adults, the use of broad-spectrum antibiotics for colds is still common in children. The need to reduce the use of antibiotics for viral conditions has important ramifications on community-wide drug resistance; in areas in which prescribing antibiotics for respiratory infections has been curtailed, reversals in antibiotic drug resistance have been observed.

Currently, the most effective symptomatic treatments are over-the-counter decongestants, the most popular of which include pseudoephedrine hydrochloride and topically applied vasoconstrictors. These agents produce short-term symptomatic relief. However, patients must be warned to use topical agents cautiously because prolonged use is associated with rebound edema of the nasal mucosa (rhinitis medicamentosa).

Several over-the-counter medications contain a mix of decongestants, cough suppressants, and pain relievers. Again, the use of these preparations will not cure the common cold but will provide symptomatic relief.

Antihistamines, with a few exceptions, have not been shown to be effective treatments. Zinc gluconate lozenges are available without a prescription, but a meta-analysis of 15 previous studies on zinc concluded that zinc lozenges were not effective in reducing the duration of cold symptoms.

Some herbal remedies are useful for treatment of the common cold. Echinacea, also known as the American coneflower, has been purported to reduce the duration of the common cold by stimulating the immune system; however, evidence for its efficacy is mixed. Echinacea should be used only for 2–3 weeks to avoid liver damage and other possible side effects that have been reported during long-term use of this herb. Ephedra, also known as ma huang, has decongestant properties that make it similar to pseudoephedrine. Ephedra is more likely than pseudoephedrine to cause increased blood pressure tachyarrhythmia. This is especially true if used in conjunction with caffeine.

Other herbal preparations that have been touted as remedies for the common cold include goldenseal, yarrow, eyebright, and elderflower. However, no systematic evidence supports the use of these herbs in treating the common cold.

Mainous AG 3rd et al: Trends in antimicrobial prescribing for bronchitis and upper respiratory infections among adults and children. Am J Public Health 2003; 93:1910. [PMID: 14600065]

Linde K et al: Echinacea for preventing and treating the common cold. Cochrane Database Syst Rev 2006;(2):CD000530. [PMID: 16437427]

SINUSITIS

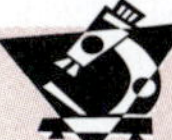

ESSENTIALS OF DIAGNOSIS

- *"Double-sickening" phenomenon.*
- *Maxillary toothache and purulent nasal discharge.*
- *Poor response to decongestants.*
- *History of discolored nasal discharge.*

General Considerations

Sinusitis is most often a complication of upper respiratory viral infections, so the incidence peaks in the winter cold season. Medical conditions that may increase the risk for sinusitis include cystic fibrosis, asthma, immunosuppression, and allergic rhinitis. Cigarette smoking may also increase the risk of bacterial sinusitis during a cold because of reduced mucociliary clearance.

Most cases of acute sinusitis are caused by viral infection. The inflammation associated with viral infection clears without additional therapy. Bacterial superinfection of upper respiratory infections (URIs) is rare and occurs in only 0.5–1% of colds. Fungal sinusitis is very rare and usually occurs in immunosuppressed individuals or those with diabetes mellitus.

Clinical Findings

Acute sinusitis has considerable overlap in its constellation of signs and symptoms with URIs. One half to two thirds of patients with sinus symptoms seen in primary care are unlikely to have sinusitis. URIs are often precursors of sinusitis and at some point symptoms from each condition may overlap. Sinus inflammation from a URI without bacterial infection is also common.

The signs and symptoms that increase the likelihood that the patient has acute sinusitis are a "double-sickening" phenomenon (whereby the patient seems to improve following the URI and then deteriorates), maxillary toothache, purulent nasal discharge, poor response to decongestants, and a history of discolored nasal discharge.

Treatment

Antibiotics are commonly prescribed for adult patients who present with complaints consistent with acute sinusitis. The effectiveness of antibiotics is unclear. If an antibiotic is used, evidence with trimethoprim-sulfamethoxazole suggests that short-duration treatment (eg, 3 days) is as effective as longer treatment. Further, a meta-analysis indicates that narrow-spectrum agents are as effective as broad-spectrum agents.

American Academy of Pediatrics. Subcommittee on Management of Sinusitis and Committee on Quality Improvement: Clinical practice guideline: Management of sinusitis. Pediatrics 2001;108:798. [PMID: 11533355]

Williams JW Jr, Simel DL: Does this patient have sinusitis: Diagnosing acute sinusitis by history and physical examination. JAMA 1993;270:1242. [PMID: 8355389]

Williams JW Jr et al: Antibiotics for acute maxillary sinusitis. Cochrane Database Syst Rev 2000;(2):CD000243. [PMID: 12804392]

OTITIS MEDIA

For discussion of otitis media, see Chapter 5.

PHARYNGITIS

ESSENTIALS OF DIAGNOSIS

- *Fever and cervical lymphadenopathy accompanying a sore throat.*
- *Rhinorrhea and cough.*
- *Positive throat culture or rapid streptococcal antigen test.*

General Considerations

The most common causes of pharyngitis are respiratory viruses. Adenovirus and the rhinoviruses account for about 80% of cases of sore throat in children who are seen by a physician. Coxsackievirus, herpesvirus, and Epstein–Barr virus (EBV) can cause tonsillitis, but are less common than adenovirus.

Group A β-hemolytic streptococci can cause an acute tonsillopharyngitis. The peak occurrence of both viral and group A streptococcal pharyngitis is winter and early spring. Streptococcal infection, in particular, can be recognized in epidemic patterns frequently affecting groups that spend considerable time together in close quarters, such as day care, school, and places of employment. Strep throat also is related to patient age. Streptococcal pharyngitis is rare in children younger than 1 year of age, but increases in early childhood with a peak occurrence for strep throat between 3 and 10 years of age. The risk of strep throat decreases in those over the age of 20.

Chlamydia and *Mycoplasma* species also have been identified in patients with acute pharyngitis. However, there have been few treatment trials that demonstrate any benefit of treating these agents; patients who received placebo had the same speed of symptom resolution as those treated with active antibiotics.

Another cause of acute pharyngitis, especially in preteen and early teenage children, is mononucleosis. Infectious mononucleosis is spread through salivary excretion of the EBV. Clinical characteristics of infectious mononucleosis include an exudative tonsillitis or pharyngitis, cervical lymph node enlargement, fever, malaise, and hepatosplenomegaly. Fever and lymphadenopathy are the most common symptoms of infectious mononucleosis and occur in over 90% of children with this infection. Tonsillitis occurs in 70–80% of children with mononucleosis. Because of the similarities in presenting symptoms with streptococcal pharyngitis, infectious mononucleosis can be mistaken for strep throat early in the course of illness.

In addition to the common causes, several other conditions can cause pharyngitis. These include infections with coxsackieviruses (herpangina), *Candida,* other bacteria (diphtheria, *Neisseria gonorrhea*), and spirochetes (leptospirosis). Retropharyngeal or peritonsillar abscesses also can present as sore throats. A complete history, including exposure to common infectious agents, risks for immunosuppression, history of smoking and alcohol use, and duration of symptoms, can be useful in distinguishing situations in which atypical causes for pharyngitis are more likely.

Clinical Findings

Table 26–2 shows some of the causes of sore throat that should be considered in the primary care setting. The findings of other symptoms suggestive of URI, such as rhinorrhea or cough, are useful in suggesting a viral cause for a sore throat. Although exudative tonsillitis is thought to signal streptococcal infection, adenovirus, coxsackievirus, and EBV also cause exudative pharyngitis that can mimic the appearance of streptococcal infection. Several clinical decision rules have been developed that help clinicians determine the risk of a strep throat based on these clinical criteria, but none has been accurate enough to replace microbiological testing in identifying a strep throat. A positive throat culture or rapid streptococcal antigen test usually confirms streptococcal pharyngitis.

Mononucleosis should be suspected when extensive adenopathy is present along with hepatomegaly or splenomegaly or when symptoms of pharyngitis persist longer than 10–14 days. The typical incubation period between exposure to EBV and the development of symptoms of infectious mononucleosis is 5–7 weeks. The diagnosis of EBV mononucleosis is usually made through the identification of immunoglobulin M (IgM) antibodies to the virus. A rapid test for the presence of these heterophil antibodies is positive in about 80% of children older than 4 years of age who have infectious mononucleosis, but is much less sensitive in children younger than 4. The IgM response can usually be detected within 3–4 weeks after the onset of symptoms. However, early in the course of the illness testing for mononucleosis is not helpful and can be confusing, because a negative heterophil antibody can be misinterpreted as excluding the diagnosis of infectious mononucleosis. A more accurate test is the VGA-IgM, which can detect IgM antibodies to EBV much earlier than the monospot test. Additional testing with a white blood count may be helpful because patients with mononucleosis often have an elevated white blood count with large numbers (> 20%) of atypical lymphocytes.

Table 26–2. Differential diagnosis for sore throat.

- Pharyngeal infection
  - Bacterial infection
    - Group A streptococcus
    - *Chlaymdia*
    - *Mycoplasma*
    - Diphtheria
    - *Mycobacterium tuberculosis*
    - *Neisseria gonorrhoeae*
  - Viral infection
    - Adenovirus
    - Respiratory syncytial virus
    - Influenza virus
    - Parainfluenza virus
    - Epstein–Barr virus (mononucleosis)
    - Coxsackievirus (herpangina)
  - Fungal infections
    - Candidiasis
- Noninfectious causes
  - Trauma
  - Smoke inhalation

Complications

The complications of pharyngitis of most concern are rheumatic fever, peritonsillar abscess, and poststreptococcal glomerulonephritis.

Post-streptococcal rheumatic fever was once a common problem in industrialized countries. Treatment with antibiotics reduces the likelihood that rheumatic fever will develop even when strains carrying the M antigen are responsible for the infection.

Peritonsillar abscess is a more common complication of streptococcal pharyngitis. Abscesses develop most often in adolescents and young adults. The primary symptoms of an abscess include increased sore throat, fever, and difficulty swallowing and speaking. The affected tonsils are large and usually displace the palate. Visualization of the uvula deviated to the contralateral side is a useful indicator of peritonsillar abscess.

Like rheumatic fever, several subtypes of group A streptococcus can cause acute post-streptococcal glomerulonephritis (APSGN). Unlike rheumatic fever that develops after a throat infection, APSGN can result from both pharyngeal and skin infections. APSGN occurs most often in young school-aged children and is rare in those younger than 3 years. Overall, the prognosis of APSGN is excellent, and 98% of children eventually recover full renal function.

Complications also can occur with mononucleosis. Very rarely, tonsillar enlargement can be so severe that airway obstruction occurs. In these cases, prompt hospitalization and consultation with appropriate specialists is essential so that an alternate airway can be provided. Another uncommon complication of mononucleosis is splenic rupture, which occurs in about 0.1% of patients. Rupture is most common in the first 3 weeks after the onset of symptoms and may or may not be associated with trauma. In nearly all cases, the spleen is enlarged to more than twice the normal size. Consequently, careful assessment of spleen size is important in managing the patient with mononucleosis, especially in the young athlete who is contemplating return to a contact sport.

Treatment

If group A streptococcus is identified, antibiotic treatment is indicated. A 10-day course of penicillin V is currently recommended as the drug of choice by most groups, although there is no consensus on the appropriate selection of antibiotic in those patients who are allergic to penicillins. Therapy with amoxicillin at 40 mg/kg/day for 10 days appears to be very successful, resulting in excellent clinical responses and low (5–10%) post-treatment carrier rates. Treatment with other agents such as azithromycin and clarithromycin produces results no better than treatment with amoxicillin or penicillin V, but at much greater expense.

Treatment of peritonsillar abscess should be aimed at draining the infection, usually with an 18-gauge needle inserted into the tonsil, along with antibiotic therapy. Single aspiration with antibiotics has been shown to result in cure rates of 92%, which compared favorably with more aggressive surgical management. Without therapy, peritonsillar abscesses may invade into the head and neck with fatal consequences.

Although the streptococcal carrier state does not require treatment, some clinicians attempt to treat patients colonized by group A streptococcus to prevent spread to other family members and close contacts. A regimen of intramuscular penicillin V plus oral rifampin has been shown to reverse the carrier status in 93% of patients treated. No studies indicate whether this regimen remains effective with increased group A streptococcus resistance to penicillin.

EBV-associated infectious mononucleosis is a self-limited condition that usually resolves over several weeks. Fever, often the earliest manifestation of illness, abates usually after 1 or 2 weeks, but malaise and hepatosplenomegaly may take 4–6 weeks to resolve. Although the exact time to return to full activities is predicated on the degree of splenic rupture and absence of other complications, a minimum of 1 month to recuperate is suggested.

If airway obstruction is severe, administration of corticosteroids should be considered and an artificial airway should be provided. Installation of an airway is preferable to emergency tonsillectomy.

Treatment of nonbacterial sore throats should focus on alleviation of symptoms.

Burroughs KE: Athletes resuming activity after infectious mononucleosis. Arch Fam Med 2000;9:1122. [PMID: 11115218]

Gerber MA: Diagnosis and treatment of pharyngitis in children. Pediatr Clin North Am 2005;52:729. [PMID: 25935660]

LOWER RESPIRATORY TRACT INFECTIONS

ACUTE BRONCHITIS

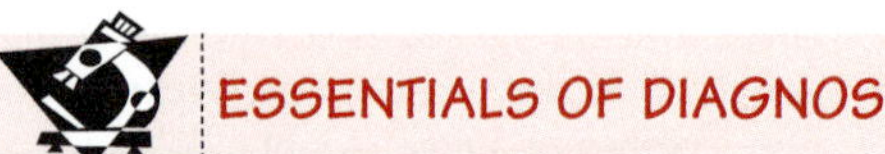

ESSENTIALS OF DIAGNOSIS

- *Cough lasting more than 3 weeks.*
- *Fever, constitutional symptoms, and a productive cough.*

General Considerations

Viral infection is the primary cause of most episodes of acute bronchitis. A wide variety of viruses has been shown to cause acute bronchitis, including influenza, rhinovirus, adenovirus, coronavirus, parainfluenza, and respiratory syncytial virus. Nonviral pathogens, including *M pneumoniae* and *Chlamydia pneumoniae* (TWAR), have also been identified as causes.

The etiologic role of bacteria such as *H influenzae* and *S pneumoniae* in acute bronchitis is unclear because these bacteria are common upper respiratory tract flora. Sputum cultures for acute bronchitis are therefore difficult to evaluate because it is unclear whether the sputum has been contaminated by pathogens colonizing the nasopharynx.

Clinical Findings

Patients with acute bronchitis may have a cough for a significant time. Although the duration of the condition is variable, one study showed that 50% of patients had a cough for more than 3 weeks and 25% had a cough for more than 4 weeks. Other causes of chronic cough are shown in Table 26–3.

Both acute bronchitis and pneumonia can present with fever, constitutional symptoms, and a productive cough. Although patients with pneumonia often have rales, this finding is neither sensitive nor specific for the illness. When pneumonia is suspected on the basis of the presence of a high fever, constitutional symptoms, severe dyspnea, and certain physical findings or risk factors, a chest radiograph should be obtained to confirm the diagnosis.

Table 26–3. Causes of chronic cough.

Pulmonary causes
- ***Infectious***
  - Postobstructive pneumonia
  - Tuberculosis
  - *Pneumocystis carinii*
  - Bronchiectasis
  - Lung abscess
- ***Noninfectious***
  - Asthma
  - Chronic bronchitis
  - Allergic aspergillosis
  - Bronchogenic neoplasms
  - Sarcoidosis
  - Pulmonary fibrosis
  - Chemical or smoke inhalation

Cardiovascular causes
- Congestive heart failure/pulmonary edema
- Enlargement of left atrium

Gastrointestinal tract
- Reflux esophagitis

Other causes
- Medications, especially angiotensin-converting enzyme (ACE) inhibitors
- Psychogenic cough
- Foreign body aspiration

Differential Diagnosis

Asthma and allergic bronchospastic disorders can mimic the productive cough of acute bronchitis. When obstructive symptoms are not obvious, mild asthma may be diagnosed as acute bronchitis. Further, because respiratory infections can trigger bronchospasm in asthma, patients with asthma that occurs only in the presence of respiratory infections resemble patients with acute bronchitis.

Finally, nonpulmonary causes of cough should enter the differential diagnosis. In older patients, congestive heart failure may cause cough, shortness of breath, and wheezing. Reflux esophagitis with chronic aspiration can cause bronchial inflammation with cough and wheezing. Bronchogenic tumors may produce a cough and obstructive symptoms.

Treatment

Clinical trials of the effectiveness of antibiotics in treating acute bronchitis have had mixed results. Meta-analyses indicated that the benefits of antibiotics in a general population are marginal and should be weighed against the impact of excessive use of antibiotics on the development of antibiotic resistance.

Data from clinical trials suggest that bronchodilators may provide effective symptomatic relief to patients with acute bronchitis. Treatment with bronchodilators demonstrated significant relief of symptoms, including faster resolution of cough and return to work. The effect of albuterol in a population of patients with undifferentiated cough was evaluated and no beneficial effect was found. Because a variety of conditions presents with cough, there may have been some misclassification in generalizing this finding to acute bronchitis.

Bent S et al: Antibiotics in acute bronchitis: A meta-analysis. Am J Med 1999;107:62. [PMID: 10403354]

Smucny JJ et al: Are antibiotics effective treatment for acute bronchitis? A meta-analysis. J Fam Pract 1998;47:453. [PMID: 9866671]

COMMUNITY-ACQUIRED PNEUMONIA

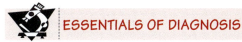

- *Fever and cough (productive or nonproductive).*
- *Tachypnea.*
- *Rales or crackles.*
- *Positive chest radiograph.*

General Considerations

Pneumonia is the cause of over 10 million visits to physicians annually, accounts for 3% of all hospitalizations, and is the sixth leading cause of death in the United States. A variety of factors, including increasing age, increase the risk of pneumonia. Among the elderly, institutionalization and debilitation further increase the risk for acquiring pneumonia. Patients aged 55 years or older, smokers, and patients with chronic respiratory diseases are more likely to require hospitalization for pneumonia. Those with congestive heart failure, cerebrovascular diseases, cancer, diabetes mellitus, and poor nutritional status are more likely to die. Thus, age and comorbidities are important factors to consider when deciding whether to hospitalize a patient with pneumonia. These risk factors are summarized in Table 26–4.

Prevention

Pneumococcal pneumonia may be prevented through immunization with multivalent pneumococcal vaccine. Pneumococcal vaccination is indicated for individuals older than 65 years, and for those 2 years of age or older with diabetes mellitus, chronic pulmonary or cardiac disease, or without a spleen. Additionally, people in certain high-risk populations such as Native Americans,

Table 26–4. Risk factors associated with mortality in community-acquired pneumonia.

Category	Characteristics	Mortality	Location of Care
Very low risk	Age <60, no comorbidities	<1%	Outpatient
Low risk	Age >60, but healthy Age <60, mild comorbidity	3%	80% can be cared for as outpatient (depending on comorbidity)
Moderate risk	Age >60 with comorbidity	13–25%	Hospitalization
High risk	Serious compromise present on presentation (hypotension, respiratory distress, etc) regardless of age	50%	Intensive care unit

Alaska Native populations, and anyone older than 50 years of age who lives in a chronic care facility should be vaccinated. Immunosuppressed patients, including those with HIV infection, alcoholism, cirrhosis, chronic renal failure, sickle cell disease, or multiple myeloma, may benefit from immunization, but the evidence is less convincing.

In addition to initial vaccination, clinicians should advise patients that the duration of protection is uncertain. For those at particularly high risk of mortality from pneumococcal pneumonia, such as patients older than 75 years of age and those with chronic pulmonary disease or lacking a spleen, revaccination every 5 years is a worthwhile precaution.

A conjugated pneumococcal vaccination is effective for children younger than 2 years of age. Current recommendations are to immunize all children younger than 2 years and high-risk children younger than 7 years.

Clinical Findings

The most common presenting complaints for patients with pneumonia are fever and a cough that may be either productive or nonproductive. As an example, in one study, 80% of patients with pneumonia had a fever. Other symptoms that may be suggestive of pneumonia include dyspnea and pleuritic chest pain. However, none of these symptoms is specific for pneumonia.

Symptoms of pneumonia may be nonspecific in older patients. Elderly individuals who suffer a general decline in their function, who become confused or have worsening dementia, or experience more frequent falls should receive a chest x-ray even if no pulmonary symptoms or physical findings are present. Elderly patients who have preexisting cognitive impairment or depend on someone else for support of their daily activities are at highest risk for not exhibiting typical symptoms of pneumonia.

The most consistent sign of pneumonia is tachypnea. In one study of elderly patients, tachypnea was observed to be present 3–4 days before the appearance of other physical findings of pneumonia. Rales or crackles are often considered the hallmark of pneumonia, but these may be heard in only 75–80% of patients. Other signs of pneumonia such as dullness to percussion or egophony, which are usually believed to be indicative of consolidation, occur in less than a third of patients with pneumonia.

Chest radiography is the standard for diagnosing pneumonia. In rare cases, the chest x-ray may be falsely negative. This generally occurs in patients exhibiting profound dehydration, early pneumonia (first 24 hours), infection with *Pneumocystis,* and severe neutropenia.

Microbiological testing for pneumonia is not very useful in relatively healthy patients with nonsevere pneumonia. Blood and sputum cultures are most likely to be beneficial in patients with risk factors for unusual organisms or who are very ill.

Differential Diagnosis

Other conditions such as postobstructive pneumonitis, pulmonary infarction from an embolism, radiation pneumonitis, and interstitial edema from congestive heart failure all may produce infiltrates that are indistinguishable from an infectious process.

Treatment

With the emergence of other pathogens causing pneumonia and the development of resistance to penicillin and other drugs in *S pneumoniae,* treatment decisions have become more complex. The 2003 update to the Infectious Disease Society of America (ISDA) and American Thoracic Society (ATS) guidelines for the treatment of community-acquired pneumonia differ depending on the health and age of patients (ie, 65 years or older), whether they have recently been treated with an antibiotic, and whether they are at risk for an aspiration pneumonia or influenza superinfection (Table 26–5). For patients with no serious comorbidities, the ISDA/ATS recommends a respira-

Table 26–5. Recommendations for empiric treatment of community-acquired pneumonia.

Treatment of Patients Not Requiring Hospitalization
No comorbidities or comorbidities but no recent antibiotic use: respiratory flouroquinolone[1]; macrolide plus high-dose amoxicillin; or macrolide plus amoxicillin-clavulanic acid
With comorbidities and recent antibiotic use: respiratory fluoroquinolone; macrolide plus β-lactam (second- or third-generation cephalosporin or lactam-lactamase inhibitor)
Treatment of Hospitalized Patients Not Critically Ill
β-Lactam with or without a macrolide or respiratory fluoroquinolone
Treatment of Critically Ill Hospitalized Patients
Pseudomonas *not suspected*: β-lactam with or without a macrolide or respiratory fluoroquinolone
Pseudomonas *possible*: antipseudomonal cephalosporin plus ciprofloxacin or antipseudomonal cephalosporin plus aminoglycoside plus respiratory fluoroquinolone
Other Situations
Suspected aspiration: clindamycin or a β-lactam with β-lactamase inhibitor
Influenza superinfection: respiratory fluoroquinolone or β-lactam (second- or third-generation cephalosporin or lactam-lactamase inhibitor)

[1]Includes levofloxacin, sparfloxacin, and grepafloxacin.

tory quinolone or an advanced macrolide plus high-dose amoxicillin (or amoxicillin-clavulanic acid) as first-line therapy. If an antibiotic has been used recently, then either a respiratory quinolone or an advanced macrolide plus a second- or third-generation cephalosporin are recommended options. If aspiration is suspected, the ISDA/ATS guidelines include a choice of amoxicillin-clavulanic acid or clindamycin as initial treatment.

Suitable empiric antimicrobial regimens for inpatient pneumonia include an intravenous β-lactam antibiotic, such as cefuroxime, ceftriaxone sodium, or cefotaxime sodium, or a combination of ampicillin sodium and sulbactam sodium plus a macrolide. New fluoroquinolones with improved activity against *S pneumoniae* can also be used to treat adults with community-acquired pneumonia. Vancomycin hydrochloride is not routinely indicated for the treatment of community-acquired pneumonia or pneumonia caused by drug-resistant *S pneumoniae.*

Ebell MH: Outpatient vs. inpatient treatment of community-acquired pneumonia. Am Fam Physician 2006;73:1425. [PMID: 16669565]

Mandell LA et al; Infectious Diseases Society of America: Update of practice guidelines for the management of community-acquired pneumonia in immunocompetent adults. Clin Infect Dis 2003;37:1405. [PMID: 14614663]

Ramanujam P, Rathlev NK: Blood cultures do not change management in hospitalized patients with community-acquired pneumonia. Acad Emerg Med 2006;13:740. [PMID: 16766742]

NONINFECTIOUS RESPIRATORY PROBLEMS

ASTHMA

ESSENTIALS OF DIAGNOSIS

- *Recurrent wheezing, shortness of breath, or cough.*
- *Histories of allergies in children.*
- *Increase in airway secretions.*
- *Airway constriction, obstruction, or both.*
- *Bronchospasm documented on spirometry.*
- *Dyspnea.*

General Considerations

Asthma is one of the most common illnesses in childhood. Risk factors for the development of asthma include living in poverty and being in a nonwhite racial group. Part of the difference in asthma rates noted among different races may be related to increased exposure to allergens and other irritants such as air pollution, cigarette smoke, dust mites, and cockroaches in less affluent families, but racial differences persist even after adjusting for socioeconomic status.

Allergy is an important factor in asthma development in children but does not appear to be as significant a factor in adults. Although as many as 80% of children with asthma also are atopic, 70% of adults younger than 30 and less than half of all adults older than 30 have any evidence of allergy. Therefore, although an allergic component should be sought in adults it is less commonly found than in children with asthma.

Clinical Findings

In most cases, asthma is diagnosed based on symptoms of recurrent wheezing, shortness of breath, or cough. Children with recurrent cases of "bronchitis" who experience night cough or have difficulty with exercise tolerance should be suspected of having asthma. An additional history of allergies is useful, because 80% of childhood asthma is associated with atopy.

Formal spirometry testing can usually be accomplished in children as young as 5 years of age and can confirm the diagnosis of asthma. Both the forced expiratory volume in 1 second (FEV_1) and FEV_1 to forced vital capacity (FVC) ratio are useful in documenting obstruction to airway flow. Further confirmation is provided by improvement of the FEV_1 by 12% or more following the use of a short-acting bronchodilator. For a valid test, though, children should avoid using a long-acting β-agonist in the previous 24 hours or a short-acting β-agonist in the previous 6 hours.

In some patients with asthma, spirometry may be normal. When there is a high index of suspicion that asthma may still be present, provocative testing with methacholine may be necessary to make the diagnosis.

It is useful to stratify patients with asthma by the severity of their illness. The severity of asthma is based on the frequency, intensity, and duration of baseline symptoms, level of airflow obstruction, and the extent to which asthma interferes with daily activities. Stages of severity range from severe persistent (step 4), in which symptoms are chronic and limit activity, to mild intermittent (step 1), in which symptoms are present no more than twice a week and pulmonary function studies are normal between exacerbations (Table 26–6). Patients are classified as to severity based on their worst symptom and frequency, not upon having met all or the majority of the criteria in any category.

Treatment

The approach to managing asthma relies on acute management of exacerbations, treatment of chronic airway inflammation, monitoring of respiratory function, and control of the factors that precipitate wheezing episodes. For all of these, patient and family education is vital.

Treatment of persistent asthma requires daily medication to prevent long-term airway remodeling. Mild, intermittent asthma may require therapy only during wheezing episodes. Guidelines for the management of asthma are based on the child's age (6 years of age or younger) and are stratified by severity of illness. Guidelines for older children, adults, and younger children are provided in Table 26–7.

The treatment of exacerbations of asthma relies on fast-acting bronchodilators to produce rapid changes in airway resistance along with management of the late-phase changes that occur several hours after the initial symptoms are manifested. The failure to recognize the late-phase component of an acute exacerbation may lead to a rebound of symptoms several hours after the patient has left the office or emergency department. Corticosteroids are the mainstay for preventing the late-phase response.

Table 26–6. Classification of asthma severity.

Step	Symptoms	Nighttime Symptoms	Lung Function
Step 4 Severe persistent	Continual symptoms Limited physical activity Frequent exacerbations	Frequent	Forced expiratory volume in 1s (FEV_1) or peak expiratory flow (PEF) ≤60% predicted PEF variability >30%
Step 3 Moderate persistent	Daily symptoms Daily use of inhaled short-acting β_2-agonist Exacerbations affect activity Exacerbations ≥2 times a week; may last days	>1 time a week	FEV_1 or PEF >60%–<80% predicted PEF variability >30%
Step 2 Mild persistent	Symptoms >2 times a week but <1 time a day Exacerbations may affect activity	>2 times a month	FEV_1 or PEF ≥80% predicted PEF variability 20–30%
Step 1 Mild intermittent	Symptoms <2 times a week Asymptomatic and normal PEF between exacerbations Exacerbations are brief; variable intensity	≤2 times a month	FEV_1 or PEF ≥ 80% predicted PEF variability <20%

Table 26–7. Asthma drug therapy based on severity.

Ages 6 Years through Adulthood		
Step	**Daily Medications**	**Quick Relief**
Step 4 Severe persistent	Choose all needed High-dose inhaled corticosteroid Long-acting bronchodilator A leukotriene modifier Oral corticosteroid	Short-acting bronchodilator Daily or increasing use of short-acting inhaled β_2-agonist indicates need for additional long-term control therapy
Step 3 Moderate persistent	Usually need 2 Either low- to medium-dose inhaled corticosteroid Long-acting bronchodilator	Short-acting bronchodilator Daily or increasing use of short-acting inhaled β_2-agonist indicates need for additional long-term control therapy
Step 2 Mild persistent	Choose one Low-dose inhaled corticosteroid Cromolyn Sustained-release theophylline (to serum concentration of 5–15 mcg/mL) A leukotriene modifier	Short-acting bronchodilator Daily or increasing use of short-acting inhaled β_2-agonist indicates need for additional long-term control therapy
Step 1 Intermittent	No daily medication needed	Short-acting bronchodilator Use of short-acting inhaled β_2-agonist >2 times per week indicates need for additional long-term control therapy
	Step Down Review treatment every 1–6 months; a gradual stepwise reduction in treatment may be possible	**Step Up** If control is not maintained, consider step up; first, review patient medication technique, adherence, and environmental control (avoidance of allergens and/or other factors that contribute to asthma severity)
Step	**Daily Anti-inflammatory Medications**	**Quick Relief**
Step 4 Severe persistent	High-dose inhaled corticosteroid with space/holding chamber and facemask **and** if needed, add systemic corticosteroids 2 mg/kg/day and reduce to lowest daily or alternate-day dose that stabilizes symptoms	Short-acting bronchodilator as needed for symptoms By nebulizer or metered dose inhaler (MDI) with spacer/holding chamber and facemask **or** oral β_2-agonist Daily or increasing use of short-acting inhaled β_2-agonist indicates need for additional long-term control therapy
Step 3 Moderate persistent	Either medium-dose inhaled corticosteroid with spacer/holding chamber and facemask **or** low- to medium-dose inhaled corticosteroid and long-acting bronchodilator (theophylline)	Short-acting bronchodilator as needed for symptoms By nebulizer or MDI with spacer/holding chamber and facemask **or** oral β_2-agonist Daily or increasing use of short-acting inhaled β_2-agonist indicates need for additional long-term control therapy
Step 2 Mild	Young children usually begin with a trial of cromolyn **or** low-dose inhaled corticosteroid with spacer/holding chamber and facemask	Short-acting bronchodilator as needed for symptoms By nebulizer or MDI with spacer/holding chamber and facemask **or** oral β_2-agonist Daily or increasing use of short-acting inhaled β_2-agonist indicates need for additional long-term control therapy
Step 1 Intermittent	No daily medication	Short-acting bronchodilator as needed for symptoms <2 times a week By nebulizer or MDI with spacer/holding chamber and facemask **or** oral β_2-agonist Two times weekly or increasing use of short-acting inhaled β_2-agonist indicates need for additional long-term control therapy
	Step Down Review treatment every 1–6 months; a gradual stepwise reduction in treatment may be possible	**Step Up** If control is not maintained, consider step up; first, review patient medication technique, adherence, and environmental control (avoidance of allergens and/or other factors that contribute to asthma severity)

For patients with persistent symptoms (step 2 and higher), chronic therapy is required. The management of persistent asthma may include long-acting bronchodilators to control intermittent symptoms and nighttime cough, but also should provide chronic anti-inflammatory therapy to prevent long-term remodeling. Both inhaled steroids and nonsteroidal anti-inflammatory medications (ie, cromoglycates) can provide anti-inflammatory therapy. When symptoms are recurrent or large doses of anti-inflammatory agents are required, treatment with a leukotriene inhibitor can provide additional anti-inflammatory therapy and may allow a reduction in the dose of other anti-inflammatory agents such as steroids.

When drugs are selected for the treatment of asthma, the potential side effects of each agent need to be weighed against the potential benefits. For children, chronic use of inhaled steroids has been associated with a small decrease in total height attained. Although the difference in height attainment is small, it might be preferable to use nonsteroidal anti-inflammatory agents such as cromolyn and nedocromil in children.

In addition to pharmacologic management, patients with asthma should avoid known and possible airway irritants. These include cigarette smoke (including second-hand inhalation of smoke), environmental pollutants, suspected or known allergens, and cold air. Children who have difficulty participating in sports may benefit from the use of a short-acting β-agonist such as albuterol before participating in exertion to prevent wheezing or cough.

The monitoring of pulmonary function is an important component of asthma management for all patients with persistent disease. Children and adults should be provided with a peak flow meter and instructed on how to use the device reliably. The use of a peak flow meter can determine subtle changes in respiratory function that may not cause symptoms for several days. To use a peak flow meter, patients must establish a "personal best," which represents the best reading that they can obtain when they are as asymptomatic as possible. Daily or periodic recordings of peak flows are compared with this personal best to gauge the current pulmonary function. Readings between 80% and 100% of the personal best indicate that the patient is doing well. Peak flows between 50% and 80% of an individual's personal best are cause for concern even if symptoms are mild. Patients should be instructed beforehand how to respond in these instances. If a repeat of the peak flow later in the day after appropriate measures have been taken does not show improvement, patients should seek further medical attention. Patients should be told that severe decreases in peak flow to less than 50% are cause for immediate medical attention.

For patients with allergic symptoms, the use of immunotherapy should be considered. However, although immunotherapy usually results in improvements in symptoms of allergic rhinitis, it often does not improve asthma symptoms.

Namazy JA, Schatz JM: Current guidelines for the management of asthma during pregnancy. Immunol Allergy Clin North Am 2006;26:93. [PMID: 16443415]

Siwik JP et al: The evaluation and management of acute, severe asthma. Med Clin North Am 2002;86:1049. [PMID: 12428545]

CHRONIC OBSTRUCTIVE PULMONARY DISEASE

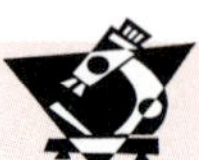

ESSENTIALS OF DIAGNOSIS

- *Productive cough featuring sputum production for at least 3 months for 2 consecutive years.*
- *Chronic dyspnea.*
- *FEV_1 below 80% predicted.*

General Considerations

Chronic airway disease is the second leading cause of disability in the United States after coronary artery disease. Symptoms of chronic bronchitis first develop when patients are between 30 and 40 years of age and progressively become more common as patients reach their 50s and 60s. The development of chronic bronchitis is associated with heavier cigarette use; those smoking over 25 cigarettes per day have a risk of chronic bronchitis that is 30 times higher than nonsmokers. Although chronic bronchitis affects both genders and all socioeconomic strata, it is more commonly observed in men and in those of lower socioeconomic classes. It is presumed that these populations may be at higher risk due to higher consumption of cigarettes observed in these groups.

In addition to smoking, air pollution may play a role in the development and exacerbation of symptoms in patients with chronic bronchitis. Patients with chronic obstructive pulmonary diseases who live in industrialized areas with heavy levels of particulate air pollution may be at increased risk of recurrent disease and death.

Only 10–15% of smokers will develop chronic obstructive pulmonary disease (COPD), so other factors must also play a role in the progression from acute to chronic lung damage. The development of chronic bronchitis is thought to include both a predisposition to inflammatory damage plus exposure to the proper stimuli that cause inflammation, such as cigarette smoke or pollutants. Genetic factors, prolonged heavy exposure to other inflammatory mediators such as environmental pollutants, preexisting lung impairment from other inflammatory processes such as recurrent infection or childhood passive smoke exposure, and other mechanisms may all predispose individuals to the development of chronic bronchitis from smoking.

α_1-Antitrypsin deficiency is a rare genetic abnormality that causes panlobular emphysema in adults and is responsible for approximately 1% of cases of COPD. This trait is inherited in an autosomal-recessive pattern. Nonsmokers with this genetic defect develop emphysema at young ages. Those with this trait who smoke develop progressive emphysema at very early ages.

Clinical Findings

COPD includes both chronic bronchitis and emphysema. Chronic bronchitis is characterized by a productive cough featuring sputum production for at least 3 months for 2 consecutive years. Emphysema causes chronic dyspnea due to destruction of lung tissue, resulting in enlargement of air space and reduced compliance. In most cases, chronic bronchitis and emphysema can be differentiated based on whether the predominant symptom is a chronic cough or dyspnea. In contrast to asthma, changes in COPD are relatively fixed and only partially reversible with bronchodilator use.

When suspected clinically, COPD can be confirmed with chest radiography and spirometry. Although chest radiographic findings occur much later in the course of the disease than alterations in pulmonary function testing, a chest x-ray may be useful in patients suspected of having COPD because it can detect several other clinical conditions often found in these patients.

Spirometry is usually used to diagnose COPD because it can detect small changes in lung function and is easy to quantify. Changes in the FEV_1 and the FVC can provide an estimate of the degree of airway obstruction in these patients. Symptoms of COPD usually develop when FEV_1 falls below 80% of the predicted rate. In addition, a peak expiratory flow rate (PEFR) less than 350 L/min in adults is a sign that COPD is likely to be present.

Spirometry also is useful in gauging the severity of COPD. Decreases in FEV_1 on serial testing are associated with increased mortality rates (ie, patients with a faster decline in FEV_1 have a higher rate of death). The major risk factor associated with an accelerated rate of decline of FEV_1 is continued cigarette smoking. Smoking cessation in patients with early COPD improves lung function initially and slows the annual loss of FEV_1. Once FEV_1 falls below 1 L, 5-year survival is approximately 50%.

Treatment

A. Nonpharmacologic Therapy

The first step in treating the patient with chronic bronchitis or COPD is promoting a healthy life-style. Regular exercise and weight control should be started and smoking stopped to maximize the patient's therapeutic options.

Smoking cessation is the first and most important treatment option in the management of chronic bronchitis or COPD. Several interventions to assist patients in smoking cessation are available. These include behavioral modification techniques as well as pharmacotherapy (see below). A combination of behavioral and pharmacologic approaches such as nicotine replacement appears to yield the best results. Even minimal counseling from the provider improves the effectiveness of the nicotine patch.

Once patients have stopped smoking, those who are hypoxemic with a PaO_2 of 55 mm Hg or less or an O_2 saturation of 88% or less while sleeping should receive supplemental oxygen. Along with smoking cessation, home oxygen is the only therapy shown to reduce mortality in COPD. Continuous long-term oxygen therapy (LTOT) should be considered in those patients with stable chronic pulmonary disease with PaO_2 less than 55 mm Hg on room air, at rest, and awake. The presence of polycythemia, pulmonary hypertension, right heart failure, or hypercapnia (PaO_2 higher than 45 mm Hg) is also an indication for use of continuous LTOT.

Exercise and pulmonary rehabilitation may also be beneficial as adjunct therapies for patients whose symptoms are not adequately controlled with appropriate pharmacotherapy. Exercise and pulmonary rehabilitation are most useful for patients who are restricted in their activities and have decreased quality of life.

B. Pharmacotherapy

1. Smoking cessation pharmacotherapy—Multiple medications are available to assist with smoking cessation. Nicotine can be substituted 1 mg (1 cigarette) per milligram with the use of the patch, gum, or inhaler to help with symptoms of nicotine withdrawal. Patches and gum are both available over the counter as well as by prescription. Some evidence suggests that use of the patch and gum simultaneously enhances quit rates, but use of both is not approved by the Food and Drug Administration. Although all these products state that patients must not smoke while using nicotine replacement because of early case reports of myocardial infarction, more recent studies show that smoking is relatively safe when using nicotine replacement and may help reduce smoking before a patient actually quits. However, even at best, the cessation rate is only about 20–30% at 1 year.

Bupropion also is approved for smoking cessation as an adjunct to behavior modification. The main effect of bupropion is to reduce symptoms of nicotine withdrawal. Bupropion should be instituted for 2 weeks before the quitting target date. Then a nicotine substitute can be used in combination to maximize alleviation of symptoms of nicotine withdrawal. Because many patients with chronic bronchitis are already taking multiple medications, potential drug interactions and adverse effects must be taken into consideration before instituting therapy with bupropion.

A third agent to assist in smoking cessation is varenicline tartrate. Varenicline is a selective nicotine receptor partial agonist. The drug stimulates nicotine receptors to produce a nicotine-replacement type effect but also blocks the receptors from additional exogenous nicotine stimulation. Use of varenicline has been reported to achieve quit rates of 40% at 12 weeks and continuous quit rates of about 22% after 1 year, which was significantly more than either bupropion or nicotine replacement alone. Adverse effects of varenicline occur in 20–30% of patients and include nausea, insomnia, headache, and abnormal dreams but necessitated discontinuation of the drug in 2–3% of patients in clinical trials.

2. Bronchodilators—An anticholinergic agent such as ipratropium bromide is the drug of choice for patients with persistent symptoms of chronic bronchitis. Anticholinergic agents such as ipratropium bromide or tiotropium have fewer side effects and a better response than intermittent β-agonists. Although both of these agents have a delayed onset of action compared with short-acting β-agonists, the beneficial effects are prolonged. Ipratropium requires dosing several times a day; in contrast, tiotropium can be used once a day.

For patients with mild to moderately severe symptoms, intermittent use of a β-agonist inhaler such as albuterol is sometimes beneficial even without significant changes in their FEV_1. Adverse effects of β-agonist agents include tachycardia, nervousness, and tremor. Short-acting β-agonists may not last through the night; when nighttime symptoms develop, long-acting β-agonists such as salmeterol may be more useful. Levalbuterol, the active agent of racemic albuterol, has recently been studied and appears to have greater efficacy than albuterol with fewer side effects.

Combination inhalers of ipratropium bromide and albuterol have also been used in the treatment of patients with chronic bronchitis but have demonstrated only minimal changes in outcomes compared with single agents.

3. Antibiotics—Patients with acute exacerbations of chronic bronchitis pose a more difficult therapeutic dilemma. Many of these exacerbations are probably due to viral infections. However, a meta-analysis of studies using a wide range of antibiotics (ampicillin, sulfamethoxazole-trimethoprim, and tetracyclines) demonstrated some benefit from empiric use of antibiotics for exacerbations of chronic bronchitis.

4. Other agents—As symptoms increase, addition of inhaled β-agonists, theophylline, and corticosteroids may provide symptomatic relief of symptoms of chronic bronchitis. In a multicenter randomized placebo-controlled trial, patients who used inhaled fluticasone had improved peak expiratory flows, FEV_1, FVC, and midexpiratory flow. At the end of treatment patients also showed increased exercise tolerance compared with the placebo group. Corticosteroids at a therapeutic dose of 60 mg/day for 5 days have been shown to provide some symptomatic relief for severe exacerbations.

Mucolytics have not been shown to be beneficial. Iodinated glycerol has not been shown to improve any objective outcome measurements.

Newer agents such as aerosolized surfactant also have been used to treat stable chronic bronchitis. A prospective randomized controlled trial showed a minimal but statistically significant improvement in spirometry and sputum clearance. However, the cost of such a treatment regimen is high and may not add any advantage to the underlying treatment.

For the treatment of cough, agents that may be of benefit for patients with chronic bronchitis include ipratropium bromide, guaimesal, dextromethorphan, and viminol.

Anabolic steroids have recently been used for patients who have severe malnutrition and in those in whom weight loss is a concern. These agents show some beneficial effects.

Bach PB et al; American College of Physicians—American Society of Internal Medicine; American College of Chest Physicians: Management of acute exacerbations of chronic obstructive pulmonary disease: A summary and appraisal of published evidence. Ann Intern Med 2001;134:600. [PMID: 11281745]

Snow V et al; Joint Expert Panel on Chronic Obstructive Pulmonary Disease of the American College of Chest Physicians and the American College of Physicians–American Society of Internal Medicine: Evidence base for management of acute exacerbations of chronic obstructive pulmonary disease. Ann Intern Med 2001;134:595. [PMID: 11281744]

EMBOLIC DISEASE

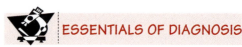

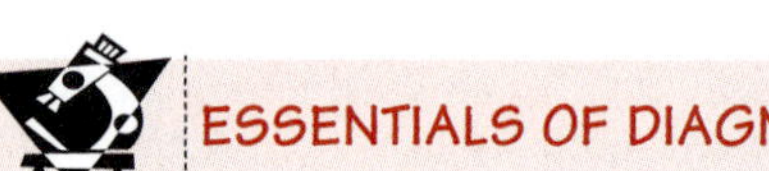

- *Dyspnea.*
- *Hypoxia.*
- *Pleuritic pain.*

General Considerations

Pulmonary embolism usually results from the mobilization of blood clots from thromboses in the lower extremities or pelvis. However, embolization of other materials including air, fat, and amniotic fluid also can obstruct the pulmonary vasculature. The symptoms of pulmonary embolism range from mild, intermittent shortness of breath or pleuritic chest pain to complete circulatory collapse and death.

The most common source of embolism is the disruption of thrombi formed in the deep veins. Mortality in untreated cases is 30% but can be reduced to 2% with prompt recognition and appropriate management. Recurrent pulmonary embolism carries a very high mortality in the range of 45–50%.

Risk factors for pulmonary embolism include venous stasis, trauma, abnormalities in the deep veins, and hypercoagulable states. Hypercoagulability occurs with some cancers as well as with inherited conditions such as factor V Leiden mutation that results in resistance to the anticoagulant effects of protein C. Other congenital hypercoagulation disorders include protein C deficiency, protein S deficiency, and antithrombin III deficiency.

Hypercoagulation states also exist with the use of certain medications. Use of estrogens either as part of hormone replacement therapy or for contraception increases the risk by a factor of three. The effects of these drugs are compounded in patients with factor V Leiden mutation.

In addition, smoking appears to be an independent risk factor for deep vein thrombosis and pulmonary embolism.

Prevention

Because pulmonary emboli usually arise from lower extremity thromboses, prophylactic anticoagulation can be used to reduce the incidence of these thrombi in high-risk individuals. Both low-molecular-weight heparin products and unfractionated heparin are effective in preventing deep venous thrombosis. Selection of the agent and the dose is based on the risk factor and other characteristics of the patient as shown in Table 26–8.

In addition to preventing initial thrombi, the pulmonary embolism can be reduced through the use of a venacaval filter in patients with known thrombi and contraindications to long-term anticoagulation. The long-term impact of intravenacaval (IVC) filters has not been studied extensively. One study showed a complication rate, such as thrombi trapped in the filter or the filter tilting, malpositioning, or migrating, in nearly 50% of those who survived 3 years. However, given the high mortality rates from recurrent pulmonary embolism, the complication rates from long-term IVC filter insertion appear to be a worthwhile trade-off in high-risk patients.

Table 26–8. Strategies to prevent venous thromboembolism.

Condition or Procedure	Prophylaxis
General surgery	Unfractionated heparin, 5000 units two or three times a day
	Enoxaparin, 40 mg/day subcutaneously
	Dalteparin, 2500 or 5000 units/day subcutaneously
	Nadroparin, 3100 units/day subcutaneously
	Tinzaparin, 3500 units/day subcutaneously, with or without graduated-compression stockings
Total hip replacement	Warfarin (target INR, 2.5)
	Intermittent pneumatic compression
	Enoxaparin, 30 mg subcutaneously twice daily
	Danaparoid, 750 units subcutaneously twice daily
Total knee replacement	Enoxaparin, 30 mg subcutaneously twice daily
	Ardeparin, 50 units/kg subcutaneously twice daily
General medical condition requiring hospitalization	Graduated-compression stockings, intermittent pneumatic compression, or unfractionated heparin, 5000 units two or three times daily
Condition requiring hospitalization in the intensive care unit	Graduated-compression stockings and intermittent pneumatic compression, with or without unfractionated heparin, 5000 units two or three times daily
Pregnancy in high-risk patient[1]	Dalteparin, 5000 units/day subcutaneously
	Enoxaparin, 40 mg/day subcutaneously

[1]High risk includes patients with previous pulmonary embolism or deep venous thrombosis.
Reprodiced with permission from Goldhaber SZ: Pulmonary embolism. New Engl J Med 1998;339:93.

Clinical Findings

Patients with pulmonary emboli usually exhibit dyspnea and hypoxia, and often have pleuritic chest pain. However, other than hypoxia, most routine studies including chest radiographs may be normal. Suspicious signs of embolism on a chest radiograph include a wedge-shaped infiltrate resulting from lobar infarction, new pleural effusion, or both. Confirmation of a pulmonary embolism is based on either demonstrating obstruction of vascular flow through pulmonary angiography, finding a mismatch of perfusion and ventilation, or visualization of a clot on spiral (helical) computed tomography (CT) scanning. Although pulmonary angiography is considered the gold standard, because of its invasiveness spiral CT and ventilation-perfusion scan are usually employed to make the diagnosis. Of the noninvasive tests available, spiral CT has the best sensitivity for detecting pulmonary artery thrombi (95–100%), although it is not as useful in identifying subsegmental emboli.

D-Dimer testing has been evaluated as a serum marker for pulmonary embolism or deep vein thrombosis. The presence of D-dimer is not specific for thrombotic disease because D-dimer also rises in other conditions such as recent surgery, congestive heart failure, myocardial infarction, and pneumonia. Although the presence of D-dimer is not useful in diagnosing thrombosis or embolism, the negative predictive value of the absence of D-dimer is very high (97–99%), so this test can be useful in ruling out embolism.

Treatment

Options for management of the patients with an acute pulmonary embolism include anticoagulation to prevent further embolism from occurring, clot lysis with thrombolytic agents, or surgical removal of the clot.

Patients without life-threatening embolism can be managed with acute anticoagulation with heparin followed by long-term maintenance on warfarin. Heparin may be administered either as unfractionated heparin or as low-molecular-weight heparin. Unfractionated heparin is generally administered intravenously with the dosage rate titrated to produce a suitable anticoagulation state. The use of a weight-based nomogram for loading and maintenance dosing can improve the time to achieve adequate anticoagulation and reduce the risks of bleeding. The drawbacks of unfractionated heparin include the need for hospitalization to monitor coagulation status and administer the intravenous drug plus the possibility of thrombocytopenia associated with the use of this agent.

In contrast, low-molecular-weight heparin can be administered as a daily intramuscular dose without titration or frequent anticoagulation monitoring. As a result, low-molecular-weight heparin therapy usually can be provided in the patient's home.

To achieve long-term anticoagulation, warfarin should be started promptly at a dose of 5 mg/day. Starting with a higher dose of warfarin does not appear to achieve oral anticoagulation any faster or reduce the days that heparin is needed. Heparin can be discontinued when a prothrombin time indicates that the international normalized ratio (INR) has reached 2.0–3.0.

The duration of anticoagulation for pulmonary embolism depends on whether the precipitating event is known and reversible or whether the cause is unknown. In situations in which the thrombosis and embolism are the result of an acute event such as an injury or surgery, treatment for 6 months is recommended. If the risk factor associated with the embolic event is not reversible, such as cancer or coagulation disorder, then lifetime anticoagulation is advisable. When a risk factor or event causing the embolism is not known, so-called idiopathic embolism, treatment with anticoagulants for 6 months is indicated.

The use of thrombolytic agents for pulmonary embolism is usually reserved for patients with extensive embolism who show hemodynamic instability. Thrombolytic agents available for use in this situation include urokinase, streptokinase, tissue plasminogen activator (tPA), and reteplase. Embolectomy is rarely performed and is reserved for patients in whom embolism is rapidly diagnosed and a very large embolism is suspected that completely occludes the pulmonary arteries. In most situations, this is treated as a "last ditch" effort to save the patient.

Piazza G, Goldhaber SZ: Acute pulmonary embolism: Part I: Epidemiology and diagnosis. Circulation 2006;114:e28. [PMID: 16831989]

Piazza G, Goldhaber SZ: Acute pulmonary embolism: Part II: Treatment and prophylaxis. Circulation 2006;114:e42. [PMID: 16847156]

Takagi H, Umemoto T: An algorithm for managing suspected pulmonary embolism. JAMA 2006;295:2603. [PMID: 16772621]

Headache

27

C. Randall Clinch, DO, MA

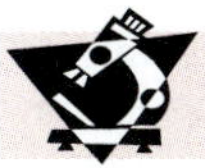

ESSENTIALS OF DIAGNOSIS

- *Migraine:*
  - — *Headache lasting 4–72 hours.*
  - — *Unilateral onset often spreading bilaterally.*
  - — *Pulsating quality and moderate or severe intensity of pain.*
  - — *Aggravated by or inhibiting physical activity.*
  - — *Nausea and photophobia.*
  - — *May present with an aura.*
- *Cluster headache:*
  - — *Strictly unilateral orbital, supraorbital, or temporal pain lasting 15–180 minutes.*
  - — *Explosive excruciating pain.*
  - — *One attack every other day to eight attacks per day.*
- *Tension-type headache:*
  - — *Pressing or tightening (nonpulsating) pain.*
  - — *Bilateral bandlike distribution of pain.*
  - — *Not aggravated by routine physical activity.*

General Considerations

Headache is among the most common pain syndromes presenting in primary care. Each year over 10 million patients visit their primary care provider's office or the emergency department with a complaint of headache. Up to $17 billion is spent annually on the direct medical and indirect costs of migraine headache alone; the cost of lost work days and medical benefits is more than $50 billion annually in the United States. The main task before the primary care provider is to determine if the patient has a potentially life-threatening headache disorder and, if not, to provide appropriate management to limit disability from headache.

A distinction between primary headaches (benign, recurrent headaches having no organic disease as their cause) and secondary headaches (those caused by an underlying, organic disease) is practical in primary care. Over 90% of patients presenting to primary care providers have a primary headache disorder (Table 27–1). These disorders include migraine (with and without aura), tension-type headache, and cluster headache. Secondary headache disorders comprise the minority of presentations; however, given that their underlying etiology may range from sinusitis to subarachnoid hemorrhage, these headache disorders often present the greatest diagnostic challenge to the practicing clinician (Table 27–2).

Lipton RB et al: Migraine in the United States: Epidemiology and patterns of health care use. Neurology 2002; 58:885. [PMID: 11914403]

Olesen J: The international classification of headache disorders, 2nd edition: Application to practice. Functional Neurol 1005; 20:61. [PMID: 15966268]

Solomon GD et al: National Headache Foundation: Standards of care for treating headache in primary care practice. Clev Clin J Med 1997; 64:373. [PMID: 9223767]

Clinical Findings

A. Symptoms and Signs

1. History—The majority of patients presenting with headache have a normal neurologic and general physical examination; for this reason, the headache history is of utmost importance (Table 27–3). A key issue in the headache history is identifying patients presenting with "red flags"—diagnostic alarms that prompt greater concern for the presence of a secondary headache disorder and a greater potential need for additional laboratory evaluation and neuroimaging (Table 27–4).

The onset of primary headache disorders is usually between 20 and 40 years of age; however, they may occur at any age. Patients without a history of headaches who present with a new-onset headache outside of this age range should be considered at higher risk for a secondary headache disorder. Serious consideration should be given to performing additional testing or neuroimaging in these patients or those complaining of their "first or worst" headache. Temporal (giant cell) arteritis should be a consideration in any patient 50 years of age or older with a new complaint of head, facial, or scalp pain, diplopia, or

Table 27–1. Primary headache disorders.

Primary headache disorders
Migraine
Migraine without aura
Migraine with aura
Childhood periodic syndromes that are commonly precursors of migraine
Retinal migraine
Complications of migraine
Probable migraine
Tension-Type Headache (TTH)
Infrequent episodic TTH
Frequent episodic TTH
Chronic TTH
Probable TTH
Cluster Headache and Other Trigeminal Autonomic Cephalalgias
Cluster headache
Paroxysmal hemicrania
Short-lasting unilateral neuralgiform headache attacks with conjunctival injection and tearing (SUNCT)
Probable trigeminal autonomic cephalalgia
Other Primary Headaches
Primary stabbing headache
Primary cough headache
Primary exertional headache
Primary headache associated with sexual activity
Hypnic headache
Primary thunderclap headache
Hemicrania continua
New daily-persistent headache (NDPH)

Source: The International Classification of Headache Disorders, 2nd edition. Cephalalgia 2004; 24(suppl 1):1.

Table 27–2. Secondary headache disorders.

Secondary headache disorders
Headache attributed to head or neck trauma
Acute post-traumatic headache
Chronic post-traumatic headache
Acute headache attributed to whiplash injury
Chronic headache attributed to whiplash injury
Headache attributed to cranial or cervical vascular disorder
Headache attributed to subarachnoid hemorrhage
Headache attributed to giant cell arteritis
Headache attributed to nonvascular intracranial disorder
Headache attributed to idiopathic intracranial hypertension
Postdural puncture headache
Headache attributed to increased intracranial pressure or hydrocephalus caused by neoplasm
Headache attributed directly to neoplasm
Postseizure headache
Headache attributed to a substance or its withdrawal
Carbon monoxide-induced headache
Medication-overuse headache
Headache attributed to infection
Headache attributed to intracranial infection
Headache attributed to bacterial meningitis
Chronic post-bacterial meningitis headache
Headache or facial pain attributed to disorder of cranium, neck, eyes, ears, nose, sinuses, teeth, mouth, or other facial or cranial structures
Headache attributed to psychiatric disorder
Cranial neuralgias and central causes of facial pain
Trigeminal neuralgia
Occipital neuralgia
Postherpetic neuralgia
Ophthalmoplegic "migraine"
Other headache, cranial neuralgia, central or primary facial pain

Source: The International Classification of Headache Disorders, 2nd edition. Cephalalgia 2004; 24(suppl 1):1.

jaw claudication. An erythrocyte sedimentation rate (ESR) should be included in the evaluation of these patients; a normal ESR makes this diagnosis very unlikely.

Symptoms suggesting a recurring, transient neurologic event, typically lasting 30–60 minutes and preceding headache onset, strongly suggest the presence of an aura and an associated migraine headache disorder (Table 27–5). Migraine without aura, the most common form of migraine (formerly called *common migraine*), may present with unilateral pain in the head (cephalalgia) with subsequent generalization of pain to the entire head. Bilateral cephalalgia is present in a small percentage of migraineurs at the onset of their headache. Nausea accompanying a migraine may be debilitating and warrant specific treatment. After excluding secondary headache disorders, the combination of either nausea, photophobia, and pulsating quality or nausea, photophobia, and worsening with physical activity in the headache history provides an 80% positive predictive value for the diagnosis of migraine headache; the absence of either of these historical combinations provides a 70% negative predictive value.

Cluster headaches are strictly unilateral in location and are typically described as an explosive, deep, excruciating pain. They are associated with ipsilateral autonomic signs and symptoms, and have a much greater prevalence in men.

Tension-type headaches, the most prevalent form of primary headache disorder, often present with pericranial muscle tenderness and a description of a bilateral bandlike distribution of the pain (Table 27–6).

Patients with chronic medical conditions have a greater possibility of having an organic cause of their headache (see Table 27–4). Patients with cancer or HIV infection may present with central nervous system metastases, lymphoma, toxoplasmosis, or meningitis as the etiology of their headache. Numerous medications have headache as a reported adverse event, and medication overuse headache (formerly drug-induced headache) may occur following frequent use of analgesics or any antiheadache medication,

Table 27–3. Questions to ask when obtaining a headache history.

H: **H**ow severe is your headache on a scale of 1–10 (1 = minimal pain, 10 = severe pain)?
How did this headache start (gradually, suddenly, other)?
How long have you had this headache?
E: **E**ver had headaches before?
Ever had a headache this bad before (first or worst headache)?
Ever have headaches just like this one in the past?
A: **A**ny other symptoms noted before or during your headache?
Any symptoms right now?
D: **D**escribe the quality of your pain (throbbing, stabbing, dull, other).
Describe the location of your pain.
Describe where your pain radiates.
Describe any other medical problems you may have.
Describe your use of medications (prescription and over-the-counter products).
Describe any history of recent trauma or any medical or dental procedures.

including the triptans. The duration and severity of withdrawal headache following discontinuation of the medication vary depending on the medication itself; withdrawal is shortest for triptans (4.1 days) compared with ergots (6.7 days) or analgesics (9.5 days), respectively. Medical or dental procedures (lumbar punctures, rhinoscopy, tooth extraction, etc) may be associated with post-procedure headaches. Any history of head trauma or loss of consciousness should prompt concern for an intracranial hemorrhage in addition to a postconcussive disorder.

2. Physical examination—Physical examination is performed to attempt to identify a secondary, organic cause for the patient's headache. Additionally, special attention should be paid to any red flags identified during the headache history (see Table 27–4). A general physical examination should be performed, including vital signs, general appearance, and examinations of the head, eyes (including a funduscopic examination), ears, nose, throat, teeth, neck, and cardiovascular regions. Particular attention should be given to palpation of the head, face, and neck.

Table 27–4. Red flags in the evaluation of acute headaches in adults.

Red Flag	Differential Diagnosis	Possible Workup
Headache beginning after 50 years of age	Temporal arteritis, mass lesion	Erythrocyte sedimentation rate, neuroimaging
Very sudden onset of headache	Subarachnoid hemorrhage, pituitary apoplexy, hemorrhage into a mass lesion or vascular malformation, mass lesion (especially posterior fossa mass)	Neuroimaging, lumbar puncture, if computed tomography is negative
Headaches increasing in frequency and severity	Mass lesion, subdural hematoma, medication overuse	Neuroimaging, drug screen
New-onset headache in patient with risk factors for HIV infection or cancer	Meningitis (chronic or carcinomatous), brain abscess (including toxoplasmosis), metastasis	Neuroimaging, lumbar puncture, if neuroimaging is negative
Headache with signs of systemic illness (fever, stiff neck, rash)	Meningitis, encephalitis, Lyme disease, systemic infection, collagen vascular disease	Neuroimaging, lumbar puncture, serology
Focal neurologic signs or symptoms of disease (other than typical aura)	Mass lesion, vascular malformation, stroke, collagen vascular disease	Neuroimaging, collagen vascular evaluation (including antiphospholipid antibodies)
Papilledema	Mass lesion, pseudotumor cerebri, meningitis	Neuroimaging, lumbar puncture
Headache following head trauma	Intracranial hemorrhage, subdural hematoma, epidural hematoma, post-traumatic headache	Neuroimaging of brain, skull, and, possibly, cervical spine

Reproduced, with permission, from Newman LC, Lipton RB: Emergency department evaluation of headache. Neurol Clin 1998;16:286.

Table 27–5. Diagnostic criteria for migraine.

Migraine without Aura

A. At least 5 attacks fulfilling criteria B–D
B. Headache attacks lasting 4–72 h (untreated or unsuccessfully treated)
C. Headache has at least two of the following characteristics:
   1. Unilateral location
   2. Pulsating quality
   3. Moderate or severe pain intensity
   4. Aggravation by or causing avoidance of routine physical activity (eg, walking or climbing stairs)
D. During headache at least one of the following:
   1. Nausea and/or vomiting
   2. Photophobia and phonophobia
E. Not attributed to another disorder

Migraine with Aura

A. At least 2 attacks fulfilling criteria B–D
B. Aura consisting of at least one of the following, but no motor weakness:
   1. Fully reversible visual symptoms including positive features (eg, flickering lights, spots, or lines) and/or negative features (ie, loss of vision)
   2. Fully reversible sensory symptoms including positive features (ie, pins and needles) and/or negative features (ie, numbness)
   3. Fully reversible dysphasic speech disturbance
C. At least two of the following:
   1. Homonymous visual symptoms and/or unilateral sensory symptoms
   2. At least one aura symptom develops gradually over ≥ 5 min and/or different aura symptoms occur in succession over ≥ 5 min
   3. Each symptom lasts ≥ 5 and ≤ 60 min
D. Headache fulfilling criteria B–D for *Migraine without aura* begins during the aura or follows aura within 60 min
E. Not attributed to another disorder

Source: The International Classification of Headache Disorders, 2nd edition. Cephalalgia 2004; 24(suppl 1):1.

Table 27–6. Diagnostic criteria for tension-type headache (TTH).

Infrequent Episodic TTH

A. At least 10 episodes occurring on < 1 day per month on average (< 12 days per year) and fulfilling criteria B–D
B. Headache lasting from 30 min to 7 days
C. Headache has at least two of the following characteristics:
   1. Bilateral location
   2. Pressing/tightening (nonpulsating) quality
   3. Mild or moderate intensity
   4. Not aggravated by routine physical activity such as walking or climbing stairs
D. Both of the following:
   1. No nausea or vomiting (anorexia may occur)
   2. No more than one of photophobia or phonophobia
E. Not attributed to another disorder

Frequent Episodic TTH

A. At least 10 episodes occurring on ≥ 1 but < 15 days per month for at least 3 months ≥ 12 and < 180 days per year and fulfilling criteria B–E.

Chronic TTH

A. Headaches happening on ≥ 15 days per month on average > 3 months ≥ 180 days per year and fulfilling criteria B–D.
B. Headache lasts hours or may be continuous
C. Headache has at least two of the following characteristics:
   1. Bilateral location
   2. Pressing/tightening (nonpulsating) quality
   3. Mild or moderate intensity
   4. Not aggravated by routine physical activity such as walking or climbing stairs
D. Both of the following:
   1. No more than one of photophobia, phonophobia, or mild nausea
   2. Neither moderate nor severe nausea or vomiting
E. Not attributed to another disorder

Source: The International Classification of Headache Disorders, 2nd edition. Cephalalgia 2004; 24(suppl 1):1.

A detailed neurologic examination should be performed and the findings well documented. Assessment includes mental status testing; level of consciousness; pupillary responses; gait; coordination and cerebellar function; motor strength; sensory, deep tendon, and pathologic reflex testing; and cranial nerve tests. The presence or absence of meningeal irritation should be sought. Examinations such as evaluation for Kernig and Brudzinski signs should be documented; both signs may be absent, however, even in the presence of subarachnoid hemorrhage.

B. Laboratory Findings and Imaging Studies

Additional laboratory investigations should be driven by the history and by any red flags that have been identified (see Table 27–4). The routine use of electroencephalography is not warranted in the evaluation of the patient with headache. Although there are different characteristics that may lead to choosing either computed tomography (CT) or magnetic resonance imaging (MRI) (Table 27–7), routine use of neuroimaging is not cost effective.

The US Headache Consortium has provided evidence-based guidelines on neuroimaging in the patient with non-acute headache. They revealed the prevalence of patients with a normal neurologic examination and migraine having a significant abnormality (acute cerebral infarct, neoplastic disease, hydrocephalus, or vascular abnormalities, eg, aneurysm or arteriovenous malformation) on a neuroimaging test is 0.2%. Their recommendations are as follows:

Table 27–7. Computerized tomographic (CT) scans versus magnetic resonance imaging (MRI) in patients with headaches.

CT Scan	MRI
Need to identify an acute hemorrhage	Need to evaluate the posterior fossa
Generally more readily available at most medical centers	More sensitive at identifying pathologic intracranial processes[1]
Generally less expensive at most medical centers	

[1]Increased sensitivity may not correlate with an improved health outcome and may be associated with identifying more clinically insignificant findings.

- Neuroimaging should be considered in patients with nonacute headache and an unexplained abnormal finding on neurologic examination.
- Evidence is insufficient to make specific recommendations in the presence or absence of neurologic symptoms.
- Neuroimaging is not usually warranted for patients with migraine and normal neurologic examination. For patients with atypical headache features or patients who do not fulfill the strict definition of migraine (or have some additional risk factor), a lower threshold for neuroimaging may be applied.
- Data were insufficient to make an evidence-based recommendation regarding the use of neuroimaging for tension-type headache.
- Data were insufficient to make any evidence-based recommendations regarding the relative sensitivity of MRI compared with CT in the evaluation of migraine or other nonacute headache.

Although the US Headache Consortium based the preceding recommendations on a review of the best available evidence, clinicians must individualize management plans to meet a variety of needs, including addressing patient fears and medicolegal concerns.

Within the first 48 hours of acute headache, CT scanning without contrast medium followed, if negative, by lumbar puncture and cerebrospinal fluid (CSF) analysis is the preferred approach to attempt to diagnose subarachnoid hemorrhage. Xanthochromia, a yellow discoloration detectable on spectrophotometry, may aid in diagnosis if the CT scan and CSF analysis are normal but suspicion of subarachnoid hemorrhage remains high. Xanthochromia may persist for up to a week following a subarachnoid hemorrhage.

In addition to CSF analysis, lumbar puncture is useful for documenting abnormalities of CSF pressure in the setting of headache. Headaches are associated with low CSF pressure (< 90 mm H_2O as measured by a manometer) and elevated CSF pressure (> 200–250 mm H_2O). Headaches related to CSF hypotension include those caused by post-traumatic leakage of CSF (ie, after lumbar puncture or central nervous system [CNS] trauma). Headaches related to CSF hypertension include those associated with idiopathic intracranial hypertension and CNS space-occupying lesions (ie, tumor, infectious, mass, hemorrhage).

Clinch CR: Evaluation of acute headaches in adults. Am Fam Physician 2001; 63:685 [PMID: 11237083]

Consortium US Headache: Evidence-based guidelines in the primary care setting: Neuroimaging in patients with nonacute headache, 2000.

Ekbom K, Hardebo JE: Cluster headache: Aetiology, diagnosis and management. Drugs 2002; 62:61. [PMID: 11790156]

Katsarava Z et al: Clinical features of withdrawal headache following overuse of triptans and other headache drugs. Neurology 2001; 57:1694. [PMID: 11706113]

Katsarava Z et al: Medication overuse headache: A focus on analgesics, ergot alkaloids and triptans. Drug Safety 2001; 24:921. [PMID: 11735648]

Martin VT et al: The predictive value of abbreviated migraine diagnostic criteria. Headache 2005; 45:1102. [PMID: 16178941]

Schulman EA: Overview of tension-type headache. Curr Pain Headache Rep 2001; 5:454. [PMID: 11560811]

Zakrzewska JM: Cluster headache: Review of the literature. Br J Oral Maxillofac Surg 2001; 39:103. [PMID: 11286443]

Differential Diagnosis

The differential diagnosis for acute headaches in adults is presented in Table 27–4.

Treatment

Treatment of headache is best individualized based on a thorough history, physical examination, and the interpretation of appropriate ancillary testing. Secondary headaches require accurate diagnosis and therapy directed at the underlying etiology (see Tables 27–2 and 27–4). Nonpharmacologic measures and cognitive–behavioral therapy (CBT) are worth consideration in most patients with primary headache disorders. CBT may have a prophylactic effect in migraine similar to propranolol (an approximate 50% reduction). Cluster headache, chronic tension-type headache, and medication overuse headache respond poorly to CBT as monotherapy. A randomized controlled trial of up to 12 (median of 9) acupuncture treatments over a 3-month period in addition to usual care for chronic headache in primary care patients (primarily those with migraine) revealed fewer headache days (the equivalent of 22 fewer than controls in a 12-month period), a 15% decrease in medication use, and 25% fewer visits to physicians among the acupuncture group. However, a randomized controlled trial of acupuncture versus minimal acu-

Table 27–8. Acute therapies for migraine.

Group 1[1]	Group 2[2]	Group 3[3]	Group 4[4]	Group 5[5]
Specific	Acetaminophen plus codeine PO	Butalbital, aspirin, plus caffeine PO	Acetaminophen PO	Dexamethasone IV
Naratriptan PO[5]	Butalbital plus aspirin plus caffeine, plus codeine PO	Ergotamine PO	Chlorpromazine IM	Hydrocortisone IV
Rizatriptan PO	Butorphanol IM	Ergotamine plus caffeine PO	Granisetron IV	
Sumatriptan SC, IN, PO	Chlorpromazine IM, IV	Metoclopramide IM, PR	Lidocaine IV	
Zolmitriptan PO	Diclofenac K, PO			
DHE SC, IM, IV, IN	Ergotamine plus caffeine plus pentobarbital plus Bellafoline PO			
DHE IV plus antiemetic				
Nonspecific	Flurbiprofen PO			
Acetaminophen plus aspirin plus caffeine PO	Isometheptene compound PO			
Aspirin PO	Ketorolac IM			
Butorphanol IN	Lidocaine IN			
Ibuprofen PO	Meperidine IM, IV			
Naproxen sodium PO	Methadone IM			
Prochlorperazine IV	Metoclopramide IV			
	Naproxen PO			
	Prochlorperazine IM, PR			

PO, orally; IN, intranasally; SC, subcutaneously; IM, intramuscularly; IV, intravenously; PR, rectally; DHE, dihydroergotamine.
[1]Proven pronounced statistical and clinical benefit (at least two double-blind, placebo-controlled clinical studies plus clinical impression of effect).
[2]Moderate statistical and clinical benefit (one double-blind, placebo-controlled study plus clinical impression of effect).
[3]Statistically but not proven clinically **or** clinically but not proven statistically effective (conflicting or inconsistent evidence).
[4]Proven to be statistically or clinically ineffective (failed efficacy vs. placebo).
[5]Clinical and statistical benefits unknown (insufficient evidence available).
Reproduced, with permission, from Silberstein SD for the US Headache Consortium: Practice Parameter: Evidence-based Guidelines for Migraine Headache (An Evidence-based Review), 2000. Available at: http://www.neurology.org/reprint/55/6/754.pdf.

puncture versus no acupuncture among patients with tension-type headache revealed a difference only between no treatment and acupuncture and not between either of the active treatment strategies. A systematic review of nine randomized clinical trials involving 683 patients with chronic headache showed moderate evidence that spinal manipulative therapy has short-term efficacy in prophylactic treatment of chronic tension-type headache and migraine; it is also more efficacious than massage for cervicogenic headache. Caution should be used, however, in applying the results of this review, given the small number of studies available for analysis.

A. Migraine

The US Headache Consortium lists the following general management guidelines for treatment of migraine patients:

- Educate migraine sufferers about their condition and its treatment, and encourage them to participate in their own management.
- Use migraine-specific agents (triptans, dihydroergotamine [DHE], ergotamine, etc) in patients with more severe migraine and in those whose headaches respond poorly to nonsteroidal anti-inflammatory drugs (NSAIDs) or combination analgesics such as aspirin plus acetaminophen plus caffeine.
- Select a nonoral route of administration for patients whose migraines present early with nausea or vomiting as a significant component of the symptom complex.
- Consider a self-administered rescue medication for patients with severe migraine who do not respond well to (or fail) other treatments.
- Guard against medication-overuse headache (the terms *rebound headache* and *drug-induced headache* are sometimes used interchangeably with *medication-overuse headache;* however, the latter is the currently recommended terminology).

Pharmacologic treatment options are numerous in the management of migraine headache. Table 27–8 details a hierarchy of evidence-based treatment options during acute migraine episodes. Of those therapies sup-

Table 27–9. Preventive therapies for migraine.

Therapies	Quality of Evidence[1]	Scientific Effect[2]	Clinical Impression of Effect[3]	Adverse Effects	Group[4]
Antiepileptics					
Carbamazepine	B	++	0	Occasional to frequent	5
Divalproex sodium/sodium valproate	A	+++	+++	Occasional to frequent	1
Gabapentin	B	++	++	Occasional to frequent	2
Topiramate	C	?	++	Occasional to frequent	3a
Antidepressants					
Tricyclic antidepressants					
Amitriptyline	A	+++	+++	Frequent	1
Nortriptyline	C	?	+++	Frequent	3a
Protriptyline	C	?	++	Frequent	3a
Doxepin, imipramine	C	?	+	Frequent	3a
Selective serotonin reuptake inhibitors					
Fluoxetine	B	+	+	Occasional	2
Fluvoxamine, paroxetine, sertraline	C	?	+	Occasional	3a
Monoamine oxidase inhibitors					
Phenelzine	C	?	+++	Frequent	3b
Other antidepressants					
Bupropion, mirtazapine, trazodone, venlafaxine	C	?	+	Occasional	3a
β-Blockers					
Atenolol	B	++	++	Infrequent to occasional	2
Metoprolol	B	++	+++	Infrequent to occasional	2
Nadolol	B	+	+++	Infrequent to occasional	2
Propranolol	A	++	+++	Infrequent to occasional	1
Timolol	A	+++	+	Infrequent to occasional	1
Calcium Channel Blockers					
Diltiazem	C	?	0	Infrequent to occasional	3a
Nimodipine	B	+	++	Infrequent to occasional	2
Verapamil	B	+	++	Infrequent to occasional	2
Nonsteroidal Anti-Inflammatory Drugs					
Aspirin Fenoprofen Flurbiprofen Mefenamic acid	B	+	+	Infrequent	2
Ibuprofen	C	?	+	Infrequent	3a
Ketoprofen	B	+	+	Infrequent	2
Naproxen/naproxen sodium	B	+	+	Infrequent	2
Serotonin Antagonists					
Cyproheptadine	C	?	+	Frequent	3a
Methysergide	A	+++	+++	Frequent	4

(continued)

Table 27–9. Preventive therapies for migraine. *(Continued)*

Therapies	Quality of Evidence[1]	Scientific Effect[2]	Clinical Impression of Effect[3]	Adverse Effects	Group[4]
Other					
Feverfew	B	++	+	Infrequent	2
Magnesium	B	+	+	Infrequent	2
Vitamin B_2	B	+++	++	Infrequent	2

[1]*Grade A:* Multiple well-designed randomized clinical trials, directly relevant to the recommendation, yielded a consistent pattern of findings. *Grade B:* Some evidence from randomized clinical trials supported the recommendation, but the scientific support was not optimal; for instance, few randomized trials existed, the trials that did exist were somewhat inconsistent, or the trials were not directly relevant to the recommendation. An example of the last point would be the case where trials were conducted using a study group that differed from the target group of the recommendation. *Grade C:* The US Headache Consortium achieved consensus on the recommendation in the absence of relevant randomized controlled trials.

[2]0: The medication is ineffective or harmful. +: The effect of the medication is either not statistically or not clinically significant (ie, less than the minimal clinically significant benefit). ++: The effect of the medication is statistically significant and exceeds the minimally clinically significant benefit. +++: The effect is statistically significant and far exceeds the minimally clinically significant benefit.

[3]0, Ineffective: most people get no improvement. +, Somewhat effective: few people get clinically significant improvement. ++, Effective: Some people get clinically significant improvement. +++, Very effective: Most people get clinically significant improvement.

[4]*Group 1:* Medications with proven high efficacy and mild to moderate adverse events. *Group 2:* Medications with lower efficacy (ie, limited number of studies, studies reporting conflicting results, efficacy suggesting only "modest" improvement) and mild to moderate adverse events. *Group 3:* Medication use based on opinion, not randomized controlled trials; *a:* Low to moderate adverse events; *b:* Frequent or severe adverse events (or safety concerns) or complex management issues. *Group 4:* Medication with proven efficacy but frequent or severe adverse events (or safety concerns), or complex management issues. *Group 5:* Medications proven to have limited or no efficacy.

Reproduced, with permission, from Silberstein SD for the US Headache Consortium: Practice Parameter: Evidence-based Guidelines for Migraine Headache (An Evidence-based Review), 2000. Available at: http://www.neurology.org/cgi/reprint/55/6/754.pdf.

ported by the best evidence (Table 27–8, group 1), DHE and the triptans are migraine specific. In addition to the triptans listed in Table 27–8, almotriptan, eletriptan, and frovatriptan have demonstrated efficacy in migraine treatment.

The goal of therapy in migraine prophylaxis is a reduction in the severity and frequency of headache by 50% or more. Table 27–9 details pharmacologic management options for prevention of migraine. The strongest evidence surrounds the use of amitriptyline (10 mg at bedtime, titrated slowly over 2–3 weeks to a maximum 150 mg daily), propranolol (beginning at 80 mg divided three to four times daily; maximum 240 mg daily), timolol (10 mg orally twice daily), and divalproex sodium (200–500 mg orally twice daily with food) for migraine prevention. Topirimate (beginning at 25 mg nightly for the first week then following a defined upward titration schedule) also has proven prophylactic effects in migraine treatment. There are conflicting results among randomized controlled trials regarding the efficacy of botulinum toxin A as a migraine preventive treatment.

B. Tension-Type Headache

Initial medical therapy of episodic tension-type headache often includes aspirin, acetaminophen, or NSAIDs. Avoidance of habituating, caffeine-containing over-the-counter or prescription drugs as well as butalbital-, codeine-, or ergotamine-containing preparations (including combination products) is recommended given the significant risk of developing drug dependency or medication-overuse headache.

Similar general management principles for treatment of migraine headaches can be applied to the treatment of chronic tension-type headaches. In a randomized placebo-controlled trial of tricyclic antidepressant use (amitriptyline hydrochloride, up to 100 mg/day, or nortriptyline hydrochloride up to 75 mg/day) and stress management (eg, relaxation, cognitive coping) therapy, combined therapy produced a statistically and clinically greater reduction (≥ 50%) in headache activity. A meta-analysis of antidepressant treatment (eg, tricyclic antidepressants, serotonin antagonists, and selective serotonin reuptake inhibitors) of chronic headache (eg, migraine, tension-type, or both) revealed treated study participants were twice as likely to report headache improvement and consumed less analgesic medication than untreated patients. Other considerations for prophylaxis of chronic tension-type headaches include calcium channel blockers and β-blockers. Five of six randomized controlled trials conducted since 2000 report no impact on pain reduction in tension-type headache with the use of botulinum toxin type A.

C. Cluster Headache

Acute management of cluster headache involves 100% oxygen at 6 L/min, DHE, and the triptans. Other agents under investigation for acute therapy include subcutaneous octreotide and intranasal civamide. Verapamil, lithium, divalproex sodium, methysergide, and prednisone may be considered for prophylaxis. Due to side effects related to chronic use, methysergide and prednisone should be used with caution.

D. Referral

Referral to a headache specialist should be considered for patients whose findings are difficult to classify into a primary or secondary headache disorder. Additionally, referral is often warranted in cases of daily or intractable headache, drug-rebound, habituation, or medication-overuse headache, or in any scenario in which the primary care provider feels uncomfortable in making a diagnosis or offering appropriate treatment. Patients who request referral, who do not respond to treatment, or whose condition continues to worsen should be considered for referral.

Brandes JL et al: Topiramate for migraine prevention: A randomized controlled trial. JAMA 2004; 291:965. [PMID: 14982912]

Bronfort G et al: Efficacy of spinal manipulation for chronic headache: A systematic review. J Manipulative Physiol Ther 2001; 24:457. [PMID: 11562654]

Dalessio DJ: Relief of cluster headache and cranial neuralgias. Promising prophylactic and symptomatic treatments. Postgrad Med 2001; 109:69. [PMID: 11198259]

Dodick DW, Capobianco DJ: Treatment and management of cluster headache. Curr Pain Headache Rep 2001; 5:83. [PMID: 11252143]

Evers S et al: Botulinum toxin A in the prophylactic treatment of migraine—a randomized, double-blind, placebo-controlled trial. Cephalalgia 2004; 24:838. [PMID: 15377314]

Holroyd KA et al: Management of chronic tension-type headache with tricyclic antidepressant medication, stress management therapy, and their combination: A randomized controlled trial. JAMA 2001; 285:2208. [PMID: 11325322]

Lake AE 3rd: Behavioral and nonpharmacologic treatments of headache. Med Clin North Am 2001; 85:1055. [PMID: 11480258]

Melchart D et al: Acupuncture in patients with tension-type headache: Randomized controlled trial. BMJ 2005; 331:376. [PMID: 16055451]

Schulte-Mattler WJ et al: Treatment of chronic tension-type headache with botulinum toxin A: A randomized, double-blind, placebo-controlled multicenter study. Pain 2005; 116:166. [PMID: 15082132]

Silberstein S et al: Botulinum toxin type A as a migraine preventive treatment. Headache 2000; 40:445. [PMID: 10849039]

Tomkins GE et al: Treatment of chronic headache with antidepressants: a meta-analysis. Am J Med 2001; 111:54. [PMID: 11448661]

US Headache Consortium: Evidence-based guidelines for migraine headache in the primary care setting: Pharmacological management of acute attacks, 2000.

US Headache Consortium: Evidence-based guidelines for migraine headache in the primary care setting: Pharmacological management for prevention of migraine, 2000.

Vickers AJ et al: Acupuncture for chronic headache in primary care: Large, pragmatic, randomized trial. BMJ 2004; 328:744. [PMID: 15023828]

Osteoporosis

28

Jeannette E. South-Paul, MD

General Considerations

Osteoporosis is a public health problem affecting more than 40 million people, one third of postmenopausal women and a substantial portion of the elderly in the United States, and almost as many in Europe and Japan. An additional 54% of postmenopausal women have low bone density measured at the hip, spine, or wrist. Osteoporosis results in more than 1.5 million fractures annually in the United States alone. At least 90% of all hip and spine fractures among elderly women are a consequence of osteoporosis. The direct expenditures for osteoporotic fractures have increased during the past decade from $5 billion to almost $15 billion per year. Thus, family physicians and other primary care providers will (1) frequently care for patients with subclinical osteoporosis, (2) recognize the implications of those who present with osteoporosis-related fractures, and (3) determine when to implement prevention for younger people.

Of the 25 million women in the United States thought to have osteoporosis, 8 million have a documented fracture. The female-to-male fracture ratios are reported to be 7:1 for vertebral fractures, 1.5:1 for distal forearm fractures, and 2:1 for hip fractures. Approximately 30% of hip fractures in persons aged 65 years and older occur in men. Osteoporosis-related fractures in older men are associated with lower femoral neck bone mineral density (BMD), quadriceps weakness, higher body sway, lower body weight, and decreased stature. Osteoporotic fractures are more common in whites and Asians than in African Americans and Hispanics, and more common in women than in men. Little is known regarding the influence of ethnicity on bone turnover as a possible cause of the variance in bone density and fracture rates among different ethnic groups. Significant differences in bone turnover in premenopausal and early perimenopausal women can be documented. The bone turnover differences do not appear to parallel the patterns of BMD. Other factors, such as differences in bone accretion, are likely responsible for much of the ethnic variation in adult BMD.

Finkelstein JS et al: Ethnic variation in bone turnover in pre- and early perimenopausal women: Effects of anthropometric and lifestyle factors. J Clin Endocrinol Metab 2002; 87:3051. [PMID: 12107200]

Pathogenesis

Osteoporosis is characterized by microarchitectural deterioration of bone tissue that leads to decreased bone mass and bone fragility. The major processes responsible for osteoporosis are poor bone mass acquisition during adolescence and accelerated bone loss during the perimenopausal period (mid-50s to the sixth decade in women and the seventh decade in men) and beyond. Both processes are regulated by genetic and environmental factors. Reduced bone mass, in turn, is the result of varying combinations of hormone deficiencies, inadequate nutrition, decreased physical activity, comorbidity, and the effects of drugs used to treat various medical conditions.

Primary osteoporosis, deterioration of bone mass not associated with other chronic illness, is related to increasing age and decreasing gonadal function. Therefore, early menopause or premenopausal estrogen deficiency states may hasten its development. Prolonged periods of inadequate calcium intake, a sedentary lifestyle, and tobacco and alcohol abuse also contribute to primary osteoporosis.

Secondary osteoporosis results from chronic conditions that contribute significantly to accelerated bone loss. These include endogenous and exogenous thyroxine excess, hyperparathyroidism, cancer, gastrointestinal diseases, medications, renal failure, and connective tissue diseases. Secondary forms of osteoporosis are listed in Table 28–1. If secondary osteoporosis is suspected, appropriate diagnostic workup may identify a different management course.

Harper KD, Weber TJ: Secondary osteoporosis. Diagnostic considerations. Endocrinol Metab Clin North Am 1998;27:325. [PMID: 9669141]

Prevention

A. Nutrition

Bone mineralization is dependent on adequate nutritional status in childhood and adolescence. Therefore, measures to prevent osteoporosis should begin with increasing the milk intake of adolescents to improve bone mineralization. Nutrients other than calcium are also essential for bone health. Adolescents must, there-

Table 28–1. Secondary forms of osteoporosis.

Endocrine or Metabolic Causes	Drugs
Acromegaly	Cyclosporine
Anorexia nervosa	Excess thyroid medication
Athletic amenorrhea	Glucocorticoids
Type 1 diabetes mellitus	Prolonged heparin Rx
Hemochromatosis	Phenytoin
Hyperadrenocorticism	Methotrexate
Hyperparathyroidism	Phenobarbital
Hyperprolactinemia	Gonadotropin-releasing hormone agonists
Thyrotoxicosis	Phenothiazines
Collagen/Genetic Disorders	**Nutritional**
Ehlers–Danlos syndrome	Alcoholism
Glycogen storage disease	Calcium deficiency
Marfan syndrome	Chronic liver disease
Osteogenesis imperfecta	Gastric operations
Homocystinuria	Malabsorptive syndromes
Hypophosphatasia	Vitamin D deficiency

fore, maintain a balance in calcium intake, protein intake, other calorie sources, and phosphorus. Substituting phosphorus-laden soft drinks for calcium-rich dairy products and juices compromises calcium uptake by bone and promotes decreased bone mass.

Eating disorders are nutritional conditions that affect BMD. Inability to maintain normal body mass promotes bone loss. The body weight history of women with anorexia nervosa has been found to be the most important predictor of the presence of osteoporosis as well as the likelihood of recovery. The BMD of these patients does not increase to a normal range, even several years after recovery from the disorder, and all persons with a history of an eating disorder remain at high risk for osteoporosis in the future.

Major demands for calcium are placed on the mother by the fetus during pregnancy and lactation. The axial spine and hip show losses of BMD during the first 6 months of lactation, but this bone mineral loss appears to be completely restored 6–12 months after weaning. Risk factors for osteoporosis are summarized in Table 28–2.

B. Life-style

Sedentary life-style or immobility (being confined to bed or a wheelchair) increases the incidence of osteoporosis. Low body weight and cigarette smoking negatively influence bone mass. Excessive alcohol consumption has been shown to depress osteoblast function and, thus, to decrease bone formation. Those at risk for low BMD should avoid drugs that negatively affect BMD (see Table 28–1).

Table 28–2. Risk factors for osteoporosis.

Female gender
Petite body frame
White or Asian race
Sedentary life-style/immobilization
Nulliparity
Increasing age
High caffeine intake
Renal disease
Lifelong low calcium intake
Smoking
Excessive alcohol use
Long-term use of certain drugs
Postmenopausal status
Low body weight
Impaired calcium absorption

C. Behavioral Measures

Behavioral measures that decrease the risk of bone loss include eliminating tobacco use and excessive consumption of alcohol and caffeine. A balanced diet with adequate calcium and vitamin D intake and a regular exercise program (see below) retard bone loss. Medications, such as glucocorticoids, that decrease bone mass should be avoided if possible. The importance of maintaining estrogen levels in women should be emphasized. Measurement of bone density should be considered in the patient who presents with risk factors, but additional evidence is needed before instituting preventive measures.

D. Exercise

Regular physical exercise can reduce the risk of osteoporosis and delay the physiologic decrease of BMD. Short-term and long-term exercise training (measured up to 12 months; eg, walking, jogging, stair climbing) in healthy, sedentary, postmenopausal women results in improved bone mineral content. Bone mineral content increases more than 5% above baseline after short-term, weight-bearing exercise training. With reduced weight-bearing exercise, bone mass reverts to baseline levels. Similar increases in BMD have been seen in women who participate in strength training. In the elderly, progressive strength training has been demonstrated to be a safe and effective form of exercise that reduces risk factors for falling and may also enhance BMD.

Estrogen deficiency results in diminished bone density in younger women as well as in older women. Athletes who exercise much more intensely and consistently than the average person usually have above-average bone mass. However, the positive effect of exercise on the bones of young women is dependent on normal levels of endogenous estrogen. The low estrogen state of exercise-induced amenorrhea outweighs the positive effects of exercise and results in diminished bone density. When mechanical stress or gravitational force on the skeleton is removed, as in bed rest, space flight, immobilization of limbs, or paralysis, bone loss is rapid and extensive. Weight-bearing exercise can significantly increase the BMD of menopausal women. Furthermore, weight-bearing exercise and estrogen replacement therapy have independent and additive effects on the BMD of the limb, spine, and Ward's triangle (hip).

No randomized prospective studies have systematically compared the effect of various activities on bone mass. Recommended activities include walking and jogging, weight training, aerobics, stair climbing, field sports, racquet sports, court sports, and dancing. Swimming is of questionable value to bone density (because it is not a weight-bearing activity) and there are no data on cycling, skating, or skiing. It should be kept in mind that any increase in physical activity may have a positive effect on bone mass for women who have been very sedentary. To be beneficial, the duration of exercise should be between 30 and 60 minutes and the frequency should be three times per week.

Cadogan J et al: Milk intake and bone mineral acquisition in adolescent girls: Randomized, controlled intervention trial. Br Med J 1997;315:1255. [PMID: 9390050]

Ernst E: Exercise for female osteoporosis. A systematic review of randomized clinical trials. Sports Med 1998;25:359. [PMID: 9680658]

Clinical Findings

A. Symptoms and Signs

The history and physical examination are neither sensitive enough nor sufficient for diagnosing primary osteoporosis. However, they are important in screening for secondary forms of osteoporosis and directing the evaluation. The goals of the evaluation should be (1) to establish the diagnosis of osteoporosis by assessing bone mass, (2) to determine fracture risk, and (3) to determine whether intervention is needed. A medical history provides valuable clues to the presence of chronic conditions, behaviors, physical fitness, and the use of long-term medications that could influence bone density. Those already affected by complications of osteoporosis may complain of upper or midthoracic back pain associated with activity, aggravated by long periods of sitting or standing, and easily relieved by rest in a recumbent position. The history should also assess the likelihood of fracture. Other indicators of increased fracture risk are low bone density, a propensity to fall, taller stature, and the presence of prior fractures.

The physical examination should be thorough for the same reasons. For example, lid lag and enlargement or nodularity of the thyroid suggest hyperthyroidism. Moon facies, thin skin, and a buffalo hump suggest hypercortisolism. Cachexia mandates screening for an eating disorder or cancer. A pelvic examination is one aspect of the total evaluation of hormonal status in women and a necessary part of the physical examination in women. Osteoporotic fractures are a late physical manifestation. Common fracture sites are the vertebrae, forearm, femoral neck, and proximal humerus. The presence of a "dowager's hump" in elderly patients indicates multiple vertebral fractures and decreased bone volume.

B. Laboratory Findings

Basic chemical analysis of serum is indicated when the history suggests other clinical conditions influencing bone density. The tests presented in Tables 28–3 and 28–4 are appropriate for excluding secondary causes of osteoporosis. These tests provide clues to serious illnesses that may otherwise have gone undetected and that, if treated, could result in resolution or modification of the bone loss. Specific biochemical markers (human osteocalcin, bone alkaline phosphatase, immunoassays for pyridinoline cross-links and type 1 collagen-related peptides in urine) that reflect the overall rate of bone formation and bone resorption are now available. These markers are primarily of

Table 28–3. Abnormalities in routine laboratory studies and suggested pathology.

Abnormal Study	Suggested Pathology
↑Creatinine	Renal disease
↑Hepatic transaminases	Hepatic disease
↑Calcium	Primary HPT or malignancy
↓Calcium	Malabsorption, vitamin D deficiency
↓Phosphorus	Osteomalacia
↑Alkaline phosphatase	Liver disease, Paget disease, fracture, other bone pathology
↓Albumin	Malnutrition
↓TSH	Hyperthyroidism
↑ESR	Myeloma
Anemia	Myeloma
↓24 h calcium excretion	Malabsorption, vitamin D deficiency

HPT, hyperparathyroidism; TSH, thyroid-stimulating hormone; ESR, erythrocyte sedimentation rate; ↑, increased; ↓, decreased. Reproduced, with permission, from Harper KD, Weber TJ: Secondary osteoporosis. Diagnostic considerations. Endocrinol Metab Clin North Am 1998;27:325.

Table 28–4. Directed laboratory assessment for secondary osteoporosis.

Hypogonadism	↓Testosterone in men
	↓Estrogen in women
	↑Gonadotropins (LH and FSH)
Hyperthyroidism	↓TSH
	↑T_4
Hyperparathyroidism	↑PTH
	↑Serum calcium
	↑1,25(OH)D
Vitamin D deficiency	↓25-Hydroxycalciferol
Hemochromatosis	Serum iron
	Ferritin
Cushing syndrome	24-h urine free cortisol excretion
	Overnight dexamethasone suppression test
Multiple myeloma	Serum protein electrophoresis—M spike and Bence–Jones proteinuria
	↑ESR
	Anemia
	Hypercalcemia
	↓PTH

LH, luteinizing hormone; FSH, follicle-stimulating hormone; TSH, thyroid-stimulating hormone; T_4, thyroxine; PTH, parathyroid hormone; 1,25(OH)D, 1,25-hydroxyvitamin D; ESR, erythrocyte sedimentation rate; ↑, increased; ↓, decreased.

Modified from Harper KD, Weber TJ: Secondary osteoporosis. Diagnostic considerations. Endocrinol Metab Clin North Am 1998;27:325.

research interest and are not recommended as part of the basic workup for osteoporosis. They suffer from a high degree of biological variability and diurnal variation and do not differentiate causes of altered bone metabolism. For example, measures of bone turnover increase and remain elevated after menopause but do not necessarily provide information that can direct management.

C. Imaging Studies

Plain radiographs are not sensitive enough to diagnose osteoporosis until total bone density has decreased by 50%, but bone densitometry is useful for measuring bone density and monitoring the course of therapy (see Table 28–5). Single or dual photon absorptiometry (SPA, DPA) has been used in the past but provides poorer resolution, less accurate analysis, and more radiation exposure than x-ray absorptiometry. The most widely used techniques for assessing bone mineral density are dual-energy x-ray absorptiometry (DXA) and quantitative computerized tomography (CT). These methods have errors in precision of 0.5–2%. Quantitative CT is the most sensitive, but results in substantially greater radiation exposure than DXA. For this reason, DXA is the diagnostic measure of choice.

Table 28–5. Indications for measuring bone density.

Concerned perimenopausal women willing to start therapy
Radiographic evidence of bone loss
Patient on long-term glucocorticoid therapy (more than 1 mo at ≥ 7.5 mg of prednisone/day)
Asymptomatic hyperparathyroidism where osteoporosis would suggest parathyroidectomy
Monitoring therapeutic response in women undergoing treatment for osteoporosis if the result of the test would affect the clinical decision

Smaller, less-expensive systems for assessing the peripheral skeleton are now available. These include DXA scans of the distal forearm and the middle phalanx of the nondominant hand and a variety of devices for performing quantitative ultrasound (QUS) measurements on bone. Recent prospective studies using QUS of the heel have predicted hip fracture and all nonvertebral fractures nearly as well as DXA at the femoral neck. Both of these methods provide information regarding fracture risk and predict hip fracture better than DXA at the lumbar spine. Clinical trials of pharmacologic agents have used DXA rather than QUS, so it is unclear whether the results of these trials can be generalized to patients identified by QUS to have high risk of fracture.

Bone densitometry reports provide a *T* score (the number of standard deviations above or below the mean BMD for sex and race matched to young controls) or *Z* score (comparing the patient with a population adjusted for age as well as for sex and race). The BMD result enables the classification of patients into three categories: normal, osteopenic, and osteoporotic. Normal patients receive no further therapy; osteopenic patients are counseled, treated, and followed so that no further bone loss develops; osteoporotic patients receive active therapy aimed at increasing bone density and decreasing fracture risk. Osteoporosis is indicated by a *T* score of more than 2.5 standard deviations below the sex-adjusted mean for normal young adults at peak bone mass. *Z* scores are of little value to the practicing clinician.

There is little evidence from controlled trials that women who receive bone density screening have better outcomes (improved bone density or fewer falls) than women who are not screened. The US Preventive Services Task

Force suggests the primary argument for screening is that postmenopausal women with low bone density are at increased risk for subsequent fractures of the hip, vertebrae, and wrist, and that interventions can slow the decline in bone density after menopause. The presence of multiple risk factors (age of 80 years or older, poor health, limited physical activity, poor vision, prior postmenopausal fracture, psychotropic drug use, and others) seems to be a stronger predictor of hip fracture than low bone density. The patient who is not asymptomatic but may have only one or two risk factors can benefit from BMD screening. Indications for BMD screening are outlined in Table 28–5.

Kroger H, Reeve J: Diagnosis of osteoporosis in clinical practice. Ann Med 1998;30:278. [PMID: 9677014]

National Institutes of Health Consensus Development Conference Statement: Osteoporosis prevention, diagnosis, and therapy. March 27–29, 2000;17(1). Available at: http://home.mdconsult.com/das/article/body/52216227-2.

Differential Diagnosis & Screening

The approach to the patient is governed by the presentation. The greatest challenge for clinicians is to identify which asymptomatic patients would benefit from screening for osteoporosis, rather than determining a treatment regimen for those with known disease (see Table 28–2). All women and girls should be counseled about appropriate calcium intake and physical activity. Assessment of osteoporosis risk is also important when following a patient for a chronic disease known to cause secondary osteoporosis (see Table 28–1). Figure 28–1 presents an algorithm to assist in the evaluation. Preventive measures are always the first step in therapy.

Should there be a suspicion of osteoporosis in a man or evidence of a pathologic fracture in a man or a woman, assessment of risk via medical history and determination of BMD should be completed. BMD measurement and laboratory evaluation are necessary to document the extent of bone loss and to rule out secondary causes of osteoporosis. Should there be clinical evidence of a particular condition, the evaluation can focus on the suspected condition once the basic laboratory work has been completed as described in Table 28–3 and Figure 28–1.

Recognizing the variety of conditions conferring risk of osteoporosis, the National Osteoporosis Foundation makes the following recommendations to physicians:

1. Counsel all women on the risk factors for osteoporosis. Osteoporosis is a "silent" risk factor for fracture just as hypertension is for stroke; one of two white women will experience an osteoporotic fracture at some point in her lifetime.
2. Perform evaluation for osteoporosis on all postmenopausal women who present with fractures, using BMD testing to confirm the diagnosis and determine the disease severity.
3. Recommend BMD testing to postmenopausal women younger than 65 years who have one or more additional risk factors for osteoporosis in addition to menopause.
4. Recommend BMD testing to all women aged 65 years and older regardless of additional risk factors.
5. Advise all patients to obtain an adequate intake of dietary calcium (at least 1200 mg/day, including supplements if necessary).
6. Recommend regular weight-bearing and muscle-strengthening exercise to reduce the risk of falls and fractures.
7. Advise patients to avoid tobacco smoking and to keep alcohol intake moderate.
8. Consider all postmenopausal women who present with vertebral or hip fractures candidates for treatment of osteoporosis.
9. Initiate therapy to reduce fracture risk in women with BMD *T* scores below –2 in the absence of risk factors and in women with *T* scores below –1.5 if other risk factors are present.
10. Pharmacologic options for prevention and treatment of osteoporosis include hormone replacement therapy, alendronate, raloxifene, and ibandronate (prevention), and calcitonin (treatment).

Treatment

Decisions to intervene when osteoporosis is diagnosed reflect a desire to prevent early or continuing bone loss, a belief that there can be an immediate impact on the patient's well-being, and a willingness to comply with the patient's desires. Bone densitometry can assist in the decision-making process if the patient's age confers risk, there are no manifestations of disease, and the decision point is prevention rather than treatment. BMD measurements can also assist in therapy when there are relative contraindications to a specific agent and demonstrating efficacy could encourage continuation of therapy. Medicare currently reimburses costs of bone densitometry according to the conditions outlined in Table 28–6. The decision to intervene with pharmacotherapy involves clinical judgment based on a global assessment, rather than BMD measurement alone. All currently approved therapeutic agents for the prevention and treatment of osteoporosis work by inhibiting or decreasing bone resorption.

A. Estrogen

Adequate estrogen levels remain the single most important therapy for maintaining adequate bone density in women. Prior to 2003, estrogen replacement therapy was considered for all women with decreased bone density, absent contraindications. However, in July 2002, the Women's Health Initiative randomized controlled

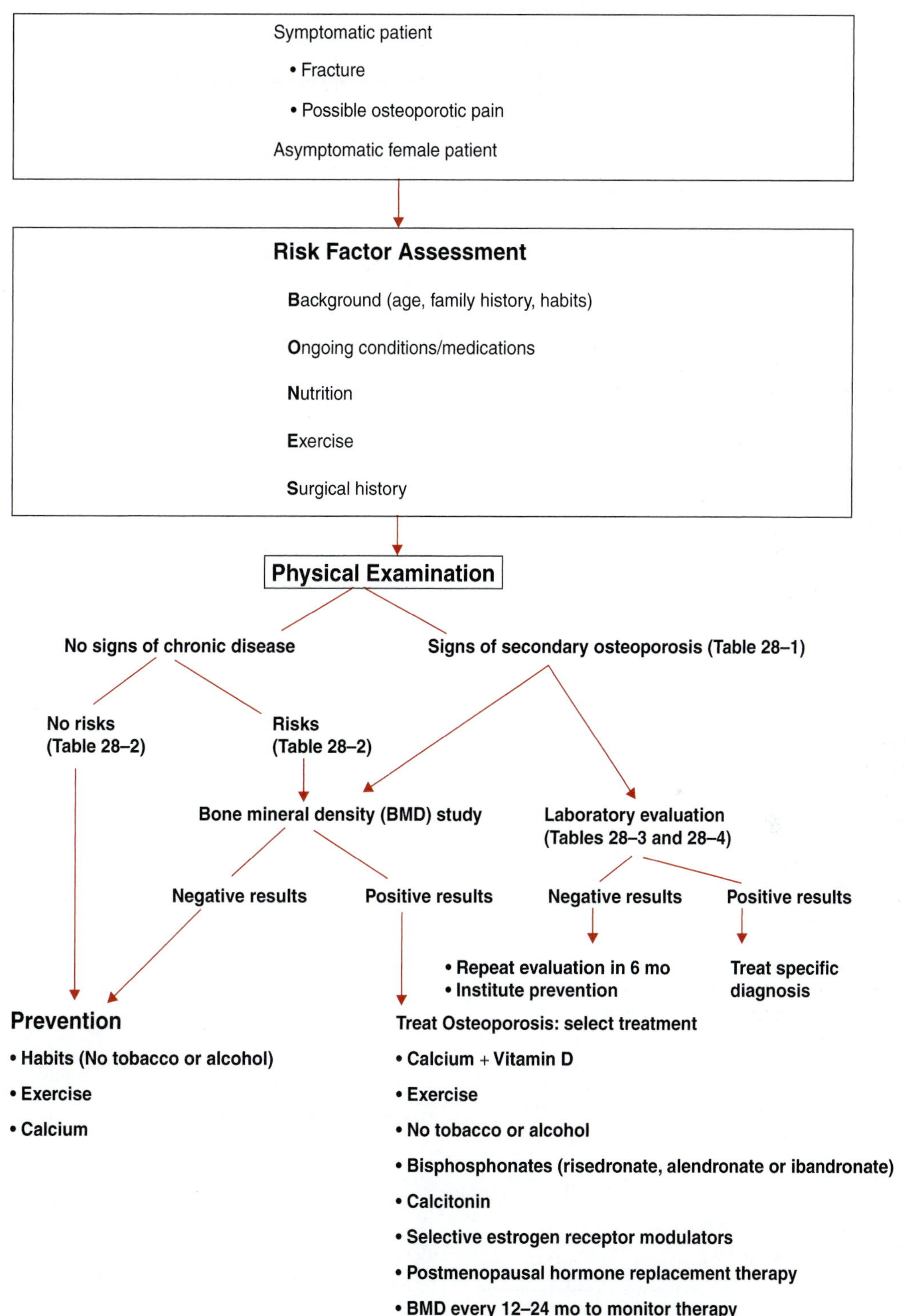

Figure 28–1. Algorithm for evaluation, prevention, and management of osteoporosis.

Table 28–6. Conditions qualifying for Medicare coverage of densitometry.

Estrogen-deficient woman at clinical risk for osteoporosis
Individual with vertebral abnormalities (eg, osteopenia, vertebral fractures, osteoporosis)
Individual receiving long-term (more than 3 mo) glucocorticoid therapy
Primary hyperparathyroidism
Individual being monitored to assess response to osteoporosis drug therapy

primary prevention trial was stopped at a mean 5.2 years of follow-up by the data and safety monitoring board because the test statistic for invasive breast cancer exceeded the stopping boundary for the adverse effect of estrogen and progesterone versus placebo. Estimated hazard ratios were excessive for coronary heart disease, breast cancer, and strokes, but were less than 1.0 for colorectal cancer, endometrial cancer, and hip fracture. Therefore, careful risk assessment is needed for each patient to determine whether the improvement of risk for hip fracture (0.66) balances the risk for cardiovascular and breast disease. Contraindications to estrogen replacement therapy are listed in Table 28–7.

Several studies have examined the effect of the timing of initiation and the duration of postmenopausal estrogen therapy on BMD. Current users who started estrogen therapy at menopause had the highest BMD levels, which were significantly higher than those of women who never used estrogen therapy or past users who started at menopause (with a duration of use of at least 10 years). BMD was similar for women using unopposed estrogen or estrogen plus progestin, for women younger or older than 75 years, and for current smokers or nonsmokers. Current users who started estrogen within 5 years of menopause had a decreased risk of hip, wrist, and all nonspinal fractures compared with those who never used estrogen. Long-term users who initiated therapy 5 years after menopause had no significant reduction in risk for all nonspinal fractures, despite an average duration of use of 16 years. Therefore, early initiation of estrogen with respect to menopause may be more important than the total duration of use. Estrogen initiated early in the menopausal period and continued into late life appears to be associated with the highest bone density.

Table 28–7. Contraindications to estrogen replacement therapy.

Absolute
History of breast cancer
Estrogen-dependent neoplasia
Undiagnosed or abnormal genital bleeding
History of or active thromboembolic disorder
Relative
Migraine
History of thromboembolism
Familial hypertriglyceridemia
Uterine leiomyomas
Uterine cancer
Gallbladder disease
Strong family history of breast cancer
Chronic hepatic dysfunction
Endometriosis

Source: Scientific Advisory Board, Osteoporosis Society of Canada: Clinical practice guidelines for the diagnosis and management of osteoporosis. Can Med Assoc J 1996;155:1113.

As more and more women utilize estrogen therapy, there has been increasing concern regarding its impact on breast cancer risk. The relation between the use of hormones and the risk of breast cancer in postmenopausal women was assessed in a follow-up survey of participants in the Nurses' Health Study in 1992. The risk of breast cancer was significantly increased among women who were currently using estrogen alone or estrogen plus progestin, as compared with postmenopausal women who had never used hormones. Women currently taking hormones who had used such therapy for 5–9 years had an adjusted relative risk of breast cancer of 1.46, as did those currently using hormones who had done so for a total of 10 or more years (RR = 1.46). The addition of progestins to estrogen therapy does not reduce the risk of breast cancer among postmenopausal women.

The only randomized trial of estrogen–progesterone therapy describes secondary prevention of coronary heart disease in postmenopausal women (HERS) and included only women who had a prior history of cardiovascular disease. Women received either estrogen or estrogen and progesterone. There was an excess of deaths from coronary heart disease and a threefold excess risk of venous thrombosis during the first year of the trial in women on estrogen and a small risk of stroke in women on estrogen and progesterone. Recommendations at the conclusion of the trial included not starting women who already have clinical cardiovascular disease on estrogen and progesterone therapy (ie, secondary prevention).

B. Calcium and Vitamin D

Calcium supplementation produces small beneficial effects on bone mass throughout postmenopausal life and may reduce fracture rates by more than the change in BMD would predict—possibly as much as 50%. Postmenopausal women receiving supplemental calcium over a 3-year period in a placebo-controlled, randomized clinical trial had stable total body calcium and BMD in the lumbar spine, femoral neck, and trochanter compared with the placebo group.

Table 28–8. Calcium-rich foods.[1]

Milk (skim, lowfat, or whole), 8 oz
Plain yogurt, 8 oz
Frozen yogurt, fruit, 8 oz
Swiss cheese, 1 oz
Ricotta cheese, part skim, 4 oz
Sardines, canned, 3 oz
Cooked greens, collards, or mustard, 8 oz
Firm cheeses (Edam, Brick, Cheddar, Gouda, Colby, Mozzarella), 1 oz
Calcium-fortified orange juice, 8 oz

[1]Approximately 300 mg.

Vitamin D increases calcium absorption in the gastrointestinal tract, so that more calcium is available in the circulation and is subsequently reabsorbed in the renal proximal tubules. There is now evidence of significant reductions in nonvertebral fracture rates from physiologic replacement of vitamin D in the elderly. Vitamin D supplementation is important in those of all ages with limited exposure to sunlight.

Dietary calcium augmentation should be recommended to maintain lifetime calcium levels and to help prevent early postmenopausal bone loss (Table 28–8). Adults should ingest 1000 mg of elemental calcium per day for optimal bone health. Teenagers, pregnant or lactating women, women older than 50 years of age taking estrogen replacement therapy, and everyone older than 65 years of age should ingest 1500 mg of elemental calcium per day for optimal bone health. If this cannot be achieved by diet alone, calcium supplementation is recommended. Calcium preparations should be compared relative to elemental calcium content. Therefore, attention to which form the patient is ingesting is important.

C. Calcitonin

Calcitonin, a hormone directly inhibiting osteoclastic bone resorption, is an alternative for patients with established osteoporosis in whom estrogen replacement therapy is not recommended. A unique characteristic of calcitonin is that it produces an analgesic effect with respect to bone pain and, thus, is often prescribed for patients who have suffered an acute osteoporotic fracture. The American College of Rheumatology recommends treatment until the pain is controlled, followed by tapering of medication over 4–6 weeks. Calcitonin decreases further bone loss at vertebral and femoral sites in patients with documented osteoporosis but has a questionable effect on fracture frequency. Calcitonin has been shown to prevent trabecular bone loss during the first few years of menopause, but it is unclear whether it has any impact on cortical bone. Calcitonin is also thought to be effective in decreasing the fracture rate of vertebrae and peripheral bones.

The PROOF (Prevent Recurrence of Osteoporotic Fractures) trial—a 5-year double-blind study that randomized 1255 postmenopausal women with osteoporosis to receive placebo or one of three dosages of intranasal calcitonin (100, 200, or 400 IU/day)—demonstrated a 36% reduction in the relative risk of new vertebral fractures compared with placebo. There was no effect with 100 IU/day and no significant change in the reduction seen with 400 IU/day.

For reasons that are poorly understood, the increase in BMD associated with administration of calcitonin may be transient or there may be the development of resistance. Calcitonin can be provided in two forms. Nasal congestion and rhinitis are the most significant side effects of the nasal form. The injectable formulation has gastrointestinal side effects and is less convenient than the nasal preparation. The increase in bone density observed by this therapy is significantly less than that achieved by bisphosphonates or estrogen and may be limited to the spine, but it still has recognized value in reducing risk of fracture.

D. Bisphosphonates

Bisphosphonates are antiresorptive agents and effective for preventing bone loss associated with estrogen deficiency, glucocorticoid treatment, and immobilization. Antiresorptive agents improve the quality of bone by preserving trabecular architecture. They may increase bone strength by methods other than by increasing BMD. All bisphosphonates act similarly on bone in binding permanently to mineralized bone surfaces and inhibiting osteoclastic activity. Thus, less bone is degraded during the remodeling cycle. First-, second-, and third-generation bisphosphonates are now available (etidronate, alendronate, risedronate, and ibandronate). Because food and liquids can reduce the absorption of bisphosphonates, they should be given with a glass of plain water 30 minutes before the first meal or beverage of the day. Patients should not lie down for at least 30 minutes to lessen the chance of esophageal irritation. In addition, patients should consider taking supplemental calcium and vitamin D if their dietary intake is inadequate.

Bisphosphonates are of comparable efficacy to hormone replacement therapy in preventing bone loss and have a demonstrated positive effect on symptomatic and asymptomatic vertebral fracture rate as well as on nonvertebral fracture rate (forearm and hip). More than 4 years of treatment would be needed in women with low bone density (*T* score > –2.0), but without preexisting fractures, to substantially reduce the risk of clinical fracture.

In clinical trials, alendronate was generally well tolerated and no significant clinical or biological adverse experiences were observed. Alendronate appears to be effective at doses of 5 mg daily in preventing osteoporosis induced by long-term glucocorticoid therapy. In placebo-controlled studies of men and women aged 17–83 years who were receiving glucocorticoid therapy, femoral neck bone density and the bone density of the trochanter and total body increased significantly in patients treated with alendronate.

Alendronate appears to be a safe and well-tolerated agent for the treatment of osteoporosis. Some small studies suggest an additional benefit of adding alendronate to hormone replacement therapy, and ongoing studies should provide additional information. However, all of the bisphosphonates accumulate over time in bone, and further research is needed to determine their long-term impact as well as their potential for use in premenopausal women and men.

Risedronate is a pyridinyl bisphosphonate approved as treatment for several metabolic bone diseases in 2000. In doses of 5 mg daily, risedronate reduces the incidence of vertebral fractures in women with two or more fractures by rapidly increasing BMD at sites of cortical and trabecular bone. In a randomized trial of 2458 postmenopausal women with diagnosed osteoporosis, participants were treated with either 2.5 mg or 5 mg of risedronate or placebo as well as calcium supplementation and cholecalciferol if they had low baseline 25-hydroxyvitamin D levels. The 2.5-mg dose was found to be ineffective in other trials and was discontinued. After 3 years of treatment, the 5-mg risedronate group showed a 41% reduction in risk of new vertebral fractures and a 39% reduction in incidence of nonvertebral fractures. In a large, prospective, trial of hip fracture prevention in elderly women, risedronate was shown to significantly reduce the risk of hip fracture in women with osteoporosis. Bisphosphonates should be prescribed for 3–4 years in women with osteoporosis and low bone density.

Ibandronate is currently approved by the Food and Drug Administration (FDA) for the treatment and prevention of osteoporosis in postmenopausal women. Over a 3-year period, ibandronate was shown to decrease the incidence of new vertebral fractures by 52% and to increase BMD at the spine by 5%. It can be administered daily or once a month.

E. Selective Estrogen Receptor Modulators

Raloxifene is the first drug to be studied from a new class of drugs termed *selective estrogen receptor modulators.* This drug has a mixed agonist-antagonist action on estrogen receptors: estrogen agonist effects on bone and antagonist effects on breast and endometrium. Its discovery evolved from a structural rearrangement of the antiestrogen tamoxifen, although it is structurally very different. It blocks estrogen in a manner similar to tamoxifen, while also binding and stimulating other tissue receptors to act like estrogen. Raloxifene inhibits trabecular and vertebral bone loss in a manner similar, but not identical, to estrogen (ie, by blocking the activity of cytokines that stimulate bone resorption).

Raloxifene therapy results in decreased serum total and low-density lipoprotein (LDL) cholesterol without any beneficial effects on serum total high-density lipoprotein (HDL) cholesterol or triglycerides. Reported side effects of raloxifene are virginities and hot flashes. Investigators in the Multiple Outcomes of Raloxifene (MORE) trial of more than 7000 postmenopausal, osteoporotic women over 3 years showed a decreased risk of breast cancer in those already at low risk for the disease. The study results were analyzed separately for women presenting with preexisting fracture. Although treatment effectiveness was similar in both groups, the absolute risk of fractures in the group with preexisting fractures was 4.5 times greater than in the group with osteoporosis, but no preexisting fracture (21% vs. 4.5%). Thus, it is important to identify and treat patients at higher risk. Studies of women at higher risk for breast cancer are currently underway.

A summary of overall treatment strategies is given in Table 28–9 and guidelines for dosing the pharmacologic

Table 28–9. Treatment strategies.

Overall

- Calcium-rich diet ± vitamin D supplements
- Weight-bearing exercise
- Avoidance of alcohol, tobacco products, excess caffeine, and drugs
- Estrogen replacement within 5 y of menopause, and used for 10+ y
- Alendronate
- Raloxifene
- Calcitonin

For Patients on Glucocorticoids

- Lowest dose of a short-acting glucocorticoid or topical preparations whenever possible
- Maintain a well-balanced, 2- to 3-g sodium diet
- Weight-bearing and isometric exercise to prevent proximal muscle weakness
- Calcium intake of 1500 mg/day and vitamin D intake of 400–800 IU/day after hypercalciuria is controlled
- Gonadal hormones in all postmenopausal women, premenopausal women with low levels of estradiol, and men who have low levels of testosterone (unless contraindicated)
- Thiazide diuretic to control hypercalciuria
- Measure bone mineral density at baseline and every 6–12 mo during the first 2 y of therapy to assess treatment efficacy
- If bone loss occurs during treatment or hormone replacement therapy is contraindicated, treat with calcitonin or bisphosphonate

Source: Lane NE, Lukert B: The science and therapy of glucocorticoid induced bone loss. Endocrinol Metab Clin North Am 1998;27:465.

Table 28–10. Pharmacotherapy for osteoporosis.

Drug	Dosage	Route
Estradiol patch	0.05 mg every wk	Topical
Conjugated estrogens	0.625–1.25 mg/day	Oral
Elemental calcium	1000–1500 mg/day	Oral
Calcitonin	200 IU/day	Intranasal
	50–100 IU/day	Subcutaneous or intramuscular
Vitamin D	400 IU/day (800 IU/day in northern locations)	Oral
Alendronate	5 mg/day (prevention) 10 mg/day (treatment)	Oral
	70 mg every wk	Oral
Risedronate	5 mg/day or 35 mg every wk	Oral
Ibandronate	2.5 mg/day or 150 mg every mo	Oral or 30 mg intramuscularly every 3 mos
Raloxifene	60 mg/day	Oral

agents are given in Table 28–10. Table 28–11 summarizes the risks and benefits of osteoporosis therapy.

F. Other Modalities

Fluoride increases bone formation by stimulating osteoblasts and increasing cancellous bone formation in patients with osteoporosis. However, the bone is formed only in the spine and is abnormal—irregularly fibrous and woven with lacunae of low mineral density. Cessation of therapy resulted in rapid loss of much of the bone formed during treatment. The major side effect of fluoride therapy is gastric distress, an effect that is thought to be related to the direct effect of hydrofluoric acid on the gastric mucosa. Fluoride is also associated with joint pain and swelling. For these reasons, sodium fluoride is not routinely used for treatment of osteoporosis and does not have FDA labeling for this indication.

Anabolic therapy produces some increase in bone mass. Teriparatide (PTH 1–34), marketed under the trade name Forteo or recombinant parathyroid hormone, is FDA approved for the treatment of osteoporosis in perimenopausal women who are at high risk for fracture. Teriparatide also has FDA labeling for increasing bone mass in men with primary or hypogonadal osteoporosis who are at high risk for fracture. Unlike antiresorptive agents, teriparatide stimulates new bone formation. There are some concerns regarding extended use of teriparatide because of the long-term effects on multiple organ systems (ie, significant hepatotoxicity, reduced HDL, and elevated LDL cholesterol).

Teriparatide is the first approved agent for the treatment of osteoporosis that stimulates new bone formation. It is administered once a day by injection (20 mcg/day) in the thigh or abdomen. Patients treated with 20 mcg/day of teriparatide, along with calcium and vitamin D supplementation, had statistically significant increases in BMD at the spine and hip when compared with patients receiving only calcium and vitamin D supplementation. Clinical trials also demonstrated that teriparatide reduced the risk of vertebral and nonvertebral fractures in postmenopausal women. The effects of teriparatide on fracture risk have not been studied in men.

Of note, osteosarcoma developed in animals in early studies, and the possibility that humans treated with teriparatide may face an increased risk of developing this cancer cannot be ruled out. This safety issue is highlighted in a black box warning in the drug label for health professionals and explained in a brochure for patients. Children and adolescents with growing bones and patients with Paget disease of the bone have a higher risk for developing osteosarcoma and should not be treated with this agent. Because the effects of long-term treatment with teriparatide are not known, therapy for more than 2 years is not recommended.

Testosterone replacement is acceptable therapy for many of the causes of hypogonadism in men (eg, Klinefelter syndrome, isolated gonadotropin deficiency [Kallmann syndrome]).

G. Complementary and Alternative Therapies

Evidence from animal studies suggests a beneficial effect of phytoestrogens on bone, but long-term human studies are lacking. Epidemiologic evidence that Asian women have a lower fracture rate than white women even

Table 28–11. Risks and benefits of osteoporosis therapy.

	Estrogen	Raloxifene	Calcitonin	Alendronate	Risedronate	Ibandronate
Reduction of vertebral fracture	Yes	Yes	Yes	Yes	Yes	Yes
Reduction of non-vertebral fracture	Yes	No	No	Yes	Yes	Yes
Experience with long-term use	Large epidemiologic studies over decades	RCT 3 y in length	RCT 5 y in length	RCT 4 y in length	RCT 3 y in length	RCT 3 y in length
Administration	Orally: once daily any time	Orally: once daily any time	Intranasally: once daily any time	Once daily in morning, 30 min before eating, with water while upright; or weekly	Once daily (or weekly) in morning, 30–60 min before eating, with water, while upright	Orally: once monthly in morning, 30–60 min before eating, with water, while upright, or intravenously every 3 mo
Adverse effects	Breast tenderness, vaginal bleeding, thromboembolic disorders	Increased risk of venous thrombosis, hot flashes, leg cramps	Nasal irritation	Dyspepsia; esophagitis; avoid in patients with esophageal disorders	Dyspepsia	Dyspepsia
Effect on CV mortality	Increased in those with preexisting CV disease	No final outcome data	None	None	None	None
Breast cancer	Increased	Possibly decreased risk of estrogen receptor-positive breast cancer	None	None	None	None
Endometrial cancer	Increased if unopposed estrogen used	None	None	None	None	None

RCT, randomized clinical trial; CV, cardiovascular.
Modified from *Managing Osteoporosis—Part 3: Prevention and Treatment of Postmenopausal Osteoporosis.* AMA CME Program, 2000.

though the bone density of Asian women is less than that of African-American women promotes consideration of the impact of nutrition. It is possible that high soy intake contributes to improved bone quality in Asian women. A comparison study of a soy protein and high isoflavone diet versus a milk protein diet or medium isoflavone and soy protein diet demonstrated that only those receiving the higher isoflavone preparation were protected against trabecular (vertebral) bone loss.

A topical form of natural progesterone derived from diosgenin in either soybeans or Mexican wild yam has been promoted as a treatment for osteoporosis, hot flashes, and premenstrual syndrome, and a prophylactic against breast cancer. However, eating or applying wild yam extract or diosgenin does not produce increased progesterone levels in humans because humans cannot convert diosgenin to progesterone.

H. Glucocorticoid-Induced Osteoporosis

Glucocorticoids are widely used in the treatment of many chronic diseases, particularly asthma, chronic lung disease, and inflammatory and rheumatologic disorders, and in those who have undergone organ transplantation. The risk oral steroid therapy poses to bone mineral density, among other side effects, has been known for some time. As a result clinicians have eagerly substituted inhaled steroids in an endeavor to protect the patient from unwanted negative steroid effects. Recent evaluations of the effects of inhaled glucocorticoids on bone density in premenopausal women demonstrated a dose-related decline in bone density at both the total hip and the trochanter. Women with asthma were enrolled and were divided into three groups: those using no inhaled steroids, those using four to eight puffs per day, and those using more than eight puffs per day at 100 mcg per puff. No dose-related effect was noted at the femoral neck or the spine. Serum and urinary markers of bone turnover or adrenal function did not predict the degree of bone loss. To achieve the best possible outcome for the patient, given the potentially devastating effects of systemic steroids, therapy to combat the steroids should begin as soon as the steroids are begun. See Table 28–9 for specific guidelines.

Col NF et al: Patient-specific decisions about hormone replacement therapy in postmenopausal women. JAMA 1997;277:1140. [PMID: 9087469]

Ettinger B et al: Reduction of vertebral fracture risk in postmenopausal women with osteoporosis treated with raloxifene: Results from a 3-year randomized clinical trial. Multiple Outcomes of Raloxifene Evaluation (MORE) Investigation. JAMA 1999;282:637. [PMID: 10517716]

Harris ST et al: Effects of risedronate treatment on vertebral and nonvertebral fractures in women with postmenopausal osteoporosis: A randomized controlled trial. Vertebral Efficacy with Risedronate Therapy (VERT) Study Group. JAMA 1999;282:1344. [PMID: 10527181]

Israel E et al: Effects of inhaled glucocorticoids on bone density in premenopausal women. N Engl J Med 2001;345:941. [PMID: 11575285]

Potter SM et al: Soy protein and isoflavones: Their effects on blood lipids and bone density in postmenopausal women. Am J Clin Nutr 1998;68 :(Suppl):1375S. [PMID: 9848502]

Rossouw JE et al: Risks and benefits of estrogen plus progestin in healthy postmenopausal women: Principal results from the Women's Health Initiative randomized controlled trial. JAMA 2002;288:321. [PMID: 12117397]

Saag KG et al: Alendronate for the prevention and treatment of glucocorticoid-induced osteoporosis: Glucocorticoid-Induced Osteoporosis Intervention Study Group. N Engl J Med 1998; 339:292. [PMID: 9682041]

Web Sites

Food and Drug Administration:

http://www.accessdata.fda.gov/scripts/cder/drusatfda

National Osteoporosis Foundation:

http:/www.nof.org

Osteoporosis management, American Medical Association CME On-Line:

http://www.ama-cmeonline.com/osteo_mgmt

Abdominal Pain 29

Cindy Barter, MD, & Laura Dunne, MD

General Considerations

Abdominal pain is the chief complaint in 5–10% of patients presenting to emergency departments and one of the top 10 outpatient complaints. Accurate diagnosis is difficult, because the array of possible problems associated with abdominal pain is wide. For this reason, a detailed history, thorough physical examination, and laboratory and radiologic evaluations are necessary.

Clinical Findings

A. History

The history is one of the most important components in the evaluation of abdominal pain and can help direct the subsequent workup. The first priority is to determine whether the pain is acute or chronic. The sudden or severe onset of abdominal pain, particularly pain associated with hemodynamic changes, leads toward an emergent evaluation and intervention.

A thorough and accurate history requires effective communication skills on the part of the clinician. Physicians are more likely to collect the full history when implementing the "engage, empathize, educate, and enlist" method. Patients should be allowed to tell their story, which usually takes 1 or 2 minutes and often answers the questions regarding onset, intensity, location, and frequency of the problem that can help focus the physical examination.

1. Onset—Sudden and severe onset of abdominal pain is often seen in appendicitis, leaking or ruptured abdominal aortic aneurysm, perforated ulcer, pancreatitis, obstruction, and some nongastrointestinal sources of pain (eg, ectopic pregnancy, myocardial infarction, sickle cell crisis, and kidney stones). Gastroesophageal reflux disease (GERD), chronic pancreatitis, functional bowel disease (irritable bowel syndrome), abdominal wall pain, celiac disease, constipation, chronic diarrhea, and other nongastrointestinal sources (eg, prostatitis, ovarian cyst, and pelvic inflammatory disease) can all be characterized by a more gradual onset of abdominal pain and by abdominal pain that is chronic in nature (Table 29–1).

2. Quality of pain—The patient's description of the quality of the pain provides clues to the etiology of the problem. For example, "burning" is often used to describe GERD. A pressure-like description ("there's an elephant sitting on me") suggests cardiac ischemia. Patients suffering from peptic ulcer disease (PUD) often describe their pain as a gnawing or hunger-like sensation.

3. Location—The location of the pain coupled with any radiation can be helpful. For example, pain from acute appendicitis may start as epigastric or periumbilical pain prior to setting in the right lower quadrant (RLQ) of the abdomen. Pain that starts in the midepigastric region and then radiates to the back suggests pancreatitis. Gallbladder pain typically radiates to the scapula. Pain from the lower esophagus may be referred higher in the chest and is often confused with pain associated with cardiac conditions, such as an acute myocardial infarction.

4. Frequency—The frequency and pattern of the pain are particularly useful in identifying abdominal pain that is gradual in onset. Pain that worsens nocturnally upon lying down suggests GERD. Pain occurring after the consumption of high-fat meals increases the probability of gallbladder disease. Pain that is relieved after a bowel movement is indicative of functional bowel symptoms.

5. Other diagnostic clues—Physicians need to determine if other associated symptoms are present. Fever and chills suggest an infectious etiology. Nausea and vomiting are associated with pancreatitis. Hematemesis can indicate a Mallory–Weiss tear or PUD. Feculent emesis is correlated with bowel obstruction. The presence of blood and melena in the stool requires further evaluation due to the possibility of gastrointestinal (GI) bleeding. Emotional stress can exacerbate functional bowel disease. However, it should not be used as a primary diagnostic discriminator between functional and organic disease because many organic diseases can be accentuated by emotional stress.

Past medical history can provide important clues to the etiology of abdominal pain. A history of previous episodes can help direct further evaluation. Previous abdominal surgery increases the risk for bowel obstruction secondary to adhesions, strangulation, or hernia. Patients with a history of cardiovascular disease are at greater risk for bowel infarction. A history of tobacco or alcohol use

Table 29–1. Common causes of abdominal pain by location.

Localized
- Midepigastric
  - Dyspepsia
  - GERD
  - Pancreatitis
  - PUD
- RUQ
  - Gallbladder diseases
  - Hepatitis
  - Hepatomegaly
- RLQ
  - Appendicitis
  - Crohn disease
  - GYN-related diseases
    - Ruptured ovarian cyst
    - Ectopic pregnancy
    - PID
    - Pregnancy
  - Meckel diverticulitis
- LUQ
  - MI
  - Pneumonia
  - Sickle cell crisis
  - Lymphoma
  - Splenomegaly—EBV
  - Gastritis
- LLQ
  - Diverticulitis
  - Bowel obstruction
  - Ischemic colitis
  - Ulcerative colitis
  - Urinary calculi
- Suprapubic
  - Cystitis
  - Prostatitis
  - Urinary retention

Generalized
- Abdominal wall pain—multiple causes
- Celiac disease
- Constipation
- Chronic diarrhea
- IBS
- Gastroenteritis/infectious diarrhea
- Mesenteric lymphadenitis
- Perforated colon
- Ruptured aortic aneurysm
- Trauma

GERD, gastroesophageal reflux disease; PUD, peptic ulcer disease; GYN, gynecologic; PID, pelvic inflammatory disease; MI, myocardial infarction; EBV, Epstein–Barr virus; IBS, inflammatory bowel disease; RUQ, right upper quadrant; RLQ, right lower quadrant; LUQ, left upper quadrant; LLQ, left lower quadrant.

is associated with an increased incidence of GERD and PUD. Alcohol abuse is also a common cause of pancreatitis. Multiparity, obesity, and diabetes mellitus all increase the risk of gallbladder disease. Tubal ligation or a history of pelvic inflammatory disease (PID) indicates a greater risk for an ectopic pregnancy.

No medical history is complete without a medication history that also includes both over-the-counter drugs and herbal supplements. Aspirin, nonsteroidal anti-inflammatory drugs (NSAIDs), and warfarin increase the risk of GI bleeding. Alendronate sodium increases the probability that the patient's symptoms of abdominal pain include epigastric pain, which further indicates erosive esophagitis. Antibiotics can be associated with nausea, diarrhea, or both.

Advancing age can change the patient's presentation and perception or abdominal pain. There is a 10–20% reduction in intensity of pain per decade of age over 60 years. One study found that only 22% of elderly patients with appendicitis presented with the classic symptom pattern. Young patients with PUD are twice as likely to present with epigastric pain as are elderly patients.

B. Physical Examination

The history obtained dictates the focus of the abdominal examination. In addition to the abdominal examination, a pelvic examination is frequently indicated in women and girls who present with abdominal pain.

An effective physical examination of the abdomen has many steps that flow intuitively. The physician should begin by positioning the patient supine with the knees slightly bent. From this position many different aspects of the abdomen can be assessed.

1. Inspection—An inspection for distention, discoloration, scars, and striae should then be conducted. Distention suggests ascites, obstruction, or other masses increasing the abdominal contents. Discoloration may include bruising as in the case of hemoperitoneum, found in the central portion of the abdomen, especially following abdominal trauma. The presence and location of scars help clarify and confirm the history previously obtained. Striae suggest rapid growth of the abdomen. Old striae tend to be white, whereas new striae or those related to endocrine abnormalities tend to be purplish or dark pink. In persons of color, this may appear to be a darkening of the skin. The abdomen should also be inspected when the patient is upright, as many hernias resolve when the patient is in a supine position.

2. Auscultation—Auscultation should be performed prior to palpation. The physician should listen for the quality of bowel sounds: normal, hypoactive, hyperactive, or high pitched. Hypoactive and hyperactive bowel sounds can both be present in the case of total or partial bowel obstruction, or ileus. It is also necessary to listen for bruits over the aorta, renal arteries, and femoral arteries when auscultating. Bruits may be suggestive of aneurysms in those areas. Palpating gently while auscultating decreases the likelihood of guarding, embellishment, or symptom magnification on the part of the patient.

3. Palpation—Palpation of the abdomen should be done in several steps, beginning with the lightest of touches away from the area of greatest pain, and moving closer to the tender area as the examination progresses. There are several aspects to palpation, including consistency, tenderness, masses, and organ size. Consistency can range from soft to rigid; increased rigidity is indicative of an acute abdomen needing more emergent intervention.

Tenderness can be separated by location, radiation, and associated rebound or guarding. Murphy sign, sudden cessation of the patient's inspiratory effort during deep palpation of the right upper quadrant (RUQ), is suggestive of acute cholecystitis. In appendicitis, rebound tenderness and sharp pain upon palpation of McBurney point is usually elicited 2 inches from the anterior superior iliac spine on a line drawn from this process through the umbilicus. However, the size of the appendix (and therefore the location of pain with palpation) varies, and pain may occur some distance from the classic McBurney point.

Pain stemming from visceral organs may appear to radiate secondary to other areas being innervated by the same nerve. For example, the pain caused by pancreatitis often radiates to the back. Kehr sign, abdominal pain radiating to the left shoulder, is indicative of splenic rupture, renal calculi, or ectopic pregnancy. Radiation of pain can also be caused by inflammation of surrounding tissues.

It is difficult to palpate the deep muscles of the abdomen, but the same effect can be obtained by examining pain with motion of muscles. For example, the iliopsoas muscle test can assess for inflammation within the psoas muscle or inflammation of overlying structures such as the appendix. The test is performed by having the patient lie supine, then lift the right leg, flexing at the hip. Resistance is applied to the leg. Pain with this maneuver is suggestive of appendicitis or retroperitoneal dissection.

Rebound tenderness indicates peritoneal irritation, which can come from perforation along the GI tract or from the non-GI sources such as a ruptured ovarian cyst or PID. When there is peritoneal irritation the patient will often demonstrate guarding. Guarding can be voluntary or involuntary. Voluntary guarding can occur when the patient anticipates the pain. The "closed eye" sign has been shown to help differentiate the etiology of the pain. Patients whose pain has an organic etiology will keep their eyes open and watch as the examiner approaches the abdomen. Patients who close their eyes are more likely to have psychosocial factors contributing to their abdominal pain.

Involuntary guarding is caused by flexion of the abdominal wall muscle as the body attempts to protect the internal organs. This protective reflex can be used to differentiate visceral pain from abdominal wall or psychogenic pain, demonstrated with the Carnett test. The test is performed by finding the area of greatest tenderness. The patient then flexes the abdominal wall and the point is palpated again. Pain that is less severe with palpation of the flexed abdomen wall has a high probability of being visceral. Pain that remains the same or is worsened with this maneuver likely stems from the abdominal wall or from nonorganic causes.

Palpation of the abdomen of a ticklish patient can be difficult. Two approaches can help the physician palpate these patients more thoroughly. One method is to first use the stethoscope for light palpation and then curl the fingers past the edge of the stethoscope to create a less sensitive tough. In an alternative technique, the patient places his or her hands on the abdomen and the examiner palpates through the patient's hands and just over the edge of the patient's fingers. This permits deep palpation without contraction of the abdominal muscles from laughing.

In addition to feeling for tenderness with palpation, the physician should examine the abdomen for masses and organ size. Palpable masses include colon cancer masses, kidney abnormalities, non-GI tumors, aneurysms, or other organ abnormalities. Most are found on deep palpation. This palpation can be facilitated by having the patient in the supine position with the knees slightly bent, to allow for relaxation of the abdominal muscles. If a mass is palpated it should be examined for location, size, shape, consistency, pulsations, mobility, and movement with respiration.

When palpating for organ size, the liver and spleen should be examined. Before trying to palpate the lower border of the liver or spleen, the examiner should ask the patient take a deep breath and then exhale while he or she palpates deeper. The normal liver span at the midclavicular line is 6–12 cm. The liver in men and taller individuals tends to be larger than the liver in women and shorter individuals. Additionally, the liver span in the midsternal line can be helpful. This span is normally 4–8 cm. Anything larger than 8 cm should be considered enlarged. The size of the liver may better be appreciated by percussing along the midclavicular line. The examiner should start in an area of tympany and progress to an area of dullness, both from above the liver and below the liver. The upper border generally sits at the fifth to seventh intercostal space. Inferior displacement is suggestive of emphysema or other pulmonary disease.

The spleen may not be palpable or just a tip of the spleen may be palpable. Both of these findings are normal. The actual span of the spleen can be determined by percussion. The area of dullness related to the spleen is generally from the sixth to the tenth rib. It should be percussed in the left midaxillary line.

4. Percussion—Percussion can be helpful to determine both the size of the organs and other information about the abdomen. Percussion over the liver or spleen should be slightly dull. A change in the character of the sound can indicate that the edge of the organ is reached. This can also be determined by the scratch test, a gentle form of percussion. It is performed by placing the stethoscope over the liver, then gently scratching the surface of the skin beginning above the upper border of the liver and progressing down below the lower border of the liver. The quality of the sound changes as the examiner's scratch travels from the lung field to the liver and then to the abdomen. These changes in sound help to identify the borders of the liver.

After determining the size of organs, the rest of the abdomen can be examined for other abnormalities. Tympany should be present over the stomach bubble because of the air present. Tympany related to the stomach should be found in the area of the left lower border of the rib cage and left epigastrium. However, any increased tympany throughout the rest of the abdomen suggests dilation or perforation of the bowel. Dullness can be stationary, as with solid masses, or shifting as with mobile fluid. Shifting dullness is generally present with significant ascites.

C. Laboratory Findings

Frequently indicated tests include complete blood count (CBC), liver function tests (LFTs), electrolytes, blood urea nitrogen (BUN), creatinine, erythrocyte sedimentation rate (ESR), C-reactive protein, stool studies, pregnancy test, urinalysis, amylase, and lipase.

Hemoglobin and hematocrit should be examined for evidence of blood loss. However, rapid blood loss can result in normal-appearing values until the patient is fluid resuscitated. The white blood cell count (WBC) is helpful in identifying infection, as in appendicitis, diverticulitis, peritonitis, and PID. Elevated amylase often indicates pancreatitis, but this value can be elevated in many abdominal processes. Lipase and trypsin are both more specific to pancreatitis and can be helpful in clarifying the etiology of pain. Electrolytes, BUN, and creatinine can help identify dehydration, kidney failure, and acidotic or alkalotic states. Patients with inflammatory bowel disease tend to have elevated ESR and C-reactive protein, especially during the times of exacerbation of the disease. The urinalysis can indicate confusing results. Evidence of red or white blood cells in the urine may suggest a kidney stone or urinary tract infection. However, these findings can occur in any inflammatory process in proximity to the bladder, such as prostatitis, appendicitis, PID, and diverticulitis. A pregnancy test should be performed on any female patient of childbearing age. If a patient has abdominal pain, prior history that includes a tubal ligation does not rule out the possibility of pregnancy and increases the risk of ectopic pregnancy.

D. Imaging Studies

Computed tomography (CT) of the abdomen and pelvis with and without contrast is usually the most helpful imaging study. CT scans provide an adequate view of many of the causes of abdominal pain and can reveal a wide range of problems. Vascular lesions such as abdominal aortic aneurysms or aortic ruptures are well visualized using CT scans, as are diverticulitis, pancreatitis, appendicitis, and bowel obstruction. A CT scan is superior to simple radiographs in detecting pneumoperitoneum specifically and perforated viscus generally. A spiral CT scan of the urinary tract is comparable to intravenous pyelography (IVP) for imaging kidney stones and urinary obstructions. With certain exceptions, a CT scan is the single most effective way to confirm a diagnosis or, upon its failure to confirm a suspected diagnosis, to dictate the need for additional testing.

Ultrasonography is another useful diagnostic tool for the examination and measurement of internal body structures and the detection of bodily abnormalities. The advantages of ultrasound include low cost, low risk (due to the absence of contrast materials), reliable imaging of biliary systems, and more reliable imaging of the female pelvic organs compared with CT. Ultrasound is the most reliable method to diagnose biliary disease. Because as many as 25% of biliary stones are isodense to bile, these stones cannot be visualized on CT scan. Exceptions to the general rule exist in the cases of obese individuals, where the study can be technically difficult, and those instances in which the skill and experience of the operator are substandard. Ultrasound has been used for the focused study of the appendix, but spiral CT scans have been shown to be more accurate for diagnosing appendicitis. An exception to this general rule is pregnant women, for whom ultrasound is the test of choice. Ultrasound can also be helpful in children who are unable to remain still for the duration of a CT scan.

Magnetic resonance imaging (MRI) is a useful test in certain situations. The magnetic resonance cholangiopancreatography (MRCP) is a noninvasive way to obtain high-quality images of the biliary tree and the liver parenchyma. MRCP is uniquely effective for patients who are unable to tolerate the administration of contrast or who are obese and patients for whom CT or ultrasound has shown lesions that need further characterization or for whom endoscopic retrograde cholangiopancreatography (ERCP) poses a significant risk. MRI has recently been used to visualize pancreatic cancer, but is has not proven to be any more useful than CT scans in this regard.

In some cases endoscopy, colonoscopy, or angiography may be indicated. Further discussion of these tests can be found in the individual sections later in this chapter.

DYSPEPSIA

ESSENTIALS OF DIAGNOSIS

- *Chronic or recurrent discomfort centered in the upper abdomen.*
- *May be associated with PUD (15–25%) or GERD (5–15%), but etiology is nonspecific in 50–60% of patients.*
- *Symptoms do not correlate with findings on endoscopy.*

General Considerations

The word *dyspepsia* was first used in the early 18th century to describe a person's ill humor, indigestion, or disgruntlement. The modern family practitioner uses the term to describe a set of symptoms that can encompass several different diseases and the etiology associated with them. Chronic or recurrent discomfort centered in the upper abdomen is the description most commonly used by clinicians for dyspepsia. Dyspepsia can be associated with heartburn, belching, bloating, nausea, or vomiting. Common etiologies include PUD and GERD. Rare causes include gastric and pancreatic cancers.

Although dyspepsia is reported to affect 40% of the world's adult population and accounts for 2–3% of all visits to primary care providers, only about 10% of affected adults seek medical advice. Approximately 15–25% of dyspepsia is caused by PUD and 5–15% by GERD.

No specific etiology is found for approximately 50–60% of patients who present with epigastric pain. When a patient has suffered at least 3 months of dyspepsia without a definitive structural or biochemical explanation, the clinical term applied is *nonulcer dyspepsia* and, less commonly, *functional dyspepsia.* Other etiologies that occur infrequently include gastric or esophageal cancer, biliary tract disease, gastroparesis, pancreatitis, carbohydrate malabsorption, medication-induced symptoms, non-GI diseases affecting the stomach (sarcoidosis, diabetes, and thyroid and parathyroid diseases), metabolic disturbances (hypercalcemia and hyperkalemia), hepatoma, intestinal parasites, and other cancers, particularly pancreatic cancer.

The history is often similar, whether the symptoms are from PUD, GERD, or nonulcer dyspepsia. Studies have shown that the symptoms and the degree of symptoms do not correlate with the findings on endoscopy.

The physical examination is also similar. There may be tenderness in the midepigastric area. Unless an ulcer has perforated, causing signs of peritonitis, the rest of the abdominal examination is unremarkable.

The treatment for dyspepsia depends on the etiology and will be discussed in the different sections on PUD, GERD, and nonulcer dyspepsia.

Talley NJ et al: American Gastroenterological Association technical review on the valuation of dyspepsia. Gastroenterology 2005; 129:1756. [PMID: 16285971]

1. *Peptic Ulcer Disease*

ESSENTIALS OF DIAGNOSIS

- *Gnawing pain with a sensation of hunger; melena.*
- *Prior history of ulcers or tobacco use.*
- *EGD visualization of an ulcer and biopsy evaluation for* H pylori.

General Considerations

The four major causes of ulcers include *Helicobacter pylori*–induced ulcers, NSAIDs, acid hypersecretory conditions, and idiopathic ulcers.

There is clear evidence to support the eradication of *H pylori* in patients who have documented ulcers. In the 1980s *H pylori* was associated with 90% of peptic ulcers. In the late 1990s *H pylori* was associated with 60–70% of all peptic ulcers. This decrease is related to increased treatment of *H pylori* infections. *H pylori* infections have been commonly associated with low income, low educational levels, and overcrowded living conditions. African Americans and Hispanics have about a one-third higher rate of infection than white Americans. In the United States, 40% of all adults are infected with *H pylori* by the time they reach 50 years of age, compared with only 5% of all children aged 6–12 years. In developing countries, children are more commonly infected at a younger age and there is a higher incidence of infection throughout the entire population.

Pathogenesis

Infection with *H pylori* is the leading cause of peptic ulcers and use of NSAIDs is the second leading cause. In the United States, one in seven individuals uses NSAIDs. Of long-term NSAID users who undergo an upper endoscopy, 5–20% are found to have an ulcer. Risk factors for developing an ulcer due to NSAID use are a personal history of ulcer, age older than 65 years, current steroid use, use of anticoagulants or a history of cardiovascular disease, and the impairment of another major organ. NSAIDs are prescribed to nearly

Table 29–2. Evaluation for *Helicobacter pylori*–related disease.

Clinical Scenario	Recommended Test	Levels of Evidence[1] and Comments
Dyspepsia[2] in patient with alarm symptoms for cancer or complicated ulcer (eg, bleeding, perforation)	Promptly refer to a gastroenterologist for endoscopy	A
Known PUD, uncomplicated	Serology antibody test; treat if result is positive	A—Best evidence for eradication in presence of documented gastric or duodenal ulcer
Dyspepsia in patient with previous history of PUD not previously treated with eradication therapy	Serology antibody test; treat if result is positive	A
Dyspepsia in patient with PUD previously treated for *H pylori* results	Stool antigen or urea breath test; if positive, treat with regimen different from the one previously used; retest to confirm eradication; consider endoscopy	B—Urea breath test should be delayed for 4 weeks following treatment, as acid suppression can lead to false-positive results
Undifferentiated dyspepsia (without endoscopy)	Serology antibody test; treat if result is positive	B—Supported by cost–benefit analyses and recent small RCTs
Documented nonulcer dyspepsia (after endoscopy)	Unnecessary	B—RCTs and meta-analyses on this topic are mixed but indicate that few patients benefit from treatment
GERD	Unnecessary	B—GERD is not associated with *H pylori* infection
Asymptomatic with history of documented PUD not previously treated with eradication therapy	Serology antibody test; treat if result is positive	C
Asymptomatic	Screening unnecessary	C

PUD, peptic ulcer disease; GERD, gastroesophageal reflux disease; RCT, randomized controlled clinical trial.
[1]Levels of evidence: A, strong evidence, based on good-quality RCTs or meta-analysis of RCTs; B, moderate evidence, based on high-quality cohort studies, case-control studies, or systematic reviews of observational studies or lower-quality RCT; C, based on consensus or expert opinion.
[2]Defined as pain or discomfort centered in the upper abdomen and persisting or recurring for more than 4 weeks.

40% of all persons older than 65 years. Elderly patients who commence a course of treatment with NSAIDs have a 1–8% chance of being hospitalized within the first year of therapy for GI complications caused by NSAIDs. Patients who are *H pylori* positive and who are taking NSAIDs have a higher risk of complications.

Prevention

Eradication of *H pylori* infection before starting a course of treatment with NSAIDs reduced the risk of developing an ulcer early in the treatment.

Clinical Findings

As with most cases of abdominal pain, the history obtained provides the majority of information used to focus the differential diagnosis. Factors pointing toward PUD include a gnawing pain with the sensation of hunger, a prior personal or family history of ulcers, tobacco use, and a report of melena.

The diagnostic test of choice is esophagogastroduodenoscopy (EGD), which allows both visualization and biopsy of the ulcer as well as testing for *H pylori* (Table 29–2).

Complications

In the elderly (aged 80 years and older) who have ulcers, the incidence of complications is much higher in patients who are taking aspirin and are *H pylori* infected. A hypersecretory condition, such as Zollinger–Ellison syndrome, is suspected in patients who have multiple ulcers and is caused by a gastrin-producing tumor. To complicate matters further, there is an increasing incidence of idiopathic ulcers in the US population at large.

Treatment

Treatment of PUD requires the initial eradication of *H pylori* if present, stopping or reducing the dose of NSAIDs, and treatment with an H_2 blocker or a proton pump inhibitor (PPI). Many Food and Drug Administration (FDA)–approved treatment regimens exist to eradicate *H pylori*. They usually include two or three antibiotics plus a PPI or an H_2 blocker for 10–14 days. Because antibiotic resistance changes and subsequently recommended treatment options change it is necessary to refer to current guidelines either locally or from the Centers for Disease Control and Prevention (CDC). Treatment of the *H pylori* infection facilitates the healing of the ulcer and decreases the rate of recurrence in the first year from 75% to only 10%. Medical treatment of peptic ulcer has become very effective and surgical intervention needs to occur less frequently. When surgery is performed it is more commonly done with a laparoscopic repair.

Ford AC et al: *Helicobacter pylori* "test and treat" or endoscopy for managing dyspepsia: An individual patient data meta-analysis. Gastroenterology 2005; 128:1838. [PMID: 15940619]

Meurer LN, Bower DJ: Management of *Helicobacter pylori* infection. Am Fam Physician 2002; 65:1327. [PMID: 11996414]

Smoot DT et al: Peptic ulcer disease. Prim Care 2001;28:487. [PMID: 11483440]

2. Gastroesophageal Reflux Disease

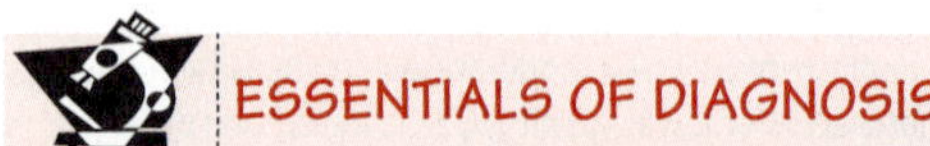

- *Heartburn (most common symptom); multiple extraesophageal symptoms may also be present.*
- *Symptoms are exacerbated by changes in body position.*
- *Diagnosis is made on the basis of history and symptomatic improvement following treatment.*

Clinical Findings

Heartburn is the single most common symptom of GERD. Ten percent of the US population experiences heartburn at least once per day and almost 50% experience symptoms at least once per month. Other common symptoms include regurgitation, belching, and dysphagia. GERD can also be associated with multiple extraesophageal symptoms and conditions. Pulmonary conditions that can be caused by GERD include asthma, chronic bronchitis, aspiration pneumonia, sleep apnea, atelectasis, and interstitial pulmonary fibrosis. Ear, nose, and throat manifestations of GERD include chronic cough, sore throat, hoarseness, halitosis, enamel erosion, subglottic stenosis, vocal cord inflammation, granuloma, and possibly cancer. Noncardiac chest pain, chronic hiccups, and nausea are also associated with GERD.

Changes in body position tend to exacerbate the symptoms of GERD, particularly lying down or bending forward. Complications include Barrett esophagus, esophageal strictures, ulceration, hemorrhage, and, rarely, perforation. Of all patients who undergo an upper endoscopy for GERD, 8–20% are found to have Barrett esophagus.

The esophagus has three mechanisms in place to try to prevent mucosal injury. The lower esophageal sphincter creates a barrier to acid reflux. Peristalsis, gravity, and saliva provide acid clearance mechanisms. The third defense mechanism is epithelial resistance.

Diagnosis is made using the medical history and treatment with H_2 receptor antagonists, prokinetic agents, or PPIs. Symptomatic improvement following treatment can be indicative of GERD. Upper endoscopy fails to reveal 36–50% of all patients who have been diagnosed via esophageal pH monitoring. Endoscopy should always be performed if alarming symptoms are present such as bleeding, weight loss, or dysphagia, especially if the alarm symptoms occur in an elderly patient.

Treatment

Treatment of GERD involves life-style modification and medication. Life-style modifications that have the greatest impact in reducing symptoms of GERD and that also provide positive health benefits include cessation of smoking, temperance in the consumption of alcohol, weight loss in the case of overweight patients, and reduction of dietary fat intake. Certain foods that decrease lower esophageal sphincter (LES) pressure (chocolate), stimulate acid secretion (coffee, tea, and cola beverages), or produce symptoms by their acidity (orange or tomato juice) should be avoided. In addition, elevating the head of the bed by 6 inches, avoiding bedtime snacks, and reducing meal size, particularly the evening meal, can all help ameliorate symptoms of GERD.

Medication treatment options are designed to decrease the acid or increase the defense mechanisms. Commonly used over-the-counter medications include antacids, Gaviscon, and H_2 blockers. Prescription medicines include prescription strength H_2 blockers, PPIs, prokinetic agents (Reglan), bethanechol, and sucralfate. Agents that can irritate the mucosa (eg, aspirin and NSAIDs) should be avoided or used only sparingly. Other agents to avoid if possible include α-adrenergic antagonists, anticholinergics, β-adrenergic agonists, calcium channel blockers, diazepam, narcotics, progesterone, and theophylline.

If the patient's symptoms have resolved or significantly improved with the preceding treatment measures, then no further evaluation is needed. If the symptoms have not improved, usually within 1–2 weeks, then endoscopy is the next step. Symptoms do not always correlate with the pathologic findings seen at the time of endoscopy. Even as symptoms improve over time there still may be a risk of developing long-term complications. Patients who have developed Barrett esophagus need closer follow-up and monitoring because they have a 50- to 100-fold increased risk of developing esophageal cancer.

Moayyedi P, Talley NJ: Gastro-oesophageal reflux disease. Lancet 2006;367:2086. [PMID: 16798392]

Richter JE: Beyond heartburn: Extraesophageal manifestations of gastroesophageal reflux disease. Am J Manag Care 2001;7:S6. [PMID: 11225351]

3. Nonulcer Dyspepsia

ESSENTIALS OF DIAGNOSIS

- *Minimum of 12 weeks of persistent or recurrent dyspepsia without evidence of organic disease and without disturbed defecation.*
- *Diagnosis is made by excluding other causes of dyspepsia.*
- *EGD is the diagnostic gold standard but should be preceded by testing for* H pylori.

General Considerations

Nonulcer dyspepsia, also referred to as *idiopathic* or *functional dyspepsia,* is defined as a minimum of 12 consecutive or nonconsecutive weeks of persistent or recurrent dyspepsia without evidence of organic disease, not relieved by defecation, and not associated with the onset of change in stool frequency or form (which would indicate irritable bowel syndrome [IBS]). Nonulcer dyspepsia is divided into four groups based on symptoms: ulcer-like dyspepsia, reflux-like dyspepsia, dysmotility-like dyspepsia, and nonspecific dyspepsia.

There is overlap among the four different groups and IBS. It has been suggested that separating the functional GI symptoms of dyspepsia and IBS may be inappropriate.

Pathogenesis

The pathophysiology of nonulcer dyspepsia is not entirely clear and is probably multifactorial. Suggested causes include changes in gastric physiology, nociception, motor dysfunction, central nervous system dysfunction, and psychological and environmental factors (see the discussion of IBS, later). *H pylori* and its effects on nonulcer dyspepsia are highly controversial. A percentage of patients with nonulcer dyspepsia and *H pylori* have significant improvement in their symptoms after using eradication therapy, yet improvement cannot be guaranteed. Approximately 50% of patients with nonulcer dyspepsia are *H pylori* positive.

Clinical Findings

Nonulcer dyspepsia is diagnosed by excluding other causes of dyspepsia. The gold standard is the EGD. Cost-effectiveness data indicate that testing for *H pylori* and treating the patient if it is found decrease the number of EGDs performed by approximately one third.

Treatment

Management of nonulcer dyspepsia is multifactorial and includes making a diagnosis early and explaining as much of the relevant physiology as possible to the patient. It is important for the physician neither to investigate excessively nor to investigate the presenting symptoms alone. New investigation in a patient who has been previously diagnosed with nonulcer dyspepsia should be done whenever alarm symptoms are present or if a new objective symptom arises. (Alarm symptoms are highlighted by the mnemonic VBAD: vomiting, evidence of bleeding or anemia, presence of abdominal mass or weight loss, and dysphagia.) It is important for the physician to determine why the patient with chronic symptoms presented at this particular time.

Psychosocial factors can exacerbate symptoms, so it is important for physicians to address these issues and offer counseling. A mainstay of management is postevaluation reassurance of the patient concerning the diagnosis and the absence of alarm symptoms. Patients should avoid any food or substance that tends to exacerbate symptoms (NSAIDs, alcohol, tobacco, and certain foods). Not all patients want or need to take prescription medicine. For these patients other treatment options should be explored. If symptoms of bloating or postprandial fullness are present, the patient should eat six small meals per day, which may help ameliorate symptoms.

A remarkable number of different medicines have been used in studies of nonulcer dyspepsia. The results are confounded by the fact that the studies do not use the same definition for the disorder and do not differentiate among the different symptom types. For example, PPIs appear to have some benefit in ulcer-like dyspepsia whereas patients with dysmotility-like dyspepsia do not respond. Medicines that have been used include antacids, H_2 blockers, PPIs, bismuth, and sucralfate. Prokinetic agents such as metoclopramide have been poorly studied. Cisapride, which was taken off the market, showed a twofold decrease in symptoms over placebo. Domperidone, which is not available in the United States, has been shown to be superior to placebo and does not produce central nervous system side effects because it does not cross the blood–brain barrier. Peppermint oil and caraway oil have been compared to cisapride with similar results. Motilin agonists such as erythromycin increase the rate of gastric emptying. Visceral analgesics such as fedotozine reduce gastric hypersensitivity. Buspirone and 5-HT_1 agonists such as sumatriptan have shown promise in studies performed to date. Antispasmodics such as dicyclomine have not been shown to be more effective than placebo in patients with dyspepsia. Antinausea agents such as ondansetron and perchlorperazine have been shown to provide modest symptom improvement, with perchlorperazine having more side effects. Antihistamines such as dimenhydrinate and cyclizine decrease gastric dysrhythmias. Promethazine has been used to treat mild nausea. Of the antidepressants, only tricyclic antidepressants have been studied in functional dyspepsia. Selective serotonin reuptake inhibitors have had some promising results with other functional bowel diseases (IBS).

Other approaches that are being used include acupuncture, acupressure, and gastric electrical stimulation. However, no randomized, double-blind controlled trials have been performed to evaluate their effectiveness. After discussing whether medications are needed and writing a prescription if necessary, physicians should schedule a follow-up appointment to assess the patient's function and to determine any responses to the treatment.

Cremonini F et al: Functional dyspepsia: Drugs for new (and old) therapeutic targets. Best Pract Res Clin Gastroenterol 2004;18:717. [PMID: 15324710]

Dickerson LM, King DE: Evaluation and management of nonulcer dyspepsia. Am Fam Physician 2004;70:107. [PMID: 15259526]

DISEASES OF THE GALLBLADDER & PANCREAS

The three main causes of abdominal pain related to the gallbladder and pancreas are biliary colic, gallstones, cholecystitis, and pancreatitis. Gallbladder-related pain is usually located in the midepigastric region and may radiate to the right shoulder, right scapula, right clavicular area, or back. Pancreatitis tends to produce pain throughout the entire upper abdomen with frequent radiation to the back. For detailed discussion of these and other diseases of the biliary tract and pancreas, see Chapter 31.

IRRITABLE BOWEL SYNDROME

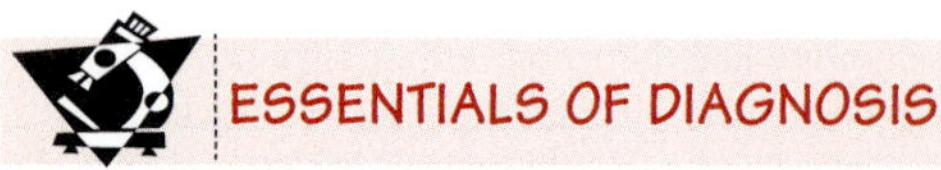

- *Symptoms of abdominal pain or discomfort associated with disturbed defecation.*
- *Diagnosis is symptom-based, once alarm features (weight loss, refractory diarrhea, family history of colon cancer) are excluded.*

General Considerations

Estimates indicate that symptoms consistent with a diagnosis of IBS are present in from 3% to 20% of adults in the western world. Although IBS occurs worldwide, cultural and social factors affect its presentation. In western countries, women have a higher incidence of the condition and are more likely to consult a physician. In India and Sri Lanka men have a higher incidence of IBS. In black South Africans, IBS symptoms are common in people who live in urban zones and are unusual in people who live in rural areas. In the United States, prevalence is similar between blacks and whites and some studies show a lower prevalence in Hispanics from Texas and Asians from California.

A large percentage of individuals (up to 50%) with symptoms consistent with a diagnosis of IBS never seek a physician's care. Those who do seek care have often had a major life event (eg, a death in the family or loss of job) before presenting with GI complaints. Primary care providers see a larger percentage of these patients than do GI specialists.

Pathogenesis

Physiologic alterations contributing to symptoms of IBS have not been elucidated. Many theories exist, including disturbance in motility, altered perception either locally in the GI tract or in the central nervous system, visceral hypersensitivity, mucosal inflammation, autonomic nerve dysfunction, and psychological disturbance, but no theory is applicable to every patient who has symptoms of IBS. In one study a positron emission tomography (PET) scan was used to examine the activity of the brain when GI symptoms were induced. Patients with IBS did not activate the anterior cingulate cortex that is associated with opiate binding but did activate the prefrontal cortex that is associated with hypervigilance and anxiety. Studies to determine whether patients with IBS have a lower threshold of pain with colonic distention are inconclusive. All that can be stated with reasonable certainty is that studies have not clarified whether symptoms of IBS are a normal perception of an abnormal function or an abnormal perception of a normal function.

Clinical Findings

A. Symptoms and Signs

IBS belongs to a group of functional bowel disorders (ie, no organic cause can be identified) in which

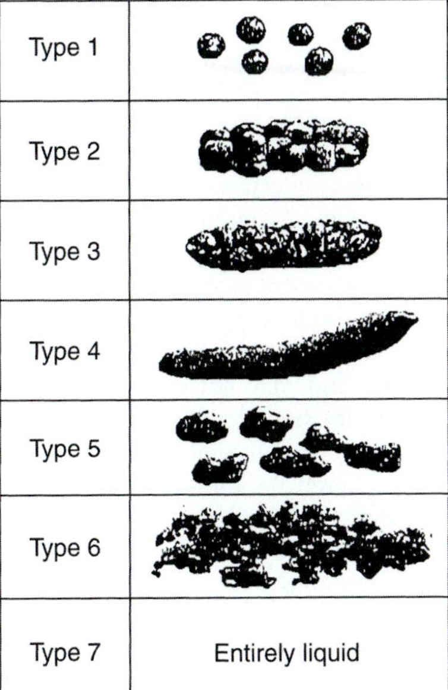

Figure 29–1. Bristol Stool Form Scale. See Table 29–3 for standard description for each of the seven types.

abdominal discomfort or pain is associated with defecation or a change in bowel habits and with features of disordered defecation. Diagnostic criteria developed by the Rome Consensus Committee for IBS are at least 12 or more weeks, not necessarily consecutive, in the preceding 12 months of abdominal discomfort or pain that is characterized by two of the following three features: (1) it is relieved with defecation, (2) its onset is associated with a change in frequency of stool, and (3) its onset is associated with a change in the form or appearance of the stool.

The Bristol Stool Form Scale (Figure 29–1 and Table 29–3) is used as a standard description for seven types of stool forms. Other symptoms that support the diagnosis of IBS include abnormal stool frequency (more than three per day or less than three per week), abnormal stool form (lumpy/hard or loose/watery), abnormal stool passage (straining, urgency, or a feeling of incomplete evacuation), passage of mucus, and a sensation of bloating or feeling of abdominal distention.

Stool form has been demonstrated to be reflective of GI transit time. Using the Bristol Stool Form Scale and frequency of bowel movements is more diagnostically precise and useful than using the imprecise terms diarrhea and constipation, which can have different meanings to different patients. Patients may complain of feeling constipated, attributable to a feeling of incomplete evacuation despite having just passed soft or watery stool.

B. History

The patient history is the single most useful tool in diagnosing IBS. Continuity of care and a well-established rapport contribute significantly to obtaining an accurate and exhaustive history. A positive physician-patient interaction, including a psychosocial history, precipitating factors, and a discussion of diagnosis and treatment with patients, results in fewer return visits for IBS and lower utilization of health care resources. Chronic or recurrent abdominal pain indicates a need to assess quality of life. In one study undergraduate students with IBS had quality of life scores that were similar to patients with congestive heart failure, indicating a significant impact by IBS symptoms.

A history of abuse should be sought in patients with chronic abdominal pain. A study at a tertiary care gastroenterology clinic reported that 60% of the overall study population, all female, reported a history of physical or sexual abuse. The self-reported history of abuse was highest for those with functional bowel disease (up to 84%) and lowest for those with organic bowel disease, such as ulcerative colitis (38%). It is therefore worthwhile to overtly assess a patient's psychosocial stressors as they can affect the success of the course of treatment. A physician should always assess for abuse when considering referral to a gastroenterologist. Family physicians are uniquely positioned to assess and address issues associated with abuse.

Patients with IBS have not been demonstrated to have a higher incidence of psychiatric diagnosis such as depression, anxiety, somatization, stress, lack of social support, or abnormal illness behavior compared with other patients presenting with abdominal pain of organic origin. However, patients presenting with abdominal pain do have more psychosocial abnormalities than control subjects without abdominal pain. Psychosocial factors have not been shown to be helpful in differentiating between organic and functional abdominal disease, but they have been helpful in understanding some of the health-seeking behavior.

Stressful life events such as the death of a family member or loss of a job often precede the onset of symptoms of

Table 29–3. The Bristol Stool Form Scale.

Type	Description
1	Separate hard lumps like nuts (difficult to pass)
2	Sausage shaped but lumpy
3	Like a sausage but with cracks on its surface
4	Like a sausage or snake, smooth and soft
5	Soft blobs with clear-cut edges (passed easily)
6	Fluffy pieces with ragged edges, a mushy stool
7	Watery, no solid pieces, entirely liquid

IBS. Although such stressful life events may not be the cause of IBS, they might factor into the decision by patients to seek care for their symptoms. In women who have symptoms of IBS, the decision to seek care has been shown to have a significant and positive correlation between daily stress levels and daily symptoms of IBS.

In gathering the history of a patient with IBS, signs or symptoms of an anatomic disease should be absent. These include fever, GI bleeding, unintentional weight loss, anemia, and abdominal mass. Physicians should assess for laxative use as laxatives could be a significant cause of IBS-like symptoms.

Patients with IBS may have had surgery, particularly appendectomy, or women may have had a hysterectomy or ovarian surgery. The most common discharge diagnosis of patients admitted to the hospital for abdominal pain is "nonspecific abdominal pain." A study of patients discharged with this diagnosis showed that 37% of women and 19% of men met the criteria for IBS 1–2 years after discharge. Of such patients 70% had other prior attacks of abdominal pain and at the initial admission only 6% of patient charts listed IBS in the differential diagnosis. Of patients presenting with acute pain of less than 1 week's duration, 50% had symptoms of IBS at the time of admission. It appears that assessing for diagnostic criteria of IBS symptoms can reduce the length of hospitalization, reduce the extent of testing, and thus decrease the cost of treatment of patients presenting with acute abdominal pain who do not need immediate surgical intervention.

C. Physical Examination

The physical examination is usually fairly unremarkable, except for some abdominal tenderness and an increased likelihood of abdominal scars.

D. Special Tests

No specific testing is required for diagnosis of IBS, although some physicians would be reassured by a normal CBC and ESR. Patients who meet the criteria to screen for colon cancer (older than 50 years or a family history of colon cancer) should be examined using either flexible sigmoidoscopy or colonoscopy. A colonoscopy should always be performed if there is a family history of colon cancer. Other tests to consider are *Clostridium difficile* toxin if the patient has recently taken antibiotics, stool evaluation for giardiasis in endemic areas (eg, Rocky Mountains), and serologic testing or gluten elimination diet for evaluation for celiac disease.

Treatment

A. Therapeutic Relationship

A therapeutic relationship is critical to the effective management of IBS. The therapeutic relationship is achieved by obtaining the history through a nondirective, patient-centered interview, being nonjudgmental, eliciting the patient's understanding of the illness and his or her concerns, identifying and responding realistically to the patient's expectation for improvement, setting consistent limits, and involving the patient in the treatment approach. The most effective treatment option is explanation and reassurance. A confident diagnosis based on the previously outlined clinical criteria helps convey that symptoms of IBS are not associated with a higher risk of other diseases (eg, cancer or GI bleeding) and that these symptoms are chronic in nature, are very likely to wax and wane over time, and may not ever completely go away. Patients' reasons for seeking care at the time they did and the possibility that psychosocial issues are contributing to the symptoms should be assessed. Counseling regarding psychosocial stressors in patients' lives may not resolve all the symptoms of IBS, but it may help patients to better cope with the symptoms.

B. Diet

Many different dietary approaches have been tried. Patients in whom gas-forming vegetables, lactose, caffeine, or alcohol exacerbate symptoms should be counseled to minimize their exposure to the offending substance. Food intolerance and elimination diets have not been proven to be effective. Dietary fiber has been shown to improve symptoms of constipation, hard stools, and straining, particularly if 30 g of fiber is consumed each day. Patients often need to gradually increase the amount of fiber to improve adherence, as a sudden increase can lead to increased symptoms of bloating and gas. The most common reason for failure of a high-fiber diet is insufficient dose. Fiber is safe and inexpensive and should be routinely recommended, particularly to patients for whom constipation is a component of their IBS symptoms.

C. Complementary and Alternative Therapies

A meta-analysis of five double-blind, placebo-controlled randomized trials suggested a significant ($P < .001$) positive effect of peppermint oil compared with placebo. Peppermint oil was given as a monopreparation in a dosage range of 0.2–0.4 mL. A randomized controlled trial of Chinese herbal medicine indicated that both a standardized herbal formulation as well as individualized Chinese herbal medicine treatment improved symptoms of IBS compared with placebo.

D. Hypnotherapy and Psychotherapy

Hypnotherapy has been studied regarding its effectiveness in treating patients with symptoms of IBS. Dramatic improvements in a high proportion of patients with poorly controlled IBS symptoms were seen for both individual and group hypnotherapy. Therapeutic audiotapes are easy to use and low cost, although somewhat inferior to hypnotherapy.

Psychotherapy relies on the relationship between the therapist and the patient and can vary according to that relationship, which makes these approaches difficult to evaluate in a randomized, controlled way.

E. Pharmacotherapy

Drugs have been used for the treatment of IBS without proven benefit and with some troublesome side effects. A meta-analysis that concluded that smooth muscle relaxants and anticholinergics were better than placebo has been criticized for methodologic inadequacies. The most frequently used drugs and most common complaints that they are used to treat include the following:

Constipation: psyllium, methylcellulose, calcium polycarbophil, lactulose; 70% sorbitol and polyethylene glycol (PEG) solution, partial 5-HT_4 agonists (Tegaserod) for female patients with constipation-predominant IBS symptoms.

Diarrhea: loperamide, cholestyramine.

Gas, bloating, or flatus: simethicone, β-D-galactosidase (Beano).

Abdominal pain: anticholinergics and antispasmodics.

Chronic pain: tricyclic antidepressants, selective serotonin reuptake inhibitors.

Encouraging patients to see their family physician on a consistent and regular basis for the purpose of reassurance, reinforcement, and explanation, combined with communication in a positive therapeutic relationship, can prevent the continual quest by patients for a "miracle" cure for IBS.

Cash BD, Chey WD: Irritable bowel syndrome: A systematic review. Clin Fam Pract 2004;6:647.

Chang L et al: Gender, age, society, culture, and the patient's perspective in the functional gastrointestinal disorders. Gastroenterology 2006;130:1435. [PMID: 16678557]

Levy RL et al: Psychosocial aspects of the functional gastrointestinal disorders. Gastroenterology 2006;130:1447. [PMID: 16678558]

Lewis SJ, Heaton KW: Stool Form Scale as a useful guide to intestinal transit time. Scand J Gastroenterol 1997;32:920. [PMID: 9299672]

Talley NJ, Spiller R: Irritable bowel syndrome: A little understood organic bowel disease? Lancet 2002;360:555. [PMID: 12241674]

APPENDICITIS

ESSENTIALS OF DIAGNOSIS

- *Rapid onset of severe abdominal pain accompanied by anorexia, nausea, and fever.*
- *Pain is periumbilical initially, then migrates to the right lower quadrant (RLQ).*
- *Rebound tenderness in RLQ with guarding.*
- *CT scan is usually the best radiologic study.*

General Considerations

Appendicitis can occur in people of any age, but is most common in later childhood through young adulthood. When appendicitis occurs in young children or in the elderly, the presentation is often not classic. There does not seem to be any race or gender predilection, although diagnosis in female patients can be more difficult.

Pathogenesis

The appendix is a long diverticulum that extends from the cecum. When its long lumen is occluded, appendicitis results. Proliferation of lymphoid tissue—often associated with viral infections, Epstein–Barr virus, upper respiratory infection, or gastroenteritis—is the most common cause of obstruction of the lumen and subsequent appendicitis in young adults. Other causes of occlusion include tumors, foreign bodies, fecaliths, parasites, or complications of Crohn disease.

Clinical Findings

A. Symptoms and Signs

The most important component in the diagnosis of appendicitis is the history. It is a critical component, because a missed diagnosis of appendicitis can have severe sequelae. The presence of the following historical indicators should be elicited: (1) abdominal pain, usually RLQ pain, often preceded by periumbilical pain (~ 100% of patients); (2) anorexia (~ 100%); (3) nausea (90%), with vomiting (75%); (4) progression of abdominal pain from periumbilical to RLQ (50%); and (5) the classic progression from vague abdominal pain to anorexia, nausea, vomiting to RLQ pain to low-grade fever (50%).

B. Physical Examination

Careful examination of the abdomen—inspection followed by palpation and then percussion—can often identify the cause of abdominal pain. Peritoneal signs, rigidity, rebound tenderness, guarding, and low-grade fever (38°C [100.4°F]) are characteristic findings in appendicitis.

A pelvic examination should be performed in all women who present with RLQ pain to rule out multiple gynecologic causes. A thorough respiratory and genitourinary examination is often helpful as well. A rectal examination is useful only when the diagnosis remains unclear, and thus should not be performed unless necessary.

There is some debate about the use of analgesics during the evaluation of possible appendicitis. Traditional practice suggested that pain medication may mask important signs or symptoms, although a recent study showed that the use of analgesic, specifically tramadol, did not compromise the ability to identify acute appendicitis. In fact, although pain was decreased in many patients, specific signs related to appendicitis were more clearly evident with the use of analgesic. Additional studies suggest that informed consent is compromised by not using adequate pain medication. An observational unit can be helpful, as well, to examine the progression of signs and symptoms.

C. Laboratory Findings

Although many laboratory studies are performed routinely on patients with abdominal pain, few if any are truly helpful in the diagnosis and management of the patient with possible appendicitis. In fact, laboratory studies can often be misleading and delay diagnosis in cases of appendicitis. The WBC count has classically been used, but studies suggest it is seldom helpful diagnostically. If the WBC count is less than 7000/mm^3, it is unlikely that the patient has appendicitis. If it is greater than 19,000/mm^3, the patient has a more than 80% chance of having appendicitis. The presence of neutrophilia makes the diagnosis of appendicitis more likely but is not diagnostic. The presence of increased WBCs with neutropenia is generally accompanied by increased C-reactive protein levels. The presence of all three is not diagnostic, but the absence of all three rules out appendicitis.

The routine use of a chemistry examination is helpful only to determine the level of dehydration. Urinalysis commonly shows some leukocytosis and some increased red blood cells. Despite these common findings, it is more often misleading than helpful. The most important use of urinalysis is as a screening test for urinary tract infection. All women of childbearing age should have a pregnancy test.

D. Imaging Studies

The CT scan is the single best test for diagnosing appendicitis. Plain radiographs can be misleading, are not diagnostic in most cases, and the cost of a complete abdominal series is about the same as that of a CT. Ultrasound is less invasive than CT, is cost efficient, and can be useful in situations in which CT is not possible. Findings can be considered "normal" only if a normal appendix is seen. If the appendix is located retroperitoneally or in the pelvis, it can be difficult to visualize. Ultrasound is most helpful in women in whom other pathologies can be identified, and it can be used in the evaluation of pregnant patients. It is also a good choice in children because of the lack of contrast and easier patient compliance with the test. However, CT is more sensitive, more specific, and provides visualization of many other possible problems. If the diagnosis of appendicitis is suspected, a focused spiral CT without contrast can be performed in less than an hour and can be very specific for appendicitis.

Treatment

Treatment consists of surgical removal of the inflamed appendix using either laparotomy or laparoscopic-assisted technique. Laparotomy is faster, simpler, and less-expensive, with a lower rate of complications, but laparoscopy allows visualization of other possible causes. Recent advances in surgical technology have shown other benefits of laparoscopic procedures: faster recovery, shorter hospital stay, and decreased postoperative pain.

Hardin DM: Acute appendicitis: Review and update. Am Fam Physician 1999;60:2027. [PMID: 10569505]

Old JL et al: Imaging for suspected appendicitis. Am Fam Physician 2005;71:71. [PMID: 15663029]

Paulson EK et al. Suspected appendicitis. N Engl J Med 2003;348: 236. [PMID: 12529465]

INFLAMMATORY BOWEL DISEASE

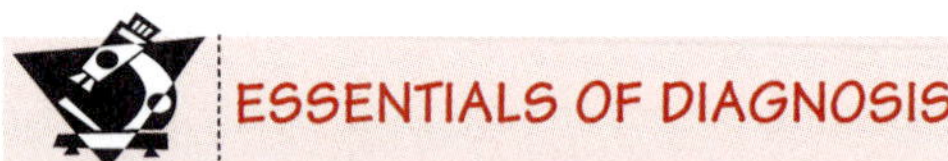

- *Abdominal pain (more common in ulcerative colitis [UC] than in Crohn disease [CD]).*
- *Bloody diarrhea and rectal pain (UC).*
- *RLQ pain (CD).*
- *Growth delay (children); malnutrition (adults and children).*
- *Episodic pain exacerbated by stress and other environmental factors.*

General Considerations

Inflammatory bowel disease (IBD) is a broad category that encompasses several disease subtypes, the most common of which are ulcerative colitis (UC) and Crohn disease (CD). The role of genetics in both of these disorders has become more clear as the human genome project has advanced, and there is now clear evidence of a genetic predisposition to both UC and CD. Prevalence of CD is much higher in Caucasians, especially in those of Jewish descent. Specific gene loci have been identified that show a correlation with susceptibility to either CD or UC. This susceptibility seems to be affected by environmental factors such as smoking and microflora of the gut.

Environmental factors may make IBD more prevalent in people who work indoors and less prevalent in manual laborers who work outdoors. There is a 20–50% increase in the prevalence of IBD in first-degree relatives, and a 50- to 100-fold increase in the offspring of patients with IBD.

Risk factors seem to include work environment and diet, but there is a difference among the subtypes of IBD. Smoking appears to decrease the risk of UC but to increase the risk of CD. Birth control pills seem to increase the risk of CD.

Pathogenesis

As more is known about which genes create susceptibility, more is understood about pathogenesis of these disease processes. Environmental factors seem to allow for an altered immunologic response to normal intestinal flora, causing destruction within the mucosa of the GI tract. CD appears to be related to altered macrophage function; whereas UC more likely represents a pathologic inflammatory response to normal intestinal microflora. Decreases in bifidobacteria and lactobacilli are noted in patients with active CD when compared with healthy controls and in those with CD in remission. *Fusobacterium varium* may be a factor in pathogenesis of UC. Changes within the microflora, combined with the immune response, result in altered mucosal barriers, luminal antigens, and macrophage function.

Clinical Findings

A. Symptoms and Signs

Although both UC and CD can present with abdominal pain, this finding is more common in patients with CD. Patients with UC almost always present with perirectal pain and bloody diarrhea, and have abdominal pain only during acute exacerbations of disease such as toxic megacolon. CD can be more difficult to differentiate from other diseases based on history and physical examination alone. RLQ pain is present in most patients with CD, reflecting involvement of the terminal ileum in 85% of cases.

B. Physical Examination

Physical examination findings are not very specific. Evaluation of the rectum for evidence of fissures, ulceration, or abscess can be helpful. Fullness or a palpable mass can suggest associated abscess. But generally, the examination reveals nonspecific generalized tenderness, with focal findings depending on the extent and activity of the disease. Skin examination may be useful because CD is associated with erythema nodosa and aphthous stomatitis, whereas UC is associated with pyoderma gangrenosa. Growth retardation and delayed sexual maturation can occur both from the disease process and from the medications used to treat the disease.

C. Laboratory Findings

Recommended laboratory tests include ESR, C-reactive protein, CBC, LFTs, albumen, electrolytes, vitamin B_{12} level, folate level, and stool studies. The ESR is elevated in 80% of patients with CD and 40% of patients with UC. In 95% of cases, patients with symptomatic CD have an elevated C-reactive protein. Anemia is common as a result of iron deficiency and blood loss. Leukocytosis with increased eosinophilia is often noted. LFTs can identify liver involvement in patients with CD (eg, sclerosing cholangitis, autoimmune hepatitis, and cirrhosis). Albumen is an indicator of malnutrition associated with malabsorption. Stool studies are important to rule out infectious etiologies of colitis. Additionally, a perinuclear antineutrophil antibody (pANCA) titer is useful to differentiate between CD and UC. Approximately 6% of patients with CD have pANCA, in contrast to 70% of patients with UC. *Saccharomyces cervisiae* (ASCA) is found in about 50% of individuals with CD and correlates closely with involvement of the small bowel, stenosing lesions, and perforating disease.

D. Imaging Studies

There are many imaging options for IBD. The most accurate test is the colonoscopy, which allows direct visualization of the mucosa and biopsy. Use of colonoscopy is not recommended in the setting of acute active disease due to the risk of perforation. Plain films can be most helpful when looking for toxic megacolon, or if "thumbprinting" is seen, as with bowel wall edema. The classic string sign can be seen on barium enema. Abdominal CT can be useful for diagnosis and management of IBD. CT is most helpful in identifying abscesses, fistulas, bowel wall thickening, and fat stranding. In patients undergoing CD, plain films can be helpful to identify strictures, skip lesions (areas of the mucosa not affected by the disease process), or perforation. The use of video capsule endoscopy is controversial due to the high risk of impaction behind strictures.

Treatment

Management of IBD includes medical therapy, nutritional support, psychological support, and surveillance for cancer. Medications include aminosalicylates, corticosteroids, immunomodulators, antibiotics, probiotics, and biological therapy. Patients with severe disease require hospital admission with bowel rest, parenteral nutritional support, and corticosteroids. Immunomodulators have been used with increasing frequency, allowing for less use of systemic steroids. Infliximab is a biological agent that is used in refractory CD.

Nutritional therapy is helpful to maintain remission and decrease likelihood of nutritional deficiency due to malabsorption. It can be as effective as medications, especially in children.

Surgical therapy is often required. Approximately 85% of patients with persistent elevation of C-reactive protein and frequent liquid stools require total colectomy. Strictures and abscess formation in CD may necessitate surgical excision of small segments of bowel or strictureplasty.

The risk of adenocarcinoma is increased in any patient with chronic colon disease. The risk of development of cancer in UC is equivalent to that of CD with colon involvement. Therefore, current guidelines recommend colonoscopy with biopsy biannually after disease is present 10 or more years. The risk of other types of cancer, such as adenocarcinoma of the jejunum and ileum (when involved in disease), lymphoma, and squamous cell carcinoma of the vulva and rectum, is increased in CD.

Familial counseling is important to help family members cope with exacerbations of the disease. Genetic counseling is needed because of the strong inheritance factor in this disease.

Bai A-P, Ouyang Q: Probiotics and inflammatory bowel disease. Postgrad Med J 2006;82:376. [PMID: 16754706]

Chutkan RK: Inflammatory bowel disease. Prim Care 2001;128:539. [PMID: 11483443]

Hyams J: Inflammatory bowel disease. Pediatr Rev 2005;26:314. [PMID: 16150873]

Nayar M, Rhodes JM: Management of inflammatory bowel disease. Postgrad Med J 2004;80:206. [PMID: 15082841]

DIVERTICULITIS

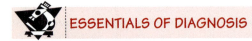

ESSENTIALS OF DIAGNOSIS

- *Left-sided abdominal pain.*
- *Constipation.*
- *Painless rectal bleeding.*

General Considerations

Changes in the epidemiology of diverticulitis over the past 100 years are directly related to the increase in cases noted today. Diverticulitis occurs in 10–25% of patients with diverticulosis. In the 20th century, the incidence of diverticulosis increased as fiber intake decreased. In addition to insufficient fiber, age is the single greatest risk factor contributing to diverticulosis. Typically, diverticulosis is seen in patients 60 years of age and older. It is uncommon before age 40, and is present in 50% of people over the age of 90 years. There is an increased prevalence of left-sided diverticula in patients of western European descent and an increased prevalence of right-sided diverticula in people of Asian descent.

Pathogenesis

The pathology of diverticulitis is directly related to the anatomy of the bowel wall. A true diverticulum consists of an outpouching of all three layers of the wall: mucosa, submucosa, and muscular layer. Most cases of diverticulitis, however, involve only pseudodiverticula. These consist of a herniation of the mucosa and submucosa through the muscular layer. The diverticula tend to form in rows between the mesenteric and lateral teniae. The area of penetration of the vasa recta has the greatest muscular weakness. This area is therefore the most common site of herniation. Lack of dietary fiber contributes to development of diverticula. As fiber content of the stool decreases, the colonic pressure increases and the transit time decreases. These changes result in high pressure in the colon, which essentially blows out areas of weakness in the colon wall.

Diverticulitis occurs when there is infection associated with one or more of these diverticula. Micro- or macroperforations of diverticula may occur, resulting in bowel contents contacting the peritoneum and infecting the pericolonic fat, mesentery, and associated organs. This process can be localized and can result in the development of an abscess, peritonitis, or a fistula. The most common fistula is a colovesical fistula, connecting the colon and the urinary bladder.

Clinical Findings

A. Symptoms and Signs

Left lower quadrant (LLQ) pain occurs in 93–100% of patients. However, pain can be right sided, especially in patients of Asian descent. When RLQ pain occurs, a duration of 3 or more days is suggestive of diverticulitis rather than appendicitis. Commonly, patients have nausea, vomiting, constipation, or diarrhea. Dysuria and urinary frequency may also be present. Complicated diverticulitis, as with a colovesical fistula, can present with recurrent urinary tract infections. In macroperforation, diffuse abdominal pain is present.

Vital signs give some evidence supportive of the diagnosis of diverticulitis. Temperature at or greater than 38.1°C (100.7°F) and the presence of tachycardia are consistent with diverticulitis. Fever is present in most patients.

B. Physical Examination

The examination should include a complete abdominal examination. Signs suggestive of diverticulitis include tender LLQ (or RLQ in more infrequent right-sided cases), signs of peritoneal irritation such as guarding or tenderness to percussion, and occasionally the presence of a tender mass, which is suggestive of abscess. The rectal examination may demonstrate rectal tenderness or occasionally a tender rectal mass.

C. Laboratory Findings

Patients suspected of having diverticulitis should have a CBC and urinalysis. The WBC count is often increased, with a high prevalence of polymorphonuclear leukocytes; leukocytosis is present in more than two thirds of patients. Anemia may be noted if there is associated diverticular bleeding. Urinalysis can show evidence of inflammation if there is irritation of the peritoneum surrounding the bladder or evidence of infection if a fistula is present.

D. Imaging Studies

Flat and upright abdominal films, or CT of the abdomen and pelvis if the diagnosis is less clear, should be obtained. The abdominal films can show evidence of free air, ileus, or mass. If the diagnosis is in doubt, a CT scan of the abdomen and pelvis can help clarify the cause of pain. In cases of diverticulitis, CT shows a thickened colonic wall and can show an abscess if present. These same findings can be seen on ultrasound, but CT best confirms diverticulitis because it reveals the presence and location of an abscess more easily. Ureteral obstruction, fistula, or air in the bladder can also be seen. CT will show and allow for percutaneous drainage of an abscess. Ultrasound can also be used to identify inflammation in the colon and allow for percutaneous drainage of an abscess. Colonoscopy should be reserved for evaluation 4–6 weeks after resolution of diverticulitis to evaluate for concomitant cancerous lesions. Colonoscopy has a role if diagnosis is not clear from CT scan and IBD is suspected.

Treatment

Treatment depends on the severity of the disease and the health of the patient. Outpatient treatment includes a clear liquid diet and oral broad-spectrum antibiotics. Current recommendations include ciprofloxacin and metronidazole for 7–10 days. Due to the ever-changing nature of antibiotic treatment and variations of resistance in different areas, the CDC guidelines or Sanford antibiotic recommendations should be followed. Pain medications such as morphine should be avoided as they increase colonic pressure and contribute to the problem. Meperidine is the best choice for pain control as it has been shown to decrease colonic pressure. Steroids and NSAIDs should be avoided due to the increased risk of GI bleeding and perforation associated with these medications.

Patients who have signs and symptoms of inflammation, such as fever and leukocytosis, require hospitalization. Patients should have complete bowel rest, intravenous fluids, and intravenous broad-spectrum antibiotics such as cefoxitin. Meperidine can be used if needed, as it decreases intraluminal pressure. A nasogastric tube is not needed unless there is significant ileus or obstruction. Most patients should improve in 48–72 hours, at which time they can resume diet, change to oral antibiotics, and be discharged home with close follow-up. If needed, invasive studies, such as colonoscopy, should be delayed 4–6 weeks. A high-fiber diet is recommended for all patients. Surgical resection is recommended for some.

Surgery usually is not recommended after the first attack because the recurrence rate is only 20–30%; however, this rate increases with each subsequent attack, as does the risk of morbidity associated with each attack. Therefore, surgery should be considered after the second or third attack. An exception is patients younger than 40 years of age, who tend to have more aggressive disease and more complications; surgery for these patients should be considered after the first attack.

Meckel Diverticulum

Meckel diverticulum is a congenital anomaly of the GI tract in which an outpouching portion of the intestine, derived from the fetal yolk stalk, contains gastric or pancreatic tissue. Patients can present with abdominal pain, nausea, vomiting, or intestinal bleeding. Meckel diverticulum can cause complications that include diverticulitis, intussusception, perforation, and obstruction. The best test for diagnosis is the technetium-99m pertechnetate scan, and treatment is surgical.

Marinella MA, Mustafa M: Acute diverticulitis in patients 40 years of age and younger. Am J Emerg Med 2000;18:140. [PMID: 10750916]

Salzman H, Lillie D: Diverticular disease: Diagnosis and treatment. Am Fam Physician 2005;72:1229. [PMID: 16225025]

ABDOMINAL WALL PAIN

There are many presentations of abdominal wall pain because there are many different causes of abdominal wall pain. Several examination findings might suggest the abdominal wall as the source of pain. The lack of evidence for an intra-abdominal process is a good first indicator. When visceral problems have been ruled out, the physician should look for abdominal wall abnormalities. The pain is usually not related to meals or bowel function, but is related to posture. Often a trigger point can be found. Most of the time there is a positive Carnett sign.

Carnett sign is elicited by having the patient tense the abdominal muscles and then examining the patient's abdomen. Places that are tender prior to tensing the abdomen and that are still tender afterward are considered positive and are suggestive of the abdominal wall as the source of pain. Most visceral pain will decrease with this maneuver. Causes of abdominal wall pain include hernias, herpes zoster, neuromas, hematomas of the abdominal wall or rectus sheath, desmoid tumor, endometriosis, myofascial tears, intra-abdominal adhesions, neuropathies, slipping rib syndrome, and general myofascial pain.

Hernias

Types of hernias include inguinal, femoral, umbilical, epigastric, spigelian, and Richter hernias. These are more commonly identified on examination rather than from the history. The history can be suggestive of many types of hernias, although it can be confusing if there is herniation of the bowel wall or omentum. Bowel herniation will cause visceral pain and obstruction, whereas omentum herniation will cause visceral pain with no signs of obstruction. A history of prior surgery, especially laparoscopic surgery, increases the likelihood that a hernia is present.

Certain hernias are more common in certain patients. Men more typically develop inguinal hernias, whereas women tend to develop femoral hernias. Umbilical and epigastric hernias are more common in obese or gravid patients. The spigelian hernia, a hernia along the border of the arcuate ligament, is most common in athletes.

Richter hernia is defined by the pathology rather than the location of the hernia. The side of the bowel wall herniates rather than the entire bowel segment. Often the hernia produces a slight bulge that may be confused with adenopathy or fat tissue. Because this type of hernia results in subtle findings, there is often a delay in diagnosis and therefore a higher fatality rate. Richter hernia is generally found in women older than 50 years of age, but it is increasing in frequency in young men, primarily due to the increased frequency of laparoscopic procedures. Because the size of the instruments used for laparoscopy is small, the abdominal wall defect left after surgery may allow only a portion of the bowel wall to herniate. The resultant tight hernia causes strangulation of the tissue that passes through. On examination, prior surgical sites must be examined. Erythema at these sites can be a sign of local infection, fistula formation, or an inflammatory process at an area of scarring.

Although a CT scan can identify hernias, they are often overlooked unless the radiologist is focused on thorough examination of the abdominal wall.

Hernias are best treated surgically. If surgery is contraindicated, hernias that cause pain or pose a risk of bowel obstruction can be treated with a truss or other restrictive garment.

Rectus Sheath Hematoma

Rectus sheath hematoma can be equally difficult to diagnose. They tend to occur more commonly in elderly or pregnant patients. The epigastric vessels are sheared, resulting in intramuscular bleeding. The shearing can occur from trauma or twisting motions. Again, the history is the most important factor in helping to direct the clinician. A history of unilateral midabdominal pain, use of anticoagulants such as aspirin or warfarin, and abdominal trauma are all important risk factors for hematoma. The pain is unilateral and is worse when patients tense their abdominal muscles. There is often a palpable mass within the rectus sheath.

Coagulation studies and blood count are the most useful laboratory studies. Helpful imaging studies include CT, ultrasound, and MRI. Ultrasound is the cheapest and most useful study if the diagnosis is highly suspected. CT is more useful for identifying other possible causes. MRI is sometimes helpful if the diagnosis remains unclear. Treatment is generally expectant, but severe cases may warrant reversal of coagulation abnormalities, administration of fluids, or even surgical evacuation and ligation or coagulation of vessels.

Herpes Zoster

Any time there is an abrupt onset of severe abdominal wall pain, herpes zoster should be suspected. The pain associated with zoster can precede the rash by more than 1 week, although commonly it is only 2–4 days. Zoster occurs most frequently in patients older than 50 years of age. Postherpetic neuralgia (PHN) can cause similar pain in patients with a history of zoster—most often patients older than 60 years. A thorough history and close follow-up are the best measures to establish this diagnosis. Prophylactic treatment includes the varicella vaccine. Treatment of acute herpes zoster with acyclovir, valacyclovir, or famciclovir in combination with a prednisone taper seems to decrease the incidence and severity of PHN. Treatment of PHN has proven difficult, and many modalities have been tried with only minor success. These include analgesics, narcotics, nerve stimulation, antidepressants, capsaicin, biofeedback, and nerve blocks.

Other Causes of Abdominal Wall Pain

Surgical scars are the location of many causes of abdominal wall pain. Hernias are frequently present at the site of scars, as previously discussed. Endometriosis can recur at the site of surgical scars, and neuromas often form at the border of scars. Other unusual causes include desmoid tumors, myofascial tears, and intra-abdominal adhesions. The desmoid tumor is a dysplastic tumor of the connective tissue that tends to form in young adults and can be identified only after surgical removal. Myofascial tears and intra-abdominal adhesions occur most frequently in athletes.

Treatment

Most abdominal wall pain has a trigger point that reproduces the pain. Finding this point can help in both diagnosis and treatment. These trigger points are often found along the lateral border of the rectus abdominis muscle where nerve roots can become stretched, compressed, and irritated. These points are also found at areas of tight-fitting clothing or at insertion points of muscles. The Carnett sign, described earlier, is useful for diagnosis of trigger points.

Management of this type of pain can be difficult. Patient education and reassurance are both very important. Preventing further unnecessary testing can be helpful to patients by decreasing their concerns about the pain. Explaining the nature of the pain and its origins helps patients deal with the pain. Tricyclic antidepressants can be useful at low doses.

Treatment of many causes of abdominal wall pain can be achieved by injection of lidocaine or its equivalent. This treatment can be both diagnostic and therapeutic. It is necessary to find the point of greatest tenderness, usually an area less than 2 cm. Insertion of the needle into the correct point should elicit intense pain, but the pain should improve dramatically with injection. For areas that require more than one injection, a small amount of steroid can be used as well. Steroids should be avoided in areas near hernias or into fascia, as they can cause hernia formation. Dry needling has been shown to be as useful, but the initial treatment is followed by more pain at first. For patients with severe needle aversion, a therapeutic trial of a transcutaneous lidocaine patch can be considered. Pain clinics can help patients with more difficult cases.

Edlow JA et al: Rectus sheath hematoma. Ann Emerg Med 1999; 34:671. [PMID: 10533018]

Suleiman S, Johnston DE: The abdominal wall: An overlooked source of pain. Am Fam Physician 2001;64:431. [PMID: 11515832]

Web Sites

American Academy of Pain Management:
http://www.aapainmanage.org
American Pain Society:
http://www.ampainsoc.org

GYNECOLOGIC CAUSES OF ABDOMINAL PAIN

Gynecologic causes of abdominal pain can be separated into three categories: acute causes in the nonpregnant patient, chronic problems in the nonpregnant patient, and acute causes in the pregnant patient. Acute causes include PID, adnexal torsion, ruptured ovarian cyst, hemorrhagic corpus luteum cyst, endometriosis, and tuboovarian abscess. Chronic causes in the nonpregnant patient include dysmenorrhea, mittelschmerz, endometriosis, obstructive müllerian duct abnormalities, leiomyomas, cancer, and pelvic congestion syndrome. In the pregnant patient causes include ectopic pregnancy, retained products of conception, septic abortion, and ovarian torsion. Psychological factors can greatly contribute to pain related to the abdomen and pelvis. Patients can present with acute pain after a sexual assault.

Because of the wide differential, a careful history and a pregnancy test are both very important when evaluating women and girls with abdominal pain. The history should include the last menstrual period, a detailed menstrual history, a sexual history including possible assault, and a family history. The physical examination should include careful abdominal, pelvic, and rectovaginal examinations. Laboratory evaluation is based on specific findings from the physical examination. In evaluating PID, LFTs can identify possible Fitz–Hughes–Curtis syndrome, especially in the presence of RUQ pain.

PID occurs in 11% of US women of reproductive age, although it is rare in pregnancy. Numerous biological factors contribute to a higher incidence of PID in adolescents, including a lower prevalence of protective chlamydial antibodies, more penetrable cervical mucus, and larger zones of cervical ectopy with more columnar cells that are more vulnerable to bacterial and viral agents. Other risk factors that increase the likelihood of PID include early age at first sexual intercourse, a higher number of lifetime partners, or a new partner within the last 30–60 days. Diagnosis of PID requires the presence of abdominal pain, adnexal pain, cervical motion tenderness, and at least one of the following: temperature greater than 38.3°C (101°F), vaginal discharge, leukocytosis greater than 10,500/mm^3, positive cervical cultures, intracellular diplococci, or WBCs on vaginal smear. Treatment varies, depending on whether the patient requires inpatient or outpatient treatment. Inpatient treatment is required in the following cases: surgical emergency, pregnancy, no response to outpatient therapy in 72 hours, nausea and vomiting, or immunodeficiency.

Endometriosis is found in 15–32% of women undergoing laparoscopy for evaluation of abdominopelvic pain. This type of pain is generally cyclical but can present acutely with rupture of an ovarian endometrioma. On physical examination, a retroverted, fixed uterus with ash spots on the cervix suggests endometriosis. Conservative treatment includes the use of NSAIDs and oral contraceptive pills.

Most gynecologic causes of abdominal pain are best evaluated with pelvic ultrasound. Sometimes laparoscopy is needed, which is often therapeutic as well, as in the case of ovarian torsion. CT can help delineate unclear findings seen on ultrasound. Consultation or follow-up with a gynecologist is often warranted.

Baines PA, Allen GM: Pelvic pain and menstrual related illnesses. Emerg Med Clin North Am 2001;19:763. [PMID: 11554286]

Anemia 30

Brian A. Primack, MD, EdM, & Kiame J. Mahaniah, MD

General Considerations

A. Adults

Anemia is defined as an abnormally low circulating red blood cell (RBC) mass, reflected by low serum hemoglobin (Hb). However, the normal range of Hb varies among different populations. For menstruating women, anemia is present if the Hb level is at or below 12 g/dL. In men and postmenopausal women, anemia is present if the Hb level is at or below 13–14 g/dL. Other factors, such as age, race, altitude, and exposure to tobacco smoke, can also alter Hb levels.

Anemia is usually classified by cell size (Table 30–1). Microcytic anemias, or those with mean corpuscular volume (MCV) below 80 fL, are usually due to iron deficiency, chronic inflammation, or thalassemia. Macrocytic anemias, those with MCV above 100 fL, are classified as megaloblastic or nonmegaloblastic. Megaloblasts, which are large, immature, nucleated precursors to RBCs, are seen with vitamin B_{12} deficiency and folic acid deficiency. Nonmegaloblastic causes of macrocytosis include alcoholism, hypothyroidism, and chronic liver disease. Normocytic anemia (MCV between 80 and 100 fL) can be due to hemolytic or nonhemolytic causes. Hemolysis can result from hereditary abnormalities of the cell contents or cell membrane. Hemolysis can also result from acquired insults caused by autoantibodies, alloantibodies (in, for instance, transfusion reactions), or a nonimmune process such as malaria or hypersplenism. Important nonhemolytic causes of normocytic anemia include poor production of RBCs due to aplastic anemia, renal insufficiency, and bone marrow infiltration.

B. Children

Normal Hb levels vary with age. At birth, mean Hb is about 16.5 g/dL. This level increases to 18.5 g/dL during the first week of life, followed by a drop to 11.5 g/dL by 1–2 months of age. This physiologic anemia of infancy is mediated by changes in erythropoietin levels. By 1–2 years of age, the Hb level begins to rise, to 14 g/dL in adolescent girls and 15 g/dL in adolescent boys. Other relevant laboratory values also vary in children. The median MCV, for example, can be as high as 120 fL in premature infants and as low as 78 fL in 1-year-old infants. Thus, laboratory values in children should always be compared with age-appropriate norms.

Many inherited causes of anemia are discovered in infancy and childhood. It is therefore important to obtain a careful family history in an anemic child, especially if the episodes of anemia are intermittent. Sickle cell anemia, thalassemia, glucose-6-phosphate dehydrogenase deficiency, and spherocytosis are examples of inherited forms of anemia. When only male members of a family are affected, glucose-6-phosphate dehydrogenase deficiency, which is X-linked, should be particularly considered.

Other elements of the history are also important when evaluating a child for anemia. Because infants with anemia can exhibit poor feeding, irritability, and tachycardia rather than classic adult symptoms and signs, these atypical features should be explored with the family. Nutrition should be evaluated carefully, with attention to dietary sources of vitamin B_{12}, folic acid, and iron. Potential sources of lead poisoning must also be considered. Finally, adolescents often require additional support and explanation. For instance, adolescent girls may not know what constitutes a normal menstrual period, so the specific number of tampons and pads used should be obtained.

Gabrilove J: Anemia and the elderly: Clinical considerations. Baillieres Clin Haematol 2005; 18:417. [PMID: 15792915]

Little DR: Ambulatory management of common forms of anemia. Am Fam Physician 1999; 59:1598. [PMID: 10193599]

Mehta BC: Approach to a patient with anemia. Indian J Med Sci 2004;58:26. [PMID: 14960799]

Onega T: Sorting out the common anemias. JAAPA 2000;13:30. [PMID: 11521621]

Scott S et al: Clinical inquiries. How should we follow up a positive screen for anemia in a 1-year old? J Fam Pract 2005;54:272. [PMID: 15755383]

Smith DL: Anemia in the elderly. Am Fam Physician 2000;62: 1565. [PMID: 11037074]

Woodman R et al: Anemia in older adults. Curr Opin Hematol 2005;12:123. [PMID: 15725902]

Table 30–1. Anemia classification by cell size.

Microcytic	Macrocytic
Iron deficiency	Megaloblastic
Anemia of chronic disease	Vitamin B_{12} deficiency
Thalassemias	Folic acid deficiency
Sideroblastic anemia	Drug related
	Nonmegaloblastic
	Hypothyroidism
	Liver disease
	Alcoholism
	Myelodysplastic syndromes
Normocytic	
Hemolytic	**Nonhemolytic**
Intrinsic	Acute blood loss
Membrane defects (spherocytosis)	Aplastic anemia
Enzyme deficiencies (G6PD deficiency)	Anemia of chronic disease
Hemoglobinopathies (sickle cell disease)	Chronic renal insufficiency
Extrinsic	Myelophthisis
Autoimmune	
Warm antibody mediated (chronic lymphocytic leukemia, systemic lupus erythematosus, idiopathic)	
Cold antibody mediated (*Mycoplasma*, idiopathic)	
Alloimmune	
Nonimmune	
Splenomegaly	
Physical trauma (thrombotic thrombocytopenic purpura, disseminated intravascular coagulation, burns)	
Infections (malaria)	

G6PD, glucose-6-phosphate dehydrogenase.

MICROCYTIC ANEMIA

IRON DEFICIENCY ANEMIA

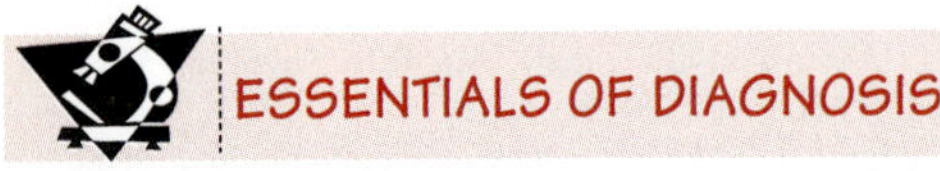

- *Low iron and serum ferritin levels, and elevated total iron-binding capacity (TIBC).*
- *Response to therapeutic trial of iron.*
- *In adults, nearly always due to blood loss.*
- *Can also be due to poor iron intake or poor absorption.*

General Considerations

Iron deficiency is the most common cause of anemia. Up to 11% of women and 4% of men have iron deficiency; however, only about 2% of women and 1% of men develop anemia due to the deficiency.

The average adult has 2–4 g of stored iron. About 65% of this reserve is located in the RBCs, with the remainder in the bone marrow, liver, spleen, and other body tissues. Iron deficiency occurs when there is a net imbalance resulting from either excessive loss or poor intake.

Pathogenesis

Extracorporeal blood loss is the most common cause of iron deficiency anemia. When RBCs are destroyed within the body, the reticuloendothelial system usually adequately recycles iron into the next generation of RBCs. Poor iron uptake, due either to poor nutrition or inadequate absorption, is a less common cause of iron deficiency anemia.

Women develop iron deficiency more readily than men because of increased potential for iron loss. On average, women lose an additional 1 mg of iron each day due to menstruation. Pregnancy, lactation, and delivery additionally cost a woman an average of 1000 mg of iron each.

Prevention

The US Preventive Services Task Force (USPSTF) recommends primary prevention of iron deficiency anemia by encouraging parents to breast-feed their infants and to include iron-enriched foods in the diet of infants and young children.

Although there is insufficient evidence to recommend for or against the routine use of iron supplements for healthy infants or pregnant women, the USPSTF does currently recommend screening for iron deficiency anemia—using Hb or hematocrit—for both pregnant women and high-risk infants.

Finally, the USPSTF suggests that although there is insufficient evidence to recommend for or against routine screening for iron deficiency anemia in other asymptomatic persons, screening may be indicated based on other clinical information.

Clinical Findings

A. Symptoms and Signs

Iron deficiency can be asymptomatic, especially in the early stages. However, patients can present with varying degrees of any of the common symptoms associated with anemia, such as weakness, fatigue, dizziness, headaches, exercise intolerance, or palpitations. Possible signs on physical examination include tachycardia, tachypnea, and pallor, especially of the palpebral conjunctivae.

One symptom associated with iron deficiency in particular is pica—the craving for ice, clay, or other unusual substances that may or may not contain iron. Rare symptoms include koilonychia (spoon nails), blue sclerae, and atrophic glossitis. Esophageal webs, dysphagia, and iron deficiency characterize the Plummer–Vinson syndrome, a disease of unknown pathophysiology that can increase the risk of squamous cell carcinoma of the pharynx and esophagus.

B. Laboratory Findings

Hb levels can be normal in early iron deficiency. Mild deficiency yields Hb levels of 9–11 g/dL, whereas in severe deficiency levels can fall as low as 5 g/dL.

Serum iron levels below 60 mcg/dL indicate iron deficiency. As iron stores are depleted, serum ferritin falls below 30 ng/dL. TIBC therefore rises above 400 mcg/dL. Percent iron saturation, which is inversely proportional to TIBC, falls below about 15%.

Although serum ferritin levels are often useful in differentiating iron deficiency from other forms of microcytic anemia, it should be noted that ferritin is an acute phase reactant that can be elevated during acute illnesses, chronic inflammatory states, or cancer.

The peripheral blood smear is also a useful test. Iron-deficient RBCs manifest varying degrees of hypochromia and microcytosis. However, the gold standard of iron deficiency is bone marrow examination, which shows absent iron reserves in affected patients. A Prussian blue stain is used to examine marrow iron stores.

Another method of diagnosis involves measuring a patient's response to oral iron therapy. Increased reticulocytosis several days after institution of oral iron treatment can be diagnostic.

Treatment

Iron can be increased in the diet. Foods particularly rich in iron include meats (especially liver) and fish. Whole grains, green leafy vegetables, nuts, seeds, and dried fruit also contain iron. Cooking with iron pots and pans also increases iron intake.

Oral iron therapy is available in the form of iron salts. One 300-mg tablet of iron sulfate, for example, delivers 60 mg of elemental iron. One 300-mg tablet of iron gluconate delivers 34 mg of elemental iron and may be better tolerated by some patients. Up to 180 mg of elemental iron can be given each day, depending on the degree of deficiency. Absorption of oral iron is dependent on many environmental factors. An acidic environment increases absorption; thus iron tablets are often given with ascorbic acid. For this same reason, antacids should be avoided within several hours of iron ingestion. Other substances that impair the absorption of iron include calcium, soy protein, tannins (found in tea), and phytate (found in bran). Side effects of oral iron therapy include gastrointestinal distress and constipation. For this reason, some physicians routinely prescribe an as-necessary stool softener along with each iron prescription.

Iron can be given intramuscularly or intravenously to patients who cannot tolerate oral iron due to gastrointestinal upset. This route may also be convenient for patients who have concurrent gastrointestinal malabsorption or ongoing blood loss, such as those with severe inflammatory bowel disease. Phlebitis, muscle breakdown, anaphylaxis, and fever are possible side effects of parenteral iron.

Leung AK, Chan KW: Iron deficiency anemia. Adv Pediatr 2001; 48:385. [PMID: 11480764]

ANEMIA OF CHRONIC DISEASE

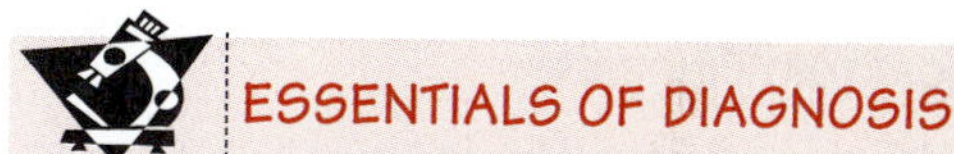

- *Presence of a chronic disease or chronic inflammation.*
- *Shortened RBC survival but poor compensatory erythropoiesis.*
- *High or normal serum ferritin level and low TIBC.*

General Considerations

Many chronic diseases—such as cancer, collagen vascular disease, chronic infections, diabetes mellitus, and coronary artery disease—can be associated with anemia (Table 30–2).

Pathogenesis

In spite of shortened RBC survival, bone marrow RBC production is low. This is thought to be due to (1) trapping of iron stores in the reticuloendothelial system, (2) a mild decrease in erythropoietin production, and (3) impaired response of the bone marrow to erythropoietin.

Clinical Findings

A. Symptoms and Signs

The anemia of chronic disease (ACD) is often mild and therefore general anemic symptoms, such as fatigue, dizziness, and palpitations, can be low grade or nonexistent. Signs such as pallor of the palpebral conjunctivae are only sometimes present. The condition must therefore be suspected and investigated in patients known to

Table 30–2. Selected causes of anemia of chronic disease.

Chronic infections
Abscesses
Subacute bacterial endocarditis
Tuberculosis
Collagen vascular disease
Rheumatoid arthritis
Systemic lupus erythematosus
Temporal arteritis
Neoplasia
Hodgkin and non-Hodgkin lymphomas
Adenocarcinoma
Squamous cell carcinoma

have underlying conditions such as collagen vascular diseases, cancers, or chronic infections.

B. Laboratory Findings

Hb levels are generally mildly decreased (10–11 g/dL), but levels can occasionally be below 8 g/dL. RBCs are often hypochromic. MCV can be either normal (80–100 fL) or low (< 80 fL). Because RBC production is poor, the absolute reticulocyte count is often low (< 25,000/μL). Acute phase reactants such as erythrocyte sedimentation rate (ESR), platelets, and fibrinogen can be elevated.

Because ACD is associated with decreased production of transferrin, serum iron level and TIBC are often both low. Calculated percent saturation, however, remains normal. This is to be distinguished from iron deficiency anemia, in which TIBC is often high, resulting in low percent saturation. Serum ferritin level is high or normal in ACD but low in iron deficiency anemia.

Treatment

Treatment of ACD should be aimed at the underlying condition. Symptomatic patients or heart patients often require packed transfusions of RBCs, especially if the HBG count is below 10 mg/dL. Erythropoietin is also used to correct anemia associated with certain chronic diseases, especially cancer.

Corwin HL: Anemia and blood transfusion in the critically ill patient: Role of erythropoietin. Crit Care (London) 2004;8 (suppl 2):S42. [PMID: 15196323]

Fink MP: Pathophysiology of intensive care unit–acquired anemia. Crit Care (London) 2004;8(suppl 2):S9. [PMID: 15196314]

Knight K et al: Prevalence and outcomes of anemia in cancer: A systematic review of the literature. Am J Med 2004;116(suppl 7A):11S. [PMID: 15050883]

Thomas C, Thomas L: Anemia of chronic disease: Pathophysiology and laboratory diagnosis. Lab Hematol 2005;11:14. [PMID: 15790548]

Weiss G, Goodnough LT: Anemia of chronic disease. N Engl J Med 2005;352:1011. [PMID: 15758012]

THALASSEMIA

ESSENTIALS OF DIAGNOSIS

- *Elevated RBC count despite decreased Hb level.*
- *Exaggerated microcytosis.*
- *Positive family history.*
- *Mediterranean or African heritage.*
- *Pattern of inheritance.*

General Considerations

One normal adult Hb molecule, also known as HbA, consists of a heme moiety, two α Hb chains, and two β Hb chains. The thalassemias are the diverse group of genetic diseases resulting from abnormal Hb due to defective α or β chains.

Other Hb chains exist, such as γ and δ chains. Fetal Hb consists of two α chains and two γ chains ($\alpha_2\gamma_2$), and HbA_2 consists of two α chains and two δ chains ($\alpha_2\delta_2$). Although ordinarily these lesser types of Hb comprise no more than 5% of the total amount of Hb, the thalassemias are characterized by increased proportions of non-A Hb because of defective α or β chains. These disorders are classified as α-thalassemias or β-thalassemias, based on the abnormal gene.

Thalassemia traits are more common in those with Mediterranean, African, and South Asian ancestry. This is at least in part because these parts of the world are inhabited by *Plasmodium* species, and heterozygous thalassemic traits confer survival advantage to those afflicted with malaria.

Pathogenesis

Because there are four α Hb genes per individual (two on each copy of chromosome 16), there are four major types of α-thalassemia. If only one α Hb gene is damaged, the result is called α-thalassemia minima, an essentially asymptomatic condition. Damage to two different α Hb genes results in α-thalassemia minor, which has only mild clinical significance. Three damaged α Hb genes can lead to a relative abundance of α Hb, causing an abundance of Hb β_4, also known as HbH. This disorder, also called *hemoglobin H disease,* is characterized by severe clinical manifestations of chronic hemolysis, hospitalizations, and decreased lifespan. Absence of normal α Hb chains causes Hb Barts disease and is fatal *in utero.*

The two β Hb genes are found on chromosome 11. If one is damaged, β-thalassemia minor results, with few clinical effects. Infants with two damaged copies of β Hb will be phenotypically normal at birth due to the predominance of fetal Hb ($\alpha_2\gamma_2$). Affected infants become severely symptomatic in the first year of life, however, and usually die before age 5.

Clinical Findings

A. Symptoms and Signs

α-Thalassemia minima is almost always asymptomatic. α-Thalassemia minor can be accompanied by occasional mild symptoms of anemia, including headaches, fatigue, and dizziness. Patients with HbH disease, however, can exhibit severe clinical manifestations of chronic hemolytic anemia, including hepatosplenomegaly and cholelithiasis (due to bilirubin gallstones). These patients often require chronic transfusions, usually beginning in late childhood and adolescence. Patients with no normal α Hb develop tetramers of γ Hb *in utero,* known as Hb Barts, which are inefficient at delivering oxygen to the tissues. The accompanying hypoxia results in high-output congestive heart failure, severe edema, and hydrops fetalis.

The clinical appearance of β-thalassemia minor often mimics that of mild or moderate iron deficiency, and often laboratory findings are necessary to distinguish the two. β-Thalassemia major, however, results in a severe phenotype. Widespread hemolysis in these patients causes pallor, irritability, jaundice, and hepatosplenomegaly. Eighty percent of patients die in the first 5 years of life due to severe anemia, high-output congestive heart failure, or infection.

B. Laboratory Findings

As with iron deficiency, Hb levels and MCV are often low with the thalassemias. In contrast to iron deficiency, however, thalassemias are usually characterized by an elevated RBC count. Furthermore, the decrease in MCV is often more exaggerated in the thalassemias; levels as low as 50–60 fL are not unusual. The red cell distribution width (RDW) can also be used to distinguish the two conditions. With iron deficiency, the RDW is elevated due to a variety of cell sizes, whereas the RDW is usually normal in thalassemic patients because RBCs are uniformly small.

Hb electrophoresis should be ordered for any patient with suspected thalassemia. Although some patients with α-thalassemia minima or media can have normal electrophoresis patterns, abnormalities are often seen in other thalassemic patients. In β-thalassemia minor, for example, relative proportions of fetal Hb ($\alpha_2\gamma_2$) and HbA_2 are increased.

Treatment

Patients with α-thalassemia minor, α-thalassemia minima, and β-thalassemia minor are generally asymptomatic and should be treated only if necessary. These patients may require blood transfusions under certain conditions, such as after vaginal delivery or surgery.

Patients with β-thalassemia major and HbH disease, however, require the care of a hematologist. These patients may require frequent transfusions, splenectomy, or both. Iron overload is a frequent complication in these patients, both those with and without transfusion therapy. Chelation therapy is often required to avoid end-organ damage in the heart, endocrine organs, and liver. Patients with a personal or family history of thalassemia should be offered genetic counseling when planning a family.

Schrier SL: Pathophysiology of thalassemia. Curr Opin Hematol 2002;9:123. [PMID: 11844995]

Shine JW: Microcytic anemia. Am Fam Physician 1997;55:2455. [PMID: 9166144]

MACROCYTIC ANEMIA

VITAMIN B_{12} DEFICIENCY

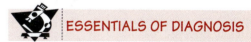

- *Macrocytosis.*
- *Serum vitamin B_{12} level below 100 pg/mL.*
- *Hypersegmented neutrophils.*

General Considerations

Vitamin B_{12} (cobalamin) is involved in two important enzymatic reactions: the conversion of methylmalonyl-coenzyme A (CoA) to succinyl-CoA and the methylation of homocysteine to methionine. This latter reaction is required for synthesis of thymidine, a component of DNA.

Because vitamin B_{12} is present in all animal products, only people with unusual diets (vegans, fad dieters) receive inadequate intake. Some special populations, such as pregnant women, require increased levels of vitamin B_{12}.

Pathogenesis

Vitamin B_{12} deficiency usually reflects a defect in the B_{12} absorption and transport chain. Vitamin B_{12} is transported from the stomach to the jejunum by intrinsic factor (IF), a protein produced in gastric parietal cells. Pernicious anemia occurs when autoantibodies against parietal cells are produced, resulting in a lack of intrinsic factor and inadequate uptake of vitamin B_{12}.

Clinical Findings

A. Symptoms and Signs

Many clinical features are common to all megaloblastic anemias: anemia, pallor, weight loss, fatigue, glossitis, lightheadedness, jaundice, and abdominal symptoms. Neurologic symptoms are specific to vitamin B_{12} deficiency, however, beginning with paresthesias in the hands and feet. Disturbances in vision, taste, smell, proprioception, and vibratory sense can also occur. Untreated, vitamin B_{12} deficiency can lead to posterior spinal column demyelination, resulting in spastic ataxia and dementia mimicking that of Alzheimer disease. These changes are often irreversible. Vitamin B_{12} deficiency can also lead to psychotic depression and paranoid schizophrenia.

B. Laboratory Findings

The MCV is usually above 100 fL, and vitamin B_{12} levels are usually below 100 pg/mL. The higher the MCV, the more likely the diagnosis. Lactate dehydrogenase and indirect bilirubin can be modestly elevated because of increased RBC destruction. The reticulocyte count can be depressed. Because DNA synthesis affects all cell lines, pancytopenia can occur. Peripheral blood smear can show markedly abnormal RBCs along with hypersegmented neutrophils, which are pathognomonic for megaloblastic anemia. There is evidence suggesting that early vitamin B_{12} deficiency can be diagnosed by elevated levels of homocysteine or methylmalonic acid. These metabolite levels are most useful in cases where diagnosis is suspected but not supported by other laboratory values. Increased levels of methylmalonic acid confirm B_{12} deficiency.

Although examination of the bone marrow is usually unnecessary for diagnosis, if performed it shows erythroid hyperplasia and marked asynchrony in maturation between cytoplasmic components and nuclear material.

The Schilling test, although not often used today, has historically been used to confirm the diagnosis of pernicious anemia. In the first stage, a large dose of intramuscular vitamin B_{12} is given, followed by oral ingestion of radiolabeled vitamin B_{12}. Patients with intact vitamin B_{12} absorption will have at least 7% of the oral dose present in urine. In the second stage, radiolabeled vitamin B_{12} is administered with intrinsic factor. If pernicious anemia is the cause of vitamin B_{12} deficiency, a poor absorption rate in the first stage will be corrected by the combination of vitamin B_{12} and intrinsic factor in the second stage.

Treatment

Treatment requires monthly parenteral treatment of vitamin B_{12} in doses of 100–1000 mcg, usually administered daily or every other day for the first few weeks, followed by maintenance doses every 1–3 months. Once vitamin B_{12} levels have been reestablished, oral therapy (1 mg/day) can then be substituted. Oral therapy alone may be sufficient. Treatment often also consists of concurrent administration of folate, 1–5 mg each day.

Oh R, Brown DL: Vitamin B12 deficiency. Am Fam Physician 2003;67:979. [PMID: 12643357]

Spoelhof GD: Reliability of serum B12 levels in the diagnosis of B12 deficiency. Am Fam Physician 1996;54:465. [PMID: 8701832]

FOLIC ACID DEFICIENCY

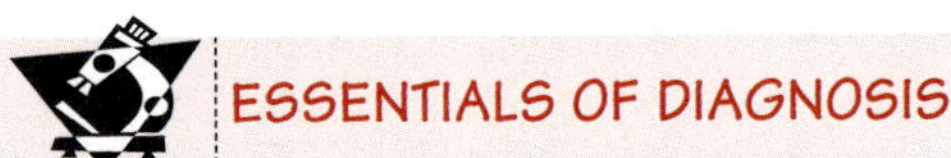

- *Reduced RBC or serum folate levels.*
- *Macrocytic anemia.*
- *Normal vitamin B_{12} levels.*
- *Hypersegmented neutrophils.*

General Considerations

In contrast to vitamin B_{12} reserves, which can last 3–5 years, folate reserves last only 4–5 months. The human body requires about 75–100 mcg/day of folic acid, which is present in leafy green vegetables, fruits, nuts, beans, wheat germ, and liver. Like vitamin B_{12}, folate is involved in the synthesis of thymidine.

Pathogenesis

Folic acid deficiency can occur as a result of decreased intake. In spite of supplementation of US wheat products with folate, nutritional deficiencies still occur, especially in alcoholics and patients with atypical diets. Malabsorption can also affect intake of folate. Because small intestine microvilli convert the ingested complex folic acid molecule into an absorbable one, diseases of the small intestine, such as gluten enteropathy and Crohn disease, can cause deficiency. Drugs such as anticonvulsants and oral contraceptives also predispose to folate malabsorption. Other medications (e.g., antineoplastic agents, trimethoprim, and certain antimalarial drugs) inhibit the enzyme necessary for the replenishment of intracellular folate and can affect folate levels.

Folate deficiency can also result if increased requirements are not met. Pregnancy, for instance, increases folate requirements 5- to 10-fold by the third trimester. Patients with hemolytic anemia and exfoliative skin diseases also have increased requirements and should receive supplementation. Because folate is dialyzable, patients on dialysis can suffer from folate deficiency if they do not receive supplementation.

Folate deficiency is common among alcoholics for several reasons. First, although some folic acid is present in beer, alcoholics tend to consume less of other foods rich in folic acid, such as leafy green vegetables. Alcohol can also adversely affect intracellular processing of folate. Finally, alcohol may suppress bone marrow function. Although alcoholics commonly present with macrocytosis, only those who are folate or vitamin B_{12} deficient will have accompanying megaloblastic anemia with its associated clinical features.

Clinical Findings

A. Symptoms and Signs

Patients with mild folate deficiency often present with anemia on a routine blood screening. Those with more severe disease can present with pallor, weight loss, fatigue, glossitis, lightheadedness, jaundice, or abdominal symptoms, as in vitamin B_{12} deficiency. In contrast to vitamin B_{12} deficiency, however, neurologic symptoms are absent.

B. Laboratory Findings

Many laboratory findings are similar to those of vitamin B_{12} deficiency: Hb levels can be variably depressed, pancytopenia can occur, and hypersegmented neutrophils can be seen on the peripheral blood smear. Also as with vitamin B_{12} deficiency, examination of the bone marrow can show erythroid hyperplasia and marked asynchrony in maturation between cytoplasmic components and nuclear material.

With folate deficiency, however, serum and RBC folate levels are low, whereas vitamin B_{12} levels are normal. RBC folate—which is low at less than 150 pg/L—is thought to be a more precise indicator of chronic folate deficiency than serum folate. The latter is thought to reflect more recent dietary intake. In cases where diagnosis remains in doubt, an elevated homocysteine level, in spite of a normal methylmalonic acid level, suggests folate deficiency.

Treatment

Foods rich in folic acid should be consumed, which include leafy green vegetables, fruits, nuts, beans, wheat germ, and liver. Supplementation with oral folic acid—from 1 to 5 mg daily—is used to treat deficiency. Total correction occurs within 6–8 weeks. Patients with increased folate requirements, such as pregnant women, should receive supplementation. Some authorities recommend treating all patients with macrocytic anemia, regardless of cause, with empirical addition of folic acid.

Abramson SD, Abramson N: "Common" uncommon anemias. Am Fam Physician 1999;59:851. [PMID: 10068709]

Barney-Stallings RA, Heslop SD: What is the clinical utility of obtaining a folate level in patients with macrocytosis or anemia? J Fam Pract 2001;50:544. [PMID: 11401743]

Davenport J: Macrocytic anemia. Am Fam Physician 1996;53:155. [PMID: 8546042]

Hebert PC et al: Physiologic aspects of anemia. Crit Care Clin 2004;20:187. [PMID: 15135460]

Irwin JJ, Kirchner JT: Anemia in children. Am Fam Physician 2001;64:1379. [PMID: 11681780]

NORMOCYTIC ANEMIA

HEMOLYTIC ANEMIA

1. Hereditary Spherocytosis

ESSENTIALS OF DIAGNOSIS

- *Autosomal-dominant inheritance pattern (in most cases).*
- *Spherocytes on peripheral blood smear.*
- *Hemolysis.*

General Considerations & Pathogenesis

Hereditary spherocytosis (HS) is the most common inherited defect of the RBC membrane. Patients with this condition inherit one of a series of mutations of the structural proteins of the RBC membrane, such as spectrin and ankyrin. The resulting decreased membrane elasticity causes loss of the normal biconcave shape of the RBC. These deformed, spherical RBCs are then detained and phagocytosed in the narrow fenestrations of the splenic cords. Less common related defects also exist, including hereditary elliptocytosis and hereditary stomatocytosis.

Prevention

For patients who have required splenectomy, immunization against *Pneumococcus* and *Meningococcus* is recommended for secondary prevention of sepsis.

Clinical Findings

A. Symptoms and Signs

HS can be classified as mild, moderate, or severe. Individuals with mild disease rarely manifest symptoms and signs. Increased erythropoietin levels compensate for early destruction of RBCs. These patients often present as adolescents or adults on routine blood screenings. Individuals with moderate disease comprise 60–75% of HS patients and can develop intermittent episodes of jaundice, dark urine, abdominal pain, and splenomegaly in infancy or early childhood. Individuals with severe disease have more marked jaundice and splenomegaly.

If bilirubin levels are chronically elevated, bilirubin gallstones can form, leading to right upper quadrant abdominal pain and tenderness, nausea, and a positive Murphy sign.

B. Laboratory Findings

Patients with mild disease may or may not be anemic. Patients with moderate and severe disease often have low Hb, reticulocyte counts between 5% and 20%, and elevated serum bilirubin level.

The mean corpuscular Hb concentration (MCHC) is a useful test in diagnosing HS. It is generally elevated to 36 g/dL in patients with HS, reflecting decreased membrane surface area and increased Hb concentration in the RBC.

The peripheral blood smear of a patient with HS shows characteristic spherocytes—small RBCs that have lost their central pallor. Although a patient with mild disease may have only a few spherocytes, patients with moderate or severe disease can have 30 or more spherocytes per high-power field.

Special tests can also be used to evaluate patients for HS. The osmotic fragility test involves suspending a patient's RBCs in increasingly dilute salt solutions and observing for cell lysis. RBCs from patients with HS will be more sensitive to hypotonic solutions because of membrane instability. The newer acidified glycerol lysis test is also used.

Treatment

Individuals with mild disease rarely require treatment. For patients with moderate disease blood transfusions may be necessary, and for patients with severe disease regular transfusions are required. Folic acid supplementation is useful for patients with this and other hemolytic diseases.

The definitive treatment is splenectomy, which leads to significantly increased RBC life span. Patients post-splenectomy are at risk for overwhelming sepsis with encapsulated organisms, however, and immunization against *Pneumococcus* and *Meningococcus* is recommended for these patients. Cholecystectomy may be necessary for patients with bilirubin gallstones.

2. Glucose-6-Phosphate Dehydrogenase Deficiency

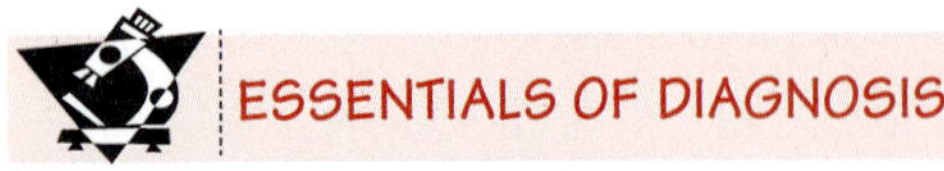

- *X-Linked inheritance pattern.*
- *African or Mediterranean heritage.*
- *Recent exposure to oxidizing substances such as primaquine, sulfa drugs, naphthalene (mothballs), or fava beans.*

General Considerations

The World Health Organization classifies glucose-6-phosphate dehydrogenase (G6PD) deficiency into five variants, from class I (the most severe enzyme deficiency) to class V (no clinical significance). The deficiency is most common in people of African and Mediterranean heritage and, like thalassemia and sickle cell disease, is thought to protect against malaria. Although it is primarily seen in men, as are most X-linked disorders, women who carry the defective gene can also manifest symptoms due to inactivation of their normal X chromosomes.

Overall, G6PD deficiency is the most common enzymatic disorder of RBCs in humans and affects 200–400 million people. Less common enzymatic deficiencies also exist. Pyruvate kinase deficiency, for example, has a similar clinical presentation.

Pathogenesis

G6PD is a cytoplasmic enzyme that prevents oxidative damage to RBCs by reducing nicotinamide adenine dinucleotide phosphate (NADP) to NADPH. Individuals who are deficient in this enzyme are more susceptible to damage from oxidative substances such as superoxide anion (O_2^-) and hydrogen peroxide. In addition to being normal by-products of cell metabolism, these substances are produced by certain drugs, household chemicals, and foods.

Clinical Findings

Persons affected with G6PD deficiency are often asymptomatic. However, a spectrum of clinical manifestations can occur, from infrequent mild episodic hemolysis to severe chronic hemolysis.

A. Symptoms and Signs

The most common clinical manifestations are jaundice, dark urine, pallor, abdominal pain, and back pain. These symptoms usually occur hours to days after an oxidative insult, which can be caused by a number of different agents (Table 30–3). Chemicals that can cause such an insult include primaquine, sulfa drugs, dapsone, nitrofurantoin, and naphthalene (found in mothballs). Aspirin and acetaminophen can precipitate hemolysis in certain individuals as well. Attacks can also be associated with infections (such as pneumonia, viral hepatitis, and *Salmonella*), and diabetic ketoacidosis. Finally, foods such as fava beans have been implicated. These beans are common in the Mediterranean and are harvested in late spring.

Table 30–3. Selected sources of oxidative damage.

Medications
Aspirin, nonsteroidal anti-inflammatory drugs
Antimalarial agents
Nitrofurantoin, sulfonamides
Quinidine
Infections
Naphthalene
Fava beans

Infants with G6PD deficiency can also present with jaundice. Again a spectrum of disease exists, from mild transient jaundice to severe jaundice, kernicterus, and death. Those with class I G6PD deficiency can have life-long, life-threatening chronic hemolysis.

B. Laboratory Findings

Hb levels mirror the severity of disease. During acute attacks in highly susceptible individuals, Hb levels can be as low as 3–4 g/dL. Many asymptomatic individuals, however, have only mildly depressed levels at 11–12 g/dL.

During periods of active hemolysis, other laboratory measures can be abnormal. To compensate for the loss of RBCs, reticulocytosis occurs and the absolute reticulocyte count is elevated above 2–3%, and sometimes above 10–15%. Haptoglobin levels are often depressed below 50 mg/dL, as this plasma protein binds Hb released from fragmented RBCs.

The peripheral blood smear in G6PD deficiency shows characteristic Heinz bodies, which represent masses of denatured, damaged Hb. "Bite cells," which appear as RBCs with a small semicircular defect, can also be seen. The definitive test for G6PD deficiency is an enzymatic assay that measures in vitro production of NADPH.

Treatment

Individuals with mild disease require no treatment except for avoidance, whenever possible, of oxidative triggers. Individuals with class I disease may require inpatient treatment of acute exacerbations with transfusion, intravenous fluid support, and monitoring of renal function. Although vitamin E and splenectomy have been advocated as possible treatments in more severe cases, neither has provided consistent benefit.

3. Sickle Cell Anemia

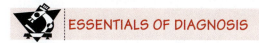

- *African, Mediterranean, or Asian heritage.*
- *Family history.*
- *Autosomal-recessive inheritance.*
- *Characteristic pattern on Hb electrophoresis.*

General Considerations

Sickle cell anemia is a genetic condition. Traits that lead to sickle cell anemia are common in those with African and South Asian heritage, as these traits confer resistance to malaria. The gene frequency for sickle cell anemia in African Americans is about 4%.

A spectrum of other sickle cell syndromes exists. HbC results from a different mutation in the β Hb chain. Patients with HbSC disease have one of each mutation and generally experience a milder phenotype than patients with homozygous sickle cell anemia (HbSS). Other permutations of abnormal Hb genes can cause similar syndromes. Patients with one sickle cell gene and one β-thalassemia gene, for example, can have significant clinical manifestations of hemoglobinopathy.

Pathogenesis

Patients with sickle cell anemia are homozygous for a mutation in the β Hb chain; the sixth amino acid is valine instead of glutamate. The resulting HbS, which consists of two normal α Hb chains and two abnormal β Hb chains, is poorly soluble when deoxygenated. The polymerization of HbS within the RBC leads to the characteristic "sickle" shape. These abnormal RBCs occlude capillary beds and lead to the many clinical manifestations of sickle cell disease.

Prevention

Several prophylactic measures can reduce the likelihood of pain crises and other manifestations of disease in patients with sickle cell anemia (ie, secondary prevention). First, adequate hydration and oxygenation are required at all times to reduce the risk of Hb polymerization and subsequent vasoocclusive crises. Folic acid should be supplemented, 1 mg orally every day. Some physicians recommend hydroxyurea, which seems to reduce the likelihood of RBC sickling by stimulating production of fetal Hb. Infectious complications can be reduced by immunization against *Streptococcus pneumoniae, Haemophilus influenzae* type B, hepatitis B, and influenza. Daily oral penicillin prophylaxis should be given until age 5 years.

Clinical Findings

A. Symptoms and Signs

Patients with homozygous sickle cell anemia manifest disease early. About 30% of patients are discovered by 1 year of age and over 90% by 6 years of age. Acute pain episodes are the most common presentations; they can occur in the extremities, abdomen, back, or chest. Many patients have several hospitalizations each year for acute episodes of pain. Although generally no inciting factor is found, stresses such as cold, infection, and dehydration can precipitate attacks. Fever, joint swelling, vomiting, and tachypnea can accompany pain episodes.

Most patients experience autoinfarction of the spleen by early childhood due to occlusion of splenic capillary beds. For this and other reasons, patients with sickle cell anemia are significantly vulnerable to infection, especially from encapsulated pathogens such as *S pneumoniae* and *H influenzae.* Pneumonia, meningitis, osteomyelitis, and bacteremia are causes of significant morbidity and mortality in these patients.

Pulmonary complications are the most common causes of death in patients with sickle cell disease. RBCs in the pulmonary system are particularly vulnerable to sickling because of its low Po_2 and relatively low blood pressure. "Acute chest syndrome" refers to the clinical triad of chest pain, pulmonary infiltrate on x-ray, and fever, which can be due to pulmonary infarction, pneumonia, or both.

Sickled RBCs can occlude vasculature and cause infarction of nearly any tissue in the body. Other serious manifestations of sickle cell disease, therefore, include stroke, myocardial infarction, bone infarction, retinopathy, leg ulcers, and priapism. Depression, low self-esteem, and social withdrawal are common, especially when adequate coping mechanisms are not in place.

B. Laboratory Findings

Laboratory findings often reflect the chronic hemolysis that accompanies sickle cell anemia. Classically the patient has a reticulocyte count increased to 3–15%, Hb mildly or moderately decreased to 7–11 g/dL, elevated direct bilirubin and lactate dehydrogenase, and a depressed haptoglobin level.

The peripheral blood smear shows sickling of half of the RBCs. Howell–Jolly bodies and target cells are also present on the smear, indicating hyposplenism. The white blood cell count can be elevated at 12,000–15,000/mm^3, even in the absence of infection.

Treatment

Despite the preventive measures discussed earlier, most patients with sickle cell anemia require frequent hospitalization for acute vasoocclusive crises or infectious complications. During acute exacerbations, patients often require hydration and oxygenation, analgesia with nonnarcotic or narcotic medications, antibiotics if appropriate, and blood transfusions.

4. Autoimmune Hemolytic Anemia

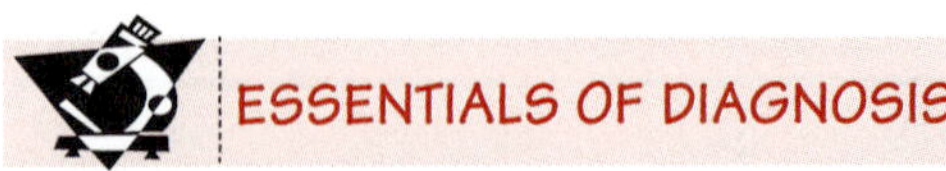

- *Positive direct Coombs test.*
- *Elevated indirect bilirubin and decreased serum haptoglobin.*
- *Inciting factor such as medication or illness.*

General Considerations

Autoimmune hemolytic anemia (AIHA) results when a patient produces antibodies directed against the body's RBCs (Table 30–4). AIHA can be classified by the temperature at which the antibodies are most reactive. "Warm" autoantibodies bind most strongly near 37°C (98.6°F), whereas "cold" autoantibodies bind RBCs near 0–4°C (32–39.2°F). Occasionally, a mixture of both types of autoantibodies is present.

Pathogenesis

Although in nearly half of cases the production of autoantibodies is idiopathic, at other times an inciting factor can be found. Lymphoproliferative disorders such as chronic lymphoblastic leukemia and autoimmune disorders such as rheumatoid arthritis, for example, can induce production of either warm or cold autoantibodies. Infections such as *Mycoplasma* and syphilis have been implicated, primarily in cold AIHA.

Medications can induce a warm antibody autoimmune reaction. Some drugs, such as methyldopa, alter RBC antigens so that they become targets of the host immune system. Other drugs bind with RBC antigens to form immunogenic complexes. This "hapten" reaction can occur with penicillin as well as a variety of other drugs.

Prevention

Any patient who receives a splenectomy should also receive secondary prevention in the form of immu-

Table 30–4. Causes of immune hemolytic anemia.

Idiopathic
Transfusion reaction
Drugs (methyldopa, penicillin, quinidine)
Connective tissue disorders
Hematologic malignancies (chronic lymphocytic leukemia, non-Hodgkin lymphoma)
Infections (*Mycoplasma*, syphilis)

nizations against *Pneumococcus, Haemophilus,* and *Meningococcus.*

Clinical Findings

A. Symptoms and Signs

Overall, a wide spectrum of possible manifestations exists. A typical patient with autoimmune hemolytic anemia presents with pallor, fatigue, or headaches due to loss of circulating RBCs. Jaundice may also be present, due to elevation of indirect bilirubin resulting from the release and breakdown of RBC heme. A patient may also have splenomegaly due to increased sequestration of damaged RBCs within the splenic cords of Billroth. In some cases, hemoglobinuria can lead to renal failure. The rate of disease progression depends on the underlying cause of hemolysis. Although in some patients clinical manifestations progress slowly, in others severe symptoms can develop in a matter of hours.

B. Laboratory Findings

A positive direct Coombs test helps diagnose AIHA. Direct Coombs tests involve washing RBCs and then immersing them in a solution containing antibodies against immunoglobulin G (IgG), C3d (a fragment of complement), or both. RBCs with adherent autoantibodies or complement will tend to agglutinate or burst.

Other laboratory findings reflect the general hemolytic process. Levels of bilirubin and lactate dehydrogenase are increased, haptoglobin levels tend to decrease, and the corrected reticulocyte count is increased. Other appropriate laboratory investigations specific to underlying causes—such as collagen vascular diseases, cancer, and infections—may be warranted.

Treatment

Although further hemolysis can result, blood transfusion should be given when the Hb level is significantly low (5–7 g/dL). Corticosteroids are often considered the treatment of choice, especially when autoantibodies are warm. Those who need long-term treatment and cannot take steroids can use other immunomodulating agents such as azathioprine, cyclosporine, and rituximab. Intravenous immunoglobulin is advocated for the acute treatment of adults with AIHA, but it is not as effective in children. Exchange transfusion, which not only delivers new RBCs but also removes destructive autoantibodies and complement, can also be useful. Splenectomy should be considered in refractory cases; as previously noted, any patient who receives a splenectomy should also receive immunizations against *Pneumococcus, Haemophilus,* and *Meningococcus.* Finally, underlying disorders should be treated as appropriate.

Gehrs BC, Friedberg RC: Autoimmune hemolytic anemia. Am J Hematol 2002;69:258. [PMID: 11921020]

5. Extrinsic Nonimmune Hemolytic Anemia

ESSENTIALS OF DIAGNOSIS

- *Negative Coombs test.*
- *Negative family history.*
- *Known mechanical trauma to RBCs, hemolytic infection, or drug or toxin exposure.*

There are many causes of extrinsic hemolysis not related to immunity (Table 30–5). The first group of conditions results from mechanical damage to RBCs. Any process that enlarges the spleen, for instance, can lead to an acquired hemolytic process because the spleen is the major organ recycling RBCs. Mechanical damage can also occur as RBCs rush past a prosthetic valve or other internal machinery. Disseminated intravascular coagulation and thrombotic thrombocytopenic purpura can result in hemolysis of RBCs that flow through areas of intravascular coagulation. Mechanical destruction of RBCs can also be due to exposure to heat, burns, or even repeated trauma such as that encountered in the feet while marching long distances.

Infectious diseases such as malaria, babesiosis, and leishmaniasis can also cause an acquired hemolysis. This is due both to direct parasitic action and to increased activity of macrophages within the spleen.

Finally, drugs and toxins can lead to hemolysis. Medications such as primaquine, dapsone, nitrites, and

Table 30–5. Nonimmune causes of hemolysis.

Hypersplenism
Microangiopathy
Disseminated intravascular coagulation
Thrombotic thrombocytopenic purpura
Physical destruction
Prosthetic valve
March hemoglobinuria
Burns
Infection
Malaria, babesiosis
Leishmaniasis
Medications
Primaquine
Dapsone
Nitrates
Toxins
Lead, copper
Arsine gas
Snake, spider venom

even topical anesthesia can induce oxidative stress, damaging RBCs. This can occur even in patients without G6PD deficiency. Toxins such as lead, copper, and arsine gas, as well as venom from snakes, insects, and spiders, can also cause hemolysis.

Symptoms and signs, laboratory findings, and treatments will be based upon the specific diagnosis made. Rather than a specific disorder, extrinsic nonimmune hemolytic anemia is a general categorization of heterogeneous disease processes.

NONHEMOLYTIC ANEMIA

1. Aplastic Anemia

ESSENTIALS OF DIAGNOSIS

- *Pancytopenia.*
- *Hypocellular bone marrow.*
- *Normal hematopoietic cells.*

General Considerations

Aplastic anemia represents the suppression of all bone marrow lines—erythroid, granulocytic, and megakaryocytic—leading to pancytopenia. Most commonly the disorder is idiopathic. However, drugs, toxins, radiation, infections (hepatitis, parvovirus), and pregnancy can all induce aplastic anemia.

Pathogenesis

The etiology is unclear. Although some causative agents have been shown to be directly toxic to the bone marrow, others seem to induce an autoimmune process. The prognosis depends on many factors. The specific etiology plays a role: drug-induced aplastic anemia carries a more favorable prognosis than idiopathic aplastic anemia. The more severe the pancytopenia, the worse is the prognosis. Age and gender do not seem to play a role.

Clinical Findings

A. Symptoms and Signs

Anemia leads to pallor, fatigue, and weakness. Neutropenia increases susceptibility to bacterial infections. Thrombocytopenia can present as mucosal bleeding, easy bruising, or petechiae. Splenomegaly is common in advanced disease.

B. Laboratory Findings

Pancytopenia is the hallmark of aplastic anemia. The associated anemia can be severe and is generally normocytic. The reticulocyte count is often low. The white blood cell count can be lower than 1500/mm^3 and the platelet count is generally less than 150,000/mL. The peripheral blood smear shows RBCs, neutrophils, and platelets that are normal in morphology but decreased in number. Bone marrow aspirate, which reveals marrow hypocellularity, is essential to the diagnosis of aplastic anemia and important in distinguishing it from other causes of pancytopenia.

Treatment

Patients with aplastic anemia should avoid sick contacts and razors. Other means of decreasing risk of infection include the use of stool softeners and antiseptic soaps. Fever or other signs of infection should be aggressively investigated. Often, empiric broad-spectrum antibiotics should be used. Menstrual blood loss can be suppressed with oral contraceptive pills. Although replacement of blood products is often necessary, it should be used as little as possible to avoid sensitizing potential candidates for bone marrow transplantation. Hematopoietic growth factors (erythropoietin and granulocyte colony-stimulating factor) are not routinely used due to transient or nil effect.

In a patient younger than 50 years of age with an HLA-matched sibling, immediate bone marrow transplantation is the treatment of choice. The toxicity associated with treatment increases with age, along with the risk of graft-versus-host disease. If successful, transplantation is curative. The 5-year survival rate is approximately 70%.

In those lacking matched siblings or those older than 50 years, treatment consists of immunosuppression with antithymocyte globulin, augmented with high-dose cyclosporine. Most patients relapse, but remission rates with additional antithymocyte globulin treatments are encouraging. Survival at 5 years is about 75%.

Young NS, Maciejewski J: The pathophysiology of acquired aplastic anemia. N Engl J Med 1997;336:1365. [PMID: 9134878]

2. Anemia of Chronic Renal Insufficiency

ESSENTIALS OF DIAGNOSIS

- *Elevated serum creatinine level.*
- *Clinical presentation consistent with renal insufficiency.*

General Considerations

Although anemia of chronic renal insufficiency (CRI) commonly occurs in patients with a creatinine clearance of 30 mL/min/1.73 m^2 or less, it can appear in patients with serum creatinine as low as 2 mg/dL.

Pathogenesis

Anemia of CRI is caused in part by a decrease in renal production of erythropoietin. The milieu of CRI also adversely affects RBC function. Studies show that RBCs from healthy patients die prematurely when injected into patients with CRI, but RBCs from CRI patients have a normal life span when injected into healthy individuals. Platelets are also affected. Platelet count is decreased and function is impaired.

Clinical Findings

A. Symptoms and Signs

Patients may exhibit bleeding or bruising due to thrombocytopenia and platelet dysfunction. Pallor and fatigue are also common. Early symptoms of uremia include nausea, vomiting, weight loss, malaise, and headache. As the blood urea nitrogen (BUN) level rises, paresthesias, decreased urine output, and waning level of consciousness can be seen. Other signs and symptoms depend on the etiology of the patient's renal insufficiency.

B. Laboratory Findings

BUN and serum creatinine are generally both elevated, above 30 and 3.0 mg/dL, respectively. The anemia tends to be normocytic and normochromic, but in some cases it can be microcytic. Hyperphosphatemia, hypocalcemia, and hyperkalemia can occur, as can metabolic acidosis. Reticulocyte count tends to be normal or decreased. The blood smear in the uremic patient can reveal acanthocytes, which are grossly deformed RBCs. Bone marrow is inappropriately normal for the degree of anemia.

Treatment

Given that the primary cause is insufficient production of erythropoietin by the affected kidneys, treatment involves erythropoietin replacement. Erythropoietin or darbepoetin is indicated when the Hb level is 11 g/dL or less. Both are recombinant products. Darbepoetin has a longer half-life and more predictable bioavailability. Prior to initiation of therapy, the patient should be screened for deficiency of iron, folate, and vitamin B_{12} as well as for occult blood loss. Intravenous iron replacement may be necessary to ensure iron stores adequate to support erythropoiesis.

Erythropoietin is given at 80–120 units/kg/week. The most common side effect of erythropoietin therapy is hypertension. There is growing evidence that treatment with erythropoietin has a favorable effect on the progression of renal disease, underscoring the importance of early diagnosis and treatment. The target Hb level is 11–12 g/dL.

3. Anemia Associated with Marrow Infiltration

ESSENTIALS OF DIAGNOSIS

- *Anemia with abnormally shaped RBCs on peripheral smear, along with abnormalities of other cell lines.*
- *Bone marrow study showing infiltration or a "dry tap."*
- *Underlying neoplastic, inflammatory, or metabolic disease with nonspecific systemic signs and symptoms.*

General Considerations

The bone marrow can tolerate fairly extensive infiltration. When marrow infiltration causes anemia or pancytopenia, however, it is referred to as *myelophthisic anemia.* The most common cause of myelophthisis is metastatic carcinoma of the lung, breast, or prostate. Other causes include hematologic malignancies (leukemia, lymphoma), infections (tuberculosis, fungi), and metabolic diseases (Gaucher disease, Niemann–Pick disease).

Pathogenesis

As the marrow is infiltrated by one of these disease processes, hematopoietic precursor cells are unable to mature and differentiate. Eventually, the normal marrow becomes replaced by collagen, reticulin, and other fibrotic cells. The severity of the resulting pancytopenia reflects the degree of infiltration. Myelophthisis occurs in less than 10% of patients with metastatic disease. The prognosis in patients with marrow metastases is generally poor.

Clinical Findings

A. Symptoms and Signs

Anemia is most commonly manifested by pallor or fatigue. Thrombocytopenia can cause petechiae, bleeding, or bruising. Neutropenia can lead to frequent or atypical infections. Fractures, bony pain, bony tenderness, hepatomegaly, and splenomegaly may occur. Other presenting signs and symptoms are usually related to the underlying cause of marrow infiltration.

B. Laboratory Findings

The anemia tends to be normocytic and mild to moderate. White blood cells and platelets may also be decreased. The peripheral blood smear is characterized by abnormal cells, particularly tear-shaped RBCs. The smear may also show poikilocytes and anisocytes. "Leukoerythroblastosis" refers to the presence of immature nucleated RBCs, immature white blood cells, and megakaryocyte fragments on the peripheral blood smear—findings that are highly suggestive of infiltration. Because of the hypocellular marrow, aspirate often yields few cells ("dry tap").

Treatment

Treatment targets the underlying disease. Successful treatment of the malignancy, through radiation, chemotherapy, or bone marrow transplantation, can resolve the anemia. Erythropoietin or blood transfusion may be used to augment the RBC count. Platelet transfusions may be needed.

Brill JR, Baumgardner DJ: Normocytic anemia. Am Fam Physician 2000;62:2255. [PMID: 11126852]

Corwin HL: Anemia and blood transfusion in the critically ill patient: Role of erythropoietin. Crit Care (London) 2004;8(suppl 2):S42. [PMID: 15196323]

Hellstrom-Lindberg E: Management of anemia associated with myelodysplastic syndrome. Semin Hematol 2005;42(suppl 1):S10. [PMID: 15846579]

Rao M et al: Management of anemia. Contrib Nephrol 2004;145:69. [PMID: 15496793]

Waltzman RJ: Treatment of chemotherapy-related anemia with erythropoietic agents: Current approaches and new paradigms. Semin Hematol 2004;41(suppl 7):9. [PMID: 15768474]

Hepatobiliary Disorders

31

Rodrick McKinlay, MD, & Samuel C. Matheny, MD, MPH

BILIARY TRACT DISEASES

Rod McKinlay, MD

APPROACH TO THE PATIENT WITH RIGHT UPPER QUADRANT PAIN

General Considerations

Patients complaining of right upper quadrant (RUQ) or epigastric abdominal pain usually have a disorder of the hepatobiliary or upper gastrointestinal system. Pain that is acute in onset, persists longer than 6 hours, and is associated with significant abdominal tenderness often signals a condition requiring surgical (or interventional endoscopic) attention. Such conditions include acute cholecystitis, perforated duodenal or gastric ulcer, pyogenic liver abscess, choledocholithiasis with or without cholangitis, perforated diverticulitis, perforated appendicitis leaking into the RUQ, or severe acute pancreatitis. Other nonsurgical conditions to consider include mild to moderate pancreatitis, perihepatitis from pelvic inflammatory disease (Fitz–Hugh–Curtis syndrome), right lower lobe pneumonia, right-sided pyelonephritis, nephroureterolithiasis, acute hepatitis, and myocardial infarction.

Laboratory & Imaging Evaluation

Cost-effective laboratory tests in working up acute RUQ pain stem from the history and physical examination, but in general, they should include a complete blood count, liver function tests, and serum amylase and lipase levels. An ultrasonography of the RUQ should be the first imaging study to rule out gallstones and related conditions. If a perforated viscus is suspected, an abdominal series should be ordered to rule out free air. Such a finding necessitates surgery. Computed tomography (CT) scans should be reserved for patients whose diagnosis is unclear following laboratory studies, ultrasonography, and plain abdominal radiographs.

Ultrasonography is cost-effective in confirming the presence of gallstones and biliary-related pathology. A complete blood count, liver function tests, amylase and lipase levels, thyroid-stimulating hormone, and erythrocyte sedimentation rate are cost-effective tests in the workup of chronic abdominal pain. For patients without gallstones, endoscopy and nuclear medicine studies (eg, hepatic iminodiacetic acid [HIDA] scan) may be beneficial. Endoscopic retrograde cholangiopancreatography (ERCP) should be reserved for patients with ultrasound evidence of bile duct dilation in whom an obstructing stone, stricture, or neoplasm is suspected, or to enable diagnosis in difficult cases.

Differential Diagnosis

The differential diagnosis for patients with subacute or chronic RUQ pain is extensive and consists of symptomatic cholelithiasis (biliary colic), peptic ulcer disease, gastroesophageal reflux, pancreatitis, chronic hepatitis, inflammatory bowel disease, porphyria, intestinal angina, pancreatic cancer, large and small bowel cancer, endometriosis, and right-sided diverticulitis.

Silen W: *Cope's Early Diagnosis of the Acute Abdomen,* 20th ed. Oxford University Press, 2000:128.

CHOLELITHIASIS

General Considerations

Between 16 and 25 million (about 1 in 13) Americans harbor gallstones. The prevalence of gallstones is related to many factors, including gender, age, and ethnic background. Gallstones are more common in women than men and increase in both sexes with age. By age 70 about 25% of women and 10% of men in the United States have gallstones. Gallstones are more prevalent in Native Americans and Caucasians and less prevalent in African Americans. Gallstones affect more than 70% of Pima Indians older than 30 years. In addition to age, gender, and ethnicity, other risk factors for gallstones include obesity, high estrogen levels, cholesterol-lowering drugs, diabetes, rapid weight loss, fasting, prolonged parenteral nutrition, and conditions of the terminal ileum, such as Crohn disease.

Avoidance or control of these conditions helps to prevent gallstones and their sequelae.

Pathogenesis

Gallstones may be divided pathologically into cholesterol stones and pigment stones. Cholesterol stones develop when the balance of cholesterol, bile salts, and lecithin within the gallbladder bile tips in favor of cholesterol supersaturation. This state allows the formation of solid cholesterol crystals, which then grow into stones by further deposition of cholesterol and calcium salts. Pigment stones are classified into black and brown stones. Black pigment stones are associated with hemolytic states in which the concentration of unconjugated bilirubin increases and precipitates with calcium. Brown stones are often formed in the setting of infection, in which bacteria secrete enzymes that hydrolyze bilirubin glucuronide to free bilirubin, which then precipitates with calcium.

Clinical Findings

Asymptomatic gallstones may be found incidentally on plain abdominal radiography, but most gallstones are composed largely of cholesterol, rendering them radiolucent. Ultrasonography is the most sensitive and cost-effective test to detect gallstones (> 90% sensitivity).

Treatment

Most people with gallstones remain asymptomatic. The risk of developing biliary colic or other complications is about 1–2% per year. Therefore, the incidental finding of asymptomatic gallstones should generally not prompt surgical referral, except in cases in which an elevated risk for gallbladder carcinoma exists (gallstones associated with a calcified, or "porcelain," gallbladder, and possibly those with stones > 3 cm). Patients with diabetes, although more likely to have complications from symptomatic disease, still do not require prophylactic cholecystectomy for asymptomatic gallstones. The longer a patient's gallstones remain clinically silent, the less likely the stones will ultimately become symptomatic.

Del Favero G et al: Natural history of gallstones in non-insulin-dependent diabetes mellitus: A prospective 5-year follow-up. Dig Dis Sci 1994;39:1704. [PMID 8050321]

Sheth S et al: Primary gallbladder cancer: Recognition of risk factors and the role of prophylactic cholecystectomy. Am J Gastroenterol 2000;95:1402. [PMID 10894571]

SYMPTOMATIC CHOLELITHIASIS (BILIARY COLIC)

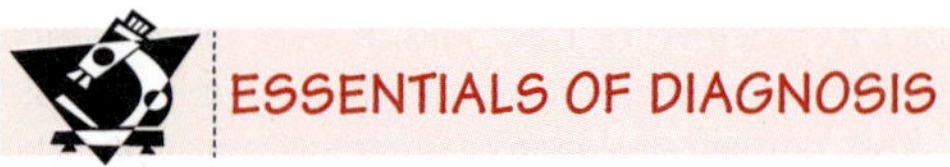

- *Episodic RUQ pain.*
- *Nausea.*
- *Ultrasound evidence of gallstones.*

Pathogenesis

Biliary colic develops when a gallstone or biliary sludge transiently obstruct the gallbladder neck, creating gallbladder distention and pain through visceral afferent fibers.

Clinical Findings

Patients typically complain of RUQ pain after eating a fatty meal. The pain often radiates to the back or to the right scapula and lasts between 30 minutes and several hours. Nausea may accompany symptoms of pain, but vomiting is uncommon in uncomplicated biliary colic. On physical examination, mild RUQ tenderness may be present. Laboratory values are normal. Ultrasonography demonstrates gallstones, with or without gallbladder wall thickening or pericholecystic fluid.

Differential Diagnosis

Other painful disorders of the RUQ include peptic ulcer disease, pancreatitis, hepatitis, gastritis, duodenitis, right-sided diverticulitis, pneumonia of the right lower lobe, or myocardial infarction.

Treatment

Elective laparoscopic cholecystectomy is the gold standard for treatment of symptomatic cholelithiasis. Patients who are young (< 60 years) and otherwise healthy can generally expect outpatient treatment with a rapid recovery, returning to work within 1–2 weeks. Older patients also do well after laparoscopic cholecystectomy but may take longer to recover. Conversion rates to open surgery are rare for elective laparoscopic cholecystectomy (< 5%) but are more likely to occur in obese, elderly, and diabetic patients. In the case of conversion, a 2- to 4-day hospital stay is customary. Contraindications for laparoscopic surgery include severe comorbid disease precluding general anesthesia and uncontrolled coagulopathy.

Cheno- and ursodeoxycholic acids may be used to treat symptomatic gallstones in patients who are not candidates for or refuse cholecystectomy, but biliary colic is more likely to recur in these patients than in those treated with cholecystectomy.

Extracorporeal shock wave lithotripsy has a relatively high rate of stone recurrence and is not approved by the Food and Drug Administration (FDA) in the United States.

Prognosis

More than 95% of patients treated with laparoscopic cholecystectomy have no further symptoms related to gallstones. The most feared complication of laparoscopic cholecystectomy is injury to the common bile duct (0.1–0.6%), which may require endoscopic intervention (eg, stent placement) or further surgery, such as hepaticojejunostomy, to correct. Retained common duct stones and cystic duct leaks occur in 2–3% of cases and are usually amenable to endoscopic therapy.

Pregnancy is a risk factor for gallstones. Pregnant patients should generally be treated conservatively, because most attacks will abate after the birth of the infant. However, in severe attacks or in acute cholecystitis, laparoscopic cholecystectomy is safe. The best time to perform surgery is during the second trimester, thus avoiding potential teratogenic effects during the first trimester and preterm labor in the third trimester.

Gadacz TR: An update on laparoscopic cholecystectomy, including a clinical pathway. Surg Clin North Am 2000;80:1127. [PMID 10987028]

Gilat T, Konikoff F: Pregnancy and the biliary tract. Can J Gastroenterol 2000;14(suppl D):55D. [PMID 11110613]

CHOLECYSTITIS

1. Acute

ESSENTIALS OF DIAGNOSIS

- *Persistent severe RUQ pain (> 4–6 hours).*
- *RUQ tenderness.*
- *Fever, leukocytosis.*
- *Ultrasound evidence of gallstones.*

Pathogenesis

Persistent gallbladder outlet obstruction by a stone or sludge causes distention of the gallbladder with resultant significant pain. Engorgement of the gallbladder leads to further inflammation and possible gangrene.

Clinical Findings

A. Symptoms and Signs

Patients with acute cholecystitis complain of persistent RUQ pain, typically lasting more than 4–6 hours, which may radiate to the back and right shoulder. Nausea and vomiting are frequently associated with the pain. RUQ tenderness is present on physical examination. The classically described Murphy sign (arrest of inspiration with RUQ palpation) is not always present, but if it can be elicited, the diagnosis of acute cholecystitis is confirmed.

B. Laboratory Findings

Laboratory values include an elevated white blood cell (WBC) count and frequently an elevated alkaline phosphatase level. The total bilirubin and liver transaminases (alanine aminotransferase [ALT], aspartate aminotransferase [AST]) may also be elevated. A total bilirubin greater than 3 mg/dL or significantly elevated alkaline phosphatase or γ-glutamyltransferase (GGT) should prompt a search for a common duct stone (see Cholangitis/Choledocholithiasis, later). Elevation of amylase and lipase should lead to suspicion of gallstone pancreatitis. A significantly elevated WBC count (> 17,000/mm^3) is associated with an increased likelihood of gallbladder gangrene.

C. Imaging Studies

RUQ ultrasonography typically shows gallstones, a thickened gallbladder wall, and pericholecystic fluid, although the latter two findings may not be present in all cases. If the diagnosis of acute cholecystitis is strongly suspected in the absence of gallstones, a HIDA scan should be performed. Failure to visualize the gallbladder (secondary to obstruction) is indicative of acute cholecystitis.

Differential Diagnosis

Perforated peptic ulcer disease, acute pancreatitis, acute hepatitis, appendicitis, or right-sided diverticulitis may mimic acute cholecystitis.

Treatment

Patients diagnosed with acute cholecystitis should be admitted to the hospital for intravenous antibiotics, analgesics, and bowel rest followed closely by laparoscopic cholecystectomy, which is the definitive treatment of choice for acute cholecystitis. Most studies favor performing surgery during the same hospitalization rather than several weeks after the resolution of the acute episode. Conversion to open surgery for acute cholecystitis occurs more frequently than for biliary colic, but still occurs in only 5–10% of cases.

For patients who are not candidates or refuse cholecystectomy, percutaneous cholecystostomy under radiologic guidance is indicated to drain potentially infected bile from the gallbladder. Antibiotic coverage is essential before and after the procedure.

Prognosis

Cholecystectomy alleviates gallstone-related pain and complications in 90% of patients with acute cholecystitis, although complications are more frequent when surgery is performed urgently for acute disease than electively for chronic disease. Post-cholecystectomy syndrome—persistent RUQ pain following cholecystectomy—occurs in a small percentage of patients and usually is due to a faulty diagnosis. A small subset of patients may have disordered functioning of the ampulla of Vater requiring further workup and treatment.

2. Chronic

When patients endure multiple episodes of biliary colic or acute cholecystitis without intervention, they may present later with chronic cholecystitis. Keys to diagnosis include a history of multiple episodes of RUQ pain, absence of RUQ tenderness, and gallstones on ultrasonography. Treatment consists of laparoscopic cholecystectomy. The gallbladder may be contracted and partially intrahepatic secondary to scarring from previous inflammatory episodes.

Gadacz TR: An update on laparoscopic cholecystectomy, including a clinical pathway. Surg Clin N Am 2000;80:1127. [PMID 10987028]

Lo CM et al: Early versus delayed laparoscopic cholecystectomy for treatment of acute cholecystitis. Ann Surg 1996;223:37. [PMID 8554416]

Merriam LT et al: Gangrenous cholecystitis: Analysis of risk factors and experience with laparoscopic cholecystectomy. Surgery 1999;126:680. [PMID 10520915]

Wang CH et al: Rapid diagnosis of choledocholithiasis using biochemical tests in patients undergoing laparoscopic cholecystectomy. Hepatogastroenterology 2001;48:619. [PMID 11462888]

GALLSTONE PANCREATITIS

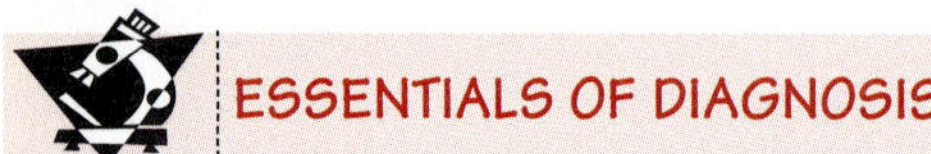

- *RUQ or epigastric pain.*
- *Elevated serum amylase and lipase.*
- *Ultrasound evidence of gallstones.*

General Considerations

Gallstones are the most frequent cause of pancreatitis in the United States, accounting for more than 50% of cases of acute pancreatitis. Transient or persistent occlusion by a gallstone of the common channel between the common and pancreatic ducts results in pancreatitis.

Clinical Findings

A. Symptoms and Signs

Patients present with RUQ and epigastric pain, which often radiates to the back. Nausea and vomiting often accompany the pain. Physical examination reveals epigastric tenderness.

B. Laboratory Findings

Depending on the degree of pancreatitis, the WBC count may be significantly elevated. Amylase and lipase levels are high. Total bilirubin, alkaline phosphatase, AST, and ALT may be elevated as well.

C. Imaging Studies

Ultrasonography demonstrates gallstones, with or without gallbladder wall thickening and pericholecystic fluid. It is not sensitive for detecting stones in the common bile duct (30–50%). For patients with severe pancreatitis, CT is a helpful adjunct to determine the degree of pancreatic inflammation and necrosis, if present. CT is also more sensitive than ultrasonography in detecting common bile duct stones (> 50%). Magnetic resonance cholangiopancreatography (MRCP) is more than 90% sensitive for common duct stones but is very expensive and is not cost-effective for typical cases of gallstone pancreatitis. In patients with elevated bilirubin (> 3–4 mg/dL), consideration should be given to preoperative ERCP to clear the pancreatic or common bile duct of stones.

Treatment

To cure a patient of gallstone pancreatitis, cholecystectomy is necessary. The timing of cholecystectomy depends on the severity of the pancreatitis. In mild to moderate pancreatitis, current recommendations are to perform laparoscopic cholecystectomy early in the initial hospitalization, provided evidence exists that pancreatitis is resolving (ie, amylase and lipase are falling toward normal levels). This resolution of pancreatitis typically occurs within 1–2 days of admission with the patient on bowel rest. Intravenous analgesics should be administered. Antibiotics are not always necessary but may be given when there is concomitant evidence of acute cholecystitis (fever, persistent leukocytosis). Many surgeons perform intraoperative cholangiography for patients who present with acute cholecystitis to ensure that the common bile duct is cleared of stones. In cases of severe pancreatitis (ie, necrotizing), endoscopic clearance of a common duct stone is usually required preoperatively. Laparoscopic or open cholecystectomy should then be performed toward the end of the patient's hospital stay, when pancreatitis is nearly resolved.

Evidence-based management supports early ERCP (within 24–72 hours of hospital admission) to extract the stone(s) responsible for pancreatic duct obstruction in patients who are predicted to have a severe attack of pancreatitis. Anytime ERCP is performed, a small risk (1–5%) of post-ERCP pancreatitis exists.

Complications of pancreatitis may occur before or after cholecystectomy, including necrotizing pancreatitis, infected pancreatic necrosis, or hemorrhagic pancreatitis. Supportive care in the intensive care unit may be necessary in these cases.

Barkun AN: Early endoscopic management of acute gallstone pancreatitis—an evidence-based review. J Gastrointest Surg 2001;5:243. [PMID 11419450]

Ferucci JT: Non-invasive imaging of the biliary ducts. J Gatrointest Surg 2001;5:232. [PMID 11419447]

Schirmer B: Timing and indications for biliary tract surgery in acute necrotizing pancreatitis. J Gastrointest Surg 2001;5: 229. [PMID 11419446]

CHOLANGITIS/CHOLEDOCHOLITHIASIS

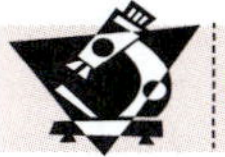

ESSENTIALS OF DIAGNOSIS

- *Persistent RUQ pain.*
- *Jaundice.*
- *Fever.*
- *Hypotension, mental status changes (acute suppurative cholangitis).*

General Considerations

Common bile duct stones (choledocholithiasis) are present in 10–15% of patients with gallstones. Common duct stones may be symptomatic or asymptomatic. Symptomatic stones cause obstruction of the biliary tract leading to jaundice, pancreatitis, or cholangitis. Biliary stasis predisposes to infection of bile and cholangitis. Pus under pressure in the biliary tract is known as acute suppurative cholangitis and requires emergent decompression of the biliary tree.

Common duct stones are classified into primary stones and secondary stones. Primary stones are those arising in the common duct *de novo* and are rare (5%). Secondary stones are those that pass into the common duct from the gallbladder and are the most common type of stone (95%).

Clinical Findings

Patients with cholangitis classically present with Charcot triad: jaundice; acute, severe RUQ pain; and fever. If pus is under pressure in the biliary tree, patients exhibit the additional signs of hypotension and mental status changes (creating the so-called Raynaud pentad).

Laboratory studies indicate elevated WBC count, hyperbilirubinemia, and elevated alkaline phosphatase. Liver transaminase levels may also be high.

Although ultrasonography has poor sensitivity for detecting a common duct stone, it may provide convincing indirect evidence of a choledocholithiasis, such as common bile duct dilation and stones in the gallbladder. To confirm the diagnosis, a CT scan, ERCP, or MRCP may be necessary.

Differential Diagnosis

The differential diagnosis includes periampullary cancer (pancreas, bile duct, or duodenum), liver metastases, cholestatic liver diseases, or hepatocellular jaundice.

Treatment

Patients should be aggressively hydrated and given broad-spectrum antibiotics upon presentation. ERCP is effective in extracting the causative stone in the majority of cases and is preferable to surgery on initial presentation. If ERCP fails, the biliary system may be decompressed with a percutaneous transhepatic drain. Failing that, surgery should be undertaken to extract the stone and drain the biliary system. If ERCP or transhepatic cholangiography is successful, patients should undergo cholecystectomy within several days to weeks as tolerated to eliminate the source of stones. This may be performed laparoscopically or as an open procedure. If surgery is needed to explore the common bile duct, a T tube draining bile from the duct to a skin level bag is left in place for 2–6 weeks. Prior to removing the T tube, a cholangiogram is performed through the T tube to ensure that the duct is clear of stones.

Prognosis

Cholangitis is a serious illness that carries a significantly greater risk of morbidity and mortality than acute cholecystitis, with mortality rates ranging from 13% to 88%. Poor prognostic indicators include advanced age, female sex, acute renal failure, concomitant medical illnesses, pH less than 7.4, preexisting cirrhosis, hepatic abscess, and malignant obstruction.

Lillemoe KD. Surgical treatment of biliary tract infections. Am Surg 2000;66:138. [PMID 10695743]

Soetikno RM et al: Endoscopic management of choledocholithiasis. J Clin Gastroenterol 1998;27:296. [PMID 9955257]

ACUTE ACALCULOUS CHOLECYSTITIS

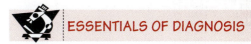

ESSENTIALS OF DIAGNOSIS

- *RUQ tenderness.*
- *Critically ill patient.*
- *Diagnosis of exclusion.*

General Considerations

Patients may develop cholecystitis without gallstones. So-called acute acalculous cholecystitis represents between 5% and 10% of all episodes of cholecystitis and typically takes a more fulminant course than calculous cholecystitis. The underlying etiology in this instance is ischemia and bile stasis as opposed to stones. Acute acalculous cholecystitis generally develops in patients who are critically ill, such as those who have sustained major burns, multiple trauma, or major nonbiliary operations, including cardiopulmonary bypass; however, outpatient cases have been documented, especially among elderly men with vascular disease.

Clinical Presentation

RUQ pain and tenderness may be present but difficult to detect secondary to the patient's critically ill state. Laboratory results show leukocytosis with or without elevation of liver function tests. Ultrasonography reveals a distended gallbladder, often with wall thickening or emphysematous changes. Cholescintigraphy (HIDA scan) shows nonfilling of the gallbladder, but the false-positive rate may be as high as 40% because of the common underlying finding of biliary stasis.

Differential Diagnosis

Perforated peptic ulcer disease, acute or necrotizing pancreatitis, ischemic bowel, or any perforated viscus may mimic acute acalculous cholecystitis.

Treatment

Treatment consists of cholecystectomy, which is usually performed open but may be performed laparoscopically in selected cases. If a patient is unable to tolerate a general anesthetic or is coagulopathic, percutaneous cholecystostomy may be necessary, with interval cholecystectomy after systemic improvement.

Kalliafas S et al: Acute acalculous cholecystitis: Incidence, risk factors, diagnosis, and outcome. Am Surg 1998; 64:471–5. [PMID 9585788]

Lillemoe KD: Surgical treatment of biliary tract infections. Am Surg 2000;66:138. [PMID 10695743]

BILIARY DYSKINESIA

ESSENTIALS OF DIAGNOSIS

- *Chronic, intermittent RUQ pain.*
- *Absence of gallstones on ultrasonography.*
- *HIDA scan demonstrating gallbladder ejection fraction < 35%.*

General Considerations

Biliary dyskinesia, which may also be referred to as chronic acalculous cholecystitis, follows a much less fulminant course than acute acalculous cholecystitis. Patients often have undergone esophagogastroduodenoscopy (EGD), upper gastrointestinal studies, or even ERCP by the time they reach HIDA scanning in an attempt to diagnose their RUQ pain. Most patients with this disorder are women younger than 50 years.

Clinical Findings

Patients typically present with episodic RUQ pain, intolerance to fatty meals, and mild nausea. Laboratory values and ultrasound studies generally are normal. A HIDA scan performed with cholecystokinin showing less than 35% gallbladder ejection fraction at 20 minutes is diagnostic of biliary dyskinesia. Reproduction of RUQ pain with sincalide injection during HIDA scan may aid in the diagnosis of biliary dyskinesia.

Treatment

Laparoscopic cholecystectomy effectively cures 80–90% of patients with biliary dyskinesia demonstrated by abnormally low gallbladder ejection fraction. In most cases the pathology report shows evidence of chronic cholecystitis.

Jones-Monahan K, Gruenberg JC: Chronic acalculous cholecystitis: Changes in patient demographics and evaluation since the advent of laparoscopy. JSLS 1999;3:221. [PMID 10527335]

Zeissman HA: Functional hepatobiliary disease: Chronic acalculous gallbladder and chronic acalculous biliary disease. Semin Nucl Med 2006;36:119. [PMID: 16517234]

BILIARY TRACT NEOPLASIA

ESSENTIALS OF DIAGNOSIS

- *RUQ pain.*
- *Jaundice.*
- *Weight loss.*

General Considerations

Cancer of the gallbladder is relatively uncommon, with 5000 new cases diagnosed each year in the United States. Women are affected more than two to three times as often as men. More than 75% of affected individuals are older than 65 years of age. The incidence of gallbladder cancer is higher among Native Americans and is particularly high in Chile.

Cholangiocarcinoma, or cancer of the bile ducts, is even less common than gallbladder cancer, with 2500 to 3000 new cases per year in the United States. Men and women are affected equally. The incidence rises with increasing age.

Clinical Findings

A. Gallbladder Cancer

Patients with gallbladder cancer may present in a number of ways. Most commonly patients present with biliary colic, complaining chiefly of chronic RUQ pain and mild nausea. However, they also can present with malignant biliary obstruction (jaundice, weight loss) or simply with weight loss and vague abdominal pain. A small subset of patients with gallbladder cancer presents with acute cholecystitis (acute RUQ pain, fever, and leukocytosis). Ultrasonography demonstrates a mass replacing the gallbladder or an irregular gallbladder wall. CT is an effective diagnostic tool for patients in whom ultrasonography is not helpful.

B. Bile Duct Cancer

Patients with bile duct cancer most commonly present with painless jaundice. Other symptoms may include pruritus, fever, vague abdominal pain, anorexia, and weight loss. Besides the finding of jaundice, the physical examination is usually unremarkable. Total bilirubin may exceed 10 mg/dL, and alkaline phosphatase is substantially elevated. CA 19-9 may also be high, helping to distinguish malignant from benign biliary obstruction. Ultrasonography and CT are the initial diagnostic studies, followed by cholangiography to evaluate for possible surgical resection.

Treatment

Patients with gallbladder cancer frequently present at a late stage and often are not candidates for surgical resection. For the small number of patients who present with early gallbladder cancer (stage T1a—mucosal involvement only), cholecystectomy is curative and survival approaches 100%. For others (stages T1b and 2–4—extension into gallbladder muscularis and beyond), extended cholecystectomy is the treatment of choice for resectable tumors, and prognosis is poor. For unresectable tumors, palliative treatment for pain and obstruction is indicated.

Tumors of the bile duct may be curatively resected in a limited number of cases. In very select cases, parenchymal cholangiocarcinoma may be treated by liver transplantation. Like gallbladder cancer, presentation is usually late and treatment is palliative.

Heimbach JK et al: Liver transplantation for perihilar cholangiocarcinoma after aggressive neoadjuvant therapy: A new paradigm for liver and biliary malignancies? Surgery 2006;140:331. [PMID 16934588]

Rumalla A, Petersen BT: Diagnosis and therapy of biliary tract malignancy. Semin Gastrointest Dis 2000;11:168. [PMID 10950465]

Sheth S et al: Primary gallbladder cancer: Recognition of risk factors and the role of prophylactic cholecystectomy. Am J Gastroenterol 2000;95:1402. [PMID 10894571]

References for Biliary Tract Diseases

Ahmed A et al: Management of gallstones and their complications. Am Fam Physician 2000;61:1673. [PMID 10750875]

Custis K et al: Common biliary tract disorders. Clin Fam Pract 2000;2:141.

Gore RM et al: Imaging benign and malignant disease of the gallbladder. Radiol Clin North Am 2002;40:307. [PMID 12479713]

Kalloo AN, Kantsevoy SV: Gallstones and biliary disease. Prim Care 2001;28:591. [PMID 11483446]

Web Sites for Biliary Tract Diseases

http://home.mdconsult.com/das/stat/view/24748043/ctt (For those with access to mdconsult.com, a clinical topic tour updated June 5, 2006, with overview of gallstone diseases and links to related texts and recent journal articles.)

http://www.emedicine.com/EMERG/topic97.htm (Cholelithiasis and choledocholithiasis.)

http://www.ssat.com/cgi-bin/chole7.cgi (Treatment guidelines for cholelithiasis and related diseases.)

http://www.aafp.org/afp/20000701/tips/16.html (Gallstone pancreatitis.)

http://www.cancer.gov/cancerinfo/pdq/treatment/gallbladder/healthprofessional (Gallbladder cancer.)

http://brighamrad.harvard.edu/Cases/bwh/hcache/95/full.html (Acute acalculous cholecystitis.)

LIVER DISEASE

Samuel C. Matheny, MD, MPH

VIRAL HEPATITIS

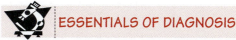

ESSENTIALS OF DIAGNOSIS

- *Variable prodromal signs and symptoms.*
- *Positive specific viral hepatitis tests.*
- *Elevation of serum AST and ALT.*

Acute viral hepatitis is a worldwide problem, and in the United States alone there are probably between 200,000 and 700,000 cases per year according to the Centers for Disease Control and Prevention (CDC).

Over 32% of cases are caused by hepatitis A virus (HAV), 43% by hepatitis B virus (HBV), 21% by hepatitis C virus (HCV), and the remainder are not identified. Although few deaths (~250) are reported yearly from acute hepatitis, considerable morbidity can result from chronic hepatitis caused by HBV and HCV infections, and mortality from complications can be pronounced for years to come.

1. Hepatitis A

General Considerations

Hepatitis A first identified in 1973, is the prototype for the former diagnosis of *infectious hepatitis.* Over the past several decades, the incidence of HAV infection has varied considerably, and a high number of cases are unreported. HAV is a very small viral particle that is its own unique genus (hepatovirus).

Most individuals infected worldwide are children. In general, there are four patterns of HAV distribution (high, moderate, low, and very low), which roughly correspond to differing socioeconomic and hygienic conditions. Countries with poor sanitation have the highest rates of infection. Most children younger than 9 years of age in these countries have evidence of HAV infection. Countries with moderate rates of infection have the highest incidence in later childhood; food and waterborne outbreaks are more common. In countries with low endemicity, the peak age of infection is likely to be at early adulthood, and in very low endemic countries, outbreaks are uncommon.

HAV is usually transmitted by ingestion of contaminated fecal material of an infected person by a susceptible individual. Contaminated food or water can be the source of infection, but occasionally infection can occur by contamination of different types of raw shellfish from areas contaminated by sewage. The virus can survive 3–10 months in water. Other cases of infection by blood exposures have been reported but are less common. The incubation period for HAV averages 30 days, with a range of 15–50 days.

In countries of low endemicity, persons at greatest risk for infection include travelers to intermediate and high HAV-endemic countries, men who have sex with men (MSM), intravenous drug users, and persons with chronic liver disease, including those who have received transplants. In areas of high endemicity, all young children are at increased risk.

Prevention

Currently in the United States, the CDC recommends that certain populations at increased risk be considered for preexposure vaccination; these include the groups listed above. In addition, the CDC now recommends universal immunization for all children older than 1 year of age. The immunization schedule consists of three doses for children and adolescents, and two for adults. In groups with the potential for high risk of exposure, including any adult over the age of 40, prevaccination testing for prior exposure may be cost effective. The appropriate test should evaluate the total anti-HAV. Travelers who receive the vaccine may assume to be protected 4 weeks after receiving the first dose, although the second dose is needed for long-term protection. If travel is anticipated in less than 4 weeks, immunoglobulin may be given in a different site for additional protection. A combination vaccine with HBV is available for persons over 18 years of age and is used on the same three-dose schedule as HBV.

Immunoglobulin may also be used for postexposure prophylaxis if given within 14 days and would most often be used for household or intimate contacts of an infected person, in some institutional settings, or if a common source is identified.

Clinical Findings

A. Symptoms and Signs

The symptoms and signs of acute viral hepatitis are quite similar regardless of type and are difficult to distinguish based on clinical findings. The prodrome for viral hepatitis is variable and may be manifested by anorexia, including changes in olfaction and taste, as well as nausea and vomiting, fatigue, malaise, myalgias, headache, photophobia, pharyngitis, cough, coryza, and fever. Dark urine and clay-colored stools may be noticed 1–5 days before jaundice.

Clinical jaundice varies considerably and may range from an anicteric state to rare hepatic coma. In acute HAV infection, jaundice is usually more pronounced in older age groups (ie, 70–80% in those older than 14 years) and rare in children younger than 6 years (< 10%). Weight loss may also be present, as well as an enlarged liver (70%) and splenomegaly (20%). Spider angiomata may be present without acute liver failure. Patients may also report a loss of desire for cigarette smoking or alcohol.

B. Laboratory Findings

Usually, the onset of symptoms coincides with the first evidence of abnormal laboratory values. Acute elevations of ALT (SGPT) and AST (SGOT) are seen, with levels as high as 4000 units or more in some patients. The ALT level is usually higher than the AST. When the bilirubin level is greater than 2.5, jaundice may be obvious. Bilirubin levels may go from 5 to 20, with usually an equal elevation of conjugated and unconjugated forms. The prothrombin time is usually normal. If significantly elevated, it may signal a poor prognosis. The complete blood count may demonstrate a relative neutropenia, lymphopenia, or atypical lymphocytosis. Urobilinogen may be present in urine in the late preicteric stage.

Serum IgM antibody (anti-HAV) is present in the acute phase and usually disappears within 3 months, although occasionally it persists longer. IgG anti-HAV is used to detect past exposure and persists for the lifetime of the patient. The more commonly available test for IgG anti-HAV is the total anti-HAV.

Treatment

Treatment for the most part is symptomatic, with many clinicians prohibiting only alcohol during the acute illness phase. Most patients can be treated at home.

Prognosis

In the vast majority of patients with HAV, the disease resolves uneventfully within 3–6 months. Rarely, fulminant hepatitis may develop, with acute liver failure and high rates of mortality. Rare cases of cholestatic hepatitis, with persistent bilirubin elevations, have also been reported. Some patients develop relapsing hepatitis, in which HAV is reactivated and shed in the stool. Affected patients demonstrate liver function test abnormalities, but virtually all recover completely. HAV does not progress to chronic hepatitis.

2. Hepatitis B

General Considerations

HBV is a double-shelled DNA virus. The outer shell contains the hepatitis B surface (HBsAg). The inner core contains several other particles, including hepatitis core antigen (HBcAg) and hepatitis B e antigen (HBeAg). These antigens and their subsequent antibodies are described in more detail later.

Worldwide, the distribution of HBV is quite varied. More than 45% of the global population live in areas of high incidence (infections in > 8% of population). There, the lifetime risk of infection is over 60%, and early childhood infections are very common. Intermediate risk areas (infections in 2–7% of population) represent 43% of the global population. The lifetime risk of infection in these areas is between 20% and 60%, and infections occur in various age groups. In low-risk areas (infections in < 2%), which represent about 12% of the global population, the lifetime risk of infection is less than 20% and is usually limited to specific adult risk groups.

In the United States, HBV is normally a disease of young adults. The largest numbers of cases are reported in adults between the ages of 20 and 39 years, but many cases in younger age groups may be asymptomatic and go unreported. Of the specific risk groups in the United States, over 50% in recent studies are those with sexual risk factors (more than one sex partner in the past 6 months, sexual relations with an infected person, or MSM transmission). Over 15% had a history of injection drug use, and 4% had other risk factors such as a household contact with HBV, or a health care exposure. The mode of transmission can thus be sexual, parenteral, or perinatal, by contact of the infant's mucous membranes with maternal infected blood at delivery.

Body fluids with the highest degree of concentration of HBV are blood, serum, and wound exudates. Moderate concentrations are found in semen, vaginal fluid, and saliva, and low or nondetectable amounts are found in urine, feces, sweat, tears, or breast milk. Saliva can be implicated in transmission through bites, but not by kissing.

The average incubation period for HBV is between 60 and 90 days, with a range of 45–180 days. Although the incidence of jaundice increases with age (< 10% of children younger than 5 years demonstrate icterus compared with 30–50% of those older than 35 years), the likelihood of chronic infection with HBV is greater when infection is contracted at a younger age. Between 30% and 90% of all children who contract HBV before the age of 5 years develop chronic disease compared with 2–10% of those older than 35 years.

Prevention

Current immunization recommendations in the United States call for routine immunization of all infants, children, adolescents, and adults in high-risk groups. Acknowledgement of a specific risk factor is not a requirement for immunizations. These recommendations include immunizing all children at birth, 1, and 6 months. Additionally, all high-risk groups should be screened, as well as all pregnant women. Prevaccination testing of patients in low risk areas is probably not necessary, but in high-risk groups, this may be cost-effective. As illustrated in the first test scenario of Table 31–1, a negative HBsAg titer and a negative anti-HBs titer are evidence of susceptibility to HBV.

The vaccine contains components of HBsAg. Pretesting with anti-HB core antibody (anti-HBc) is probably the single best test, because it would identify those who are infected and those who have been exposed. Posttesting for vaccine is not usually recommended, except for individuals who may have difficulty mounting an immune response (eg, immunocompromised patients). In these patients, the HB surface antibody (anti-HBs) would be the appropriate test. Some authorities recommend revaccinating high-risk individuals if titer levels have fallen below 10 IU/L after 5–10 years.

Children born to women of unknown hepatitis B status should receive a first dose of hepatitis B vaccine at birth, and hepatitis B immune globulin (HBIG) within 7 days of birth if maternal blood is positive. Repeat testing of all infants born to HBV-infected mothers should be repeated at 9–15 months with HBsAg and anti-HBs. Infants born to HBV-infected mothers should receive both the first dose of hepatitis B vaccine at birth as well as 0.5

Table 31–1. Interpretation of the hepatitis B panel.

Tests	Results	Interpretation
HBsAg Anti-HBc Anti-HBs	Negative Negative Negative	Susceptible
HBsAg Anti-HBc Anti-HBs	Negative Positive Positive	Immune due to natural factors
HBsAg Anti-HBc Anti-HBs	Negative Negative Positive	Immune due to hepatitis B vaccination
HBsAg Anti-HBc IgM anti-HBc Anti-HBs	Positive Positive Positive Negative	Acutely infected
HBsAg Anti-HBc IgM anti-HBc Anti-HBs	Positive Positive Negative Negative	Chronically infected
HBsAg Anti-HBc Anti-HBs	Negative Positive Negative	Four interpretations possible[1]

[1](1) May be recovering from acute HBV infection. (2) May be distantly immune and the test is not sensitive enough to detect very low levels of anti-HBs in serum. (3) May be susceptible with a false-positive anti-HBc. (4) May be an undetectable level of HBsAg present in the serum and the person is actually a carrier.

mL of HBIG in separate sites within 12 hours after birth. Recommendations for postexposure prophylaxis of HBV can be reviewed in the current CDC recommendations.

Clinical Findings

Acute infection may range from an asymptomatic infection to cholestatic hepatitis to fulminant hepatic failure. HBsAg and other markers usually become positive about 6 weeks after infection and remain positive into the clinical signs of illness. Other biochemical abnormalities begin to show abnormalities in the prodromal phase and may persist several months, even with a resolving disease process. Anti-HB core IgM becomes positive early, with onset of symptoms, and both anti-HB core IGM and anti-HB core IgG may persist for many months or years. Anti-HBs is the last antibody to appear and may indicate resolving infection. The presence of HBeAg indicates active viral replication and increased infectivity (Figure 31–1). Liver function tests should be obtained early in the course of infection, and evidence of prolonged prothrombin time (> 1.5 INR) should raise concern for hepatic failure. Patients who remain chronically infected may demonstrate HBsAg and HBeAg for at least 6 months, with a usual trend in liver function tests towards normal levels, although results may remain persistently elevated (Figure 31–2). Extrahepatic manifestations of HBV infection may occur and include serum sickness, polyarteritis nodosa, and membranoproliferative glomerulonephritis.

Complications

Complications of chronic infection may include progression to cirrhosis and hepatocellular carcinoma (HCC). Patients with active viral replication are at highest risk of chronic disease, with 15–20% developing progressive disease over a 5-year period. Continued positivity for HBeAg is associated with an increased risk of HCC. Most patients who are chronically infected remain HBsAg positive for their lifetime. There is no general agreement concerning the appropriate screening for patients with chronic infection for HCC. Some experts would not screen carriers if all laboratory tests are normal but would screen with ultrasonography and α-fetoprotein for evidence of chronic active hepatitis every 2–3 years, and more frequently in patients with cirrhosis. It appears that the incidence of progression of disease is greater in countries with high endemicity, and clinicians in these countries screen as frequently as every 6 months.

Treatment

Treatment for chronic disease depends on evidence of viral activity, HBeAg status, HIV and HCV comorbidity, histologic evidence of liver injury, and elevated liver function tests. Currently approved treatment modalities include interferon-alfa, lamivudine, and, most recently, abacavir and entecavir. Other new antiviral agents are currently being tested. Sensitive tests for determination of response to therapy, such as covalently closed circuit (ccc) DNA and others may be more readily available in the future.

3. Hepatitis C

General Considerations

HCV has become the most common blood-borne infection and the leading cause of chronic liver disease in the United States. It is also the leading cause of liver transplantation in the United States. Worldwide, more than 170 million people are infected, but the infection rates vary considerably. In the United States, it is estimated that around 3.8% of the population may be infected with HCV. The responsible virus is an RNA virus of the Flaviviridae family. Six major genotypes, numbered 1 through 6, are known, with additional subtypes. There are varying distributions of these genotypes, and they may affect the progression of disease and the response to treatment regimens.

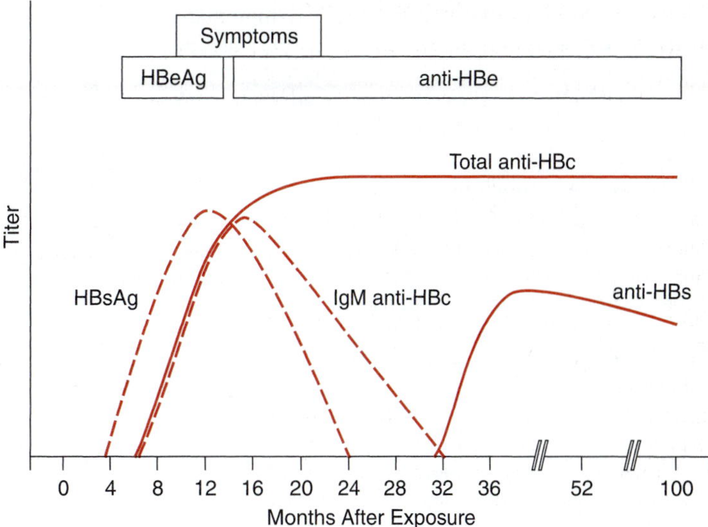

Figure 31–1. Acute hepatitis B virus infection with recovery.

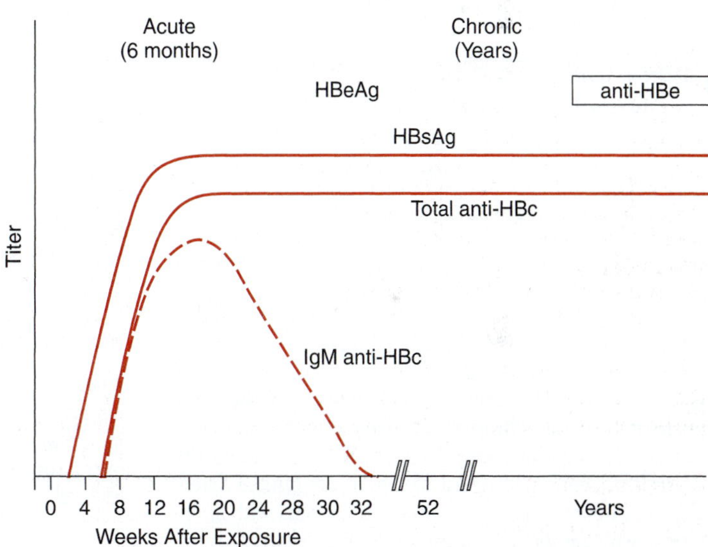

Figure 31–2. Progression to chronic hepatitis B virus infection.

HCV is spread primarily through percutaneous exposure to blood. Since 1992, all donated blood has been screened for HCV. Intravenous drug use is responsible for over 50% of new cases. Within 1–3 months after a first incident of needle sharing, 50–60% of intravenous drug users are infected. Other risk factors include use of intranasal cocaine, hemodialysis, tattooing (debatable), and vertical transmission, which is rare. Breast-feeding carries a low risk of transmission. Sexual transmission is uncertain but is probably 1–3% over the lifetime of a monogamous couple. Health care workers are at particular risk following a percutaneous exposure (1.8% average incidence).

Prevention

No immunizations are currently available for HCV infections. Prevention consists mainly of reduction of risk factors, including screening of blood and blood products, caution to prevent percutaneous injuries, and reduction in intravenous drug use.

Clinical Findings

A. Symptoms and Signs

1. Acute hepatitis—The incubation period for HCV varies between 2 and 26 weeks but most commonly is

6–7 weeks. Most patients with HCV are asymptomatic at the time of infection. However, over 20% of all recognized cases of acute hepatitis in the United States are caused by HCV, and as many as 30% of adults who are infected may present with jaundice. Acute, fulminant hepatic failure is rare.

2. Chronic hepatitis—In contrast to HAV and HBV, most people infected with HCV (85%) develop a chronic infection. The incidence of significant liver disease is 20–30% for cirrhosis and 4% for liver failure; over 1–4% of patients with chronic infection develop HCC annually, or 11–19% over 4–11 years in one study. It appears that certain risk factors increase the likelihood of progression to serious disease. These include increased alcohol intake, age greater than 40 years, HIV coinfection, and possibly male gender and other liver coinfections.

Extrahepatic manifestations of chronic infection are fairly common and are similar to those of HBV, including autoimmune conditions and renal conditions such as membranous glomerulonephritis.

B. Laboratory Findings

Patients should be first tested with an approved anti-HCV screening test. A positive test should be confirmed by a recombinant strip immunoblot assay (RIBA) test for anti-HCV or a reverse transcriptase polymerase chain reaction (RT-PCR) for HCV RNA. (Diagnosis of acute infection may require the use of the RT-PCR, because anti-HCV may not be positive for several weeks.)

Treatment

Treatment for both acute and chronic HCV has undergone significant strides in the past few years. A recent study documents the conversion of a significant number of patients to negative serology when treated in the acute phase of infection. Chronic HCV treated with a combination of pegylated interferon 2b (PEG-IFN) or 2a and ribavirin is the current standard of care in the United States, although poorer responses are seen in patients with genotype 1, which is the most common in this country.

It is important to immunize patients with chronic HCV infection for HAV, because the incidence of fulminant hepatitis A has been shown to be significantly increased in this population. Patients infected with HCV should also abstain from alcohol. It has also been recommended that HCV-infected individuals be vaccinated for HBV owing to the poor prognosis of coinfected individuals.

4. Other Types of Infectious Hepatitis

Over 97% of the viral hepatitis in the United States is either A, B, or C. Other types of viral hepatitis occur much less frequently, although worldwide, they may be more important.

Hepatitis D

Hepatitis D virus (HDV) is a virus that can replicate only in the presence of HBV infection. HDV infection can occur either as a coinfection with HBV or as a superinfection in a chronically infected individual with HBV. Although coinfection can produce more severe acute disease, a superinfection poses the risk of more significant chronic disease, with 70–80% of patients developing cirrhosis. The mode of transmission is most commonly percutaneous. The only tests commercially available in the United States are IgG–anti-HDV. Prevention of HDV depends on prevention for HBV. There are no products currently available to prevent HDV infection in patients infected with HBV.

Hepatitis E

Hepatitis E virus (HEV) is the most common cause of enterically transmitted non-A, non-B hepatitis. Acute HEV infection is similar to other forms of viral hepatitis; no chronic form is known. Severity of illness increases with age, and for reasons that are unclear, case fatality rates are particularly high in pregnant women. Most cases of HEV reported in the United States have occurred in travelers returning from areas of high endemicity. In certain areas of the world (North Africa, the Middle East, and Asia) epidemics of HEV may be common. Prevention includes avoidance of drinking water and other beverages of unknown purity, uncooked shellfish, and uncooked vegetables and fruits. No vaccines are currently available, and pooled gamma globulin does not appear to be effective.

Hepatitis F & G

The existence of a hepatitis F has been debated, and very rare cases of another newly identified virus have been reported, labeled *hepatitis G*. Very little is currently known of transmission or patterns of illness, although the infectivity level in the United States may be significant.

5. Acute Hepatitis: A Cost-Effective Approach

Because the vast majority of cases of viral hepatitis are caused by HAV, HBV, or HCV, tests to determine the precise etiology are necessary for appropriate primary and secondary prevention for the patient, as well as potential for therapy. Figure 31–3 outlines one cost-effective approach. If these tests fail to indicate a diagnosis, the etiology may be due to less frequent causes of viral hepatitis such as Epstein–Barr virus, in which jaundice can rarely accompany infectious mononucleosis; cytomegalovirus or herpesvirus in immunocompromised patients; or other nonviral etiologies, such as alcoholic hepatitis, drug toxicity, Wilson disease, or an autoimmune hepatitis.

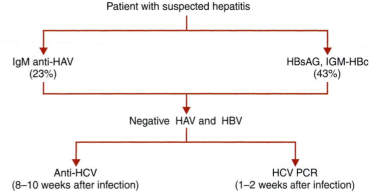

Patient with suspected hepatitis

IgM anti-HAV (23%)

HBsAG, IGM-HBc (43%)

Negative HAV and HBV

Anti-HCV (8–10 weeks after infection)

HCV PCR (1–2 weeks after infection)

Figure 31–3. **Cost-effective workup for acute viral hepatitis.** (Reproduced, with permission, from Ahmed A, Keefe E: Cost-effective evaluation of acute viral hepatitis. West J Med 2000;172:29.)

Advisory Committee on Immunization Practices (ACIP); Fiore AE et al: Prevention of hepatitis A through active or passive immunization: Recommendations of the Advisory Committee on Immunization Practices (ACIP). MMWR Recomm Rep 2006;55(RR-7):1. [PMID 16708058]

Ahmed A, Keefe E: Cost-effective evaluation of acute viral hepatitis. West J Med 2000;(179):29.[PMID 10695442]

Hughes CA, Shafran SD: Chronic hepatitis C virus management, 2000–2005 update. Ann Pharmacother 2006;40:74. [PMID: 16368925]

United Kingdom National Guideline on the Management of the Viral Hepatitis A, B and C, 2005. British Association for Sexual Health and HIV (BASHH), 2005.

US Public Health Service: Updated U.S. Public Health Service guidelines for the management of occupational exposures to HBV, HCV, and HIV and recommendations for postexposure prophylaxis. MMWR Morb Mortal Wkly Rep 2001;50(RR-11):1. [PMID 11442229]

Web Sites

American Liver Foundation, Liver Update: Function and Disease (excellent survey of issues pertaining to hepatitis):

http://www.liverfoundation.org

Centers for Disease Control National Center for Infectious Diseases, hepatitis information (references for immunization and testing, as well as patient information in several languages): http://www.cdc.gov/ncidod/diseases/hepatitis

National Institutes of Health, *Consensus Statement: Management of Hepatitis C: 2002.* June 10–12, 2002, Vol. 19, No. 1:

http://consensus.nih.gov/cons/116/116cdc_intro.htm

ALCOHOLIC LIVER DISEASE

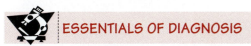

ESSENTIALS OF DIAGNOSIS

- *History of alcohol use.*
- *Mildly elevated serum ALT and AST.*
- *Variable clinical signs (may include jaundice, hepatomegaly).*

General Considerations

Alcoholic liver disease includes several different disease entities, spanning a large clinical spectrum. These diseases range from the syndrome of acute fatty liver to severe liver damage as manifested by cirrhosis. **Fatty liver** is usually asymptomatic except for occasional hepatomegaly and is the histologic result of excessive use of alcohol over a several-day period. In **perivenular fibrosis,** fibrous tissue is deposited in the central areas of the liver, particularly the central veins; this is an indication that the individual may then rapidly progress to more severe forms of liver disease. Patients can progress from this stage directly to cirrhosis. **Alcoholic hepatitis** is a condition in which necrosis of hepatic cells occurs as part of an inflammatory response, which includes polymorphonuclear cells, along with evidence of fibrosis. **Cirrhosis** may result from continued progression of disease from alcoholic hepatitis or may occur without evidence of prior alcoholic hepatitis. Cirrhosis is characterized by distortion of the liver structure, with bands of connective tissue forming between portal and central zones. Changes in hepatic blood circulation may also occur, resulting in portal hypertension. Additionally, evidence of abnormal fat metabolism, inflammation, and cholestasis may be seen. Progression to **hepatocellular carcinoma (HCC)** may also occur, although the exact risk of cirrhosis itself in the progression to HCC is not clear.

It is known that women are more likely than men to develop alcoholic liver disease, although the reasons for this phenomenon are only now being clarified. There may be additional genetic factors, most notably in specific enzyme systems, such as the metabolism of tumor necrosis factor (TNF) and alcohol-metabolizing systems, which affect the development of disease. Concomitant disease, such as HCV infection, is also a risk factor. Other factors (eg, obesity) may also play a role in the progression of disease.

Clinical Findings

A. Symptoms and Signs

A history of drinking alcohol in excess of 80 g/day (six to eight drinks) is seen with the development of more advanced forms of the disease, although there is considerable individual variation. Numerous questionnaires have been designed for detection of excessive drinking, but the CAGE questionnaire (Cut down, Annoyed by criticism, Guilty about drinking, Eye-opener drinks) is probably the most useful.

Clinical findings may be limited at this stage to occasional hepatomegaly. Patients with alcoholic hepatitis may present with classic signs and symptoms of acute hepatitis, including weight loss, anorexia, fatigue, nausea, and vomiting. Hepatomegaly may be evident, as well as other signs of more advanced disease, such as cirrhosis, because the development of cirrhosis may occur concomitant with a new episode of alcoholic hepatitis. These signs include jaundice, splenomegaly, ascites, spider angiomas, and signs of other organ damage secondary to alcoholism (eg, dementia, cardiomyopathy, or peripheral neuropathy).

B. Laboratory Findings

Various commercially available laboratory tests have been used to detect excessive alcohol intake in the early stages. The sensitivity and specificity of these tests vary. Liver function tests for elevations of AST, ALT, and GGT are frequently used. Elevation of mean corpuscular volume (MCV) has also been noted in patients with early-stage disease.

Transaminase levels are usually only mildly elevated in pure alcoholic hepatitis unless other disease processes, such as concomitant viral hepatitis, or acetaminophen ingestion are present (Figure 31–4). AST elevation is usually greater than ALT. Elevated prothrombin time and bilirubin levels have a significant negative prognostic indication. *The presence of jaundice may have special significance in any actively drinking person and should be carefully evaluated.* Several instruments have been used for evaluation of severity, but the most common is the Maddrey discriminant function (DF):

$$DF = 4.6 \times (\text{prothrombin time in seconds} - \text{control}) + \text{serum bilirubin (mg/dL)}$$

A score higher than 32 is indicative of high risk of death.

Treatment

Initial treatment centers on ensuring adequate volume replacement, with concern for the ability to handle normal saline. Diuretics should be avoided. Adequate nutrition should be given, parenterally if necessary. There is no indication that avoidance of protein is helpful in patients with encephalopathy. Broad-spectrum antibiotics should be considered early in the treatment course. Many patients develop spontaneous peritonitis, pneumonia, or cellulitis, which should be treated aggressively. Abstinence from alcohol is essential. Recovery from the acute episode is associated with an 80% 7-year survival rate versus 50% survival in those who continue drinking. Corticosteroids have been suggested as beneficial, but considerable debate still ensues. A subgroup of patients with hepatic encephalopathy may benefit.

Liver transplantation may be an option. Alcoholic liver disease is currently the second most common reason for liver transplantation in the United States. To be considered for transplantation, patients should not have active alcoholic hepatitis, should have remained sober for more than 6 months, and should have had addictive treatment. The prognosis is excellent if relapse from drinking can be avoided. Relapse occurs in 15–30% of patients.

Other treatment methodologies in various stages of testing include modification of TNF with pentoxifylline; antioxidant therapy with agents such as S-adenosyl-L-methionine (SAMe), silymarin, or vitamin E; and antifi-

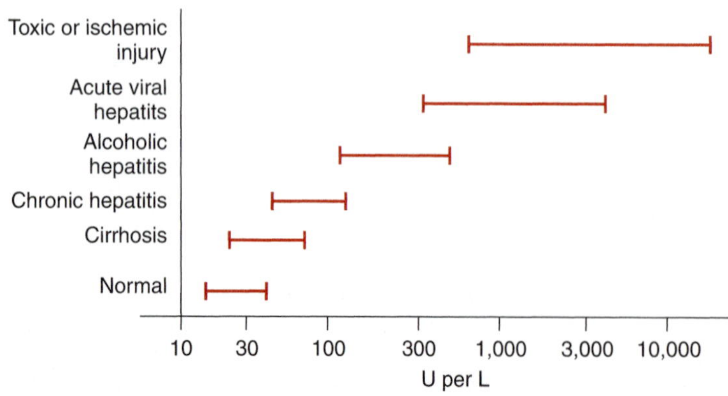

Figure 31–4. Typical AST or ALT values in disease. (Reproduced, with permission, from Johnson D: Am Fam Pract 1999.)

brotics such as polyenylphosphatidylcholine (PPC). Further studies are needed before these therapies can be recommended.

Maher J: Advances in liver disease: Alcoholic hepatitis, non-cirrhotic portal fibrosis, and complications of cirrhosis. Treatment of alcoholic hepatitis. J Gastroenterol Hepatol 2002;17:448. [PMID 11987726]

Yeung E, Wong FS: The management of cirrhotic ascites. Medscape Gen Med 2002;4(4). Available at: http://www.medscape.com/viewarticle/44236454.

OTHER LIVER DISEASES

1. Nonalcoholic Fatty Liver Disease

A new condition described around 1980, nonalcoholic fatty liver disease (NAFLD) encompasses a wide clinical spectrum of patients whose liver histology is similar to patients with alcohol-induced hepatitis, but without the requisite history. Women are affected more frequently than men. Many of these patients progress to cirrhosis. NAFLD is now the most common liver disease in the United States, occurring in up to 20% of the population in some studies. This condition is common in obese patients, as well as in patients with type 2 diabetes mellitus. It may be a part of the syndrome X, which includes obesity, diabetes mellitus, dyslipidemia, and hypertension. Clinical features include hepatomegaly (75%) and splenomegaly (25%), but no pathognomonic laboratory markers. Elevations of ALT and AST may be up to five times normal, with the AST:ALT ratio less than 1. Treatment includes weight reduction, treatment of diabetes, lipid disorders, and, possibly, ursodeoxycholic acid or vitamin E.

2. Wilson Disease

Wilson disease, which is characterized by hepatolenticular degeneration, is caused by abnormal metabolism of copper. It is inherited in an autosomal-recessive pattern and has a prevalence in the general population of about 1 in 30,000. Although patients in asymptomatic stages may manifest only transaminasemia or Kayser–Fleisher rings (golden-greenish granular deposits in the limbus), hepatomegaly or splenomegaly may already be present. In most symptomatic patients (96%), the serum ceruloplasmin level is less than 20 mg/dL. In patients with more advanced disease, symptoms of acute hepatitis or cirrhosis may be present. Neurologic signs include dysarthria, tremors, abnormal movements, and psychological disturbances. HCC may occur in patients with advanced disease. Treatment includes penicillamine, trientine, or zinc salts.

3. Hemochromatosis

An inborn error of iron metabolism leading to increased iron absorption from the diet, hemochromatosis is associated with diabetes, bronze skin pigmentation, hepatomegaly, loss of libido, and arthropathy. Patients may also show signs of cardiac or endocrine disorders. Symptoms usually first manifest between 40 and 60 years of age, and men are 10 times more likely than women to be affected. Hemochromatosis is the most common inherited liver disease in people of European descent. Physical signs include hepatomegaly (95% of symptomatic patients), which precedes abnormal liver function tests. Cardiac involvement includes congestive heart failure and arrhythmias. Many patients have cirrhosis by the time they are symptomatic (50–70%), 20% have fibrosis, and 10–20% have neither. HCC is very common in patients with cirrhosis (30%) and is now the most common cause of death. Laboratory findings include elevated serum iron concentration, increased serum ferritin, and increased transferrin saturation. Treatment involves treating the complications of hemochromatosis, removing excess iron by phlebotomy, and in patients with cirrhosis, surveillance for HCC and treatment of hepatic and cardiac failure.

4. Autoimmune Hepatitis

Autoimmune hepatitis is a hepatocellular inflammatory disease of unknown etiology. Diagnosis is based on histologic examination, hypergammaglobulinemia, and presence of serum autoantibodies. The condition may be difficult to discern from other causes of chronic liver disease, which need to be excluded in making the diagnosis. Immunoserologic tests that are essential for diagnosis are assays for antinuclear antibodies (ANA), smooth muscle antibodies (SMA), and antibodies to liver and kidney microsome type 1 (anti-LKM1), as well as perinuclear antineutrophil cytoplasmic antibodies (aANCAs).

5. Drug-Induced Liver Disease

More than 600 drugs or other medicinals have been implicated in liver disease. Worldwide, drug-induced liver disease represents about 3% of all adverse drug reactions; in the United States, more than 20% of cases of jaundice in the elderly are caused by drugs. Acetaminophen and other drugs account for 25–40% of fulminant hepatic failure. Diagnosis is based on the discovery of abnormalities in hepatic enzymes or the development of a hepatitis-like syndrome or jaundice. Most cases occur within 1 week to 3 months of exposure, and symptoms rapidly subside after cessation of the drug, returning to normal within 4 weeks of acute hepatocellular injury. Hepatic damage may manifest as acute hepatocellular injury (isoniazid, acetaminophen), cholestatic injury (contraceptive steroids, chlorpromazine), granulomatous hepatitis (allopurinol, phenylbutazone), chronic hepatitis (methotrexate), vascular injury (herbal tea preparations with toxic plant alkaloids), or neoplastic lesions (oral contraceptive steroids).

6. Primary Biliary Cirrhosis

This autoimmune disease of uncertain etiology is manifested by inflammation and destruction of interlobular and septal bile ducts, which can cause chronic cholestasis and biliary cirrhosis. It is predominantly a disease of middle-aged women (female-to-male ratio of 9:1) and is particularly prevalent in northern Europe. The condition may be diagnosed on routine testing or be suspected in women with symptoms of fatigue or pruritus, or in susceptible individuals with elevated serum alkaline phosphatase, cholesterol, and IgM levels. Antimitochondrial antibodies are frequently found. Ursodeoxycholic acid is the only therapy currently available, although some patients may benefit from liver transplantation.

7. Hepatic Tumors & Cysts

HCC is the most common malignant tumor of the liver; it is the fifth most common cancer in men, and the eighth most common in women. Incidence increases with age, but the mean age in ethnic Chinese and black African populations is lower. Signs of worsening cirrhosis may alert the clinician to consideration of HCC, but in many cases, the onset is subtle. There are no specific hepatic function tests to detect HCC, but elevated serum tumor markers, most notably α-fetoprotein, are useful. Ultrasonography can detect the majority of HCC but may not distinguish it from other solid lesions. CT and MRI are also helpful in making the diagnosis. Risk factors for HCC include HBV, HCV, all etiologic forms of cirrhosis, ingestion of foods with aflatoxin B_1, and smoking. In these patients, ultrasonography and α-fetoprotein measurements every 4–6 months are recommended. In moderate-risk patients (ie, with later-onset HBV), measurement of α-fetoprotein every 6 months and annual ultrasound study is suggested.

8. Benign Tumors

Benign tumors include hepatocellular adenomas, which have become more common with the use of oral contraceptive steroids, and cavernous hemangiomas, which may occur with pregnancy or oral contraceptive steroid use and are the most common benign tumor of the liver.

9. Liver Abscesses

Liver abscesses can be the result of infections of the biliary tract or can have an extrahepatic source such as diverticulitis or inflammatory bowel disease. In about 40% of cases, no source of infection is found. The most common organisms are *Escherichia coli, Klebsiella, Proteus, Pseudomonas,* and *Streptococcus* species. Amebic liver abscesses are the most common extraintestinal manifestation of amebiasis, which occurs in over 10% of the world's population and is most prevalent in the United States in young Hispanic adults. Amebic abscesses may have an acute presentation, with symptoms present for several weeks; few patients report typical intestinal symptoms such as diarrhea. Ultrasonography or CT scans with serologic tests such as enzyme-linked immunosorbent assay (ELISA) or indirect fluorescent antibody tests help confirm the diagnosis.

Alvarez F et al: International Autoimmune Hepatitis Group report: Review of criteria for diagnosis of autoimmune hepatitis. J Hepatol 1999;31:929. [PMID: 10580593]

Lewis JH: Drug-induced liver disease. Med Clin North Am 2000;84:1275. [PMID 11026929]

Powell LW, Yapp TR: Hemochromatosis. Clin Liver Dis 2000;4;211. [PMID 11232185]

Yu AS, Keeffe EB: Nonalcoholic fatty liver disease. Rev Gastroenterol Disord 2002;2:11. [PMID 12122975]

PANCREATIC DISEASE

Samuel C. Matheny, MD, MPH

ACUTE PANCREATITIS

ESSENTIALS OF DIAGNOSIS

- *Sudden, severe, abdominal pain in epigastric area, with frequent radiation to the back.*
- *Elevated serum amylase and lipase.*
- *Elevated ALT (biliary pancreatitis).*
- *Evidence of etiology on ultrasound (biliary causes) or CT and MRI (other causes).*

General Considerations

Hospital admissions for acute pancreatitis are fairly frequent, and the most common causes vary with the age and sex of the patient. In the United States, gallstones and alcohol abuse are the most frequent etiologies (20–30%), but infectious causes such as mumps virus or parasitic disease should be considered, as well as medications, tumors, and trauma. About 20% of cases are idiopathic. A more detailed discussion of gallstone pancreatitis appears earlier in this chapter.

Clinical Findings

A. Symptoms and Signs

Abdominal pain—usually epigastric, which may radiate to the back—is the common presenting sign. However, the pain may not be significant, and some cases of acute pancreatitis are missed or diagnosed after more significant complications have occurred. Abdominal tenderness ranging from rigidity to mild tenderness may be present. Lack of a specific diagnostic test may affect the accuracy of an early diagnosis.

B. Laboratory Findings

Useful laboratory tests include serum amylase (elevated 3–5 times above normal), serum lipase (more than twice normal), and, for determining the etiology, liver function tests, especially ALT. Serum amylases that are significantly elevated in the presence of epigastric pain are strong indicators of pancreatitis. However, amylase clears rapidly from the blood and levels may be normal even in patients with severe pancreatitis. A urine dipstick test for trypsinogen-2 may also be useful.

C. Prognostic Tests

Over 20% of patients have a severe case of pancreatitis and of these, a significant number die. It is therefore important to accurately stage the severity of the illness and treat accordingly. Attempts to quantify severity of disease have lead to certain scoring criteria, such as the Acute Physiology and Chronic Health Evaluation (APACHE) II score (> 7 on admission is indicative of severe illness), or the Ranson or Glasgow scores. All are complicated and have varying degrees of sensitivity and specificity. Peritoneal lavage has also been used, but it is difficult to justify in patients with mild symptoms. C-reactive protein scores that exceed 150 mg/L in the first 48 hours, interleukin-6 values greater than 400 pg/mL, and interleukin-8 values greater than 100 pg/mL on admission have also been suggested as indicators of severe pancreatitis. Other prognostic tests that may indicate severe illness include the following: urine trypsinogen activation peptide (TAP) greater than 35 nmol/L, urine trypsinogen-2 greater than 2000 mcg/L, and polymorphonuclear elastase (PMN-e) greater than 300 mcg/L, all measured within the first 24 hours of hospitalization.

D. Imaging Studies

Although ultrasonography is helpful in identifying the etiology of pancreatitis, it has limited value in staging the severity of disease. Contrast-enhanced CT is the most common currently available imaging technique for staging the severity of pancreatitis and can determine the presence of glandular enlargement, intra- and extrapancreatic fluid collections, inflammation, necrosis, and abscesses. This study may not be necessary for patients with mild disease. Magnetic resonance cholangiopancreatography (MRCP) may be as accurate as and has some advantages over contrast-enhanced CT in certain patients.

Complications

Complications include organ failure, cardiovascular collapse, and fluid collections around the pancreas. The latter may be asymptomatic or they may enlarge, causing pain, fever, and infection. Pancreatic pseudocysts may occur in patients with very high amylase levels and obstruction of the pancreatic duct. Pancreatic necrosis may also occur, and can be fatal. Infection of necrotic tissue should be suspected in patients with unexpected deterioration, fever, and leukocytosis, and confirmed by CT scan and fine-needle aspiration. Sterile necrosis should probably be managed nonoperatively unless progressive deterioration occurs. Septic necrosis usually requires surgical debridement.

Treatment

Patients who have the potential to develop severe pancreatitis, or who already have severe pain, dehydration, or vomiting, should be hospitalized and their hydration needs monitored closely. These patients should receive nothing by mouth and should be given intravenous pain medication. Patients should be monitored carefully to assess adequate renal function, because renal failure is a major cause of morbidity and mortality. Signs of worsening condition include rising hematocrit, tachycardia, and lack of symptom improvement in 48 hours.

Nutritional treatment has evolved in recent years, but areas of controversy remain. Increasing evidence indicates that in cases of mild pancreatitis, there is no benefit to nasogastric suction, and patients who are not vomiting may continue oral fluids or resume oral fluids after the first week. There is also growing evidence that in severe pancreatitis, early enteral feeding within the first week may lower endotoxin absorption and reduce other complications. If patients cannot absorb adequate quantities via the enteric route, then parenteral feeding may be necessary.

The use of antibiotics is also controversial. Prophylactic antibiotics have been used in severe pancreatitis, but some concern exists that they may predispose patients to fungal infections. General consensus is to use antibiotics, preferably broad-spectrum agents, for severe pancreatitis and for as brief a period as possible (ie, < 7 days).

Rettally CA et al. The usefulness of laboratory tests in the early assessment of severity of acute pancreatitis. Crit Rev Clin Lab Sci 2003;40:117. [PMID: 12755453]

Whitcomb D: Clinical practice. Acute pancreatitis. N Engl J Med 2006;354:2142. [PMID: 16707751]

Yousaf M et al: Management of severe acute pancreatitis. Br J Surg 2003;90:407. [PMID: 12673741]

PANCREATIC CANCER

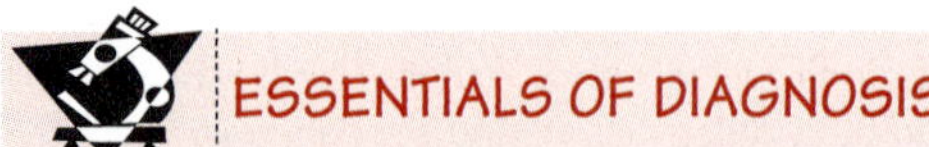

- *Anorexia, jaundice, weight loss, epigastric pain radiating to back, dark urine, and light stools.*
- *Spiral CT of the abdomen or endoscopic ultrasonography showing evidence of tumor.*
- *CA 19-9 serum tumor marker.*

General Considerations

Although pancreatic cancer is diagnosed in only 30,000 patients each year in the United States, it is the fourth most common cause of death from cancer and the second most common gastrointestinal malignancy. Pancreatic cancer has a very poor prognosis: over 80% of patients die within the first year, and the 5-year survival rate is less than 4%. In the vast majority of patients, the cancer is discovered at too late a stage to benefit from resection, and the response to chemotherapy is very poor. Over 90% of pancreatic cancers are ductal adenocarcinoma.

Cigarette smoking is the major risk factor established to date. Diet may also be a factor, with high intake of fat or meat and obesity associated with an increased risk, and fruits, vegetables, and exercise being protective. Likewise, a history of chronic pancreatitis is considered a risk factor, along with surgery for peptic ulcer disease, hereditary pancreatitis, and some genetic mutations (eg, *BRAC2,* associated with hereditary breast cancer). No guidelines currently exist regarding screening of the general population for pancreatic cancer, although some experts feel that patients with a family history of hereditary pancreatitis should be screened.

Clinical Findings

A. Symptoms and Signs

The clinical presentation of pancreatic cancer can vary widely; tumors that occur in the head of the pancreas (two thirds of all pancreatic cancer) may produce early signs of obstructive jaundice. Tumors in the body and tail of the pancreas may grow quite large and cause fewer signs of obstruction. Symptoms more likely to be associated with pancreatic cancer include abdominal pain, jaundice, dark urine, light-colored stools, and weight loss. Pain may be worse when the patient is lying flat or eating. Other physical signs associated with pancreatic cancer include Courvoisier sign (palpable, nontender gallbladder in a patient with jaundice).

B. Laboratory Findings

Laboratory evaluation should include liver function tests. The serum tumor antigen CA 19-9 may be useful in confirming a diagnosis but is not an appropriate screening tool. Other markers such as human chorionic gonadotropin (β-hCG) and CA 72-4 are under consideration.

C. Imaging Studies

There is some debate as to the best imaging study. Dual-phase spiral CT with a pancreatic protocol has a high rate of sensitivity and can also assist in staging of the tumor, which is important for clinical management. Endoscopic ultrasonography may become the most accurate test for diagnosis.

Treatment

Because the only hope for a cure is surgical resection, staging of pancreatic tumors is important for management. The difficulty lies in identifying the small fraction of patients who will benefit from surgery from those who will not—patients with metastatic disease who would otherwise be subjected to unnecessary invasive procedures and the resultant increased morbidity and mortality.

For patients with metastatic disease, chemotherapy and palliative care should be offered; surgery is avoided. Patients with advanced local disease but no metastases may benefit from radiotherapy and chemotherapy, and those without invasion or metastases may be candidates for resection. Even with resection, the outlook is poor (5-year survival rates of < 25%). Radiation therapy may be useful in some patients with localized but nonresectable tumors, and chemotherapy (5-fluorouracil and gemcitabine) has some limited success.

Pain management can be a significant problem, and various modalities may need to be utilized. Biliary decompression may be required for jaundice.

Freelove R, Walling A: Pancreatic cancer: Diagnosis and management. Am Fam Physician 2006;73:485. [PMID: 16477897]

Holly EA et al: Signs and symptoms of pancreatic cancer. A population-based case-control study in the San Francisco Bay area. Clin Gastroenterol Hepatol 2004;2:510. [PMID: 15181621]

Lowenfels A, Maisonneuve P: Epidemiology and prevention of pancreatic cancer. Jpn J Clin Oncol 2004:34;238. [PMID: 15231857]

Vaginal Bleeding

32

Patricia Evans, MD, MA

General Considerations

Abnormal bleeding affects up to 30% of women at some time during their lives. Evaluating vaginal bleeding involves an examination of the patient's menstrual cycle. The normal menstrual cycle is generally 21–35 days in length with a menstrual flow lasting 2–7 days and a total menstrual blood loss of 20–60 mL. During the normal menstrual cycle the endometrium is exposed initially to estrogen, followed by ovulation and production of progesterone as well as estrogen, and finally the withdrawal of estrogen and progesterone, causing menstruation.

Different diseases are associated with certain patterns of vaginal bleeding, although there is a wide variation in presentation within each. Common terminology used to discuss vaginal bleeding includes menorrhagia, metrorrhagia, menometrorrhagia, hypermenorrhea, polymenorrhea, and oligomenorrhea. The bleeding patterns associated with each term are listed in Table 32–1.

There are normal changes in most women's menstrual patterns throughout their lifetimes. Just as anovulation is common during the years following menarche, the perimenopausal patient usually experiences changes in her menstrual cycle related to decreasing, irregular anovulation. Although age plays an important role in constructing a differential diagnosis in a patient presenting with vaginal bleeding, many of the causes can occur in any adult woman.

Albers JR: Abnormal uterine bleeding. Am Fam Physician 2004; 69:1915. [PMID: 15117012]

Clinical Findings

A. Symptoms and Signs

1. History—Taking a history of a patient who presents with vaginal bleeding should begin with an exploration of the patient's usual bleeding pattern. The physician should try to establish whether the patient's pattern is cyclic or anovulatory. If the patient menstruates every 21–35 days her cycle is consistent with an ovulatory pattern of bleeding. To confirm ovulation patients can check their basal body temperature, cervical mucus, and luteinizing hormone (LH) levels. Basal body temperature can be checked using a basal body temperature thermometer, which allows for a precise measurement of the patient's temperature within a narrower range than a standard thermometer. The patient takes her temperature orally as soon as she awakens in the morning and records it on a chart. After ovulation the ovary secretes an increased amount of progesterone, causing an increase in temperature of approximately 0.5°F over the baseline temperature in the follicular phase. The luteal phase is often accompanied by an elevation of temperature that lasts 10 days. In addition, patients can be taught to check the consistency of their cervical mucus, watching for a change from the sticky, whitish cervical mucus of the follicular phase to the clear, stretching mucus of ovulation. Finally, the patient can use an enzyme-linked immunosorbent assay, available as a home testing kit, to check for the elevation of LH over baseline that occurs with ovulation.

The patient should then be asked by the physician to describe the current vaginal bleeding in terms of onset, frequency, duration, and severity. This history will help the physician to focus the differential diagnosis. For example, if the patient reports a long-standing history of anovulatory bleeding the workup can focus on causes for chronic hyperandrogenicity such as polycystic ovarian syndrome (PCOS) and congenital adrenal hyperplasia (CAH). Age, parity, sexual history, previous gynecologic disease, and obstetric history further assist the physician in focusing the evaluation of the woman with vaginal bleeding. These questions help in evaluating the likelihood of pregnancy-related causes of vaginal bleeding, infectious disease, and cancer.

The physician should ask about medications, including contraceptives, prescription medications, and over-the-counter medications and supplements. Contraception is a common cause of vaginal bleeding in women. Specifically, the patient should be asked about any over-the-counter preparations she may be taking. Patients may not be aware that herbal preparations may contribute to vaginal bleeding. Ginseng, which has estrogenic properties, can cause vaginal bleeding and St John's Wort can interact with oral contraceptives to cause breakthrough bleeding. A review of symptoms should include questions regarding fever, fatigue, abdominal pain, hirsutism, galactorrhea, changes in bowel movements, and intolerance to heat or cold. A

Table 32–1. Patterns of vaginal bleeding.

Descriptive Term	Bleeding Pattern
Menorrhagia	Regular cycles, prolonged duration, excessive flow
Metrorrhagia	Irregular cycles
Menometrorrhagia	Irregular cycles, prolonged duration, and excessive flow
Hypermenorrhea	Regular cycles, normal duration, and excessive flow
Polymenorrhea	Frequent cycles
Oligomenorrhea	Infrequent cycles

careful family history will aid in identifying patients with a predisposition to PCOS, CAH, thyroid disease, premature ovarian failure, fibroids, and cancer. Physicians should also keep in mind that women usually present complaining of vaginal bleeding when symptoms deviate from the patient's normal bleeding pattern. Patients with chronic anovulatory bleeding patterns or lifelong heavy menses secondary to von Willebrand disease may not perceive their underlying menses pattern as abnormal. Therefore, the physician should avoid asking the patient if her periods have been "normal" and instead should ask for specific details regarding the patient's bleeding pattern.

2. Physical examination—The physical examination for women complaining of vaginal bleeding should begin with an evaluation of the patient's vital signs. Does the patient have a fever (indicating possible infection), increased pulse, low blood pressure, or significant orthostatic changes in blood pressure (indicating significant acute blood loss)? Has she had a significant weight change and an enlarged or tender thyroid gland, indicating thyroid disease? The physician should also evaluate the patient's weight for obesity and hair distribution for hirsutism. These can indicate possible chronic anovulation syndromes. The pelvic examination will aid in identifying other causes of bleeding, including anatomic abnormalities such as cervical polyps; signs of infections such as cervical discharge, cervical motion tenderness, and uterine or adnexal tenderness; signs of pregnancy such as changes in the cervix and a symmetrically enlarged uterus; and signs of fibroids such as an enlarged but irregular uterus.

B. Evaluation

The evaluation of patients presenting with vaginal bleeding includes a combination of laboratory testing, imaging studies, and sampling techniques. The evaluation is directed both by patient presentation and a risk evaluation for endometrial cancer. For example, a patient who presents with a history and physical examination consistent with pelvic inflammatory disease (PID) will obviously be tested for gonorrhea and chlamydia. If the physician feels an enlarged uterus on physical examination the initial evaluation will include a pregnancy test followed by a pelvic ultrasound. If the results are inconclusive a sonohysterogram can aid in detecting a focal versus a diffuse lesion. This in turn can lead to a hysteroscopy for further evaluation of a focal lesion or an endometrial biopsy for a diffuse lesion.

The choice of evaluation is also based on the risk of endometrial cancer. For a patient who is at risk, an endometrial biopsy should be included in the evaluation. Patients having prolonged exposure to unopposed estrogen (either iatrogenically or because of chronic anovulation) for more than 1 year, regardless of age, should also have an endometrial biopsy. In addition, because the incidence of endometrial cancer begins to increase after the age of 35, any patient older than this should also have an endometrial biopsy during an evaluation for unexplained vaginal bleeding.

C. Laboratory Studies

Most patients presenting with vaginal bleeding should be evaluated with a complete blood count. In addition, every woman of reproductive age should have a urine or serum pregnancy test. Thyroid-stimulating hormone should be evaluated in women whose symptoms are consistent with hypo- or hyperthyroidism and in those who present with a change from a normal menstrual pattern.

Adolescents presenting with menorrhagia at menarche should have an evaluation for coagulopathies, including a prothrombin time, partial thromboplastin time, and bleeding time.

There is no general agreement on the diagnostic criteria for PCOS. In patients with symptoms suggestive of PCOS it is reasonable to check for elevated LH, testosterone, and androstenedione. These values may be elevated in patients with PCOS, but due to the large variation among individual women these tests are not definitive. Therefore, the physician needs to interpret test results in conjunction with the clinical picture to make a diagnosis of PCOS.

Overall, the incidence of adult-onset CAH is about 2% in women with hyperandrogenic symptoms. The incidence is higher in individuals of Italian, Ashkenazi, and Yugoslav heritage. Deciding on screening for adult-onset CAH should be based on both the patient's clinical presentation and the patient's ethnic background. A basal 17-hydroxyprogesterone (17-HP) level should be drawn in the early morning to screen for adult-onset CAH. Patients with an abnormal result can have another 17-HP level drawn after receiving a dose of adrenocorticotropic hormone (ACTH).

D. Imaging Studies

1. Ultrasonography—A pelvic ultrasound study can be used to evaluate the ovaries, uterus, and endometrial lining for abnormalities. An evaluation of the ovaries can assist in the diagnosis of PCOS, because many women with PCOS have enlarged ovaries with multiple, small follicles. As with laboratory testing, this study does not provide a definitive diagnosis.

Pelvic ultrasonography is also useful for evaluating an enlarged uterus for the presence of fibroids. Fibroids appear as hypoechoic, solid masses seen within the borders of the uterus. Subserosal fibroids can be pedunculated and therefore can be seen outside the borders of the uterus.

An endovaginal ultrasound study can be used to evaluate the thickness of the endometrial stripe. The results need to be interpreted based on whether a patient is pre- or postmenopausal. For all women, the thicker the endometrial stripe, the more likely it is that the patient has an endometrial abnormality.

Endovaginal ultrasonography is a sensitive test for patients with postmenopausal bleeding whether or not they are using hormone replacement therapy. Therefore, postmenopausal patients with an endometrial stripe thicker than 4–5 mm should have a histologic biopsy. Hormone replacement therapy can cause proliferation of a patient's endometrium, making an endovaginal evaluation less specific.

Endovaginal ultrasonography is also useful in evaluating the endometrial stripe in premenopausal patients. Whereas the normal endometrial stripe is thicker in the premenopausal patient than in the postmenopausal patient, the median thickness of an abnormal endometrium is similar for both. The endovaginal ultrasound examination is less likely to detect myomas and polyps.

2. Sonohysterography—Sonohysterography involves performing a transvaginal ultrasound following installation of saline into the uterus. Performed after an abnormal vaginal ultrasound, the study is most useful in differentiating focal from diffuse endometrial abnormalities. Detection of a focal abnormality indicates the need for evaluation by hysteroscopy, and detection of an endometrial abnormality indicates the need to perform an endometrial biopsy or dilation and curettage (D&C). This can be considered as a study of first choice in premenopausal women with abnormal uterine bleeding.

3. Magnetic resonance imaging—Magnetic resonance imaging (MRI) can be used to evaluate the uterine structure. The endometrium can be evaluated with an MRI scan, but the endometrial area seen on MRI does not correspond exactly to the endometrial stripe measured with ultrasound. In most situations, transvaginal ultrasound is the preferred imaging modality, but if the patient cannot tolerate the procedure MRI provides an option for evaluation. MRI is better than ultrasound in distinguishing adenomyosis from fibroids, so if the history and examination suggest either of these, an MRI may be the best first choice. MRI is also sometimes used to evaluate fibroids prior to uterine artery embolization.

E. Endometrial Sampling

The workup for endometrial cancer should be pursued most aggressively with patients at greatest risk for the disease, such as postmenopausal patients who present with vaginal bleeding. In patients younger than 40 years, endometrial cancer is usually seen in obese patients, patients who are chronically anovulatory, or both. Therefore, a patient who presents with an anovulatory pattern of bleeding for more than 1 year should be evaluated for hyperplasia and neoplasm with an endometrial sample. In addition, the evaluation of women older than 35–40 years who present with a new onset of menorrhagia should include endometrial sampling, because the incidence of endometrial cancer increases after age 35.

Findings from the initial workup and response to treatment will determine the need for additional studies, including sonohysterography, diagnostic hysterography, and MRI.

1. Dilation and curettage—D&C provides a blind sampling of the endometrium, of less than half the uterine cavity. Because an endometrial biopsy can be completed in the office setting, it has generally replaced the D&C as the initial method of obtaining an endometrial sample. D&C is useful in patients with cervical stenosis or other anatomic factors that prevent an adequate endometrial biopsy. It is not effective as the sole treatment for menorrhagia.

2. Endometrial biopsy—An endometrial biopsy is an adequate method of sampling the endometrial lining to identify histologic abnormalities. Several devices can be used. Early devices were hooked to an external suction source. More commonly clinicians use one of the clear, flexible endometrial curettes with an inner plunger or piston that generates suction during the procedure. The different devices available (eg, Pipelle, Explora, Z-Sampler, and Endosampler) provide similar biopsy results. The rates of obtaining an adequate endometrial sample depend on the age of the patient. Because many postmenopausal women have an atrophic endometrium, sampling in this group more often results in an inadequate endometrial specimen for examination. In this situation, the clinician must use additional diagnostic studies to fully evaluate the cause of the vaginal bleeding.

3. Diagnostic hysteroscopy—Hysteroscopes are available in a variety of forms, including rigid, semirigid, and flexible. Diameters range from less than 3 mm to 6 mm. All hysteroscopes uses a light source, camera, and dilating medium to visualize the uterine cavity.

The direct exploration of the uterus is useful in identifying structural abnormalities such as fibroids and endometrial polyps. Small-caliber hysteroscopes allow the endometrium to be evaluated without the need for cervical dilation. Currently these instruments are limited by the fact that instruments cannot be passed through the endoscope and by their limited field of view. Hysteroscopes with larger diameters allow specific biopsy of lesions. In general, the diagnostic hysteroscopy is combined with a D&C or endometrial biopsy to maximize identification of abnormalities.

Bradley LD et al: Radiographic imaging techniques for the diagnosis of abnormal uterine bleeding. Obstet Gynecol Clin North Am 2000;27:245. [PMID: 10857118]

Burkman RT et al: Current perspectives on oral contraceptive use. Am J Obstet Gynecol 2001;185:4. [PMID: 1152117]

Cooper JM, Erickson ML: Endometrial sampling techniques in the diagnosis of abnormal uterine bleeding. Obstet Gynecol Clin 2000;27:235. [PMID: 10857117]

Hatasaka H: The evaluation of abnormal uterine bleeding. Clin Obstet Gynecol 2005;48:258. [PMID: 15805785]

Mol BW: Saline contrast hysterosonography is an accurate diagnostic test in women with abnormal bleeding—meta-analysis. Evidence-based Obstet Gynecol 2004;6:17.

Klein A, Schwartz ML: Uterine artery embolization for the treatment of uterine fibroids: An outpatient procedure. Am J Obstet Gynecol 2001;184:1556. [PMID: 11408880]

Laing FC et al: Gynecologic ultrasound. Radiol Clin North Am 2001;39:523. [PMID: 11506091]

Differential Diagnosis

The differential diagnosis of vaginal bleeding encompasses a wide range of possible etiologies. The patient's history and physical examination will determine the direction of the workup. Age and ovulatory status play important roles in determining the direction of the workup once relatively straightforward causes of vaginal bleeding such as pregnancy and infection have been eliminated.

The history and physical examination often lead to a narrowing of the differential diagnosis (Table 32–2). The physician should not narrow the differential diagnosis too quickly, because a patient can have more than one possible cause of vaginal bleeding. For example, a patient on oral contraceptives could also present with PID or hypothyroidism. Generating the differential diagnosis will aid the physician in deciding how to further evaluate and treat the patient.

A. Pregnancy-Related Bleeding

The initial evaluation of any patient presenting with vaginal bleeding should include testing for pregnancy. In recent years urinary assays for β-human chorionic gonadotropin have become so sensitive that they are a viable alternative to serum testing. The differential diagnosis for vaginal bleeding for pregnancy varies depending on the estimated gestational age. Early in pregnancy it includes spontaneous miscarriage, ectopic pregnancy, and trophoblastic disease. Later in pregnancy the appearance of bleeding should lead the physician to investigate the possibilities of placenta previa and placental abruption.

B. Bleeding Secondary to Hormone Medications

1. Contraception—Vaginal bleeding is a common side effect of many forms of contraception. Many women starting oral contraceptive pills (OCPs) experience breakthrough bleeding in the initial months. Lower dose OCPs have higher rates of spotting and breakthrough bleeding. Possible causes of vaginal bleeding in patients taking OCPs include inadequate estrogenic or progestogenic stimulation of the endometrium, skipped pills, or altered absorption and metabolism of the pills.

Vaginal bleeding is also frequent with Depo-Provera, and is the most commonly cited reason women discontinue taking it, as well as OCPs. For this reason, when initiating either form of contraception the expected course of possible bleeding should be discussed with the patient. After the initial dose of Depo–Provera, 50% of women experience irregular bleeding or spotting; this decreases to 25% after 1 year of use.

2. Hormone replacement therapy—The indications for hormone replacement therapy (HRT) have been greatly decreased since the findings of the Women's Health Initiative study were released. Nonetheless, some women continue to receive HRT. Bleeding is common with HRT, and can occur with both the sequential and continuous regimens. With sequential administration of estrogen and progesterone, most women experience bleeding near the end or right after taking the progesterone therapy. Although most women taking sequential therapy continue to bleed every month, women can experience abnormal bleeding patterns, including heavy or prolonged bleeding during the regular cycle or bleeding between cycles.

Theoretically patients taking continuous estrogen and progesterone therapy should not experience any bleeding, because the therapy is meant to result in an atrophic endometrium. In reality, about 40% of women who start continuous regimens experience bleeding within 4–6 months of initiating treatment. To avoid higher rates of irregular bleeding many physicians use sequential HRT for 12 months after the start of menopause to avoid the effects of endogenous ovarian function.

C. Anatomic Causes

1. Fibroids—Fibroids or leiomyomas are benign uterine tumors that are often asymptomatic. The most common

Table 32–2. Differential diagnosis of vaginal bleeding.

Diagnosis	Clinical Presentation	Most Commonly Associated Bleeding Pattern
Contraception	Known OCP/Depo use	OCP: spotting Depo: irregular or continuous bleeding
HRT	Known HRT use	Sequential: menorrhagia or spotting Continuous: irregular spotting
Fibroids	Asymptomatic, pelvic pain, and/or dysmenorrhea	Menorrhagia
Adenomyosis	Dysmenorrhea	Menorrhagia
Endometrial polyps	Asymptomatic	Intermenstrual spotting, metrorrhagia and/or menorrhagia
Cervical polyps	Asymptomatic	Intermenstrual and/or postcoital bleeding
PID	High-risk sexual behavior, fever, pelvic pain, tenderness	Menorrhagia and/or metrorrhagia
PCOS, Adult-onset CAH	Hirsutism, acne, central obesity, or asymptomatic	Oligomenorrhea, menometrorrhagia
Hyperthyroidism	Nervousness, heat intolerance, diarrhea, palpitations, weight loss	Oligomenorrhea, amenorrhea, polymenorrhea, or menorrhagia
Hypothyroidism	Fatigue, cold intolerance, dry skin, hair loss, constipation, weight gain	Menorrhagia, polymenorrhea, oligomenorrhea, amenorrhea
Bleeding disorder	Asymptomatic mucocutaneous bleeding, easy bruising	Menorrhagia
Endometrial hyperplasia	Asymptomatic	Menorrhagia and/or metrorrhagia
Endometrial cancer	Asymptomatic	Postmenopausal: irregular spotting Perimenopausal: menometrorrhagia
Cervical cancer	Asymptomatic	Irregular spotting, postcoital bleeding

OCP, oral contraceptive pills; HRT, hormone replacement therapy; PID, pelvic inflammatory disease; PCOS, polycystic ovarian syndrome; CAH, congenital adrenal hyperplasia.

symptoms associated with fibroid tumors are pelvic discomfort and abnormal uterine bleeding. Fibroids can be subserosal, intramural, or submucosal. Fibroids located subserosally may be felt on the physical examination as an irregular enlargement of the surface. Depending on the size of the fibroid, intramural and subserosal fibroids can be more difficult to palpate on examination. Most commonly, women with symptomatic fibroids experience either heavy or prolonged periods. In the past, theories about possible mechanisms of uterine bleeding included increased vascularity, interference with uterine contractility, endometrial ulceration, and increased endometrial surface area. More recently, there is evidence to suggest that fibroids involve abnormalities of growth factors that in turn have direct effects on vascular function and angiogenesis.

2. Adenomyosis—Adenomyosis is defined as the presence of endometrial glands within the myometrium. This is usually asymptomatic, but women can present with heavy or prolonged menstrual bleeding as well as dysmenorrhea. The dysmenorrhea can be severe and begin up to 1 week prior to menstruation. The appearance of symptoms usually occurs after age 40.

3. Endometrial and cervical polyps—Endometrial polyps can cause intermenstrual spotting, irregular bleeding, and menorrhagia. In contrast, cervical polyps usually cause intermenstrual spotting or postcoital bleeding. Other cervical lesions such as condyloma and herpes simplex virus ulcerations can present with similar abnormal bleeding patterns.

D. Infectious Causes

Microorganisms, including sexually transmitted microorganisms, respiratory pathogens, and endogenous vaginal bacteria, can ascend into the endometrium and fallopian tubes, causing PID. Factors that increase endocervical accessibility increase a patient's risk for

PID. This occurs during menstruation, and with alterations in the cervical mucus secondary to alterations in the vaginal flora due to bacterial vaginosis. PID in its classic form presents with fever, pelvic discomfort, cervical motion tenderness, and adnexal tenderness. Patients can present atypically with nothing but a change in their bleeding pattern. PID can cause menorrhagia or metrorrhagia, so the patient presenting with abnormal vaginal bleeding should be fully evaluated for PID.

The squamous epithelium of the ectocervix is a continuation of the vaginal epithelium. Therefore, cervical inflammation occurs in the ectocervix when invaded by microorganisms causing vaginitis. The physician will see a bright red cervix ("strawberry" cervix) in patients with severe cases of trichomonas. The pathogens causing mucopurulent endocervicitis (*Neisseria gonorrhoeae* and *Chlamydia trachomatis*) invade the glandular epithelium of the endocervix. Both kinds of cervical inflammation can cause intermenstrual spotting and postcoital bleeding.

E. Anovulatory Bleeding

When a woman does not ovulate she does not produce a corpus luteum, and then does not produce any progesterone. As a result, the endometrium of the uterus continues to proliferate. Eventually the growth of the endometrium cannot be sustained, resulting in irregular sloughing of the uterine lining. This irregular sloughing causes the bleeding pattern associated with anovulatory bleeding: irregular, heavy periods.

There are multiple causes of anovulation, including physiologic and pathologic etiologies. During the first year following menarche, anovulation is a normal result of an immature hypothalamic–pituitary–gonadal axis. Irregular ovulation also is a normal physiologic result of declining ovarian function during the perimenopausal years, and the hormonal changes associated with lactation.

Hyperandrogenic causes of anovulation include PCOS, adult-onset CAH, and androgen-producing tumors. The etiology of PCOS is uncertain, and its clinical features vary. Most recently research has focused on the underlying disorder of insulin resistance in these patients, and the possibility that hyperinsulinemia stimulates excess ovarian androgen production. Making the diagnosis of PCOS involves the evaluation of clinical features and endocrine abnormalities, and the exclusion of other etiologies. Women with PCOS can present with oligomenorrhea or dysfunctional uterine bleeding from prolonged anovulation. In addition, these women can have hirsutism, acne, and central obesity. Endocrinologically they can have increased testosterone activity, elevated LH concentration with a normal follicle-stimulating hormone level, and hyperinsulinemia due to insulin resistance. PCOS usually has its onset during puberty, and so these women often report a long history of irregular periods.

Adult-onset CAH results from an enzyme defect in the adrenal gland, most commonly a deficiency of 21-hydroxylase. There are three hypothesized allelic variants of the 21-hydroxylase deficiency gene: a normal variant, a mild variant, and a severe variant. Patients with adult-onset CAH are either homozygous for the mild allele or have one mild and one severe allele. The genetic defect causes an abnormality in steroid synthesis of glucocorticoids. The hypothalamic–pituitary axis compensates by increasing secretion of ACTH. This in turn causes a hyperplastic adrenal cortex, which produces increased androgens as well as corticoid precursors. Phenotypically women can present in a variety of ways: with PCOS symptoms, with hirsutism alone, or with hyperandrogenic laboratory work but no hyperandrogenic symptoms. Typically patients present at or after puberty. As a result, these women also report a long history of irregular periods.

Other causes of anovulation, including androgen-producing tumors, hypothalamic dysfunction, hyperprolactinemia, pituitary disease, and premature ovarian failure, are more likely to present as amenorrhea than vaginal bleeding.

F. Endocrine Abnormalities

Both hyper- and hypothyroidism can cause changes in a woman's menstrual cycle. Hyperthyroidism can cause amenorrhea, oligomenorrhea, hypermenorrhea, or polymenorrhea. Of all the menstrual abnormalities, oligomenorrhea is the most common in patients with hyperthyroidism. Patients who smoke and have higher total thyroxine (T_4) levels tend to have more menstrual disturbances.

A patient with hypothyroidism may experience changes in her menstrual cycle including amenorrhea, oligomenorrhea, polymenorrhea, or menorrhagia. Menstrual abnormalities occur more frequently with severe than with mild hypothyroidism. Hypothyroidism most likely causes menorrhagia through a combination of anovulation and subsequent breakthrough bleeding as well as decreased levels of coagulation factors.

G. Bleeding Disorders

Formation of a platelet plug is the first step of homeostasis during menstruation. Patients with disorders that interfere with the formation of a normal platelet plug can experience menorrhagia. The two most common disorders are von Willebrand disease and thrombocytopenia. Bleeding can be particularly severe at menarche, due to the dominant estrogen stimulation causing increased vascularity. Patients with von Willebrand disease usually present with a long history of heavy periods. Patients with thrombocytopenia may have menorrhagia at the onset of their disease.

Bleeding disorders resulting from coagulation deficiencies cause impaired formation of fibrin from fibrinogen. These deficiencies are more common in men. They more often cause bleeding in soft tissues and mucocutaneous tissues. Cases of menorrhagia in women with coagulation deficiencies have been reported.

H. Endometrial Hyperplasia

Endometrial hyperplasia is an overgrowth of the glandular epithelium of the endometrial lining. This usually occurs when a patient is exposed to unopposed estrogen, either estrogenically or because of anovulation. Retrospectively, we know that the rate of neoplasms found with simple hyperplasia is 1% and that the rate with complex hyperplasia is much higher, reaching almost 30% when atypia is present. It is not known whether the different types of hyperplasia reflect a spectrum, what percentage progress to invasive cancer, and over what time period this occurs. Most patients without atypia respond to progestin therapy. Patients having hyperplasia with atypia should have a hysterectomy due to the high incidence of subsequent endometrial cancer.

I. Neoplasms

Uterine cancer is the fourth most common cancer in women. Risk factors for endometrial cancer include nulliparity, late menopause (after age 52), obesity, diabetes, unopposed estrogen therapy, tamoxifen, and a history of atypical endometrial hyperplasia. Endometrial cancer most often presents as postmenopausal bleeding in the sixth and seventh decade, although when investigated only 10% of patients with postmenopausal bleeding have endometrial cancer. In the perimenopausal period endometrial cancer can present as menometrorrhagia.

Vaginal bleeding is the most common symptom in patients with cervical cancer. The increased cervical friability associated with cervical cancer usually results in postcoital bleeding, but also can appear as irregular or postmenopausal bleeding.

Amant F: Endometrial cancer. Lancet 2005;366:491. [PMID: 16084259]

Kaunitz AM: Injectable long-acting contraceptives. Clin Obstet Gynecol 2001;44:73. [PMID: 11219248]

Lethaby A et al: Hormone replacement therapy in postmenopausal women: Endometrial hyperplasia and irregular bleeding. Cochrane Database Syst Rev 2004;(3):CD000402. [PMID: 15266429]

Montgomery BE: Endometrial hyperplasia: A review. Obstet Gynecol Surv 2004;59:368. [PMID: 15097798]

Richardson MR: Current perspectives in polycystic ovary syndrome. Am Fam Physician 2003;68:697. [PMID: 12952386]

Scrager S: Abnormal uterine bleeding associated with hormonal contraception. Am Fam Physician 2002;65:2073. [PMID: 12046776]

Stovall DW: Clinical symptomatology of uterine leiomyomas. Clin Obstet Gynecol 2001;44:364. [PMID: 11344999]

Wallach EE, Vlahos NF: Uterine myomas: An overview of development, clinical features and management. Obstet Gynecol 2004;104:393. [PMID: 15292018]

Warren MP: A comparative review of the risks and benefits of hormone replacement therapy regimens. Am J Obstet Gynecol 2004;190:1141. [PMID: 15118656]

Treatment

The treatment for vaginal bleeding depends on the underlying cause. When the vaginal bleeding is found to have a specific cause, such as an infectious agent or thyroid disease, the treatment should obviously be directed at the specific underlying disease. The primary care physician can also initiate many other treatments for vaginal bleeding. When initial treatment fails, patients can be referred for treatment with surgical options.

A. Bleeding from Contraception

Physicians often change formulations of OCPs to try to decrease the incidence of intermenstrual bleeding, although conflicting study results make it difficult to determine whether different formulations actually make a difference. All formulations share the characteristic of a higher incidence of intermenstrual bleeding during the first cycle of use. Therefore, one of the most important things physicians can do is to reassure the patient and encourage continued use. The physician can try adding exogenous estrogen daily for 7—10 days to control prolonged intermenstrual bleeding, but no clinical trials support this strategy. Physiologically, this approach makes sense, as OCPs cause endometrial atrophy.

Similarly, bleeding is common with Depo-Provera, especially early during the treatment. Reassurance and patience should be the initial treatment of any bleeding. With continued bleeding physicians can consider the unstudied practice of adding low-dose estrogen supplementation for 1–3 months.

B. Fibroids

Medical management of fibroids is fairly limited. OCPs have not been found to be efficacious in the treatment of fibroid symptoms. They also have not been found to increase fibroid size and therefore can be used in women with fibroids for other reasons. Recently some evidence has shown that depot medroxyprogesterone acetate (DMPA) may significantly improve menorrhagia attributed to fibroids. Mifepristone and selective estrogen receptor modulators may be available as treatment options after further study. Administration of a gonadotropin-releasing hormone (GnRH) agonist can greatly reduce the volume of a patient's fibroids. Unfortunately this effect is temporary. As a result, this treatment is largely reserved for preoperative therapy to facilitate the removal of the uterus or fibroid. Pretreatment can also improve the patient's hematologic parameters by decreasing vaginal bleeding prior to surgery. The exception to these restrictions is the perimenopausal patient. If a woman is close to menopause, treatment with a GnRH agonist is a reasonable approach. To achieve success, this approach depends on the woman beginning menopause during treatment. This reduces the chance that myomas will increase in size after the cessation of treatment. Because it is impossible to predict the start of menopause, the number of patients benefiting from this approach is limited.

Treatment with nonsteroidal anti-inflammatory drugs may be effective in decreasing abnormal uterine bleeding, but randomized trials examining this treatment are lacking. Ibuprofen at doses of 1200 mg daily effectively reduces bleeding in patients with primary menorrhagia, but this may not be as effective in women with fibroids. If patients fail these ambulatory approaches, surgical options include myomectomy, hysterectomy, or uterine embolization. Although the primary care physician will refer the patient for these procedures, patients often want to discuss possible treatment options with their physicians. Myomectomy is a good option for the patient who does not want her uterus removed or desires future childbearing. The risk exists for the growth of new fibroids and the growth of fibroids too small for removal at the time of surgery. Women undergoing hysterectomy may have the option of an abdominal or vaginal hysterectomy. Vaginal hysterectomies involve fewer complications and shorter hospital stays. The size of the uterus at the time of surgery determines the feasibility of this approach, because the surgeon must be able to remove the uterus completely through a vaginal incision.

Women wanting to avoid hysterectomy now have the option of uterine fibroid embolization. In this procedure an interventional radiologist injects tiny polyvinyl alcohol particles into the uterine arteries. Because the hypervascular fibroids have no collateral vascular supply, they undergo ischemic necrosis. Women with pedunculated or subserosal fibroids are not considered ideal candidates for this procedure. In addition, because the effects of uterine artery embolization on childbearing are not well known, the procedure is generally not performed on women desiring future fertility. Menorrhagia is improved in over 90% of women undergoing uterine artery embolization.

C. Anovulatory Bleeding

In general, medical management is the preferred treatment for anovulatory bleeding. Treatment goals should include alleviation of any acute bleeding, prevention of future noncyclic bleeding, a decrease in the patient's future risk of long-term health problems secondary to anovulation, and improvement in the patient's quality of life. Treatment options include prostaglandin synthetase inhibitors, estrogen, OCPs, and cyclic progesterones. Those who fail medical management have surgical options, including hysterectomy and endometrial ablation.

Blood loss can be reduced by 50% in women treated with prostaglandin synthetase inhibitors, including mefenamic acid, ibuprofen, and naproxen. Because many of the studies evaluating the role of prostaglandin synthetase inhibitors were completed in women with ovulatory cycles, the results cannot be directly applied to women with anovulatory bleeding; women with anovulatory bleeding may not find this approach as effective. In addition, this treatment does not address the issues of future noncyclic bleeding and decreasing future health risks due to anovulation.

Estrogen alone is usually used to treat an acute episode of heavy uterine bleeding. Premarin used intravenously will temporarily stop most uterine bleeding, regardless of the cause. The dose commonly used is 25 mg of conjugated estrogen every 4 hours. Nausea limits using high doses of estrogen orally, but lower doses can be used in a patient with acute heavy bleeding who is hemodynamically stable. One suggested regimen is 2.5 mg of conjugated estrogen every 4–6 hours.

After acute bleeding is controlled, the physician should add a progestin to the treatment regimen to induce withdrawal bleeding. A combination of estrogen and progesterone is given for 7–10 days and then stopped, inducing withdrawal bleeding. To decrease the risk of future hyperplasia or endometrial cancer, a progestin is continued for 10–14 days each cycle. Traditionally, treatment has been with medroxyprogesterone acetate (Provera), 10 mg. Other progestational agents include norethindrone acetate (Aygestin), norethindrone (Micronor), norgestrel (Ovrette), and micronized progesterone (Prometrium, Crinone). The micronized progesterones are natural progesterones that have been modified to have a prolonged half-life and cause less destruction in the gastrointestinal tract. Women who experience mood changes with synthetic progestins may better tolerate treatment with a micronized progesterone.

OCPs provide an option for treatment of both the acute episode of bleeding and future episodes of bleeding, as well as prevention of long-term health problems from anovulation. Acutely, one option to control bleeding is to use a 50-mcg estrogen OCP four times a day until bleeding ceases, then continue the OCP for a week. This may not be as effective as estrogen alone for quick stoppage of bleeding but is very convenient and easy. Long term, OCPs are effective in treating all patterns of dysfunctional uterine bleeding. Although the triphasic norgestimate-ethinyl estradiol combination has been studied in a double-blind, placebo-controlled study, various OCPs have been used for decades to control uterine bleeding. Patients with a history of thromboembolism, cerebrovascular disease, coronary artery disease, estrogen-dependent neoplasias, or liver disease should not be started on an OCP. Relative contraindications include migraine headaches, hypertension, diabetes, age greater than 35 years in a smoking patient, and active gallbladder disease.

When evaluating various treatment regimens for dysfunctional uterine bleeding the clinician should realize that few studies have evaluated the most effective type, dose, regimen, and administrative route. This contributes to a wide range of suggested treatment options, none of which has been proven to be superior to another.

Patients who are unable to tolerate hormonal management can consider endometrial ablation. Using electrocautery, laser, cryoablation, or thermoablation, these techniques all result in destruction of the endometrial lining. Initially used exclusively in patients with menorrhagia, these treatments are now also used in women with anovulatory bleeding, although outcomes are not well studied for this indication. Because endometrial glands often persist after ablative treatment, most women do not experience long-term amenorrhea after treatment. Also, because endometrial glands persist, the risk of endometrial cancer is not eliminated after treatment. Women at risk for endometrial cancer from long-term unopposed estrogen exposure still need preventive treatment. This procedure should be used only in women who choose not to preserve future fertility. Because pregnancies have occurred after endometrial ablation, some form of contraception may be needed after the procedure.

D. Alternative Therapies

Although no controlled studies have been completed, small studies suggest that acupuncture may be an option for young women with dysfunctional bleeding and for women with PCOS.

The nomenclature used in traditional Chinese medicine differs from western medicine, so making a direct comparison of treatments is difficult. Again, no controlled studies have been completed, but smaller studies suggest a possible role in certain situations for patients interested in pursuing alternative therapies. Keishi-bukuryo-gan (KBG) is a traditional herbal remedy that may act as an LH-releasing hormone antagonist and a weak antiestrogen. It has been used successfully in the treatment of uterine fibroids. A smaller number of patients have been treated for acute bleeding and then induction of ovulation.

Agency for Healthcare Research and Quality: Management of uterine fibroids. Summary, evidence report/technology assessment: Number 34. Publication No. 01-E051. AHRQ, January 2001.

American College of Obstetricians and Gynecologists: ACOG practice bulletin: Management of anovulatory bleeding. ACOG Pract Bull 2000;14;1.

Apgar BS, Greenberg G: Using progestins in clinical practice. Am Fam Physician 2000;8:1839. [PMID: 11057840]

Chavez NF, Stewart EA: Medical treatment of uterine fibroids. Clin Obstet Gynecol 2001;44:372. [PMID: 11347559]

Guarnaccia MM, Rein MS: Traditional surgical approaches to uterine fibroids: Abdominal myomectomy and hysterectomy. Clin Obstet Gynecol 2001;44:385. [PMID: 11345000]

Hickey M et al: Progestogens versus oestrogens and progestogens for irregular uterine bleeding associated with anovulation. Cochrane Database Syst Rev 2000;(2):CD001895. [PMID: 10796833]

Kammerer-Doak DN, Rogers RG: Endometrial ablation: Electrocautery and laser techniques. Clin Obstet Gynecol 2000;43:561. [PMID: 10949759]

Smith SJ: Uterine fibroid embolization. Am Fam Physician 2000; 61:3601. [PMID: 10892632]

Hypertension 33

Maureen O'Hara Padden, MD, & Bernhard Stepke, MD, PhD, LCDR, MC, USN

General Considerations

At least 65 million Americans have hypertension, defined as systolic blood pressure greater than or equal to 140 mm Hg or diastolic blood pressure greater than or equal to 90 mm Hg, or both. This translates to one in four adults and more than half of those older than 60 years of age. The incidence of hypertension increases with age. If an individual is normotensive at age 55, the lifetime risk for hypertension is 90%. High blood pressure resulted in the death of 52,602 Americans in 2003. From 1993 to 2003, the death rate from hypertension rose 29.3% and the actual number of deaths rose 56.1%. Of persons with high blood pressure roughly one third are not aware of their diagnosis. Hypertension is most prevalent among the black population, affecting one of every three African Americans. Non-Hispanic blacks and Mexican Americans are also more likely to suffer from high blood pressure than non-Hispanic whites.

The National High Blood Pressure Education Program (NHBPEP), which is coordinated by the National Heart, Lung, and Blood Institute (NHBLI) of the National Institutes of Health, was established in 1972. The program was designed to increase awareness, prevention, treatment, and control of hypertension. Data from the National Health and Nutrition Examination Survey (NHANES), conducted between 1976 and 2000, revealed that of patients aware of their high blood pressure and under treatment, the number who had achieved control of their high blood pressure had increased (Table 33–1). Coincident with these positive changes was a dramatic reduction in morbidity and mortality (40–60%), including stroke and myocardial infarction secondary to hypertension. However, the most recent NHANES III survey, conducted in 1999–2000, showed a leveling off of improvement.

High blood pressure is easily detected and usually controlled with appropriate intervention. However, among persons with high blood pressure, only 70% are aware of their condition, 59% are being treated, and 34% achieve adequate control. In addition, the incidence of end-stage renal disease and the prevalence of heart failure continue to increase. Both conditions have been linked to uncontrolled hypertension.

In 2003, the seventh report of the Joint National Committee on Prevention, Detection, Evaluation, and Treatment of High Blood Pressure (JNC VII) was released. It provided updated recommendations based on recent studies, including more concise clinical guidelines and a simplified blood pressure classification (Table 33–2).

Abbott KC, Bakris GL: What have we learned from the current trials? Med Clin North Am 2004; 88:189. [PMID: 14871059]

Chobanian AV et al: Seventh report of the Joint National Committee on Prevention, Detection, Evaluation, and Treatment of High Blood Pressure: The JNC 7 report. JAMA 2003; 289:2560. [PMID: 12748199]

Fields LE et al: The burden of adult hypertension in the United States 1999 to 2000: A rising tide. Hypertension 2004:1. [PMID: 15326093]

Kaplan NM: What can we expect from the new guidelines? Med Clin North Am 2004; 88:141. [PMID: 14871056]

Magill MK et al: New developments in the management of hypertension. Am Fam Physician 2003; 68:853. [PMID: 13678132]

Pathogenesis

A. Primary or Essential Hypertension

In 90–95% of cases of hypertension, no cause can be identified. A role for genetics has been implicated in the development of high blood pressure (eg, hypertension is more prevalent in some families and in African Americans). Additional risk factors include increased salt intake, excess alcohol intake, obesity, sedentary lifestyle, and certain personality traits, including aggressiveness and poor stress coping skills.

B. Secondary Hypertension

In only 5% of cases can a cause for hypertension be found; however, it is reasonable to look for an underlying cause in patients diagnosed with hypertension. History or physical examination may suggest an underlying etiology, or the first clue may come later when patients fail to respond appropriately to standard drug therapy. In addition, secondary hypertension should be considered in those with sudden onset of hypertension, in those with suddenly uncontrolled blood pressure that had previously

Table 33–1. Trends in awareness, treatment, and control of high blood pressure in adults aged 18–71 years.[1]

	NHANES (%)			
	II (1976–80)	III (Phase 1, 1988–91)	III (Phase 2, 1991–94)	1999–2000
Awareness	51	73	68	70
Treatment	31	55	54	59
Control[2]	10	29	27	34

NHANES, National Health and Nutrition Examination Survey.

[1]High blood pressure is systolic blood pressure (SBP) ≥ 140 mm Hg or diastolic blood pressure (DSP) ≥ 90 mm Hg or taking antihypertensive medication.

[2]SBP < 140 mm Hg and DBP < 90 mm Hg.

Sources: Unpublished data from 1999–2000 computed by M. Wolz, National Heart, Lung, and Blood Institute; and *Seventh Report of the Joint National Committee on Prevention, Detection, Evaluation, and Treatment of High Blood Pressure.* NIH Publication No. 03-5233. US Department of Health and Human Services, 2003.

been well controlled, and in patients younger than 30 years of age without a family history of hypertension.

Etiologies of secondary hypertension that must be considered in the appropriate patient include use of certain medications such as oral contraceptives, sympathomimetics, decongestants, nonsteroidal anti-inflammatory drugs, appetite suppressants, antidepressants, adrenal steroids, cyclosporine, and erythropoietin. All of these medications can contribute to an elevation in blood pressure. Hypertension can also be related to excessive use of caffeine, ingestion of licorice, or use of illicit drugs such as cocaine or amphetamines.

Hypertension can also occur secondary to acute and chronic kidney disease, which might be suggested by a flank mass, elevated creatinine level, or abnormal findings such as proteinuria, hematuria, or casts on routine

Table 33–2. Classification and management of blood pressure in adults.[1]

BP Classification	SBP[1] (mm Hg)	DBP[1] (mm Hg)	Life-style Modification	Initial Drug Therapy: Without Compelling Indication	Initial Drug Therapy: With Compelling Indication (see Table 33–5)
Normal	< 120	and < 80	Encourage	No antihypertensive drug indicated	Drug(s) for compelling indications[2]
Prehypertension	120–139	or 80–90	Yes		
Stage 1 hypertension	140–159	or 90–99	Yes	Thiazide-type diuretics for most; may consider ACE inhibitor, ARB, β-blocker, calcium channel blocker, or combination	Drug(s) for compelling indications[3]; other antihypertensive drugs (diuretics, ACE inhibitors, β-blockers, calcium channel blockers) as needed
Stage 2 hypertension	≥ 160	or ≥ 100	Yes	Two-drug combination for most[3] (usually thiazide-type diuretic and ACE inhibitor or ARB or β-blocker or calcium channel blocker)	

BP, blood pressure; SBP, systolic blood pressure; DBP, diastolic blood pressure; ACE, angiotensin-converting enzyme; ARB, angiotensin II receptor blocker.

[1]Treatment determined by highest BP category.

[2]Treat patients with chronic kidney disease or diabetes to BP goal of < 130/80 mm Hg.

[3]Initial combined therapy should be used cautiously in those at risk for orthostatic hypotension.

Source: Seventh Report of the Joint National Committee on Prevention, Detection, Evaluation, and Treatment of High Blood Pressure. NIH Publication No. 03-5233. US Department of Health and Human Services, 2003.

urinalysis. Rarely, hypertension may be related to renal artery stenosis, particularly if onset is before the age of 20 or after the age of 50 years. Abdominal bruits with radiation to the renal area may be heard. Other causes to consider in the differential diagnosis include hypo- or hyper-thyroidism, primary hyperaldosteronism, Cushing syndrome, coarctation of the aorta, pheochromocytoma, and sleep apnea syndrome in the appropriate clinical presentation. When such causes are entertained, appropriate evaluation should be undertaken.

Prevention

A healthy life-style is hailed both as prevention and as initial therapy for hypertension (Table 33–3). Clinical trials assessing both prevention (Trials of Hypertension Prevention–Phase II, TONE) and nonpharmacologic treatment of mild hypertension (TOMHS, DASH, low-sodium DASH, PREMIER) support the positive impact of maintaining optimal weight, a regular aerobic exercise program, and a diet low in sodium, saturated fat, and total fats and rich in fruits and vegetables. Excessive alcohol intake should be reduced and smoking cessation encouraged.

Clinical Findings

Before patients with hypertension can be offered adequate treatment, they must be properly diagnosed. Because patients are often asymptomatic, the risk factors for hypertension must be understood and appropriate patients screened. In addition to the modifiable risk factors noted earlier, there are nonmodifiable factors, including African-American race, family history of hypertension, and increasing age.

A. Symptoms and Signs

There are usually no physical findings early in the course of hypertension. In some patients, the presence of hypertension may be signaled by early morning headaches or, in those with severe hypertension, by signs or symptoms associated with target organ damage. Such symptoms might include nausea, vomiting, visual disturbance, chest pain, or confusion. More typically, the first indication is an elevated blood pressure measurement taken with a sphygmomanometer during a routine visit to a medical provider or after the patient has had a stroke or myocardial infarction.

For proper measurement of blood pressure, the patient should be seated in a chair with his or her back supported and the arm bared and supported at heart level. Caffeine and tobacco should be avoided in the 30 minutes preceding measurement, and measurement should begin after 5 minutes of rest. The cuff size should be appropriate for the patient's arm, defined by a cuff bladder that encircles 80% of the arm. It is important that the diagnosis be made after the elevation of blood pressure is documented with three separate readings, on three different occasions, unless the eleva-

Table 33–3. Life-style modifications to manage hypertension.[1]

Modification	Recommendation[2]	Approximate SBP Reduction (range)
Weight reduction	Maintain normal body weight (BMI 18.5–24.9 kg/m^2)	5–20 mm Hg/10 kg weight loss
Adopt DASH eating plan	Consume a diet rich in fruits, vegetables, and low-fat dairy products with a reduced content of saturated and total fat	8–14 mm Hg
Dietary sodium reduction	Reduce dietary sodium intake to no more than 100 mmol/d (2.4 g sodium or 6 g sodium chloride)	2–8 mm Hg
Physical activity	Engage in regular aerobic physical activity such as brisk walking (at least 30 min/d, most days of the week)	4–9 mm Hg
Moderation of alcohol consumption	Limit consumption to no more than 2 drinks (1 oz or 30 mL ethanol; eg, 24 oz beer, 10-oz wine, or 3 oz 80-proof whiskey) per day in most men and to no more than 1 drink per day in women and lighter weight persons	2–4 mm Hg

SBP, systolic blood pressure; BMI, body mass index; DASH, Dietary Approaches to Stop Hypertension.

[1]For overall cardiovascular risk reduction, stop smoking.

[2]The effects of implementing these modifications are dose and time dependent, and could be greater for some individuals.

Source: Seventh Report of the Joint National Committee on Prevention, Detection, Evaluation, and Treatment of High Blood Pressure. NIH Publication No. 03-5233. US Department of Health and Human Services, 2003.

tion is severe or is associated with symptoms requiring immediate attention (hypertensive urgency or emergency). Transient elevation of blood pressure secondary to pain or anxiety, as experienced by some patients when they enter a physician's office ("white coat syndrome"), does not require treatment. In cases in which the diagnosis is in question, properly taken home blood pressure measurements can be useful.

1. Classification of blood pressure—A goal of JNC VII was to simplify blood pressure classification when making the diagnosis of hypertension (see Table 33–2). A new category, designated *prehypertension,* was added, and stages 2 and 3 from JNC VI were combined to form a single category (stage 2). These classifications are based on the average of two or more provider-obtained blood pressure measurements from a seated patient.

2. Self-monitoring—Patients should be encouraged to do self-monitoring of their blood pressure at home. Many easy-to-use blood pressure monitors are commercially available at reasonable cost for use at home. Validated electronic devices are recommended, and independent reviews of available devices, such as that published by Consumer Reports, are available to assist the consumer. These devices should be periodically checked for accuracy. Self-measurement can be helpful, not only in establishing the diagnosis of hypertension, but also in assessing response to medical therapy, and in encouraging patient compliance with therapy by providing regular feedback on therapy response.

B. Evaluation

Patients with documented hypertension must undergo a thorough evaluation that includes objectives advanced by JNC VII: assessment of life-style and identification of cardiovascular risk factors, identification of comorbidities that would guide therapy, and surveillance for identifiable causes of high blood pressure and to establish whether the patient already manifests evidence of target end-organ damage.

1. History—A thorough history should be obtained. Any prior history of hypertension should be elicited as well as response and side effects to any previous hypertension therapy. It is important to inquire about any history or symptoms suggestive of coronary artery disease or other significant comorbidities, including diabetes mellitus, heart failure, dyslipidemia, renal disease, and peripheral vascular disease. The family history should also be reviewed, with special attention to the presence of hypertension, premature coronary artery disease, diabetes, renal disease, dyslipidemia, or stroke. Use of tobacco, alcohol, or illicit drugs should be documented, as well as dietary intake of sodium, saturated fat, and caffeine. Recent changes in weight and exercise level should be queried. Current medications used by the patient should be reviewed, including over-the-counter medications and herbal formulations.

2. Physical examination—The initial physical examination should be comprehensive and should pay careful attention to the areas outlined in Table 33–4.

C. Laboratory and Diagnostic Studies

JNC VII specifically recommends that the following tests be performed: electrocardiogram (ECG), urinalysis, fasting blood glucose level, potassium level, creatinine level, calcium level, and fasting lipid panel. Urinalysis should be assessed for evidence of hematuria, proteinuria, or casts suggestive of intrinsic renal disease. The complete blood count is helpful to rule out anemia or polycythemia. Potassium levels help assess for hyperaldosteronism, and creatinine levels reflect renal function. The fasting blood glucose level is used to assess for

Table 33–4. Physical examination: hypertension.

Component of Examination	Assessment Focus
General	Baseline height, weight, and waist circumference Upper and lower extremity blood pressure measurement to assess for coarctation of the aorta Features of Cushing syndrome
Eyes	Funduscopic examination for signs of hypertensive retinopathy (eg, arteriolar narrowing, focal arteriolar constriction, atrioventricular nicking, hemorrhages, exudates)
Neck	Carotid bruits Neck vein distention or thyroid gland enlargement
Heart	Abnormalities in rate, rhythm, murmurs, or extra heart sounds
Lungs	Rales, rhonchi, or wheezes
Abdomen	Abdominal bruits suggestive of renal artery stenosis Enlargement of kidneys (mass) or aortic pulsation suggesting aneurysm
Extremities	Diminished or absent peripheral arterial pulsations Edema Signs of vascular compromise
Neurologic	Neurologic deficits

diabetes mellitus, and the lipid profile is an indicator of cardiovascular risk. Further testing is warranted if blood pressure control is not achieved. Additional tests to consider include hemoglobin A_{1c}, thyroid-stimulating hormone, urine microalbumin, creatinine clearance, and 24-hour urine for protein. Echocardiograms and chest x-rays are not routinely recommended for evaluation of hypertensive patients. In certain cases, however, an echocardiogram may prove useful in guiding therapy when baseline abnormalities are found on the ECG (eg, left ventricular hypertrophy or signs of previous silent myocardial infarction). A chest radiograph may be useful if there are abnormal findings on physical examination. Tests that evaluate for rare causes of hypertension, such as renal artery stenosis (renal ultrasound) or pheochromocytoma (24-hour urine for catecholamines), should only be ordered in patients whose history and physical examination findings raise suspicion.

Treatment

A. Cardiovascular Risk Stratification

In treating hypertension, the public health goal is reduction of cardiovascular and renal morbidity and mortality. Hypertension is clearly important, but it is not the only risk factor. JNC VII defines specific components of cardiovascular risk and recommends evaluation of patients for evidence of target organ damage in performing risk stratification and in considering recommendations for therapy (Table 33–5).

The JNC VII guidelines include an algorithm for use when considering initial therapy for patients with hypertension (Figure 33–1). It is recognized that most patients, especially those aged 50 years and older, will reach their diastolic blood pressure goal once the systolic blood pressure goal is reached. Life-style modification may be used initially if blood pressure is in the prehypertensive range (< 140/90 mm Hg). When no risk factors, no target organ damage, and no evidence of cardiovascular disease are identified in a patient, the target blood pressure for treatment is less than 140/90 mm Hg. If diabetes mellitus or renal disease is present, the blood pressure target for treatment is less than 130/80 mm Hg.

When life-style modification is used as initial therapy but successful control is not achieved, drug therapy should be initiated (see later discussion). Further reassessments should consider optimization or titration of the drug regimen in terms of dosage or use of combinations, as well as reinforcing adherence to life-style modification. Follow-up visits should occur at approximately monthly intervals until the blood pressure goal is reached, or more frequently in patients with significant comorbidities. Once patients reach their goal, 3- to 6-month intervals for visits are appropriate.

Table 33–5. Components of cardiovascular risk stratification in patients with hypertension.

Major Risk Factors
Hypertension[1]
Age (> 55 y for men, 65 y for women)[2]
Diabetes mellitus[1]
Elevated LDL (or total) cholesterol, or low HDL cholesterol[1]
Estimated GFR < 60 mL/min
Family history of premature CVD (men < 55 y of age or women < 65 y of age)
Microalbuminuria
Obesity[1] (BMI ≥ 30 kg/m^2)
Physical inactivity
Tobacco usage, particularly cigarettes
Target Organ Damage
Heart
Left ventricular hypertrophy
Angina or prior myocardial infarction
Prior coronary revascularization
Heart failure
Brain
Stroke or transient ischemic attack
Dementia
Chronic kidney disease
Peripheral arterial disease
Retinopathy

LDL, low-density lipoprotein; HDL, high-density lipoprotein; GFR, glomerular filtration rate; CVD, cardiovascular disease; BMI, body mass index.

[1]Components of the metabolic syndrome. Reduced HDL, elevated triglycerides, and abdominal obesity also are components of the metabolic syndrome.

[2]Increased risk begins at approximately 55 and 65 y of age for men and women, respectively. Adult Treatment Panel III used earlier age cut points to suggest the need for earlier action.

Source: Seventh Report of the Joint National Committee on Prevention, Detection, Evaluation, and Treatment of High Blood Pressure. NIH Publication No. 03-5233. US Department of Health and Human Services, 2003.

If the blood pressure goal is not achieved with triple-drug therapy (ie, agents from different classes, including a diuretic), further investigation must ensue. A lack of motivation on the patient's part can undo the most effective regimen; however, this outcome can be minimized through positive experiences with the clinician to address misunderstandings about the condition and treatment. Poor response to therapy by patients receiving a triple regimen of antihypertensive drugs should also prompt consideration of referral to a hypertension

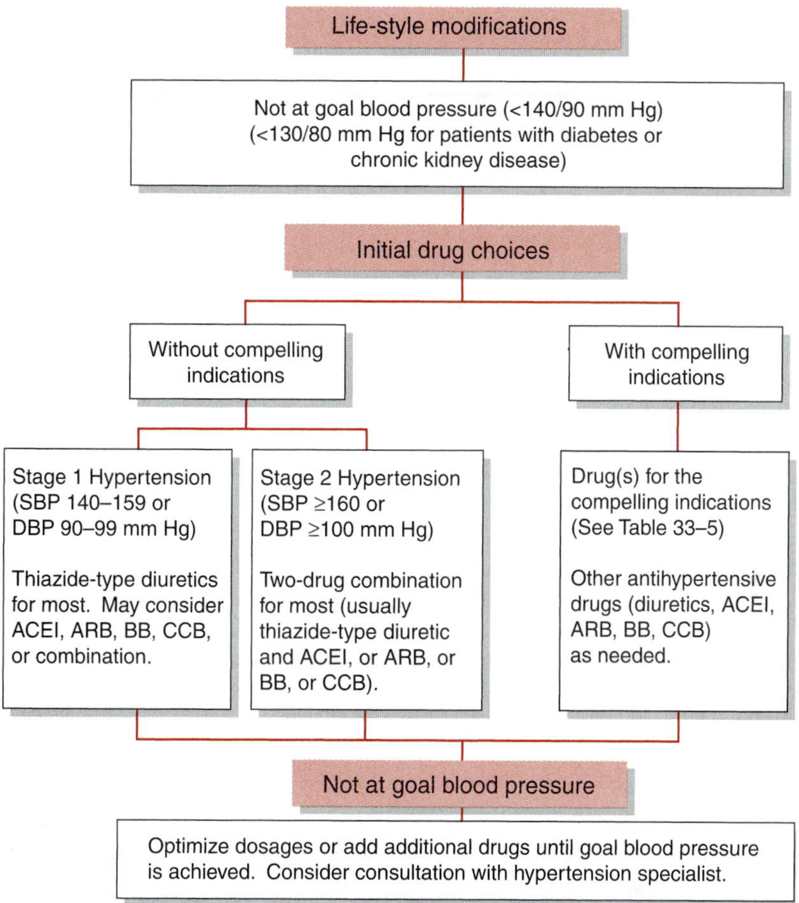

Figure 33–1. **Algorithm for treatment of hypertension. ACE, angiotensin-converting enzyme; ARB, angiotensin II receptor blocker; BB, β-blocker; CCB, calcium channel blocker; DBP, diastolic blood pressure; SBP, systolic blood pressure.** (From the *Seventh Report of the Joint National Committee on Prevention, Detection, Evaluation, and Treatment of High Blood Pressure.* NIH Publication No. 03-5233. US Department of Health and Human Services, 2003.)

specialist for evaluation and recommendations concerning treatment.

Dickerson LM, Gibson MV: Management of hypertension in older persons. Am Fam Physician 2005;71:469. [PMID: 15712622]

B. Life-style Modification

JNC VII cites the adoption of life-style modifications as critical, not only for the prevention of hypertension but also in the treatment thereof. Major recommendations include encouraging the overweight patient to lose weight. Even small amounts of weight loss (10 pounds [4.5 kg]) can improve blood pressure control and reduce cardiovascular risk. Weight loss can be facilitated through dietary changes and increased exercise. Patients should be encouraged to set their exercise goal for 30–45 minutes of aerobic activity most days of the week. Adoption of the Dietary Approaches to Stop Hypertension (DASH) eating plan is also recommended. This plan promotes potassium and calcium intake, reduced sodium and fat intake, exercise, and moderation of alcohol consumption. The blood pressure reduction gained is roughly equivalent to that of single-drug therapy. However, patients taking angiotensin-converting enzyme (ACE) inhibitors or angiotensin II receptor blockers should be cautioned regarding potassium intake, because these medications can result in potassium retention. Any use of tobacco should be discouraged, and patients currently using tobacco should be counseled to quit, as this may help lower blood pressure.

C. PHARMACOTHERAPY

Many medications are available to treat hypertension. Medication should be initiated at a low dose and titrated slowly to achieve desired blood pressure control. When available, formulations available in once-daily dosing are preferred due to increased patient compliance. Also useful are the many combination formulations now available that incorporate two different classes of drugs. Good clinical outcomes trial data exist demonstrating reduction in complications of hypertension with blood pressure lowering by β-blockers, calcium channel blockers, thiazide diuretics, ACE inhibitors, and angiotensin II receptor blockers. When selecting a medication, side effect profile and patient comorbidities should help guide choice.

Favorable effects of selective antihypertensive agents may increase interest in their use. Thiazide diuretics slow demineralization in osteoporosis. β-Blockers are useful for atrial arrhythmias and fibrillation, migraine headache prophylaxis, thyrotoxicosis, and essential tremor. Calcium channel blockers are useful in Raynaud syndrome and some arrhythmias, and α-blockers are helpful in prostatism.

Unfavorable effects include cautions for the use of thiazide diuretics in patients with gout or a history of hyponatremia. β-Blockers should be avoided in patients with asthma or with second- or third-degree heart block. ACE inhibitors and angiotensin II receptor blockers have the potential to cause birth defects and thus should be avoided in women likely to become pregnant and discontinued in those who do become pregnant. Hyperkalemia may be caused by aldosterone antagonists and potassium-sparing diuretics.

Ethnic differences have been noted in the blood pressure response to monotherapy. African Americans, who have increased prevalence and severity of hypertension, have demonstrated blunted response to β-blockers and ACE inhibitors versus diuretics or calcium channel blockers. This effect is eliminated by combination therapy.

The recommendations that follow are based on JNC VII (Table 33–6). If a single drug does not achieve control, a second drug from a different class should be added. If the blood pressure remains more than 20/10 mm Hg above goals, two-drug therapy should be considered. Effective and timely control for most patients will be accomplished with at least two antihypertensive medications. The clinician should advise patients—especially those who are diabetic, have autonomic dysfunction, or are elderly—of the risk for orthostatic hypotension.

1. Diuretics—JNC VII recommends initially treating uncomplicated hypertension with diuretics, in the absence of a compelling reason to use another agent. This strong recommendation is based on the many ran-

Table 33–6. Clinical trial guideline basis for compelling indications for individual drug classes.

Compelling Indication[1]	Recommended Drugs						Clinical Trial Basis[2]
	D	BB	ACEI	ARB	CCB	Aldo ANT	
Heart failure	•	•	•	•		•	ACC/AHA Heart Failure Guideline, MERIT-HF, COPERNICUS, CIBIS, SOLVD, AIRE, TRACE, ValHEFT, RALES
Post–myocardial infarction		•	•			•	ACC/AHA Post-MI Guideline, BHAT, SAVE, Capricorn, EPHESUS
High coronary disease risk	•	•	•		•		ALLHAT, HOPE, ANBP2, LIFE, CONVINCE
Diabetes mellitus	•	•	•	•	•		NKF-ADA Guideline, UKPDS, ALLHAT
Chronic kidney disease			•	•			NKF Guideline, Captopril Trial, RENAAL, IDNT, REIN, AASK
Recurrent stroke prevention	•		•				PROGRESS

D, diuretic; BB, β-blocker; ACEI, angiotensin-converting enzyme inhibitor; ARB, angiotensin II receptor blocker; CCB, calcium channel blocker; Aldo ANT, aldosterone antagonist.

[1]Compelling indications for antihypertensive drugs are based on benefits from outcome studies or existing clinical guidelines; the compelling indication is managed in parallel with the blood pressure.

[2]Conditions for which clinical trials demonstrate benefit of specific classes of antihypertensive drugs.

Source: Seventh Report of the Joint National Committee on Prevention, Detection, Evaluation, and Treatment of High Blood Pressure. NIH Publication No. 03-5233. US Department of Health and Human Services, 2003.

domized controlled trials that have demonstrated a superior response for diuretics in reduction in morbidity—including stroke, coronary artery disease, and congestive heart failure—and total mortality. ALLHAT (Antihypertensive and Lipid-Lowering Treatment to Prevent Heart Attack Trial) was one of the largest such trials. It compared diuretics, calcium channel blockers, and ACE inhibitors as initial therapies in a population with a large number of African-American participants. The authors concluded that regardless of age, sex, or race, the use of diuretics in hypertensive, high-cardiovascular-risk patients was associated with similar risk of cardiovascular events equivalent to that of calcium channel blockers and ACE inhibitors, but was superior in performance in patients with underlying heart conditions including heart failure.

Diuretics should be used cautiously in patients with gout, as worsening hyperuricemia can result. They may also cause muscle cramps or impotence in some individuals. Diuretics may be effective at lower doses in patients with dyslipidemia and diabetes mellitus, but patients placed on higher doses must be observed closely for worsening hyperglycemia or hyperlipidemia. The thiazide diuretics are most commonly used in the treatment of hypertension, because loop diuretics are more likely to lead to electrolyte abnormalities such as hypokalemia and to have a shorter duration of action. However, loop diuretics can sometimes be useful in the treatment of hypertension in patients with chronic renal disease and a serum creatinine level greater than 2.5 mg/dL. The loop diuretics have found most utility in the treatment of congestive heart failure.

ALLHAT Officers Coordinating for the ALLHAT Collaborative Research Group: Major outcomes in high-risk hypertensive patients randomized to angiotensin-converting enzyme inhibitor or calcium channel blocker vs diuretic: The Antihypertensive and Lipid-Lowering Treatment to Prevent Heart Attack Trial (ALLHAT). JAMA 2002;288:2981. [PMID: 12479763]

2. β-Blockers—Whether used as first-line agents in the case of compelling indications or in a drug therapy combination, β-blockers have favorable effects on migraine headache, hyperthyroidism, and anxiety. Patients should be informed that β-blockers may cause sexual dysfunction. These agents should be used with caution, if at all, in patients with a history of depression, asthma or reactive airway disease, second- or third-degree heart block, or peripheral vascular disease. In patients with mild to moderate reactive airway disease, β-blockers do not produce adverse effects in the short term. The United Kingdom Prospective Diabetes Study (UKPDS) demonstrated that β-blockers can be used safely and effectively for type 2 diabetes mellitus, although there is concern that hypoglycemic episodes might be masked. Any patient with diabetes mellitus placed on a β-blocker should, therefore, be carefully monitored. Although previously not recommended, patients with congestive heart failure are now being successfully treated with β-blockers lacking intrinsic sympathomimetic activity, including two of the most studied agents, carvedilol and metoprolol. Careful use of these agents has shown promise in reducing mortality and improving ejection fraction in patients with New York Heart Association class II or III congestive heart failure.

Ko DT et al: Beta-blocker therapy and symptoms of depression, fatigue, and sexual dysfunction. JAMA 2002; 288:351. [PMID: 12117400]

Salpeter S et al: Cardioselective beta-blockers for reversible airway disease. Cochrane Database Syst Rev 2002;(4):CD002992. [PMID: 12519582]

3. Calcium channel blockers—There are two classes of calcium channel blockers: the dihydropyridine calcium channel blockers, which vasodilate (nifedipine, amlodipine, felodipine), and the rate-lowering calcium channel blockers (verapamil, diltiazem). They have relatively few side effects but may cause headache, nausea, rash, or flushing in some patients. Calcium channel blockers are not recommended as first-line therapy by JNC VII, although the guidelines suggest use of long-acting dihydropyridine calcium channel blockers as an alternative to β-blockers in patients with stable angina in ischemic heart disease, and in diabetics. Nondihydropyridines, with their negative inotropic and chronotropic actions, have a beneficial role in atrial fibrillation and supraventricular tachyarrhythmias. Data for the use of calcium channel blockers in the elderly are mixed. The Systolic Hypertension in Europe (SYSEUR) trial, released in 1997, randomized 5000 elderly patients with isolated systolic hypertension to treatment with either placebo or the long-acting dihydropyridine calcium channel blocker nitrendipine. In 2 years of follow-up there was significant reduction in stroke and cardiovascular events. Similar benefits were reported in elderly patients with hypertension and diabetes using nitrendipine, although the findings were not superior to other antihypertensive agents. In African Americans, response to monotherapy using β-blockers, ACE inhibitors, and angiotensin II receptor blockers is blunted. This is not the case when using calcium channel blockers or diuretics. Use of combination regimens with a diuretic eliminates these differential responses.

Tuomilehto J et al: Effects of calcium-channel blockade in older patients with diabetes and systolic hypertension: Systolic Hypertension in Europe Trial Investigators. N Engl J Med 1999;340:677. [PMID: 10053176]

4. ACE inhibitors—The ACE inhibitors stimulate vasodilation by blocking the renin–angiotensin–aldosterone system and inhibiting degradation of bradykinin. In several randomized, controlled clinical trials, these agents have been shown to reduce cardiovascular events in hypertensive patients (CAPPP trial), including particular subgroups (high-risk patients older than 55 years [HOPE study], older men [ANBP study], and diabetic patients [FACET and ACAPP trials]). Compelling indications exist for ACE inhibitor use in patients with diabetes mellitus, congestive heart failure, and chronic kidney disease, and in patients who have had a myocardial infarction with systolic dysfunction. ACE inhibitors have been shown to reduce progression of renal disease in African Americans (AASK trial) and diabetics but may increase the risk of stroke when used as monotherapy in African Americans (ALLHAT trial). These agents have also been shown to be more effective in promoting regression of left ventricular hypertrophy than diuretics, β-blockers, or calcium channel blockers. Left ventricular hypertrophy is considered one of the best predictors of cardiovascular events in patients with hypertension.

ACE inhibitors have relatively few side effects and are well tolerated by most patients. A dry cough may be reported in as many as 25% of patients. Because hyperkalemia may occur, particularly in patients who are also receiving potassium-sparing diuretics, periodic monitoring of electrolytes and serum creatinine should be performed.

ACE inhibitors must be used cautiously in patients with known renovascular disease and, when used, may need dose adjustment due to reduced drug clearance. When creatinine elevations exceed 30% above baseline, temporary cessation or reduction of dose is warranted. These agents should be used with extreme caution, if at all, in patients whose serum creatinine level exceeds 3.0 mg/mL. ACE inhibitors should not be used in patients with bilateral renal artery stenosis. Angioedema may occur with these agents, and this complication is two to four times more frequent in African Americans.

Agodoa LY et al: Effect of ramipril vs amlodipine on renal outcomes in hypertensive nephrosclerosis: A randomized controlled trial. JAMA 2001;285:2719. [PMID: 11386927]

Hansson L et al: Effect of angiotensin-converting-enzyme inhibition compared with conventional therapy on cardiovascular morbidity and mortality in hypertension: The Captopril Prevention Project (CAPPP) randomized trial. Lancet 1999;353:611. [PMID: 10030325]

Tatti P et al: Outcome results of the Fosinopril Versus Amlodipine Cardiovascular Events Randomized Trial (FACET) in patients with hypertension and NIDDM. Diabetes Care 1998;21:597. [PMID: 9571349]

Wing LM et al; Second Australian National Blood Pressure Study Group: A comparison of outcomes with angiotensin-converting-enzyme inhibitors and diuretics for hypertension in the elderly. N Engl J Med 2003;348:583. [PMID: 12584366]

Wright JT et al; African American Study of Kidney Disease and Hypertension Study Group: Effect of blood pressure lowering and antihypertensive drug class on progression of hypertensive kidney disease: Results from the AASK trial. JAMA 2002;288:2421. [PMID: 12435255]

Yusuf S, et al: Effects of an angiotensin-converting-enzyme inhibitor, ramipril, on cardiovascular events in high-risk patients: The Heart Outcomes Prevention Evaluation Study Investigators. N Engl J Med 2000;342:145. [PMID: 10639539]

5. Angiotensin II receptor blockers (ARBs)—ARBs selectively block angiotensin II activation of AT_1 receptors, which are responsible for mediating vasoconstriction, salt and water retention, and central and sympathetic activation among others. Angiotensin II is still able to activate AT_2 blockers, facilitating vasodilation and production of bradykinin, which aids in reduction of blood pressure. This class of medication is well tolerated and has a favorable side effect profile. ARBs are a good alternative for patients who cannot tolerate ACE inhibitor–associated cough but should be avoided in patients with ACE inhibitor–associated angioedema. JNC VII does not recommend that ARBs be used for initial therapy in treatment of hypertension; however, compelling indications for use include heart failure, diabetes mellitus, and chronic kidney disease. ARBs have been shown to be more effective than β-blockers in preventing cardiovascular events in hypertensive patients with left ventricular hypertrophy, both with and without diabetes (LIFE trial). Renal protective effects of ARBs have been shown clinically to reduce the progression of nephropathy in diabetic hypertensive patients (RENAAL trial) and to reduce the incidence of new-onset diabetes (VALUE trial). Recently, it has been demonstrated that ARBs reduce subsequent events in patients with acute ischemic stroke (ACCESS study).

Brenner BM et al; RENAAL Study Investigators: Effects of losartan on renal and cardiovascular outcomes in patients with type 2 diabetes and nephropathy. N Engl J Med 2001;345:861. [PMID: 11565518]

Julius S et al: Outcomes in hypertensive patients at high cardiovascular risk treated with regimens based on valsartan or amlodipine: The VALUE randomized trial. Lancet 2004;363:2022. [PMID: 15207952]

Lewis EJ et al: Renoprotective effect of the angiotensin-receptor antagonist irbesartan in patients with nephropathy due to type 2 diabetes. N Engl J Med 2001;345:851. [PMID: 11565517]

Lindholm LH et al; LIFE Study Group: Cardiovascular morbidity and mortality in patients with diabetes in the Losartan Intervention for Life Endpoint reduction in hypertension study (LIFE): A randomized trial against atenolol. Lancet 2002;359:1004. [PMID: 11937179]

Parving HH et al: The effect of irbesartan on the development of diabetic nephropathy in patients with type 2 diabetes. N Engl J Med 2001;345:870. [PMID: 11565519]

Schrader J et al: The ACCESS Study: Evaluation of Acute Candesartan Cilexetil Therapy in Stroke Survivors. Stroke 2003;34:1699. [PMID: 12817109]

6. Other drugs—Other drugs, including α-blockers and direct vasodilators, are used to treat hypertension, although less commonly than the other classes of drugs. They are typically used as second- or third-line agents because of increased side effects. The ALLHAT trial suggested that α-blockers and direct vasodilators such as doxazosin may increase the risk of stroke and congestive heart failure when used in the treatment of hypertension, resulting in discontinuation of that arm of the trial. Eplenerone (Inspra), a selective aldosterone receptor antagonist, was recently approved for the treatment of hypertension. Interest is focused on its use in patients with congestive heart failure or in combination with other antihypertensives; however, data on morbidity and mortality are not yet available.

D. Special Considerations

The drug selections noted in Table 33–6 are based on favorable outcome data from clinical trials and should be considered in light of current medications, tolerability, and blood pressure target goal.

1. Ischemic heart disease—β-Blockers are the first-line drug for patients with stable angina; alternatively, long-acting calcium channel blockers may be considered. ACE inhibitors should be added in patients with acute coronary syndromes, and consideration should be given to aldosterone antagonists post–myocardial infarction.

2. Heart failure—ACE inhibitors and β-blockers are recommended for asymptomatic patients with ventricular dysfunction. Symptomatic or end-stage heart disease should be treated with ACE inhibitors, β-blockers, ARBs, aldosterone blockers, and loop diuretics.

3. Diabetes mellitus—All classes of antihypertensive medications have proven beneficial in reducing the incidence of cardiovascular disease and stroke in diabetic patients. The progression of diabetic nephropathy is reduced with ACE inhibitors or ARBs.

4. Chronic kidney disease—Goals for these patients include slowing deterioration of renal function and preventing cardiovascular disease. Typically a combination of three drugs is needed to accomplish aggressive blood pressure management. ACE inhibitors and ARBs should be used and may be continued in patients with an increase in serum creatinine clearance of 35% above baseline, unless hyperkalemia develops. Increasing doses of loop diuretics are usually needed once the creatinine level reaches 2.5–3.0 mg/dL.

5. Cerebrovascular disease—The combination of an ACE inhibitor and thiazide diuretic has been shown to lower recurrent stroke rates.

E. Hypertensive Urgency and Emergency

Hypertensive urgencies are situations in which the blood pressure must be lowered within several hours, either due to an asymptomatic, severely elevated blood pressure (> 240/130 mm Hg) or a moderately elevated blood pressure (> 200/120 mm Hg) with associated symptoms, including angina, headache, and congestive heart failure. When such symptoms are present, even lower blood pressures may warrant more urgent treatment. Oral therapy can often be utilized with good response.

Hypertensive emergencies require treatment of elevated blood pressures within 1 hour to avoid significant morbidity and mortality. The symptomatology with which the patient presents warrants the immediate attention, not the actual blood pressure value itself. Such patients show evidence of end-organ damage from the elevated blood pressure, including encephalopathy (headache, irritability, confusion, coma), renal failure, pulmonary edema, unstable angina, myocardial infarction, aortic dissection, and intracranial hemorrhage. Hypertensive emergency is an indication for hospital admission, and such patients typically require intravenous therapy with antihypertensives.

The goal of therapy is reduction of systolic pressure by 20–40 mm Hg and diastolic pressure by 10–20 mm Hg. The initial blood pressure target is a systolic blood pressure in the range of 180–200 mm Hg and a diastolic blood pressure in the range of 110–120 mm Hg. Blood pressure should not be lowered too quickly, because doing so can result in hypoperfusion of the brain and myocardium. Once initial treatment goals are achieved, blood pressure can subsequently be reduced gradually to more appropriate levels.

Nitroprusside is the preferred agent in emergencies such as hypertensive encephalopathy, because the infusion can be titrated easily to effect. When myocardial ischemia is present, intravenous nitroglycerin or intravenous β-blockers such as labetalol or esmolol are preferred. Once blood pressure has been brought under control using intravenous therapy, oral agents should be initiated slowly as intravenous therapy is gradually withdrawn. Whether a patient is being treated for hypertensive urgency, emergency, or benign hypertension, long-term therapy and life-style modification are essential. Patients must receive regular follow-up and meet the treatment goals established by JNC VII to prevent unnecessary morbidity and mortality.

Diabetes Mellitus

34

Belinda Vail, MD

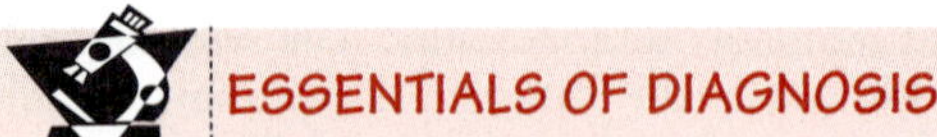

ESSENTIALS OF DIAGNOSIS

- *Two separate measurements of any combination of the following:*
  - *Random plasma glucose ≥ 200 mg/dL, with polydipsia, polyuria, polyphagia, or weight loss.*
  - *Fasting plasma glucose ≥ 126 mg/dL.*
  - *Two-hour oral glucose tolerance test ≥ 200 mg/dL after a 75-g glucose load.*

General Considerations

The increasing acquisition of processed food combined with decreasing physical activity has led to an explosion in worldwide obesity and type 2 diabetes mellitus, with the greatest rate of increase in the young. Diabetes is now the sixth leading cause of death in the United States, and one in every seven health care dollars goes to its treatment, with 63% spent on inpatient care. It is a major cause of blindness, renal failure, lower extremity amputations, cardiovascular disease, and congenital malformations. With 90% of patients receiving their care from primary care physicians, diabetes is the epitome of a chronic disease requiring a multidisciplinary management approach.

Narayan KM et al: Diabetes—a common, serious, costly, and potentially preventable public health problem. Diabetes Res Clin Pract 2000; 50:77. [PMID: 11024588]

Pathogenesis

Diabetes develops from a complex interaction of environmental and genetic factors. In type 1 diabetes this leads to destruction of the pancreatic beta cells and loss of the body's ability to produce insulin. Type 2 diabetes is the result of increasing cellular resistance to insulin. Obesity and inactivity accelerate this process. A very small percentage of diabetic patients may have latent-onset autoimmune diabetes with an onset similar to type 2 but destruction of the beta cells, and a more rapid progression to insulin dependence.

Pietropaolo M, Le Roith D: Pathogenesis of diabetes: Our current understanding. Clin Cornerstone 2001; 4:1. [PMID: 11838323]

Pradhan AD et al: C-reactive protein, interleukin 6, and risk of developing type 2 diabetes mellitus. JAMA 2001;286:327. [PMID: 11466099]

Prevention

It is unknown if significant life-style change can prevent diabetes, but it does delay its development. Diet and exercise intervention have been shown to reduce the risk of progression to type 2 diabetes by 58%. Metformin and pioglitazone also delay its onset by a more modest percentage. Tight control of hyperglycemia and blood pressure significantly reduce the complications of diabetes, and a sustained reduction in hemoglobin A_{1c} (HbA_{1c}) is associated with significant cost savings within 1–2 years.

Motivating individuals to make life-style changes is difficult but cost-effective and safe and can result in reduced obesity and hypertension and improvement of lipid profiles. A low-fat, high-fiber diet, modest exercise, and smoking cessation are modalities vastly superior to the complexities of the care of patients with diabetes and its complications.

The effect of intensive treatment of diabetes on the development and progression of long-term complications in insulin dependent diabetes mellitus. Diabetes Control and Complications Trial Research Group. N Engl J Med 1993;329:977. [PMID: 8366922]

Tuomilehto J et al; Diabetes Prevention Study Group: Prevention of type 2 diabetes mellitus by changes in lifestyle among subjects with impaired glucose tolerance. N Engl J Med 2001; 344:1343. [PMID: 11333990]

Turner R et al: UK Prospective Diabetes Study 17: A nine-year update of a randomized, controlled trial on the effect of improved metabolic control on complications in non-insulin dependent diabetes mellitus. Ann Intern Med 1996;124:136. [PMID: 8554206]

Screening

Fasting glucose is the screening method of choice, although a random glucose is acceptable. HbA_{1c} is not recommended as a screening test due to the lack of standardization and experience with its use in screening.

The US Preventive Services Task Force (USPSTF) recommends screening for diabetes in adults with hypertension or hyperlipidemia. The American Diabetes Association (ADA) recommends screening every 3 years beginning at age 45 or sooner and more frequently in those with the following risk factors:

1. Family history of diabetes.
2. Hypertension.
3. Dyslipidemia (especially high triglyceride level and low high-density lipoprotein [HDL] level).
4. Obesity.
5. High-risk ethnic or racial groups (African American, Hispanic, Native American).
6. Previous history of impaired glucose tolerance.
7. Gestational diabetes, or birth of a child weighing more than 9 pounds (4 kg).
8. Habitually physically inactive.
9. Cardiovascular disease.
10. Polycystic ovarian disease.

A consensus panel has recommended screening of overweight children (body mass index [BMI] or weight for height > 85th percentile or weight > 120% of ideal) every 2 years beginning at age 10 years or onset of puberty if the following risk factors are present:

1. Family history of diabetes in first- or second-degree relatives.
2. High-risk racial or ethnic group (Native Americans, African Americans, Hispanics, or Pacific Islanders).
3. Signs of, or conditions associated with, insulin resistance (eg, acanthosis nigricans, hypertension, dyslipidemia, and polycystic ovarian disease).

The USPSTF found insufficient evidence to recommend for or against universal screening for gestational diabetes. Women with the following risk factors usually require screening:

1. Age older than 25 years.
2. High-risk racial or ethnic group.
3. BMI of 25 or higher.
4. History of abnormal glucose tolerance test.
5. Previous history of adverse pregnancy outcomes usually associated with gestational diabetes.
6. Diabetes in a first-degree relative.

Initial screening is done with a 1-hour glucose tolerance test (GTT) consisting of a 50-g glucose load performed between 10 and 28 weeks' gestation, depending on severity of risk. If the 1-hour GTT is 130–140 mg/dL or higher, it is followed by a diagnostic 3-hour GTT consisting of a 100-g glucose load administered after an overnight fast. Two of the following must be abnormal to meet the diagnostic criteria:

1. Fasting level: ≥ 95 mg/dL.
2. One hour: ≥ 190 mg/dL.
3. Two hour: ≥ 165 mg/dL.
4. Three hour: ≥ 140 mg/dL.

American Diabetes Association: Gestational diabetes mellitus (position statement). Diabetes Care 2003;26(suppl 1):S103. [PMID: 12502639]

Type 2 diabetes in children and adolescents. American Diabetes Association. Diabetes Care 2000;23:381. [PMID: 10868870]

US Preventive Services Task Force: *Guide to Clinical Preventive Services,* 3rd ed*: Periodic Updates.* USPSTF, 2003. Available at: http://www.achcpr.gov/clinic/uspstf/supsdiab.htm.

Wareham NJ, Griffin SJ: Should we screen for type 2 diabetes? Evaluation against National Screening Committee criteria. Br Med J 2001;322:986. [PMID: 11312236]

Clinical Findings

A. Symptoms and Signs

The classic signs of diabetes are polyuria, polydipsia, and polyphagia, but initial signs may be subtle and nonspecific. Patients with type 1 diabetes exhibit fatigue, malaise, nausea and vomiting, irritability, and weight loss. Abdominal pain is common in children. Patients with type 1 diabetes present early in the disease process but usually are quite ill at presentation, often already ketoacidotic. Signs and symptoms of ketoacidosis include those associated with dehydration (dry skin and mucous membranes, decreased skin turgor, tachycardia, and hypotension), tachypnea and labored respirations with the classic "fruity" breath, abdominal pain, and confusion.

In type 2 diabetes symptoms are seen well after onset of the disease and may be due to complications. The classic signs are still prominent, but patients may also complain of fatigue, irritability, drowsiness, blurred vision, numbness or tingling in the extremities, slow wound healing, and frequent infections of the skin, gums, or genitourinary tract, including candidal infections.

Expert Committee on the Diagnosis and Classification of Diabetes Mellitus: Report of the expert committee on the diagnosis and classification of diabetes mellitus. Diabetes Care 2003;26(suppl 1):S5. [PMID: 12502614]

B. History and Physical Examination

The initial assessment for newly diagnosed diabetic patients is extensive because diabetes has a truly systemic effect. (Table 34–1). The use of written checklists or questionnaires, electronic health records, or the assistance of a trained nurse or assistant can decrease physician time. Standing orders are an excellent way to make the visit more efficient (Table 34–2). It is important to

Table 34–1. Necessary elements of the initial history and physical examination in patients with diabetes mellitus.

History
Current and previous symptoms consistent with diabetes
Weight changes; history of obesity
Eating patterns; nutritional status (growth and development in children)
Exercise history and ability to exercise
Details of previous treatment; prior HbA_{1c} records and monitoring
Current treatment (medications, diet)
Previous acute or severe complications (ketoacidosis, hypoglycemia)
Previous and current infections particularly of skin, feet, and GU systems
History of hypertension, hyperlipidemia, coronary artery disease, and insulin resistance
Chronic complications (eg, retinopathy, nephropathy, neuropathy, GI problems, vascular problems, sexual dysfunction, foot problems)
History of gestational diabetes, large-for-gestational-age infants, or miscarriages
Medications and allergies
Family history of diabetes, endocrine disorders, or heart disease
Tobacco, alcohol, and drug use
Life-style, cultural, psychosocial, education, and economic factors influencing control
Physical Examination
Height, weight, and BMI
Blood pressure (including orthostatic)
Ophthalmoscopic examination
Oral examination
Thyroid palpation
Cardiac examination
Evaluation of pulses, including carotid
Abdominal examination
Skin examination (including injection sites, if applicable)
Neurologic examination with particular attention to reflexes, vibratory senses, light tough (monofilament examination of both feet), and proprioception

HbA_{1c}, hemoglobin A_{1c}; GU, genitourinary; GI, gastrointestinal; BMI, body mass index.

update routine screening examinations (Papanicolaou [Pap], mammogram, colonoscopy) and ensure all immunizations are current (pneumococcal vaccine, tetanus, and yearly influenza vaccine).

Interim visits focus attention on compliance and patients' special issues with management. Any history of hypoglycemia or hyperglycemia, results of self-monitoring, and adjustments by patients in their therapeutic regimen are of particular importance. A brief history of complications, medications, psychosocial issues, and life-style changes should be obtained, and patients' goals—and their motivation for achieving them—assessed. The examination includes determination of weight and blood pressure and ophthalmoscopic, cardiac, and brief skin examinations. Shoes and socks are removed to allow visualization of the skin, palpation of pulses, and a monofilament examination of the feet. This examination uses a standardized length of 10-gauge nylon monofilament. When the line is touched to the bottom of the foot and bends, the patient should be able to detect its presence. It is also important to assess the status of yearly ophthalmology visits, semiannual dental examinations (because of the increased risk of periodontal disease), and any other required specialist visits.

Visit frequency is based on control of diabetes and the patient's understanding and comfort. Patients initiating insulin therapy may require daily contact, by phone or e-mail. Patients with poor control or making frequent changes may require weekly to monthly visits. Patients with well-controlled diabetes usually need visits only quarterly. Novel approaches to patient visits have also been described. These include visits in which multiple providers are seen, one after another, keeping physician time low; or group visits in which multiple patients are seen by the provider at the same time, sharing ideas and information among the group.

Table 34–2. Standing orders for diabetic patients.

1. Place the flowsheet in the patient's record and update with information from the patient and his/her chart (or update the electronic health record)
2. Monitor and record blood pressure in the same arm at each visit
3. Measure and record the patient's weight
4. If HbA_{1c} has not been evaluated in the past 6 months, complete a requisition and attach to the patient's chart
5. If urinalysis and microalbumin testing have not been done in the past year
   a. Perform a urine dipstick and record the results on the flowsheet
   b. Complete a requisition for urine microalbumin test and attach it to the patient's chart
6. If a lipid profile has not been obtained in the past year, complete a requisition and attach it to the patient's chart
7. If a dilated eye examination has not been performed in the past year, complete a referral for an ophthalmology examination and attach it to the patient's chart
8. Ask the patient to remove his/her shoes and socks
   a. Palpate dorsalis pedis and posterior tibial pulses
   b. Inspect the skin for any skin breakdown
   c. Record the findings on the patient's flowsheet

Physician Signature: _______________ Date: __________

Smith SA, Poland GA; American Diabetes Association: Immunization and the prevention of influenza and pneumococcal disease in people with diabetes. Diabetes Care 2003;26(suppl

1):S126. [PMID: 12502639]

Smith SA, Poland GA: The use of influenza and pneumococcal vaccines in people with diabetes. Diabetes Care 2000;23:95. [PMID: 10857977]

C. Laboratory Findings

Initial and yearly laboratory studies include fasting glucose, fasting lipid profile, serum electrolytes, blood urea nitrogen (BUN)/creatinine, urinalysis, and microalbumin. Evaluation of thyroid-stimulating hormone may be indicated. Depending on age and duration of disease, an electrocardiogram (ECG) should be performed, but because microalbuminuria is a marker for cardiovascular disease, an ECG should be performed at the onset of microalbuminuria. HbA_{1c} is measured every 3 months. Random microalbumin levels or microalbumin/creatinine ratios may be used for screening or monitoring, but patients may require a 24-hour urine collection for protein and creatinine clearance when there are significant changes.

Sacks DB et al: Guidelines and recommendations for laboratory analysis in the diagnosis and management of diabetes mellitus. Clin Chem 2002;48:436. [PMID: 11861436]

Complications

Preventing and delaying progression of all complications in patients with diabetes is dependent on life-style modification, tight control of blood glucose and blood pressure (< 130/80 mm Hg), and smoking cessation. Aspirin has no effect on microvascular complications but is important in the prevention of cardiovascular complications. Consider low-dose oral contraceptives in adolescent girls with type 1 diabetes who are older than 16 years and amenorrheic, although data on their effectiveness are limited.

A. Ketoacidosis

Ketoacidosis occurs when there is insufficient insulin to meet the body's needs, due either to a deficiency of insulin or to an increase in the body's needs (ie, illness or stress). In this state, gluconeogenesis and fatty acid oxidation increase, osmotic diuresis occurs, and the patient develops dehydration. This is accompanied by ketogenesis from fatty acid oxidation, resulting in a metabolic acidosis. The incidence of ketoacidosis in children is about 8 per 100 person-years; it increases with age in girls and is highest for children with poor control, inadequate insurance, or psychiatric disorders.

Treatment involves rehydration with normal saline and an insulin drip. Potassium is replaced when it starts to fall. Glucose is added to fluids when serum glucose approaches 250 mg/dL. Laboratory values are monitored every 1–2 hours, and the insulin drip is continued until acidosis is resolved and ketones are cleared.

B. Infections

Patients with diabetes are at greater risk for infections, including community-acquired pneumonia (particularly pneumococcal), influenza, cholecystitis, urinary tract infections, and pyelonephritis. Persistent fever and flank pain lasting more than 3–4 days despite appropriate antibiotic treatment should elicit an evaluation (preferably by computed tomography) for a perinephric abscess. Fungal infections are frequently seen, especially vaginal candidiasis, but also mucormycosis, and infections of the eye or skin. Foot infections include cellulitis, osteomyelitis, plantar abscesses, and necrotizing fasciitis.

C. Nephropathy

Diabetic nephropathy is the most common cause of end-stage renal disease (ESRD) in the United States. The incidence is much higher in patients with type 1 diabetes, but the prevalence is higher in those with type 2. It is more common in Native Americans, Asians, and Mexican Americans, and among African Americans the rate is four times that of whites. Risk factors include poor glycemic control, smoking, hypertension, family history, and glomerular hyperfiltration. All patients should be screened yearly with a microalbumin test. Microalbuminuria is defined as 30–300 mg protein in a 24-hour urine collection, a more accurate but significantly more cumbersome test. More than 300 mg/24 h constitutes macroalbuminuria or nephropathy.

Intensive therapy, reduces the incidence of microalbuminuria, and patients treated early maintain better renal function that those who gain tight control later. The risk of microalbuminuria increases by 25% for each 10% rise in HbA_{1c}. Angiotensin-converting enzyme (ACE) inhibitors are the drug of choice in patients with microalbuminuria. Ramipril has been shown to reduce ESRD and death by 41% and proteinuria by 20% compared with amlodipine. Angiotensin II receptor blockers (ARBs) have shown comparable efficacy, and a combination of the two may be highly effective. Referral to a nephrologist is indicated in the presence of rising creatinine level or increasing microalbuminuria.

American Diabetes Association: Diabetic nephropathy (Position Statement). Diabetes Care 2003;26(suppl 1):S94. [PMID: 12502639]

Barnett A: Prevention of loss of renal function over time in patients with diabetic nephropathy. Am J Med 2006;119:S40. [PMID: 16563947]

D. Retinopathy

About 20% of diabetic patients show signs of retinopathy at the time of diagnosis, and progression is orderly, from mild abnormalities (small retinal hemorrhages) to proliferative retinopathy with growth of new vessels on the retina and into the vitreous, culminating in vision loss. The risk of retinopathy increases with increasing HbA_{1c} level and duration of the disease, so improving glycemic control may delay onset. Patients with type 1 diabetes may begin yearly ophthalmology visits 5 years after diagnosis, but those with type 2 should begin yearly office visits as soon as the diagnosis is made. Laser photocoagulation therapy is currently the only treatment option once the disease progresses.

American Diabetes Association: Diabetic retinopathy (position statement). Diabetes Care 2003;26(suppl 1):S99. [PMID: 12502639]

E. Neuropathy

Peripheral neuropathy leads to a loss of sensation and pain in the hands and feet and is the major cause of foot problems in diabetic individuals. Treatment of peripheral neuropathy remains symptomatic. Pregabalin (Lyrica), indicated for diabetic neuropathy, is available in multiple strengths from 25 to 300 mg and is taken two to three times a day. It should be taken with caution in patients using pioglitazone or rosiglitazone. Other treatment options with some efficacy include nonsteroidal anti-inflammatory drugs (NSAIDs), tricyclic antidepressants (amitriptyline, 10–150 mg/day), several anticonvulsants (gabapentin, 900–3600 mg/day; carbamazepine, 200 mg twice a day), newer selective serotonin reuptake inhibitors (duloxetine and venlafaxine), and topical capsaicin cream.

Autonomic neuropathy may be more difficult to detect, and patients should be asked intermittently about symptoms of orthostatic hypotension, diarrhea or constipation, incontinence, impotence, and heat intolerance. It is also important to check for any of the following findings: resting tachycardia, orthostatic hypotension, dependent edema (to assess impaired venoarteriolar reflex), and decreased diameter of dark-adapted pupils. Gastrointestinal motility may be improved with metoclopramide or erythromycin.

Attal N et al: EFNS guidelines on pharmacological treatment of neuropathic pain. Eur J Neurol 2006;13:1153 [PMID: 17038030]

Jensen TS: New perspectives on the management of diabetic peripheral neuropathic pain. Diab Vasc Dis Res 2006;3:108. [PMID:17058631]

F. Cardiovascular Disease

Heart disease is the leading cause of death in patients with diabetes, and recent advances in cardiac care have not reduced mortality in diabetics. Half of diabetic patients have coronary disease at the time of diagnosis, and their prevalence of coronary events is 2–20 times higher than in the general population. Men have double, and women four to five times the risk for myocardial infarction (MI), with a higher incidence of diffuse, multivessel disease, plaque rupture, superimposed thrombosis, and in-hospital mortality. Five-year survival following angioplasty or coronary artery bypass graft (CABG) is lower in patients with diabetes; however, survival rates are significantly higher with CABG.

ACE inhibitors are the first-line choice for treatment of hypertension in diabetic patients, producing a significant decrease in stroke, MI, cardiac death, post-MI mortality, and ischemic events following revascularization procedures. They have been shown to reduce left ventricular mass by as much as 40%, thereby decreasing the risk of sudden death, congestive heart failure, and ventricular dysrhythmias. In the Heart Outcomes Prevention Evaluation (HOPE) trial the use of ACE inhibitors correlated with a 34% reduction in the onset of new cases of diabetes and a mild improvement in lipid profiles. These agents may be used in all diabetic patients with systolic blood pressure greater than 100 mm Hg and for hypertension in patients with signs of insulin resistance. Although compelling, the body of data is insufficient to recommend prophylactic ACE inhibitor therapy for all diabetics. The drugs can be used irrespective of creatinine level, but potassium level must be carefully monitored as creatinine rises. ACE inhibitors are contraindicated in pregnancy. The most troublesome side effects are a bradykinin-induced dry cough and angioedema. There appears to be a nonsynergistic effect between aspirin and ACE inhibitors that may be reduced by using 81 mg of aspirin or giving the two medications 12 hours apart. Increasing data support the use of ARBs for cardiovascular risk reduction as well, and they are better tolerated than ACE inhibitors.

Thiazide diuretics and β-blockers are effective in lowering blood pressure and have been shown to reduce cardiovascular morbidity and mortality. Although they can have some effect on glucose control, they are acceptable for use in patients with diabetes if used judiciously. (For further information about treatment of hypertension in patients with diabetes, see Chapter 33.)

Aspirin therapy at doses of 81–325 mg/day is indicated for all diabetic individuals older than 40 years of age or with known cardiovascular disease, and smoking cessation must be emphasized.

Gerstein HC et al: Albuminuria and risk of cardiovascular events, death, and heart failure in diabetic and nondiabetic individuals. JAMA 2001;286:421. [PMID: 11466120]

O'Keefe JH et al: Improving the adverse cardiovascular prognosis of type 2 diabetes. Mayo Clin Proc 1999;74:171. [PMID: 10069357]

Tight blood pressure control and risk of macrovascular and microvascular complications in type 2 diabetes: UKPDS 38. UK Prospective Diabetes Study Group. BMJ 1998;317:703. [PMID: 9732337]

Yusuf S et al: Effects of an angiotensin-converting-enzyme inhibitor, ramipril, on death from cardiovascular causes, myocardial infarction, and stroke in high-risk patients. The Heart Outcomes Prevention Evaluation Study Investigators. New Engl J Med 2000;342:145. [PMID: 10639539]

G. Hyperlipidemias

Patients with type 2 diabetes often have a distinct triad of elevated triglyceride and low-density lipoprotein (LDL) levels, and decreased HDL level. Each of these abnormalities has been shown to be an independent factor in atherogenesis. Current recommendations are to maintain total cholesterol below 200 mg/dL, triglycerides below 150 mg/dL, and LDL cholesterol below 100 mg/dL or below 70 mg/dL in the presence of cardiovascular disease.

Hydroxymethylglutaryl coenzyme A (HMG-CoA) reductase inhibitors (statins) are the drugs of choice in treating hyperlipidemia in diabetic patients. Most outcome studies on lipid management have excluded patients with diabetes, but subgroup analysis shows a reduction in cardiovascular events of 25–37% with the use of statins to improve the lipid profile. These drugs are contraindicated in pregnancy and must be used with extreme caution in adolescents. Most patients who have an insufficient response or cannot tolerate statins can now be managed with ezetimibe (Zetia). Other medications are used less frequently in diabetic patients. (See Chapter 20 for further information.)

H. Diabetic Feet

Diabetes is the leading nontraumatic cause of foot amputation and Charcot foot in the United States. These complications are caused by a combination of neuropathy, altered foot structure, and vasculopathy. Fifteen percent of diabetics will have a foot ulcer at some time and 20% of these will lead to amputation. Feet should be examined at every office visit and patients instructed in good foot care. Prevention of skin breakdown and infections is the best treatment. Medicare will pay for special shoes and the fitting of these shoes by a podiatrist or orthotist. However, careful attention to foot care by primary providers was found to be more effective at preventing ulcers than special shoes or inserts.

Treatment of diabetic foot ulcers requires removing pressure or unloading the ulcer and good wound care with deep debridement and appropriate dressings. Betadine is not appropriate for cleaning, and antibiotics should be used only if infection is clearly present, as they have been shown to retard healing in the noninfected foot. Wound cultures almost always yield multiple organisms and usually are helpful only if taken from the bone in cases of osteomyelitis. Becaplermin (Regranex) aids in healing but is expensive and is usually not necessary. The best indication of ability to heal is an intact pulse. The test of choice for diagnosis of osteomyelitis is magnetic resonance imaging, although bone scans are a good alternative. Treatment efficacy can be followed by monitoring the sedimentation rate.

Treatment

A. Overall Management

Glycemic control is cost effective in minimizing microvascular complications, and blood pressure control independently affects the progression of microvascular and macrovascular complications. There is good clinical evidence to support aggressive management of hyperglycemia, hypertension, and hyperlipidemia to reduce nephropathy, retinopathy, neuropathy, and cardiovascular events.

The management goals are to maintain fasting glucose levels of 80–100 mg/dL, bedtime levels below 120 mg/dL, and HbA_{1c} levels below 7%; the American College of Endocrinology and the American Association of Clinical Endocrinologists have set a goal for HbA_{1c} of less than 6.5%. The American Kidney Association recommends that blood pressure be maintained below 130/80 mm Hg. Less stringent treatment goals may be appropriate in patients with limited life expectancies, in the very young, in older adults at risk for hypoglycemia, or in patients with comorbid conditions. Several evidence-based recommendations are available to guide management of patients with diabetes mellitus (Table 34–3).

B. Patient Education

Education is the cornerstone of diabetes management. Because the most important management tool is life-style alteration, it is imperative that the patient take ownership of the disease and develop skills for managing it. Clinicians, nurse practitioners, nurses, diabetes educators, dietitians, and others can all contribute to the educational process using didactic discussions, reading materials, Internet sites, and self-tests. Patients need to have a basic understanding of diabetes and the complications of both the disease and the treatments. This includes the interrelationship of life-style changes, smoking cessation, home monitoring, management of blood pressure and lipids, and foot and skin care. Additionally they need to know and understand their medication and insulin regimens and how to recognize problems with medications. Some patients will need instruction in special situations that may involve work or travel. Time should be devoted to the psychological aspects of the disease, including family and other outside support, self-image, and relationships. Finally, as they gain a better understanding of their disease patients will be able to set treatment goals in conjunction with the care team.

C. Nutritional Therapy

The goal of nutritional therapy in diabetes is to maintain a near-normal blood glucose level and optimal serum lipid levels. Weight loss in obese individuals of 10–15% significantly improves glucose control and insulin sensitivity and decreases mortality. A reduction of 300–400 kcal/day will induce a modest weight loss in most individuals. Surgery for weight loss can lead to a significant weight loss and normalization of blood

Table 34–3. Evidence-based recommendations for diabetes.

Recommendation	Source
1. In patients with type 2 diabetes, the risk of diabetic complications was strongly associated with previous hyperglycemia. Any reduction in HbA_{1c} is likely to reduce the risk of complications, with the lowest risk being in those with HbA_{1c} values in the normal range (<6.0%).	**SOR-B:** http://www.icsi.org/knowledge/detail.asp?catID=29&itemID=182
2. Both vigorous exercise and moderate exercise reduce the risk of type 2 diabetes in women. The more exercise is taken, the greater the risk reduction.	RCT: http://www.jr2.ox.ac/bandolier/booth/hliving/excer2diab.html
3. Metformin should be considered as the first-line oral hypoglycemic agent in overweight patients with diabetes.	SOR-A: http://www.guideline.gov/summary/summary.aspx?doc_id=3078
4. Patients with microalbuminuria or proteinuria should be considered for angiotensin II antagonist therapy.	SOR-A: http://www.guideline.gov/summary/summary.aspx?doc_id=3078
5. For patients with type 2 diabetes mellitus, low-dose aspirin therapy (81–325 mg daily) should be initiated in patients 40 years of age and older unless there is a contraindication to aspirin therapy.	Class A, B: http://www.icsi.org/knowledge/detail.asp?

HbA_{1c}, hemoglobin A_{1c}; SOR, strength of recommendation (A: randomized controlled trials [RCT]; B: other types of trials [retrospective, cohort]).

glucose. The shift in nutrition is toward individualization and achievement of goals, health, and well-being. Structured programs designed to promote life-style changes that include education, decreased fat and overall calorie intake, regular exercise, and regular follow-up have been shown to produce long-term weight loss of about 5–7%.

The recommended intake of carbohydrates is 55–60% of total calories, with the greatest percentage coming from fruits and vegetables (5 servings per day), whole grains, and low-fat dairy products. Increasing low-fat dairy consumption in overweight adults leads to decreased insulin resistance. A high-fiber diet (particularly soluble type) improves glycemic control, decreases hyperinsulinemia, and lowers plasma lipid concentrations in patients with type 2 diabetes. Nonnutritive sweeteners are safe when used within the acceptable intake levels recommended by the Food and Drug Administration (FDA). Patients should also be advised to limit alcohol.

Less than 10% of energy intake should be derived from saturated fats, with a maximum of 30% for total fat, and dietary cholesterol of less than 300 mg/day. Long-term maintenance of low-fat diets contributes to modest weight loss and improvement of dyslipidemia.

Diabetic patients may consume 10–20% of total calories as protein. There is no evidence that further restriction protects against renal disease but with the onset of microalbuminuria restriction to 10–15% will help delay progression. Patients with hypertension should restrict sodium intake to less than 2400 mg/day. Individuals receiving fixed daily doses of insulin should try to maintain a consistent daily caloric intake.

American Diabetes Association: Evidence-based nutrition principles and recommendations for the treatment and prevention of diabetes and related complications (position statement). Diabetes Care 2003;26(suppl 1):S51. [PMID: 12502639]

Knowler WC et al; Diabetes Prevention Program Research Group: Reduction in the incidence of type 2 diabetes with lifestyle intervention or metformin. N Engl J Med 2002;346:393. [PMID: 11832527]

D. Exercise

Exercise improves self-esteem, reduces stress, lowers heart rate and blood pressure, improves circulation, lowers lipid levels, improves digestion, controls appetite, lowers blood glucose, increases strength and endurance, reduces risk of cardiovascular disease, improves sleep and energy level, may increase HDL cholesterol and insulin sensitivity, and can contribute to weight loss. When combined with dietary therapy, a daily walking program has been shown to decrease weight and improve insulin sensitivity. Exercise programs alone decrease HbA_{1c} levels by 0.66% with no significant changes in body mass. Benefit seems greatest prior to or early in the disease course, and exercise may help delay or even prevent the onset of type 2 diabetes. A regular exercise program adapted to complications for all patients should be prescribed, including moderate aerobic or physical activity for 20–60 minutes at least every 48 hours. Older patients and those at increased risk of coronary artery disease should have a careful physical examination and an exercise stress test before beginning or significantly advancing an exercise program and should avoid sudden strenuous exercise. Athletes with type 1 diabetes may not participate in strenuous exercise when their blood glucose level is greater than 300 mg/dL or greater than 250 mg/dL with urine ketones present. Treatment consists of insulin and careful monitoring without increasing exercise.

E. Home Glucose Monitoring

The consensus panel of the ADA recommends that all patients with diabetes perform home glucose monitoring. Eighty-four percent of patients who monitor their blood glucose are within 20% of their target range. Home monitors should be checked if values obtained by patients do not correspond with office-obtained values. Newer glucose monitors are smaller, require less blood, and calculate serum glucose more rapidly. They also have the ability to store previous readings, and many have systems that can download the memory onto a personal computer. Medicare and some insurance companies cover the cost of monitoring, so choice of machine may be influenced by insurance coverage. A wristwatch-style device and a continuing monitoring system are available but are very expensive.

Type 1 diabetics should monitor blood glucose at least four times a day. Patients with type 2 diabetes can monitor once or twice a day based on their degree of control, but they need to include fasting, bedtime, and pre- and 2-hour post-prandial readings. Patients taking intermediate-acting insulin (neutral protamine Hagedorn [NPH]) may also need to obtain readings at 2–3 AM. In general, fasting and 2-hour post-prandial values are the most helpful and predictive of long-term control and minimization of complications.

F. Pharmacotherapy

There are now six categories of oral medications, two subcutaneous medications, and increasing choices for insulin. In most cases, therapy is begun with one agent and dosage is increased before adding a second, but two may be synergistic. Table 34–4 lists trade names and available dosages of current oral agents.

Table 34–4. Oral agents for treatment of diabetes.

Drug	Available Dosage (mg)	Dosage Range (mg/day)
Biguanides		
Metformin (Glucophage)	500, 850, 1000	500–2500
Metformin XR (Glucophage XR)	500, 750	500–2000
Sulfonylureas		
Glimepiride (Amaryl)	1, 2, 4	1–8
Glipizide (Glucotrol)	5, 10	5–40
Glipizide XL (Glucotrol XL)	2.5, 5, 10	2.5–20
Glyburide (DiaBeta, Micronase)	1.25, 2.5, 5	1.25–20
Glyburide, micronized (Glynase)	1.5, 3, 6	
Meglitinides		
Nateglinide (Starlix)	60, 120	60–120 (three times daily)
Repaglinide (Prandin)	0.5, 1, 2	0.5–4 (two to four times daily)
Thiazolidinediones		
Pioglitazone (Actos)	15, 30, 45	15—45
Rosiglitazone (Avandia)	2, 4, 8	15—45
α-Glucosidase Inhibitors		
Acarbose (Precose)	25, 50, 100	25–100 (three times daily)
Miglitol (Glyset)	25, 50, 100	25–100 (three times daily)
Dipeptidyl Peptidase-4 Inhibitor		
Sitagliptin (Januvia)	25, 50, 100	100 (25–50 renal impairment)
Combination		
Glyburide/Metformin	1.25/250, 2.5/500, 5/500	1.25/250–20/2000
Actoplus Met	15/500, 15/850	15/500–45/2550
Avandamet	1/500, 2/1000, 2/500,4/500	1/500–8/2000

1. Biguanides—Metformin is a potent oral antihyperglycemic, lowering HbA_{1c} levels by 1.5–2.0%, and is the preferred first-line agent in treating type 2 diabetes. It decreases gluconeogenesis in the liver, improves insulin sensitivity in the liver and in muscle tissue, and may decrease intestinal glucose absorption. It also lowers insulin levels, has a beneficial effect on lipids, and improves endothelial function. This leads to a decrease in cardiovascular events, a reduction in diabetes end points, a decrease in diabetes-related deaths, and a reduction in all-cause mortality. Metformin does not cause hypoglycemia and may contribute to some weight loss by decreasing appetite.

Gastrointestinal side effects, particularly nausea and diarrhea, are common but are reduced by using the recommended starting dose of 500 mg twice a day, or once a day with the largest meal. Metformin should not be used in patients with congestive heart failure requiring medication or with renal insufficiency (creatinine > 1.5 mg/dL), due to the slight possibility of lactic acidosis. Although rare, lactic acidosis has a 50% mortality rate. Metformin should be used with caution in the elderly and in patients with hepatic dysfunction. It must be stopped when giving intravenous contrast dye and is restarted 48 hours after the procedure. A category B drug, it may be used in pregnancy but not during lactation. It is, however, the drug of choice in children with type 2 diabetes and has been used successfully in children 10 years of age and older. There is no evidence for its safety in younger children. Metformin is used in patients with impaired glucose tolerance to prolong or prevent the onset of diabetes.

2. Sulfonylureas—Sulfonylureas are insulin secretagogues that stimulate the pancreatic beta cells to increase insulin production. Hypoglycemia and weight gain are the most common side effects. They are safe for use in the elderly at lower doses. Sulfonylureas should be taken 1 hour before meals to induce insulin secretion or at bedtime, which helps limit hepatic glucose production. They are efficacious, lowering HbA_{1c} levels up to 2.0%, but about 20% of patients who start on sulfonylureas will not respond. Because these agents tend to lose efficacy over time, doses must be increased or other medications added. Glyburide is the most commonly used agent but also has the greatest propensity to cause hypoglycemia. Glimepiride is the newest and most expensive agent. It has a more rapid onset and longer duration of action than other sulfonylureas, but induces less hypoglycemia, and may be the best choice in patients with known coronary disease.

3. Meglitinides—The meglitinides, repaglinide and nateglinide, are short-acting insulin secretagogues. They have a rapid onset of action, and a half-life of less than an hour, so they may be taken immediately before meals. If a meal is skipped, the dose is skipped as well. Nateglinide has a more rapid onset and shorter duration of action than repaglinide and is indicated for combination therapy with metformin. The meglitinides have been reported to reduce HbA_{1c} levels from 0.5% to 2.0%, but are significantly more expensive than sulfonylureas. They are particularly useful in patients whose fasting glucose levels are well controlled but who have high post-prandial values or for patients who eat few or irregular meals. These medications should be used with caution in patients with hepatic dysfunction but can be used in renal failure.

4. Thiazolidinediones—The thiazolidinediones (TZDs), rosiglitazone and pioglitazone, work primarily by improving target cell response to insulin in muscle and adipose tissue, thereby decreasing insulin resistance. They also decrease hepatic gluconeogenesis and increase peripheral glucose disposal. Pioglitazone has been shown to decrease triglyceride levels and increase HDL levels, but the TZDs cause an increase in LDL cholesterol levels and are associated with weight gain, water retention and edema, and congestive heart failure. They can delay the onset of diabetes, but their long-term effects on cardiovascular outcomes and mortality remain controversial. TZDs are metabolized by the liver, so they may be used in patients with renal failure, but liver function tests must be monitored. They increase ovulation and, therefore, increase the chance of pregnancy in obese diabetic women, but they can also be used in pregnancy. They are not currently recommended for children. They have been shown to increase extremity fracture risk in females.

Initiating therapy with TZDs requires patience. It may take 12 weeks for the medication to reach its maximum potential. Increases in dosage should be made only after several weeks on the same dose.

5. α-Glucosidase inhibitors—The α-glucosidase inhibitors, acarbose and miglitol, interfere with disaccharide metabolism and delay carbohydrate absorption in the gut by inhibiting α-glucosidase in the brush border of the small intestine and blunting post-prandial hyperglycemia. This mechanism produces a modest and relatively expensive reduction in HbA_{1c} of 0.7–1.0%. They work only when taken with food, so they do not cause hypoglycemia when used alone. They are particularly useful in patients with erratic or poor eating habits, because they are taken only with meals.

If α-glucosidase inhibitors are used with a sulfonylurea or insulin and hypoglycemia occurs, the patient must be treated with simple sugars (glucose or lactose), not with sucrose. Therapy should be initiated at a low dose and increased slowly to minimize side effects as gastrointestinal side effects are frequent and objectionable. Flatulence is caused by continued disaccharide decomposition in the large intestine. α-Glucosidase inhibitors should not be used in patients with inflammatory bowel disease or other chronic intestinal disorders and are contraindicated in those with ketoacidosis or cirrhosis. Efficacy is altered with digestive enzymes, antacids, or cholestyramine. In addition, these agents are not recommended when serum creatinine exceeds 2.0 mg/dL. Serum transaminase levels must be followed every 3 months for the first year.

6. Incretin mimetics—The newest drug in this category is the dipeptidyl peptidase-4 (DDP-4) inhibitor sitagliptin (Januvia). Glucagon-like peptide 1 (GLP-1) stimulates insulin secretion and biosynthesis and inhibits glucagon secretion and gastric emptying. This peptide is normally degraded by DDP-4. Sitagliptin's inhibition of DDP-4 increases plasma insulin and decreases plasma glucagon. It is dosed at 100 mg/day and is indicated for monotherapy or in combination with metformin or a thiazolidinedione.

Exenatide (Byetta) suppresses inappropriate glucagon secretion and slows gastric emptying. It is indicated for use with metformin or a sulfonylurea and is given as a subcutaneous injection (5–10 mcg) before breakfast and dinner. Side effects include nausea and weight loss.

Pramlintide acetate (Symlin) is an analog of human amylin, a neuroendocrine hormone synthesized by the pancreatic beta cells that facilitates glucose control during the post-prandial period. It is given as a separate, subcutaneous injection with insulin prior to meals. Starting dose is 15 mcg and may be doubled weekly to a maximum of 120 mcg. Both exenatide and pramlintide may contribute to significant weight loss.

7. Combination therapy—Insulin, sulfonylureas, and meglitinides all increase insulin levels. They can be used together but are more efficiently used with metformin, a TZD, or an α-glucosidase inhibitor. Combining drugs with different mechanisms of action is most efficacious. Caution must be exercised in combining drugs with similar side effects. The best results in the UKPDS trial were achieved with the combination of insulin and metformin. Metformin can be combined with any of the other medications and is available combined with two sulfonylureas and both TZDs. Rosiglitazone is combined with glimepiride. α-Glucosidase inhibitors should be used with caution with the TZDs because both can be hepatotoxic. They also must be carefully monitored with sulfonylureas, meglitinides, and insulin because treatment of hypoglycemia can be difficult. In addition, the similar target of post-prandial hyperglycemia and the three-times-daily dosing of the meglitinides and α-glucosidase inhibitors make them a poor combination. Patients with long-standing diabetes may require the addition of insulin as they age and beta cell function is depleted.

8. Insulin—The UKPDS trial did not show any increase in cardiovascular disease due to the use of insulin but did demonstrate a significant improvement in all complications of diabetes with tight control. A long-acting insulin provides a basal rate that minimizes hepatic glucose production. A short-acting insulin is used with meals to minimize the post-prandial insulin peak. In normal patients circulating insulin returns to the basal level as soon as post-prandial blood glucose levels normalize.

The new synthetic insulins more closely mimic the pharmacokinetics of human insulin in vivo (Table 34–5). Regular insulin has a slower onset and peak and longer duration, leading to a blood glucose nadir several hours after meals and often necessitating the use of a snack to maintain blood glucose levels. It is also given about 30 minutes before meals, making any delay in eating a hazard. The synthetic insulin analogs—lispro, aspart, and glulisine—have a shorter onset and peak and duration of only 2–4 hours, corresponding to a normal fall in post-

Table 34–5. Current insulins.

	Onset of Action	Peak (h)	Duration (h)
Rapid Acting			
Lispro (Humalog)	15 min	0.5–1.5	2–4
Aspart (NovoLog)	15 min	1–3	3–5
Glulisine (Apidra)	15 min	1–1.5	5
Insulin human inhalation powder (Exubera)	10 min	0.5–1.5	6
Short Acting			
Regular	30 min	2–4	5–8
Intermediate			
NPH or N	1–3 h	5–7	16–18
Long Acting			
Glargine (Lantus)	1 h	None	24
Detemir (Levemir)	1 h	None	20

prandial blood glucose. These insulins are given immediately before the meal and disappear with the normalization of blood glucose, decreasing post-prandial hypoglycemia. Humalog mix 75/25 is a mixture of 75% lispro protamine suspension and 25% lispro (it has the same onset and peak as lispro but has a longer duration of action).

Human insulin is available as an orally inhaled powder (Exubera). This insulin has a rapid onset and peak but a duration similar to regular insulin. It is dosed by body weight and is available in blister packs of 1 mg and 3 mg, roughly equivalent to 3 units and 8 units of regular insulin, respectively. It can not be used in smokers or in patients with significant lung disease (chronic obstructive pulmonary disease, asthma). All patients must have pulmonary function tests prior to initiation of therapy because inhaled insulin produces mild deterioration in lung function.

The intermediate acting insulin, neutral protamine Hagedorn (NPH) is usually given twice a day, with peaks occurring in the afternoon and early morning, although it is occasionally given once a day in patients with type 2 diabetes. Dosage changes are made based on fingersticks taken about 8 hours following the dose. The long-acting insulin analogs, glargine and detemir, are peakless insulins with a consistent 24-hour duration. They are less soluble in subcutaneous tissue, prolonging absorption, and can be used with any of the short-acting insulins and oral medications. They cannot, however, be mixed in the same syringe with other insulins. They are usually taken once a day but may be divided (especially helpful when giving more than 100 units). When converting to these insulins, total all insulin that they are replacing and multiply by 0.8. If no episodes of severe hypoglycemia occur after monitoring for two consecutive days, the dose may be increased two units for every 20 mg/dL rise in glucose above 100 mg/dL, but do not increase more than 8 units at a time.

Bioavailability of insulin changes with the site of injection. Abdominal injection (especially above the umbilicus) produces the quickest response; using the arm is slower, but is faster than using the hip or thigh. The ADA now recommends rotating injections within the same area instead of rotating between areas.

When initiating insulin therapy in patients with type 1 diabetes, their total insulin requirement for 24 hours (from insulin infusion or sliding scale regular) should be estimated. Half of this amount will be given as an intermediate- or long-acting insulin and the other half as a short-acting insulin. If using an intermediate form, its portion is divided, with two thirds given in the morning and one third in the evening. The short-acting portion is divided, with 40% given before breakfast, 40% before dinner, and the remaining 20% prior to lunch.

9. Insulin pump—Continuous subcutaneous insulin infusion (CSII) was first reported in the 1970s. Since then, these "insulin pumps" have become smaller and easier to use, with more safety features. Current pumps weigh about 4 ounces and are about the size of a beeper. CSII allows for continuous use of short-acting insulin and produces a more consistent absorption rate because the site of injection is not rotated. The newer short-acting insulin analogs (lispro and aspart) appear to be more beneficial in the CSII system than regular insulin. Patients can achieve tighter control with the pump while gaining more flexibility in eating habits and a more normal life-style. Used correctly there are fewer episodes of severe hypoglycemia, a reduction of total insulin usage, and less weight gain. Particularly good candidates for insulin pump therapy include patients who have difficulty achieving control of blood glucose, wide glucose swings, erratic schedules, or a significant dawn phenomenon; pregnant women; and teenagers with poor control or frequent episodes of ketoacidosis.

When initiating pump therapy in adults the total dose of insulin may be reduced by 25–30%. In children the total dose usually remains the same. In general, the average adult requires about 0.7 units/kg/day. Older individuals may require only 0.5 units/kg/day; adolescents may need 1.0 unit/kg/day. Half of the insulin is given continuously as a basal dose and the other half is divided into mealtime boluses. Only short- or rapid-acting insulin is used. A sample calculation of insulin dosage for pump therapy is included in Table 34–6.

10. Transplantation—During the 1990s more than 250 brittle, insulin-dependent diabetics received islet cell transplants, but only 12% remained insulin independent for more than 1 week. A new method of islet cell injection that also uses an immunosuppressive combination that does not include steroids looks promising. Seven patients who received these transplants remained insulin independent for 4–15 months. Although each transplant requires only two cadaver donors, the limited supply of donated organs will continue to make this an option only for patients whose diabetes is extremely difficult to control.

Table 34–6. Sample calculation of insulin dosage for pump therapy.

Calculation for 70-kg individual:
- 70 kg × 0.7 = 49 units regular or lispro/aspart insulin
- 49 ÷ 2 = 24.5
- 24 units as basal dose ÷ 24 hours = 1 unit/h basal dose
- 25 units are then available for bolus dosing (10 units for breakfast, 5 units for lunch, and 10 units for dinner)

When plasma glucose is high:
- 1500 ÷ 49 = ~30 mg/dL drop per unit of insulin (if blood glucose is 200 mg/dL, 3 units will decrease plasma levels by 90)

Effect of intensive blood-glucose control with metformin on complications in overweight patients with type 2 diabetes (UKPDS 34). UK Prospective Diabetes Study (UKPDS) Group. Lancet 1998;352:854. [PMID: 9742977]

Inzucchi SE: Oral antihyperglycemic therapy for type 2 diabetes: Scientific review. JAMA 2002;287:360. [PMID: 11790216]

Mayfield JA, White RD: Insulin therapy for type 2 diabetes: Rescue, augmentation, and replacement of beta-cell function. Am Fam Physician 2004;70:489. [PMID: 15317436]

Pereira MA et al: Dairy consumption, obesity, and the insulin resistance syndrome in young adults: The CARDIA study. JAMA 2002;287:2081. [PMID: 11966382]

Ratner RE: Glycemic control in the prevention of diabetic complications. Clin Cornerstone 2001;4:24. [PMID: 11838325]

Richter B et al: Pioglitazone for type 2 diabetes mellitus. Cochrane Database Syst Rev 2006;(4);CD006060. [PMID: 17054272]

G. Alternative and Complementary Therapies

Much of the conventional therapy for diabetes falls under the category of integrative medicine. Diet, exercise, and a multidisciplinary approach are all extremely important. There are no large randomized-controlled trials on alternative therapies, but a number of small studies have shown some promise.

1. **Chromium.** Chromium may augment the action of insulin and have a beneficial effect on mild glucose intolerance. Chromium picolinate is available over the counter, but questions have been raised concerning possible chromosomal damage with long-term, high-dose therapy. The current recommendation is 200 mcg/day. It seems to be most efficacious in patients with a low chromium level due to poor dietary intake, but there is no readily available assay to detect these patients.
2. **Magnesium.** Observations have been made that patients with well-controlled diabetes have magnesium levels in the normal range, and those with poorly controlled diabetes have low levels. It is not known if magnesium influences glucose levels or if elevated glucose levels cause magnesium levels to fall. No significant studies show improved glycemic control with magnesium supplementation, but it might decrease complication rates.
3. **Other substances.** There is some evidence for the use of vanadium to lower blood glucose, but no studies have been performed to establish a safe dose of this element. Recently cinnamon was reported to lower glucose levels. Biotin, vitamin B_6, fenugreek seeds (found in curry), American ginseng, and bitter melon are other substances that are reputed to lower blood glucose level, but evidence for all is minimal.

Alternative therapies that are used in the treatment of complications of diabetes include acupuncture and biofeedback. Both may be used to decrease pain from peripheral neuropathy or vascular disease. α-Lipoic acid and γ-linolenic acid (evening primrose oil), and zinc may decrease the symptoms of peripheral neuropathy, and ginkgo biloba may decrease symptoms from peripheral vascular disease.

H. Cultural Considerations

Diabetes is a disease that affects all races and nationalities. Indigenous peoples who have come later to a western life-style are protected primarily when they maintain their native diet. Many have unique beliefs when dealing with western medicine. Helping them to maintain a healthy life-style consistent with their heritage is the best way to avoid cultural gaffes and to affect long-term results.

Systems Approach to Care

Numerous studies have looked at the health care system and the delivery of health care for diabetes. Several approaches have been shown to dramatically improve glycemic control. Development of guidelines helps practitioners to cover all areas of diabetes care in an efficient manner. Diabetes improvement models that target education and quality review of providers have been shown to improve provider compliance. Use of electronic medical records or computerized registry systems can provide recurrent review for all aspects of diabetes care, and can be used for call-back and reminder systems so fewer patients are lost to care. Most importantly, patients must become empowered and take ownership of their disease. The health care team is a resource for assisting them in the care of their disease. Diabetes is a complicated, chronic disease with a complex management requiring a multidisciplinary team approach.

The evidence is clear that life-style change is the most efficacious and cost-effective therapy for this deadly disease.

WEB SITES

American Association of Diabetes Educators:

http://www.aadenet.org

American Diabetes Association (ADA):

http://www/diabetes.org

Centers for Disease Control and Prevention (CDC), Division of Diabetes:

http://www.cdc.gov.diabetes

Joslin Diabetes Center:

http://www.joslin.harvard.edu

National Diabetes Education Program:

http://ndep.nih.gov

National Institute of Diabetes and Digestive and Kidney Diseases:

http://www.niddk.nih.gov

Endocrine Disorders 35

William J. Hueston, MD, Peter J. Carek, MD, MS, & Pamela Allweiss, MD, MSPH

THYROID DISORDERS

Thyroid disorders affect 1 in 200 adults but are more common in women and with advancing age. The incidence of hypothyroidism, for instance, is 0.3–5 cases per 1000 individuals per year, including 7% of women and 3% of men aged 60 to 89 years. Hypothyroidism is much more common than hyperthyroidism, nodular disease, or thyroid cancer. Thyroid nodules occur in 4–8% of all individuals and, like other thyroid problems, increase in incidence with age.

Thyroid disease is more common in people who have conditions such as diabetes or other autoimmune diseases (eg, lupus); in those with a family history of thyroid disease or a history of head and neck irradiation; and in patients who use certain medications, including amiodarone and lithium. Recent guidelines from the American Thyroid Association suggest that all adults have their serum thyroid-stimulating hormone (TSH) concentrations measured, beginning at age 35 and every 5 years thereafter.

HYPOTHYROIDISM

General Considerations

Causes of hypothyroidism are outlined in Table 35–1. The most common noniatrogenic condition causing hypothyroidism in the United States is Hashimoto thyroiditis. Other common causes are post–Graves disease, thyroid irradiation, and surgical removal of the thyroid. Hypothyroidism may also occur secondary to hypothalamic or pituitary dysfunction, most commonly in patients who have received intracranial irradiation or surgical removal of a pituitary adenoma. In addition, some patients may have mild elevations of TSH despite normal thyroxine levels, a condition termed *subclinical hypothyroidism.*

Clinical Findings

A. Symptoms and Signs

Patients with hypothyroidism present with a constellation of symptoms that can involve every organ system. Symptoms include lethargy, weight gain, hair loss, dry skin, slowed mentation or forgetfulness, depressed affect, cold intolerance, constipation, hair loss, muscle weakness, abnormal menstrual periods (or infertility), and fluid retention. Because of the range of symptoms seen in hypothyroidism, clinicians must have a high index of suspicion, especially in high-risk populations. In older patients, hypothyroidism can be confused with Alzheimer disease or other conditions that cause dementia. In women, hypothyroidism is often confused with depression.

Physical findings that can occur with hypothyroidism include low blood pressure, bradycardia, nonpitting edema, generalized hair thinning along with hair loss in the outer third of the eyebrows, skin drying, and a diminished relaxation phase of reflexes. The thyroid gland in a patient with chronic thyroiditis may be enlarged, atrophic, or of normal size. Thyroid nodules are common in patients with Hashimoto thyroiditis.

B. Laboratory Findings

The most valuable test for hypothyroidism is the sensitive TSH assay. Measurement of the free thyroxine (T_4) level may also be helpful. TSH is elevated and free T_4 decreased in overt hypothyroidism (Table 35–2). Other laboratory findings may include hyperlipidemia and hyponatremia. Hashimoto thyroiditis, an autoimmune condition, is one of the most common causes of hypothyroidism. Testing for thyroid autoantibodies (antiperoxidase, antithyroglobulin) is positive in 95% of patients with Hashimoto thyroiditis.

Patients with associated subclinical hypothyroidism have a high TSH level (usually in the 5–10 μIU/mL range) in conjunction with normal free T_4 level. Between 3% and 20% of these patients will eventually develop overt hypothyroidism. Patients who test positive for thyroid antibodies are at increased risk.

Treatment

In patients with primary hypothyroidism, therapy should begin with thyroid hormone replacement. In patients with secondary hypothyroidism, further investigation with provocative testing of the pituitary can be performed to determine if the cause is a hypothalamic or pituitary problem.

Table 35–1. Causes of hypothyroidism.

Primary Hypothyroidism (95% of cases)
Idiopathic hypothyroidism (probably old Hashimoto thyroiditis)
Hashimoto thyroiditis
Post-thyroid irradiation
Postsurgical
Late-stage invasive fibrous thyroiditis
Iodine deficiency
Drugs (lithium, interferon)
Infiltrative diseases (sarcoidosis, amyloid, scleroderma, hemochromatosis)
Secondary Hypothyroidism (5% of cases)
Pituitary or hypothalamic neoplasms
Congenital hypopituitarism
Pituitary necrosis (Sheehan syndrome)

Most healthy adult patients with hypothyroidism require about 1.6 mcg/kg of thyroid replacement, with requirements falling to 1 mcg/kg for the elderly. The initial dosage may range from 12.5 mcg to a full replacement dose of 100–150 mcg of levothyroxine (0.10–0.15 mg/day). Doses will vary depending on age, weight, cardiac status, duration, and severity of the hypothyroidism. Therapy should be titrated after at least 6 weeks following any change in levothyroxine dose. The serum TSH level is the most important measure to gauge the dose, and a free T_4 estimate may be included as well.

Treatment of subclinical hypothyroidism remains controversial. The American Association of Clinical Endocrinologists (AACE) guidelines suggest treating patients with TSH levels higher than 10 μIU/mL as well as those with TSH levels between 5 and 10 μIU/mL in conjunction with goiter or positive antithyroid peroxidase antibodies, or both.

Once the TSH level reaches the normal range, the frequency of testing can be decreased. Each patient's regimen must be individualized, but the usual follow up after TSH is stable is at 6 months; the history and physical examination should be repeated on a routine basis thereafter.

Thyroid hormone absorption can be affected by malabsorption, age, and concomitant medications such as cholestyramine, ferrous sulfate, sucralfate, calcium, and some antacids containing aluminum hydroxide. Drugs such as anticonvulsants affect thyroid hormone binding, whereas others such as rifampin and sertraline hydrochloride may accelerate levothyroxine metabolism, necessitating a higher replacement dose. The thyroid dose may also need to be adjusted during pregnancy. There has been some interest in using a combination of T_4 and triiodothyronine (T_3) or natural thyroid preparations in pregnant women with hypothyroidism, but studies to date have been small and findings inconsistent.

Bunevicius R et al: Effects of thyroxine as compared with thyroxine plus triiodothyronine in patients with hypothyroidism. New Engl J Med 1999; 340:424. [PMID: 9971866]

Grebe SK et al: Treatment of hypothyroidism with once weekly thyroxine. J Clin Endocrinol Metab 1997; 82:870. [PMID: 9062499]

Gussekloo J et al: Thyroid status, disability and cognitive function, and survival in old age. JAMA 2004; 292:2591. [PMID: 15572717]

HYPERTHYROIDISM

General Considerations

Hyperthyroidism has several causes. The most common is toxic diffuse goiter (Graves disease), an autoimmune

Table 35–2. Laboratory changes in hypothyroidism.

TSH	Free T_4	Free T_3	Likely Diagnosis
High	Low	Low	Primary hypothyroidism
High (> 10 μIU/mL)	Normal	Normal	Subclinical hypothyroidism with high risk for future development of overt hypothyroidism
High (6–10 μIU/mL)	Normal	Normal	Subclinical hypothyroidism with low risk for future development of overt hypothyroidism
High	High	Low	Congenital absence of T_4–T_3-converting enzyme or amiodarone effect
High	High	High	Peripheral thyroid hormone resistance
Low	Low	Low	Pituitary thyroid deficiency or recent withdrawal of thyroid replacement after excessive replacement

TSH, thyroid-stimulating hormone; T4, thyroxine; T3, triiodothyronine.

disorder caused by immunoglobulin G (IgG) antibodies that bind to TSH receptors initiating the production and release of thyroid hormone. Other causes include toxic adenoma; toxic multinodular goiter (Plummer disease); painful subacute thyroiditis; silent thyroiditis, including lymphocytic and postpartum thyroiditis; iodine-induced hyperthyroidism (eg, related to amiodarone therapy); oversecretion of pituitary TSH; trophoblastic disease (very rare); and excess exogenous thyroid hormone secretion.

Clinical Findings

A. Symptoms and Signs

Patients with hyperthyroidism usually present with progressive nervousness, tremor, palpitations, weight loss, dyspnea on exertion, fatigue, difficulty concentrating, heat intolerance, and frequent bowel movements or diarrhea. Physical findings include a rapid pulse and elevated blood pressure, with the systolic pressure increasing to a greater extent than the diastolic pressure, creating a wide pulse-pressure hypertension. Exophthalmos (in patients with Graves disease), muscle weakness, sudden paralysis, dependent low-extremity edema, or pretibial myxedema may also be present. Cardiac arrhythmias such as atrial fibrillation may be evident on physical examination or electrocardiogram, and a resting tremor may be noted on physical examination.

In patients with subacute thyroiditis, symptoms of hyperthyroidism are generally transient and resolve in a matter of weeks. There may be a recent history of a head and neck infection, fever, and severe neck tenderness. Postpartum thyroiditis may occur in the first few months after delivery. Both types of thyroiditis may have a transient hyperthyroid phase, a euthyroid phase, and occasionally a later hypothyroid phase.

B. Laboratory and Imaging Evaluation

Hyperthyroidism is detected by a decreased sensitive TSH assay and confirmed, if necessary, by the finding of an elevated free T_4 level. Testing for thyroid autoantibodies, including TSH receptor antibodies (TRAb) or thyroid-stimulating immunoglobulins (TSI), may be done as necessary. Once hyperthyroidism is identified, radionucleotide uptake and scanning of the thyroid, preferably with iodine-123, is useful to determine whether hyperthyroidism is secondary to Graves disease, an autonomous nodule, or thyroiditis (ie, by showing activity and anatomy of the thyroid). In scans of patients with Graves disease, there is increased uptake on radionucleotide imaging with diffuse hyperactivity. In contrast, nodules demonstrate limited areas of uptake with surrounding hypoactivity, and in subacute thyroiditis, uptake is patchy and decreased overall.

Complications

Thyroid storm represents an acute hypermetabolic state associated with the sudden release of large amounts of thyroid hormone. This occurs most often in Graves disease but can occur in acute thyroiditis. Individuals with thyroid storm present with confusion, fever, restlessness, and sometimes with psychotic-like symptoms. Physical examination shows tachycardia, elevated blood pressure, and sometimes fever. Cardiac dysrhythmias may be present or develop. Patients will have other signs of high-output heart failure (dyspnea on exertion, peripheral vasoconstriction) and may exhibit signs of cardiac or cerebral ischemia. Thyroid storm is a medical crisis requiring prompt attention and reversal of the metabolic demands from the acute hyperthyroidism.

Treatment

A. Radioactive Iodine

Radioactive iodine is the treatment of choice for Graves disease in adult patients who are not pregnant. It has also been used on an individual basis in patients younger than 20 years of age. To date, studies have shown no evidence of adverse effects on fertility, congenital malformations, or increased risk of cancer in women who were treated with radioactive iodine during their childbearing years or in their offspring. Patients should be advised to postpone pregnancy for at least 6 months postablation therapy.

Radioactive iodine should not be used in breastfeeding mothers. There is also concern that the administration of radioactive iodine in patients with active ophthalmopathy may accelerate progression of eye disease. For this reason, some experts initially treat Graves disease with oral suppressive therapy until the ophthalmologic disease has stabilized.

B. Pharmacotherapy

Antithyroid drugs are well tolerated and successful at blocking the production and release of thyroid hormone in patients with Graves disease. These drugs work by blocking the organification of iodine. Propylthiouracil (PTU) also prevents peripheral conversion of T_4 to the more active T_3. PTU must be given in divided doses (two or three times a day), whereas methimazole and carbimazole can be administered once a day. PTU can be used during pregnancy. The most serious side effect of these drugs is agranulocytosis, which occurs in 3 per 10,000 patients per year. Antithyroid drugs are especially useful in adolescents, in whom Graves disease may go into spontaneous remission after 6–18 months of therapy.

If it has been determined that symptoms of hyperthyroidism are due to thyroiditis, symptomatic treatment with a β-blocker can be used temporarily with little need for long-term therapy.

C. Surgical Intervention

Surgery is reserved for patients in whom medication and radioactive iodine ablation are not acceptable treatment strategies or in whom a large goiter is present that compresses nearby structures or is disfiguring.

D. Treatment of Thyroid Storm

For patients with thyroid storm, aggressive initial therapy is essential to prevent complications. Treatment should include the administration of high doses of PTU (100 mg every 6 hours) to quickly block thyroid release and reduce peripheral conversion of T_4 to T_3. In addition, high doses of β-blockers (propranolol, 1–5 mg intravenously or 20–80 mg orally every 4 hours) can be used to control tachycardia and other peripheral symptoms of thyrotoxicosis. Hydrocortisone (200–300 mg/day) is used to prevent possible adrenal crisis.

E. Postablation Follow-up

Follow-up is necessary to evaluate possible hypothyroidism postablation. Follow-up can begin 6 weeks after therapy and continue on a regular basis until there is evidence of early hypothyroidism, as confirmed by an elevated TSH level. Therapy should then be started as described earlier in the discussion of hypothyroidism.

American Association of Clinical Endocrinologists: American Association of Clinical Endocrinologists medical guidelines for clinical practice for the evaluation of hyperthyroidism and hypothyroidism. Endocr Pract 2002;8:457. [PMID: 15260011]

Adlin V: Subclinical hypothyroidism: Deciding when to treat. Am Fam Physician 1998;57:776. [PMID: 9491000]

Haddow JE et al: Maternal thyroid deficiency during pregnancy and subsequent neuropsychological development of the child. N Engl J Med 1999;341:549. [PMID: 10451459]

Singer PA et al: Treatment guidelines for patients with hyperthyroidism and hypothyroidism. JAMA 1995;273:808. [PMID: 75432241]

THYROID NODULES

General Considerations

Thyroid nodules are a common clinical finding, reported in 3–7% of patients based on palpation. The prevalence of diagnosed thyroid nodules has increased dramatically in the past 20 years because of the widespread use of ultrasonography for the evaluation of thyroid and nonthyroid neck conditions. Autopsy data indicate that thyroid nodules may be present in 50% of the population. Thyroid nodules are more common in women, the elderly, patients with a history of head and neck irradiation, and those with a history of iodine deficiency.

Pathogenesis

Thyroid nodules may be associated with benign or malignant conditions. Benign causes include multinodular goiter, Hashimoto thyroiditis, simple or hemorrhagic cysts, follicular adenomas, and subacute thyroiditis. Malignant causes include carcinoma (papillary, follicular, Hürthle cell, medullary, or anaplastic), primary thyroid lymphoma, and metastatic malignant lesion.

Clinical Findings

A. Symptoms and Signs

Many patients with thyroid nodules are asymptomatic. Often the nodule is discovered incidentally on physical examination or by imaging studies ordered for unrelated reasons. Evaluation is needed to rule out malignancy. A thorough history should be obtained, including any history of benign or malignant thyroid disease (as discussed under hyper- and hypothyroidism, earlier) and head or neck irradiation. Patients should be asked about recent pregnancy, characteristics of the nodule, and any neck symptoms (eg, pain, rate of swelling, hoarseness, swelling of lymph nodes).

Several features of the history are associated with an increased risk of malignancy in a thyroid nodule. These include prior head and neck irradiation, family history of medullary carcinoma or multiple endocrine neoplasia syndrome type 2, age younger than 20 years or older than 70 years, male gender, and rapid growth of a nodule. Physical findings that should raise clinical suspicion of malignancy include firm consistency, cervical adenopathy, and symptoms such as persistent hoarseness, dysphonia, dysphagia, or dyspnea.

B. Laboratory and Diagnostic Findings

Laboratory and diagnostic evaluation relies on ultrasound, measurement of TSH level, and fine-needle aspiration (FNA). Ultrasound is not useful as a universal screening tool but can be helpful in screening patients whose history places them at high risk for developing thyroid cancer (see Symptoms and Signs, earlier).

1. Workup of a palpable thyroid nodule—If the nodule is palpable, TSH assay and ultrasonography of the thyroid should be performed. These two modalities will help guide clinical decision making. If the nodule appears suspicious on ultrasound (based on position, shape, size, margins, or echogenic pattern), FNA should be done irrespective of whether the patient's TSH level is elevated, normal, or suppressed. For instance, it has been reported that nodules in patients with Graves disease may be malignant in 9% of the cases. If the nodule on ultrasound does not appear suspicious, the clinician can proceed with workup of the abnormal TSH level. For example, if the TSH level is suppressed, the patient may have hyperthyroidism caused by either a single autonomous nodule or a multinodular goiter. The patient would then be evaluated for hyperthyroidism and therapy initiated, as appropriate.

In patients with an elevated TSH level suggestive of hypothyroidism, the next steps would be based on the ultrasound findings. If the nodule does not appear suspicious, thyroid peroxidase antibodies (useful for diagnosing Hashimoto thyroiditis) can be measured and treatment of hypothyroidism initiated (ie, using levothyroxine therapy). If the nodule appears suspicious, FNA should be performed.

2. Workup of an "incidental" thyroid nodule— If the thyroid nodule is found incidentally by ultrasonography, the next step is to obtain a TSH level. If the TSH level is normal, the nodule is less than 10 mm, the patient does not have risk factors for thyroid malignancy, and the ultrasound findings do not appear suspicious, clinical follow-up is done. If the nodule is greater than 10 mm or the patient has risk factors for thyroid malignancy, FNA should be performed.

About 70% of FNA specimens are classified as benign, 5% are malignant, 10% are suspicious, and 10–20% are nondiagnostic. If FNA reveals malignant cells, surgical intervention is indicated and further treatment will be based on the characteristics noted at surgery (pathologic findings, positive lymph nodes, etc).

Treatment

Patients with malignant thyroid nodules should be referred to surgical and medical oncologists familiar with the management of these tumors. The remainder of this discussion focuses on follow up and management of patients with FNA-negative thyroid nodules.

Use of exogenous levothyroxine therapy in a euthyroid patient in an effort to "suppress the TSH" (decrease TSH level below 0.1 IU/mL) and "shrink" the nodule is of benefit in only a few patients with palpable nodules. The side effects of exogenous thyroid therapy (cardiac arrhythmias, osteoporosis, etc) must be considered, especially in older patients and in postmenopausal women; its use in these populations is thus relatively contraindicated.

Patients with very large nodules may require surgery, especially if symptoms secondary to the size (eg, dysphagia) are present. If there is a change in size of the nodule, a repeat FNA should be performed.

Ultrasound-guided percutaneous ethanol injection (PEI) is a therapeutic option for patients with benign nodules that have a large fluid component (thyroid cysts). Aspiration (eg, during FNA) itself may drain a cyst and shrink the size, but recurrences are common. Surgery is sometimes needed if the cyst is very large. Some data show that PEI is more effective in decreasing the size of a nodule than aspiration alone.

AACE/AME Task Force on Thyroid Nodules: American Association of Clinical Endocrinologists and Associazione Medici Endocriniologi guidelines for clinical practice for the diagnosis and management of thyroid nodules. Endoc Pract 2006;12:63. [PMID: 16596732]

ADRENAL DISORDERS

ADRENAL INSUFFICIENCY

General Considerations

The most common cause of primary adrenal insufficiency is autoimmune adrenalitis (Addison disease). Other possible causes include AIDS and the antiphospholipid syndrome. Secondary adrenal insufficiency may result from pituitary or hypothalamic disease. Iatrogenic tertiary adrenal insufficiency caused by suppression of hypothalamic–pituitary–adrenal function secondary to glucocorticoid administration is a more common secondary cause of adrenal insufficiency (Table 35–3).

Clinical Findings

A. Symptoms and Signs

Adrenal insufficiency presents with a wide range of symptoms and signs, including weakness, malaise, anorexia, hyperpigmentation (especially of the gingival mucosa, scars, and skin creases), vitiligo, postural hypotension, abdominal pain, nausea and vomiting, diarrhea, constipation, myalgia, and arthralgia. The most specific sign of primary adrenal insufficiency is hyperpigmentation of the skin and mucosal surfaces. Another specific symptom of adrenal insufficiency is a craving for salt. Autoimmune adrenal disease can be accompanied by other autoimmune endocrine deficiencies, such as thyroid disease, diabetes mellitus, pernicious anemia, hypoparathyroidism, and ovarian failure.

In acute adrenal failure, adrenal crisis occurs. Adrenal crisis is characterized by hypotension, bradycardia, fever, hypoglycemia, and a progressive deterioration in

Table 35–3. Causes of adrenal insufficiency.

Primary
Autoimmune adrenalitis
Tuberculosis
Adrenomyeloneuropathy
Systemic fungal infections
AIDS
Metastatic carcinoma
Isolated glucocorticoid deficiency
Adrenal hemorrhage, necrosis, or thrombosis
Secondary
Pituitary or metastatic tumor
Craniopharyngioma
Pituitary surgery or radiation
Lymphocytic hypophysitis
Sarcoidosis
Histiocytosis
Empty-sella syndrome
Hypothalamic tumors
Long-term glucocorticoid therapy
Postpartum pituitary necrosis (Sheehan syndrome)
Necrosis or bleeding into pituitary macroadenoma
Head trauma, lesions of the pituitary stalk
Pituitary or adrenal surgery for Cushing syndrome

Reproduced, with permission, from Oelkers W: Adrenal insufficiency. New Engl J Med 1996;335: 1206.

mental status. Abdominal pain, vomiting, and diarrhea also may be present. In the patient with spontaneous adrenal insufficiency, acute adrenal hemorrhage and adrenal-vein thrombosis should be considered.

B. Laboratory Findings

Laboratory abnormalities occur in nearly all patients and include hyponatremia, hyperkalemia, acidosis, slightly elevated plasma creatinine concentrations, hypoglycemia, hypercalcemia, mild normocytic anemia, lymphocytosis, and mild eosinophilia. The diagnosis of adrenal insufficiency relies on a finding of inadequate cortisol production. Plasma cortisol concentration fluctuates throughout the day in a diurnal pattern that is normally high in the early morning and low in the late afternoon. Cortisol levels also increase with stress. A low plasma cortisol level of less than 3 mcg/dL (83 nmol/L) either in the morning or at a time of stress provides presumptive evidence of adrenal insufficiency. Conversely, a level of 20 mcg/dL (550 nmol/L) or greater rules out adrenal insufficiency. An intermediate plasma cortisol level of 3–19 mcg/dL (83–525 nmol/L) is not diagnostic.

For most patients in whom adrenal insufficiency is considered, a short adrenocorticotropic hormone (ACTH) stimulation test should be performed. In this test, a low-dose of ACTH (1 g or 0.5 g/1.73 m^2 surface area) is given and the patient's blood is tested 30 and 60 minutes later to confirm a corresponding increase in plasma cortisol. A rise in plasma cortisol concentration after 30 or 60 minutes to a peak of 20 mcg/dL (55 nmol/L) or more is considered normal. No increase in serum cortisol or a blunted response after ACTH administration confirms adrenal insufficiency. If the test is slightly abnormal, an insulin or a metyrapone test using 30 mg/kg of metyrapone with a snack at midnight should be performed.

C. Imaging Studies

In patients with adrenal insufficiency, radiologic studies may be indicated. In patients having headaches and visual disturbances, a magnetic resonance imaging (MRI) scan should be performed to investigate for a possible pituitary or hypothalamic tumor. In patients with suspected primary adrenal insufficiency, a computed tomography (CT) scan of the adrenal glands should be performed to rule out hemorrhage, adrenal vein thrombosis, or metastatic disease as the cause of the adrenal dysfunction.

Treatment

For patients with symptomatic adrenal insufficiency, attention needs to be paid to fluid management, correction of other metabolic abnormalities such as hypoglycemia and hyperkalemia as well as the administration of corticosteroids. An approach to managing this condition is shown in Table 35–4.

While providing fluid resuscitation and addressing other metabolic emergencies, emergency doses of hydrocortisone should be given. Once the patient is stabilized, corticosteroid maintenance should be provided in divided doses early in the morning and afternoon to simulate the diurnal release of cortisol by the adrenal gland. The smallest dose that relieves the patient's symptoms should be used to minimize weight gain and risk of osteoporosis. During febrile illnesses, acute injury, or other periods of physiologic stress, the dose of hydrocortisone should be doubled or tripled temporarily. Patients with primary adrenal insufficiency should also receive fludrocortisone as a substitute for aldosterone.

August GP: Treatment of adrenocortical insufficiency. Pediatr Rev 1997;18:59. [PMID: 9029933]

Malchoff CD, Carey RM: Adrenal insufficiency. Curr Ther Endocrinol Metab 1997;6:142. [PMID: 9174724]

CUSHING SYNDROME

General Considerations

Cushing syndrome refers to overproduction of cortisol due to any cause (eg, adrenal hyperplasia, exogenous

Table 35–4. Approach to treating acute adrenal insufficiency.

1. Stabilize blood pressure and replace fluids	Administer bolus with normal saline (500 mL/m^2) over 1 h then adequate fluids to maintain sufficient urine output
2. Correct other metabolic problems	
• Hypoglycemia	Give 25% glucose if hypoglycemia
• Hyperkalemia	Treat with polystyrene sulfonate (Kayexalate) oral suspension every 3–4 h; give 10% calcium gluconate for dangerously high potassium levels, monitoring heart rate for bradycardia
3. Emergency corticosteroid replacement therapy	
• Hydrocortisone	Adults: 100 mg bolus dose followed by infusion of 100–200 mg/24 h Children: 25–50 mg/m^2/24 h
4. Chronic corticosteroid replacement	
• Hydrocortisone	Adults: 25 mg (divided into doses of 15 and 10 mg) Children: 25 mg/m^2/day in 3 divided doses
• Cortisone	Adults: 37.5 mg (divided into doses of 25 and 12.5 mg) Children: 32 mg/m^2/day divided 3 times daily
5. Evaluate for mineralocorticoid deficiency and replace if needed	
• Fludrocortisone (substitute for aldosterone)	Adults: 50–200 mcg (single daily dose) Children: 50–150 mcg (single daily dose)

Adapted, with permission, from August GP: Treatment of adrenocortical insufficiency. Pediatr Rev 1997;18:59.

steroid use). *Cushing disease* is a more specific term that refers to excessive cortisol resulting from excessive ACTH produced by pituitary corticotrophic tumors. ACTH-producing tumors account for 80% of cases of Cushing syndrome. The remaining 20% are caused by adrenal tumors, such as adenomas, carcinomas, and micronodular and macronodular hyperplasia, associated with autonomous production of glucocorticoids.

Cushing syndrome is rare, with a prevalence estimated at about 10 per one million persons. Cushing disease is four to six times more prevalent in women than in men, whereas ectopic ACTH secretion is more common in men, largely due to the higher incidence in men of bronchogenic lung cancers that produce ACTH.

Clinical Findings

A. Symptoms and Signs

The most common signs of Cushing syndrome are sudden onset of central weight gain, often accompanied by thickening of the facial fat, which rounds the facial contour ("moon facies"), and a florid complexion due to telangiectasia. Other concomitant signs include an enlarged fat pad ("buffalo hump"), hypertension, glucose intolerance, oligomenorrhea or amenorrhea in premenopausal women, decreased libido in men, and spontaneous ecchymoses (Table 35–5).

B. Laboratory Findings

The evaluation of suspected excessive glucocorticoid production includes screening and confirmatory tests for the diagnosis and localization of the source of hormone excess. Tests that can be used to confirm excessive glucocorticoid production include a 24-hour urinary free cortisol test, an overnight dexamethasone suppression test, and a midnight cortisol level determination. The 1-mg overnight dexamethasone suppression test has been considered the screening test of choice, but problems associated with its low specificity have led to the use of the urinary free cortisol excretion rate as the preferred test for many patients.

Affective psychiatric disorders (ie, major depression) and alcoholism can be associated with the biochemical features of Cushing syndrome and, therefore, may decrease the reliability of test results.

C. Imaging Studies

Following confirmation of Cushing syndrome, imaging studies should be performed to look for adenomas

Table 35–5. Clinical symptoms and signs of Cushing syndrome.

General:
- Central obesity
- Proximal muscle weakness
- Hypertension
- Headaches
- Psychiatric disorders

Skin
- Wide (>1 cm), purple striae
- Spontaneous ecchymoses
- Facial plethora
- Hyperpigmentation
- Acne
- Hirsutism
- Fungal skin infections

Endocrine and metabolic derangements
- Hypokalemic alkalosis
- Osteopenia
- Delayed bone age in children
- Menstrual disorders, decreased libido, impotence
- Glucose intolerence, diabetes mellitus
- Kidney stones
- Polyuria

Elevated white blood cell count

Reprinted, with permission, from Meier CA, Biller BM: Clinical and biochemical evaluation of Cushing's syndrome. Endocrinol Metab Clin North Am. Elsevier. 1997;26:741.

(MRI scan) or adrenal tumors (CT scan). If both of these studies are negative, chest radiography or CT scanning should be performed to look for ectopic sources of ACTH production.

Treatment

For patients with a pituitary adenoma (Cushing disease) in whom a circumscribed microadenoma can be identified and resected, the treatment of choice is transsphenoidal microadenomectomy. If an adenoma cannot be clearly identified, patients should undergo a subtotal (85–90%) resection of the anterior pituitary gland. Patients who wish to preserve pituitary function (ie, in order to have children) should be treated with pituitary irradiation. If radiation does not decrease exogenous ACTH production, bilateral total adrenalectomy is a final treatment option. For adult patients not cured by transsphenoidal surgery, pituitary irradiation is the most appropriate choice for the next treatment.

Patients who have a nonpituitary tumor that secretes ACTH are cured by resection of the tumor. Unfortunately, most nonpituitary tumors that secrete ACTH are not amenable to resection. In these cases, cortisol excess can be controlled with adrenal enzyme inhibitors, alone or in combination, with the proper dose determined by measurements of plasma and urinary cortisol.

For patients with adrenal hyperplasia, bilateral total adrenalectomy is required. Patients with an adrenal adenoma or carcinoma can be managed with unilateral adrenalectomy. Patients with hyperplasia or adenomas almost invariably have recurrences that are not amenable to either radiation or chemotherapy.

Patients who are taking corticosteroids for prolonged periods of time may exhibit signs or symptoms of Cushing syndrome. Once the primary problem for which steroids are being prescribed is controlled, patients should be withdrawn from their corticosteroid treatment slowly to avoid symptoms from adrenal suppression. There are few studies evaluating methods of withdrawal from chronic steroid use, however. Clinicians should be guided by the severity of the underlying condition, the duration that steroids have been used, and the dosage of steroids in determining how quickly dosages of steroids should be reduced.

Meier CA, Biller BM: Clinical and biochemical evaluation of Cushing's syndrome. Endocrinol Metab Clin North Am 1997;26:741. [PMID: 9429858]

Newell-Price J et al: Cushing's syndrome. Lancet 2006;367:1605. [PMID: 16698415]

Nieman LK, Ilias I: Evaluation and treatment of Cushing's syndrome. Am J Med 2005;118:1340. [PMID: 16378774]

HYPERALDOSTERONISM

General Considerations

Primary hyperaldosteronism accounts for 70–80% of all cases of hyperaldosteronism and is usually caused by a solitary unilateral adrenal adenoma. Other causes of hyperaldosteronism include bilateral adrenal hyperplasia, so-called idiopathic hyperaldosteronism, and glucocorticoid-remediable hyperaldosteronism. Adrenal carcinoma and unilateral adrenal hyperplasia are rare causes.

Clinical Findings

A. Symptoms and Signs

Patients with hyperaldosteronism present with hypertension and hypokalemia. Other complaints include headaches, muscular weakness or flaccid paralysis caused by hypokalemia, or polyuria. Inappropriate hypersecretion of aldosterone is an uncommon cause of hypertension, accounting for fewer than 1% of cases. Any patient presenting with hypertension and unprovoked hypokalemia should be considered for the evaluation of hyperaldosteronism. Hypertension may be severe, although malignant hypertension is rare. The peak incidence occurs between 30 and 50 years of age, and most patients are women.

B. Laboratory Findings

Initially, laboratory evaluation is used to document hyperaldosteronemia and suppressed renin activity. Further diagnostic tests, including imaging procedures, are used to determine whether the etiology is amenable to surgical intervention or requires medical management.

Screening aldosterone measurements can be made on plasma or 24-hour urine collection. Plasma aldosterone is usually measured after 4 hours of upright posture. Plasma renin activity should be measured in the same sample. A ratio of plasma aldosterone concentration to plasma renin activity greater than 20:25 is very suspicious for hyperaldosteronism.

In the hypertensive patient with hypokalemia or kaliuresis or with an elevated plasma aldosterone-renin ratio, the diagnosis of hyperaldosteronism is confirmed by demonstrating failure of normal suppression of plasma aldosterone. Urine aldosterone excretion of more than 30 nmol (14 mcg)/day after oral sodium loading over 3 days establishes the diagnosis.

The intravenous saline suppression test is also widely used to confirm hyperaldosteronism. In this test, isotonic saline is infused intravenously at a rate of 300–500 mL/h for 4 hours, after which plasma aldosterone and renin activity are measured. Aldosterone levels normally fall to less than 0.28 nmol/L (10 ng/dL) and renin activity is suppressed. Failure to suppress normally identifies patients with aldosterone-producing adenomas, because most patients with secondary forms of hyperaldosteronism suppress normally. False-negative results are most often seen in patients with bilateral hyperplasia.

Once the diagnosis is established, it is necessary to distinguish between aldosterone-producing adrenal adenoma and bilateral adrenal hyperplasia. A widely used test is based on the less complete suppression of renin activity in hyperaldosteronism caused by bilateral hyperplasia. Plasma renin activity rises slightly and aldosterone concentration increases significantly after the stimulation of 2–4 hours of upright posturing in these patients. In contrast, renin remains suppressed and aldosterone does not rise in patients with adenomas, in whom plasma aldosterone level may fall.

C. Imaging Studies

Imaging procedures can assist in differentiating causes of hyperaldosteronism and lateralizing adenomas. The diagnostic accuracy of high-resolution CT scans is only about 70% for aldosterone-producing adenomas, largely because of the occurrence of nonfunctioning adenomas. MRI is no better than CT in differentiating aldosterone-secreting tumors from other adrenal tumors. Scintigraphic imaging with iodine-131–labeled cholesterol derivatives during dexamethasone suppression provides an image based on functional properties of the adrenal gland. Asymmetric uptake after 48 hours indicates an adenoma, whereas symmetric uptake after 72 hours indicates bilateral hyperplasia. Diagnostic accuracy is 72%. However, if the adrenal CT scan is normal, iodocholesterol scanning is unlikely to be helpful.

Treatment

For adrenal adenoma, total unilateral adrenalectomy is the treatment of choice and provides a cure in most cases. Although some patients with primary bilateral hyperplasia may benefit from subtotal adrenalectomy, these patients cannot be accurately identified preoperatively. Following surgery, the electrolyte imbalances usually correct rapidly, whereas blood pressure control may take several weeks to months.

Medical therapy is indicated for most patients with bilateral adrenal hyperplasia or for patients with adrenal adenomas who are unable to undergo adrenalectomy. Spironolactone controls the hyperkalemia, although it is not a very potent antihypertensive agent. Amiloride and calcium channel blockers are often used to control blood pressure.

Bravo EL: Primary aldosteronism. Issues in diagnosis and management. Endocrinol Metab Clin North Am 1994;23:271. [PMID: 8070422]

PARATHYROID DISORDERS

HYPERPARATHYROIDISM

General Considerations

Hyperparathyroidism refers to excessive production of parathyroid hormone (PTH). Primary hyperparathyroidism is the overproduction of PTH in an inappropriate fashion, resulting usually in hypercalcemia. Primary hyperparathyroidism is more common in postmenopausal women. The most common cause is a benign solitary parathyroid adenoma (80% of all cases). Another 15% of patients have diffuse hyperplasia of the parathyroid glands, a condition that tends to be familial. Carcinoma of the parathyroid occurs in less than 1% of cases.

In secondary hyperparathyroidism, patients have appropriate additional production of PTH because of hypocalcemia related to other metabolic conditions such as renal failure, calcium absorption problems, or vitamin D deficiency.

Clinical Findings

A. Symptoms and Signs

Most patients have nonspecific complaints that may include aches and pains, constipation, muscle fatigue, generalized weakness, psychiatric disturbances, polydipsia, and polyuria. The hypercalcemia can cause nausea and vomiting, thirst, and anorexia. A history of peptic ulcer disease or hypertension may be present, as well as accompanying constipation, anemia, and weight loss. Precipitation of calcium in the corneas may produce a band keratopathy, and patients may also experience recurrent pancreatitis. Finally, skeletal problems can result in pathologic fractures.

B. Laboratory Findings

Hypercalcemia (serum calcium level > 10.5 mg/dL when corrected for serum albumin level) is the most important clue to the diagnosis. In patients who have an elevated calcium level with no apparent cause, serum PTH should be determined using a two-site immunometric assay. An elevated PTH level in the presence of hypercalcemia confirms the diagnosis of primary hyperparathyroidism.

Other findings may include a low serum phosphate level (< 2.5 mg/dL) with excessive phosphaturia. Urine calcium excretion may be high or normal. Alkaline phosphatase levels are elevated only in the presence of bone disease, and elevated plasma chloride and uric acid levels may be seen.

C. Imaging Studies

With chronic hyperparathyroidism, diffuse bone demineralization, loss of the dental lamina dura, and subperiosteal resorption of bone (particularly in the radial aspects of the fingers) may be apparent on x-rays. Cysts may be noted throughout the skeleton, and "salt-and-pepper" appearance of the skull may be seen. Pathologic fractures can occur, and renal calculi and soft tissue calcification may be visualized.

Imaging studies are usually reserved for patients with resistant or recurrent disease. In these cases, ultrasonography, CT scanning, MRI, and thallium-201–technetium-99m scanning may help locate ectopic parathyroid tissue.

Treatment

Treatment of severe hypercalcemia and parathyroidectomy are the mainstays for therapy. When hypercalcemia is severe, treatment includes aggressive hydration. Correction of any underlying hyponatremia and hypokalemia should be initiated, along with administration of a loop diuretic to accelerate calcium clearance. Other medications that can be effective in reducing hypercalcemia include etidronate, plicamycin, and calcitonin. Any medications or other products that increase calcium levels, such as estrogens, thiazides, vitamins A and D, and milk, should be avoided.

In addition to management of acute hypercalcemia, surgical removal of parathyroid tissue should be undertaken. Surgical resection provides the most rapid and effective method of reducing serum calcium in these patients. Hyperplasia of all glands requires removal of three glands along with subtotal resection of the fourth. Surgical success is directly related to the experience and expertise of the operating surgeon.

For mild cases and poor surgical candidates, conservative therapy with adequate hydration and long-term pharmacologic therapy is recommended. Patients should avoid drugs and products that elevate calcium and should have their serum calcium monitored closely.

HYPOPARATHYROIDISM

General Considerations

Hypoparathyroidism results from underproduction of PTH. The most common cause is the removal of the parathyroid glands during a thyroidectomy or following surgery for primary hyperparathyroidism. Less commonly, hypoparathyroidism is idiopathic, familial, or the result of a congenital absence of the parathyroid glands (DiGeorge syndrome). Patients with idiopathic hypoparathyroidism often have antibodies against parathyroid and other tissues, and an autoimmune component may play a role. Other unusual causes of hypoparathyroidism include previous neck irradiation, magnesium deficiency, metastatic cancer, and infiltrative diseases.

Clinical Findings

A. Symptoms and Signs

The lack of PTH results in hypocalcemia, which produces most of the symptoms associated with hypoparathyroidism. Symptoms associated with hypocalcemia include tetany, carpopedal spasms, paresthesias of the lips and hands, and a positive Chvostek sign or Trousseau sign. Patients may also exhibit less specific symptoms such as anxiety, depression, or fatigue. Additionally, hyperventilation, respiratory alkalosis with or without respiratory compromise, laryngospasm, hypotension, and seizures may occur with severe hypocalcemia.

B. Laboratory Findings

On laboratory evaluation, patients with hypoparathyroidism have low serum calcium and elevated serum phosphate levels, with a normal alkaline phosphatase level. Urinary levels of calcium and phosphate are decreased. The key finding is a low to absent PTH value.

Treatment

Acute hypocalcemia with tetany requires aggressive therapy with multiple drugs. Therapy should be started with calcium gluconate administered intravenously in a 10% solution. The infusion is given slowly until tetany resolves. Oral calcium along with vitamin D supplementation should be given after the acute crisis has resolved. Hypomagnesemia should be corrected with intravenous magnesium sulfate administered at a dose of 1–2 g every 6 hours. Chronic replacement of magnesium can be accomplished using 600-mg magnesium oxide tablets once or twice daily.

For the maintenance of normal calcium, vitamin D supplementation along with oral calcium should be given. Calcium in the form of calcium carbonate (40% elemental calcium) is the drug of choice, administered in a dose of 1–2 g of calcium a day. Serial calcium levels should be obtained regularly (every 3–6 months), and "spot" urine calcium levels should be maintained below 30 mg/dL.

Acute Musculoskeletal Complaints 36

Anne S. Boyd, MD, & Ronica A. Martinez, MD

Approximately 20% of all office visits to primary care providers involve musculoskeletal complaints. The purpose of this chapter is to survey the most common presenting complaints of the upper and lower extremities, highlighting the etiology, clinical findings, differential diagnosis, and evidence-based treatment options for each.

UPPER EXTREMITY

ROTATOR CUFF IMPINGEMENT

General Considerations

The term *subacromial impingement* defines any entity that compromises the subacromial space and irritates the enclosed rotator cuff tendons. Impingement can involve any of the structures within the subacromial space, and the term encompasses various entities from subacromial bursitis to rotator cuff calcific tendonitis and tendinosis. Often these entities arise in a similar fashion and are difficult to differentiate.

Impingement syndrome is classified into external, internal, and secondary impingement. The most common form is *external impingement,* which is caused by compression of the rotator cuff tendons as they pass under the coracoacromial arch. Subacromial bursitis can develop subsequently and intensify the compression. *Internal impingement* is caused by fraying of the infraspinatus tendon where it contacts the posterior glenoid. This occurs while the arm is maximally abducted and externally rotated and is seen in athletes who participate in overhead and throwing activities. Lastly, *secondary impingement* is caused by glenohumeral instability. Diagnosis is made with a meticulous history and physical examination, and appropriate imaging.

Clinical Findings

A. Symptoms and Signs

Diagnosis of subacromial impingement is primarily clinical. The patient complains of dull shoulder pain of insidious onset over weeks to months. Less often, these symptoms arise after a traumatic experience. Pain is typically localized to the anterolateral acromion and radiates to the lateral deltoid. Pain is aggravated at night, by sleeping with the arm overhead or lying on the involved shoulder. Overhead activities, throwing motions, and activities in which the humerus is flexed with an inward rotation also aggravate symptoms.

Physical examination usually reveals normal range of motion (ROM), although the patient may experience a painful arc of motion or pain upon approaching maximum internal rotation and forward flexion. Muscular weakness is sometimes seen in the supraspinatous muscle or the internal and external rotators of the shoulder. Supraspinatous strength (empty can test) is tested with the arm in 90 degrees of abduction and 30 degrees of forward flexion, with the thumb pointing downward. Decreased strength indicates a positive test. To differentiate weakness due to pain from actual loss of strength, it may be necessary to perform a subacromial injection with an anesthetic to alleviate the pain variable.

B. Imaging Studies

Radiographs that may aid in diagnosis include anteroposterior (AP), outlet, and axillary views of the affected shoulder. Curvature of the acromion or acromial spurs can be seen on an outlet view and may contribute to compression of the rotator cuff musculature or subacromial impingement.

C. Special Tests

Provocative testing includes the Neers test and the Hawkins–Kennedy test. The Neers test involves passive elevation of an internally rotated, forward-flexed arm. In the Hawkins–Kennedy test, the arm is positioned in 90 degrees of forward flexion and is internally rotated with a bent elbow. This causes impingement of the supraspinatus tendon against the anterior inferior acromion. Pain with either maneuver is considered a positive test; however, these tests may also be positive in patients with other pathologic entities.

Differential Diagnosis

Differential diagnosis includes acromioclavicular joint arthritis, osteolysis of the distal clavicle, rotator cuff tear, cervical disc herniation, adhesive capsulitis, supraspinatous nerve entrapment, glenohumeral instability, and arthritis.

Treatment

Treatment is initially conservative, using modified activity and nonsteroidal anti-inflammatory drugs (NSAIDs). The goal is to relieve inflammation, reestablish pain-free ROM, prevent atrophy, and enable return to previous activity. Current evidence supports the use of physical therapy to initiate rotator cuff and scapular musculature strengthening and joint mobilization techniques. A subacromial corticosteroid injection also can offer relief of symptoms when used with muscular strengthening. Surgical intervention is considered only after failure of conservative treatment.

Chang WK: Shoulder impingement syndrome. Phys Med Rehabil Clin N Am 2004; 15:493. [PMID: 15145427]

Desmeules F et al: Therapeutic exercise and orthopedic manual therapy for impingement syndrome: A systemic review. Clin J Sports Med 2003; 13:176. [PMID: 12792213]

Go moll AH et al: Rotator cuff disorders: Recognition and management among patients with shoulder pain. Arthritis Rheum 2004; 50:3751. [PMID: 15593187]

Koester MC et al: Shoulder impingement syndrome. Am J Med 2005; 118:452. [PMID: 15866244]

Michener LA et al: Effectiveness of rehabilitation for patients with subacromial impingement syndrome: A systemic review. J Hand Ther 2004; 7:152. [PMID: 15162102]

CALCIFIC TENDONITIS

General Considerations

Calcific tendonitis of the shoulder is an acute or chronic condition caused by inflammation around calcium deposits adjacent to the rotator cuff tendons. It affects about 10% of the population and is more common in women and in individuals older than 30 years.

Clinical Findings

Onset is usually abrupt and severely limits activities. It is theorized that the disease becomes painful only when the calcium is undergoing resorption; therefore, the patient may be pain free initially. Diagnosis is clinical and is based on a history of shoulder pain similar to impingement along with abrupt onset and tenderness over the greater tuberosity.

Radiographic evidence of a calcified tendon is best seen on plain films. To localize the calcification, it is recommended that the radiographic views include AP, internal and external rotation, scapular Y (or outlet), and axillary views. Magnetic resonance imaging (MRI) is not routinely indicated.

Treatment

Initial treatment consists of NSAIDs for a few weeks. A referral for physical therapy should be made to maintain ROM, and therapeutic ultrasound may be effective in reducing pain. In patients with signs of impingement, a corticosteroid injection into the subacromial may also be beneficial.

Hurt G, Baker CL: Calcific tendinitis of the shoulder. Orthop Clin North Am 2003; 34:567. [PMID: 14984196]

ROTATOR CUFF TEAR

General Considerations

Rotator cuff tears have been noted in 5–39% of people examined in cadaver and MRI studies. Their prevalence increases with age. The exact cause and best treatment are still being explored.

The rotator cuff complex is made up of four muscles: the subscapularis, supraspinatus, infraspinatus, and teres minor. Biomechanically, the rotator cuff abducts the arm with the assistance of the deltoid and also acts to rotate the humerus with respect to the scapula. The supraspinatus, infraspinatus, and teres minor externally rotate the humerus, whereas the subscapularis is a strong internal rotator. Together the rotator cuff muscles contract to maintain the humeral head in the glenoid during movement and thus maintain shoulder stability.

Clinical Findings

A. Symptoms and Signs

Many rotator cuff tears are asymptomatic. If symptoms are present, patients describe pain, stiffness, and occasional weakness around the shoulder. The pain is located at the front of the shoulder and radiates down the arm. It may be aggravated by overhead activity or sleeping on the affected side. Generally, pain is worse with resisted muscle activity in patients with a partial-thickness rotator cuff tear; whereas in those with a full-thickness tear, there is often only muscular weakness without pain.

Careful examination may demonstrate subtle atrophy of the supraspinatous and infraspinatus muscles, which is a sign of advanced disease. Tenderness at the insertion site of the supraspinatous tendon (just below anterior lateral acromion) is common. Occasionally in a complete tear, a defect can be palpated.

Limitations in ROM are due to muscle weakness and pain. Full-thickness tears are characterized by a decrease in active abduction, but normal passive ROM. Although quite variable, classically there is pain and slight weakness in patients with a partial-thickness rotator cuff tear, and weakness without pain in a full-thickness tear. The supraspinatus muscle often shows weakness in patients with a tear (positive empty can test).

Often a patient demonstrates a "painful arc" (pain or weakness between 60 and 120 degrees of abduction). With a complete tear, patients may also demonstrate a "drop arm sign" (the arm dropping from abduction) because there is no muscle to control the arm as the patient brings the raised arm back to the side.

B. Imaging Studies

Plain films can be useful to rule out other causes of shoulder pain (eg, calcific tendonitis or osteoarthritis). Changes seen on plain films that may be consistent with rotator cuff disease include decreased spacing between the humeral head and acromion, acromial spurs, and sclerosis with cystic changes in the greater tuberosity. Ultrasound can diagnose a rotator cuff tear (91% sensitive) if read by a skilled radiologist, but MRI is considered the gold standard in diagnostic imaging of rotator cuff disease.

Treatment

Treatment focuses on pain management using NSAIDs. Patients should be referred for physical therapy early in the diagnosis to take advantage of pain-reducing modalities such as heat, cold, and ultrasound. Flexibility and strengthening of the shoulder (rotator cuff muscles), scapula, and surrounding musculature are also helpful with treatment. Patients should be advised to avoid movements and activities that worsen symptoms.

Once a rotator cuff tear has been confirmed, referral should be made to an orthopedic surgeon. There is some evidence of improved results with surgical repair for both partial- and full-thickness tears. Patients with acute tears tend to have better outcomes than patients who have had pain for more than 6 months.

Barr KP: Rotator cuff disease. Phys Med Rehabil Clin North Am 2004; 15:475. [PMID: 15145426]

BICEPS TENDONITIS & INSTABILITY

General Considerations

Disorders of the biceps tendon have been labeled as either a tendonitis or an overuse syndrome (tendinosis). *Biceps tendonitis* is an inflammatory process involving the portion of the tendon located in the intertubercular groove. *Tendinosis* is an overuse injury that begins with an influx of inflammatory cells and progresses to exudation of fluid into the tendon sheath. In either case, this tissue thickens and becomes more painful. Many investigators believe that biceps tendonitis is secondary to shoulder impingement and rarely occurs alone. Alternately, some consider biceps tendonitis to be secondary to biceps tendon instability in the bicipital groove which, if present, is usually associated with subscapularis tendon pathology.

Clinical Findings

A. Symptoms and Signs

Patients usually complain of pain in the bicipital groove in the anterior aspect of the shoulder. The pain can radiate toward the deltoid insertion and it may be difficult to distinguish biceps tendon pathology from shoulder impingement or rotator cuff disease. Usually there is a history of repetitive overhead activity, which either initiates or aggravates symptoms. There may also be an audible or palpable "snap" at the bicipital groove during the arc of motion if instability is present.

The most common finding on physical examination is tenderness over the tendon within the bicipital groove. It is localized best when the arm is internally rotated to 10 degrees; at this angle, the biceps tendon is about 3 inches below the acromion.

B. Imaging Studies

Plain standard radiographs of the shoulder (AP, outlet, axillary views) are most often normal. For this reason, MRI should be considered (98% sensitive). An MRI arthrogram should be ordered if there is high suspicion of an associated cartilaginous tear of the labrum.

C. Special Tests

Data demonstrating the sensitivity and specificity of provocative special tests of the biceps tendon are limited. The Speed and Yergason tests may, however, be used to assist with the diagnosis of biceps tendinopathy. In the Speed test, the patient is asked to flex the arm against resistance with the elbow extended and forearm supinated. In the Yergason test, the patient supinates against resistance with the elbow flexed at 90 degrees. With either test, the presence of pain at the bicipital groove indicates a positive test.

Biceps instability is elicited by fully abducting and then externally rotating the patient's arm. An audible or palpable snap detected at the bicipital groove as the tendon subluxates or dislocates is a positive result indicating biceps instability.

An injection of anesthetic into the subacromial space (not the biceps tendon sheath) can be used to aid in diagnosis and to help rule out rotator cuff tendonitis. Pain caused by biceps tendonitis should remain postinjection.

Treatment

Initial treatment of biceps tendonitis is conservative, consisting of NSAIDs, rest, and modified activity. Physical therapy is useful to strengthen the rotator cuff but should not be aggressive during the acute pain stage. Subacromial corticosteroid injections are also useful in the treatment of biceps tendonitis, but direct injection into the biceps tendon should be avoided.

Treatment of biceps instability is similar. Older, sedentary patients may benefit from conservative therapy, including injections; however, younger, more active patients should be referred promptly for surgical repair.

Patton WC, McCluskey GM 3rd: Biceps tendinitis and subluxation. Clin Sports Med 2001; 20:505. [PMID: 11494838]

Paynter KS: Disorders of the long head of the biceps tendon. Phys Med Rehabil Clin N Am 2004; 15:511. [PMID: 15145428]

RUPTURE OF THE LONG HEAD OF THE BICEPS

General Considerations

Ruptures of the proximal biceps tendon are most often found in association with rotator cuff tears, but isolated ruptures can occur.

Clinical Findings

A. Symptoms and Signs

History includes pain in the anterior shoulder just prior to a complete tendon rupture. At the time of rupture, the patient usually hears an audible "pop" followed by immediate relief of symptoms. There is commonly an associated tear of the cartilaginous labrum, so the patient may also complain of catching, popping, or locking of the shoulder.

Physical examination may reveal pain over the bicipital groove, bruising in the anterior aspect of the arm, and a "Popeye muscle" (particularly with biceps flexion) due to the distal retraction of the muscle mass.

B. Imaging Studies

Radiographs are usually normal. MRI can confirm biceps tendon rupture. Gadolinium-enhanced MRI is preferred if a labral tear is also suspected.

Treatment

Treatment of an isolated rupture of the biceps long head is conservative and not surgical if the patient is inactive or would not be hindered significantly by loss of strength in the injured arm. Pain is managed with NSAIDs and modified activity, and activity is slowly increased as tolerated. Physical therapy is useful to improve rotator cuff strength, if an associated rotator cuff tear is not present. If a labral or rotator cuff tear is suspected along with the rupture of the biceps long head, referral to an orthopedic surgeon is warranted.

SHOULDER INSTABILITY

General Considerations

Shoulder instability can be viewed as any condition in which the balance of various stabilizing structures in the shoulder is disrupted, resulting in increased joint translation subluxation, or dislocation. Most dislocations are anterior, but they can also be posterior, and on rare occasion, inferior. In younger patients, dislocations are most often caused by trauma and sports injuries, whereas in the elderly, falls are the predominant cause (usually accompanied by a fracture). This discussion focuses on anterior subluxations and dislocations.

Anterior instability is categorized using two acronyms: TUBS (traumatic, unidirectional, Bankart surgery) and AMBRI (traumatic, multidirectional, bilateral, rehabilitation, inferior capsular surgery). The acronym for TUBS describes the cause and the direction of instability. An avulsion of the anteroinferior glenohumeral ligament and tear of the labrum (Bankart lesion) is also commonly seen. Treatment for this type of instability is surgical repair. AMBRI describes an atraumatic mechanism and instability that is usually multidirectional and bilateral. This type of injury usually responds well to rehabilitation. If rehabilitation does not improve symptoms, surgical repair (inferior capsular shift) is warranted.

Clinical Findings

A. Symptoms and Signs

The patient with an acute shoulder dislocation generally presents with shoulder pain, an unwillingness to move the affected arm, and a tendency to cradle the arm. The history usually includes a traumatic event, and a detailed description of the trauma—including arm position, energy level, and subsequent treatment adherence—is essential for diagnosis. Most subluxations and dislocations occur during abduction and maximum external rotation. On inspection, a bulge due to the displaced location of the humeral head may be noticeable, along with a dimpling inferior to the acromion where the humeral head should be.

If the patient's shoulder is not dislocated at the time of the examination, but the history describes episodes of subluxation, the apprehension test should be performed. In this test, the patient is supine with the arm in 90 degrees of abduction; the examiner then applies an external rotation stress. Patient apprehension due to subluxation of the humeral head is considered a positive test. Posterior pressure on the proximal humeral head can relieve symptoms if shoulder instability is the cause of pain (relocation test).

B. Imaging Studies

Radiographs are required to confirm shoulder dislocations. AP and outlet views are standard; however, an axillary view shows the relationship of the humeral head to the glenoid fossa and is more accurate when assessing for dislocation. Occasionally a bony defect in the posterolateral portion of the humeral head (Hil–Sachs lesion) is seen radiographically.

Treatment

Treatment for a shoulder dislocation consists of pain management and relocation. After relocation, the shoulder must be immobilized for 7–10 days to permit capsular healing. ROM exercises are then started, along with rotator cuff strengthening. Because younger patients with shoulder dislocations tend to have a high recurrence rate, surgical repair is warranted and early referral should be made in this population.

If the patient has signs of AMBRI, the standard treatment is a rehabilitation program to strengthen the rotator cuff and scapular musculature. If no improvements occur after rehabilitation, the patient should be referred for possible surgical repair.

Levine WN et al: Arthroscopic treatment of anterior shoulder instability. Instr Course Lect 2005; 54:87. [PMID: 15948437]

Wang VM, Flatow EL: Pathomechanics of acquired shoulder instability: A basic science perspective. J Shoulder Elbow Surg 2005; 14:2S. [PMID: 15726083]

Woodward TW, Best TM: The painful shoulder: Part II. Acute and chronic disorders. Am Fam Physician 2000; 61:3291. [PMID: 10865925]

DE QUERVAIN TENOSYNOVITIS

General Considerations

De Quervain stenosing tenosynovitis involves the abductor pollicis longus and the extensor pollicis brevis of the thumb. Although once thought to be an inflammatory condition, recent evidence has shown that degeneration of the tendon is present. The condition can arise with repetitive activity that requires grasping with ulnar deviation or repetitive thumb use.

Clinical Findings

Diagnosis is mainly clinical. Patients may complain of difficulty gripping items and often rub the area over the radial styloid. Pain is located on the radial side of the wrist and thumb, and occasionally radiates proximally.

There is tenderness to palpation just distal to the radial styloid. Pain can also be reproduced with resisted thumb abduction and extension, or with thumb adduction into a closed fist and passive ulnar deviation (Finklestein test). Pain over the tendons represents a positive test; however, the test may also be positive in patients with an arthritic flare of the first carpometacarpal joint.

Radiographs are not needed for diagnosis but may be useful to rule out osteoarthritis of the first carpometacarpal joint or a scaphoid fracture.

Treatment

The goals of treatment are to decrease inflammation, prevent adhesion formation, and prevent recurrent tendonitis. Brief periods of icing and use of NSAIDs are helpful initially, and the patient should be placed in a thumb restricting splint (thumb spica splint). If pain continues, a corticosteroid injection should be considered. In most patients, symptoms resolve after a single steroid injection. Steroid injection may be repeated after 4–6 weeks if symptoms are not 50% improved. If no improvement occurs after two injections within the year, a referral for surgical consultation should be obtained.

Ashe MC et al: Tendinopathies in the upper extremity: A paradigm shift. J Hand Ther 2004;17:329. [PMID: 15273673]

Hong E: Hand injuries in sports medicine. Prim Care 2005;32:91. [PMID: 15831314]

Richie CA 3rd, Briner WW: Corticosteroid injection for treatment of de Quervain's tenosynovitis: A pooled quantitative literature evaluation. J Am Board Fam Pract 2003;16:102. [PMID: 12665175]

Tallia AF, Cardone DA: Diagnostic and therapeutic injection of the wrist and hand region. Am Fam Physician 2003;67:745. [PMID: 12613728]

LATERAL & MEDIAL EPICONDYLITIS

General Considerations

For many years epicondylitis was thought to be caused by inflammation at the origin of the tendon bundle; however, recent evidence shows it is actually due to a breakdown of collagen from aging, microtrauma, or vascular compromise. Although properly termed *tendinosis,* the condition is referred to by its long-standing name, "epicondylitis," throughout this discussion to avoid confusion. Lateral and medial epicondylitis occur at the elbow and are primarily overuse or repetitive stress disorders.

Clinical Findings

A. Symptoms and Signs

Lateral epicondylitis is a tendinosis at the origin of the extensor tendons on the lateral epicondyle of the humerus. It is commonly known as "tennis elbow" because it is seen in activities that involve repetitive wrist extension. Patients complain of pain over the lateral elbow that may radiate down the forearm. There is tenderness to palpation over the origin of the extensor carpi radialis brevis tendon, which is anterior and distal to the lateral epicondyle. Pain is aggravated with resisted wrist extension or forearm supination.

Medial epicondylitis ("golfer's elbow") is seen after repetitive use of the flexor and pronator muscles of the wrist and hand (as occurs when playing golf, using a screwdriver, or hitting an overhead tennis stroke). Pain is insidious at the medial elbow and is worse with resisted forearm pronation and wrist flexion. Patients may also complain of a weak grasp. Tenderness to palpation occurs just distal and anterior to the medial epicondyle.

B. Imaging Studies

Imaging is not warranted for diagnosis of either lateral or medial epicondylitis; however, plain films of the elbow should be considered prior to any injections.

Differential Diagnosis

Differential diagnosis of lateral epicondylitis includes radial tunnel syndrome and posterior interosseous nerve syndrome. The differential for medial epicondylitis should include ulnar neuritis (cubital tunnel syndrome) and ulnar ligament injury.

Treatment

Initial treatment for either entity consists of activity modification and pain management with NSAIDs. A counterforce brace may be used during activities. In addition, biomechanics should be evaluated (ie, racquet grip, golf swing technique, etc). Physical therapy can be prescribed once acute symptoms have been controlled to establish pain-free ROM and strengthen muscles around the wrist and elbow. If pain is refractory, a steroid injection can be administered for either medial or lateral epicondylitis. Surgical treatment is recommended if no improvement occurs after 3–6 months of nonoperative treatment.

Ciccotti MC et al: Diagnosis and treatment of medial epicondylitis of the elbow. Clin Sports Med 2004; 23:693. [PMID: 15474230]

Sellards R, Kuebrich C: The elbow: Diagnosis and treatment of common injuries. Prim Care 2005;32:1. [PMID: 15831310]

LOWER EXTREMITY

PATELLAR TENDINOPATHY

General Considerations

The patellar tendon is an extension of the quadriceps femoris tendon and traverses from the inferior pole of the patella to its anchor point at the tibial tuberosity. Patellar tendinopathy, formerly known as "jumper's knee," is a painful condition at the inferior pole of the patella.

Pathogenesis

Traditionally, pain at the patellar tendon was thought to originate from inflammation. However, evidence now indicates that, as with other chronic tendinopathies, patellar tendinopathy is caused primarily by tendon overload. Repeated strain causes microtears, tenocyte death, fibrosis, and neovascularization, creating a zone of tendinosis within the tendon. Therefore, the term *patellar tendinopathy* should be encouraged over former terms such as *patellar tendinitis,* and treatment should also be directed toward more evidence-based and pathology-focused management.

Clinical Findings

A. Symptoms and Signs

Clinically, patellar tendinopathy presents with the insidious onset of localized anterior knee pain, primarily at the inferior pole of the patella. Pain is exacerbated by activity, prolonged knee flexion, and ascending or descending stairs. Discomfort often manifests when there has been an increase in intensity or frequency of activity. Pain may be present initially only after activity but will generally progress to the point where it occurs during or even between periods of activity.

Diagnosis of patellar tendinopathy is primarily clinical. On examination, the most consistent finding is tenderness over the tendon at the inferior pole of the patella with the leg in extension. Although radiographs may show associated bony anomalies such as Osgood–Schlatter disease or tendinous calcification, the clinical relevance of these changes is debatable.

Treatment

With the understanding that patellar tendinopathy is more accurately a degenerative tendinosis caused by overload than an inflammatory tendonitis, treatment strategies have moved away from the traditional anti-inflammatory approach to a focus on diminishing tendon stress and on muscle strengthening. Recommendations include use of eccentric strengthening exercises, improving quadriceps and hamstring flexibility, proprioception, evaluation of biomechanics, and modification of aggravating activities. Patients with acute tendon pain may benefit from NSAIDs, but their widespread use in tendinopathy is not evidence based. The utility of other modalities, including ultrasound and extracorporeal shock wave therapy, is promising but requires further confirmation. Depending on the chronicity of symptoms, recovery may require from 2 to 6 months.

Khan KM et al: Histopathology of common tendinopathies: Update and implications for clinical management. Sports Med 1999;27:393. [PMID: 10418074]

Peers KH, Lysens RJ: Patellar tendinopathy in athletes: Current diagnostic and therapeutic recommendations. Sports Med 2005;35:71. [PMID: 15651914]

Warden SJ, Brukner P: Patellar tendinopathy. Clin Sports Med 2003;22:743. [PMID: 14560545]

PATELLOFEMORAL PAIN SYNDROME

General Considerations

Patellofemoral pain syndrome (PFPS) is a broad term used to define anterior knee pain not related to intra-articular pathology, bursitis, tendonitis, fracture, patellar subluxation, or Osgood–Schlatter disease.

The patella normally sits comfortably in a groove with its posterior cartilaginous surface "molded" to complement the trochlea of the femur. The patella is held in place by its natural shape, by the trochlea, and by the tension of the medial and lateral patellar retinacula (Figures 36–1 and 36–2). When flexing or extending the knee, the muscles of the hamstring and quadriceps function like reins to direct the patella within the trochlea and to rotate the tibia. In extension, the patella sits at the proximal aspect of the trochlea. As the knee flexes, the posterior patella becomes engaged in the trochlea. Compressive forces at the posterior cartilaginous surface of the patella intensify with increasing flexion and can reach impressive levels at 90 degrees of flexion.

Pathogenesis

Although the cartilage itself does not possess pain fibers, the pain of PFPS is associated with friction between the subpatellar chondral surface and the trochlea of the femur. Three major contributing factors have been evaluated in relation to PFPS: malalignment of the lower extremity, muscular imbalances, and overactivity. Lower extremity alignment factors associated with PFPS include torsion of the femur or tibia, genu valgum, genu recurvatum, increased Q angle, femoral anteversion, and foot pronation. Additionally, various patterns of muscle weakness have been reported in the quadriceps. It seems logical that each of these factors has the potential to draw the patella laterally and contribute to disturbed patellar tracking. However, research has not been convincing in showing significant biomechanical differences between asymptomatic individuals and those with symptoms of PFPS, or that the muscular imbalances observed are a cause or an effect of PFPS. Nonetheless, the most recent theory embraces the idea that each individual has an independent "comfort zone" based on his or her own specific biomechanics, joint history, and activity level. Exceeding this comfort zone via overuse surpasses the reserve of the joint and creates patellofemoral symptoms. Therefore, the

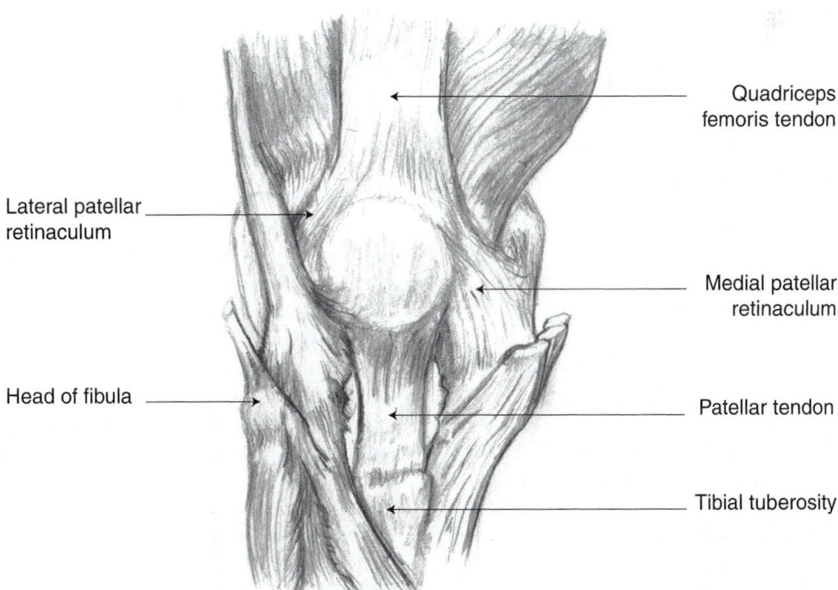

Figure 36–1. Anatomy of the anterior knee. (Illustration by Anne Boyd, MD.)

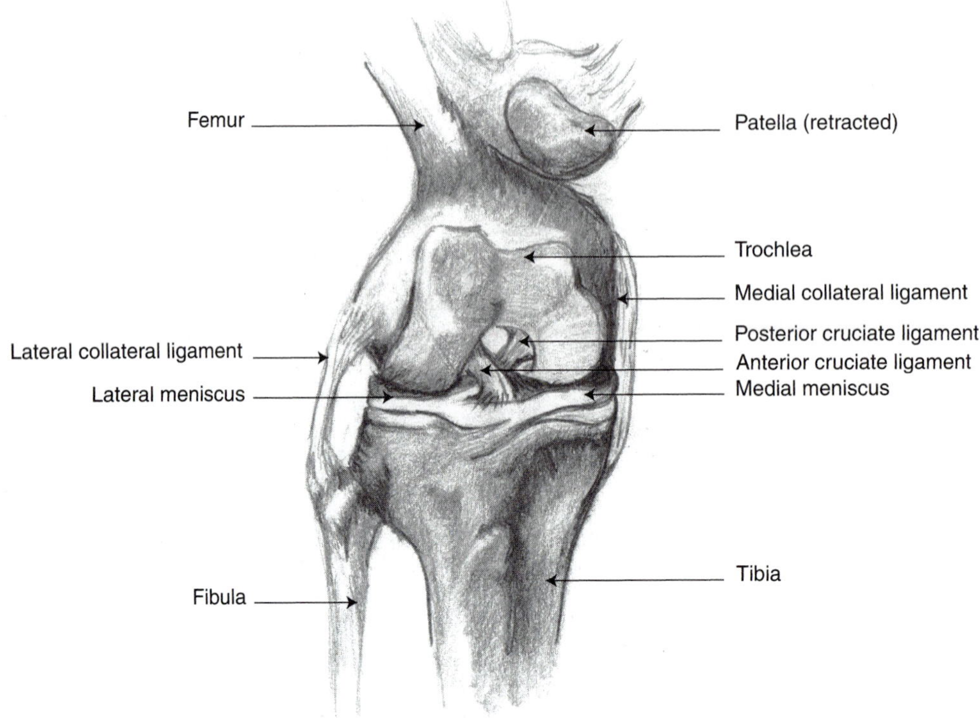

Figure 36–2. Intra-articular structures of the knee. (Illustration by Anne Boyd, MD.)

same person may be asymptomatic when not training but become symptomatic with increased activity despite the consistency of the individual's joint biomechanics.

Clinical Findings

A. Symptoms and Signs

Historically, patients with PFPS are young patients who present with insidious onset of diffuse, aching, anterior knee pain. Pain is often bilateral and is aggravated by climbing stairs, ascending a hill, squatting, or sitting with the knee flexed for a prolonged period of time (theater sign).

Although the extent of their contribution is unclear, alignment, gait, and stance should be assessed and gross abnormalities addressed. Maltracking of the patella and chronic irritation of the patellar cartilage often produce tenderness at the posteromedial or posterolateral patellar facets, and also a positive "patellar grind" or Clarke sign (pain with slight compression of the patella that is exacerbated by quadriceps contraction). It is paramount to note that children may have significant hip pathology that presents solely as knee pain; pediatric patients must therefore be considered as a distinct population with a broader differential.

B. Imaging Studies

Radiographs are usually not indicated unless pain is prolonged or associated with trauma, or if bony pathology is suspected.

Treatment

Treatment is directed at altering patellar tracking, correcting biomechanical factors that lead to overuse, and decreasing the intensity of the aggravating activity. Exercises designed to strengthen the medial quadriceps, hip abductors, adductors, and internal rotators have proven helpful as well as stretching exercises for the hamstrings, iliotibial band, and lateral patellar retinaculum. The use of foot orthotics is promising acutely for those with structural foot problems. Bracing and taping may be effective in some patients. Limited evidence exists for the effectiveness of NSAIDs, and their utility is questioned in patients with this disorder. Surgery is reserved for patients with damage to the chondral surface and those who have failed prolonged therapy.

Adams WB: Treatment options in overuse injuries of the knee: Patellofemoral syndrome, iliotibial band syndrome, and degenerative meniscal tears. Curr Sports Med Rep 2004;3:256. [PMID: 15324592]

Calmbach WL, Hutchens M: Evaluation of patients presenting with knee pain: Part I. History, physical examination, radiographs, and laboratory tests. Am Fam Physician 2003;68:907. [PMID: 13678139]

Scuderi G, McCann P: *Sports Medicine: A Comprehensive Approach.* Elsevier/Mosby, 2005.

Thomee R et al: Patellofemoral pain syndrome: A review of current issues. Sports Med 1999;28:245. [PMID: 10565551]

LIGAMENTOUS INJURIES TO THE KNEE

General Considerations

The knee is a modified hinge joint that is stabilized by the anterior cruciate ligament (ACL), posterior cruciate ligament (PCL), medial collateral ligament (MCL), lateral collateral ligament (LCL), menisci, capsule, and surrounding musculature (see Figure 36–2).

1. Anterior Cruciate Ligament Injury

Pathogenesis

An intact ACL prevents anterior translation of the tibia on the femur. Injury to the ACL may occur with forced hyperextension; however, more often injury occurs when the foot is planted and the knee twisted, forcing the tibia forward. There is often a component of valgus stress, but no direct blow is required.

Clinical Findings

A. Symptoms and Signs

These injuries frequently occur when an athlete "cuts" or stops abruptly, and the patient often hears or feels a "pop." Swelling is rapid (minutes to hours) as a large hemarthrosis develops within the joint.

Without the restraint of an intact ACL, the tibia displaces anteriorly as the patient ambulates and causes a sensation of instability or giving way with walking, particularly with pivoting motions.

An acute ACL injury can often be diagnosed acutely; however, the majority of patients present a day or more after the injury. By that time, muscle spasm and pain have set in. Because muscle relaxation is critical for an accurate examination, this may complicate or delay the examination.

The most sensitive test in the setting of an acutely swollen knee is the Lachman test. With the patient supine and the relaxed knee in 30 degrees of flexion, the examiner stabilizes the distal femur with one hand, grasps the proximal tibia with the other, and attempts to sublux the tibia anteriorly. The anterior drawer test also assesses the integrity of the ACL. With the knee flexed to 90 degrees, the examiner stabilizes the relaxed leg by sitting on the patient's foot, grasps the calf with both thumbs on the tibial tubercle, and applies an anterior force. With either test, significant anterior translation of the tibia or lack of a discrete endpoint is considered a positive test and indicates a compromised ACL.

B. Imaging Studies

Although radiographs are of limited value in diagnosing ACL tears, a *standard knee series*—including a bilateral standing AP view, a lateral view, a bilateral posteroanterior (PA) flexion weight-bearing or tunnel view (45 degrees of flexion), and a patellar profile (Merchant or skyline) view—is recommended to rule out other bony pathology. MRI is the imaging modality of choice to confirm clinical suspicion.

Treatment

Initial treatment includes a brief period of immobilization, protected weight bearing with crutches for 7–10 days, cryotherapy, and early ROM exercises. Thereafter, physical therapy is initiated to restore motion and strength. Bracing may provide some subjective benefit. There is insufficient evidence to recommend conservative over operative treatment of ACL tears. General consensus holds that, in relatively inactive individuals, nonoperative treatment is a viable option. These patients, however, may have to accept some degree of chronic instability and acknowledge the potential for further meniscal and articular surface injuries. Younger patients, those with chronic instability, those failing conservative therapy, and athletic individuals who wish to participate in activities involving running, jumping, or pivoting should be referred for possible surgical intervention.

Fithian DC et al: Fate of the anterior cruciate ligament-injured knee. Orthop Clin North Am 2002;33:621. [PMID: 12528905]

Linko E et al: Surgical versus conservative interventions for anterior cruciate ligament ruptures in adults. Cochrane Database Syst Rev 2005:(2):CD001356. [PMID: 15846618]

Solomon DH et al: The rational clinical examination. Does this patient have a torn meniscus or ligament of the knee? Value of the physical examination. JAMA 2001;286:1610. [PMID: 11585485]

Torg JS et al: Clinical diagnosis of anterior cruciate ligament instability in the athlete. Am J Sports Med 1976;4:84. [PMID: 961972]

2. Posterior Cruciate Ligament Injury

Pathogenesis

The PCL limits posterior displacement of the tibia on the femur. PCL tears occur less often than ACL tears, may be asymptomatic, and often go undetected. The usual mechanism of injury is a posteriorly directed force on the proximal tibia with a flexed knee, such as a fall on a bent knee with the foot plantar flexed, or a bent knee striking a dashboard in a motor vehicle accident.

Clinical Findings

Patients with PCL injuries, unlike those with ACL tears, often do not report a "pop." The initial trauma may be subtle, and subsequent symptoms are frequently vague. Limping, a moderate knee effusion, difficulty with the last 10–20 degrees of flexion, and posterior knee pain often accompany this injury. Unsteadiness may be a complaint, but significant instability is more likely to be reported with combined injuries.

The posterior drawer test is the most accurate test for PCL integrity. Imaging preferences are the same as for suspected ACL injuries.

Treatment

Nonoperative management is acceptable for chronic and for isolated, low-grade, acute PCL tears. Acutely, treatment is similar to ACL treatment, except crutches are utilized for 14 days and physical therapy emphasizes quadriceps strengthening. Indications for expeditious surgical referral include combined ligamentous injury, significant laxity, and avulsion fractures.

Harner C, Hoher J: Evaluation and treatment of posterior cruciate ligament injuries. Am J Sports Med 1998;26:471. [PMID: 9617416]

Wind W et al: Evaluation and treatment of posterior cruciate ligament injuries: Revisited. Am J Sports Med 2004;32:1765. [PMID: 15494347]

3. Injuries of the Medial Collateral & Lateral Collateral Ligaments

Pathogenesis

Of the main stabilizing ligaments of the knee, the MCL is the most commonly injured. A medially directed valgus force, as occurs with a noncontact twisting injury or a blow to the lateral side of the knee, is the most common cause of MCL disruption. Isolated LCL disruption is relatively rare and occurs with a blow to the anteromedial knee.

Clinical Findings

Patients with an isolated collateral ligament tear generally present with a classic mechanism of injury and may report the sensation of a "pop" with the trauma. Patients complain of localized pain and tenderness over the damaged ligament but rarely report significant instability or locking. Localized swelling may be seen with isolated tears, but significant effusion is rare.

Valgus and varus stress testing to evaluate the MCL and LCL, respectively, is performed at full extension (0 degrees) and 30 degrees. Laxity that is apparent only at 30 degrees of flexion suggests an isolated MCL or LCL injury. Additional laxity in full extension suggests concomitant soft tissue injury.

Radiographs are helpful in ruling out concomitant bony pathology but are usually not necessary to diagnose a pure tear of the MCL or LCL. MRI is useful when examination findings are equivocal.

Treatment

Treatment of isolated collateral tears is primarily conservative. Ice and use of a compression wrap assist with local swelling. Crutches and toe-touch weight bearing may be all that a patient with a higher grade sprain may tolerate initially. However, regardless of grade, the patient needs to be encouraged to gradually increase weight bearing as soon as possible. Although hinged bracing does not speed healing, it provides some protection and a subjective sense of stability. Prior to full return to sports, athletes should have achieved full ROM and completed a functional rehabilitation program, and should have minimal pain and nearly complete quadriceps and hamstring strength. Recovery may vary from days to weeks, but nonoperative management is still favored.

Quarles JD, Hosey RG: Medial and lateral collateral injuries: Prognosis and treatment. Prim Care 2004;31:957. [PMID: 15544829]

Reider B: Medial collateral ligament injuries in athletes. Sports Med 1996;21:147. [PMID: 8775518]

MENISCAL TEARS

General Considerations

The lateral and medial menisci are C-shaped wedges of fibrocartilaginous tissue with attachments at the anterior and posterior aspects of the tibial plateau (see Figure 36–2). The menisci have many functions, including load bearing and distribution, shock absorption, passive stabilization, and proprioception.

Meniscal tears tend to involve the medial meniscus, because it is more fixed than the lateral meniscus and therefore more susceptible to injury. Younger patients tend to have an associated injury, whereas adults over age 40 tend toward atraumatic tears related to degeneration.

Clinical Findings

A. Symptoms and Signs

Acute, isolated tears primarily occur due to shearing forces during a twisting or hyperflexion injury. Pain is moderate and may subside, allowing some return to activity following the tear. Effusion is slower to develop (24–36 hours) and is generally moderate. Occasionally, large, bucket-handle tears displace and lodge in the joint, preventing full extension and creating a "locked knee." This presentation requires early surgical referral. More often, patients present days to weeks after the original injury and have full ROM. They complain of pain with squatting and of painful locking or catching, reflecting the meniscal fragment within the joint. Patients with degenerative tears tend to present with an atraumatic history, insidious onset, mechanical symptoms, and mild, intermittent swelling.

Physical examination may demonstrate an effusion. ROM should be assessed to ensure that there is no loss of extension or flexion. Joint line tenderness over the affected meniscus is the best clinical indicator of a meniscal tear (74% sensitivity; 50% positive predictive value). Several provocative maneuvers have been developed to recreate impingement of the torn fragment. These tests include the McMurray test and the Apley test, which are helpful but marginally sensitive or specific.

B. Imaging Studies

Although radiographs cannot confirm a diagnosis of meniscal tear, a standard knee series (see earlier discussion of ACL injury) is obtained to rule out additional bony pathology and to examine joint space narrowing. MRI is the confirmatory imaging modality of choice.

Treatment

Initial treatment for isolated meniscal pathology includes cryotherapy, rest, NSAIDs, crutches and weight bearing as tolerated for 7–10 days, and early ROM exercises. If full ROM is attained, and neither pain nor effusion recurs, the patient may gradually return to activity. Partial response to conservative measures warrants physical therapy. Indications for surgical referral include failure to respond to nonoperative treatment or recurrent episodes of catching or giving way.

Greis PE et al: Meniscal injury: I. Basic science and evaluation. J Am Acad Orthop Surg 2002;10:168. [PMID: 12041938]

ANKLE SPRAINS

General Considerations

Ankle ligament sprains are the most common ankle injuries and account for 19–23% of all sports injuries. The overwhelming majority of these sprains are inversion injuries affecting the lateral ligamentous complex, including the anterior talofibular ligament (ATFL), the calcaneofibular ligament (CFL), and the posterior talofibular ligament (Figure 36–3). Medially, the deltoid ligament provides eversion restraint.

Clinical Findings

A. Symptoms and Signs

Patient history is the key to assessing ankle trauma. Generally, patients with a lateral ankle sprain report an inversion, internal rotation injury with the foot in plantar flexion. Pain over the involved ligaments is common. Discomfort with weight bearing and ecchymosis

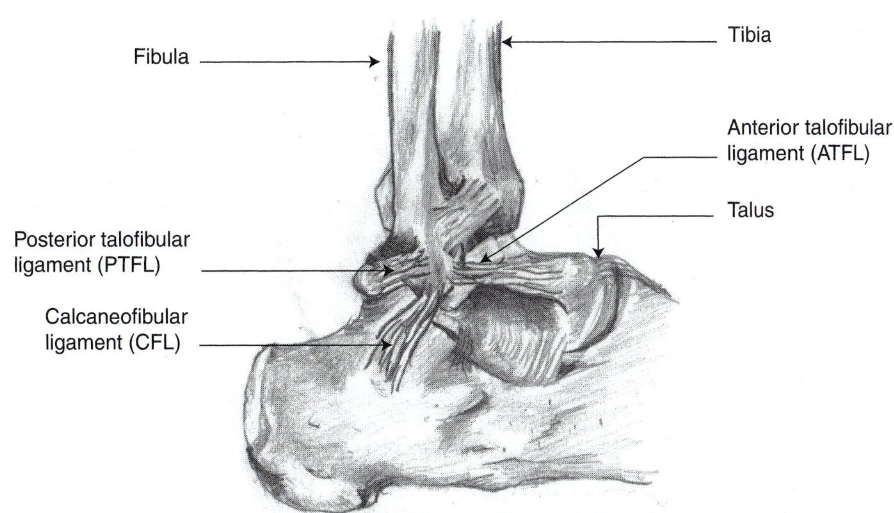

Figure 36–3. Lateral ankle joint anatomy. (Illustration by Anne Boyd, MD.)

are variable. Often after an acute injury, the ankle is too swollen or the patient too guarded to permit a diagnostic examination, and a repeat physical examination may be necessary several days after the initial injury.

Observation of the patient's gait, inspection, palpation, and the anterior drawer and talar tilt tests are the cornerstones of the physical examination. Inspection demonstrates variable swelling, and palpation yields focal tenderness over the involved ligaments, generally the ATFL and CFL. The anterior drawer test is performed with the patient's foot relaxed off the edge of the table. The examiner stabilizes the distal tibia with one hand, then grasps the calcaneus in the palm of the other hand and applies an anterior force. Excessive anterior motion or a "clunk" suggests disruption of the ATFL. The talar tilt test is performed by stabilizing the tibia with one hand, then grasping the calcaneus in the palm of the opposite hand and inverting or everting the hindfoot. Significant laxity with inversion suggests disruption of the ATFL and CFL, whereas laxity with eversion suggests disruption of the deltoid ligament.

B. Imaging Studies

The Ottawa ankle rules provide high-yield criteria for ordering radiographs (level of evidence C). Indications for radiographs include bony tenderness at the posterodistal portion of the lateral or medial malleolus, or inability to bear weight immediately and during the examination. Routine radiographs include anterior, lateral, and mortise views.

Treatment

Initial treatment of isolated, acute ankle sprains consists of rest, ice, compression or support, and elevation (RICE). Occasionally, crutches, a posterior splint, cast, or walking boot are required initially. Regardless, rest is relative and temporary. Early protected mobilization and weight bearing have been shown to facilitate return to activity and should be encouraged. Application of ice works as well as or better than heat to speed recovery at any stage of the injury (strength of recommendation B). Options for supportive devices for ankle sprains are numerous. Although the use of an elastic bandage has fewer complications, the use of a semirigid ankle support (such as an Aircast Stirrup) appears to be associated with less subjective instability and more rapid return to work and to sports. A lace-up ankle support appears to significantly reduce swelling and is also a reasonable option. NSAIDs may increase bleeding and swelling acutely, so acetaminophen or mild narcotics may be used for pain within the first 48 hours. Rehabilitation follows the initial therapy with the goals of restoring motion, strengthening the ankle everters and dorsiflexors, stretching the Achilles tendon, and gradually progressing to proprioceptive and functional conditioning.

Worsening symptoms or lack of improvement in the first several weeks after a lateral ankle sprain should prompt the physician to consider other causes of ankle pain. Differential diagnosis should include fracture or osteochondral lesion of the talus; peroneal tendon subluxation; fractures of the calcaneus, distal fibula, fifth metatarsal, or navicular; and subtalar or Lisfranc sprain.

Medial sprains are caused by eversion and dorsiflexion and involve sequential tearing of the deltoid ligament, the anterior tibiofibular ligaments, and the interosseous membrane. These significant injuries are beyond the scope of this chapter; however, readers are cautioned that symptoms are prolonged and treatment is significantly more aggressive with these types of injury.

Boyce SH et al: Management of ankle sprains: A randomized controlled trial of the treatment of inversion injuries using an elastic support bandage or an Aircast ankle brace. Br J Sports Med 2005;39:91. [PMID: 15665204]

Cohen RS, Balcom TA: Current treatment options for ankle injuries: Lateral ankle sprain, Achilles tendonitis, and Achilles rupture. Curr Sports Med Rep 2003;2:251. [PMID: 12959705]

Kerkhoffs GM et al: Different functional treatment strategies for acute lateral ankle ligament injuries in adults. Cochrane Database Syst Rev 2002;(3):CD002938. [PMID: 12137665]

Stiell IG et al: Implementation of the Ottawa ankle rules. JAMA 1994;271:827. [PMID: 8114236]

Thompson C et al: Clinical inquiries. Heat or ice for acute ankle sprain? J Fam Pract 2003;52:642. [PMID: 12899822]

MEDIAL TIBIAL STRESS SYNDROME

General Considerations

Medial tibial stress syndrome (MTSS) is a common overuse injury that causes activity-related pain over the posteromedial aspect of the distal two thirds of the tibia. The term *MTSS* has replaced the previously favored term *shin splints,* as it is far less generic and more accurately reflects the etiology and location of the pain. Runners are most commonly affected, but MTSS is also quite prevalent in athletes who participate in jumping sports such as basketball and gymnastics, and in military recruits.

Pathogenesis

Although multiple muscle groups have been implicated and the roles of inflammation versus bone remodeling have been investigated, the precise pathophysiologic mechanism of MTSS remains an enigma. The most recent theory implicates the fascial insertion of the medial soleus as the probable source of pathology. Theory holds that during activity the medial soleus contracts to plantar flex and invert the foot, disrupting the fascial fibers at the muscle insertion onto the tibial periosteum.

Clinical Findings

A. Symptoms and Signs

Patients present with complaints of dull pain along the middle or distal posteromedial tibia. Pain often coincides with a significant increase in the intensity, frequency, or duration of the patient's activity, or with a change in the patient's footwear or running surface. Initially, pain may be present only at the beginning or the end of activity, and symptoms are promptly relieved with rest. If training continues, however, pain may become more severe and persistent.

Physical examination reveals diffuse tenderness along the posteromedial border of the middle and distal tibia. Provocative maneuvers include passive dorsiflexion, active plantar flexion, standing toe raises, and one- or two-legged hop. Excessive foot pronation, hindfoot or forefoot varus, and heel cord tightness are thought to be risk factors for MTSS.

B. Imaging Studies

Radiographic findings are frequently normal. A bone scan, however, is particularly useful for distinguishing MTSS from a stress fracture. In contrast to the focal uptake seen with a stress fracture, MTSS demonstrates diffuse, longitudinal uptake at the posteromedial tibia only on the delayed phase of the scan.

Differential Diagnosis

The differential of exertional leg pain includes MTSS, deep venous thrombosis, fascial herniations, muscle strains, nerve or artery entrapment, chronic compartment syndrome, and stress fracture.

Treatment

Initial treatment of MTSS consists of activity modification and avoidance of aggravating factors. If normal ambulation causes pain, crutches may be used to eliminate weight bearing temporarily. Activities that do not cause discomfort may be continued. Activities that induce pain must be discontinued and resumed only when the activity can be performed pain free. Thereafter, training level may be increased gradually over a 3- to 6-week period as long as the patient remains asymptomatic with each advancing stage. Although unproven, several adjuvant treatments may be beneficial, including ice massage, NSAIDs, shock-absorbent inserts, heel cord stretching, and correction of malalignment. Surgical referral for fasciotomy is reserved for patients with extremely resistant, painful symptoms.

Edwards PH et al: A practical approach for the differential diagnosis of chronic leg pain in the athlete. Am J Sports Med 2005;33:1241. [PMID: 16061959]

Kortebein PM et al: Medial tibial stress syndrome. Med Sci Sports Exerc 2000;32:S27. [PMID: 10730992]

PLANTAR FASCIITIS

General Considerations

Plantar fasciitis is extremely common in young runners, and is reportedly the most common cause of heel pain in adults as well. The peak incidence in the general population is between the ages of 40 and 60 years.

Pathogenesis

The plantar fascia is a fibrous aponeurosis that extends from the medial calcaneus to the metatarsal heads. It provides static support of the longitudinal arch of the foot and dynamic shock absorption. The etiology of plantar fasciitis is likely multifactorial. Although data are limited, several risk factors have been identified, including obesity, pes planus, pes cavus, and a tight Achilles tendon. In athletes, the primary risk factor is thought to be overactivity. Athletes commonly report a change in the intensity, distance, or duration of their activity or an alteration in their running surface or footwear that accompanied the onset of symptoms.

Although the term *fasciitis* implies inflammation, histologic specimens from patients undergoing plantar fascia release have shown predominantly degenerative and chronic inflammatory changes in the tissue. Therefore, this entity may more appropriately be considered a fasciosis.

Clinical Findings

A. Symptoms and Signs

Classically, patients present with insidious onset of pain on the plantar surface of the heel that is worse with the first steps in the morning or when standing after a prolonged period of rest. Pain usually diminishes with rest but may recur at the end of the day. Athletes report that running, hill climbing, and sprinting exacerbate the pain. Pain is bilateral in up to one third of cases.

Physical examination generally demonstrates tenderness along the anteromedial aspect of the calcaneus which intensifies with stretching of the plantar fascia by passive dorsiflexion of the toes. Limitation of ankle dorsiflexion associated with a tight heel cord may also be noted.

B. Imaging Studies

Radiographs are rarely indicated for initial diagnosis and treatment of plantar fasciitis. Heel spurs on the anterior calcaneus can be misleading; these are present in 15–25% of the general population without symptoms, and many symptomatic patients do not have spurs. Therefore, the detection of heel spurs is of no value in either confirming or ruling out the diagnosis of plantar fasciitis.

Differential Diagnosis

The differential diagnosis of heel pain includes calcaneal stress fracture, plantar fascia rupture, fat pad atrophy, retrocalcaneal bursitis, nerve entrapment syndromes, spondyloarthropathies, infection, tumor, and Paget disease.

Treatment

Fortunately, in 80% of patients with plantar fasciitis, regardless of therapy, the injury is self-limited. However, resolution of symptoms can take 6–18 months, and there is limited evidence concerning the value of many of the treatments. Regardless, initially it seems reasonable to recommend conservative, low-risk interventions. These include activity modification, NSAIDs, heel cushions or arch supports, and an aggressive Achilles and plantar fascia stretching program. Support for the use of ice, heat, massage, or strengthening of the intrinsic muscles of the foot is predominantly anecdotal. Corticosteroid injections may provide short-term benefit. More intensive treatments, including custom orthotics, night splints, and cast immobilization, may be beneficial in patients with recalcitrant symptoms. Extracorporeal shock wave therapy is a promising option on the horizon, but its efficacy is still controversial in the literature. Surgical release is generally reserved for patients who have not responded to appropriate conservative treatment of at least 6–9 months' duration.

Aldrige T: Diagnosing heel pain in adults. Am Fam Physician 2004;70:332. [PMID: 15291091]

Buchbinder R: Clinical practice. Plantar fasciitis. N Engl J Med 2004;350:2159. [PMID: 15152061]

Young CC et al: Treatment of plantar fasciitis. Am Fam Physician 2001;63:467. [PMID: 11272297]

Common Upper & Lower Extremity Fractures

37

David A. Nikovits, MD, Richard E. Rodenberg, Jr., MD, Thomas D. Armsey, MD, & Robert G. Hosey, MD

UPPER EXTREMITY FRACTURES

CLAVICLE FRACTURES

Clinical Findings

A. Symptoms and Signs

A direct blow to the clavicle or a fall on the lateral shoulder may cause a clavicular fracture. Fractures of the clavicle occur in the middle (80%), distal (15%), and medial (5%) thirds. Patients hold the affected arm adducted and resist motion. Typically, there is swelling and tenderness over the fracture site and a visible and palpable deformity.

B. Imaging Studies

Imaging studies should include an anteroposterior (AP) view. Sometimes an apical lordotic view (AP view 45 degrees cephalad) helps visualize the clavicle without rib interference. A distal third fracture with articular involvement may require cone views or a lateral view. Likewise, at times a medial third fracture is seen with cone and lateral views. A computed tomography (CT) scan helps visualize articular fractures.

Complications

Complications may include subclavian vascular injuries and nerve root avulsion or contusion. Middle third fractures may develop malunion, excessive callus formation, and nonunion. Displaced distal third fractures with torn coracoclavicular ligaments may lead to delayed union. It may require years for a large callus to remodel. Articular surface involvement in either the medial or distal third can lead to degenerative arthritis.

Treatment

Treatment includes ice, analgesics, sling immobilization, and physical therapy. Initial radiographs, may show early callus formation. At 2-week follow-up, radiographs should be obtained to evaluate for displacement and angulation. Significant callus typically forms between 4 and 6 weeks, along with disappearance of the fracture line. If the fracture is not clinically healed, repeat radiographs at 6–8 weeks are indicated. Once the fracture is clinically and radiographically healed, radiographs can be discontinued. The patient may return to normal activity when the clavicle is painless, the fracture is healed on radiograph, and the shoulder has a full range of motion and near-normal strength.

Displaced fractures, open fractures, nonunion, and persistent pain 6–8 weeks post-fracture are indications for referral.

Eiff MP: Management of clavicle fractures. Am Fam Physician 1997; 55:121. [PMID:9012272]

COLLE FRACTURES (DISTAL RADIUS FRACTURE)

Clinical Findings

A. Symptoms and Signs

A fall-on-outstretched-hand (FOOSH) injury can lead to a Colle fracture. Patients typically present with pain, swelling, and tenderness at the distal forearm. On examination a "dinner fork" deformity (dorsal displacement of the distal fragment and volar angulation of the distal intact radius with radial shortening) may be identified.

B. Imaging Studies

Imaging studies consist of AP and lateral radiographs (Figure 37–1). Concomitant fracture of the ulnar styloid process may be present. With immobilization, the fracture becomes stable in 6–8 weeks.

Complications

There are early and late complications of Colle fractures. Early complications include median nerve compression,

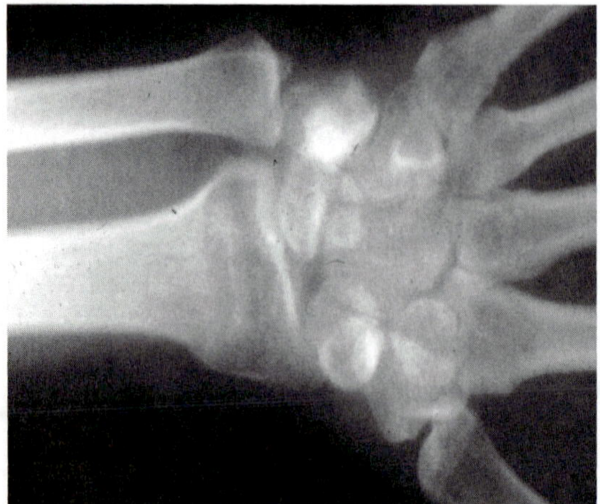

Figure 37–1. Distal radius fracture. (Courtesy of Kentucky Sports Medicine, Dr. Mary Lloyd Ireland.)

tendon damage, ulnar nerve contusion or compression, compartment syndrome, and fragment displacement with loss of reduction. Patients may develop a decreased range of motion of the wrist and prolonged swelling. Possible late complications include stiffness of the fingers, shoulder, or radiocarpal joint, shoulder–hand syndrome, cosmetic defects, rupture of the extensor pollicis longus, malunion, nonunion, flexor tendon adhesions, and chronic pain of the radioulnar joint with supination. If there is distal radial ulnar joint disruption and radial shortening, decreased grip strength, decreased range of motion with supination, and difficulty writing may develop.

Treatment

A nondisplaced distal radial fracture or minimally displaced fracture with little comminution can be managed by the primary care provider. Treatment steps include anesthesia, reduction of the fracture with traction and manipulation, and immobilization with casting. Afterward, postreduction radiographs are taken to ensure proper alignment.

Reduction is necessary to maintain radial length and volar tilt. A short arm cast may be used in an elderly patient and for others with a nondisplaced fracture. All others should be placed in a long arm cast for 3–6 weeks followed by a short arm cast. Physical therapy is helpful for maintaining elbow range of motion. The cast should extend to the proximal palmar crease volarly and to the metacarpophalangeal (MCP) prominences dorsally to allow finger and MCP motion and allow opposition. Care should be taken to ensure there is adequate padding around the edges of the cast.

At 2 weeks, AP and lateral radiographs may show little or no callus formation. These should be compared with the original radiographs. Rereduction may be necessary. At the 4- to 6-week follow-up visit, radiographs may show a bridging callus. If there is adequate callus and no tenderness or motion at the fracture site, then cast immobilization may be discontinued. Physical therapy for wrist and elbow range of motion should be started. At 6–8 weeks bridging callus should be visualized. Radiographs should be checked to assess for malunion, radial shortening, and delayed union as well as for functionality of the wrist. The cast should be discontinued if criteria at the 4- to 6-week follow-up are met. At the 8- to 12-week follow-up, additional callus should be seen. Nonunion occurs with no healing at 4–6 months postinjury.

Indications for referral include fractures with radiocarpal or radioulnar joint involvement, significantly comminuted fractures, and displaced articular fractures.

SCAPHOID FRACTURES

Clinical Findings

A. Symptoms and Signs

Scaphoid fractures are caused by a forceful hyperextension of the wrist. This is typically due to a FOOSH with the wrist dorsiflexed and radially deviated. Fracture locations are the distal pole, waist, proximal pole, and tubercle. Another important factor is stability of the fracture. A scaphoid fracture is stable unless there is (1) displacement greater than 1 mm, (2) scapholunate angulation greater than 60 degrees, or (3) radiolunate angulation greater than 15 degrees. Associated injuries to look for include perilunate dislocation, lunate dislocation, trapezium fractures, triquetrum fractures, radial styloid fractures, distal radius fractures (Colle fractures), fractures of metacarpals 1 and 2, and capitate fractures. Patients present with a painful wrist and may report swelling or paresthesias of the affected hand. On examination, there is maximal tenderness in the anatomic snuff box, pain with radial deviation of the wrist, and pain with axial compression of the thumb.

Bone healing occurs at different rates depending on the location of the fracture. A tuberosity fracture usually heals in 4–6 weeks, and a scaphoid waist fracture in 10–12 weeks. A proximal pole fracture can require 16–20 weeks for healing.

B. Imaging Studies

Imaging studies include AP (hand in neutral position), AP (tube tilted 40 degrees distally), lateral (distal arm elevated 15 degrees), and oblique (hand in 10 degrees of supination and maximal ulnar deviation) radiographic views. Occasionally, right and left oblique views or a scaphoid view may be necessary. Further imaging with a magnetic resonance imaging (MRI) scan is appropriate when a fracture is clinically suspected but radiographs are negative and the patient needs to return to activity as early as possible.

Complications

Several complications are associated with a scaphoid fracture: delayed union (no healing, no trabeculae crossing the fracture line, at 3 months), avascular necrosis (radiographs show sclerosis and cyst development), compartment syndrome (rarely), and compression neuropathy (rarely). Of utmost concern is malunion or nonunion (absence of evidence of healing at 4–6 months). Malunion resulting in a humpback deformity can lead to carpal instability, loss of wrist extension, weakness of grip, carpal collapse, and degenerative changes in the wrist.

Treatment

Nondisplaced or minimally displaced (< 1 mm) scaphoid fractures are placed in a thumb spica cast. A short arm cast is used for tuberosity fractures and long arm casts for all other nondisplaced or minimally displaced scaphoid fractures. When casting, the wrist should be in a neutral flexion-extension, neutral to radial deviation with the thumb included. A long arm cast is used for 6 weeks and is then replaced with a short arm cast for another 6 weeks.

Follow-up should occur at 2 weeks with AP, lateral, and oblique radiographic views, checking for step-offs, angulation, and displacement. At this point no callus and possible fracture site resorption are seen. Later, at 4–6 weeks, there is no callus because there is no periosteal membrane. However, trabecular bone may be visible across the fracture line. At 8–12 weeks the fracture line begins to disappear. The normal trabecular bone pattern returns in 12–16 weeks. Rehabilitation takes 3–6 months. Union rates vary; for a nondisplaced fracture the rate is 100%. Angulated fracture union rates are 65% and displaced rates are 45%. The proximal one third fracture union rate range is 60–70% with immobilization.

Consultation is required for open reduction and internal fixation for displaced, delayed union, and nonunion scaphoid fractures. Referral is also appropriate for a patient initially presenting more than 3 weeks after the injury.

Web Sites

http://www.physsportsmed.com/issues/1996/06_96/gutierez.htm

METACARPAL FRACTURES

Clinical Findings

A. Symptoms and Signs

Metacarpal fractures are caused by direct trauma to the hand. These fractures can be stable or unstable. Stable fractures can be impacted or isolated fractures with little or no displacement. Unstable fractures are comminuted, displaced, oblique, or spiral, often multiple fractures. Patients present with tenderness and swelling.

Special fractures include the following:

- Bennett fracture (two-part intra-articular fracture of the base of the first metacarpal).
- Rolando fracture (three-part intra-articular fracture of the base of the first metacarpal).
- Reverse Rolando fracture (three-part intra-articular fracture of the base of the fifth metacarpal).
- Boxer fracture (fifth metacarpal neck fracture).

B. Imaging Studies

AP and lateral radiographs are needed and comparison views are sometimes helpful. However, it is recommended that initial radiographs of fractures of the fourth and fifth metacarpals be AP and oblique pronated views. Additional lateral radiographs are helpful only after confirmation of a proximal comminuted fracture or signs of a pronounced AP dislocation. A CT scan may be helpful for fractures of the metacarpal head and base.

Complications

Complications are many and include decreased grip strength, arthritis if the articular surface is involved, prolonged swelling, reflex sympathetic dystrophy, compartment syndrome, decreased MCP prominence with metacarpal shaft dorsal prominence, and decreased range of motion.

Treatment

Treatment depends on a variety of factors. Casting is appropriate in the following situations: no degree of rotational deformity; an intra-articular fracture, with no more than a 1- to 2-mm step-off; stable neck and shaft fractures; extra-articular metacarpal base fractures; comminuted metacarpal head fractures; and second, third, and fourth intra-articular metacarpal base fractures. Certain angular restrictions must be adhered to.

For shaft fractures:

- First digit—no more than 30 degrees of apex dorsal angulation.
- Second and third digits—no more than 10 degrees of apex dorsal angulation.
- Fourth and fifth digits—no more than 20 degrees of apex dorsal angulation.

For neck fractures:

- Second digit—no more than 10 degrees of apex dorsal angulation.

- Third digit—no more than 20 degrees of apex dorsal angulation.
- Fourth digit—no more than 30 degrees of apex dorsal angulation.
- Fifth digit—no more than 40 degrees of apex dorsal angulation.

If the metacarpal fracture meets the preceding conditions it may be casted or splinted. The affected digit is buddy taped. The wrist is casted in 30 degrees of extension. The MCP joints are flexed 60–90 degrees. The distal and proximal interphalangeal joints are placed in 5–10 degrees of flexion. The cast should be trimmed to allow visualization of the tip of the injured digit and the adjacent buddy-taped digit. This step facilitates checking capillary refill. Recheck for loss of correction after casting.

At 2 weeks postcasting, a radiograph should be checked for loss of correction. Bridging callus should be seen at 4–6 weeks. If there is tenderness, motion, or inadequate callus formation, the digit should be recasted and rechecked every 2 weeks. If there is no tenderness, no motion at the fracture site, and adequate callus formation is noted, a protective splint can be considered for an additional 1–2 weeks. If symptoms continue beyond 6 weeks, cast immobilization and reassessment at 2-week intervals should be continued until radiographic and clinical healing is achieved.

Unstable fractures of the metacarpal neck or shaft should be referred to an orthopedic surgeon. Most intra-articular fractures of the base of the first and fifth metacarpals also need referral. These fractures will likely be treated by closed reduction and percutaneous pinning. Open reduction and internal fixation are indicated for intra-articular fractures of the metacarpal base that cannot be maintained by closed reduction and for fractures of the metacarpal head with mild comminution.

RADIAL HEAD FRACTURES

Clinical Findings

A. Symptoms and Signs

Radial head fractures can be caused by a FOOSH while the arm is pronated or partially flexed. Another mechanism of injury is a valgus force on the elbow, forcing the humeral capitellum into the radial head. Patients present with elbow pain and swelling. Physical findings are tenderness over the radial head, pain that is increased with supination, reduced range of motion, and swelling secondary to a hemarthrosis. Swelling in the center of a triangle formed by the lateral epicondyle, olecranon, and radial head may occur. The patient should be evaluated for neurovascular compromise, checking capillary refill, sensation, and posterior interosseous nerve function. The medial collateral ligament should be evaluated for tenderness and opening with valgus stress.

B. Imaging Studies

AP and lateral views of the wrist should be obtained to rule out disruption of the distal radial ulnar joint. Imaging studies of the elbow include AP, lateral (Figure 37–2), and radiocapitellar (45 degrees from the lateral toward the radial head) views. Look for the radiocapitellar line and a fat pad sign. Follow-up radiographs at 2 weeks will not show a callous; however, at 4–6 weeks a bridging callous should be noted. Bone healing is visible between 6 and 8 weeks. Rehabilitation should begin as soon as the fracture is stable, to maintain functional range of motion. At 8–12 weeks there should be abundant bridging callous and a resolving fracture line. In the rare case of nonunion, the patient will report pain and examination will reveal tenderness.

Complications

Possible complications include reflex sympathetic dystrophy, compartment syndrome of the elbow and forearm, heterotropic ossification, increased carrying angle of the elbow, arthritis with restricted range of motion, deformity, valgus instability, decreased grip strength, posterior interosseous or median nerve injury, and brachial artery injury.

Classification (Mason)

Type I—Nondisplaced.

Type II—Marginal fractures with displacement, depression, or angulation.

Type III—Comminuted fractures of the entire head or completely displaced fractures of the radial head.

Type IV—Type I, II, or III with elbow dislocation.

Treatment

The primary care physician can treat type I (nondisplaced radial head) fractures. Treatment includes aspiration (to decrease the hematoma and capsular distention; injection of anesthetic may aid in evaluation), early range of motion, and a sling for 5–7 days. Bone healing typically occurs in 6–8 weeks. Range of motion rehabilitation should be started as soon as possible, when the fracture is stable.

Based on the Mason classification, type II fractures (displacement of 2–3 mm, greater than 25-degree involvement of the articular surface) require open reduction with internal fixation. Additionally, type III fractures (nonreparable comminuted) may require radial head excision. Patients with type IV fractures (posterior dislocation) should be referred.

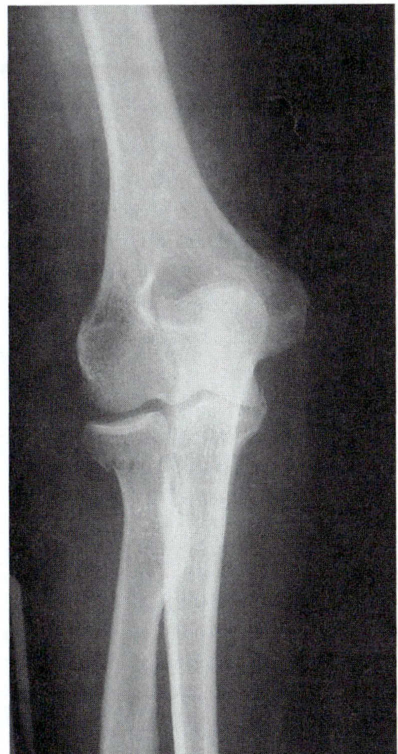
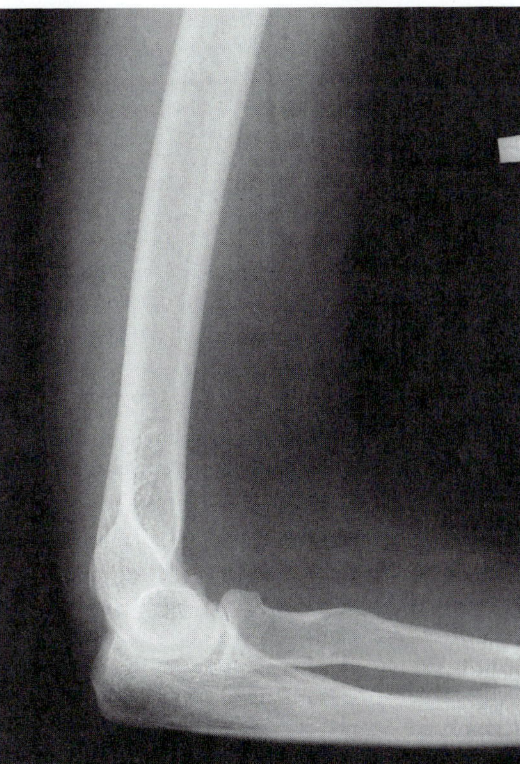

Figure 37–2. AP and lateral view of radial head fracture.

Web Sites

http://www.orthoseek.com/articles/fractman.html
http://www.physsportsmed.com/issues/1996/06_96/cordas.htm
http://www.worldortho.com/database/sgt/tr4a.pdf

LOWER EXTREMITY FRACTURES

STRESS FRACTURES

General Considerations

Management of traumatic fractures of the lower extremity long bones is relatively straightforward if a few simple rules are recognized. Orthopedic referral is required for any traumatic fracture that is displaced or involves a joint line. The physician who seeks to obtain competence in acute traumatic fracture management, requiring casting, should seek other references. The goal of this section is to guide the primary care physician through a basic understanding of concepts surrounding bone stress pathogenesis, including epidemiology, clinical signs and symptoms, physical examination, radiographic diagnostic aids, and treatment of four difficult-to-treat areas of stress reaction in the lower extremities. The population most at risk for stress reaction is athletes. This population presents therapeutic challenges secondary to their increased activity, predilection to overuse injury, and desire to return to competition as quickly as possible, which may lead them to compete before the stress injury fully resolves.

Stress fractures are estimated to make up 10% of all athletic injuries. Ninety-five percent of stress injuries occur in the lower extremities secondary to the extreme repetitive weight-bearing loads placed on these bones. The peak incidence occurs in people 18–25 years of age. However, with recent emphasis on exercise for the elderly, the diagnosis of stress fracture should not be neglected in this population. There is a decreased incidence of stress fracture in men secondary to greater lean body mass and overall bone structure. It has been estimated that women military recruits have a relative risk of stress fracture that is 1.2–10 times greater than men while engaging in the same level of training. In athletic populations a gender difference is not as evident, possibly because athletic women are more fit and better conditioned. Incidence is estimated to be comparable for all races.

Stress fracture is most common after changes in an athlete's training regimen. Injury is especially prevalent in unconditioned runners who increase their training regimen. Training error, which can include increased quantity or intensity of training, introduction of a new activity, poor equipment, and change in environment (ie, surface), is the most important risk factor for stress injury. Low bone density, dietary deficiency, abnormal body composition, menstrual irregularities, hormonal imbalance, sleep deprivation, and biomechanical abnormalities also place athletes at risk. Keeping this in mind and recognizing the increasing incidence of female athletic triad (amenorrhea, eating disorder, and osteoporosis), it is easy to understand why women can have an increased risk for stress injury.

Clinical Findings

A. Symptoms and Signs

Stress fractures are related to a maladaptive process between bone injury and bone remodeling. Bone reacts to stress by early osteoclastic activity (old bone resorption) followed by strengthening osteoblastic activity (new bone formation). With continued stress, bone resorption outpaces new bone formation and a self-perpetuating cycle occurs, with continued activity allowing weakened bone to be more susceptible to continued microfracture and ultimately progressing to frank fracture. The initiation of stress reaction is unclear. It has been postulated that excessive forces are transmitted to bone when surrounding muscles fatigue. The highly concentrated muscle forces act across localized area of bone, causing mechanical insults above the stress-bearing capacity of bone. These insults occur at the insertion of tendons and lead to insults in the bone that may propagate into a stress fracture.

Athletic stress fracture follows a crescendo process. Symptoms start insidiously with dull, gnawing pain at the end of physical activity. Pain increases over days to the point where the activity cannot be continued. At first pain decreases with rest, then shorter and shorter duration of activity causes pain. More time is then needed for pain to dissipate until it is present with minimal activity and at night. After a few days of rest, pain resolves, only to return once again with resumption of activity. More specific historical and physical examination findings are discussed below in conjunction with specific anatomic regions.

B. Imaging Studies

The diagnosis of stress fracture is primarily clinical and is based on history and physical examination. It is prudent to start with plain radiographs, which have poor sensitivity but high specificity, as the initial study. The presence of stress reaction is confirmed by the presence of periosteal reaction, intramedullary sclerosis, callus, or obvious fracture line. Plain films typically fail to reveal a bony abnormality unless symptoms have been present for at least 2–3 weeks.

The technetium triple-phase bone scan is often employed to improve diagnostic power. Stress reactions can often be visualized within 48–72 hours from symptom onset. Triple-phase bone scan can differentiate soft tissue and bone injury. The first phase flow image, taken immediately after intravenous injection of tracer, shows perfusion in bone and soft tissue. The second phase (static blood pool phase), taken 1 minute after injection, reflects the degree of hyperemia and capillary permeability of bone and soft tissue showing acute inflammation. In the third phase (delayed image), taken 3–4 hours after injection of tracer, approximately 50% of the tracer has concentrated in the bone matrix. All three phases can be positive in an acute fracture. In soft tissue injuries, with no bony involvement, the first two phases are often positive, whereas the delayed image shows minimal or no increased uptake. In conditions such as medial tibial stress syndrome (MTSS), in which there is early bony stress reaction, the first two phases are negative and the delayed image is positive. Bone scan does not visualize the fracture and is not used to monitor healing secondary to delayed images showing uptake 12 months after initial studies.

CT scans can identify conditions that mimic stress fracture on bone scan, confirm fracture suspected on bone scan, or help to make treatment decisions as with navicular stress fractures.

MRI offers the advantage of visualizing soft tissue changes in anatomic regions in which the soft tissue structures often cloud the differential diagnosis. Bone stress is identified as marrow edema, whereas frank stress fracture can be visualized as a line at the cortex surrounded by an intense zone of edema in the medullary cavity. Clinically the high sensitivity of bone scan and MRI is necessary only when the diagnosis of stress fracture is in question or the exact location or extent of injury must be known in order to determine treatment.

Brukner P et al: Managing common stress fractures: Let risk level guide treatment. Physician Sportsmed 1998;26:39.

Knapp TP, Garrett WE: Stress fractures: General concepts. Clin Sports Med 1997;16:339. [PMID: 9238314]

Perron AD et al: Management of common stress fractures: When to apply conservative therapy, when to take an aggressive approach. Postgrad Med 2002;111:95. [PMID: 11868316]

1. Femoral Stress Fractures

General Considerations

Stress fractures involving the femur can occur in a variety of locations, most commonly the femoral shaft and neck. One study that looked at 320 athletes with bone scan–positive stress fractures revealed the femur to be the fourth most frequent site of injury.

Differential Diagnosis

The symptom most commonly encountered with stress fractures of the femur is pain at the anterior aspect of the hip. Differentiating the diagnosis can be difficult secondary to the multiple number of structures in the hip that have the potential to produce similar pain syndromes and the deep nonpalpable structures of the anatomic region. The differential diagnosis is broad but must include consideration of disease processes such as apophyseal and epiphyseal injury in adolescents, arthritis in adults, along with inflammatory arthritides, muscle strains, tendinitis, stress fractures, sports hernia with nerve entrapment, osteitis pubis, and acetabular labral tears across all age groups. Diagnosis can be made complex by the multitude of structures in this region from which pain may emanate; thus, the physician must be attuned to the history to narrow the differential down to a list in which stress fracture is prominent. This is important in order to avoid severe complications associated with fractures of the femoral neck.

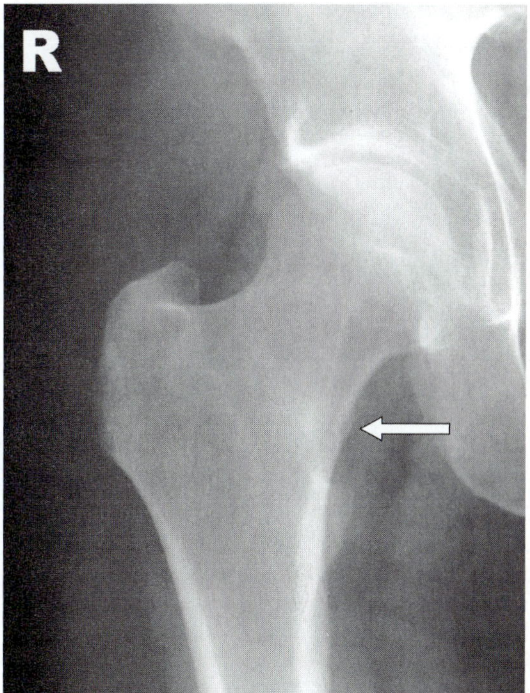

Figure 37–3. Compression-sided stress fracture of the right femoral neck indicated by the white arrow at the site of periosteal reaction.

Femoral Shaft Fractures

Femoral shaft stress fractures are more common than expected, with an incidence in athletes of 3.7%. Onset of pain can be gradual over a period of days to weeks. Average time from symptom onset to diagnosis is approximately 2 weeks. The fulcrum test is well suited to act as a guide for ordering radiologic tests and thereby decreasing time to diagnosis. It is also a useful clinical test to assess healing. For this test, the athlete is seated on the examination table with legs dangling as the examiner's arm is used as a fulcrum under the thigh. The examiner's arm is moved from the distal to proximal thigh as gentle pressure is applied to the dorsum of the knee with the opposite hand. A positive test is elicited by sharp pain or apprehension at the site of the fracture. Plain films usually are not sensitive in detecting stress fractures within the first 2–3 weeks of symptoms. Bone scan or MRI may be useful in this time period to aid in diagnosis. The most common site of injury in athletes is the midmedial or posteromedial cortex of the proximal femur.

Once diagnosis is confirmed, treatment depends on the underlying causes responsible for the injury. If the fracture is consistent with a compression-sided fracture, treatment consists of rest with gradual resumption of activity (Figures 37–3 and 37–4). This usually is adequate for healing of nondisplaced fractures. Treatment protocols are based on empiric data gathered from clinical observation. An example of a treatment protocol may consist of rest for a period of 1–4 weeks of toe-touch weight bearing progressing to full weight bearing. This would be followed by a phase of low-impact activity (ie, biking, swimming). Once patients are able to perform low-impact activity for a prolonged time without pain, they may gradually advance to high impact. Resumption of full activity averages between 8 and 16 weeks. Surgical treatment should be considered if there is displacement of the fracture, delayed union, or nonunion following conservative therapy.

Femoral Neck Fractures

Stress fractures of the femoral neck are uncommon but carry a high complication rate if the diagnosis is missed or the fracture is improperly treated. The primary presenting symptom is pain at the site of the groin, anterior thigh, or knee. Pain is exacerbated by weight bearing or physical activity. The athlete may have an antalgic gait or painful, limited hip range of motion in internal rotation or external rotation. MRI is the diagnostic modality of choice for evaluating femoral neck stress fractures.

Stress fractures of the femoral neck are divided into two categories: compression and tension type. Compression fractures are more common in younger patients. The frac-

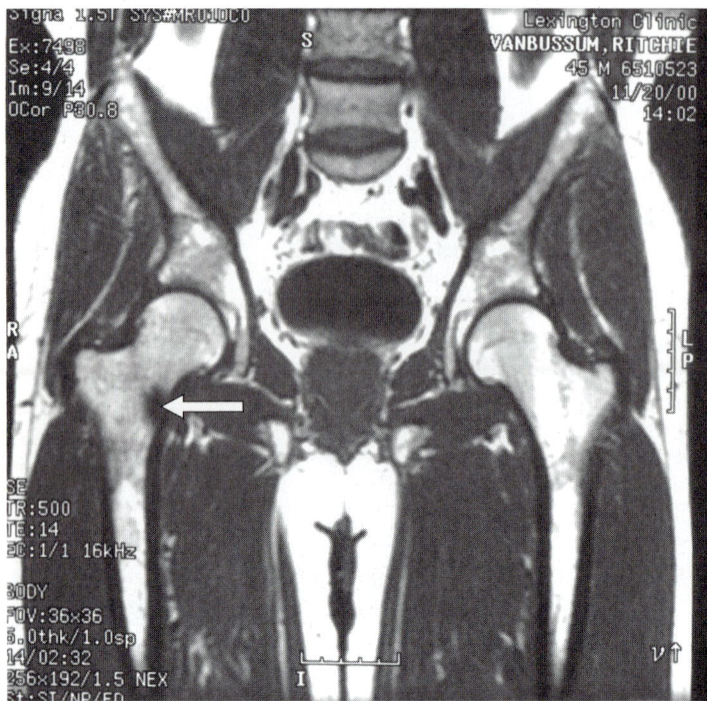

Figure 37–4. Compression-sided stress fracture of the right femoral neck as indicated on MRI by the white arrow.

ture line, if seen on the radiograph, can propagate across the femoral neck. A nondisplaced, incomplete compression fracture is treated with rest until the patient is pain free with full motion. Non–weight-bearing ambulation with the patient on crutches follows until radiographic healing as shown on plain films is complete. Frequent radiographs may need to be obtained to monitor propagation of the fracture. If the compression fracture becomes complete, or fails to heal with rest, then internal fixation may be necessary (Figure 37–5). Patients treated nonsurgically may not achieve full activity for several months. Tension (distraction)-sided femoral neck fractures are an emergency because of the potential for complications (ie, nonunion or avascular necrosis). The patient is immediately made non–weight-bearing and will acutely need internal fixation. If the fracture is displaced the patient will need open reduction and internal fixation urgently.

Boden BP, Speer KP: Femoral stress fractures. Clin Sports Med 1997;16:307. [PMID: 9238312]

O'Kane JW: Anterior hip pain. Am Fam Physician 1999;60:1687. [PMID: 10537384]

2. Tibial Stress Fractures

General Considerations

Tibial stress fractures account for half of all stress fractures diagnosed. Most tibial stress fractures in athletes are secondary to running. An average of 3–6 weeks of overtraining has been shown to be associated with increased incidence of tibial stress fractures.

Two sites located within the tibia are most commonly associated with stress fractures. The first of these is located between the middle and distal third of the tibia along the posteromedial border. This type of injury is most often associated with running. The second site is along the middle third of the anterior cortex. This injury is most commonly associated with activities involving a great deal of jumping (ie, dancing, basketball, gymnastics).

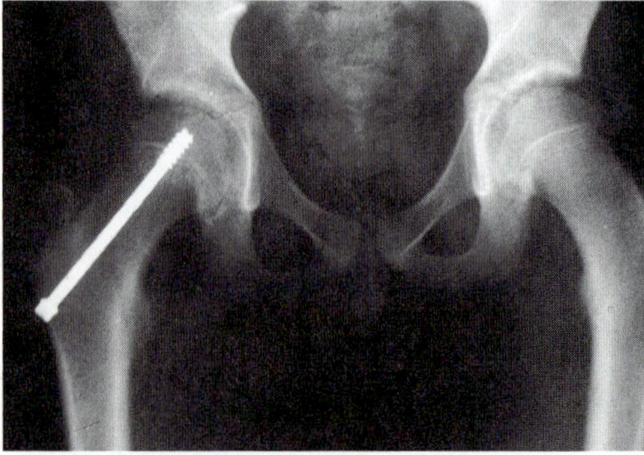

Figure 37–5. Intramedullary screw fixation of a femoral neck stress fracture.

Clinical Findings

A. Symptoms and Signs

On history the patient commonly describes pain occurring in the region of the fracture with activity (ie, running or jumping) and resolving with rest. The pain eventually progresses and lasts longer after the activity until the patient is symptomatic at rest. Physical examination often reveals localized pain to palpation. Sometimes persistent thickening, secondary to periosteal reaction, can be appreciated by palpation along the tibia.

B. Imaging Studies

Diagnosis by radiographic plain film may be possible if symptoms have been present for at least 4–6 weeks. Triple-phase bone scan is very sensitive and may allow diagnosis within 48–72 hours of symptom onset. Tibial stress fractures can be seen clearly on MRI with sensitivity comparable to triple-phase bone scan. Both bone scan and MRI allow differentiation of medial tibial stress syndrome and stress fracture.

Differential Diagnosis

Medial tibial stress syndrome (MTSS) is the most commonly confused diagnosis in the classification of tibial stress injuries with stress fracture. MTSS usually occurs diffusely along the middle and distal third of the posteromedial tibia and is commonly seen in runners. This condition, however, can also be seen with activities involving persistent jumping. The symptom spectrum commonly progresses, as does that of stress fractures, with continued activity. MTSS represents a stress reaction within bone whereby the usual remodeling process becomes maladaptive. This injury responds well to rest in a shorter time period as compared with stress fracture and is easily differentiated from stress fracture on triple-phase bone scan. If symptoms do not resolve or are consistent with distal numbness or in a region of nerve traversing one of the four involved compartments of the lower leg, the diagnosis of chronic compartment syndrome must be considered.

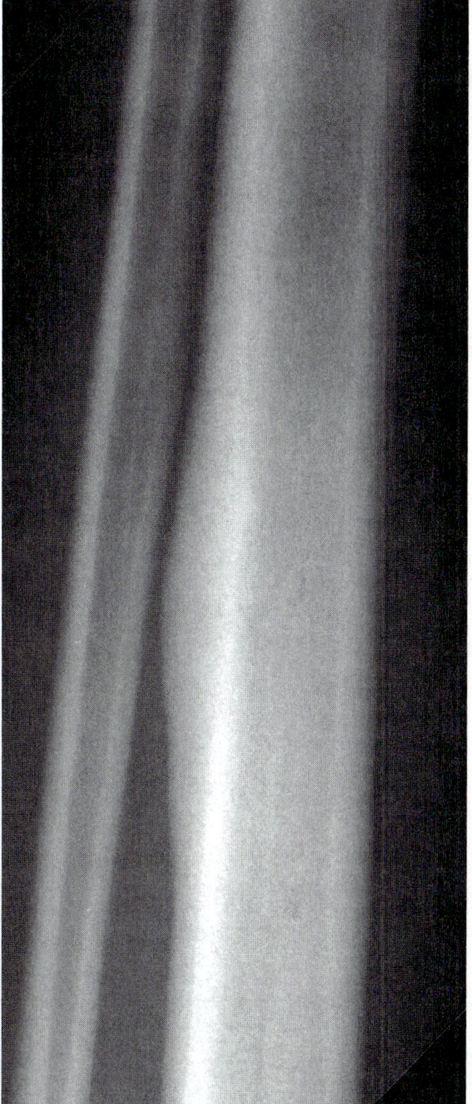

Figure 37–6. Periosteal stress reaction at the posterior medial aspect of the tibia.

Treatment

Once the diagnosis of tibial stress fracture has been made, a distinction between a compression versus tension-sided injury must be made. Fractures along the posteromedial border are considered compression stress injuries and respond well to conservative therapy (Figure 37–6). The average recovery time for this injury is approximately 12 weeks when the patient is treated with rest alone. Most guidelines for treatment of this injury involve relative or absolute rest. These stress fractures can be effectively treated in a pneumatic leg brace. Athletes treated in the pneumatic brace (long leg air cast) showed decreased time to pain-free symptoms (14 ± 6 days) and time to competitive participation (21 ± 2 days) versus traditional mode non-weight-bearing treatment (77 ± 7 days). Athletes in the brace may continue exercising, but modifications of the training routine must be made to maintain pain-free activities. Patients are progressed based on a functional activity progression as outlined by Swenson and colleagues.

Tibial stress fractures of the midanterior cortex, also known as "the dreaded black line," radiographically (Figure 37–7), are very difficult to manage conservatively. This fracture occurs at the tension side of the tibial cor-

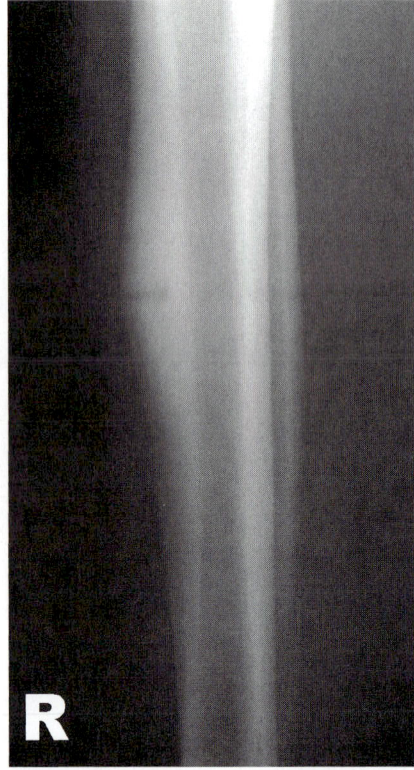

Figure 37–7. Dreaded black line at the anterior medial aspect of the tibia.

tex, most commonly in athletes who jump. Two significant complications—delayed union and complete fracture—plague this fracture site, and average time to symptom-free return to activity from symptom onset is more than 12 months with conservative care. Conservative treatment revolves around rest, or immobilization, or both. Patients who do not respond to conservative treatment or are involved in activities (career or competitive athletics) are individuals in whom surgical treatment with tibial intramedullary nailing would be beneficial (Figure 37–8). Patients with these fractures, secondary to the prolonged treatment and risk of complication, should be referred to a sports medicine specialist.

Beck BR: Tibial stress injuries: An aetiological review for the purpose of guiding management. Sports Med 1998;26:265. [PMID: 9820925]

Couture CJ, Karlson KA: Tibial stress injuries: Decisive diagnosis and treatment of "shin splints." Physician Sportsmed 2002; 30:29.

Perron AD et al: Management of common stress fractures: When to apply conservative therapy, when to take an aggressive approach. Postgrad Med 2002;111:95. [PMID: 11868316]

Rettig AC et al: The natural history and treatment of delayed union stress fractures of the anterior cortex of the tibia. Am J Sports Med 1988;16:250. [PMID: 3381982]

Swenson EJ et al: The effect of a pneumatic leg brace on return to play in athletes with tibial stress fractures. Am J Sports Med 1997;25:322. [PMID: 9167811]

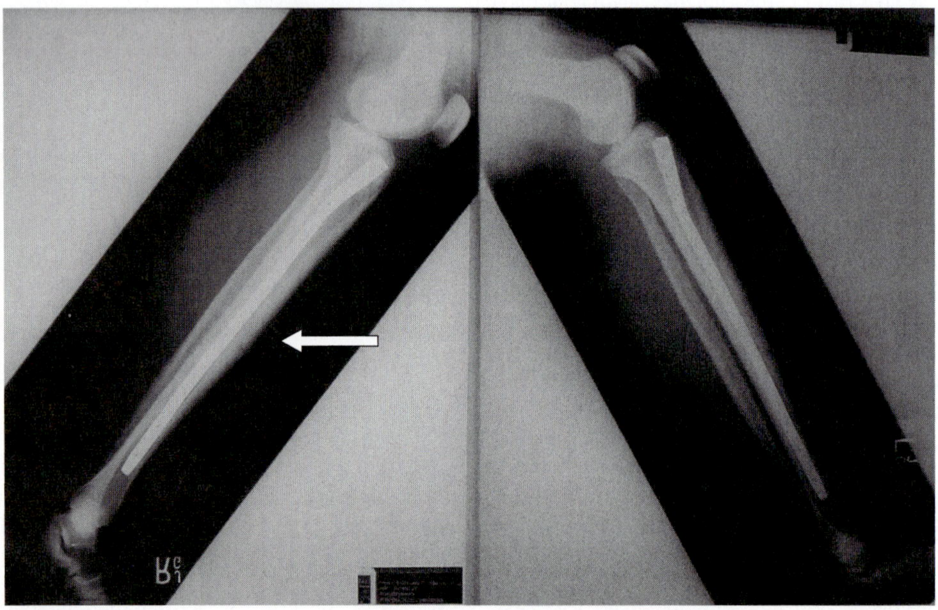

Figure 37–8. Intramedullary screw (white arrow) fixation of bilateral anterior medial tibial stress fractures.

3. *Tarsal Navicular Stress Fractures*

General Considerations

Tarsal navicular stress fractures are an underdiagnosed source of prolonged, disabling foot pain predominantly seen in active athletes involved in sprinting and jumping. One study, involving 111 competitive track and field athletes, found that navicular stress fractures are the second most common lower extremity stress fracture.

Clinical Findings

A. Symptoms and Signs

These fractures are prone to misdiagnosis secondary to the vague nature of pain. The pain may radiate along the medial arch and not directly over the talonavicular joint. Sometimes pain radiates distally, causing the physician to suspect a Morton neuroma or metatarsalgia. The pain often disappears with a few days of rest, often tricking the athlete into not believing the potential seriousness of the diffuse foot pain. The diagnosis is also clouded because the fractures are rarely seen on plain film.

B. Imaging Studies

A retrospective multicenter study by Khan and colleagues looking at 86 fractures of the tarsal navicular bone, all with CT confirmation of clinical diagnosis, reported a range in time of diagnosis from symptom onset to be 3–60 months (average 4 months). Symptoms suggesting a clinical diagnosis consisted of (1) insidious onset of vague pain over the dorsum of the medial midfoot or over the medial aspect of the longitudinal arch, (2) ill-defined pain, soreness, or cramping aggravated by activity and relieved by rest, (3) well-localized tenderness to palpation over the navicular bone or medial arch, and (4) little swelling or discoloration. Certain foot abnormalities, including short first metatarsal and metatarsus adductor and limited dorsiflexion of the ankle, may concentrate stress on the tarsal navicular region, predisposing to stress reaction.

Treatment

The retrospective study by Khan and colleagues confirmed that the best treatment modality is 6–8 weeks of non–weight-bearing cast immobilization. This study also offered guidelines for treatment, the CT appearance of the fracture after conservative treatment, and parameters used to follow fracture healing. When seriously considering diagnosis of tarsal navicular stress fractures, plain film radiographs should be obtained in an AP, lateral, and oblique standing position (Figure 37–9). If the radiograph is normal, a bone scan should be obtained. If the bone scan is positive and the radiograph is negative, a CT scan to confirm stress fracture as opposed to stress reaction should be obtained. The CT slices must be no wider than 1.5 mm apart and must include the dorsal proximal cortical surface. Most fractures are located in the sagittal plane and in the central third of bone along the proximal articular surface corresponding to angiographic studies indicating this to be a relatively avascular region (Figure 37–10).

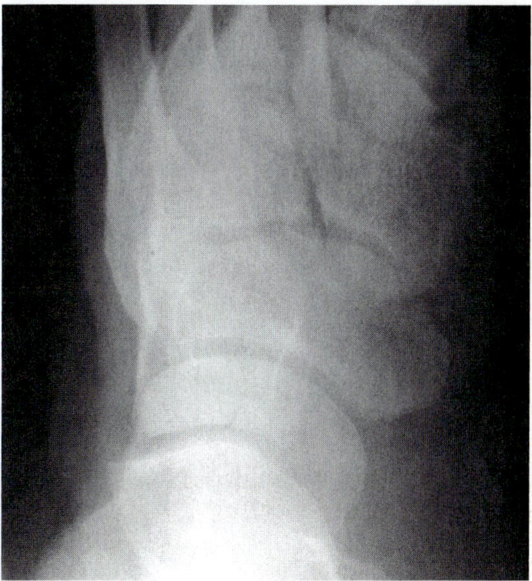

Figure 37–9. **Radiograph revealing stress fracture of the tarsal navicular.** (Courtesy of Kentucky Sports Medicine, Dr. Mary Lloyd Ireland.)

Data indicate that 6–8 weeks of non–weight-bearing cast immobilization compares favorably with surgical treatment for failed weight-bearing treatment. Surgery is recommended for a displaced, complete fracture with a small transverse fragment (ossicle), or failure of conservative management. Conservative management, however, may be warranted initially for patients with these fractures. Surgical treatment often consists of either bone graft or screw fixation (Figure 37–11) followed by non–weight-bearing cast immobilization for 6 weeks.

After 6 weeks of non–weight-bearing cast immobilization, fracture healing is followed clinically by palpation of the fracture site along the dorsal proximal region of the navicular bone. Persistent tenderness over this "N" spot requires an additional 2 weeks of non–weight-bearing immobilization before reassessment. If the fracture site is not tender after casting, the patient may begin weight bearing. Plain films do not provide a reliable indication of fracture healing secondary to low sensitivity. Bone scan often remains positive long after clinical union. A CT scan up to 3–6 months following

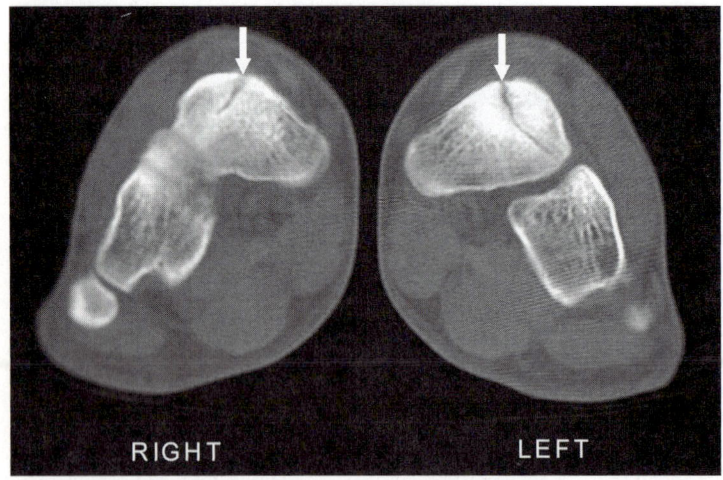

Figure 37–10. CT scan of bilateral tarsal navicular stress fractures (white arrows). (Courtesy of Kentucky Sports Medicine, Dr. Mary Lloyd Ireland.)

therapy, although asymptomatic, can show blurring of the fracture line and cortical bridging. The CT scan may not show complete obliteration on 3-month repeat films. For this reason the recommendation is not to repeat the CT scan but instead to rely on clinical examination (palpation of the "N" spot).

Of note is the topic of "bone strain." During this phenomenon the bone scan may be positive but the patient is asymptomatic. This can be seen when the bone scan is ordered to assess MTSS and activity is picked up in the navicular bone. The CT scan remains normal. Persistent training results in progression to stress fracture. Treatment of bone strain does not require cast immobilization. This condition can be managed successfully with 6 weeks of strict limitation of activity with weight bearing.

Khan KM et al: Outcome of conservative and surgical management of navicular stress fracture in athletes: Eighty-six cases proven with computerized tomography. Am J Sports Med 1992;20:657. [PMID: 1456359]

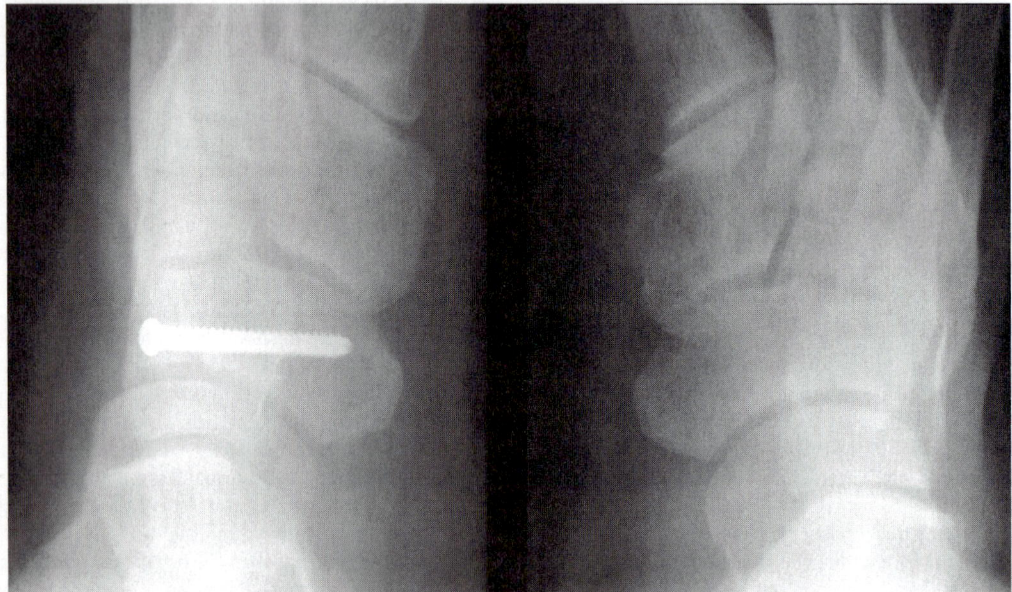

Figure 37–11. Radiograph of screw fixation of a tarsal navicular stress fracture. (Courtesy of Kentucky Sports Medicine, Dr. Mary Lloyd Ireland.)

4. Metatarsal Stress Fractures

General Considerations

Metatarsal stress fractures in athletes are very common. Depending on the study referenced they are either third or fourth in incidence. These fractures are also known as "March fractures" because of the large numbers of military recruits who obtained these fractures after sudden increases in their level of activity. The second metatarsal is the most common location followed by the third and fourth metatarsals. The second metatarsal is subjected to three to four times body weight during loading and push-off phases of gait.

Clinical Findings

A. Symptoms and Signs

Clinical suspicion for this injury is raised when the athlete complains of forefoot or midfoot pain of insidious onset. On examination these injuries present as areas of point tenderness overlying the metatarsal shaft.

B. Imaging Studies

Radiographs are usually sufficient to document stress fracture, which is visualized as a frank fracture or periosteal reaction at the affected site. As with most stress fractures the patient may be symptomatic 2–4 weeks prior to visualizing the fracture on radiograph. If the diagnosis is in question, bone scan and MRI have significantly higher sensitivity and specificity for detecting these injuries at an earlier time frame.

Treatment

Treatment is easily managed by the primary care physician. The injury is treated symptomatically, allowing the athlete to participate in activities that are not painful. Immobilization in the form of a steel shank insole or stiff, wooden-soled type shoe may be necessary for a limited time, until no longer painful. At times the patient may benefit from a short leg walking cast or removable walking boot for severe pain. Four weeks of rest is usually sufficient for healing. During these 4 weeks, the athlete may continue modified conditioning with non–weight-bearing exercises (ie, swimming and pool running), followed by cycling and stair climbing.

Although most of these fractures heal well with conservative management, fractures of the proximal fifth metatarsal have a high incidence of delayed union and nonunion. A thorough understanding of the classification and anatomy of fractures in this location is required for proper identification to determine conservative versus surgical treatment.

FRACTURES OF THE PROXIMAL FIFTH METATARSAL

Fractures of the proximal fifth metatarsal include tuberosity avulsion fractures, acute Jones fractures, and diaphyseal stress fractures. Diaphyseal stress fractures in this area can further be classified as early, delayed union, and nonunion fractures.

The fifth metatarsal consists of a base tuberosity, shaft (diaphysis), neck, and head. The tuberosity protrudes plantarward from the base. The metaphysis tapers to the diaphysis. There are three articulations, including the cuboid fourth metatarsal, cuboid fifth metatarsal, and the fourth and fifth intermetatarsal articulation in this region. The proximal fifth metatarsal serves as the insertion of the lateral band of the plantar fascia, peroneus brevis tendon, and peroneus tertius tendon (Figure 37–12).

Tuberosity Fractures

Tuberosity fractures are typically known as dancer fractures because they are usually associated with an ankle

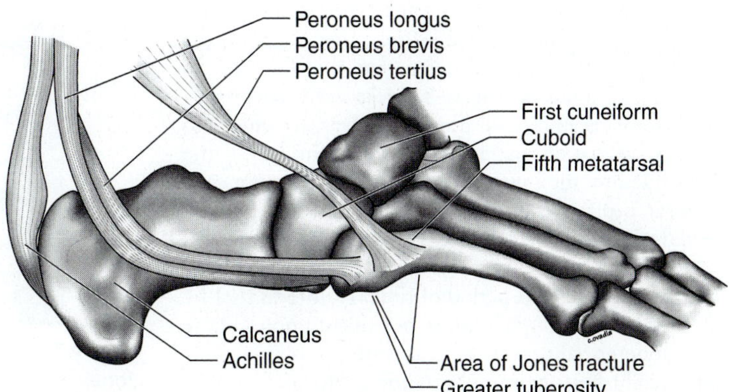

Figure 37–12. Anatomy of the proximal fifth metatarsal. (Courtesy of Ellsworth C. Seeley, MD.)

inversion plantar flexion injury. It was commonly thought that these injuries were associated with tearing of the peroneus brevis tendon insertion. However, this injury is more likely secondary to the plantar aponeurosis pulling from the base of the fifth metatarsal. Nondisplaced fracture carries an excellent prognosis, almost always healing in 4–6 weeks with conservative therapy. The athlete's treatment consists of limited weight bearing to pain with modified activity such as that used with second, third, and fourth metatarsal injuries. If needed the athlete can be immobilized in a walking cast, wooden (or steel shank)–soled shoe, or walking boot. The immobilization can usually be removed by 3 weeks (average 3–6 weeks) in favor of modified footwear if pain has diminished. The patient then gradually may return to vigorous activity, with most athletes returning to full sports activity in 6–8 weeks. Bony union usually takes place by 8 weeks. Orthopedic referral is needed for displaced fractures or comminuted fractures involving more than 30% of the cubometatarsal articular surface or step-off greater than 2 mm. Sometimes small displaced fractures at this site may require surgical removal if bony union does not occur secondary to chronic irritation. As a side note, the physician should be aware that certain conditions, such as apophysis of the tuberosity and accessory ossicles (os peroneum and os vesatranium), may radiographically mimic an avulsion fracture. Usually, these entities have smooth radiolucent lines on radiograph as compared with that of a fracture.

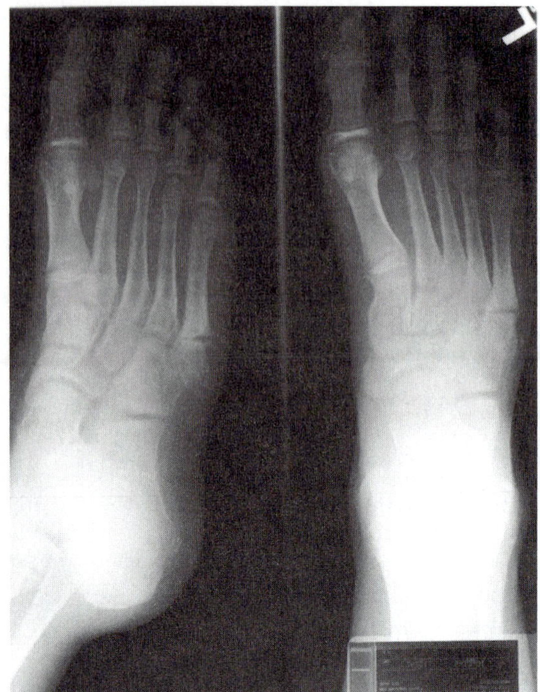

Figure 37–13. The Jones fracture.

Jones Fractures

Jones fractures consist of a transverse fracture at the junction of the diaphysis and metaphysis corresponding to the area between the insertion of the peroneus brevis and tertius tendons without extending past the fourth and fifth intermetatarsal articulation (Figure 37–13).

The Jones fracture is believed to occur when the ankle is in plantar flexion and a large adduction force is applied to the forefoot. It is important to realize this is a midfoot injury with no prodromal symptoms. Therefore, the injury is classified as acute.

Torg and colleagues showed that this fracture, in nonathletes, could heal in 6–8 weeks with strict non–weight-bearing immobilization. However, secondary to low vascularization and high stresses at the site of the Jones fracture, the injury is associated with a poor outcome; it is plagued by delayed union and nonunion if treated conservatively in athletic patients. Many athletes are unwilling to tolerate non–weight-bearing ambulation for this extended period of time. Failure to heal by 12 weeks in this population is not uncommon. Those who undergo conservative treatment are placed on a non–weight-bearing immobilization protocol, in a plaster cast, for 6–8 weeks. If there is lack of clinical healing by 6–8 weeks, therapy is individualized. If clinical healing is present by 6–8 weeks, immobilization is continued in a fracture brace with range of motion and gradual weight bearing. If there are no signs of clinical healing, treatment must be individualized either with continued cast immobilization or surgical intervention. Surgical intervention for Jones fracture consists of either intramedullary screw fixation (first choice; Figure 37–14) or bone grafting.

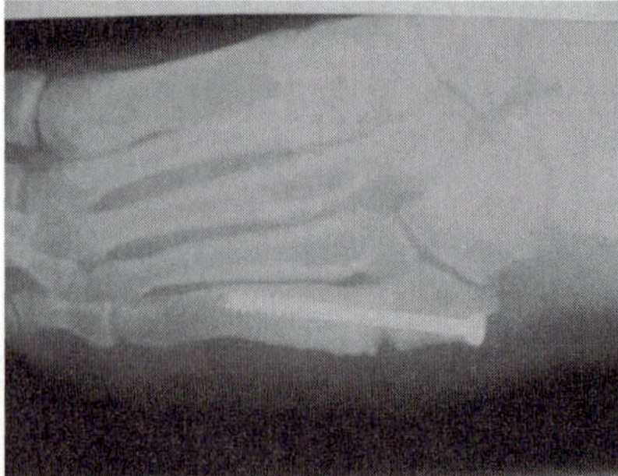

Figure 37–14. Intramedullary screw fixation for the Jones fracture. (Courtesy of Kentucky Sports Medicine, Dr. Mary Lloyd Ireland.)

Diaphyseal Fractures

Stress fractures distal to the site of Jones fractures and acute-on-chronic fractures occurring in the same position as Jones fractures are commonly seen in athletes who run. Pain is usually over the lateral aspect of the foot, over the fifth metatarsal base. Usually no significant trauma has been associated with these fractures. Prodromal symptoms occurring weeks to months in advance of an acute injury can often be elicited in the history.

Torg and colleagues classified these stress fractures into three types based on radiographic appearance. By adhering to this classification, much of the guesswork for determining treatment can be avoided. Type I can show minimal periosteal reaction, indicating early stress reaction with no intramedullary sclerosis. Type II shows features of delayed union represented by a fracture line involving both cortices with associated periosteal bone union, a widened fracture line with adjacent radiolucency related to bone reabsorption, and, most importantly, evidence of intramedullary sclerosis. Type III represents nonunion fractures revealing a widened fracture line, new periosteal bone and radiolucency, and complete obliteration of the medullary canal by sclerotic bone. Acute or chronic injuries show a fracture line at the same site as a Jones fracture but also evidence of stress injury, as previously described. Careful history reveals the patient had a prodrome of symptoms consisting of intermittent pain.

Treatment of choice for acute nondisplaced diaphyseal stress fracture is non–weight-bearing immobilization. Ninety-three percent of the patients in Torg's series healed within 7 weeks. Treatment for type II stress fractures is individualized. Conservative treatment may take up to 20 weeks and result in nonunion. Complications of prolonged immobilization include recurrence of fracture and significant dysfunction from muscle atrophy and loss of range of motion. For athletes, surgical options are recommended. Symptomatic nonunion fracture or type III fractures require surgical treatment. Casting and prolonged immobilization of acute or chronic fractures frequently fail, giving rise to delayed or nonunion fractures. Surgery is often needed and is the recommended procedure of choice.

The difference between screw fixation and bone grafting is recovery time. It takes up to 12 weeks to return to prefracture activity with grafting versus 6–8 weeks with screw fixation. Grafting carries a higher failure rate. Screw fixation is now recommended first and bone grafting if fixation fails.

Nunley JA: Fractures of the base of the fifth metatarsal: The Jones fracture. Orthoped Clin North Am 2001;32:171. [PMID: 11465126]

Strayer SM et al: Fractures of the proximal fifth metatarsal. Am Fam Physician 1999;59:2516. [PMID: 2891450]

Torg JS et al: Overuse injuries in sport: The foot. Clin Sports Med 1987;6:298. [PMID: 2891450]

Yu WD, Shapiro MS: Fractures of the fifth metatarsal. Physician Sportsmed 1998;26:47.

SECTION IV
Geriatrics

Healthy Aging & Assessing Older Adults

38

Cynthia M. Williams, DO, MA, FAACP

The population of the United States, like that of other industrialized nations, is aging. In 1900 4% of the US population was 65 years of age or older; that segment is now more than 13% and it is projected to be over 20% by 2030. These changing demographics also reveal that the "oldest old"—persons aged 85 years and older—are the most rapidly growing group within the population.

The aging population is heterogeneous. Researchers group this population by ages, with 65–74–year-olds considered "young-old," 75–84-year-olds considered "old," and those 85 years and older, "old-old." Those with the poorest health are identified as "frail" or "at-risk" elders. These divisions, however, are arbitrary and do not take into account functional abilities, comorbidities, or the presence of other infirmities.

In the rapidly changing fields of health care financing and delivery, services that promote or improve functional abilities, prevent or delay disease progression, and improve the overall health status of this aging population are needed. Little information and evidence are available about what constitutes the best practices in health promotion, prevention, and counseling for older adults. This chapter defines successful and healthy aging, provides recommendations for prevention and health promotion, and describes how to assess for at-risk elders.

Federal Interagency Forum on Aging-Related Statistics: *Older Americans 2004: Key Indicator of Well-being. Federal Interagency Forum on Aging-Related Statistics.* Government Printing Office, 2004. Available at: https:\\www.agingstats.gov.

CHARACTERISTICS OF HEALTHY AGING

In a highly heterogeneous population, some individuals are ravaged early by a multitude of chronic conditions and disabilities, whereas others appear to have excellent health and a high level of functioning. Aging is a process, and the term *healthy aging* does not imply an absence of limitations, but rather an adaptation to the changes associated with the aging process that is acceptable to the individual. Successful or healthy aging appears to include three factors: (1) low probability of disease and disability, (2) higher cognitive and physical functioning, and (3) an active engagement with life. This active engagement (interpersonal relations and productive activity) appears to represent the concept of successful aging most fully. Embedded in the construct of healthy aging is active engagement in living or "going and doing something meaningful" (Table 38–1). Older adults actively engaged in life who are involved in such endeavors as volunteer activities enjoy a better quality of life. Health care providers can promote healthy aging by assisting the older adult in developing competence in directing and managing future roles, thereby maintaining autonomy and a sense of self-worth.

Bryant LL et al: In their own words: A model of healthy aging. Soc Sci Med 2001; 53:927. [PMID: 11522138]

Kyle L: A concept analysis of healthy aging. Nurs Forum 2005; 40:45.

EPIDEMIOLOGY OF AGING

Most older adults are healthy and independent, and contribute to the society in which they live. The epidemiol-

Table 38–1. Factors associated with healthy aging.

"Going and doing" is worthwhile and desirable to the individual
Social activities
Reading
Travel
Housework
Fishing
Creative outlets: music, arts, dance, needlework
Sufficient abilities to accomplish valued activities
Mobility
Vision
Cognitive functioning
Coping
Independence
Having appropriate resources to support the activity
Valued relationships: friends and family
Health care and health information
Optimistic attitude
Self-esteem, self-efficacy, self-confidence

Source: Bryant LL et al: In their own words: A model of healthy aging. Soc Sci Med 2001;53:927.

ogy of aging evaluates not only the demographic changes associated with aging but also those diseases causing excess morbidity and mortality as well as the conditions that cause disability and decline in independent function. Many epidemiologic studies on aging focus on prevention in an attempt to establish a scientific basis for minimizing the illnesses associated with aging and their related burden. Health status in the elderly is a function of the chronic diseases associated with aging as well as the "geriatric syndromes" most commonly associated with this population (Table 38–2).

Table 38–2. Most common conditions associated with aging.

Arthritis
Hypertension
Heart disease
Hearing loss
Influenza
Injuries
Orthopedic impairments
Cataracts
Chronic sinusitis
Depression
Cancer
Diabetes mellitus
Visual impairments
Urinary incontinence
Varicose veins

The overall health status and well-being of older adults is highly complex and results from many interacting processes, including risk factor exposure (tobacco, alcohol, drugs, diet, sedentary life-style), underlying biological age-related changes, progressive development of impairments, the consequences of these impairments, the risk that changes in health and function confer, and the interactions of underlying health status with acute clinical conditions. Many of the conditions previously thought of as "normal aging" are now known to be modifiable or even preventable if disease prevention and health promotion strategies are taken seriously not only by health care providers but also by the patients for whom they care.

Fried LP: Epidemiology of aging. Epidemiol Rev 2000;22:95. [PMID: 10939013]

PREVENTION & HEALTH PROMOTION

Prevention in geriatrics attempts to delay morbidity and disability until the last years of life and is a primary goal of any medical practice caring for older individuals. The primary strategy for prevention lies in the alteration of life-style and environmental factors that contribute to the development of chronic disease. In attempting to delay or prevent the onset of chronic, disabling disease, a strategy to promote health must become part of the provider-patient contract.

Health promotion does not necessarily equate with disease prevention. *Health promotion* is a broad term that encompasses the objective of improving or enhancing the individual's current health status. The purpose of health promotion, especially as applied to the elderly, is the prevention of avoidable decline, frailty, and dependence, thereby promoting healthy aging

Frailty as a concept is beyond the scope of this chapter, but it is important to understand that the purpose of health promotion is to delay or prevent eventual frailty. Frailty is a multifaceted condition. It is the midway point between independence and near-death in which the older adult becomes more vulnerable and is at greatest risk for adverse health outcomes. The trajectory of frailty is one in which an older adult goes from independence, to coping and needing assistance, to "the dwindles" and functional decline. This progression leads to "frailty," with its attendant failure to thrive, disability, failure to cope, dependence, taking to bed, cachexia, and eventual death. Frailty has been associated with numerous conditions, many of which may be preventable if recognized early (Table 38–3). Prevention for older adults needs to be addressed within the framework of disability (frailty) prevention or, put another way, of function preservation.

For health promotion to be effective with older adults, it must be individualized in terms of patient age, functional status, patient preference, and culture. Culture is important in understanding the older adult's health belief

Table 38–3. Conditions associated with frailty.

Advanced age, usually 85 y and older
Functional decline
Falls and associated injuries (hip fracture)
Polypharmacy
Chronic disease
Dementia and depression
Social dependency
Institutionalization or hospitalization
Nutritional impairment

Source: Hammerman D: Toward an understanding of frailty. Ann Intern Med 1999;130:945.

Table 38–5. Preventable major causes of death associated with aging.

Cause of Death	Percentage of All Deaths
Cardiovascular disease	47
Cancer	20
Stroke	11
Lung disease	6
Accidents/falls	2
Diabetes mellitus	2

Source: Rubenstein LZ: Update on preventive medicine for older adults. Generations, Winter 1996–1997;20:47.

system. Without this understanding, a health care provider may be unable to negotiate a treatment strategy (including prevention practices) that is acceptable to the patient and the provider. Another important factor to consider is the socioeconomic status of the older adult. Persons with a lower socioeconomic status use preventive services less often. Minority women, in particular, have higher rates of disability, indicating a vulnerable population, especially in terms of functional independence.

The benefits of secondary prevention, including cancer screening, are uncertain for older adults. There is a paucity of evidence due to the lack of randomized clinical trials in patients older than 75 years, and most prevention and health promotion recommendations are extrapolated from younger subjects. When considering a screening test for older adults, the risk of dying from the disease process, the benefits of the screening, the harm resulting from the screening, and the patient's values and preferences need to be weighed (Table 38–4). The US Preventive Services Task Force (USPSTF) has set the standard for providing recommendations for clinical practice on preventive interventions, including screening tests, counseling interventions, immunizations, and chemoprophylactic regimens. These standards were established by a review of the scientific evidence for the clinical effectiveness of each preventive service. In considering screening strategies, major causes of death (Table 38–5) and remaining life expectancy of the older adult should be considered. A healthy 65-year-old individual has a life expectancy of another 15–20 years, but an 85-year-old has a life expectancy of 5–7 years, with most averaging 3–5 years. It has therefore been recommended that for healthy older adults, screening can be stopped at 85 years, especially for individuals who have had repeated negative screenings in the past, who are frail or demented, or who have a limited quantity and quality of life remaining.

Table 38–4. Potential downside of screening tests.

There is no single operational definition for cancer
Aggressive cancers can be missed
Test results may be ambiguous requiring additional testing
Pseudodisease may be detected
Unnecessary treatments may be started
Following screening protocols may distract the physician from issues important to the patient

Source: Welch GH: Informed choice in cancer screening. JAMA 2001;285:2776.

Many of the leading causes of death in this population are amenable to both primary and secondary preventive strategies, especially if targeted early in life. The major targets of prevention should therefore be focused at the major causes of death—including coronary heart disease, cancer, and stroke—with the goals of reducing premature mortality caused by acute and chronic illness, maintaining function, enhancing quality of life, and extending active life expectancy. A priority in screening should be given to preventive services that are both easy to deliver and associated with beneficial outcomes. Tables 38–6 and 38–7 outline the recommended preventive services and screening for individuals aged 65 years and older. Details of preventive services can be found in the references listed within the tables, and frequent updates are found online at http://www.ahrq.gov and http://members.aol.com/TGoldberg/prevrecs.htm.

Physical Activity in Older Adults

A person is never too old to start a physical activity program. Exercise received a grade of "A" from the USPSTF, which recommends that older adults should be counseled on the benefits of aerobic and resistance exercise. Either exercise in the form of aerobic training, resistance training, or life-style modification has many benefits in older adults, even the oldest old.

Table 38–6. Health promotion and preventive screening for older adults.

Screening of Asymptomatic Older Adults[1,2]	Recommendation	Grade[3]	Notes
Blood pressure[a–c]	Every exam, at least every 1–2 y	A	Goal for primary prevention 140/80; treat systolic BP >160 mm Hg
Lipid disorders[d]	Screen men aged 35 and older and women aged 45 and older for total cholesterol and HDL-C; screen every 5 years until age 65	A	Those with CVD and DM need individualized management http://www.nhlbi.nih.gov.
Breast cancer screening			
Physician breast examination[4]	Annually beginning at age 40	A	
Mammogram[4,a,b,e,f]	Annually beginning at age 40 (ACS) or every 1–2 y ages 50–69 (USPSTF) or continue every 1–3 y ages 70–85 (AGS, USPSTF)	A C > 69 years old	Older women who undergo regular mammography are diagnosed with early stage disease and are less likely to die from breast cancer[g] http://www.americangeriatrics.org
Breast cancer screening			
Pap smear/pelvic examination[4,a,b,h,i]	Every 1–3 y after two or three negative exams; annual exams can be decreased or discontinued after ages 65–70	A C > 65 years old	No need to do a Pap smear in a women who had a complete hysterectomy (including cervix) http://www.americangeriatrics.org
Colon cancer screening			
Fecal occult blood testing[4,a,b,e,j,k]	Annually ≥ 50 y old	B	ACS recommends a total colon examination (air-contrast barium enema or colonoscopy) every 10 years; or fecal occult blood testing annually and sigmoidoscopy every 5 years http://www.cancer.org and http://www.gastro.org
Sigmoidoscopy	Every 5 y ≥50 years old	B	See above
Problem drinking[a,l]	Periodically	B	Counsel on drinking and driving; encourage men to limit drinking to 2 drinks per day and women to 1 drink per day (1 glass wine = 4 oz, 12 oz beer, or $1\frac{1}{2}$ oz 80-proof spirits)
Hearing impairment[a,b]	Periodically	C	Inquire; use office audioscope
Vision/glaucoma screening[a,b,m]	Periodically by eye specialist age 65 y and older	C	
Glucose[5,n]	Periodic in high-risk groups	C	Every three years starting age 45 (American Diabetic Association); http://www.diabetes.org
Thyroid function test (TSH)[a,o]	TSH every 5 y for women over age 50 y	C	American College of Physicians; http://www.acp.org
Electrocardiogram[p]	Periodically 40–50 y	C	AHA; http://www.heart.org
Cognitive impairment[q,r,s]	As needed, be alert for decline	C	Follow-up based on caregivers concerns or informal descriptions of decline; assessment may be based on individual complaint of memory loss

(continued)

Table 38–6. Health promotion and preventive screening for older adults. *(Continued)*

Screening of Asymptomatic Older Adults[1,2]	Recommendation	Grade[3]	Notes
Exam of mouth, nodes, testes, skin, heart, lung[e,p]	Annually	C	http://www.cancer.org http://www.heart.org
Bone mineral density (osteoporosis)[j,t]	If needed for treatment decision	C	Counsel perimenopausal women concerning calcium intake and hormone replacement http://www.nof.org
Prostate exam/PSA[a,e,u]	Annually age 50 and older if greater than 10-y life expectancy; not recommended by USPSTF	C–D	http://www.auanet.org; http://www.cancer.org USPSTF recommends counseling patients about potential benefits and harm of early detection and treatment
Chest x-ray[a,b]	Not recommended	D	

ACS, American Cancer Society; AGS, American Geriatric Society; AHA, American Heart Association; bp, blood pressure; CVD, cardiovascular disease; DM, diabetes mellitus; HDL-C, high-density lipoprotein cholesterol; PSA, prostate-specific antigen; TSH, thyroid-stimulating hormone; USPSTF, United States Preventive Services Task Force.

[1]References:

[a]US Preventive Services Task Force: Guide to Clinical Preventive Services, 2nd ed. Williams & Wilkins, 1996/2001. Updates available online at http://www.ahrq.gov.

[b]Institute for Clinical Systems Improvement: ICSI Health Care Guideline. Institute for Clinical Systems Improvement, 2001. http://www.ICSI.org.

[c]Smith SC et al: AHA/ACC guidelines for preventing heart attack and death in patients with atherosclerotic cardiovascular disease: 2001 update. Circulation 2001;104:1577.

[d]Agency for Healthcare Research and Quality: Screening for lipid disorders: Recommendations and rationale. Article originally in Am J Prevent Med 2001;20(3S):73. http://www.ahrq.gov/clinic/ajpmsuppl/lipidrr.htm.

[e]Smith RA et al: American Cancer Society guidelines for the early detection of cancer. CA 2000;50:34.

[f]American Geriatric Society Clinical Practice Committee: Breast cancer screening in older women. J Am Geriatr Soc 2000;48:842.

[g]McCarthey EP et al: Mammography use, breast cancer state at diagnosis, and survival among older women. J Am Geriatr Soc 2000;48:1226.

[h]Goldberg TH, Chavin SI: Preventive medicine and screening in older adults. J Am Geriatr Soc 1997;45:344.

[i]American Geriatric Society Clinical Practice Committee: Screening for cervical carcinoma in elderly women. J Am Geriatr Soc 2001;49:655.

[j]Goldberg TH: Update: Preventive medicine and screening in older adults. J Am Geriatr Soc 1999;47:122.

[k]Ransohoff DF, Sandler RS: Screening for colorectal cancer. N Engl J Med 2002;346:40.

[l]Fingerhood M: Substance abuse in older people. J Am Geriatr Soc 2000;48:985.

[m]Smeeth L, Iliffe S: Community screening for visual impairment in the elderly (Cochrane Review). In: The Cochrane Library, Issue 3: Update Software, 2001.

[n]The Expert Committee on the Diagnosis and Classification of Diabetes Mellitus: Report of the Expert Committee on the Diagnosis and Classification of Diabetes Mellitus. Diabetes Care 2002;25(Suppl 1):S5.

[o]American College of Physicians: Screening for thyroid disease: clinical guideline, part 2. Ann Intern Med 1998;129:141. http://www.acponline.org.

[p]Grundy SM et al: Assessment of cardiovascular risk by use of multiple-risk-factor assessment equations: A statement for healthcare professionals from the American Heart Association and the American College of Cardiology. Circulation 1999;100:1481.

[q]Petersen RC et al: Practice parameter: Early detection of dementia: Mild cognitive impairment (an evidence-based review). Neurology 2001;56:1133.

[r]Knopman DS et al: Practice parameter: Diagnosis of dementia (an evidence-based review). Neurology 2001;56:1143.

[s]Doody RS et al: Practice parameter: Management of dementia (an evidence-based review). Neurology 2001;56:1154.

[t]National Osteoporosis Foundation: Physicians Guide to the Prevention and Treatment of Osteoporosis.http://www.nof.org/professional/clinical/clinical.htm.

[u]American Urological Society: Prostate-specific antigen (PSA) best practice policy. Oncology 2000;14:267.

[2]Screening recommendations for asymptomatic older adults; clinical judgment should be used always, especially with regard to patients >85 years old, who are frail, or who have a limited quality and quantity of life.

[3]A–B, do; C, equivocal; D, don't.

[4]Covered by Medicare.

[5]Medicare covers diabetes self-management.

Table 38–7. Chemoprophylaxis and counseling for older adults.

Chemoprophylaxis/ Counseling[1]	Recommendation	Rating[2]	Notes[3]
Exercise[a–f]	Encourage aerobic and resistance exercise as tolerated	A	Encourage a minimum of 30 min of moderate-intensity exercise (brisk walking) daily; this may be done in intermittent or short bouts (~10 min) of activity throughout the day to total 30 min
Nutrition and weight management[a,b,f–n]	Limit intake of fat and cholesterol and maintain caloric balance; encourage a well-balanced diversified diet low in saturated fat and high in fiber	A–B	Health care providers should enlist the help of registered dietitians or qualified nutritionists; BMI = weight in kilograms divided by height in meters squared
Tobacco cessation counseling[a,b,f,g]	Complete history of tobacco use and assessment of dependence	A	The most effective clinician message is a brief, unambiguous, and informative statement on the need to stop using tobacco
Falls prevention[i]	Discuss measures to reduce the risk of falling including exercise to improve balance; environmental hazard reduction and monitoring medications	B–C	High-risk elders for falls include >75 years old or persons aged 70–74 using benzodiazepines, antihypertensives, or more than four medications; impaired cognition, strength, balance, and gait
Aspirin[g,j]	Discuss use with adults who are at increased risk of CHD including men > 40 y; post-menopausal women; and those with hypertension, diabetes, and current smokers	A	75 mg/day Discuss benefits—prevention of MI Discuss risks—GI and intracranial bleeding Most trials included men 40–75 years old Current benefits and harms may not be reliable for women and older men Older adults may derive greatest benefit because of their risk for CHD and stroke, but bleeding risks may also be greater
Tetanus–diphtheria vaccine[a,b]	Primary series then booster every 10 years	A	
Influenza vaccine[4,a,g]	Annually 65 years and older or if chronically ill	B	
23-valent pneumococcal vaccine[4,a,b]	At least once at age 65 years	B	
Zostavax (herpes zoster vaccine)	Once after 60 y		

Calcium[a,k]	800 to 1500 mg/day	B	National Osteoporosis Foundation
Estrogen/estrogen receptor-modifying agent (SERM) or bisphosphonate[k,l]	Postmenopausal women	B	Osteoporosis prevention and treatment, National Osteoporosis Foundation

BMI, body mass index; CHD, coronary heart disease; GI, gastrointestinal; MI, myocardial infarction.

[1]References:

[a]US Preventive Services Task Force: Guide to Clinical Preventive Services, 2nd ed. Williams & Wilkins, 1996/2001. Updates available online at http://www.ahrq.gov.

[b]Institute for Clinical Systems Improvement: ICSI Health Care Guideline. Institute for Clinical Systems Improvement, 2001. http://www.ICSI.org.

[c]Pate RR et al: Physical activity and public health: A recommendation from the Centers for Disease Control and Prevention and the American College of Sports Medicine. JAMA 1995;273:402.

[d]Fletcher CF et al: Statement on exercise: benefits and recommendations for physical activity programs for all Americans: a statement for health professionals by the Committee on Exercise and Cardiac Rehabilitation of the Council on Clinical Cardiology, American Heart Association. Circulation 1996;94:857.

[e]Mazzeo RS et al: American College of Sports Medicine Position Stand: Exercise and physical activity for older adults. Med Sci Sports Exerc 1998;30:992.

[f]Institute of Medicine Health and Behavior: The Interplay of Biological, Behavioral, and Societal Influences. National Academy Press, 2001.

[g]Smith SC et al: AHA/ACC guidelines for preventing heart attack and death in patients with atherosclerotic cardiovascular disease: 2001 update. Circulation 2001;104:1577.

[h]Institute of Medicine: The Role of Nutrition in Maintaining Health in the Nation's Elderly. National Academy Press, 2000.

[i]Feder G et al: Guidelines for the prevention of falls in people over 65. Br Med J 2000;321:1007.

[j]Agency for Healthcare Research and Quality: Aspirin for the Primary Prevention of Cardiovascular Events. Recommendations and Rationale, January 2002. http://www.ahrq.gov/clinic/3rduspstf/aspirin/asprr.htm.

[k]National Osteoporosis Foundation: Physicians Guide to the Prevention and Treatment of Osteoporosis.http://www.nof.org/professional/clinical/clinical.htm.

[l]Goldberg TH: Update: preventive medicine and screening in older adults. J Am Geriatr Soc 1999;47:122.

[2]A–B, do; C, equivocal.

[3]Web sites of interest: http://www.ctfphc.org (Canadian Task Force on Preventive Health Care), http://www.ahrq.gov (Agency for Health Care Research and Quality), and http://www.ICSI.org (Institute for Clinical Systems Improvement).

[4]Covered by Medicare; Medicare also covers hepatitis B vaccine.

Table 38–8. Contents of a physical activity preparticipation evaluation for older adults.

History, to include:
- Patient's lifelong pattern of activities and interests
- Activity level in the past 2–3 months to determine a current baseline
- Concerns and perceived barriers regarding exercise and physical activity:
  - Lack of time
  - Unsafe environment
  - Cardiovascular risks
  - Limitations of existing chronic diseases
  - Level of interest and motivation for exercise
  - Social preferences regarding exercise.

Physical examination, with emphasis on cardiopulmonary systems, musculoskeletal, and sensory impairments

Source: Fletcher GF et al: AHA Scientific Statement: Exercise standards for testing and training; a statement for healthcare professionals from the American Heart Association. Circulation 2001;104:1694.

Exercise and physical activity as a form of primary prevention have many benefits even for sedentary older adults. A recent meta-analysis of physical activity and well-being in advanced age concluded that physical activity had its strongest effect on self-efficacy (self-confidence), and improvements in cardiovascular status, strength, and functional capacity also improved well-being. Life-style physical activities that are more unstructured as compared with a formal exercise plan are being shown to increase levels of physical activity in sedentary populations.

DiPietro L: Physical activity in aging: Changes in patterns and their relationship to health and function. J Gerontol A Biol Sci Med Sci 2001;56(special issue 2):13. [PMID: 11730234]

Netz Y et al: Physical activity and psychological well-being in advanced age: A meta-analysis of intervention studies. Psychol Aging 2005;20:272. [PMID: 16029091]

Pescatello LS: Exercising for health: The merits of lifestyle physical activity. West J Med 2001;174:114. [PMID: 11156922]

Promoting an Active Life-style

To make an expected change in physical activity the older adult needs to understand the importance and benefit of increasing physical activity. Obtaining and documenting a detailed history and physical examination should be one of the first steps to embarking on an increased physical activity plan (Table 38–8). The American College of Sports Medicine recommends stress testing for any older adult who intends to begin a vigorous exercise program such as strenuous cycling or running (Table 38–9). Conditions that are absolute and relative contraindications to exercise stress testing or embarking on an exercise program should be evaluated (Table 38–10). Finally, an exercise prescription should be written on a prescription pad to strengthen the endorsement for increased physical activity. The prescription should include frequency, intensity, type, and time of exercise.

It is important to "start low and go slow," especially if the older adult has been relatively sedentary. It is more important to get the older adult to do any physical activity than to prescribe something that is unattainable. The health of older adults may be better served if they perform a little more exercise or activity than the previous week, attempting to incorporate the activity into their normal daily lives such as walking to a store or gardening. The goal should be for the person to feel "pleasantly" tired a few hours after the activity with the aim of increasing the activity slowly until a desired level of fitness is obtained.

Promotion of an active life-style is important at all ages and the benefits to older adults are numerous. Health care providers need to realize that for exercise to be beneficial it need not be strenuous or prolonged. Just encouraging patients to get up out of their chairs and start moving will improve not only the quality, but the quantity, of disability-free years.

Christmas C, Andersen RA: Exercise and older patients: Guidelines for the clinician. J Am Geriatr Soc 2000;48:318. [PMID: 10733061]

King A: Interventions to promote physical activity by older adults. J Gerontol A Biol Sci Med Sci 2001;56(special issue 2):36. [PMID: 11730236]

Nutrition in Older Adults

Nutrition is a priority for Healthy People 2010. As individuals age, chronic diseases, functional impairments, polypharmacy, and age-related physiologic and socioeconomic changes may all act in concert to place an older adult nutritionally at risk. Undernutrition is a major factor associated with mortality in older persons. Health care providers, however, rarely take the time to consider the diet and nutritional status of their patients.

Many disorders affecting older adults relate to nutritional status. Poor nutritional status may be the result of too little dietary intake leading to malnutrition, too much dietary content for actual expenditure leading to obesity, and inappropriate dietary intake exacerbating such conditions as diabetes, hypertension, and renal insufficiency. Weight tends to increase with aging until the seventh decade, when it stabilizes or begins to decline. Obesity tends to be a problem for patients younger than 75 years, whereas undernutrition is commonly encountered in those older than 85. Energy requirements decrease in the elderly. The recommended daily allowance (RDA) of 2300 kcal for a 77-kg man and 1900 kcal for a 65-kg woman should be

Table 38–9. Graded exercise test (GXT) recommendations according to coronary heart disease (CHD) risk factors[1] and exercise stratification.

Risk	Moderate Intensity Exercise	Vigorous Intensity Exercise
	Walking at 3–4 mph Cycling for pleasure <10 mph Moderate effort swimming Racket sports Pulling or carrying golf clubs	Walking briskly uphill or with a load Cycling fast or racing >10 mph Swimming, fast tread or crawl Singles tennis or racquetball
Low Men <45 y old and women <55 y old with ≤1 CHD risk factor and asymptomatic	GXT not necessary	GXT not necessary
Moderate Men ≥54 and women ≥55 y old or those with ≥2 CHD risk factors	GXT not necessary	GXT recommended
High Individuals with symptoms of disease or known metabolic, cardiovascular, or pulmonary disease	GXT recommended	GXT recommended

[1]CHD risk factors: family history, cigarette smoking, hypertension, dyslipidemia, impaired fasting glucose tolerance, obesity, sedentary life-style.

Source: American College of Sports Medicine: ACSM's Guidelines for Exercise Testing and Prescription, 6th ed. Lippincott Williams & Wilkins, 2000.

reduced by 10% based on basal energy expenditure between ages 51 and 75 years, with an additional 10–15% reduction after age 75. Although animal studies have indicated increased longevity with lower body weight and caloric restriction without malnutrition, studies on the relative risk of obesity to mortality in older adults are inconsistent, ranging from a protective effect for hip fractures to increased functional disability.8

Table 38–10. Absolute and relative contraindications to exercise stress testing or starting an exercise program.

Absolute Contraindications	Relative Contraindications
Acute myocardial infarction within 2 days	Left main coronary stenosis
Critical or severe aortic stenosis	Moderate stenotic valvular heart disease
Active endocarditis	Tachyarrhythmias or bradyarrhythmias
Decompensated heart failure	Atrial fibrillation with uncontrolled ventricular rate
High-risk unstable angina	Hypertrophic cardiomyopathy
Active myocarditis or pericarditis	Electrolyte abnormalities
Acute pulmonary embolism or infarction	Mental impairment leading to an inability to cooperate
Serious cardiac arrhythmias causing hemodynamic compromise	High-degree atrioventricular block
Acute noncardiac condition that may affect exercise performance or may exacerbate the condition (infection, renal failure, thyrotoxicosis)	
Physical disability that precludes safe and adequate test performance	
Inability to obtain consent	

Source: Fletcher GF et al: Exercise standards for testing and training: A statement for healthcare professions from the American Heart Association. Circulation 2001;104:1649.

Table 38–11. Nutrient requirements in older adults, with signs of excess and deficiency.

Nutrient	Requirement	Signs of Deficiency	Signs of Excess
Vitamin A	Requirements **decrease** with advancing age 3333 IU for men 2667 IU for women	Loss of bright, moist appearance of eyes; dry conjunctiva; gingivitis	Toxic effects include headache, lassitude, anorexia, reduced white blood cell count, impaired hepatic function, and bone pain with hypercalcemia; hip fracture
Vitamin B_1 (thiamine)	1.1–1.2 mg/day	Common in alcoholic elderly and institutionalized elderly; disordered cognition (delirium), neuropathies, and cardiomegaly	Liver damage and exacerbation of peptic ulcer disease especially with those using megadoses
Vitamin B_2 (riboflavin)	1.1–1.3 mg/day	Cheilosis, angular stomatitis, gingivitis; changes to tongue papillae	
Vitamin B_6 (pyroxidine)	1.5–1.7 mg/day	Glossitis, peripheral neuropathy, and dementia especially related to alcohol abuse	Liver damage and nervous system dysfunction especially with those using megadoses
Vitamin B_{12}	2.4 mcg/day	Pallor, optic neuritis, hyporeflexia, ataxia, anorexia; loss of proprioception, vibratory sense, and memory loss; megaloblastic anemia	
Vitamin C		Gingival hypertrophy, bleeding gums, petechiae, and ecchymoses	Megadose use can cause diarrhea, oxalate kidney and bladder stones; impaired absorption of vitamin B_{12}; interfere with serum and urine glucose testing; false-negative hemoccult testing
Vitamin D	10–15 mcg/day (400–600 IU/day)	Osteomalacia; severe bone pain and osteoporosis; muscular hypotonia; pulmonary macrophage dysfunction	Nausea, headache, anorexia, weakness, and fatigue; interferes with vitamin K absorption
Vitamin K	Widely distributed in food and provided by synthesis of intestinal bacteria; supplements advised for fat malabsorption syndromes and long-term antibiotic therapy	Hemorrhages in skin or gastrointestinal tract; unexplained prolongation of prothrombin time	Unknown
Folic acid	400 mcg/day	Pallor, stomatitis, glossitis, memory impairment, depression	
Vitamin E	400 IU/day	Deficiency is rare; abundant in diet	Interferes with vitamin K metabolism; thrombophlebitis; gastrointestinal (GI) distress; possible reduction in wound healing
Niacin	14–16 mg/day	Fissured tongue; dry, thickened, scaling, hyperpigmented skin; diarrhea; dementia	Histamine flush; liver toxicity
Calcium	1200–1500 mg/day	Osteoporosis	

(continued)

Table 38–11. Nutrient requirements in older adults, with signs of excess and deficiency. *(Continued)*

Nutrient	Requirement	Signs of Deficiency	Signs of Excess
Iron		Rare secondary to increased iron stores; usually secondary to pathologic blood loss	Constipation; excess iron usually given when anemia of chronic disease is misdiagnosed as iron deficiency anemia; some association between neoplasia and coronary artery disease
Zinc		Impaired wound healing; diarrhea; decreased vision, olfaction, insulin, and immune function; anorexia; impotence	GI disturbance; sideroblastic anemia from impaired copper absorption; adverse effect on cellular immunity; interfere with other vitamin absorption

Source: Johnson L: Vitamins and aging. In Morley JE, et al, eds: *The Science of Geriatrics,* Vol. 2. Springer Publishing, 2000, p. 379 and Dywer JT, et al: Assessing nutritional status in elderly patients. Am Fam Physician 1993;47:613.

A multitude of interrelated factors can place an older adult at nutritional risk (Table 38–11 and Table 38–12). An older adult with an unintentional weight loss of 10% or more or a basal metabolic index (BMI) of less than 17 kg/m^2 needs to be evaluated. Because anorexia, weight loss, and undernutrition in older persons have such deleterious effects, factors that can be treated or reversed are of major importance. Treatment with orexigenic agents to promote weight gain is controversial but should be considered. Megestrol acetate in doses up to 800 mg per day increases weight (fat mass) in older persons and must be used with caution if the individual has a history of clotting disorders. Dronabinol, a cannabis derivative, can enhance weight gain but has a tendency to cause dysphoria in the elderly, which limits its usefulness.

The significance of mild to moderate obesity in the elderly is unclear. Individual consideration is required. Height/weight charts for ideal body weight based on life insurance tables are probably relevant only to the age of 54 years. Recommending weight loss, especially to an older individual should be done with caution because weight loss in general carries a poor prognosis. For patients younger than 70 years of age who are 20% above ideal body weight, prudent weight loss should be recommended. For patients older than 70, if a medical condition is likely to be significantly improved by prudent dieting then it should be recommended. Such conditions would include severe hypertension, back pain from obesity, degenerative joint disease, gait and balance problems, and diabetes mellitus. Dietary management of hypercholesterolemia is controversial, especially if the individual is already close to or at ideal body weight. Severe restriction of fat may lead to weight loss, causing more harm than good. A dietician can assist the primary care physician in formulating a weight loss program for older patients, with a goal of 0.5–1 pound of weight loss per week.

The old adage "we are what we eat" is applicable to older adults. Promotion of a balanced, healthy diet for all older adults, including recognition and remediation of macronutrient deficiencies, should be incorporated into the health promotion strategies of all primary care physicians caring for older adults.

Alibhai SM et al: An approach to the management of unintentional weight loss in elderly people. CMAJ 2005;172:773. [PMID: 15767612]

Table 38–12. Factors associated with undernutrition in the elderly.

Depression
Dementia
Anorexia
Poor dental health
Medications
Pain
Fatigue
Sensory alterations
Impaired function
Dietary restrictions (more common in women)
Social isolation
Impecuniousness
Alcoholism
Swallowing dysfunction
Dieting (low fat, low cholesterol)

Source: Stechmiller JK: Early nutritional screen of older adults. J Infusion Nurs 2003;26:170; and Morley JE: Anorexia and weight loss in older persons. J Gerontol Med Sci 2003;58A:131.

De Castro JM: Age-related changes in the social, psychological, and temporal influences on food intake in free-living, healthy, adult humans. J Gerontol A Biol Sci Med Sci 2002;57:M368. [PMID: 12023266]

Kennedy RL et al: Obesity in the elderly: Who should we be treating, and why, and how? Curr Opin Clin Nutr Metab Care 2004;7:3. [PMID: 1509896]

Lui L et al: Undernutrition and risk of mortality in elderly patients within 1 year of hospital discharge. J Gerontol A Biol Sci Med Sci 2002;57:M741. [PMID: 12403803]

Position of the American Dietetic Association: Nutrition, aging and the continuum of care. J Am Diet Assoc 2000;100:580. [PMID: 10812387]

US Department of Health and Human Services: *Healthy People 2010: Understanding and Improving Health.* DHHS, 2000.

GERIATRIC ASSESSMENT

Geriatric assessment is a way to obtain information about functional performance in older adults in order to identify elders at risk for increasing frailty. Health care providers by clinical judgment alone can diagnose severe functional impairment but have difficulty identifying moderate impairments, which are more likely to affect a community-dwelling older population. The multitude and complexity of problems that may be experienced by a frail older adult requires more than just management of their diseases. It is important to identify elders who may be frail or vulnerable in the outpatient clinical practice because they will benefit from a coordinated and comprehensive care plan. The vulnerable elderly are adults older than 65 years of age who are at risk for functional decline and death. Family physicians assessing this population should strive to identify the conditions and clinical situations most affecting this group (Table 38–13).

In general, geriatric assessment attempts to obtain a "big picture" in order to provide quality care for the elderly (Table 38–14). Geriatric assessment is often necessary to accurately define an older person's problems, develop interventions, and serve as a baseline from which to measure outcomes of treatment.

Ensberg M, Gerstenlauer C: Incremental geriatric assessment. Prim Care Clin Office Pract 2005;32:619. [PMID: 16140119]

Who Needs Assessment?

Which older person needs assessment, and what is the best approach to implement this screening? Because geriatric assessment is an attempt to gain a complete picture of the health status of an older individual, the primary care provider must become involved not only in diagnosing and treating medical problems but also in all the factors that affect the health of older patients. A geriatric assessment is a *diagnostic tool,* not a therapeutic intervention for the cure of chronic disease and the reversal of disability. Table 38–15 details the components of a geriatric assessment.

The majority of older adults do not need an extensive evaluation; instead, assessment should be oriented toward screening to uncover problems. If screening uncovers a problem or problems, a more extensive evaluation can then be performed and a treatment plan can be implemented. Table 38–16 presents a common screening tool that can be used by nonphysician office staff to screen

Table 38–13. Common chronic syndromes among the vulnerable elderly.

Dementia
Depression
Diabetes mellitus
Falls and mobility disorders
Hearing impairment
Heart failure
Hypertension
Ischemic heart disease
Malnutrition
Osteoarthritis
Osteoporosis
Pneumonia and influenza
Pressure ulcers
Stroke and atrial fibrillation
Urinary incontinence
Vision impairment

Source: Wegner NS et al, eds: Quality indicators for assessing care of vulnerable elders. Ann Intern Med 2001;135 [suppl (8; pt. 2)]: 653. Online at http://www.acponline.org.

Table 38–14. Goals of geriatric assessment.

To define the functional capabilities and disabilities of older patients
To appropriately manage acute and chronic diseases of frail elders
To promote prevention and health
To establish preferences for care in various situations (advance care planning)
To understand financial resources available for care
To understand social networks and family support systems for care
To evaluate an older patient's mental and emotional strengths and weakness

Table 38–15. Components of geriatric assessment.

A. Functional assessment
  1. Basic activities of daily living (BADLs)—fundamental to self-care:
    Bathing
    Dressing
    Toileting
    Transfers
    Continence
    Feeding
  2. Instrumental activities of daily living (IADLs)—complex daily activities fundamental to independent community living and interactions)[1]:
    Housework—Can you do your own housework?
    Traveling—Can you get places outside of walking distance?
    Shopping—Can you go shopping for food and clothing?
    Money—Can you handle your own money?
    Meal preparation—Can you prepare your own meals?
  3. Advanced activities of daily living (AADLs)—"functional signature"
    Gait-mobility and balance
    Upper extremity evaluation
B. Cognitive and affective assessment
  Dementia
  Depression
  Suicide
  Alcohol misuse
  Sensory impairments
  Nutrition
  Incontinence
C. Social assessment (caregivers, environment, finances)
  Driving
  Sexuality
  Advance care planning

[1]In order of most difficult to least difficult—knowing a person can perform one item indicates they can perform item below it.
Source: Gallo JJ et al: *Handbook of Geriatric Assessment,* 4th ed. Jones & Bartlett, 2005; Katz S et al: Studies of illness in the aged: The index of ADL: A standardized measure of biological and psychosocial function. JAMA 1963;185:914; and Fillenbaum G: Screening the elderly: A brief instrumental activities of daily living measure. J Am Geriatr Soc 1985;33:683.

ambulatory older patients. Another validated self-administered screening tool, developed by the ACOVE (Assessing Care of Vulnerable Elders) Project, can be found online at http://www.rand.org/health/projects/acove/. The Vulnerable Elders Survey assesses functional and health status and can be used as a case finding tool before implementing more extensive screening.

Saliba D et al: The Vulnerable Elders Survey: A tool for identifying vulnerable older people in the community. J Am Geriatr Soc 2001;49:1691. [PMID: 11844005]

Functional Assessment

A. Predictors of Functional Decline

The ability to function independently in the community is an important public health and quality-of-life issue for all older adults. A recent trend toward declining disability has been noted among older persons, especially those with higher levels of education. For example, older adults who walk a mile at least once a week show decreasing decline in functional limitations and disability than their sedentary counterparts. However, these trends are not indicative of the total population. Non–Hispanic black and Mexican-American men and women generally report more functional limitations and disability and represent a vulnerable subpopulation within the United States.

Several predictors of functional decline and mortality have been reported. Health status belief and decreased abilities in activities of daily living (ADLs) appear to be important predictors of mortality. Older individuals (both men and women) with high depressive symptomatology have increased risk of ADL disability, as it appears depressive symptoms undermine efforts to maintain physical functioning. Social networks, and overdependence on these networks, may have a negative impact on ADLs by provoking dependency and a sense of "learned" helplessness, especially in older men.

Kivela SL, Pahkala K: Depressive disorder as a predictor of physical disability in old age. J Am Geriatr Soc 2001;49:290. [PMID: 11300240]

Ostchega Y et al: The prevalence of functional limitations and disability in older persons in the US: Data from the National Health and Nutrition Examination Survey III. J Am Geriatr Soc 2000;48:1132. [PMID: 10983915]

B. Evaluation of Functional Status

Assessment of function is at the core of caring for older adults. The capacity to perform functional tasks necessary for daily living can be used as a surrogate measure of independence or a predictor of decline and institutionalization. A specific evaluation of functional status is necessary in older individuals, because functional impairment cannot be predicted by an individual's medical diagnoses. Functional status needs to be assessed directly and independently of medical, laboratory, and cognitive evaluation, because specific functional loss is not disease specific and cognitive impairment does not necessarily imply inability to function independently in a familiar environment. Functional assessment can identify an older individual's capabilities and, by noting changes in these, can prompt the search for possible illness such as cognitive impairment, depression, substance abuse, adverse drug events, or sensory impairment, and then guide interventions using the appropriate support and resources.

Table 38–16. A geriatric screening for impaired ambulatory elderly.

1. Medications
   Did the patient bring in all bottles or a list of medications?
   List all medications
   Remember to ask about over-the-counter medications
   Remember to ask about supplements and herbs
2. Nutrition
   Weigh patient and record
   Have you lost more than 10 lb in the last 6 months?
   Positive screen: 10 lb weight loss or < 100 lb
   Intervention: Further evaluation with the Mini-Nutritional Assessment
3. Hearing
   Use handheld audioscope at 40 dB and screen both ears at 1000 and 2000 Hz
   Positive screen: Patient unable to hear 1000 or 2000 Hz frequency in *both* ears *or* unable to hear the 1000 and 2000 Hz frequency in *one* ear
   Intervention: Evaluate for cerumen impaction; refer to audiology
4. Vision
   Ask: "Do you have any problems driving, watching TV, reading, or doing any of your activities because of your eyesight?" If yes
   Do Snellen eye chart
   Positive screen: 20/40 or greater
   Intervention: Refer to optometry or ophthalmology
5. Mental Status
   Ask to remember three objects—"ball, car, and flag" (have them repeat objects after you)
   Positive screen: Unable to remember all three items after 1 min
   Intervention: Administer more formal mental status testing such as the 7-Minute Neurocognitive Screening Battery or MMSE; assess for causes of cognitive impairment including delirium, depression, and medications
6. Depression
   Ask: "Are you depressed?" or "Do you often feel sad or depressed?"
   Positive screen: Yes
   Intervention: Perform a more thorough depression screen (Geriatric Depression Scale); evaluate medications; consider pharmacological treatment and/or refer to psychiatry
7. Urinary Incontinence
   Ask: "In the last year have you ever lost urine or gotten wet?" if *yes*
   Ask:" Have you lost urine in at least 6 separate days?"
   Positive screen: Yes to both
   Intervention: Initiate workup for incontinence; consider urology referral
8. Physical Disability
   Ask: Are you able to do strenuous activities like fast walking or biking? Heavy work around the house like washing windows, floors, and walls? Go shopping for groceries or clothes? Get to places out of walking distance? Bathe, either sponge bath, tub bath, or shower? Dress, like putting on a shirt, buttoning and zipping, and putting on your shoes?
   Positive screen: Unable to do any of the above independently or able to do only with assistance from another
   Intervention: Corroborate responses if accuracy uncertain with caregivers; determine reason for inability to perform task; institute appropriate medical, social, and environmental interventions. Patient may benefit from physical and/or occupational therapy and a home visit
9. Mobility
   Ask: "Do you fall or feel unbalanced when walking or standing?"
   Positive Screen: Yes
   Intervention: "Get-Up and Go" test: Get up from the chair, walk 20 feet, turn, walk back to the chair, and sit down (walk at normal, comfortable pace)
   Positive screen: Unable to complete the task in 15 s
   Intervention: Refer to physical therapy for gait evaluation and assistance with use of appropriate adaptive devices; home safety evaluation. Patient may need to be instructed in strengthening of both upper and lower extremities

(*continued*)

Table 38–16. A geriatric screening for impaired ambulatory elderly. *(Continued)*

10. Home Environment
    Ask: Do you have trouble with stairs either inside or outside of your house? Do you feel safe at home?
    Positive Screen: Yes
    Intervention: Supply the older patient or caregiver with a home safety self-assessment check list; consider making a home visit or use a visiting nurse or other community resource to evaluate the home; make appropriate referrals to help remediate safety issues
11. Social Support
    Ask: Who would be able to help you in case of an illness or emergency?
    Record identified person(s) in medical record with contact information
    Intervention: Become familiar with available resources for the elderly within your community or know who can provide you with that assistance

Source: Lachs MS et al: A simple procedure for general screening for functional disability in elderly patients. Ann Intern Med 1990;112:699 and Moore AA, Siu AL: Screening for common problems in ambulatory elderly: A clinical confirmation of a screening instrument. Am J Med 1996;100:438.

Functional assessment can be seen as a hierarchy. The basic activities of daily living (BADLs) are self-care activities that are at the most basic level of functioning, such as bathing, dressing, toileting, transfers, continence, and feeding (see Table 38–15). An older adult may be fully independent, need assistance, or be fully dependent in any or all of these activities. Individuals may move in and out of needing assistance or dependence, especially at the time of and after the onset of an acute illness or disease process.

Assessment of BADL items allows the primary care provider to focus on functional abilities, thus matching services to needs. The hierarchy for loss of BADL abilities is associated with increasing age and appears to be dependent on lower extremity strength, such that bathing, mobility, and toileting are lost before dressing and feeding, which rely on upper extremity strength. Of all of the BADL measures, dependence with regard to going to the toilet has been shown to be an indicator of overall performance and the need for overall higher levels of assistance.

The next higher level of functioning is known as the instrumental activities of daily living (IADLs). These activities are required for independent living within the community and include a set of more complex and demanding tasks (see Table 38–15). Older individuals living in the community who cannot perform IADLs may have difficulty functioning at home. The more IADLs that are impaired in a community-dwelling elder, the greater the likelihood of developing dementia within 1 year.

The advanced activities of daily living (AADLs) are those tasks that may be considered the "functional signature" of a well community-dwelling older individual. These tasks include voluntary social, occupational, or recreational activities. An older person who does not successfully participate in such activities may not be dysfunctional, but an assessment that uncovers significant involuntary loss of such function may be an important risk factor for further functional losses. Globally knowing how an elderly person spends his or her days can give the physician a reference point for potential functional decline at subsequent visits. Online reference tools for completing a detailed functional assessment can be found at http://www.medicine.uiowa.edu/igec/tools/default.asp and http://www.geriatricsatyourfingertips.org/.

Gallo JJ et al: *Handbook of Geriatric Assessment,* 4th ed. Jones & Bartlett, 2005.

Sherman FT: Functional assessment: Easy-to-use screening tools to speed initial office work-up. Geriatrics 2001;56:36. [PMID: 11505859]

Other Considerations in Geriatric Assessment

The remainder of this chapter focuses on issues that need to be addressed in the evaluation of older adults. Issues relating to mobility and balance (Chapter 39), incontinence (Chapter 40), depression (Chapter 41), and sensory impairments (Chapter 44) are covered elsewhere in this book, and the reader is referred to those chapters for more detailed information.

A. Alcohol Misuse

Alcohol consumption and alcoholism are commonplace among the elderly, with 10.5% of men and 3.9% of women in one primary care practice reporting problem alcohol use. Detection of alcoholism in the elderly is difficult for numerous reasons, including the idea that elderly patients do not see alcoholism as a disease, but rather as a sign of weakness. Physicians create their own barriers to the diagnosis, including uncertainty of the diagnosis, pessimism concerning treatment, and possible subconscious hostility toward the alcoholic older patient. Preventive care should include screening all elders at least once to detect problems or hazardous drinking by taking a history of alcohol use and using a standard screening questionnaire, such as the 4-item CAGE or the 10-item AUDIT.

American Medical Association: *Alcoholism in the Elderly: Diagnosis, Treatment, and Prevention: Guidelines for Primary Care Physicians.* AMA, 1995.

B. Driving Competence

Evaluating the driving competence of an older patient is a challenge for physicians. The automobile is the ultimate symbol of freedom and the most important source of transportation for older adults. The ability to drive is closely linked to independence and self-esteem, allowing the older adult to maintain important links within the community. Those who are unable to drive or who stop driving risk social isolation, depression, and functional decline. Driving is an instrumental activity of daily living composed of complex tasks that require not only physical but mental integrity. It is estimated that by 2020, 15% of all drivers will be older than 65 years. Adults over the age of 65 are expected to account for 27% of all automobile fatalities in 2015, an increase of 373% since 1975.

In an attempt to reduce risk, many older drivers alter their driving habits by driving shorter distances, driving only during daylight, and avoiding rush hour, major highways, and inclement weather. However, not all older drivers avert risk. One study found that older adults diagnosed with Alzheimer dementia and those needing help with dressing and bathing still persisted in driving. Adults who voluntarily stop driving are usually older (over 85 years), female, nonwhite, and had driven less than 50 miles per week. Heart disease and hearing impairment are more often associated with reports of adverse driving events. Driving accidents with older adults rarely involve high speeds or alcohol. Their accidents are usually related to issues involving visual-spatial difficulties and cognitive and motor skills.

Assessment of the older driver is made all the more difficult because chronic illness, functional status, or even cognitive impairment cannot consistently predict adverse driving events. An assessment of the older driver should include a review of the driving record, medications, alcohol use, and functional measures including vision, hearing, attention (spell "world" backward), visual-spatial skills (clock drawing), muscle strength, and joint flexibility. Older drivers should be advised on the importance of safety restraints, obeying speed limits, use of a helmet if riding a motorcycle or bicycle, taking a driving refresher course, and avoidance of drinking and use of cellular telephones while driving. It is important for primary care physicians to know the laws of their state with regard to driving and reportable medical conditions. A physician's guide to assessing and talking to older drivers can be obtained from the National Traffic and Safety Board at http://www.nhtsa.dot.gov/people/outreach/media/catalog/topic.cfm.

Carr DB: The older adult driver. Am Fam Physician 2000;61:141. [PMID: 10643955]

Foley KT, Mitchell SJ: The elderly driver: What physicians need to know. Cleve Clin J Med 1997;64:423. [PMID: 9308218]

Ott BR et al: Clinician assessment of the driving competence of patients with dementia. J Am Geriatr Soc 2005;53:829. [PMID: 15877559]

C. Social Assessment

An important aspect of caring for older persons, especially vulnerable older persons, is understanding their social environment. Social assessment includes the sources and kinds of help available to the older adult and assessment of the primary caregiver, often called the "hidden patient." The social assessment is important in the development of an effective care plan and all parts of the social assessment should be covered, usually over several patient visits.

1. Social support—It is important to understand the social networks of an older person. The social networks consist of informal supports such as family and close longtime friends, formal supports such as social welfare and other social service and health care delivery agencies, and semiformal supports such as church groups, neighborhood organizations, and clubs. Relationships with family and friends are intricate and can have consequences for the vulnerable elder. The availability of assistance from family or friends frequently determines whether a functionally dependent elder remains at home or is institutionalized, and identifying who would be available to help the elder if he or she becomes ill should be documented even for healthy elders. Other important information to obtain from older persons is outlined in Table 38–17. For a more formal assessment of social support, the Norbeck Social Support Questionnaire or the Lubben Social Network Scale should be considered.

2. Caregiver burden—For individuals caring for a frail, often cognitively impaired elder, the demands can be overwhelming. Caregiver burden has been defined as the strain or load borne by the person who cares for an elderly, chronically ill, or disabled family member or other person. Caregivers are at higher risk for mortality if there is increased mental or emotional strain. Caregiver burden is linked to the caregiver's ability to cope and handle stress. The physician should be alert for

Table 38–17. Social support screening.

How many relatives do you see or hear from in the course of a month?
Tell me about the relative with whom you have the most contact.
How many relatives do you feel close to—such as to discuss private matters?
How many friends do you see or hear from in the course of a month?
Tell me about the friend with whom you have the most contact.
When you have an important decision to make, do you have someone you can talk to about it?
Do you rely on anybody to assist you with shopping, cooking, doing repairs, cleaning house, etc?
Do you help others with shopping, cooking, transportation, childcare, etc?
Do you live alone?
With whom do you live?

Source: Gallo JJ et al: Handbook of Geriatric Assessment, 4th ed. Jones & Bartlett, 2005.

signs of possible caregiver burnout, including multiple somatic complaints, increased stress and anxiety, circular thinking, social isolation, depression, and weight loss. More formal assessment tools include the Caregiver Strain Index and the Zarit Burden Interview, for which a short version and screening version are available.

Bedard M et al: The Zarit Burden interview: A short version and screening version. Gerontologist 2001;41:652. [PMID: 11574710]

Kasuya RT et al: Caregiver burden and burnout: A guide for primary care physicians. Postgrad Med 2000;108:119. [PMID: 1126138]

Schulz R, Beach SR: Caregiving as a risk factor for mortality: The Caregiver Health Effects Study. JAMA 1999;282:2215. [PMID: 10605972]

3. Economic factors—Economic factors have important consequences with respect to an older person's health, nutrition, and living environment. Understanding the impact of financial status of the elderly may provide insight into how the individual copes, such as buying food versus medications. The primary care provider should have a working knowledge of Medicare and state and local assistance programs and know where the older person could go to obtain needed assistance in applying for appropriate financial benefits. The physician can inquire by asking if older individuals have enough financial resources to meet their needs. The physician also needs to know if a proposed treatment will be an economic burden on the individual.

4. Physical environment—The physical environment of the older person, including home environment, neighborhood, and transportation system, is critical to maintaining independence. Environmental hazards within the home are high and can be a potential constraint not only on the day-to-day functioning of frail elders but also on older persons without any specific physical deficits. Common environmental hazards within the home include loose throw rugs, curled carpet edges, obstructed pathways, lack of grab bars in tub and shower, and low and loose toilet seats. These hazards could lead to an increased risk of falls and fractures. The physician should inquire about the safety of the neighborhood and ask if older persons have transportation or transportation services available in close geographic proximity to where they live. This is especially important for elders who are dependent in IADLs and still living within the community.

Older persons often have problems that are not easily detected during an office visit. A home visit either by the physician or a community agency provider such as a visiting nurse can reveal problems in the living situation, such as wandering, household and bathing hazards, social isolation and loneliness, family stress, nutrition problems, financial concerns, and even alcohol abuse. An environmental checklist that the older person or family member can use for a self-assessment can be found at the National Safety Council's web site (http://www.nsc.org).

Unwin BK, Jerant AF: The home visit. Am Fam Physician 1999;60:1481. [PMID: 10524492]

5. Sexual health—Sexuality late in life is a normal and important part of aging. Primary care providers need to be aware of their own comfort level in taking a sexual health history from older adults. Older adults prefer that the provider initiate the discussion surrounding sexual functioning. Using open-ended questions allows the individual to give as much or as little information as is comfortable. The physician needs to have an understanding of what the older adult's normal sexual patterns and interests have been and what if any changes have occurred that affect sexual functioning and intimacy such as health problems, medications, physical disabilities, or cognitive impairments.

The physician should inquire into the nature of the older person's sexual quality of life by asking about how affection is displayed and how physical intimacy is expressed. Because not all older persons are in committed heterosexual relationships, it is vitally important that the physician express openness to answers conveyed. It is important for the physician to gain an understanding of what the older adult perceives about changes that may have occurred with regard to sexual

Table 38–18. Five steps to successful advanced care planning.

Steps	Process
1. Introduce the topic	During a wellness visit or some other time when the individual is in a good state of health Explain the purpose and nature of the discussion Inquire into how familiar the individual is with advanced care planning and define terms as necessary Be aware of the comfort level of the patient—give information and be supportive Suggest that family members, friends, or even members of the community explore how to manage potential burdens Discuss the identification of a proxy decision maker Encourage the patient to bring the proxy decision maker to the next visit
2. Engage in structured discussions	Convey commitment to patients to follow their wishes and protect patients from unwanted treatment or undertreatment Involve the potential proxy decision maker in discussions and planning Allow the patient to specify the role he or she would like the proxy to assume if the patient is incapacitated—follow patient's explicit wishes or allow the proxy to decide according to the patient's best interests Elicit the patient's values and goals Use a validated advisory document available at http://www.medicaldirective.org
3. Document patient preferences	Review advanced directives with patient and proxy for inconsistencies and misunderstandings Enter the advanced directives into the medical record Recommend statutory documents be completed by the patient that comply with state statutes Distribute directives to hospital, patient, proxy decision maker, family members, and all health care providers Include advanced directives in the care plan
4. Review and update the directive regularly	
5. Apply directives to actual circumstances	Most advanced directives go into affect when the patient can no longer direct his or her own medical care Assess the patient's decision-making capacity Never assume advanced directive content without reading it thoroughly Advanced directives should be interpreted in view of the clinical facts of the case Physician and proxy decision maker will need to work together to resolve ambiguous or uncertain situations If disagreements between physician and proxy cannot be resolved—seek the assistance of an ethics consultant or committee

Source: Emanuel LL et al: Advance care planning. Arch Fam Med 2000;9:1181.

function with aging. Issues concerning the quality of erections and orgasm for men or concerns about erectile dysfunction should be discussed. Women may have concerns about their sexual cycle and issues surrounding lubrication and orgasm.

If a problem is uncovered it should be documented and a more thorough assessment and evaluation should be undertaken. Finally, issues surrounding safer sex practices should be discussed with older adults who are sexually active and not in a committed monogamous relationship.

Zeiss AM et al: Assessment of sexual function and dysfunction in older adults. In Lichtenberg PA, ed: *Handbook of Assessment in Clinical Gerontology*. Wiley, 1999:270.

6. Spirituality—Assessing an older person's spirituality is important to understanding the overall well-being of that individual. It is important to ascertain what religion or spirituality means to the older adult and what role it plays in his or her life. The spiritual assessment should include the older person's concept of God or deity, religious practices, beliefs about spirit and hell, and value and meaning in life. Older adults can suffer from spiritual distress that may be expressed as depression, crying, fear of abandonment, or hopelessness, anxiety, and despair. This distress may occur after a loss of a significant other, after a family or personal disaster, or when there is a disruption in usual religious activities. Religion and spirituality are a source of comfort for patients. Inquiring into the spirituality of patients requires empathy on the part of the physician, strong interpersonal skills, and a closely established physician-patient relationship.

7. Advanced care planning—Advanced care planning is a process of planning for the medical future in which the patient's preferences will guide the nature and intensity of future medical care, particularly if the patient is unable to make his or her own decisions. As part of the assessment of the older person it is important for the physician to learn about the patient's goals and preferences for care (Table 38–18). This is especially important for the frail elderly, because it will ultimately influence management decisions. The process of advanced care planning helps patients identify their personal values and goals about health and medical treatment. Older adults should indicate the care they would and would not want to receive in various situations. Advanced care planning is designed to ensure that the patient's wishes are known, even if the patient is unable to participate in those decisions. (For more information on advanced care planning, see Chapter 63.)

Emanuel LL et al: Advance care planning. Arch Fam Med 2000;9: 1181. [PMID: 11115227]

Kahana B et al: The personal and social context of planning end-of-life care. J Am Geriatr Soc 2004;52:1163. [PMID: 15209656]

WEB SITES

AGS Foundation for Health in Aging:
http://www.healthinaging.org
Administration on Aging:
http://www.aoa.gov
American Association of Retired Persons:
http://www.aarp.org
American Geriatrics Society:
http://www.americangeriatrics.org
American Medical Directors Association:
http://www.amda.com
American Society of Consultant Pharmacists:
http://www.ascp.com
Assisted Living Federation of America:
http://www.alfa.org
Children of Aging Parents:
http://www.caps4caregivers.org
CDC National Prevention Information Network:
http://www.cdcnpin.org
Family Caregiver Alliance:
http://www.caregiver.org
Medicare Hotline:
http://www.medicare.gov
National Adult Day Services Association:
http://www.nadsa.org
National Council on the Aging:
http://www.ncoa.org
National Institute on Aging:
http://www.nia.nih.gov

Common Geriatric Problems

39

Daphne P. Bicket, MD, MLS, Richie-Ann G. Rodriguez, MD, & Sheila Ann B. Alas, MD

The syndromes of failure to thrive, pressure ulcers, and falls, common in the elderly, share features that make them particularly challenging. Their etiologies are multifactorial; they require an interdisciplinary approach to maximize care; and they often herald disability, institutionalization, and death. Maintaining open communication with patients and caregivers is vital. It not only empowers them to play a role in care, but also focuses their expectations realistically. Clinicians should continually reassess their objectives, remembering that in elders concern is as much for independence and quality of life as it is for cure.

FAILURE TO THRIVE

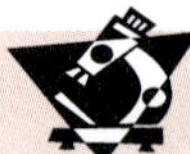

ESSENTIALS OF DIAGNOSIS

- *Weight loss of more than 5%.*
- *Anorexia.*
- *Malnutrition.*
- *Functional decline.*

General Considerations

Failure to thrive (FTT), a syndrome of community-dwelling elders, is also known as "the dwindles," wasting, or end-stage frailty. Typically the patient is brought in because of weight loss, apathy, and overall functional and social decline. The pathogenesis is unknown; FTT is not a normal part of aging.

Clinical Findings

Weight loss is only one aspect of FTT. Other features are impaired physical functioning, malnutrition, depression, cognitive impairment with or without dehydration, depression, impaired immune function, and low cholesterol. There is no underlying terminal disease. As in infants, FTT can occur from organic and nonorganic causes, necessitating an approach that includes medical, psychological, functional, and social domains.

The history provided by the patient and caregiver is key in establishing the onset and uncovering potential triggers. Common acute medical problems include infections, constipation, or peptic ulcer disease. Common chronic diseases include poorly controlled cardiac, pulmonary, or endocrine disorders; tuberculosis; dementia; depression; and rarely, hypoactive delirium. Physicians should assess, not assume, medication compliance, looking at all the patient's drugs and asking the patient to demonstrate how he or she is taking them. Levels are nonspecific; normal therapeutic levels can also have adverse effects. Anticholinergic drugs are ubiquitous and dangerous. Table 39–1 lists drugs that contribute to anorexia, weight loss, and FTT.

Substance use should be evaluated, and patients (or caregivers) asked if they have noted increased memory loss or depression. Recent changes such as death or loss of a friend, family member, or pet can trigger FTT.

A comprehensive physical examination is important. Special emphasis should be placed on the items noted in Table 39–2. Ancillary test recommendations are listed in Table 39–3.

Treatment

Once the diagnosis of FTT is made, the life expectancy of the patient should be assessed based on age and comorbidities. Reversible conditions should be addressed one at a time; physicians should not try to correct conditions that will neither improve quality of life nor impact life expectancy. Risk–benefit analysis and shared medical decision making with patient and family are essential. As medical interventions become more limited, palliative measures should be initiated. The physician can and should maintain a therapeutic relationship with the patient and the family beyond the time medical therapies are effective.

A team approach is essential. Medication regimens can be simplified with help of a PharmD. A social worker from the hospital, home health agency, or Area Agency on Aging should be involved. Concerns about neglect or abuse should be discussed openly and nonjudgmentally, and should be reported. A nutritionist should be consulted; malnutrition in the nonterminal state is correctable. A psychiatrist should be consulted if

Table 39–1. Drugs that contribute to anorexia or FTT.

Alendronate
Antibiotics
Antiarrhythmics
Antihistamines
α-Antagonists
Benzodiazepines
β-Blockers
Calcium antagonists
Digoxin
Diuretics
Glucocorticoids
Iron supplements
Metformin
Metronidazole
Neuroleptics
Nonsteroidal antiinflammatory drugs
Narcotics
Selective serotonin reuptake inhibitors
Tricyclic antidepressants
Xanthines
More than six prescription drugs

See Zhan C et al: Potentially inappropriate medication use in the community-dwelling elderly: Findings from the 1996 medical expenditure panel survey JAMA 2001;286:2823; Huffman GB: Evaluating and treating unintentional weight loss in the elders. Am Fam Physician 2002;65:640; and Verdery RB: Clinical evaluation of failure to thrive in older people. Clin Geriatr Med 1997;13:769.

there are questions about psychiatric assessment and management. Spiritual needs should be addressed. Physicians should remain committed to the patient and caregiver; home visits are key to assessment, reassessment, and management.

Robertson RG, Montagnini M. Geriatric failure to thrive. Am Fam Physician 2004:70:343. [PMID: 15291092]

Verdery RB: Clinical evaluation of failure to thrive in older people. Clin Geriatr Med 1979;13:769. [PMID: 9354754]

Web Sites

Area Agency on Aging web site, with regional and local contact numbers, and list of services:

http://www.aaa.gov.

PRESSURE ULCERS

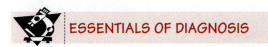

- *Skin ulcer caused by ischemia due to prolonged pressure.*

Table 39–2. Physical examination details and considerations.[1]

Vital signs: BMI < 21 or percentage of weight loss since last visit, BP and HR in two positions, pulse for 60 s; abnormal if > 88/min, respiratory rate and effort
Ears: hearing defects or tinnitus lead to social isolation
Eyes: cataracts/vision disturbance lead to depression and isolation
Oral health: tooth or gum disease impairs eating
Swallowing: aspiration and cough can negatively impact eating; have patient swallow liquid in your presence if any question of aspiration
JVD: most sensitive marker for CHF exacerbation
Breast mass: will often be unnoticed by the patient
Abdomen: masses, constipation, urinary bladder distention
Skin: sacrum and feet, axillae, panniculus, and groin for breakdown/candida/impetigo
Feet: any condition causing gait or balance disturbance
Motor: gait: bradykinesia, consider Parkinson's disease; shoulder/hip weakness, consider polymyalgia rheumatica
Mental status: test for variance from baseline and screen for depression

[1]BMI, body mass index; BP, blood pressure; HR, heart rate; JVD, jugular venous distention; CHF, congestive heart failure.

Table 39–3. Standard tests to evaluate FTT.

Test	Condition
CBC	Anemia, vitamin or iron deficiency, infection, or hematopoietic or lymphoproliforative disorder
Serum electrolytes, calcium, BUN, creatinine	Hypo- or hypernatremia or -kalemia, acid–base disorder, osmolality, renal failure, dehydration
Glucose	Diabetes
Serum bilirubin and transaminase levels	Liver failure, hepatitis
Thyroid-stimulating hormone level	Hypo- or hyperthyroidism
Fecal occult blood	Cancer
Urinalysis	Infection
ESR	Active inflammation
PPD	Tuberculosis

CBC, complete blood count; BUN, blood urea nitrogen; ESR, erythrocyte sedimentation rate; PPD, purified protein derivative.

See Huffman GB: Evaluating and treating unintentional weight loss in the elders. Am Fam Physician 2002;65:640; and Verdery RB: Clinical evaluation of failure to thrive in older people. Clin Geriatr Med 1997;13:769.

- *Occurs on weight-bearing or bony prominences (eg, sacrum, hip, heel).*

General Considerations

Pressure ulcers are serious problems: development of an ulcer is associated with increased mortality, and prevention is not always successful. Healing of stage 1 or 2 ulcers typically takes 4–8 weeks, and stage 3 or 4 ulcers may require many months to heal. There is scant evidence from randomized controlled trials to identify interventions that work. Physicians thus continue to rely on the Agency for Healthcare Research and Quality (AHRQ) guidelines, which are now more than a decade old.

Pathogenesis

Extrinsic and intrinsic factors cause pressure ulcers. The presence and duration of pressure are the most significant extrinsic factors. Contributors are friction, shear forces, moisture, and prolonged immobilization, including physical restraints and postoperative periods. Intrinsic causes are the susceptibility of aged skin, loss of sensation, circulatory compromise, immobility, weight loss, dehydration, and malnutrition.

Prevention

All patients who have an impaired ability to reposition themselves are at risk. Commonly used screening tools for ulcer risk are the Braden and Norton scales. The Braden scale contains six subscales: sensory perception, skin moisture, activity level, mobility, nutritional status, and friction and shear. The Norton scale, unlike the Braden, includes cognitive status.

All elders who are admitted to the hospital should be screened and placed on a prevention protocol within 12 hours of admission. Table 39–4 summarizes the AHRQ guidelines for pressure ulcer prevention. A baseline evaluation by the physician should document the condition of the elbows, sacrum, ischia, greater trochanters, heels, malleoli, vertebrae, and areas near casts or other orthopedic devices. Although patient repositioning remains a mainstay in clinical practice, no data support the view that it reduces the incidence of ulcers. Pressure-reducing devices are superior to standard mattresses and are used for at-risk patients. All patients at risk for malnutrition (ie, those with a body mass index [BMI] < 19; > 5% weight loss in 30 days or > 10% loss in 180 days; albumin < 3.5 g/dL) should have a dietary consult. Although no studies have shown that adequate nutrition prevents pressure ulcers, there is indirect evidence that prevention of malnutrition will reduce the risk of ulcer formation. Use of sedation is associated with significantly increased risk of multiple and severe ulcers.

Table 39–4. AHRQ guidelines for pressure ulcer prevention.

Assess risk and institute care plan within 12 h of admission
Inspect high-risk patients daily (all vulnerable sites)
Keep skin clean with mild soap and water
Keep *clean skin* dry with moisture barrier
Minimize friction and shear with lift-sheet, bed trapeze, or both
Post a turning schedule near patient
Relieve heel pressure with inflatable heel elevators
Avoid doughnut cushions
Leave head of bed flat when possible
Use pressure-relieving chair cushion; reposition frequently
Maintain and promote mobility; avoid bed rest
Address nutrition in patients who are hypoalbuminemic, anemic, or in whom BMI is abnormal

From the Agency for Healthcare Research and Quality: *Pressure Ulcer Treatment, Quick Reference Guide for Clinicians.* AHRQ, 1994.

Clinical Findings

Symptoms may include warmth over a bony prominence, redness and irritation around the ulcer, blistering, and skin loss. Each ulcer must be documented according to its stage, location, size, and depth (Figure 39–1). A stage 1 ulcer should be evaluated by palpating the ulcer to ensure the absence of fluctuance, crepitus, or soft tissue breakdown beneath the surface. An ulcer that is stage 2 or higher should be probed with a sterile cotton-tipped swab moistened with normal saline to identify and measure undermining or sinus tracts. Stage 3 or 4 ulcers should be drawn or photographed in addition to being measured. Accurate staging is not possible if necrotic tissue or eschar is present; it must first be removed. The one exception to this is the heel, which should not be debrided.

Differential Diagnosis

Among the differential diagnoses for pressure ulcers are vascular ulcers (caused by venous or arterial insufficiency), diabetic ulcers (caused by neuropathy), and cellulitis. Venous ulcers are usually located over the medial malleolus. Arterial ulcers may be located between toes, over phalangeal heads, or around the lateral malleolus. Diabetic ulcers are usually located on the plantar aspect of the foot, metatarsal heads, or under the heel. Cellulitis is an acute inflammation that blanches with palpation.

Complications

The most common complications are cellulitis, osteomyelitis, and sepsis.

Patient Name____________________Date:________________Time:________

Ulcer 1:			Ulcer 2:		
Site__________			Site__________		
Stage[a]________			Stage[a]________		
Size (cm)			Size (cm)		
Length________			Length________		
Width________			Width________		
Depth________			Depth________		
	No	Yes		No	Yes
Sinus Tract	☐	☐	Sinus Tract	☐	☐
Tunneling	☐	☐	Tunneling	☐	☐
Undermining	☐	☐	Undermining	☐	☐
Necrotic Tissue	☐	☐	Necrotic Tissue	☐	☐
Slough	☐	☐	Slough	☐	☐
Eschar	☐	☐	Eschar	☐	☐
Exudate	☐	☐	Exudate	☐	☐
Serous	☐	☐	Serous	☐	☐
Serosanguineous	☐	☐	Serosanguineous	☐	☐
Purulent	☐	☐	Purulent	☐	☐
Granulation	☐	☐	Granulation	☐	☐
Epithelialization	☐	☐	Epithelialization	☐	☐
Pain	☐	☐	Pain	☐	☐
Surrounding Skin:					
Erythema	☐	☐	Erythema	☐	☐
Maceration	☐	☐	Maceration	☐	☐
Induration	☐	☐	Induration	☐	☐

Description of Ulcer(s):

____

____

Indicate Ulcer Sites:

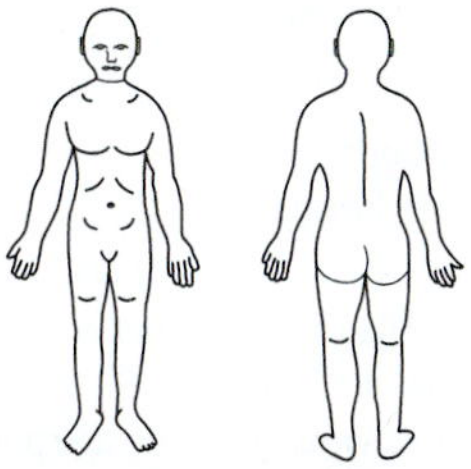

Anterior Posterior

(Attach a color photo of the pressure ulcer[s] [Optional])

[a]Classification of pressure ulcers:

Stage I: Nonblanchable erythema of intact skin, the heralding lesion of skin ulceration. In individuals with darker skin, discoloration of the skin, warmth, edema, induration, or hardness may also be indicators.

Stage II: Partial thickness skin loss, involving epidermis, dermis or both.

Stage III: Full thickness skin loss involving damage to or necrosis of subcutaneous tissue that may extend down to, but not through, underlying fascia. The ulcer presents clinically as a deep crater with or without undermining adjacent tissue.

Stage IV: Full thickness skin loss with extensive destruction, tissue necrosis, or damage to muscle, bone, or supporting structures (e.g., tendon or joint capsule).

Figure 39–1. Pressure ulcer assessment and classification. (From the Agency for Healthcare Research and Quality: *Pressure Ulcer Treatment, Quick Reference Guide for Clinicians.* AHRQ, 1994.)

If local erythema greater than 1 cm occurs around the wound, a topical antibiotic such as sulfasalazine should be used. If the erythema is rapidly expanding, and there is heat, edema, induration, fever, or leukocytosis, the patient should be treated for cellulitis with systemic antibiotics. A superficial wound culture is not helpful because the wound has already been colonized. If there is no improvement or deterioration occurs, a wound culture should be obtained by needle aspiration or punch biopsy.

Osteomyelitis should be suspected in patients with painful and nonhealing ulcers. The technetium-99m bone scan and magnetic resonance imaging (MRI) have equal sensitivity for osteomyelitis; computed tomography (CT) has good specificity, but poor sensitivity. Needle biopsy of bone is the most useful single test for osteomyelitis, with a sensitivity of 73% and a specificity of 96%. Tetanus immunity should be updated.

Finally, sepsis is a serious consequence of infected pressure ulcers and a frequent cause of death, with mortality rates as high as 48%. Currently, there are no US guidelines regarding methicillin-resistant *Staphylococcus aureus* (MRSA) colonization. MRSA has become prevalent in all settings in the United States, including the community, and is commonly found in open wounds. Many institutions currently screen patients by nasal swab. Local practice and national guidelines promulgated by the Centers for Disease Control and Prevention should be reviewed.

Treatment

A. Management of Pressure Ulcers

A stage 1 ulcer should be kept clean and dry. A protective ointment is appropriate. If exposed to friction, a thin transparent film should be used. (Refer to Table 39–5 for product descriptions.) Donut cushions and

Table 39–5. Product list and use.

Product Description	Use	Product Examples
Prevention Products		
Incontinence cleanser	Cleanse perineal area	Periwash, Aloe Vesta Cleansing Foam
Moisture barrier	Protects	Proshield, Aloe Vesta Protective Ointment
Extra protection barrier	Moderate to severe excoriation	Balmex, Desitin, Zinc Oxide, SensiCare
Emollient lotion	Protects dry skin	Lubriderm, Eucerin, Aquaphor
Condom catheters	Contain incontinence	Hollister urinary external catheter
Drainable fecal collector	Contain incontinence	Hollister drainable fecal collector
Retracted penis bag	Contain incontinence	Hollister retracted penis pouch
Wound Treatments		
Wound cleanser	Cleanse wounds	NSS, Dermal wound cleanser
Hydrogel	Moist wound healing	IntraSite, Normlgel, SoloSite, Duoderm Gel
Hydrogel sheet	Moist wound healing: skin tears	Nu-Gel, Vigilon, FlexiGel
Hydrogel-impregnated gauze	Moist wound healing in deeper wounds requiring packing	Carrasyn, Normlgel
Hydrocolloid dressing	Promote moist wound healing and autolytic debridement; should not be used in infected wound or on fragile skin	Duoderm, Thin Duoderm, Restore, Comfeel
NaCl-impregnated dressing	Absorbent dressing; aids in debridement of yellow slough	Mesalt 3×3 and rope for packing
Island dressings	Absorbent semipermeable, self-adhesive, secondary dressing	Alldress 4×4 and 6×6, Primapore
Transparent dressing	Protect from friction and promote moist wound bed; should not be used on fragile skin	Bioclusive, Op-site, Tegaderm, Polyskin
Calcium alginate/hydrofiber/absorbent dressing	Absorbent for high- exudate wounds; should be changed when saturated	Kaltostat, Sorbsan, Aquacel, Melgisorb
Secondary composite cover dressing	Cover for primary dressing	Hydrocolloid, Island Dressing, All Dress
Nonadherent dressing	Skin tears, superficial lacerations	Mepitel, Vaseline gauze, Xeroform gauze, Telfa

From University of Pittsburgh Medical Center, McKeesport Policy and Procedures Manual, 2006.

bunny boots worsen ulcers and should be avoided. Instead, a foam or gel overlay can be used for beds or chairs, and inflatable heel elevators used to protect feet.

Stage 2 ulcers involve loss of the epidermis or dermis but do not break the fascia. If the wound is superficial and clean, a transparent adhesive dressing is appropriate. For wounds involving the dermis with scant to minimal exudate, a hydrocolloid or hydrogel wafer is appropriate. Cleansing of the wound should be done with saline only; old favorites such as hydrogen peroxide, povidone-iodine (Betadine), liquid detergent, acetic acid, and hypochlorite solutions are potentially toxic to both fibroblasts and white blood cells. Cleansing around the wound with a wound cleanser (see Table 39–5) rather than normal saline has been shown to promote healing in stage 2–4 ulcers, with stage 2 gaining the greatest benefit in healing time.

Stage 3 and 4 ulcers require a staged approach. They should first be debrided of devitalized tissue. The only exception to debriding is stable heel ulcers, which should left alone and protected from pressure. Debridement is done mechanically or chemically. Mechanical methods include surgery, saline wet-to-dry dressings, whirlpool, water pic at number 1 setting, or a 35-mL syringe with a 19-gauge catheter. Chemical debridement utilizes enzymes such as collagenase (Santyl) and papain (Accuzyme).

When debridement is accomplished, dressings that maintain a moist environment should be applied (see Table 39–5). If a wound has heavy drainage, alginates such as Sorbsan can be used to absorb exudates and promote healing; the dressings are changed when they become saturated. A moist wound can be protected with hydrogel or hydrogel gauze.

The wound should be checked daily, and documentation of healing performed weekly. A tool to document healing has been developed by the National Pressure Ulcer Advisory Panel. The Pressure Ulcer Status for Healing (PUSH) tool measures three components—size, exudate amount, and tissue type—and is available on-line (see web site at the end of this discussion).

The surface on which the patient is resting affects healing. Pressure-reducing devices are categorized in three groups, and because of the complexity of their use and reimbursement, employing the help of a wound care nurse is worthwhile.

Nutrition should be maximized: 30–40 kcal/kg body weight/day, 1.0–1.5 g protein/kg body weight/day, and minimum fluid intake of 30 mL/kg body weight/day are recommended. Other members of the health team should be involved as needed (eg, dietician, occupational therapist, speech therapist, oral surgeon or dentist). Although supplementation of vitamin C and zinc is commonly recommended, there is no evidence they enhance wound healing, and zinc at 100 mg daily can cause nausea and vomiting. A daily multivitamin is sufficient in most patients.

Pain management is essential. Oral narcotics should be given prior to dressing changes and for persistent wound pain. Topical narcotics such as morphine transdermal gel are also effective and have the added advantage of producing fewer side effects (eg, sedation, constipation) because of minimal systemic absorption.

B. Alternative Therapies

Platelet-derived growth factors, therapeutic ultrasound, electromagnetic therapy, nutritional supplements, hyperbaric oxygen, and infrared, ultraviolet, low–energy, and laser irradiation have not been shown to improve healing in the elderly.

C. Cultural Considerations

Some studies have shown a higher incidence and severity of pressure ulcers in black and Native American populations. Postulated contributing factors are dark skin color and economic factors.

Prognosis

Prognosis varies depending on the stage and circumstance of ulcer formation. In frail elders who have multiple comorbidities, complications, recurrence rates, and mortality are high. Caring for a patient with pressure ulcers is extremely demanding, because the caregiver must perform all the functions of a nurse around the clock. Referral to home health, respite, or hospice services should be considered, when appropriate.

Berlowitz D: Prevention and treatment of pressure ulcers. Available at: UpToDate, http://www.uptodate.com. (This subscription service, which is updated regularly, is well worth cost; includes a detailed overview and extensive references.)

Web Sites

http://www.medicaledu.com: Good resource for professionals learning about wound care, patients and caregivers; easy to navigate.

http://www.ahrq.gov: Source for 1994 guidelines, which are still the standard of care.

http://www.npuap.org.PDF/push3.pdf: Source for the PUSH tool, with instructions on use.

http://borun.medsch.ucla.edu/modules/Pressure_ulcer_prevention: Up-to-date site with an easy-to-use training module for nurses in long-term care as well as links, including the Braden scale.

FALLS

General Considerations

Falls are a serious public health problem for older adults. More than one third of community-dwelling elders fall each year, and of those, 20–30% suffer moderate to severe injuries such as hip fractures and head trauma that reduce mobility and independence. The cost of falls was estimated at $27.3 billion in 1994 and is projected to reach $32.4 billion by 2020. In 2003, more than 1.8 million seniors aged 65 years and older were treated in emergency departments for fall-related injuries, and more than 421,000 were hospitalized. In addition to physical injuries, falls have psychological and social consequences. Fear of falling, anxiety, social isolation, and loss of self-confidence contribute to a lower quality of life, and the reduction in mobility and independence are often serious enough to result in admission to a hospital or a nursing home or even premature death.

Pathogenesis

Most falls in older people result from the interaction of multiple factors, both intrinsic (age-related physiologic changes, medications, gait or balance disturbance) and extrinsic (environmental hazards, footwear). Whether the physician is addressing falls during the acute visit for which it is the chief complaint or for those at risk identified by geriatric assessment, a multidimensional approach is warranted. A practical working construct incorporates (1) postural stability, (2) medical comorbidities, (3) overall function, and (4) environment.

Postural stability is maintained in three phases: input, processing, and output. Input includes vision, vestibular apparatus, and proprioception. Processing requires an intact nervous system: both central processing and competent efferent command. Output requires a motor system characterized by strength, flexibility, absence of pain, and cardiovascular endurance. Impairment of any one increases the risk for falls, and the risk is cumulative. Conversely, interventions to modify any of these impairments will decrease the risk for falls.

Chronic diseases, and the medications used to treat them, constitute the second key area of assessment. Conditions and drugs that affect the components of postural stability are suspect, and there are usually more than one.

Finally, the concept of functional thresholds places the data into a framework that identifies the point at which a particular patient exceeds his or her compensatory abilities. A detailed history and focused physical and performance examination will provide key information about function. For frail elders, who most commonly fall at home, a home assessment completes the evaluation.

Prevention

Falls like other syndromes of the elderly, are multifactorial and require a multidisciplinary approach. Assessment that identifies intrinsic and extrinsic causes helps focus targeted interventions. A team approach that incorporates the patient, specialists (physiatrist, ophthalmologist, optometrist, podiatrist, orthopedist), and occupational and physical therapists will maximize outcomes.

Table 39–6. Evidence-based strategies to reduce fall risk.

Muscle-strengthening and balance-retraining program prescribed by a trained health professional
Tai chi group exercise program (15 wk)
Home hazard assessment and modification prescribed for patients with history of falling
Withdrawal of psychotropic medications
Cardiac pacing for at-risk elders with cardioinhibitory carotid sinus hypersensitivity
Multidisciplinary, multifactorial, health-environmental risk factor screening and intervention programs for patients in the community
Multidisciplinary assessment and intervention program for patients in residential care facilities

A systematic review of scientific studies has identified several evidenced-based strategies, targeting both intrinsic and environmental risk factors, that are likely to be beneficial in preventing falls (Table 39–6). Risk reduction should also include advice on appropriate footwear (hard-soled, flat, closed-toed shoes), adequate lighting for all activities, and caution with any activity that requires balance. For example, elderly persons should not climb stairs without a hand on the railing, and stairs should be well lit and in good repair. Climbing ladders should be discouraged. Robust elders should be cautioned about activities (skiing, skating, etc) that increase the risk for falls, hence putting them at higher risk for fractures. Patients identified as having balance difficulties or who have had multiple falls will benefit from muscle strengthening and balance retraining. When possible, medications should be reduced and psychotropic agents eliminated. Assistive devices may prevent falls when used correctly within a targeted intervention. Hip protectors may be necessary to prevent serious injuries such as hip fractures. Environmental modification is of known benefit as part of an overall targeted intervention in the subgroup of older patients who are at known risk for falls (see later discussion).

Additional interventions that may or may not prove beneficial are listed in Table 39–7.

Clinical Findings

A. Symptoms and Signs

The history should elicit the exact details and circumstances surrounding the fall as precisely as possible. Unfortunately, patients often have vague descriptions of their fall. Additional details from a third party may

Table 39–7. Interventions of unknown effectiveness in mitigating risk of falls.

Home hazard modification in older persons without a history of falling, in association with advice on optimizing medication or in association with education on exercise and reducing falls
Individual lower limb strength training
Group exercise program
Nutritional supplementation
Vitamin D supplementation with or without calcium.[1]
Cognitive-behavioral approaches
Pharmacotherapy with raubasine-dihydroergocristine
Hormone replacement therapy
Use of restraints

[1]Authors' recommendation: Checking vitamin D in patients with decreased muscle strength is reasonable; supplementation is inexpensive and safe.

be very useful. The clinician should ask questions regarding when the fall or near-fall occurred (time of the day, pre- or post-prandial), where the patient was (indoors, outdoors), what the patient was doing (climbing stairs, turning, reaching, stooping, micturition), whether there was pain (severe arthritis) or other symptoms (chest pain, shortness of breath, dizziness or lightheadedness, vertigo, diaphoresis, numbness and weakness of extremities, loss of consciousness), what medications were taken (prescription, over the counter), and whether the patient had ingested alcohol.

The patient's subjective complaints relating to instability or the fall can be very helpful in pinpointing the cause. Light-headedness or a near-faint is consistent with cerebral ischemia and suggests orthostasis, arrhythmias, and other cardiovascular conditions as contributing factors. Muscular weakness—the sense that the legs cannot hold them up—is more consistent with deconditioning or neuromuscular disease. Dysequilibrium—the sensation of no coordination between the legs and the walking surface—is suggestive of vestibulospinal tract, proprioception, somatosensory, and cerebellar lesions. Finally, the sensation of movement within the patient or of the room spinning is true vertigo.

Table 39–8 lists chronic conditions and medications that can contribute to postural instability and falls.

Table 39–8. Conditions and drugs that increase risk for falls.

Medical Conditions	Medications
Syncope	Polypharmacy (more than four medications)
Seizures	Psychotropics
Orthostasis	Benzodiazepines, short and long acting
Dysrhythmia	Narcotics
Vertebrobasilar insufficiency	Antiarrhythmics
Cervical degeneration	Digoxin
Carotid sinus syndrome	Diuretics
Vertigo	Selective serotonin reuptake inhibitors
Parkinson disease	Tricyclic antidepressants
Movement disorder	Antihypertensives
Cerebrovascular accident	Anticholinergics
Intracranial mass or hydrocephalus	Other: alcohol
Peripheral neuropathy	
Myopathy	
Deconditioning from any cause	
Pain	
History of previous falls	
Vision impairment	
Depression	
Cognitive impairment	

B. Physical Examination

The physical examination should be problem focused as noted in Table 39–9.

C. Performance Assessment

When approaching performance assessment, it is helpful to categorize the patient as frail, intermediate, or robust. Vigorous elders usually fall outside the home, while engaging in complicated activities such as stair climbing or challenging themselves with tasks that displace the center of mass. Frail elders generally fall at home while performing activities of daily living. Most studies show equal injury rates in both, although the frail fall more often. Gait speed is currently the best predictor of mobility problems and correlates with future disability in activities of daily living.

Elderly patients who are robust should be asked to tandem walk and stand on one leg with the other leg flexed for 30 seconds. If they have no problems, risk reduction counseling is all they need. If they have difficulty, the physician's focus should be on peripheral neuropathy as a potential and remediable cause. Its onset is insidious, it affects an estimated 20% of elders, and it significantly increases risk of falling. Intermediate patients should be asked to climb stairs, step over objects, and rise from a chair with their arms folded and stand on one leg for 10 seconds. The 10-second stand is a more sensitive screening test than the Romberg test. Difficulty with these tasks may represent deconditioning, a neuromuscular disorder, or peripheral neuropathy.

Frail elders should be asked to perform the "Up and Go" and functional reach tests. The timed "Up and Go" is a simple, well-validated office tool for assessing gait and balance disturbance in frail elders. The patient sits in a straight-back chair, then rises and walks 10 meters, turns, walks back, and sits on the chair. The

Table 39–9. Focused physical examination for patients at risk of falls.

Vital signs: orthostatic blood pressure and heart rate, sitting and standing. Pulse for 1 min.

Height: loss of height and kyphosis indicate osteoporosis. Intervention may reduce fracture risk.

Body mass index: if below 21, patient is at risk of malnutrition and/or depression. Decreased padding leads to increased injury risk.

Vision: visual acuity, field testing, pupillary size, depth perception. Visual field loss and depth perception have a much greater impact on mobility and vision function than acuity. Dark adaptation time increases with age and is contingent on pupil size; lens opacification and duration and brightness of light aggravate the problem further.[1] An annual ophthalmological examination is recommended for all elders; alert the ophthalmologist to your concerns.

Vestibular function: have patient march in place with eyes closed. Abnormal response is moving more than a few degrees or moving more than a foot in any direction.[2]

Cardiovascular: assess for dysrhythmia, valvular disease, congestive heart failure.

Neuromuscular

Proximal muscle weakness suggests polymyalgia rheumatica, polymyositis, adrenal, thyroid, or parathyroid disease.

Distal muscle weakness is more suggestive of peripheral neuropathy.

Peripheral neuropathy: up to 20% of elders will have peripheral neuropathy: common causes are diabetes, alcohol, chronic lung disease, monoclonal gammopathy, neoplasm, medication (dilantin, lithium, isoniazid, vincristine), renal disease, thyroid disease, and vitamin B_{12} deficiency. Neuropathy occurs before weakness or ataxia. Further testing includes vibratory sense: patients should be able to feel a 128-Hz tuning fork at the malleolus for 10 s. Absence of position sense and heel jerk helps confirm the diagnosis.[3]

Generalized muscle weakness: consider toxic myopathy from alcohol, glucocorticoids, HMG coenzyme A reductase inhibitors, and colchicine. Atrophy suggests deconditioning; overall weakness suggests electrolyte imbalance.

Muscle tone and postural reflexes should be assessed to rule out Parkinson's disease or movement disorders.

Range of motion: joint, neck, spine, hip, knee, and ankle should be assessed; restriction impairs reflex time and precision. Cervical spondylosis is a significant cause of falls.

Feet: in addition to peripheral neuropathy, check for deformities such as bunions, calluses, ulcers, hammertoes, and nail pathology. Achilles reflex suggests peripheral neuropathy but is absent in up to 70% of normal aged individuals.[4] Note footwear; thick, soft-soled shoes increase fall risk.

Cognitive ability can be screened by three-item recall, Mini-mental status examination, or clock draw.

[1]Maino JH: Visual deficits and mobility: Evaluation and management. Clin Geriatr Med 1996;12:803.
[2]Studenski S, Rigler SK: Clinical overview of instability in the elderly. Clin Geriatr Med 1996;12:679.
[3]Richardson JK, Ashton-Miller JA: Peripheral neuropathy, an often overlooked cause of falls in the elderly. Postgrad Med 1996;99:161.
[4]Klein RB, Knoefel JE: Neurologic problems in the elderly. In: Reichel's Care of the Elderly, Clinical Aspects of Aging, ed 5. Gallo J et al (editors). Lippincott Williams & Wilkins, 1999.
See King MB, Tinetti ME: A multifactorial approach to reducing injurious falls. Clin Geriatr Med 1996;12:745; Berg K, Norman KE: Functional assessment of balance and gait. Clin Geriatr Med 1996;12:705; and Alexander N: Differential diagnosis of gait disorders in older adults. Clin Geriatr Med 1996;12:689.

patient may use whatever assistive device he or she normally uses and should be allowed one trial before being timed. Completion of the test in less than 10 seconds represents no risk and can be expected from nonfrail elders. A score of 10–19 seconds represents minimal risk; 20–29 seconds, moderate risk; and more than 30 seconds, a definite risk for falling. Referral to physical therapy is warranted for any patient whose score is 20 seconds or more.

The functional reach test can also be used to assess balance. The patient is asked to stand with one shoulder close to the wall, extend the fist along the wall directly forward, and then lean forward, fist extended in front as far as possible without taking a step or losing balance. The patient should be able to move the fist forward a distance of 6 inches. A lesser distance represents a significant risk for falls.

D. Laboratory and Imaging Evaluation

Although the role of laboratory testing in the prevention of falls has not been well established, it may be reasonable to perform the following studies on persons who are at high risk for falling: complete blood count, serum electrolyte levels, blood urea nitrogen, creatinine, glucose, vitamin B_{12}, 25-hydroxyvitamin D level and thyroid function tests. Results of these studies may identify treatable causes.

Neuroimaging can be useful in patients with head injuries or a new neurologic deficit identified by history and physical examination. Electroencephalography is rarely helpful but may be indicated if there is high suspicion of seizure. Patients with unexplained falls may benefit from ambulatory electrocardiography (Holter monitor), although this has been associated with high false-positive and false-negative results.

Table 39–10. Environmental checklist: Risk of falls.

Approach outside: uneven sidewalk or walkway, exterior lighting, steps, ease of opening screen/storm/front door, proximity of steps to front door, ease of unlocking door.
Interior lighting: especially on stairs and thresholds, loose electrical cords, accessibility of light switches.
Carpets: scatter rugs, frayed or worn or high-pile carpets.
Floors: slippery, polished, unkempt (water, oil, clutter).
Bathroom: toilet height and ease of use, grab bars or bilateral grab bars if needed, bathing site including ease of entry, lighting, surface features, visibility of shower threshold. For overall safety ask about water temperature at this time; should be no more than 120°F (48.8°C).
Kitchen: location of most commonly used items, reaching and stooping, unstable stools, chair, or pedestal or glass table. Smoke alarm.
Stairs: lighting, handrail, condition of steps, ease of use, nonskid surface.
Furnishings: sharp edges, location in trafficked areas, height of bed and chairs.
Assistive devices: good repair, appropriate height for patient, stored out of the way when not in use.

See Connell BR: Role of the environment in falls prevention. Clin Geriatr Med 1996;12:859 and Scanameo AM, Fillit H: House calls: A practical guide to seeing the patient at home. Geriatrics 1995;50(3):33.

E. Environmental Assessment

A home assessment is warranted for frail elders, and for anyone who has fallen at home. Although the evidence is mixed on the effectiveness of modifying the home environment after a fall, prudence dictates that anyone discharged from the hospital after a fall should have a home evaluation as part of a multidimensional targeted intervention. This may be done by the physician or occupational therapist and should include the environment itself as well as a replay of the circumstances of the fall (Table 39–10).

For frail patients, a review of their activities in the home can be informative. The patient should be asked to simulate daily activities, from getting out of bed to navigating the bathroom, kitchen, and basement stairs, to entering and leaving the house, including locking the door. The more frail the individual, the greater is the benefit of reducing environmental demands (eg, through redesign of the environment and use of assistive devices). Any modification that both reduces risk and allows for maintenance of the patient's activities of daily living is of benefit.

Gillespie LD et al: Interventions for preventing falls in elderly people. Cochrane Database Syst Rev 2005;(1):CD000340. [PMID: 11686957]

Maino JH: Visual deficits and mobility: Evaluation and management. Clin Geriatr Med 1996;12:803. [PMID: 8890117]

Rao SS: Prevention of falls in older patients. Am Fam Physician 2005;72:81. [PMID: 16035686]

Tinetti ME: Clinical practice. Preventing falls in elderly persons. N Engl J Med 2003;348:42. [PMID: 12510042]

Web Sites

American Geriatrics Society (an excellent resource for clinicians and patients. Provides a comprehensive toolkit to help physicians understand falls; educational materials for patients; suggested guidelines; and forms and tools for evaluation, diagnosis, and treatment):

http://www.americangeriatrics.org/staging/education/falls.shtml

National Center for Injury Prevention and Control (provides a home safety check list, fall prevention checklist, and other educational materials):

http://www.cdc.gov/ncipc/falls

US Consumer Product Safety Commission (provides a checklist that can be used by patients and clinicians to assess the presence of extrinsic, situational, and environmental factors that cause falls, with recommendations):

http://cpsc.gov/

Urinary Incontinence

40

Robert J. Carr, MD

General Considerations

Urinary incontinence is the involuntary loss of urine that is so severe as to have social or hygienic consequences. It is very common, with a prevalence in community-dwelling elderly persons as high as 35%, and significantly higher rates among institutionalized patients. Despite this high prevalence, studies have shown that about half of all incontinent persons have never discussed the problem with a physician. This is likely because of embarrassment, a belief that incontinence is normal with aging, or an assumption that nothing can be done to help. Incontinence is associated with significant medical morbidity, including infection, sepsis, pressure ulcers, and falls. It is also associated with significant psychological stress and social isolation. Incontinence causes significant caregiver burden, and is frequently cited as a reason for deciding to abandon home care efforts in favor of nursing home placement. The economic burden of incontinence is also substantial, with an estimated direct cost in the United States of $16.3 billion per year.

Because of its high prevalence, significant morbidity, and high psychosocial impact, it is important for family physicians to accurately identify, assess, and treat incontinent patients. The large majority of patients with incontinence can be diagnosed and managed effectively by family physicians in the primary care setting.

A. Physiology of Normal Urination

A basic understanding of the normal physiology of urination is important to understand the potential causes of incontinence, and the various strategies for effective treatment.

The lower urinary tract consists primarily of the bladder (detrusor muscle) and the urethra. The urethra contains two sphincters, the internal urethral sphincter (IUS), composed predominantly of smooth muscle, and the external urethral sphincter (EUS), which is primarily voluntary muscle. The detrusor muscle of the bladder is innervated predominantly by cholinergic (muscarinic) neurons from the parasympathetic nervous system, the stimulation of which leads to bladder contraction. The sympathetic nervous system innervates both the bladder and the IUS. Sympathetic innervation in the bladder is primarily β-adrenergic and leads to bladder relaxation, whereas α-adrenergic receptors predominate in the IUS, leading to sphincter contraction. Thus, in general, sympathetic stimulation of the urinary tract promotes bladder filling (relaxation of the detrusor with contraction of the sphincter), whereas parasympathetic stimulation leads to bladder emptying (detrusor contraction and sphincter relaxation).

The EUS, on the other hand, is striated muscle and primarily under voluntary (somatic) control. This allows for some ability to voluntarily postpone urination by tightening the sphincter and inhibiting the flow of urine. Additional voluntary control is provided by the central nervous system through the pontine micturition center. This allows for central inhibition of the autonomic processes previously described, and for further voluntary postponement of the need to urinate until the circumstances are more socially appropriate or until necessary facilities are available.

The physiologic factors influencing normal urination are summarized in Table 40–1 and are important considerations when discussing urinary disorders and treatment.

B. Age-Related Changes

Contrary to common perception, urinary incontinence is not inevitable with aging. Most elderly patients remain continent throughout their lifetimes, and a complaint of incontinence at any age should receive a thorough evaluation and not be dismissed as "normal for age." Nonetheless, many common age-related changes predispose elderly patients to incontinence and increase the likelihood of its development with advancing age.

The frequency of involuntary bladder contractions (detrusor hyperactivity) increases in both men and women with aging. In addition, total bladder capacity decreases, causing the voiding urge to occur at lower volumes. Bladder contractility decreases, leading to increased postvoid residuals and increased sensation of urgency or fullness. Elderly patients excrete a larger percentage of their fluid volume later in the day than younger persons. This, in addition to the other changes listed, often leads to an increase in the incidence of nocturia with aging, and more frequent nighttime awakenings.

In women, menopausal estrogen decline leads to urogenital atrophy and a decrease in the sensitivity of

Table 40–1. Physiologic factors influencing normal urination.

Bladder filling	Sympathetic nervous system	β-Adrenergic	Detrusor relaxation
		α-Adrenergic	IUS contraction
Bladder emptying	Parasympathetic nervous system	Cholinergic	Detrusor contraction
Voluntary control	Somatic nervous system	Striated muscle	EUS contraction
	Central nervous system	Pontine micturition center	Central inhibition of urinary reflex

IUS, internal urethral sphincter; EUS, external urethral sphincter.

α-receptors in the IUS. In men, prostatic hypertrophy can lead to increased urethral resistance, and varying degrees of urethral obstruction.

It is important to remember that these age-related changes are found in many healthy, continent persons as well as those who develop incontinence. It is not completely understood why the predisposition to urinary problems is stronger in some patients than in others, which emphasizes the multifactorial basis of incontinence.

Clinical Findings

A. Symptoms and Signs

1. Incontinence outside the urinary tract—Incontinence is often classified based on whether it is related to specific urogenital pathology or to factors outside the urinary tract. Terms such as *transient* versus *established, acute* versus *persistent,* and *primary* versus *secondary* have been used to highlight this distinction. The mnemonic DIAPPERS is helpful in remembering the many causes of incontinence that occur outside the urinary tract (Table 40–2). These "extraurinary" causes are very common in the elderly, and it is important to identify or rule them out before proceeding to a more invasive search for primary urogenital etiologies.

Delirium, depression, and disorders of excessive urinary output generally require medical or behavioral management of the primary cause rather than strategies relating to the bladder. Once the primary causes are corrected, the incontinence often resolves. Urinary tract infections, although easily treated if discovered, are a relatively infrequent cause of urinary incontinence in the absence of other classic symptoms (dysuria, urgency, frequency, etc). Asymptomatic bacteriuria, which is common even in well elderly, does not cause incontinence.

Pharmaceuticals are a particularly important and very common cause of incontinence. Because of the many neural receptors involved in urination (see Table 40–1), it is easy to understand why so many medications used to treat other common problems can readily affect continence. Medications frequently associated with incontinence are listed in Table 40–3. Many of these medications are available over the counter and in combination (Table 40–4). In addition, commonly used substances such as caffeine and alcohol can contribute to incontinence by virtue of their diuretic effects or the effects they have on mental status. Because of this, some medications and substances associated with a patient's incontinence may not be considered important or readily volunteered during a medication history unless the physician specifically asks about them.

Restricted mobility or the inability to physically get to the bathroom in time to avoid incontinence is also referred to as "functional" incontinence. The incontinence may be temporary or chronic, depending on the nature of the physical or cognitive disability involved. Physical therapy or strength and flexibility training may be helpful, as well as simple measures such as a bedside commode or urinal.

Stool impaction is very common in the elderly and may cause incontinence both through its local mass effect and by stimulation of opioid receptors in the bowel. It has been reported to be a causative factor in up to 10% of patients referred to incontinence clinics for evaluation. Continence can often be restored by a simple disimpaction.

2. Urologic causes of incontinence—Once secondary or transient causes have been investigated and ruled out, further evaluation should focus on specific urologic pathology that may be causing incontinence.

Table 40–2. Causes of urinary incontinence without specific urogenital pathology.[1]

D	Delirium/confusional state
I	Infection (symptomatic)
A	Atrophic urethritis/vaginitis
P	Pharmaceuticals
P	Psychiatric causes (especially depression)
E	Excessive urinary output (hyperglycemia, hypercalcemia, congestive heart failure)
R	Restricted mobility
S	Stool impaction

[1]Also known as transient, acute, or secondary incontinence.

Table 40–3. Pharmaceuticals contributing to incontinence.

Pharmaceutical	Mechanism	Effect
α-Adrenergic agonists	IUS contraction	Urinary retention
α-Adrenergic blockers	IUS relaxation	Urinary leakage
Anticholinergic agents Antidepressants Antihistamines Antipsychotics Sedatives	Inhibit bladder contraction, sedation, immobility	Urinary retention and/or functional incontinence
β-Adrenergic agonists	Inhibits bladder contraction	Urinary retention
β-Adrenergic blockers	Inhibits bladder relaxation	Urinary leakage, urgency
Calcium channel blockers	Relaxes bladder	Urinary retention
Diuretics	Increases urinary frequency, urgency	Polyuria
Narcotic analgesics	Relaxes bladder, fecal impaction, sedation	Urinary retention and/or functional incontinence

IUS, internal urethral sphincter.

The urinary tract has two basic functions: the emptying of urine during voiding and the storage of urine between voiding. A defect in either of these basic functions can cause incontinence, and it is useful to initially classify incontinence by whether it is primarily a defect of storage or of emptying. An *inability to store* urine occurs when the bladder contracts too often (or at inappropriate times), or when the sphincter(s) cannot contract sufficiently to allow the bladder to store urine and keep it from leaking. Thus the bladder rarely, if ever, fills to capacity and the patient's symptoms are generally characterized by frequent incontinent episodes of relatively small volume. An *inability to empty* urine occurs when the bladder is unable to contract appropriately, or when the outlet or sphincter(s) is partially obstructed (either physically or physiologically). Thus the bladder continues to fill beyond its normal capacity and eventually overflows, causing the patient to experience abdominal distention and continual or frequent leakage.

Determining whether the primary problem is the inability to store or the inability to empty can often be done easily during the history and physical examination based on the patient's pattern of incontinence (intermittent or continuous) and whether abdominal (bladder) distention is present. Determination of postvoid residual is also helpful in making this distinction (see Physical Examination, later). This initial classification is important in narrowing down the specific etiology of

Table 40–4. Nonprescription agents contributing to incontinence.

Agent	Mechanism	Effect	Common Examples
Alcohol	Diuretic effect, sedation, immobility	Polyuria and/or functional incontinence	Beer, wine, liquor, some liquid cold medicines
α-Agonists	IUS contraction	Urinary retention	Decongestants, diet pills
Antihistamines	Inhibit bladder contraction, sedation	Urinary retention and/or functional incontinence	Allergy tablets, sleeping pills, antinausea medications
α-Agonist/antihistamine combinations	IUS contraction *and* inhibition of bladder contraction	Marked urinary retention	Multisymptom cold tablets
Caffeine	Diuretic effect	Polyuria	Coffee, soft drinks, analgesics

IUS, internal urethral sphincter.

Table 40–5. Types and classification of urinary incontinence.

Underlying Defect	Symptomatic Classification	Most Common Urodynamics	Possible Etiologies
Inability to store urine	Urge (U)	Detrusor hyperactivity	Uninhibited contractions; local irritation (cystitis, stone, tumor); central nervous system causes
	Stress (S)	Sphincter incompetence	Urethral hypermobility; sphincter damage (trauma, radiation, surgery)
Inability to empty urine	Overflow (O)	Outlet obstruction	Physical (benign prostatic hyperplasia, tumor, stricture); neurologic lesions, medications
		Detrusor hypoactivity	Neurogenic bladder (diabetes, alcoholism, disc disease)
	Functional (F)	Normal	Immobility problems; cognitive deficits
	Mixed	U + S, U + F	

the incontinence, and in ultimately deciding on the appropriate management strategy.

3. Symptomatic classification—Once it is determined whether the primary problem is with storage or with emptying, incontinence can be further classified according to the type of symptoms that it causes in the patient. The most common categories are discussed below. The first two types, urge incontinence and stress incontinence, result from an inability to store urine. The third type, overflow incontinence, results from an inability to empty urine. A patient may have a single type of incontinence, or a combination of more than one type (mixed incontinence). Table 40–5 summarizes the major categories of incontinence, the underlying urodynamic findings, and the most common etiologies for each.

a. Urge incontinence—Urge incontinence is the most common type of incontinence in the elderly. Patients complain of a strong, and often immediate, urge to void followed by an involuntary loss of urine. It is often not possible to reach the bathroom in time to avoid incontinence once the urge occurs, and patients often lose urine while rushing toward a bathroom or trying to locate one. Urge incontinence is most frequently caused by involuntary contractions of the bladder, often referred to as *detrusor instability.* These involuntary contractions increase in frequency with age, as does the ability to voluntarily inhibit them. Although the symptoms of urgency are a hallmark feature of this type of incontinence, detrusor instability can sometimes result in incontinence without these symptoms. Although most patients with detrusor instability are neurologically normal, uninhibited contractions can also occur as the result of neurologic disorders such as stroke, dementia, or spinal cord injury. In these cases it is often referred to as *detrusor hyperreflexia.* Detrusor instability and urgency can also be caused by local irritation of the bladder as with infection, bladder stones, or tumors. The term *overactive bladder syndrome* (OABS) is now commonly used to describe the symptoms of urgency caused by detrusor instability and to emphasize that they can occur either with *or without* incontinence. OABS is described by the International Continence Society as voiding eight or more times during a 24-hour period, and awakening two or more times during the night. Treatment of OABS is similar whether or not incontinence is present.

b. Stress incontinence—Stress incontinence is much more common among women than men and is defined as a loss of urine associated with increases in intra-abdominal pressure (Valsalva maneuver). Patients complain of leakage of urine (usually small amounts) during coughing, laughing, sneezing, or exercising. In women, stress incontinence is most often caused by urethral hypermobility resulting from weakness of the pelvic floor musculature, but it can also be caused by intrinsic weakness of the urethral sphincter(s), most commonly following trauma, radiation, or surgery. Stress incontinence is rare in men, unless they have suffered damage to the sphincter through surgery or trauma. In making the diagnosis of stress incontinence, it is important to ascertain that the leakage occurs exactly *coincident with* the stress maneuver. If the leakage occurs several seconds after the maneuver, it is more likely caused by an uninhibited bladder contraction that has been triggered by the stress maneuver, and is urodynamically more similar to urge incontinence. This is sometimes known as *stress-induced detrusor instability.*

c. Overflow incontinence—Overflow incontinence is a loss of urine associated with overdistention of the bladder. Patients complain of frequent or constant leakage or dribbling, or they may lose large amounts of urine without warning. Overflow incontinence may result either from a defect in the bladder's ability to contract (*detrusor hypoactivity*) or from obstruction of the bladder outlet or urethra. Detrusor hypoactivity is most commonly the result of a *neurogenic bladder* secondary to diabetes mellitus, chronic alcoholism, or disc disease. It can also be caused by medications, primarily muscle relaxants and β-adrenergic blockers. Outlet obstruction can be physical (prostatic enlargement, tumor, stricture), neurologic (spinal cord lesions, pelvic surgery), or pharmacologic (α-adrenergic agonists). Because neurogenic bladder is relatively rare in the geriatric population, it is important to rule out possible causes of obstruction whenever the diagnosis of overflow incontinence is made.

d. Functional incontinence—The term *functional incontinence* is used to describe physical or cognitive impairments that interfere with continence even in patients with normal urinary tracts (see Restricted Mobility and Table 40–2, the DIAPPERS mnemonic, earlier).

e. Mixed incontinence—*Mixed incontinence* describes various combinations of the preceding four types. When present, it can make the diagnosis and management of incontinence more difficult. The term is most frequently used to describe patients who present with a combination of stress and urge incontinence, although other combinations are also possible. Functional incontinence, for example, can coexist with stress, urge, or overflow incontinence, further complicating the treatment of these patients. Side effects of medications being used to treat other comorbidities can also cause a mixed picture when combined with underlying incontinence of any type. Mixed stress and urge incontinence is particularly common among elderly women. When present, it is helpful to focus on the symptom that is most bothersome to the patient, and to direct the initial therapeutic interventions in that direction.

B. History and Physical Findings

The history and physical examination of a patient presenting with incontinence should have the following goals:

1. To evaluate for and rule out causes of incontinence outside the urinary tract (DIAPPERS).
2. To determine whether the primary defect is an inability to store urine or an inability to empty urine.
3. To determine the type of incontinence based on the patient's symptoms and likely etiologies.
4. To determine the pattern of incontinence episodes and its effect on the patient's functional ability and quality of life.

1. History—A thorough medical history should include a special focus on the neurologic and genitourinary history of the patient as well as any other medical problems that may be contributing factors (see Table 40–2). Information on any previous evaluation(s) for incontinence, as well as their degree of success or failure, can be helpful in guiding the current evaluation and in determining patient expectations. A careful medication history is very important, focusing on the categories of medications listed in Table 40–3 and remembering to include nonprescription substances (see Table 40–4). Finally, the pattern of incontinence is important in helping to classify its type and in planning appropriate therapy. This includes episode frequency, timing, precipitating factors, and volume of urine lost as well as a determination of the symptoms that are most bothersome to the patient and their impact on his or her life. A voiding diary or bladder record can be a very useful tool in obtaining this information. The patient or caregiver is given a set of forms and is asked to keep a written record of each incontinent episode for several days. A sample form is shown in Table 40–6. Incontinent episodes are recorded in terms of time, estimated volume (small or large), and precipitating factors. Fluid intake, as well as any episodes of urination in the toilet, is also recorded. When completed accurately, the bladder record can often elucidate the most likely type of incontinence and provide a clue to possible precipitating factors. Continuous leakage, for example, may be more consistent with overflow incontinence, whereas multiple, large-volume episodes may be more consistent with urge. Smaller volume episodes associated with coughing or exercise may be more consistent with stress incontinence, whereas incontinence occurring only at specific times each day may suggest an association with a medication or other non–urinary tract cause. Although other information from the physical and laboratory evaluations will obviously be needed, the physician can often make significant progress toward determining the type of incontinence and possible precipitating factors from the history and voiding record alone.

2. Physical examination—In addition to a thorough search for nonurologic causes of incontinence, the physical examination should focus on the abdominal, genital, and rectal areas. Evidence of bladder distention on abdominal examination should raise suspicion for overflow incontinence. Genital examination should include a pelvic examination in women to assess for evidence of atrophy or mass, as well as any signs of uterine prolapse, cystocele, or rectocele. A rectal examination is helpful in ruling out stool impaction or mass, as well as in evaluating sphincter tone and perineal sensation for evidence of a neurologic deficit. A prostate examination is usually included, but several studies have demonstrated a poor correlation between prostate size and urinary obstruction. A neurologic examination focusing on the lumbosacral area is helpful in ruling out a spinal cord lesion or other neurologic deficits.

3. Special tests—Two additional tests, specific to the diagnosis of incontinence, should be added to the general physical examination.

Table 40–6. Sample voiding record.

Bladder Record

Name:

Date:

Instructions: Place a check in the appropriate column next to the time you urinated in the toilet or when an incontinence episode occurred. Note the reason for the incontinence and describe your liquid intake (for example, coffee, water) and estimate the amount (for example, one cup).

Time interval	Urinated in toilet	Had a small incontinent episode	Had a large incontinent episode	Reason for incontinent episode	Type/amount of liquid intake
6–8 a.m.					
8–10 a.m.					
10–noon					
Noon–2 p.m.					
2–4 p.m.					
4–6 p.m.					
6–8 p.m.					
8–10 p.m.					
10–midnight					
Overnight					

Number of pads used today: ______________________

Number of episodes: ______________________

Comments:

a. Provocative stress testing—This test attempts to reproduce the symptoms of incontinence under the direct visualization of the physician and is useful in differentiating stress from urge incontinence. The patient should have a full bladder and preferably be in a standing position (although a lithotomy position is also acceptable for patients unable to stand). The patient should be told to relax, and then to cough vigorously while the physician observes for urine loss. If leakage occurs simultaneously with the cough, a diagnosis of stress incontinence is likely. A delay between the cough and the leakage is more likely caused by a reflex bladder contraction and is more consistent with urge incontinence.

b. Postvoid residual (PVR)—This measurement should be obtained for incontinent patients suspected of urinary retention and potential obstruction. PVR measurement is traditionally done by urinary catheterization; however, portable ultrasound scanners for this purpose are now available that also provide very accurate readings. These ultrasound devices minimize the risks of instrumentation and infection that are inherent in catheterization, especially in male patients. Prior to measurement, the patient should be asked to empty the bladder as completely as possible. Measurement of residual urine in the bladder should be made within a few minutes after emptying using either in-and-out catheterization or ultrasound. A PVR of less than

50 mL is normal; more than 200 mL indicates inadequate bladder emptying and is consistent with overflow incontinence. PVRs between 50 and 199 mL can sometimes be normal but may also exist with overflow incontinence, and results should be interpreted in light of the clinical picture. Patients with elevated PVRs should generally be referred for further evaluation and to rule out obstruction prior to treatment of the incontinence symptoms.

c. Other diagnostic maneuvers—Other maneuvers, or "bedside urodynamics," have often been recommended to help in the diagnosis of incontinence. The best known of these are the Q-tip test to diagnose pelvic laxity and the Bonney (Marshall) test to determine whether surgical intervention will be helpful. Although these tests may be useful in some settings, recent studies have cast doubt on their predictive value, and in the family practice setting they are unlikely to add clinically useful information to that obtained from the history and physical examination as previously described. Likewise, bedside urodynamics to assess bladder contractions and function will not likely add useful information to help in sorting out the small percentage of patients whose diagnosis remains unclear after a thorough history and physical examination.

C. Laboratory and Imaging Evaluation

Like the history and physical examination, the laboratory evaluation should be focused on ruling out the nonurologic causes of incontinence. A urinalysis is very helpful in screening for infection as well as in evaluating for hematuria, proteinuria, or glucosuria. It must be remembered, however, that asymptomatic bacteriuria is very common in the elderly and is not a cause of incontinence. Antibiotic treatment of asymptomatic bacteriuria has not been shown to reduce morbidity or to improve incontinence either in the institutionalized elderly or in ambulatory women. Thus antibiotic treatment in the face of incontinence and bacteriuria should be reserved for patients whose incontinence is of recent onset, has recently worsened, or is accompanied by other signs of infection. Hematuria, in the absence of infection, should be referred for further evaluation to rule out carcinoma.

Additional laboratory studies that are recommended and may be helpful include measurement of renal function (blood urea nitrogen and creatinine) and evaluation for metabolic causes of polyuria (hypercalcemia, hyperglycemia). Radiologic studies are not routinely recommended in the initial evaluation of most patients with incontinence; however, a renal ultrasound study is useful in patients with obstruction to evaluate for hydronephrosis.

Abrutyn E et al: Does asymptomatic bacteriuria predict mortality and does antimicrobial treatment reduce mortality in elderly ambulatory women? Ann Intern Med 1994;121:827. [PMID: 7818631]

Fantl JA et al: Urinary incontinence in adults: Acute and chronic management. Clinical Practice Guideline No. 2, 1996 Update. US Department of Health and Human Services. Public Health Service, Agency for Health Care Policy and Research. AHCPR Publication No. 96-0682, 1996.

Ouslander JG: Management of overactive bladder. N Engl J Med 2004;350:786. [PMID: 14973214]

Resnick NM: Urinary incontinence. Lancet 1995;346:94. [PMID: 7603221]

Treatment

If nonurologic or functional causes are found as major contributors to the patient's incontinence, treatment should be targeted at the underlying illnesses and improving any functional disability. In addition to medical management of the underlying disorder(s), physical therapy and the use of assistive devices may be helpful in improving the patient's level of function and his or her ability to reach the bathroom prior to having an incontinent episode. For the ambulatory patient, a home visit is often useful in assessing for environmental hazards that may be contributing to functional incontinence.

Simple life-style modifications may be helpful in mild cases of urinary incontinence. Fluid restriction and avoidance of caffeine and alcohol, especially in the evening, can be recommended as an initial step. Weight loss can be recommended if the patient is obese, and the use of a bedside commode or urinal can also be helpful. For patients with more severe incontinence, however, including most patients with urologic causes, further treatment measures usually are necessary.

Treatment for urinary incontinence is divided into three categories: behavioral and nonpharmacologic therapies, pharmacotherapy, and surgical intervention.

A. Behavioral and Nonpharmacologic Therapies

Behavioral therapies should be the first line of treatment in most patients with urge or stress incontinence, as they have the advantages of being effective in a large percentage of patients with few, if any, side effects. Behavioral therapies range from those designed to treat the underlying problem and restore continence (eg, bladder training, pelvic muscle exercises) to those designed simply to promote dryness through increased attention from a caregiver (eg, timed voiding, prompted voiding). The former category requires a motivated patient who is cognitively intact, whereas the latter category can be used even in patients with significant cognitive impairment.

1. Bladder training—This technique is designed to help patients control their voiding reflex by teaching them to void at scheduled times. The patient is asked to keep a voiding record for approximately 1 week to determine the pattern of incontinence and the interval between incontinent episodes. A voiding schedule is then developed with a scheduled voiding interval significantly shorter than the patient's usual incontinence interval. (For example, if the usual time between incontinent episodes is 1–2 hours, the patient should be scheduled to void every 30–60 minutes.) The patient is asked to empty the bladder as completely as possible at each scheduled void whether or not an urge is felt. Patients who have the urge to void at unscheduled times should try to stop the urge through relaxation or distraction techniques until the urge passes, and then void at the next scheduled time. If the urge between scheduled voids becomes too uncomfortable, the patient should go ahead and void, but should still void again as completely as possible at the next scheduled time. As the number of incontinent episodes decreases, the scheduled voiding intervals should be gradually extended each week, until a comfortable voiding interval is reached.

Fantl and colleagues, in a well-publicized albeit relatively small trial of bladder retraining, demonstrated significant improvement in both the number of incontinent episodes and the amount of fluid lost in incontinent elderly women. Although the benefit was greatest in women with urge incontinence, women with stress incontinence also demonstrated improvement. In a later study, their group also demonstrated a significant improvement in quality of life following institution of bladder training. Studies in a family practice setting, in a home nursing program, and in a health maintenance organization also demonstrated significant benefit from a program of bladder training. The latter, a randomized controlled trial published in 2002, included patients with stress, urge, and mixed incontinence. Overall, patients had a 40% decrease in their incontinent episodes with 31% being 100% improved, 41% at least 75% improved, and 52% at least 50% improved.

2. Pelvic muscle exercises—These exercises, also known as Kegel exercises, are designed to strengthen the periurethral and perivaginal muscles. They are most useful in the treatment of stress incontinence but may also be effective in urge and mixed incontinence. Patients are initially taught to recognize the muscles to contract by being asked to squeeze the muscles in the genital area as if they were trying to stop the flow of urine from the urethra. While doing this, they should be sure that only the muscles in the front of the pelvis are being contracted, with minimal or no contraction of the abdominal, pelvic, or thigh muscles. Once the correct muscles are identified, patients should be taught to hold the contraction for at least 10 seconds followed by 10 seconds of relaxation. The exercises should be repeated between 30 and 80 times per day. Patients are then taught to contract their pelvic muscles before and during situations in which urinary leakage may occur to prevent their incontinent episodes from occurring.

A recent systematic review of 43 published clinical trials concluded that pelvic muscle exercises are effective for both stress and mixed incontinence, but that their effectiveness for urge incontinence remains unclear. Biofeedback has been used effectively to improve patients' recognition and contraction of pelvic floor muscles, but required equipment and expertise can make this impractical in a primary care setting. Weighted vaginal cones and electrical stimulation have also been used to enhance pelvic muscle exercises. These modalities are provided by many physical therapy or geriatric departments and can be considered as additional options for women who are unsuccessful with pelvic muscle exercises or who have obtained only partial improvement. The Cochrane group concluded that weighted vaginal cones, electrostimulation, and pelvic muscle exercises are probably similar in effectiveness. There was not enough evidence to conclude that the effectiveness of cones plus pelvic muscle exercises is different than either one alone.

3. Timed voiding—Timed voiding is a passive toileting assistance program that is caregiver dependent and can be used for patients who are either unable or unmotivated to participate in more active therapies. Its goal is to prevent incontinent episodes rather than to restore bladder function. The caregiver provides scheduled toileting for the patient on a fixed schedule (usually every 2–4 hours), including at night. There is no attempt to motivate the patient to delay voiding or resist the urge to void as there is in bladder training. The technique can be used both for patients who can toilet independently as well as those who require assistance. It has been used with success in both male and female patients and has achieved improvements of up to 85%. Timed voiding has also been used effectively in post-prostatectomy patients as well as in patients with neurogenic bladder.

A variation of timed voiding, known as *habit training*, uses a voiding schedule that is modified according to the patient's usual voiding pattern rather than an arbitrarily fixed interval. The goal of habit training is to preempt incontinent episodes by scheduling the patient's toileting interval to be shorter than the usual voiding interval. Both timed voiding and habit training are most commonly used in nursing homes but may also be used in the home if a motivated caregiver is available.

4. Prompted voiding—Prompted voiding is a technique that can be used for patients with or without cognitive impairment; it has been studied most frequently in the nursing home setting. Its goal is to teach patients to initiate their own toileting through requests for help and positive reinforcement from caregivers. Approximately every 2 hours, caregivers prompt the patients by asking whether they are wet or dry and suggesting that they attempt to void. Patients are then assisted to the toilet if necessary and praised for trying to use the toilet and for staying dry. A recent systemic analysis of controlled trials of prompted voiding concluded that the evidence was suggestive, although inconclusive, that prompted voiding provided at least short-term benefit to incontinent patients. The addition of oxybutynin to a prompted voiding program may provide additional benefit for some patients. A recent nursing home trial demonstrated that prompted voiding is most effective for reducing daytime incontinence, and that routine nighttime toileting was not effective in reducing incontinent episodes during the night.

B. Pharmacotherapy

Medications may be used alone or in conjunction with behavioral therapy when degree of improvement has been insufficient. There are very few studies comparing drug therapy with behavioral therapy, but both have been found more effective than placebo. An accurate diagnosis of the type of incontinence is necessary in order to choose appropriate pharmacotherapy for each patient.

1. Urge incontinence—Anticholinergic medications are the drugs of choice for urge incontinence, and five medications are now available. Oxybutynin, the earliest of these medications, is now available in a transdermal patch (Oxytrol) that can be dosed twice weekly, as well as a long-acting formulation (Ditropan XL) that can be dosed once daily. It is also available in a generic formulation that is significantly less expensive, but requires dosing (2.5–5 mg) two to four times a day.

Tolterodine is also available in both short-acting (Detrol) and long-acting (Detrol LA) formulations that can be dosed either once or twice daily. No direct trial has yet been published comparing the long-acting forms of the two drugs. A study of long-acting oxybutynin versus short-acting tolterodine found oxybutynin was modestly more effective with a similar side-effect profile and cost. A meta-analysis of four comparative trials (looking mainly at the short-acting formulations) concluded that oxybutynin is superior in efficacy, but that tolterodine is better tolerated with fewer dropouts because of medication side effects. Major side effects of both drugs include dry mouth, urinary retention, and delirium. These effects are less common with tolterodine, and dry mouth seems less common with the transdermal formulation of oxybutynin due to a lower production of metabolite.

Three new anticholinergic medications have recently been released that will compete with oxybutynin and tolterodine. Trospium (Sanctura), released in 2004, offers the advantage of fewer drug–drug interactions because it is not metabolized by the cytochrome P450 system. Solifenacin (Vesicare) and darifenacin (Enablex), both released in 2005, are more selective for the M3 muscarinic receptors in the bladder than the more traditional agents. M3 receptors are found preferentially in smooth muscle, the salivary glands, and the eyes. This selectivity leads to a lower incidence of drowsiness and dizziness in some patients, with the most common side effects being dry mouth and constipation.

The tricyclic antidepressant imipramine has traditionally been widely used to treat urge incontinence, but its use has now largely been supplanted by these newer agents with more favorable side-effect profiles and better documented efficacy.

2. Stress incontinence—Medical treatment is most effective for patients with mild to moderate stress incontinence and without a major anatomic abnormality. The α-agonist pseudoephedrine, at a dosage range of 15–60 mg three times a day, is the drug of choice for patients without contraindications. Side effects include nausea, dry mouth, insomnia, and restlessness. Studies using phenylpropanolamine (now removed from the market) demonstrated improvement in 19–60% of women and cure in 9–14%. One study indicated that a significant number of patients referred for surgical intervention could avoid surgery with α-agonist therapy.

Traditionally, estrogen therapy has been used in conjunction with α-agonists to increase α-adrenergic responsiveness and improve urethral mucosa and smooth muscle tone. However, the recent Heart and Estrogen/Progestin Replacement Study (HERS) demonstrated estrogen therapy to be less effective than placebo for symptoms of urinary incontinence, with only 20.9% of the treatment group reporting improvement and 38.8% reporting worsening of their incontinence (compared with 26% improvement and 27% worsening in the placebo group). Data from the Women's Health Initiative study indicating that patients on an estrogen-progestin combination demonstrated increased risk for heart disease, stroke, breast cancer, and pulmonary embolism also cast significant doubt on the advisability of long-term estrogen use for this indication. Although the risks and benefits of topical estrogen are not completely known, it would be prudent to use caution when considering its use until more conclusive data are available.

3. Overflow incontinence—Overflow incontinence associated with outlet obstruction is generally not treated with medications because the primary therapy is removal of the obstruction. In men, outlet obstruction is most commonly caused by prostatic enlargement secondary to infection (prostatitis), benign prostatic hyperplasia, or prostate cancer. Prostatitis can be treated with a 2- to 4-week course of a fluoroquinolone or trimethoprim-sulfamethoxazole. Once prostate cancer has been ruled out, benign prostatic hyperplasia may be treated with α-blockers, finasteride, surgery, or transurethral microwave thermotherapy. α-Blockers have been shown to be ineffective in "prostatism-like" symptoms in elderly women.

Medical treatment of overflow incontinence caused by bladder contractility problems is usually not highly efficacious. The cholinergic agonist bethanechol may be useful subcutaneously for temporary contractility problems following an overdistention injury but is generally ineffective when given orally or when used long term.

C. Surgical Intervention

Surgical therapy may be indicated for patients with incontinence resulting from anatomic abnormalities (eg, cystocele, prolapse), with outlet obstruction resulting in urinary retention, or for patients in whom more conservative methods of treatment have not provided sufficient relief.

Beyond the correction of anatomic abnormalities or obstruction, surgical therapy is most effective for stress incontinence or for mixed incontinence in which stress incontinence is a primary component. Numerous surgical options are available for the management of stress incontinence, including injection of periurethral bulking agents, transvaginal suspensions, retropubic suspensions, slings, and sphincter prostheses. Choice of procedure is based on the relative contributions of urethral hypermobility versus intrinsic sphincter deficiency, urodynamic findings, the need for other concomitant surgery, the patient's medical condition and life-style, and the experience of the surgeon.

Surgical management of refractory urge incontinence is generally more difficult. Options include sacral root neuromodulation procedures and augmentation enterocystoplasty, both of which offer substantial success rates in properly selected patients.

D. Primary Care Treatment versus Referral

Once the information from the history, physical examination, voiding record, provocative stress testing, PVR measurement, and laboratory data is available, a presumptive diagnosis can be made in the large majority of patients. If the patient has uncomplicated urge or stress incontinence, or a mixture of urge and stress, primary treatment can be initiated by the family physician. If the patient has overflow incontinence, manifested by an elevated PVR, referral is indicated to rule out obstruction prior to attempting medical or behavioral management. In the minority of patients in whom the type or cause of incontinence remains unclear, referral for urodynamic testing is indicated if a specific diagnosis will be helpful in guiding therapy. Urodynamic testing in the routine evaluation of incontinence is not indicated as studies have not shown an improvement in clinical outcome between patients diagnosed by urodynamics and patients treated based on history and physical examination.

Other indications for referral include incontinence associated with recurrent symptomatic urinary tract infections, hematuria without infection, history of prior pelvic surgery or irradiation, marked pelvic prolapse, suspicion of prostate cancer, lack of correlation between symptoms and physical findings, and failure to respond to therapeutic interventions as would be expected from the presumptive diagnosis.

E. Pads, Garments, Catheterization, and Pessaries

The use of absorbent pads and undergarments is extremely common among the elderly. Although they are not recommended as primary therapy before other measures have been tried, they may be useful in patients whose incontinence is infrequent and predictable, who cannot tolerate the side effects of medications, or who are not good candidates for surgical therapy. The main purpose of these pads and garments is to contain urine loss and prevent skin breakdown. However, very few studies have compared the numerous absorbent products available and their degree of success or failure in meeting these objectives. A recent Cochrane review concluded that disposable products may be more effective than nondisposable products in decreasing the incidence of skin problems, and that superabsorbent products may perform better than fluff pulp products. More comparative studies are needed in this area to assist patients and caregivers in making better-informed decisions.

Although urethral catheterization should be avoided as a general rule, it is sometimes indicated in cases of overflow incontinence or in patients for whom no other measures have been effective. External collection devices (eg, Texas catheters) are preferable to indwelling catheters, but acceptable external devices are not widely available for women and adverse reactions such as skin abrasion, necrosis, and urinary tract infection may occur. When internal catheterization is needed, intermittent or suprapubic catheterization has been shown to be preferable to indwelling catheterization in reducing the incidence of bacteriuria and its consequent complications. Indwelling urethral catheterization should be limited to very few circumstances, including comfort measures for the terminally ill, prevention of contamination of pressure ulcers, and for patients with inoperable outflow obstruction.

Pessaries are intravaginal devices used to maintain or restore the position of the pelvic organs in patients with genitourethral prolapse. Although there are few comparative data on their use in incontinence, they can sometimes be useful in patients with intractable stress incontinence who are poor candidates for, or who do not desire, surgery.

Appell RA et al; Overactive Bladder: Judging Effective Control and Treatment Study Group: Prospective randomized controlled trial of extended-release oxybutynin chloride and tolterodine tartrate in the treatment of overactive bladder: Results of the OBJECT study. Mayo Clin Proc 2001;76:358. [PMID: 11322350]

Benson JT: New therapeutic options for urge incontinence. Curr Womens Health Rep 2001;1:61. [PMID: 12112953]

Eustice S et al: Prompted voiding for the management of urinary incontinence in adults. Cochrane Database Syst Rev 2000;(2):CD002113. [PMID: 10795861]

Fantl JA et al: Efficacy of bladder training in older women with urinary incontinence. JAMA 1991;265:609. [PMID: 1987410]

Glazener CM, Lapitan MC: Urodynamic investigations for management of urinary incontinence in adults. Cochrane Database Syst Rev 2002;(3):CD003195. [PMID: 12137680]

Godec CJ: "Timed voiding"—a useful tool in the treatment of urinary incontinence. Urology 1994;23:97. [PMID: 6691214]

Grady D et al: Postmenopausal hormones and incontinence: The Heart and Estrogen/Progestin Replacement Study. Obstet Gynecol 2001;97:116. [PMID: 11152919]

Harvey MA et al: Tolterodine versus oxybutynin in the treatment of urge urinary incontinence: A meta-analysis. Am J Obstet Gynecol 2001;185:56. [PMID: 11483904]

Hay-Smith EJ et al: Pelvic floor muscle training for urinary incontinence in women. Cochrane Database Syst Rev 2001;(1):CD001407. [PMID: 11279716]

Madersbacher H et al: Conservative management in the neuropathic patient. In Abrams P et al, eds: Incontinence: First International Consultation on Incontinence. Recommendations of the International Scientific Committee: the Evaluation and Treatment of Urinary Incontinence. Health Publication Ltd, 1999.

O'Mara NB: Antimuscarinic medications for overactive bladder. Pharmacist's Letter/Prescriber's Letter 2005;21(2):210–209.

Rossouw JE et al; Writing Group for the Women's Health Initiative Investigators: Risks and benefits of estrogen plus progestin in healthy postmenopausal women: Principal results from the Women's Health Initiative randomized controlled trial. JAMA 2002;288:321. [PMID: 12117397]

Shirran E, Brazzelli M: Absorbent products for the containment of urinary and/or faecal incontinence in adults. Cochrane Database Syst Rev 2000;(2):CD001406. [PMID: 10796783]

Subak LL et al: The effect of behavioral therapy on urinary incontinence: A randomized controlled trial. Obstet Gynecol 2002;100:72. [PMID: 12100806]

Depression in Older Patients

41

Crystal March, MD,[1] *& Charles F. Reynolds III, MD*[1,2]

General Considerations

Depression is common in elderly primary care patients, with clinically significant symptoms affecting about 15–20% of patients aged 60 years and older at any time. Depression in later life usually coexists with other chronic medical illnesses, especially hypertension, diabetes mellitus, arthritis, chronic pain, hypothyroidism, coronary artery disease, congestive heart failure, chronic obstructive lung disease, and neurodegenerative disorders such as Alzheimer or Parkinson disease. This amplifies the disability and burden of caregiving occasioned by these illnesses. Depression diminishes quality of life, leads to nonadherence with self-care (diet, exercise, taking medication as prescribed), increases use of other medical services, is a risk factor for suicide (especially in older white men), and is frequently associated with cognitive impairment. Because of time constraints and inadequate reimbursement for provision of mental health services, depression in later life often does not compete well for time in primary care practices and may go unrecognized and untreated. However, depression in the elderly is treatable, and most elderly persons prefer to be treated in the general medical sector rather than being referred to specialty care. Moreover many, if not most, primary care physicians feel that treating depression in their elderly patients is properly a part of their clinical expertise and responsibility.

Of particular clinical relevance to general medical and family medicine practice, depression in later life is very much a "family affair" in the sense that family members are critically important in getting patients to treatment and keeping them in treatment long enough to do some good. At the same time, the burden of providing care to an elderly family member with depression is considerable, with the result that family members need information about the illness and how best to care for themselves. Hence, we advocate a patient-focused and family-centered approach to care. As we elaborate below, depression in late life is usually a chronic illness, often following a relapsing course. We tell our patients that getting well is not enough—it is staying well that counts. To achieve this objective, it is usually medically appropriate to institute maintenance treatment, beyond the acute treatment of the episode, to prolong recovery and prevent recurrence. Notwithstanding the advances in the science of treatment of depression in late life, reimbursement policies are discriminatory (reflecting a view of mental health parity) and represent a major obstacle to the implementation of good care. As well, further research is very much needed on ways of improving the cultural competency of providers, practice structures, and incentives to optimize depression care in older Americans.

Pathogenesis

There are multiple pathways to depression in old age. In the clinical samples reported in many of our National Institutes of Health (NIH)–sponsored investigations, about half of the subjects report onset of depression earlier in life, with recurrences in older ages. The role of genetic liability to depression seems to figure more prominently in early-onset illness. The other half of subjects experience clinical depression for the first time after the age of 60 years. Well-identified major psychosocial risk factors for the development of late-onset and recurrent depression include bereavement, caregiver strain, social isolation, and disability. Most significantly, the loss of a spouse and loved ones can lead to complicated grief, which is more likely to lead to depression, depending on how socially isolated this leaves the individual. Also detrimental are new role transitions (such as retirement or residing in a nursing home) and severe medical problems (ie, stroke, macular degeneration, hip fractures or replacements) that accompany loss of independence and often require rehabilitation. The imbalance of the negative impact from such aforementioned factors, relative to an older adult's social support and coping style, largely influences whether or not he or she will develop depression. In other late-onset cases, depression may herald the onset of a dementing disorder or be the product of cerebrovascular disease, including but not lim-

---

[1]With the Pittsburgh Late Life Depression Research Network Development Core: Charlotte Brown, PhD, Mario Cruz, MD, Ellen G. Detlefsen, DLS, David Hall, MD, Kathy Homrok, MD, Amy Kilbourne, PhD, Brenda Lee, Eric Lenze, MD, Crystal March, MD, Mark D. Miller, MD, Jeffrey Palmer, Edward P. Post, MD, PhD, Charles F. Reynolds III, MD, Grant Shevchik, MD, Francis X. Solano, MD, Gregory Spence-Jones, PhD, and Jeannette South-Paul, MD.

[2]Supported in part by NIMH Grants P30 MH071944, R01 MH59381, and K23 MH01879. Dr Kilbourne is supported by a VA Health Service Career Development Award.

ited to stroke. Some cases of depression in old age may represent subclinical cerebrovascular disease, with white matter hyperintensities on magnetic resonance imaging scans and prominent apathy and executive dysfunction clinically. Although depression in old age can be iatrogenic and the result of inappropriate sedative hypnotic use, in some cases depression is merely an unfavorable side effect of medications such as steroids.

Arean PA et al: The impact of psychosocial factors on late-life depression. Biol Psychiatry 2005;58:277. [PMID: 16102545]

Prevention

There is increasing interest in early preventive interventions (secondary prevention) with patients who are at high risk for developing depression in the wake of medical events such as stroke, myocardial infarction, macular degeneration, interferon therapy, and arthritis. Some of these interventions could take the form of using selective serotonin reuptake inhibitors (SSRI) pharmacotherapy in patients with elevated symptoms of depression either before or after a medical insult, as well as the use of problem-solving therapies to help patients cope more effectively with increasing limitations. Efforts to research primary prevention strategies could be usefully focused on other high-risk groups of elderly, such as the recently bereaved (20–30% of spousally bereaved elderly develop clinically significant depression), those who provide care to family members with mild cognitive impairment or Alzheimer dementia, those with chronic insomnia (itself a risk factor for the subsequent development of depression), and those advancing into the final years of life with increasing frailty. In those circumstances, it seems likely that prevention plans may include multicomponent interventions such as psychoeducation about the particular challenges being confronted, stress-coping techniques, and affective self-management. As the bard of Avon noted hundreds of years ago, sleep "knits up the raveled sleeve of care." Protecting sleep quality through better sleep hygiene may be an important component of helping the elderly successfully meet the challenges of growing old, which include but are not limited to coping with bereavement, caregiving, or loss of independence.

Over the past decade, it has become clear that antidepressant treatments can have a very favorable impact on the long-term course of depressive illness, particularly in preventing recurrences of disease (ie, tertiary prevention). (For further discussion, see Treatment, later.)

Clinical Findings

A. Initial Assessment

The initial assessment procedures should include a focused psychiatric history and examination, including a brief clinical cognitive examination. In addition, a medical history, physical examination, and focused neurologic examination are preferred as part of the assessment. Primary symptoms in diagnosing depression in older patients include persistent sadness, frequent tearfulness, loss of pleasure in previously enjoyable interests or hobbies, and recurrent thoughts of death or suicide. Other important tip-offs include feelings of hopelessness, worry, guilt, or dependency; isolation from social interactions; lack of pleasure in usual activities; psychomotor agitation or retardation; difficulty making decisions; difficulties initiating new projects; numerous inexplicable somatic complaints; and increased utilization of health services.

It is also important to assess other domains, including the older adult's level of functioning or disability, loss or grief concerns, physical environment, and psychosocial situation. Several instruments are useful for screening for depressive symptoms in primary care practices. These include the Center for Epidemiologic Studies depression scale (CES-D), the Patient History Questionnaire (PHQ)-9, and, for diagnostic purposes, the mood disorders module of the PRIME-MD. Similarly, the Folstein Mini-Mental State Examination (MMSE) is a useful bedside screen for cognitive impairment. Scores of 23 or lower on the Folstein MMSE raise the possibility of impairment that should have further assessment.

Assessing risk factors for suicide is an essential part of the diagnostic process. The most important risk factors in older patients include severity of depression; the presence of psychotic depression; alcoholism and other substance abuse, including sedative hypnotics or painkillers; recent loss or bereavement; and the development of disability. Elderly white men have the highest rates of suicide, almost always related to depression. In 70% of these cases, handguns are used to commit suicide, underscoring the importance of asking about access to lethal means and working with family members to remove handguns from the home environment. Up to three quarters of suicide victims will have seen a primary care physician in the month before death, signaling an opportunity for life-saving interventions. Thus, physicians must always watch for the red flag of hopelessness when assessing suicidality.

B. Symptoms and Signs

Because depression in older patients often occurs in the context of medical and neurologic illnesses, somatic symptoms such as changes in sleep and appetite, although important, have limited diagnostic utility. More emphasis is appropriately placed on sad, downcast mood, recurrent thoughts of death or suicide, and diminished interest in pleasurable activities. Typically, these symptoms have been present for weeks, if not months, and are associated with anguish and diminished functioning. An elderly person presenting with numerous seemingly unrelated somatic complaints is likely to have an underlying depression or anxiety disorder. Those somatic symptoms often improve and distressed help-seeking decreases with effective treatment of the underlying depression or anxiety.

Although the majority of older depressed patients are treated in primary care settings, some cases are especially difficult to manage in general medical clinics. Specialized psychiatric care is strongly indicated if clinical findings support a diagnosis of psychotic depression, bipolar disorder, depression accompanied by active suicidal ideation or planning and easy access to lethal means such as handguns, depression with comorbid substance abuse, depression with comorbid dementia, or other needs for more specialized assessment.

Differential Diagnosis

The most critical comorbid conditions to assess for include alcohol and substance-use disorders, medications that can cause mood disturbances (eg, prednisone), and other central nervous system illnesses, especially Alzheimer dementia. Depending on the clinical presentation, physicians should also assess the patient for a variety of general medical problems that could be contributing to mood symptoms. Such conditions include cerebrovascular disease, chronic pain, myocardial infarction, orthostatic hypotension, hypertension, diabetes mellitus, congestive heart failure, coronary artery disease, neoplasms, hypothyroidism, and chronic obstructive pulmonary disease. Accidental misuse of medications and physical, verbal, or emotional abuse by caregivers or relatives should also be evaluated.

Depression in later life usually coexists with cognitive impairments. Based on clinical research experience, close to 50% of elderly patients treated to remission of depression qualify for a diagnosis of mild cognitive impairment (amnestic or other subtypes). The US Preventive Services Task Force has determined that the evidence is insufficient to recommend for or against routine screening for dementia in older adults. However, the task force has said that primary care physicians should be vigilant for signs of dementia whenever cognitive deterioration is suspected based on the physician's direct observation; a patient's own report; or concerns raised by family members, friends, or caregivers. The full recommendation and rationale are found at http://www.ahrq.gov/ clinic/3rduspstf/dementia/ dementrr.htm. The key practice point is that depression and dementia frequently coexist. Treating depression in the cognitively impaired elder usually benefits mood, cognition, and behavior.

Complications

If unrecognized and untreated, depression in old age generally does not resolve on its own and may in fact worsen over time with respect to symptom burden and impact on functional status and quality of life. Depression also affects cognition in many ways, for example, by reducing the speed of information processing, interfering with attentional and memory capacities, and, quite prominently, undermining executive control functions. Because depression amplifies the disability associated with coexisting medical illness, depressed elderly patients can become caught up in a "vicious cycle" of noncompliance with medical treatment, a downward spiral of disability and depression, and early mortality (including, but not limited to, suicide). Depression in old age can be viewed as a "contagious" illness—one that burdens (and burns out) family members and caregivers, and erodes social networks. Depression produces isolation no less than being the consequence of isolation, and it is now recognized as a risk factor for both coronary artery disease and Alzheimer dementia. Furthermore, given that late-life depression is a risk factor or prodrome to dementia, it is important to avoid or to minimize the use of medications that impair cognition, especially anticholinergics.

Treatment

A. Working with Minority Elders Suspected of Having Psychiatric or Cognitive Disorders

Providers must keep in mind that patients and providers have unique backgrounds that tailor how they understand the meaning of illness in their lives and what symptoms constitute disease. Providers and patients must develop a relationship of openness and trust if they are to feel comfortable exploring the unique meaning of illness in the patient's life for appropriate diagnosis and treatment plans. Ethnic diversity in the United States is increasing at a fast pace. In 2010 almost 50% of the US population is projected to be nonwhite, with Hispanic Americans as the largest minority group. With this shift in population demographics, health care providers must acquire cross-cultural competency skills to ensure optimal care for all individuals they see. Such skills involve accurate knowledge of the attributes, values, beliefs, and behaviors of certain ethnic groups; sensitivity and awareness of one's own cultural identity; and ethnic biases that are created as a result of one's own cultural background that foster the tendency to stereotype individuals from another ethnic group. The essential communication skills elicit patients' explanatory models (what patients believe is causing their illness) and agendas (what patients seek from treatment), the role of family members in their lives and how those family members will react to the patient being treated for a mental illness, and how patients perceive taking medicine for depression and sharing some of their darkest secrets with someone outside their usual group of confidants.

Providers must also have the sensitivity to recognize, particularly with the elderly, how real-world experiences of racism and prejudice have sensitized them to be suspicious of diagnoses that do not require radiologic or laboratory examinations to prescribe treatment. The communication skills of the provider to address the aforementioned issues and the capacity to convey humility, empathy, respect, and compassion, will be the deciding factors in the accurate diagnosis and treatment of depression in ethnically diverse populations.

Health communications research has shown that recognition of depression is improved if providers pursue questions related to depression early in appointments rather than saving them for later. Thus, when evaluating patients, physicians should ask questions pertaining to depressive symptoms (eg, sleep and appetite disturbances, recent losses, and anhedonia) near the beginning of the visit. This allows more time during the visit to explore any concerns related to cultural issues.

It is also of note that patients prefer office visits in which the provider balances the allotted time among symptom assessment, history gathering, health education, and discussion of the social and interpersonal influences in their lives and the effect these influences have on their psychological well-being. Often these influences are related to the person's spirituality or religious affiliation. The mere presence of a religious affiliation and, even more so, the saliency of a person's religion, has been shown to be a protective factor for depression, particularly in older adults with medical illnesses or disability. It is critical that providers take this into account, not only because it may largely influence how patients cope with their illnesses, but also because studies have proven that validating this aspect of a patient's life and incorporating it into treatment plans can positively affect the patient's adherence to treatment and even speed up rates of remission. Approaching the subject of religion and spirituality should be done with openness and respect. Despite any lack of comfort felt by the provider, it is a subject that should be discussed, as with any other social history pertinent to a patient. This balance between symptom assessment and the exploration of psychosocial beliefs will help develop an effective treatment plan to which the patient is capable of adhering (Table 41–1).

Treatment effectiveness requires the activation of the patient as a participant in his or her own treatment. Patient activation ensures that patients understand that depression is a medical and treatable illness, how depression has negatively influenced their lives, and that treatment effectiveness is contingent on adhering to the agreed-on recommendations and returning for future appointments. Overall, there have been fewer adherences to treatment recommendations in nonwhite patients in the United States. Studies have shown that providers tend to dominate discussions and have shorter visits with nonwhite patients, which limits patients' ability to actively participate in their care. This leaves patients with the impression that the provider has little interest in them, and therefore they have less interest in adhering to recommendations. To ensure that patients are motivated to participate in their care, they must have enough time to speak, ask questions, and discuss different treatment options. This approach is all the more important in minority elderly patients, who most often receive all of their health care from primary care providers. Because many nonwhite adults are even more reluctant than other adults to seek care from mental health specialists, depressive disorders are largely underdiagnosed in African Americans, Latinos, and Asian Americans.

Table 41–1. Useful strategies for working with minority elderly with suspected mental illness.

Confidentiality is even more important than usual because of the persisting stigma of mental illness (dementia falls into this category as well).
Although families will accept as normal higher levels of mental and emotional dysfunction than might be seen in the rest of the population, families may be totally unable to cope and require rescue once the threshold is reached.
Be prepared for and support sharing the management of mental disorders with the clergy. Seek information regarding faith belief models and feedback as to how such beliefs are influencing care.
Carefully elicit data regarding mental status. Minority elderly who feel questions infantilize them often become angry with how they perceive they are being treated.

Misdiagnosis can be the result of misinterpretation of illness presentation or miscommunication between physicians and patients. Latinos and Asians sometimes express distress in vivid and highly emotional narratives, particularly those individuals for whom English is not their first language. If the provider does not speak the patient's native language, a well-trained health care interpreter should be used to ensure that accurate information is exchanged.

The psychiatric diagnostic evaluation emphasizes the interpretation of the patient's appearance, behavior, language, and thought content, all of which are considered highly sensitive to cross-cultural misinterpretation. When diagnosing mental illness in individuals of ethnic groups different from his or her own, the physician must guard against "category fallacy," the application of western European categories or terms to describe a patient's presentation without ensuring that the category or term is valid in the patient's local culture. To guard against category fallacy, the *Diagnostic and Statistical Manual of Mental Disorders,* Fourth Edition, Text Revision (DSM-IV-TR), recommends that the diagnostic evaluation include a cross-cultural formulation. This would include an assessment of (1) the cultural identity of the individual, (2) cultural explanations of the individual's illness, (3) cultural factors related to psychosocial environment and level of functioning, (4) cultural elements of the relationship between the individual and the clinician, and (5) overall cultural assessment for diagnosis and care.

American Psychiatric Association: *Diagnostic and Statistical Manual of Mental Disorders,* 4th ed, text revision. APA, 2000.

Carney PA et al: How physician communication influences recognition of depression in primary care. J Fam Pract 1999;48:958. [PMID: 10628576]

Cooper-Patrick L et al: Patient-physician race concordance and communication in primary care. J Gen Intern Med 2000;15:106.

Koenig HG et al: Religiosity as a protective factor in depressive disorder. Am J Psychiatry 1999;156:810.

Koenig HG et al: Religiosity and remission of depression in medically ill older patients. Am J Psychiatry 1998;155:536. [PMID: 9546001]

Smedley BD et al, eds: *Unequal Treatment: Confronting Racial and Ethnic Disparities in Healthcare.* Institute on Medicine, National Academies Press, 2003.

Snowden LR: Bias in mental health assessment and intervention: Theory and evidence. Am J Public Health 2003;93:239. [PMID: 12554576]

B. Medications and Psychotherapy

In elderly patients with severe unipolar nonpsychotic major depression, expert consensus is to combine antidepressant medication with psychotherapy as the treatment of choice, with medication alone as another first-line strategy. Electroconvulsive treatment is an alternative strategy for severe depression, especially if the patient is actively suicidal, psychotic, or treatment resistant. Psychotherapy should not be used alone for severe depression. A combination of medication and psychotherapy is also recommended as first-line treatment for milder cases of depression, but either treatment modality could be used alone, depending partly on patient preference. SSRIs are the medications of choice for treatment of depression in old age. Venlafaxine XR (extended release) and duloxeline are other first-line options, which may be useful in patients who fail a trial with SSRIs. Second-line alternatives include bupropion and mirtazapine, as well as nortriptyline or desipramine for more severe depression.

With respect to the choice of specific medication within classes, expert opinion favors citalopram, escitalopram, sertraline, or paroxetine among the SSRIs and nortriptyline or desipramine among the tricyclic antidepressants. Antidepressants best avoided in the elderly, because of side effects and other safety concerns, include amitriptyline, imipramine, and doxepin. Table 41–2 outlines adequate dosing of commonly prescribed antidepressants in elderly patients.

Alexopoulos GS et al: Pharmacotherapy of depressive disorders in older patients. The Expert Guideline Series. *Postgraduate Medicine.* McGraw-Hill, 2001.

C. Frequently Asked Questions

1. What is a general strategy for managing depression in the context of a medical condition known to contribute to depression (eg, hypothyroidism)?— The preferred strategy is to use antidepressant medication in addition to medication for the comorbid condition from the outset. In contrast, the strategy of first treating the comorbid medical condition and prescribing an antidepressant only if depressive symptoms persist usually produces only partial remission of depression.

Table 41–2. Adequate dose of antidepressants in elderly patients.

Antidepressant	Average Starting Dose (mg/day)	Average Dose after 6 Weeks (mg/day)	Usual Highest Dose (mg/day)
Bupropion SR	100	150–300	300–400
Citalopram	10–20	20–30	30–40
Desipramine	10–40	50–100	100–150
Duloxetine	20–30	40–60	120
Escitalopram	10	20	20
Fluoxetine	10	20	20–40
Mirtazapine	7.5–15	15–30	30–45
Nortriptyline	10–30	40–100	75–125
Paroxetine	10–20	20–30	30–40
Sertraline	25–50	50–100	100–200
Venlafaxine XR	25–75	75–200	150–300

If the major depressive episode coexists with alcohol or benzodiazepine abuse, the preferred strategy is to treat the substance abuse first and then prescribe an antidepressant if depressive symptoms persist. There is less consensus on this point, however, than with respect to other comorbid medical conditions. Although drug–drug interactions are generally not problematic, if warfarin is coprescribed with SSRIs, its dosage may need to be downwardly adjusted.

2. How long should the physician wait before making a change in the treatment regimen (ie, switching to a different agent) for an older patient who is having an inadequate response to initial treatment?— If the physician has already raised the dose to the maximum level that the patient is able to tolerate, expert opinion calls for waiting 3–5 weeks if there is a partial response to a low dose and 4–7 weeks if there is a partial response to a high dose. Guidelines published by the Agency for Healthcare Research and Quality (AHRQ) recommend continuing for 6 weeks if there is little or no response or 12 weeks if there is partial response. Further consultation with a local mental health specialist on second-line treatment for poorly or partially responding patients is advisable.

3. What psychosocial interventions are preferred?— The preferred psychotherapy techniques include supportive, problem-solving, and interpersonal psychotherapy, and cognitive-behavioral therapy. Additional interventions include a range of psychoeducation, family counseling, visiting nurse services to help with medication, bereavement groups, and use of senior citizen centers.

4. How can treatment outcomes be evaluated?— The most important indicators are presence and severity of suicidal ideation, severity of depressive symptoms, and level of disability (functional deficits). Although rating scales, such as the Hamilton Depression Rating Scale, are useful for assessing response, another more practical suggestion is that the primary care physician write down two to four target symptoms (eg, "depressed 90% of the time, poor sleep almost nightly, and feelings of hopelessness"), as well as functional status (eg, unable to do housework), and document changes in these target symptoms as treatment progresses.

If an older patient is in remission after a single life-time episode of major depression, the preference is to continue with antidepressant medication for 1 year; if the patient has had two episodes, medication should be continued at least 2 years if not longer; and if the patient has had three or more episodes, there is broad agreement to continue antidepressant medication at least 3 years and probably indefinitely. The preferred strategy in any scenario is to continue using the dose of antidepressant medication that was effective during acute treatment. Lowering the dose may put the patient at risk for partial or complete relapse.

Reynold CF, et al: Maintenance treatment of major depression in old age. N Engl J Med 2006;354:1130 [PMID: 16540613]

D. Management of the Elderly in Primary Care Settings

Recent clinical trials with elderly depressed patients conducted in 20 primary care settings demonstrated the efficacy and usefulness of placing depression care managers in primary care practices to improve the recognition and treatment of depression in the elderly. In the randomized controlled Prevention of Suicide in Primary Care Elderly: Collaborative Trial (PROSPECT), depression care managers (psychiatric nurses, social workers, or psychologists) worked with primary care physicians to enable the successful implementation of guideline-based care by the AHRQ. From this study, significantly higher rates of decline and resolution were seen in suicidal ideation, in addition to the degree of depression and speed of symptom reduction, compared with responses to usual care. Better short- and long-term outcomes were seen due to the physician having more on-target and on-time input from the care managers. This model of collaborative care is more respectful of the chronic nature of depression in the elderly in that it addresses the need for family education on the illness and its treatment, which subsequently leads to better compliance with appropriate care. The challenge remains whether changes in reimbursement policies will ensue that will allow coverage of this type of service.

Thomas L et al: Response speed and rate of remission in primary and specialty care of elderly patients with depression. Am J Geriatr Psychiatry 2002;10:583. [PMID: 12213693]

Unutzer J et al; IMPACT Investigators. Improving Mood-Promoting Access to Collaborative Treatment: Collaborative care management of late-life depression in the primary care setting: A randomized controlled trial. JAMA 2002;288:2836. [PMID: 12472325]

Prognosis

The good news is that depression in later life responds to treatment. Most patients can be treated to remission, especially if medication and psychotherapy are combined. Depression in later life is a chronic, relapsing illness; however, treatment works not only to make patients well, but also to keep them well. Treatment prevents relapse and recurrence, prolongs recovery, and facilitates functional recovery as well as symptomatic relief. Effective treatment of depression also ameliorates suicidal ideation in the majority of patients; however, in about 20% of patients, suicidal ideation persists and may require additional specialized treatment beyond routine depression care.

An area of active ongoing research addresses the relationship between depression in old age and dementia. Evidence suggests that depression in old age is a risk factor for the subsequent onset of dementia and may, in some cases, be an early harbinger of dementia. Treatment of depression in old age generally improves cognitive functioning but often does not normalize it completely. Additional research is needed to determine if the coprescription of antidepressant medication and cognitive enhancers such as cholinesterase inhibitors will help further improve and stabilize cognition in late-life depression.

Bruce ML et al: Reducing suicidal ideation and depressive symptoms in depressed older primary care patients: A randomized controlled trial. JAMA 2004;291:1081. [PMID: 14996777]

Charney DS et al; Depression and Bipolar Support Alliance: Depression and Bipolar Support Alliance consensus statement on the unmet needs in diagnosis and treatment of mood disorders in late life. Arch Gen Psychiatry 2003;60:664. [PMID: 12860770]

Szanto K et al: Occurrence and course of suicidality during short-term treatment of late-life depression. Arch Gen Psychiatry 2003;60:610. [PMID: 12796224]

RESOURCES & WEB SITES

Miller MD, Reynolds CF: *Living Longer Depression Free.* Johns Hopkins University Press, 2002. (Written for consumers and family members.)

Alzheimer's Association:

http://www.alz.org

American Association for Geriatric Psychiatry:

http://www.aagpgpa.org

Depression and Bipolar Support Alliance:

http://www.dbsa.org

Intervention Research Center for Late Life Mood Disorders, University of Pittsburgh:

http://www.latelifedepression.org

National Alliance for the Mentally Ill:

http://www.nami.org

National Institute of Mental Health:

http://www.nimh.nih.gov

Elder Abuse

42

Deborah J. Bostock, MD, & Cynthia M. Williams, DO, MA, FAACP

General Considerations

As hidden as the other forms of family violence may be, domestic elder abuse is even more concealed within our society. Elder abuse was first described in the literature in 1975, when the first reports of "granny battering" appeared. Vastly underreported, only one in four domestic elder abuse incidents (excluding the incidents of self-neglect) come to the attention of authorities.

The most common reporters of abuse are family members (17%) and social services agency staff (11%). Physicians reported only 1.4% of the cases. Although physicians are mandatory reporters in all states, many physicians feel ill-equipped to address this important social and medical problem. Concerns for patient safety and retaliation by the caregiver, violation of the physician–patient relationship, patient autonomy, confidentiality, and trust issues are quoted as reasons for low reporting.

Family physicians are particularly well positioned to assist in identifying and managing elder abuse. Except for the primary caregivers, they may be the only ones to see an abused elderly patient. Older victims who suffer from neglect, self-neglect, or physical abuse are likely to seek care from their primary care physician or gain entry into the medical care system through an emergency department.

In the 2000 census, 35 million people in the United States were 65 years of age and older. Adults 85 years and older showed the highest percentage increase of any age group (38%), from 3.1 million to 4.2 million. As the baby boomers age, the number of elders in the United States will continue to increase. The societal cost for the identification and treatment of elder abuse is also projected to rise as the baby boomers enter the elder years.

Feldhaus KM: Physician's knowledge of and attitudes toward a domestic violence mandatory reporting law. Ann Emerg Med 2003;41:159. [PMID: 12526132]

Lachs MS, Pillemer K: Elder abuse. Lancet 2004;364:1263. [PMID: 15464188]

A. Definition and Types of Abuse

Elder abuse is an all-inclusive term that describes all types of mistreatment and abusive behaviors toward older adults. The mistreatment can be either acts of commission (abuse) or acts of omission (neglect). Labeling a behavior as abusive, neglectful, or exploitative can depend on the frequency, duration, intensity, severity, consequences, and cultural context. Currently, state laws define elder abuse, and definitions vary considerably from one jurisdiction to another. Research definitions also vary, making it difficult to review comparative data.

There are three basic categories of elder abuse: (1) domestic elder abuse, (2) institutional elder abuse, and (3) self-neglect or self-abuse. The National Center on Elder Abuse (NCEA) describes seven different types of elder abuse: physical abuse, sexual abuse, emotional abuse, financial exploitation, neglect, abandonment, and self-neglect (Table 42–1).

Wood EF: *The Availability and Utility of Interdisciplinary Data on Elder Abuse: A White Paper for the National Center on Elder Abuse.* American Bar Association Commission on Law and Aging for the National Center on Elder Abuse. National Center on Elder Abuse at American Public Human Services Association, 2006.

B. Prevalence

According to the 2003 National Research Council Panel to Review Risk and Prevalence of Elder Abuse and Neglect, it is estimated that approximately one to two million elders were victims of various types of domestic elder abuse, excluding abuse due to self-neglect. More than 2–10% of the nation's elderly may be victims of moderate to severe abuse, but because of underreporting, poor detection, and differing definitions, the true estimate of elder abuse may be far greater. It is estimated that for every one case of elder abuse, neglect, exploitation, or self-neglect reported to authorities, about five more go unreported. Current estimates put the overall reporting of financial exploitation at only 1 in 25 cases, suggesting that there may be at least five million financial abuse victims each year.

In reported cases of domestic elder abuse, 77% of the victims were white and 22% were African American. The proportions of Native Americans and Asian Americans/Pacific Islanders were each less than 1%. Neglect—the failure of a designated caregiver to meet the needs of a dependent elderly person—is the most

Table 42–1. Elder abuse: definitions.

Physical abuse	Use of physical force that may result in bodily injury, physical pain, or impairment
Sexual abuse	Nonconsensual sexual contact of any kind with an elderly person
Emotional abuse	Infliction of anguish, pain, or distress through verbal or nonverbal acts
Financial/material exploitation	Illegal or improper use of an elder's funds, property, or assets
Neglect	Refusal, or failure, to fulfill any part of a person's obligations or duties to an elderly person
Abandonment	Desertion of an elderly person by an individual who has physical custody of the elder or by a person who has assumed responsibility for providing care to the elder
Self-neglect	Behaviors of an elderly person that threaten the elder's health or safety

Source: Tatara T: *Understanding Elder Abuse in Minority Populations.* Brunner/Mazel, 1999.

common form of elder maltreatment in domestic settings. In almost 90% of cases the perpetrator of the abuse is known, and in two thirds of cases the perpetrators are spouses or adult children.

Elder Mistreatment: Abuse, Neglect and Exploitation in an Aging America. National Research Council Panel to Review Risk and Prevalence of Elder Abuse and Neglect, 2003.

Wolf R: The nature and scope of elder abuse. Generations 2000; 24:6.

C. Risk Factors

Several explanations have been proposed to explain the origins of elder mistreatment. These explanations have focused on overburdened caregivers, dependent elders, mentally disturbed caregivers, a history of childhood abuse and neglect, and the marginalization of elders in society. Risk factors commonly cited for elder mistreatment are listed in Table 42–2.

Table 42–2. Risk factors for elder abuse.

Overall poor health (neglect)
Living with someone (physical and verbal abuse)
Lack of access to resources (neglect and financial abuse)
Social isolation or living alone (financial abuse and neglect)
Impaired activities of daily living performance (physical abuse and neglect)

From the Indicators of Abuse (IOA) screen, a profile of the abuser has been developed that can identify abuse cases 78–85% of the time. The salient features of the profile are detailed in Table 42–3.

A typology of abusers has also been suggested to better delineate who may perpetrate abuse. Five types of offenders have been postulated:

1. *Overwhelmed offenders* are well intentioned and enter caregiving expecting to provide adequate care; however, when the amount of care expected exceeds their comfort level, they lash out verbally or physically. The maltreatment is usually episodic rather than chronic. This type of offender is often seen in long-term care settings.
2. *Impaired offenders* are well intentioned, but have problems that render them unqualified to provide adequate care. The caregiver may be of advanced age and frail, have physical or mental illness, or have developmental disabilities. This type of maltreatment is usually chronic and the caregiver is unable to recognize the inadequacy of the care. Neglect is frequently observed in these cases.
3. *Narcissistic offenders* are motivated by anticipated personal gain and not the desire to help others. These individuals tend to be socially sophisticated and gain a position of trust over the vulnerable elder. Maltreatment is usually in the form of neglect and financial exploitation and is chronic in nature. These offenders will also use psychological abuse and physical maltreatment to obtain their objective. This type of offender may work in a long-term care facility and become involved in stealing from the residents.
4. *Domineering or bullying offenders* are motivated by power and control and are prone to outbursts of rage, believing their actions are justified by rationalizing that the victim "deserved it." These offenders know where and when they can get away with abuse. This abuse is chronic, multifaceted, and ongoing with frequent outbursts of temper. Abuse takes the form of physical, psychological, and even forced sexual coercion. Their victims are fearful, and the abuser may lash out when confronted or attempt to manipulate those who confront them.
5. *Sadistic offenders* derive feelings of power and importance by humiliating, terrifying, and harming others. They have sociopathic personalities and inflict severe, chronic, and multifaceted abuse. Signs of this type of abuse include bite, burn, and restraint marks and other signs of physical and sexual assault. Their victims are fearful and experience terror. If confronted, the abuser may attempt to charm and manipulate or intimidate and threaten the accuser in an attempt to control professionals who are trying to stop the abuse.

Table 42–3. Profiles of elder abusers.

Personal Abusive Caregiver Characteristics	Interpersonal Caregiver Characteristics	Abused Elder Characteristics
Abuses alcohol or other substance	Has poor relationships generally or with the elder	Was abused in the past
Is depressed or has a personality disorder	Has current marital or family conflict	Lacks social support
Has other mental health problems	Lacks empathy and understanding for the elder	
Has behavioral problems	Is financially dependent on the elder	
Caregiving inexperience or is reluctant to give care		

Source: Reis M, Nahmiash D: Validation of the indicators of abuse (IOA) screen. Gerontologist 1998;38:471.

Ramsey-Klawsnik H: Elder-abuse offenders: A typology. Generations 2000;24:17.

Reis M: The IOA Screen: An abuse-alert measure that dispels myths. Generations 2000;24:13.

Clinical Findings

Several medical and social factors make the detection of elder abuse more difficult than other forms of family violence. Given the higher prevalence of chronic diseases in older adults, signs and symptoms of mistreatment may be misattributed to chronic disease, leading to "false negatives," such as fractures that are ascribed to osteoporosis instead of physical assault. Alternatively, sequelae of many chronic diseases may be misattributed to elder mistreatment, creating "false positives," such as weight loss because of cancer erroneously ascribed to intentional withholding of food. Another significant issue for the physician is denial that the reason for the presentation into the health care system could be attributable to abuse. Physician barriers to reporting elder abuse are listed in Table 42–4.

A. Screening

The US Preventive Services Task Force (USPSTF) found insufficient evidence to recommend for or against routine screening of older adults or their caregivers for elder abuse. The American Medical Association recommends that all older patients be asked about family violence even when evidence of such abuse does not appear to exist. A careful history is crucial to determining if suspected abuse or neglect exists. The elderly dependent patient may fear retaliation from the abuser and may be reluctant to come forward with information. The physician should interview the patient and caregiver separately and alone. General questions about feeling safe at home and who prepares meals and handles finances can open the door to more specific questions about disagreements with the caregiver and how these disagreements are handled, such as the caregiver yelling, hitting, slapping, kicking, or punching; making the elder wait for meals and medications; or confining the elder to a room. It is also important to inquire about the possibility of sexual abuse (unwanted touching), financial abuse (stolen money, signing legal documents without understanding the consequences), and finally threats of institutionalization. Table 42–5 lists important questions to ask when screening for suspected abuse.

The caregiver interview should avoid confrontation and blame. The physician needs to appear sympathetic and understanding of the abuser's perceived burden in caregiving. The physician should be alert to a caregiver who has poor knowledge of a patient's medical problems, has excessive concerns about costs, dominates the medical interview, or is verbally aggressive either to the patient or physician during the interview. A caregiver with substance abuse or mental health problems and one who is financially dependent on the elder should also alert the physician to a greater potential for abuse.

Table 42–4. Physician barriers to reporting elder abuse.

Lack of consistent definitions
Unfamiliarity with mandatory reporting laws
Lack of required training to recognize abuse
Time constraints
Concerns with offending patients
Lack of awareness of available resources
Subtle presentation
Reluctance/fear of confronting the abuser
Abused elder requests abuse not be reported
Cultural issues
Isolation of victims
Fear of jeopardizing relationship with hospital or nursing facility

Sources: Swagerty DL et al: Elder mistreatment. Am Fam Physician 1999;59:2804. Kleinschmidt KC: Elder abuse: A review. Ann Emerg Med 1997;30:463. Rosenblatt DE et al: Reporting mistreatment of older adults: The role of physicians. J Am Geriatr Soc 1996;44:65.

Table 42–5. Questions to elicit information about elder abuse.

Physical Abuse
- Are you afraid of anyone at home?
- Have you been struck, slapped, or kicked?
- Have you been tied down or locked in a room?

Psychological Abuse
- Do you ever feel alone?
- Have you been threatened with punishment, deprivation, or institutionalization?
- Have you received "the silent treatment"?
- Have you been force-fed?
- Do you receive routine news or information?
- What happens when you and your caregiver disagree?

Sexual Abuse
- Has anyone touched you without permission?

Neglect
- Do you lack aids such as eyeglasses, hearing aids, or false teeth?
- Have you been left alone for long periods?
- Is your home safe?
- Has anyone failed to help you care for yourself when you needed assistance?

Financial Abuse
- Is money stolen from you or used inappropriately?
- Have you been forced to sign a power of attorney, a will, or another document against your wishes?
- Have you been forced to make purchases against your wishes?
- Does your caregiver depend on you for shelter or financial support?

Source: Kleinschmidt K: Elder abuse: A review. Ann Emerg Med 1997;30(4):464.

US Preventive Services Task Force: Screening for family and intimate partner violence: Recommendation statement. Ann Fam Med 2004;2:156. [PMID: 15083857]

B. Physical Examination

A thorough physical examination is the initial invitation to recognizing and documenting elder abuse. Particular attention to the functional and cognitive status of the elder is important to understanding the degree of dependency that the elder may have on the caregiver. The primary care physician may be confronted with subtle forms of ongoing abuse or mistreatment in which neglect and psychological abuse predominate. Behavioral observations of withdrawal, a caregiver who treats the elder like a child, or a caregiver who insists on giving the history should heighten the clinician's suspicions. Table 42–6 lists the basic features of the physical examination for assessing suspected elder mistreatment or abuse.

Detailed documentation of the physical examination is important as it may be used as evidence in a criminal trial. Documentation must be complete and legible, with accurate descriptions and annotations on sketches or, when possible, with the use of photo documentation.

Intervention & Reporting

Once elder abuse is suspected all health care providers and administrators are legally obligated to report the abuse to the appropriate authorities. Most states have anonymous reporting and Good Samaritan laws that can offer an alternative to a direct physician report if there are significant concerns for maintaining the physician-patient relationship. As previously noted, laws differ from state to state, and physicians should become familiar with the specific reporting requirements of their state. By emphasizing the diagnosis and treatment of the health consequences of the mistreatment or the abuse, the elderly patient and caregiver may feel less threatened. Reporting should be done in a caring and compassionate manner in order to protect the autonomy and self-worth of the elder while ensuring his or her continued safety.

The victim should be told that a referral will be made to Adult Protective Services (APS). Involving the caregiver in the discussion must be carefully considered with regard to potential retaliation on the victim. The law enforcement implications of APS should be downplayed and the social support and services offered by APS should be offered as part of the medical management of the victim. Victims may deny the possibility of abuse or fail to recognize its threat to their personal safety. In the event of financial abuse the victim or the offender, or both, may not acknowledge the abuse. If the victim refuses the APS referral, the clinician may explain that he or she is bound to adhere to state laws and regulations in making the referral and that the regulations were developed to help older persons who were not receiving the care they needed for whatever reason.

The safety of the patient is the most important consideration in any case of suspected abuse. If the abuse is felt to be escalating, as may occur with physical abuse, law enforcement as well as APS should be contacted. Hospitalization of the elder may be the only temporary solution to removing the victim from the abuser.

If elders are competent and not cognitively impaired, their wishes to either accept interventions for suspected abuse or refuse those interventions must be respected. If an abused elder refuses to leave an abusive environment, the primary care physician can help by providing support and whatever interventions the older person will accept. Helping the older victim to develop a safety plan, such as when to call 911, or installing a Lifeline emergency alert system may be part of the management plan. Close follow-up should be offered.

If older victims no longer retain decision-making capacity, the courts may need to appoint a guardian or

Table 42–6. Physical examination and possible signs of abuse or mistreatment.

Focus of Examination	Possible Signs of Abuse/Mistreatment	Type of Abuse
General	Hygiene, cleanliness of clothing, weight loss, dehydration	Neglect
Skin and mucous membranes	Skin turgor and signs of dehydration Multiple skin lesions in various stages of healing Bruises, welts, bite marks, burns Pressure ulcers	Neglect Physical Neglect
Head and neck	Traumatic alopecia, scalp hematomas Lacerations or abrasions Poor oral hygiene	Physical Neglect
Trunk and extremities	Bruises and welts; wrist or ankle lesions suggesting restraint use; immersion burns	Physical
Musculoskeletal	Occult fractures, pain; observe gait	Physical
Genitorectal/urinary	Vaginal, rectal bleeding, itching, pain, or bruising; sexually transmitted disease; torn, stained, or bloody underwear Poor hygiene; inguinal rash, urine burns, fecal impaction	Sexual Neglect
Neurological and psychiatric status	Thorough cognitive evaluation; look for depression and anxiety; cognitive impairment suggesting delirium or dementia that can affect decision-making capacity Behaviors such as rocking, sucking, antisocial or borderline, or conduct disorders	All forms Psychological
Imaging/laboratory	As indicated from clinical examination; albumin, creatinine, blood urea nitrogen, possible toxicology screen	
Social and financial	Inquire about other members of social network and who can assist and about financial resources and who handles finances	

Source: Kleinschmidt KC: Elder abuse: A review. Ann Emerg Med 1997;30:463. Lachs MS, Pillemer K: Abuse and neglect of elderly persons. New Engl J Med 1997;332:437.

conservator to make decisions about living arrangements, finances, and care. This is typically coordinated through APS. The physician's role in these cases is to provide documentation not only of the physical findings of abuse but also of impaired decision-making capacity.

As the growth of the elderly population in the United States continues, physicians will need to use vigilance to identify and assist patients at risk for elder abuse. Geroff and Olshaker have provided a framework to help the physician with this potentially overwhelming task. The primary care physician's role is to recognize or suspect abuse in its various forms, treat the medical problems associated with the abuse, and provide a safe disposition for the patient. The additional evaluations, assessments, and long-term follow-up may be provided by a team of social workers, APS personnel, attorneys, and other members of the traditional health care team. The initial assessment by the primary care or emergency physician may start these crucial interventions.

Geroff AJ, Olshaker JS: Elder abuse. Emerg Med Clin North Am 2006;24:491. [PMID: 16584968]

Movement Disorders 43

Yaqin Xia, MD, MHPE, & Goutham Rao, MD

General Considerations

A movement disorder is a neurologic condition that disrupts normal voluntary body movement or is characterized by abnormal movement. Diagnosis of movement disorders can be challenging, because symptoms and signs are often subtle and presentations may be complex. Accurate diagnosis relies on a detailed history, recognition of the different phenomena of movement disorders together with a detailed neurologic examination, and appropriate supportive laboratory tests.

Family physicians should be familiar with the common presenting symptoms and signs and the management of the common movement disorders. The care of most patients will be managed by a neurologist, and the assistance of a specialist may also be helpful for the diagnosis of complex or less common movement disorders. However, family physicians can play a significant role by providing support to patients and their families, through counseling and referral to support groups and community resources, and in coordinating patients' care.

Classification of Movement Disorders

Movement disorders are classified as *hypokinesias,* characterized by overall slowness of movement (bradykinesia), lack of movement (akinesia), or difficulty in initiating movement; and *hyperkinesias,* characterized by extra or exaggerated movements (eg, tremor). Common hypokinesias and hyperkinesias are listed in Table 43–1.

The following symptom characteristics (recommended by H. Kummer and D.B. Cale) can help narrow the diagnosis in evaluating a patient with a possible movement disorder:

- Topography (distribution).
- Symmetry (asymmetric or symmetric).
- Nature (eg, stereotyped or nonstereotyped)
- Velocity (slow, intermediate, or fast).
- Rhythm (continuous or intermittent).
- Relation to voluntary movement, performance of specific tasks, posture, and sleep.
- Overflow to other body parts.
- Associated sensory symptoms.
- Suppressibility.
- Aggravating or precipitating factors (eg, stress, anxiety, alcohol, caffeine), and ameliorating factors (eg, sleep, rest, alcohol).
- Distractibility and consistency (to distinguish functional movement disorders).

HYPOKINESIA

PARKINSON DISEASE

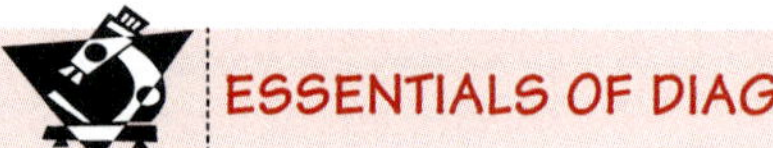

- *Two of the following cardinal features, and absence of a secondary cause:*
  - *Resting tremor.*
  - *Rigidity.*
  - *Bradykinesia.*
  - *Postural instability (late presentation).*

General Considerations

Parkinson disease (PD) is a chronic, progressive neurodegenerative disorder associated with a loss of dopaminergic nigrostriatal neurons. PD is the most common neurodegenerative disease, with a prevalence of approximately 31 to 328 per 100,000 people.

Risk factors include advanced age, family history (ie, a first-degree relative with PD), rural living, exposure to well water, and agricultural work (suggesting that pesticides or herbicides may have an etiologic role). Interestingly, factors that appear to reduce the risk for PD include cigarette smoking and caffeine consumption.

Clinical Findings

A. Symptoms and Signs

The most common initial finding is an asymmetric resting tremor in an upper extremity. The asymmetry of cardinal symptoms (ie, resting tremor, bradykinesia,

Table 43–1. Classification of movement disorders.

Hypokinetic Disorders	Hyperkinetic Disorders
Parkinson disease	Tremor
Secondary parkinsonism	Tic disorders (eg, Tourette syndrome)
Progressive supranuclear palsy (PSP)	Chorea (eg, Huntington disease)
Multisymptom atrophy (MSA)	Myoclonus
	Dystonia
	Ataxia

rigidity) typically becomes bilateral within several years although symptoms may remain more severe on the initial presenting side throughout the disease course.

1. Primary motor abnormalities—Resting tremors occur as the presenting symptom in 50–75% of patients with PD. Tremors usually have a regular rhythm (4–6 beats/s) and are lessened by sleep and voluntary movement. The most frequently affected areas are the hands, fingers, forearm, and foot, but tremors may also affect the head, face, lips, tongue, jaw, and neck.

Bradykinesia refers to an overall slowing of voluntary movement or difficulty initiating and completing movement. Patients report rapid fatigue with repetitive movements and difficulty executing sequential actions, such as buttoning their clothes. As symptoms worsen, the face takes on a masklike look (hypomimia), and speech may become softer or slurred. A soft glabellar reflex (Myerson sign) may be noted.

Rigidity refers to increased resistance to passive movement. Patients often display "cogwheel" rigidity (in which there is intermittent resistance during passive motion of a limb). Symptoms of rigidity can progress to affect breathing, eating, swallowing, and speech.

Postural instability usually occurs late in the disease course and results from the impairment or loss of reflexes. Because this finding may also occur in elderly patients without the disorder, it is only useful as an adjunct to the diagnosis. The instability may lead to frequent falls and it is the most disabling and least treatable of the motor symptoms.

Patients with advanced disease demonstrate a **parkinsonian gait** characterized by short, shuffling steps (festination), diminished arm swing, and reduced stride.

2. Secondary symptoms—Cognitive, automatic, and psychiatric disturbances may be associated with the primary motor abnormalities described above. Cognitive and behavioral symptoms include anxiety, depression, fatigue, and sleep disturbance. Dementia occurs late in the disease course in 20–30% of patients with PD. Autonomic complaints include constipation, orthostatic hypotension, impotence, and excessive salivation or sweating. Altered sensation is manifested by pain (50% of patients), cramps, paresthesias (40%), and restless legs syndrome.

B. Laboratory and Imaging Studies

Computed tomography (CT) or magnetic resonance imaging (MRI) scans, along with blood and cerebrospinal fluid analysis, may be ordered to rule out intracranial disorders. Measurement of dopamine levels in peripheral blood lymphocytes may be useful in the diagnosis of early-stage PD. Positron emission tomography (PET) scans have been investigated for use in diagnosing PD and differentiating PD from secondary parkinsonism, but results have been inconsistent and further research is needed. Further studies are also needed to clarify the utility of L-dopa challenge tests, which may improve diagnostic accuracy.

Complications

PD results in progressive disability, which interferes with the performance of daily activities. In later stages of the disease patients may have difficulty swallowing, increasing their risk of aspiration and malnutrition. Other significant complications include dysarthria, falls, and injuries; deep vein thrombosis; neuropsychiatric morbidity; and sleep disorders.

Complications also occur over the course of treatment as a result of drug therapy. Three to five years after starting medical treatment for PD, most patients begin to experience motor complications or side effects from treatment. Levodopa-induced side effects include motor fluctuations and dyskinesias. Motor fluctuations are alterations in the severity of impairment of movement that occur because of a fluctuating response to levodopa. Patients respond well to medication during "on" periods and poorly during "off" periods, and these fluctuations become more rapid as the disease progresses. Dyskinesias induced by levodopa can include choreiform movements, dystonia, and myoclonus.

Treatment

Although no treatment has been shown conclusively to slow the progression of the disease, several pharmacologic and surgical therapies are available that can successfully control patients' symptoms for many years. Numerous nonpharmacologic approaches may also be used to improve patients' quality of life.

The goals of treatment vary, depending on the disease stage. In early PD, treatment goals are to control symptoms and maintain patients' independent function; in late PD, to maximize medication effectiveness and control medication side effects.

A. Pharmacotherapy

The goals of pharmacotherapy are twofold: neuroprotection and symptomatic therapy of motor disability. Pharmacotherapy also may be needed to manage depression, anxiety, and other psychiatric symptoms if these symptoms are debilitating.

1. Neuroprotective agents—The identification of neuroprotective agents to slow disease progression remains a major focus of current research into PD. Vitamin E is probably ineffective in the treatment of PD, and there is insufficient evidence to support or refute the use of riluzole, coenzyme Q10, pramipexole, ropinirole, rasagiline, amantadine, or thalamotomy for neuroprotection. By the time of clinical diagnosis, more than 70% of dopaminergic cells have already been lost. More emphasis therefore needs to be placed on the development of methods to identify presymptomatic patients for clinical trials of potential neuroprotective therapies.

2. Symptomatic therapy—Symptomatic therapy should be started only when the patient begins to experience functional impairment. There are no strict rules as to what constitutes functional impairment, and the decision to begin treatment should be based on individual condition. This decision requires close cooperation and communication between the patient and the physician. Factors that influence decision making include:

- Degree of impairment; for example, symptoms that affect the dominant hand, or the presence of more disabling features of PD (eg, bradykinesia).
- Effect of symptoms on employment.
- Patient's attitude toward medications.

Each category of medications has its own side effects, and the choice of medication should be individualized. Table 43–2 lists the main categories of medications used in the treatment of PD.

Levodopa is the mainstay treatment. The American Academy of Neurology recommends initial therapy with levodopa in patients with prominent motor disability; however, its use early in the disease process is limited by the development of motor fluctuations and drug-induced dyskinesias.

Dopamine agonists can be used as the first-line medication in patients with early or advanced PD. These agents may be preferable in patients younger than 65 years of age, who can better tolerate the psychiatric side effects of these drugs. When introduced in early-stage PD, dopamine agonists provide adequate symptomatic benefit and delay the need for levodopa. Pergolide was removed from the market in March 2007 for its potential serious side effect of heart valve damage.

Catecholamine-*O*-methyltransferase (COMT) inhibitors, by limiting dopamine metabolism, increase levodopa bioavailability, prolong the "on" response to levodopa, reduce motor fluctuations effectively, and allow a reduction in daily levodopa dosage. Two COMT inhibitors are currently available: tolcapone and entacapone.

Selegiline, amantadine, or an anticholinergic drug may also be appropriate in the initial treatment of patients with mild symptoms. Anticholinergics may provide moderate improvement in rigidity and tremor, but the neuropsychiatric and cognitive side effects of these agents limit their clinical uses. It is prudent to start any medication at a low dosage and titrate slowly until a therapeutic dosage is reached.

3. Psychiatric treatment—Antidepressants are most often used for control of depression. Although amitriptyline is effective, it is not considered a first-line medication because of its multiple side effects, especially in elderly patients.

Cholinesterase inhibitors are effective treatments for dementia in patients with PD. Donepezil or rivastigmine also may be used for dementia treatment.

Atypical antipsychotic agents are used in management of psychotic symptoms in adult patients with PD. Commonly used agents include clozapine and quetiapine. Clozapine improves psychosis and resulted in improved motor function in some patients. Some studies have shown that olanzapine probably does not improve psychosis and worsens motor function, and is not recommended.

B. Surgical Intervention

Surgery is the mainstay of treatment in late-stage PD when medication efficacy has decreased or side effects have become intolerable. Surgical procedures are less effective in patients who are not responding to medical regimens, and only about 10% of patients are considered candidates. Three surgical procedures are currently performed.

1. Ablative or destructive surgery (thalamotomy, pallidotomy) is designed to eliminate uncontrolled dyskinesias and tremor by destroying the globus pallidus and the brain tissue in the thalamus.
2. In deep brain stimulation, an implanted electrode inactivates but does not destroy the subthalamic nucleus, globus pallidus, or thalamus. The electrode is connected via a wire running beneath the skin to a stimulator and battery pack in the patient's chest. This enables the stimulus to be turned on and off, for precise control of symptoms.
3. In transplantation surgery, dopamine-producing fetal cells are implanted into the striatum. This technique has achieved only moderate effectiveness as 90% of implanted cells usually die. Nonfetal cells (eg, pig embryo cells, stem cells) have a better survival rate.

C. Ancillary Treatment and Supportive Measures

Short-term efficacy has been demonstrated for the following therapies: allied health interventions; occupational

Table 43–2. Pharmacotherapy for Parkinson disease.

Class/Drug	Usual Daily Dosage	Clinical Use and Side Effects
Dopaminergic Agents		
Precursor amino acid: levodopa		Dyskinesia, dystonia, hallucinations, hyperkinesia, dizziness, fatigue, abdominal pain, constipation, diarrhea, nausea, vomiting, cardiac abnormalities, orthostatic hypotension, discolored urine
Carbidopa-levodopa (Sinemet)	200–2000 mg/day, divided three times daily	Increase by 1 tablet every day or every other day to a maximum of 8 tab/day
Controlled release (Sinemet CR)	200–1400 mg/day, divided twice daily	Increase by 1 tablet every 3 days to a maximum of 8 tab/day
Madopar CR 100/25mg (L-dopa and benserazide)	1–8 tabs 4–6 times daily	Introduce gradually
Carbidopa-levodopa-entacapone (Stalevo)	12.5 mg carbidopa with 50 mg levodopa and 200 mg entacapone twice daily	Used when other medications become less effective Increase slowly to a maximum of 8 tab/day
Dopamine agonists		Somnolence, sudden onset of sleep (caution with driving), confusion, hallucinations, hypotension
Bromocriptine	2.5–60 mg/day 1.25 mg twice daily	Adjust every 2 weeks
Pramipexole	0.125 mg three times daily	Adjust every week up to a maximum of 1.5 mg three times daily
Ropinirole	0.25 mg three times daily	Adjust every week up to a maximum of 12–16 mg
Monamine oxidase B inhibitors		Sleep disturbance, light-headedness, nausea, abdominal pain, confusion, hallucinations
Selegiline (deprenyl)	5 mg at breakfast and lunch	No dosage titration required
Indirect agonists		Hallucinations, dry mouth, livedo reticularis, ankle swelling, myoclonic encephalopathy in setting of renal failure
Amantadine	100–300 mg/day	Avoid in patients with cognitive impairment
Catecholamine-*O*-Methyltransferase (COMT) inhibitors		Effective only with levodopa and given in combination to reduce levodopa-induced dyskinesias; enables levodopa dosage to be reduced, increase levodopa bioavailability, and prolongs its half-life; reduces "off" time and increases "on" time
Tolcapone	300–600 mg/day, or 100 or 200 mg three times daily	Worsening of levodopa-induced dyskinesias (as evidenced by improvement with decrease in levodopa dosage), diarrhea, nausea, vivid dreams, visual hallucinations, sleep disturbances, daytime drowsiness, headache, hepatotoxicity
Entacapone[1]	200 mg, twice to eight times daily, with each dose of carbidopa-levodopa	
Other Drug Classes		
Anticholinergics[2]		Confusion, sleepiness, blurred vision, constipation
Trihexyphenidyl	2–15 mg/day	
Biperiden	1–8 mg/day	Avoid in patients with cognitive impairment or patients older than 65.
Novel neuroleptics		Used for psychosis and unusual tremor
Clozapine	12.5–100 mg/day	Fatal neutropenia, somnolence
Quetiapine	12.5–100 mg/day	Somnolence, potential aggravated parkinsonism
Miscellaneous		
Amitriptyline	10–50 mg/day at bedtime	Sleep fragmentation, dry mouth, forgetfulness, blurred vision, constipation
Baclofen	10–80 mg/day	Dystonic cramps, sleepiness, dizziness

Tab, tablet; CR, controlled release.

[1]No hepatotoxicity reported.

[2]May worsen motor symptoms on discontinuation; tapering is needed.

therapy; physical therapy; psychotherapy (counseling); and speech, swallowing, and voice therapy. Patients can be referred to various support groups, including the American Parkinson Disease Association (http://www.apdaparkinson.com), the National Parkinson Foundation (http://www.parkinson.org), the Michael J. Fox Foundation for Parkinson's Research (http://www.michaeljfox.com), and the Parkinson's Disease Foundation (http://www.parkinsons-foundation.org).

D. Monitoring the Disease Process

Caring for patients with PD involves long-term assessment of disease severity and monitoring for side effects of therapy, usually levodopa. Adjustment of medications is a complicated but unavoidable task that is necessary to minimize "off" periods, maximize "on" periods, and decrease side effects.

Clinical rating scales are used to evaluate disease severity and the efficacy of pharmacotherapy. The Unified Parkinson Disease Rating Scale is currently the most commonly used scale. Its six sections assess mood and cognition; activities of daily living in both "on" and "off" state; motor abilities; complications of therapy; disease severity; and global function (ie, level of disability, mood, and both disease- and treatment-related manifestations of PD).

Prognosis

PD is a progressive, irreversible disease. In patients with newly diagnosed PD, older age at onset and the presence of rigidity or hypokinesia as an initial symptom predict a more rapid rate of motor progression. Associated comorbidities (stroke, auditory deficits, and visual impairments), Parkinson-induced gait disturbances, and male sex also predict a faster rate of motor progression.

Agency for Healthcare Research and Quality: *Diagnosis and Treatment of Parkinson's Disease: A Systematic Review of the Literature.* AHRQ, 2003. Available at: http://www.ahrq.gov/clinic/epcsums/parksum.htm; http://www.ahrq.gov/downloads/pub/evidence/pdf/parkinsons/parkinsons.pdf.

Dickerson LM et al: Treatment of early Parkinson's disease. Am Fam Physician 2005;72:497. [PMID: 16100865]

Miyasaki JM: Practice parameter: Evaluation and treatment of depression, psychosis, and dementia in Parkinson disease: Report of the Quality Standards Subcommittee of the American Academy of Neurology. Neurology 2006;66:996. [PMID: 16606910]

Suchowersky O et al: Practice parameter: Neuroprotective strategies and alternative therapies for Parkinson disease (an evidence-based review): Report of the Quality Standards Subcommittee of the American Academy of Neurology. Neurology 2006;66:976. [PMID: 16606908]

Kumar A, Calne DB: Chapter 1: Approach to the patient with a movement disorder and overview of movement disorders. In Watts RL, Koller WC, eds: *Movement Disorders: Neurologic Principles and Practice,* 2nd ed. McGraw-Hill, 2004:3–16.

Web Site

http://www.wemove.prg/par/

SECONDARY PARKINSONISM, PROGRESSIVE SUPRANUCLEAR PALSY, & MULTISYSTEM ATROPHY

It is important to distinguish between "parkinsonism" and PD. *Parkinsonism* refers to any condition that causes any combination of the types of movement abnormalities seen in PD. About 76% of patients clinically diagnosed with *idiopathic parkinsonism* actually have PD. Atypical features and obvious triggers identified from the history should raise the suspicion of parkinsonism rather than PD (Table 43–3).

Secondary parkinsonism is caused by another illness or other etiologies (eg, drugs; infections; toxins; metabolic, structural, or vascular conditions), and shares symptoms similar to PD. Patients with secondary parkinsonism may have a positive medication or medical history (eg, patients with vascular parkinsonism generally have a history of chronic hypertension, stepwise progression, unilateral symptoms, and positive imaging findings).

The *"parkinsonism plus" syndromes* include corticobasal ganglionic degeneration, hemiparkinsonism-hemiatrophy, diffuse Lewy body disease, multiple system atrophy (MSA; which encompasses parkinsonism-amyotrophy, Shy-Drager syndrome, olivopontocerebellar atrophy, and striatonigral degeneration), and progressive supranuclear palsy (PSP). These disorders are relatively uncommon and share similar features. Corticobasal ganglionic degeneration is characterized by limb apraxia, cortical sensory abnormalities, coarse unilateral tremor, and early dementia. Patients with diffuse Lewy body disease tend to have early dementia, psychosis, agitation, and visual hallucinations. PSP is characterized by a downgaze palsy, square-wave jerks, upright posture, pseudobulbar palsy (dysarthria, dysphagia), and early gait instability; tremor is uncommon in these patients and symptoms do respond to levodopa.

Hereditary degenerative diseases, such as Wilson disease, Huntington disease, and pantothenate kinase–associated neurodegeneration (formerly Hallervorden-Spatz disease), may also produce parkinsonism.

Treatment is based on etiology. Patients with nonidiopathic parkinsonism typically do not respond well to standard anti-PD medications.

HYPERKINESIAS

TREMOR

Tremor is a rhythmic, involuntary, oscillatory movement of body parts. It is the most common movement disorder. There are several types of tremor with differing underlying physiologic or pathologic etiologies (Table 43–4). Tremors may also be caused by alcohol and by numerous drugs,

Table 43–3. Atypical features in parkinsonism.

Clinical Finding	Differential Diagnosis
Early onset	Young-onset (before age 40 y) or juvenile (before age 20 y) Parkinson disease, Wilson disease, pantothenate kinase–associated neurodegeneration
Minimal or absent tremor	Striatonigral degeneration, progressive supranuclear palsy (PSP), Shy-Drager syndrome, vascular or hydrocephalic parkinsonism
Atypical tremor	Corticobasal ganglionic degeneration (CBGD), olivopontocerebellar degeneration (OPCD)
Predominant postural instability	PSP, multisystem atrophy (MSA), vascular or hydrocephalic parkinsonism
Ataxia	MSA (particularly OPCD)
Pyramidal signs	MSA (striatonigral degeneration), CBGD, vascular or hydrocephalic parkinsonism
Neuropathy	MSA (parkinsonism-amyotrophy)
Marked motor asymmetry	Hemiparkinsonism-hemiatrophy, CBGD
Symmetric onset	Striatonigral degeneration, vascular or hydrocephalic parkinsonism
Myoclonus	CBGD, Creutzfeldt-Jakob disease
Early dementia	Diffuse Lewy body disease, Alzheimer disease, Creutzfeldt-Jakob disease, multi-infarct dementia, PSP
Focal cortical signs	CBGD
Alien limb sign	CBGD
Oculomotor deficits	PSP, OPCA, CBGD
Dysautonomia	MSA (particularly Shy-Drager syndrome)

Source: Paulson HL, Stern MB: Chapter 14: Clinicial maifestations of Parkinson's disease. In Watts RL, Koller WC, eds: *Movement Disorders: Neurologic Principles and Practice,* 2nd ed. McGraw-Hill, 2004:233–246.

including amphetamines, β-adrenergic agonists, caffeine, lithium, neuroleptic agents, steroids, and tricyclic antidepressants.

Smaga S: Tremor. Am Fam Physician 2003;68:1545. [PMID: 14596441]

ESSENTIAL TREMOR

ESSENTIALS OF DIAGNOSIS

Core criteria:

- *Bilateral action tremor (postural or kinetic) of the hands and forearms, but not rest tremor.*
- *Isolated head tremor with no signs of dystonia.*
- *Absence of other neurologic signs, with the exception of the "cogwheel" phenomenon.*

Secondary criteria:

- *Long duration (> 3 years).*
- *Positive family history.*
- *Beneficial effect of alcohol.*

General Considerations

Essential tremor is the most common movement disorder, affecting about 300 per 100,000 people annually. Eighty-five percent of affected individuals report significant changes in their livelihood and socializing as a result of the condition, and 15% report being seriously disabled by it. However, less than 10% of those affected seek treatment.

Clinical Findings

A. Symptoms and Signs

Essential tremor is characterized by a slowly progressive postural or kinetic tremor that usually affects both upper extremities. A family history is noted in 50–60% of patients. Age of onset has bimodal peaks—the first in late adolescence to early adulthood and the second in older adulthood. The mean age at presentation is 35–45 years. Both sexes are equally affected.

In Table 43–5, the classic phenomena of essential tremor are described and contrasted with features of tremor resulting from other physiologic and pathologic causes. Most patients with essential tremor have varying degrees of postural and kinetic tremor. Atypical presentations may also occur (eg, kinetic-predominant tremor with minimal or absent postural component; a primary writing tremor that is present for the duration of writing; isolated tremors of the tongue, chin, and voice). The main clinical features and supportive diagnostic tests for common differential diagnoses of essential tremor are listed in Table 43–5.

The severity of tremor can be assessed by using a tremor scale (eg, Columbia University Disability Ques-

Table 43–4. Classification of tremors.

Category of Tremor	Tremor Characteristics	Associated Medical Conditions
Rest Tremors	Frequency: low to medium (3–6 Hz) Occurs in a body part that is not voluntarily activated and is completely supported against gravity	Parkinsonism Rubral (midbrain) tremor Wilson disease Severe essential tremor
Action Tremors	Occurs during any voluntary movement	Dystonic tremor
Postural tremors	Frequency: medium to high (4–12 Hz) Occurs when a body part (limb) is maintaining a posture against the force of gravity	(Enhanced) physiologic tremor Essential tremor Orthostatic tremor Psychogenic tremor Rubral tremor Neuropathic tremor (Enhanced) physiologic tremor
Kinetic tremors		
Simple kinetic tremors	Frequency: 3–10 Hz Occurs with non–target-directed movement of extremities (eg, pronation-supination or flexion-extension wrist movements)	
Intention tremors	Frequency: < 5 Hz Occurs with target-directed movement (eg, finger-to-nose)	Cerebellar etiology (eg, multiple sclerosis, trauma, stroke, tumor, vascular disease, Wilson disease, drug- or toxin-induced) Rubral tremor
Task-specific intention tremors	Frequency: 5–7 Hz Involves skilled, highly learned motor acts (eg, writing, sewing, playing musical instruments)	Primary writing tremor Musician's tremor
Isometric tremors	Frequency: 4–6 Hz Occurs with muscle contraction against a stationary object	
Miscellaneous Tremors		Myoclonus Convulsions Asterixis Fasciculation Clonus Psychogenic

tionnaire for essential tremor, modified Klove-Matthews Motor-Steadiness Battery) or other clinical scales.

B. Imaging Studies

Imaging studies are not routinely ordered for diagnosis, and findings are typically normal. MRI is useful to exclude structural and inflammatory lesions (including multiple sclerosis) and Wilson disease, and should be performed if the tremor has an acute onset or a stepwise progression.

C. Special Tests

Electromyography or accelerometry can be used to assess frequency, rhythmicity, and amplitude of the tremor, but neither test is part of the routine evaluation.

Table 43–5. Clinical and differential diagnosis of tremors.

Condition	Characteristic Findings	Laboratory and Diagnostic Studies
Essential tremor (ET)	Age of onset has bimodal peaks Slowly progressive postural or kinetic tremor usually affects both upper extremities: in young adults, 8- to 12-Hz tremor; in elderly, 6- to 8-Hz tremor Family history; negative trauma history; no other neurologic signs Tremor is worsened by stress, fatigue, and voluntary movement Usually responds to alcohol, propranolol, and primidone	No laboratory studies are necessary if history and physical examination point to the diagnosis of ET CBC, comprehensive metabolic panel, thyroid function tests, and serum ceruloplasmin (for Wilson disease) may be ordered for differential diagnosis
Enhanced physiologic tremor	High-frequency 10- to 12-Hz tremor Most common cause of postural and action tremor Occurs under various conditions (eg, stress, fatigue, hypoglycemia, thyroid and adrenal gland dysfunction, alcohol withdrawal, and medications) No other neurologic signs Responds to reduction or removal of offending medication or toxin, treatment of endocrine disorders, and stress management Use of propranolol prior to stressful events may reduce tremor	Chemistry profile (glucose, liver function tests); thyroid function tests; review of medications
Parkinsonism	Usually late age of onset Asymmetric, slow (4- to 6-Hz), high-amplitude rest tremor; biplanar; pill-rolling; action tremor may also occur Onset in hands or legs; patient usually has other signs of Parkinson disease Tremor is worsened by stress, improves with voluntary movement, and is unaffected by alcohol	No testing is needed for patients with typical presentations For atypical presentations, obtain MRI scan; consider PET or SPECT scanning, if available
Cerebellar tremor	Kinetic tremor on ipsilateral side of the body, 3–4 Hz Ataxia, dysmetria, nystagmus, and other cerebellar signs	CT or MRI scan CSF analysis of IgG if multiple sclerosis is suspected Screening for alcohol abuse Obtain lithium level if lithium toxicity is suspected
Orthostatic tremor	Late onset; rare family history Occurs exclusively while standing Tremor is limited to legs and paraspinal muscles Responds to gabapentin, pramipexole, and clonazepam	
Neuropathic tremor	Associated with peripheral nerve pathology (eg, hereditary neuropathies, Guillain-Barré syndrome, chronic inflammatory demyelinating polyneuropathy) Does not respond to propranolol or other therapy	

(*continued*)

Table 43–5. Clinical and differential diagnosis of tremors. *(Continued)*

Condition	Characteristic Findings	Laboratory and Diagnostic Studies
Rubral or midbrain tremor	Occurs with midbrain injury Rest tremor, but slower (3–5 Hz) than that seen in parkinsonism Tremor may be variable with rest; postural, action, and kinetic	
Psychogenic tremor	Variable tremor that increases with direct observation and may decrease or disappear when patient is distracted or not under direct observation, or with psychotherapy or placebo Changes with voluntary movement of contralateral limb Somatization in past history	Electrophysiologic testing: patient is asked to tap a beat with the limb contralateral to the tremulous limb; if the tremor decreases or shifts to the frequency of the tapping (ie, entrainment), psychogenic tremor is suspected
Wilson disease	Wing-beating tremor Ascites, jaundice, signs of hepatic disease Intracorneal ring-shaped pigmentation Rigidity, muscle spasms Mental symptoms	Liver function tests; serum ceruloplasmin; urine copper; slit-lamp examination

CBC, complete blood count; MRI, magnetic resonance imaging; PET, positron emission tomography; SPECT, single photon emission computed tomography; CT, computed tomography; CSF, cerebrospinal fluid; IgG, immunoglobulin G.

Treatment

Both pharmacologic and surgical approaches have been used successfully in the treatment of essential tremor. Responses to these treatments vary, depending on the tremor variant body part affected, and individual patient characteristics.

A. Pharmacotherapy

Pharmacotherapy is the main (and most effective) therapy for essential tremor. Several categories of medication are used (Table 43–6). Essential tremor of the hand responds well to pharmacologic treatment, but this therapy is less successful for head and voice tremor.

In addition to the medications listed in Table 43–6, the use of small amounts of alcoholic beverages before meals or other events to reduce tremor is often helpful. Occasional use of alcohol in patients with essential tremor carries a low risk of alcoholism. Use of phenobarbital in patients with essential tremor is controversial; however, it may be considered in patients who do not respond well to propranolol or primidone.

Physicians Cersosimo and Koller suggest to start with primidone 50 mg at bedtime, and increase as needed up to 250 mg; then may add on or switch to long-acting propranolol in the morning, starting from 80 mg, increase as needed up to 320 mg. Alprazolam or clonazepam may be started if the control of tremor is not achieved with above medications.

B. Surgical Intervention

Surgical intervention should be considered only for patients with severe and disabling tremors who do not respond to maximally tolerated doses of propranolol, primidone, and clonazepam. Stereotaxic thalamotomy and deep brain stimulation are currently used with good results.

C. Behavioral Therapy

With limited effectiveness, psychotherapy, biofeedback, and hypnosis are also used in the management of essential tremor.

Prognosis & Complications

Essential tremor is a progressive condition: with age, tremor frequency declines and amplitude increases. Writing, drinking liquids, and occupational skills become increasingly difficult. The Sickness Impact Profile is a standardized assessment tool that can be used to measure illness-related dysfunction (see http://www.outcomes-trust.org). Significant psychosocial dysfunction, depression, anxiety, and even social phobia-like symptoms are associated with greater functional disability.

Bain P et al: Criteria for the diagnosis of essential tremor. Neurology 2000;54(suppl 4):S7. [PMID: 10854345]

Cerosimo MG, Koller WC: In Watts RL, Koller WC, eds: *Movement Disorders: Neurologic Principles and Practice,* 2nd ed. McGraw-Hill, 2004.

Table 43–6. Pharmacotherapy for essential tremor.

Class/Drug	Usual Daily Dosage	Clinical Use and Side Effects
Primidone (Mysoline)	50–1000 mg/day Low dose (250 mg) is as effective as high dose	Decreases tremor more than propranolol Tolerance may develop Mild to moderate sedation, drowsiness, fatigue, nausea, giddiness, vomiting, ataxia, malaise, dizziness, unsteadiness, confusion, vertigo, acute toxic reaction
β-Adrenergic blockers		Well tolerated Clinical response is variable and often incomplete
Propranolol	60–800 mg/day 240–320 mg/day may be optimal dose	Mild to moderate reduced arterial pressure, reduced pulse rate, tachycardia, bradycardia, impotence, drowsiness, exertional dyspnea, confusion, headache, dizziness
Propranolol (long-acting)	80–320 mg/day	
Benzodiazepines		
Alprazolam (Xanax)	0.125–3 mg/day	As effective as propranolol Mild fatigue, sedation; potential for abuse
Clonazepam	1–3 mg/day	Very effective in treating kinetic-predominant tremor and orthostatic truncal tremor
Gabapentin	1200–1800 mg/day	Mild lethargy, fatigue, decreased libido, dizziness, nervousness, shortness of breath
Topiramate (Topamax)	Up to 400 mg/day	Mild appetite suppression, weight loss, paresthesia, anorexia, concentration difficulties
Botulinum toxin injection		
For hand tremor	50–100 units per arm	Moderate hand and finger weakness, reduced grip strength, pain at injection site, stiffness, cramping, hematoma, paresthesias
For head tremor	40–400 units (has some efficacy)	Mild to moderate neck weakness, postinjection pain
For voice tremor	0.6–15 units (has some efficacy)	Mild to moderate breathiness, weak voice, difficulty swallowing

Zesiewicz TA et al: Practice parameter: Therapies for essential tremor: Report of the Quality Standards Subcommittee of the American Academy of Neurology. Neurology 2005;64:2008. [PMID: 15972843]

Manyam B: Chapter 28: Uncommon forms of tremor. In Watts RL, Koller WC, eds: *Movement Disorders: Neurologic Principles and Practice*, 2nd ed. McGraw-Hill, 2004:459–480.

Smaga S: Tremor. *Am Fam Physician.* 2003;15;68(8):1545. Review. [PMID: 14596441]

TIC DISORDERS

Tics are sudden, brief, recurrent, nonrhythmic, stereotyped, purposeless movements (motor tics) or sounds (vocal tics). Many patients with tics experience urges or somatic sensations of discomfort (sensory tics), such as burning, itching, tingling, or pain, prior to the episodes. Sensory tics are involuntary. Motor or sound tics are voluntary acts to relieve the urges. Tics can be simple and isolated (eg, blinking, grimacing, head jerking, thrpat clearing, or cough); or complex, more coordinated and seemingly purposeful (e.g., jumping, kicking, abdomen thrusting, stuttering, echolalia, or coprolalia). The discussion that follows focuses on Tourette syndrome—a serious, chronic tic disorder.

TOURETTE SYNDROME

ESSENTIALS OF DIAGNOSIS

- *Multiple motor tics and one or more vocal tics are present.*
- *Tics occur several times a day for a least 1 year without a tic-free period of more than 3 consecutive months.*

- *Disease onset before age 18.*
- *Other causes of tics ruled out (e.g., stimulants, tardive tics, encephalitis, stroke, or Huntington disease).*

General Considerations

Tourette syndrome is the most common tic disorder, affecting about 200 per 100,000 people annually. Three times as many boys as girls are affected. The average age of onset is 7 years, with most cases developing between 2 and 15 years of age.

Clinical Findings

A. Symptoms and Signs

Tourette syndrome is transmitted within families. While genes are currently considered the major factor for the development of Tourette syndrome, environment may also play an important role. Tics usually start in the upper body, especially the eyes or other parts of the face. The severity, distribution, and waves of different combinations of tic types fluctuate over days to weeks. Tics may worsen during periods of stress, excitement, boredom, or fatigue, and they may persist during sleep.

Tourette syndrome includes a spectrum of behavioral features in addition to the different clinical manifestations of tics. Half of patients with Tourette syndrome have coexisting obsessive-compulsive disorder or attention-deficit/hyperactivity disorder (ADHD). Anxiety, conduct disorder, depression, mania, stuttering, obesity, and alcoholism are also associated with Tourette syndrome.

Complications

Little or no excess mortality is associated with Tourette syndrome. However, children can experience severe social disability related to their loud vocalizations and large movements. Social stigma can cause individuals to withdraw from activities or experience prejudice in school or at work. Severe tics interrupt the individual's behavior and thought, often causing disruptive behaviors and school problems. Self-injury may occur—either intentional (from severe depression) or pseudointentional (in complex tics, from repeatedly hitting self, or in sensory tics, from impulsions). Learning disabilities are present in 20% of patients with Tourette syndrome, most often related to comorbid ADHD.

Treatment

Educating patients, families, teachers, and peers about the nature of Tourette syndrome and providing a supportive, structured environment are crucial components in the management of Tourette syndrome, which can delay the need for drug therapy and improve the patient's quality of life and self-esteem. Management should include therapy for comorbid disorders (eg, obsessive-compulsive disorder, ADHD, and other behavioral disturbances).

Pharmacotherapy should be started before symptoms become disabling and cease to respond to psychosocial interventions. The goal is to use the lowest dose of a drug that achieves satisfactory control rather than striving to eliminate tics completely (Table 43–7).

Prognosis

Patients and their families should be advised that treatment is unlikely to eliminate tics completely. However, with aging, most tics become stable or disappear.

American Psychiatric Association: *Diagnostic and Statistical Manual of Mental Disorders,* 4th ed, text revision. American Psychiatric Association, 2000.

Kurlan R: Chapter 41: Tourette's syndrome. In Watts RL, Koller WC, eds: *Movement Disorders: Neurologic Principles and Practice,* 2nd ed. McGraw-Hill, 2004:685–692.

Juncos JL: Chapter 42: Pathophysiology and differential diagnosis of tics. In Watts RL, Koller WC, eds: *Movement Disorders: Neuroloc Principles and Practice*, 2nd ed. McGraw-Hill, 2004:683–701.

Web Site

The Tourette Syndrome Association
http://www.tsa-usa.org

CHOREATIC DISORDERS: HUNTINGTON DISEASE

ESSENTIALS OF DIAGNOSIS

- *Movement abnormalities (chorea and abnormal voluntary movements).*
- *Gait disturbances, abnormal eye movements, dysarthria, dysphagia, and rigidity.*
- *Cognitive, behavioral, and mood disturbances; dementia.*

General Considerations

Huntington disease (HD) is an autosomal-dominant progressive neurodegenerative disorder caused by a

Table 43–7. Pharmacotherapy for Tourette syndrome.

Class/Drug	Usual Daily Dosage	Clinical Use
α-Agonists[1]		First-line agents
Clonidine (oral, transdermal)	0.05 mg at bedtime, increased by 0.05 mg every few days to a maximum of 0.6 mg/day Most patients respond to 1 tab (0.1 mg) three times daily	Initial treatment of Tourette syndrome
Guanfacine	0.5–1 mg at bedtime; maximum of 4 mg/day	Newer, single daily dosing, which is less sedating, is becoming the first choice for many clinicians
Antipsychotics[2]		Second-line agents: May be added to α-agonist or monotherapy First-line agents: For patients with severe tics
Risperidone	0.25–16 mg/day	
Olanzapine	2.5–15 mg/day	
Ziprasidone	20–200 mg/day	
Haloperidol	0.25–2 mg/day	Used if atypical antipsychotics listed above are ineffective

[1]Withdrawal: taper over 7–10 days if medication needs to be discontinued.
[2]Given as a single bedtime dose; pimozide or fluphenazine may be used if listed agents are ineffective.

genetic mutation of the *IT15* gene on chromosome 4. Although it affects only 4–10 of every 100,000 people, its impact can be devastating. Men and women are affected in equal numbers.

Clinical Findings

A. Symptoms and Signs

Onset of clinical symptoms is usually between 30 and 50 years of age. The disease is characterized by movement abnormalities as well as cognitive, behavioral, and emotional disturbances. HD diagnosis is based on the presence of characteristic symptoms and signs in the setting of a positive family history (Table 43–8). A detailed medical history, family history, and neurologic examination are very important.

B. Laboratory and Imaging Studies

Laboratory tests may be ordered to rule out other causes. The diagnostic workup may include liver function tests; complement levels; antinuclear antibody titers; antiphospholipid antibody titers; serum and urine evaluation for the presence of amino acids; enzymatic studies from skin fibroblasts; levels of thyroid-stimulating hormone, thyroxine (T_4), and parathormone; and a peripheral blood smear for acanthocytes.

Brain imaging studies may provide evidence of HD. CT scanning may show cerebral atrophy or atrophy of the caudate nucleus in patients with advanced disease. MRI and PET scanning may reveal reduced glucose utilization in an otherwise normal-appearing caudate nucleus.

C. Special Tests

Genetic testing can detect the gene responsible for HD, which has CAG trinucleotide repeats (repeated sequences of cytosine, adenine, and guanine). Because there is no cure for HD, counseling should be provided before and after the test regarding the possible results (positive, negative, or uninformative); the personal, family, social, and ethical issues surrounding the test; and the diagnosis. Children of patients with HD should be offered genetic counseling and genetic testing.

Complications

The most common complications are rhabdomyolysis, local trauma, and aspiration pneumonia.

Treatment

No treatment is currently available to slow or alter the progression of HD. Close and effective communica-

Table 43–8. Symptoms and signs of Huntington disease.

	Manifestations
Movement disorder	
Chorea	Excessive, spontaneous, continuous, irregular, nonrepetitive movements that are randomly distributed and abrupt in character Movements may vary in severity from restlessness with mild intermittent exaggeration of gesture and expression, fidgeting movements of the hands, and an unstable dancelike gait to a continuous flow of disabling, violent movements
Dystonia and parkinsonism	Chorea, dystonia, rigidity, and postural instability that become more severe as disease progresses
Dysarthria and dysphagia	Articulation disturbances, hypophonic, irregular rate and rhythm, to unintelligible speech
Eye movement disorder	Slowed and uncoordinated ocular saccades, impaired opticokinetic nystagmus
Other hyperkinesias	Motor and vocal tics, myoclonus
Cognitive disorder	Dementia, bradyphrenia (slow thinking), aphasia, agnosia, and apraxia, executive function loss
Behavioral disorder	Depression, suicide, psychosis, obsessive-compulsive symptoms, sleep disorder

tion with the patient and family and psychosocial support are the mainstays of HD management.

A. Monitoring the Disease Process

A multidisciplinary approach is required, including symptomatic and supportive medical management; psychosocial support; physical, occupational, or speech therapy; genetic counseling; and additional supportive services. Patients can be referred to several national support groups and organizations, including the Huntington's Disease Society of America (http://www.hdsa.org/site/PageServer), the International Huntington Association (http://www.huntington-assoc.com/), the Hereditary Disease Foundation (http://www.hdfoundation.org), and the National Institutes of Health/National Institute of Neurological Disorders and Stroke (NIH/NINDS) (http://www.ninds.nih.gov/).

B. Pharmacotherapy

Little efficacy has been found in pharmacologic treatment of HD. Patients with disabling chorea may respond to dopamine receptor antagonists (eg, phenothiazines, butyrophenones, thioxanthenes) or dopamine-depleting agents (eg, reserpine, tetrabenazine). However, the response is only temporary and these medications may exacerbate parkinsonism. Antiglutamatergic agents may also be used (eg, riluzole, amantadine, lamotrigine). Levodopa and dopamine agonists may be used in patients with bradykinesia and rigidity but will exacerbate chorea, dystonia, and behavioral disorders.

Patients with behavioral manifestations may benefit from tricyclic antidepressants, selective serotonin reuptake inhibitors (eg, fluoxetine), carbamazepine, valproate, or lithium.

The use of neuroprotective agents (eg, riluzole, coenzyme Q10, creatine, minocycline) and transplantation of fetal striatal tissue are under investigation as possible treatments to slow the progression of HD.

Prognosis

There is no cure for HD. Neuropsychological tests that are sensitive indicators of disease progression include the Unified Huntington's Disease Rating Scale (UHDRS), Trail Making Test Part B, and Wechsler Adult Intelligence Scale-Revised (WAIS-R).

Marshall F: Chapter 35: Clinical features and treatment of Huntington's disease. In Watts RL, Koller WC, eds: *Movement Disorders: Neurologic Principles and Practice,* 2nd ed. McGraw-Hill, 2004:589–601.

OTHER MOVEMENT DISORDERS

1. Myoclonus

Myoclonus refers to sudden, brief, shocklike involuntary movements. These movements may be "positive" or "negative." Positive myoclonus results in contraction of a muscle or multiple muscles. Negative myoclonus (asterixis) results in a brief loss of muscle tone and then the tightening (contraction) of other muscles, causing a flapping-type motion.

Physiologic myoclonus refers to benign movements that occur in many people (eg, sleep jerks, hiccups, or benign infantile myoclonus with feeding). No treatment is usually needed.

Essential myoclonus, which can be either hereditary or sporadic, is similar to physiologic myoclonus, but the jerking is more frequent, can occur at any time, and interferes with social or physical functioning. It is described as "essential" because myoclonus is the only neurologic manifestation. Although essential myoclonus can be disabling, it is not progressive. Electroencephalographic (EEG) and other laboratory findings are normal.

Epileptic myoclonus describes jerking that occurs with epileptic seizures. It produces EEG and electromyographic (EMG) changes.

Symptomatic (secondary) myoclonus is the most common myoclonic disorder and is caused by damage to the central nervous system from various conditions, including anoxia, trauma, drug intoxication, and metabolic problems (organ failure, electrolyte or endocrine disorders).

In any patient with clinically significant myoclonus, a careful search should be made for secondary causes. Polygraphic EMG studies, EEG or magnetoencephalography (MEG), somatosensory evoked potentials, and reflex studies can be useful in the workup of myoclonus. Measurement of electrolyte and glucose levels, tests for renal and hepatic function, and drug and toxin screening may be ordered, as necessary.

Treatment is aimed at the underlying etiology. For symptomatic control of disabling myoclonus, first-line drugs include levetiracetam, clonazepam, valproic acid, primidone, piracetam, and acetazolamide.

Caviness JN: Primary care guide to myoclonus and chorea. Characteristics, causes, and clinical options. Postgrad Med 2000; 108:163. [PMID: 11043088]

2. Dystonia

Dystonia is characterized by sustained and directional twisting, repetitive movements, or abnormal postures resulting from uncoordinated and persistent contractions of agonist and antagonist muscle groups. It is involuntary and may be triggered only by certain specific actions at the early stage of the disease, such as hand cramps with writing (writer's cramp) initially, then with other body part movements (overflow). Eventually, the dystonia may become persistent with affected body part being held in one position permanently, such as in spasmodic torticollis. Dystonic movments get worse with stress or fatigue. They may improve with rest, sleep, and occasionally alcohol. Geste antagonists (sensory tricks) is another clinical phenomenon of dystonic movements. Patients may suppress abnormal spasm or movements by touching affected or adjunct body parts. It can be primary (sporadic or inherited in an autosomal-dominant or X-linked recessive pattern) or secondary, resulting from a wide variety of neurologic diseases (eg, HD, pantothenate kinase–associated neurodegeneration, Wilson disease [hepatolenticular degeneration], parkinsonism, central nervous system infections, tumors, or stroke) and medications such as neuroleptic drugs.

A thorough history (including family history) and neurologic examination are important for diagnosis and workup of the cause. Tests to consider include CT, MRI, EEG, EMG, nerve conduction, and reflex studies; DNA testing for individuals with early-onset or limb-onset dystonia, regardless of their family history; and appropriate blood and other laboratory tests (eg, serum ceruloplasmin with slit-lamp examination in early-onset dystonia, cerebrospinal fluid analysis, antinuclear antibody titers, erythrocyte sedimentation rate, and metabolic panels).

Treatment depends on the cause. For secondary dystonia, treatment of the underlying disorder or withdrawal of medications may improve patient symptoms. Dystonia can be managed by medications such as benzodiazepines, baclofen, anticholinergics, and dopamine-blocking or dopamine-depleting agents; by injections of therapeutic agents (eg, botulinum toxin) directly into dystonic muscle; and by surgery (thalamotomy, pallidotomy, or deep brain stimulation).

Physical therapy and well-fitted braces may be used to improve posture, maintain or recover range of motion in affected joints, and prevent contractures—a substitute for the "sensory tricks" patients often use (eg, touching or stroking a particular spot on the skin) to interrupt muscle twisting.

3. Ataxia

Ataxia describes a lack of coordination while performing voluntary movements, which may appear as clumsiness, inaccuracy, or instability. Movements are not smooth and may appear disjointed or jerky. Patients may manifest a delay in movement initiation and termination (dysmetria), disturbances of smooth and repeated movement (clapping hands), or wide-based gait to compensate for instability. Ataxia is associated with cerebellar dysfunction involving input and output systems.

Causes of ataxia are varied. There are inherited forms of ataxia, associated with a positive family history (eg, Friedreich ataxia and spinocerebellar ataxia). However, the most common forms likely to be seen by family physicians are acquired. These include ataxic cerebral palsy; ataxia secondary to stroke, trauma, hypoxic injury, hydrocephalus, or central nervous system infection or tumor; drug- or toxin-induced ataxia (most commonly from phenytoin, carbamazepine, antihistamines, barbiturates, lithium, alcohol, or heavy metal poisoning); and vitamin deficiency–induced ataxia (eg, vitamins B_{12} or E; thiamine).

Initial laboratory tests include blood and urine analysis for electrolytes, glucose, amino acids, organic acids, ammonia, copper, and vitamin E. MRI of the brain should be part of the initial workup. Metabolic tests and genetic screening may be carried out as needed.

Accurate diagnosis is the key to treatment, especially for acquired forms of ataxia. Symptomatic treatment with thyrotropin-releasing hormone, clonazepam, or gabapentin may provide some relieve of patients' symptoms.

Brown P, Thompson PD: Electrophysiological aids to the diagnosis of psychogenic jerks, spasms, and tremor. Mov Disord 2001;16:595. [PMID: 11481681]

Hearing & Vision Impairment in the Elderly

44

Alan L. Williams, MD, & Pamela M. Williams, MD

Family physicians are keenly aware of the joy that comes from interacting with the world around them. Many elderly patients are deprived of parts of this world because of hearing and vision impairment. Sensory impairment affects up to two thirds of the geriatric population. Identification, evaluation, and treatment of these conditions (Table 44–1) may improve patients' quality and quantity of life.

The impact of sensory impairments is significant. The same objective level of sensory function can result in different levels of disability depending on the needs and expectations of patients. Vision and hearing impairments have been linked with the wish to die in elderly patients. Poor hearing is associated with depression as well as decreased quality of life, mental health, and physical, social, and cognitive functioning. Vision impairment increases the risk of death and is associated with an elevated risk of falling and hip fracture.

Given the functional impact of undetected and untreated sensory impairments, many arguments have been made for population-based screening. Although research has yet to demonstrate that community-based screening of asymptomatic older people results in improvements in vision or hearing, the US Preventive Services Task Force (USPSTF) and the American Academy of Family Physicians (AAFP) recommend screening geriatric patients with a Snellen visual acuity chart and questioning them about hearing difficulties. Patients should be counseled about available treatment when abnormalities are identified.

COMMON CAUSES OF HEARING IMPAIRMENT IN THE ELDERLY

PRESBYCUSIS

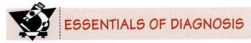

ESSENTIALS OF DIAGNOSIS

- *Age-related high-frequency sensorineural hearing loss.*
- *Difficulty with speech discrimination.*

General Considerations

Presbycusis is the most common form of hearing loss in the elderly, although it often goes unrecognized. It occurs more frequently with advancing age and in patients with a positive family history. This multifactorial disorder is due to a combination of structural and neural degeneration and genetic predisposition. Presbycusis is a diagnosis of exclusion.

Prevention

Until the exact pathophysiology of presbycusis is understood, attempts at prevention will be limited. Although several studies have evaluated the role of vitamins, antioxidants, smoking cessation, and diet in preventing presbycusis, there have been no conclusive findings in humans.

Clinical Findings

Patients with this disorder may present with a chief complaint of hearing loss and difficulty understanding speech. However, presbycusis is often diagnosed only after complaints are raised by close patient contacts, or hearing loss is noted on routine screening in a patient without hearing-related complaints. Abnormalities of the whisper test are found as the level of hearing loss increases. Results of the Weber tuning-fork test remain normal as long as the hearing loss is symmetric. Results of Rinne testing are normal, because presbycusis is a sensorineural hearing loss and not a conductive one.

An audiogram of a patient with presbycusis typically shows bilaterally symmetric high-frequency hearing loss.

Treatment

The treatment of presbycusis consists of hearing rehabilitation, which often involves fitting for binaural hearing aids. Patients are more likely to perceive benefit from hearing aids if they view their hearing loss as a problem. Cochlear

Table 44–1. Differential diagnosis of geriatric hearing and vision impairment.[1]

Hearing Impairment	Vision Impairment
Presbycusis	**Presbyopia**
Cerumen impaction	**Age-related macular degeneration**
Noise-induced hearing loss	**Glaucoma**
Central auditory processing disorder	**Senile cataract**
Otosclerosis	**Diabetic retinopathy**
Chronic otitis media	Central retinal artery or vein occlusion
Glomus tumor or vascular anomaly	Posterior vitreous or retinal detachment
Cholesteatoma	Vitreous hemorrhage
Autoimmune hearing loss	Temporal arteritis
Perilymph fistula	Optic neuritis
Ménière disease	Corneal pathology
Acoustic neuroma	Iritis

[1]The most common causes are indicated by bold type.

implantation is reserved for patients with profound hearing loss that is unresponsive to hearing aids. Additional tools include lip-reading classes; television closed captioning; sound-enhancing devices for concerts, church, or other public gatherings; and telephone amplifiers. A combined approach involving the patient, hearing loss specialist, family physician, and close contacts of the patient is likely to produce the best overall treatment plan.

Suggested topics for patient education include patient self-advocation as well as the proper use of hearing aids and other assistive devices.

Prognosis

The expectation of slow progression of this hearing loss should be communicated to the patient. Complete deafness, however, is not typical of presbycusis.

NOISE-INDUCED HEARING LOSS

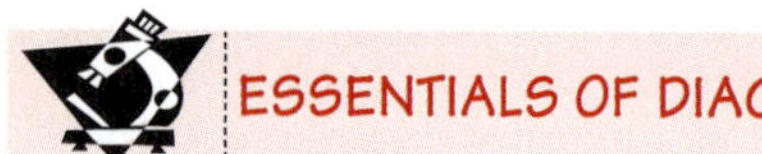

ESSENTIALS OF DIAGNOSIS

- *History of occupational or recreational noise exposure.*
- *Bilateral notch of sensorineural hearing loss between 3000 and 6000 Hz on audiogram.*
- *Problems with tinnitus, speech discrimination, and hearing in the presence of background noise.*

General Considerations

Noise-induced hearing loss is the second most common sensorineural hearing loss after presbycusis. Up to one third of patients with hearing loss have some component of their deficit that is noise induced. The degree of hearing loss is related to the level of noise and the duration of exposure. Excessive shear force from loud sounds or long exposure results in cell damage, cell death, and subsequent hearing loss.

Prevention

Hearing protection programs are prevalent in industrial settings and typically include the use of earplugs, intermittent audiograms, and limiting exposure. Patient commitment to the use of hearing protection is critical for the success of prevention programs.

Clinical Findings

Patients may present with tinnitus, decreased speech discrimination, and difficulty hearing when background noise is present. Patients identified through hearing protection programs may be asymptomatic. Results of the whisper test or office-based pure-tone audiometry may be normal or abnormal, depending on the degree of hearing loss.

Audiometric evaluation of noise-induced hearing loss reveals a bilateral notch of sensorineural hearing loss between 3000 and 6000 Hz.

Treatment

When prevention fails, treatment involves hearing rehabilitation, as previously outlined in the treatment of presbycusis. Education about the risks of loud noise exposure should begin when patients are young, because hearing loss can occur from significant recreational noise. The importance of adhering to hearing protection programs should also be emphasized.

Prognosis

Nothing can be done to reverse cell death from noise-induced hearing loss; however, some patients exposed to brief episodes of loud noise exhibit only hair cell injury and may recover hearing over time. These patients are more susceptible to noise-induced hearing loss on reexposure.

CERUMEN IMPACTION

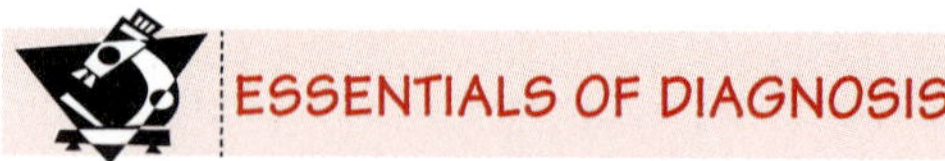

ESSENTIALS OF DIAGNOSIS

- *Mild, reversible conductive hearing loss.*

- *Cerumen buildup in ear canal, limiting sound transmission.*
- *Direct visualization of wax plug confirms diagnosis.*

General Considerations

Impaction of wax in the external auditory canal is a common, frequently overlooked problem in the elderly. Removal of cerumen has been shown to significantly improve hearing ability. The incidence of cerumen impactions increases in the elderly population. Cerumen gland atrophy results in drier wax that is more likely to become trapped by the large tragi hairs in the external ear canal. The likelihood of impaction is increased by hearing aid or earplug use.

Prevention

Cerumen impactions may be prevented by the regular use of agents that soften wax. Readily available household agents such as water, mineral oil, cooking oils, hydrogen peroxide, or glycerin may be used. Commercially available ceruminolytic compounds, such as carbamide peroxide, triethanolamine polypeptide, and docusate sodium liquid are also efficacious, but not more so than less-expensive options.

Clinical Findings

Patients presenting with cerumen impaction may complain of sudden or gradual hearing loss affecting one or both ears. Examination of the external canal reveals partial or complete occlusion of the ear canal with cerumen.

Complications

Various removal methods are associated with ear discomfort and potential for ear canal trauma. Canal trauma can result in bleeding, canal swelling, or infection. Warm water should be used for ear irrigation, because cold water can induce vertigo.

Treatment

The management of impactions may be approached in a variety of ways. When the wax is soft, gentle irrigation of the canal with warm water may be sufficient to remove the offending material. In the case of firmer wax, ceruminolytic agents may be applied, followed by irrigation. Any cerumen remaining after these maneuvers may be removed using a curette in combination with an otoscope for direct visualization. The patient may experience an improvement of symptoms even with partial removal of the impaction. Patients should be instructed about ear cleaning techniques and home use of ceruminolytics.

Prognosis

Cerumen impaction has an excellent prognosis, and hearing can be dramatically improved with relatively simple interventions. However, recurrence of impaction is common.

CENTRAL AUDITORY PROCESSING DISORDER

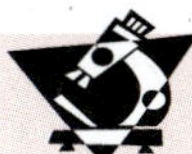

ESSENTIALS OF DIAGNOSIS

- *Hearing impairment due to insult to central nervous system.*
- *Reduction in speech discrimination exceeds hearing loss.*

General Considerations

Central auditory processing disorder (CAPD) is the general term for hearing impairment that results from central nervous system (CNS) dysfunction. Any insult to the nervous system such as stroke or dementia can cause CAPD. The disorder is characterized by a loss of speech discrimination that is more profound than the associated loss in hearing.

Prevention

It may be postulated that the protection of the CNS provided by aspirin therapy and hypertension control could reduce the incidence of CAPD.

Clinical Findings

Patients with CAPD have difficulty understanding spoken language but may be able to hear sounds well. A patient may have difficulty following verbal instructions but understand written ones. There are no specific physical findings of CAPD, but patients may have other evidence of neurologic abnormalities.

Treatment

Treatment of CAPD is limited. If CNS dysfunction is caused by a reversible entity, then treatment for the underlying cause should be initiated. Identifying and treating other causes of sensory impairment may improve the patient's level of disability; however, CAPD may decrease the effectiveness of auditory rehabilitation. Patient education efforts should focus on educating friends and family about the disorder and options for hearing rehabilitation. The prognosis for patients with CAPD is determined by the underlying disorder.

References for Hearing Impairment in the Elderly

Bogardus ST et al: Screening and management of adult hearing loss in primary care: Clinical applications. JAMA 2003;289:1986. [PMID: 12697802]

Yueh B et al: Screening and management of adult hearing loss in primary care: Scientific review. JAMA 2003;289:1976. [PMID: 12697801]

WEB SITES

National Institute on Deafness and Other Communication Disorders (patient education materials on a wide variety of hearing impairment–related topics including presbycusis and hearing aids):

http://www.nidcd.nih.gov/index.asp

National Institute on Aging (patient education handout on the hearing loss):

http://www.niapublications.org/engagepages/hearing.asp

COMMON CAUSES OF VISION IMPAIRMENT IN THE ELDERLY

PRESBYOPIA

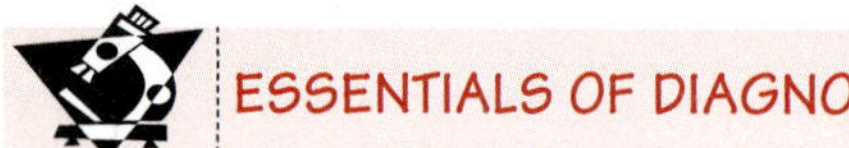

- *Age-related decrease in near vision.*
- *Distance vision remains unaffected.*

General Considerations

Presbyopia is an age-associated progressive loss of the focusing power of the lens. Its incidence increases with age. The cause of this disorder is the ongoing increase in the diameter of the lens as the result of continued growth of the lens fibers with aging. This thickened lens accommodates less responsively to the contraction of muscles in the ciliary body, limiting its ability to focus on near objects.

Clinical Findings

Patients presenting with this disorder frequently complain of eye strain or of blurring of their vision when they quickly change from looking at a nearby object to one that is far away. On examination, the only abnormality noted is a decrease in near vision.

Treatment

Because presbyopia is due to normal age-related changes of the eye, there is no proven prevention. In patients with normal distance vision, treatment for this disorder is as simple as purchasing reading glasses. For patients requiring correction of their distance vision, options include spectacle correction with bifocal or trifocal lenses, monovision contact lenses in which one eye is corrected for distance vision and the other eye for near vision, or contact lens correction of distance vision and simple reading glasses for near vision. Surgical treatment of presbyopia is an evolving science.

Prognosis

All patients should be educated to anticipate a decline in near vision with aging. When left uncorrected, problems may occur with reading, driving, or other activities of daily living.

AGE-RELATED MACULAR DEGENERATION

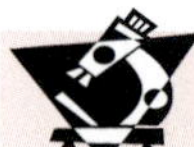

ESSENTIALS OF DIAGNOSIS

- *Slowly progressive central vision loss with intact peripheral vision.*
- *Drusen located in the macula of the retina.*

General Considerations

Age-related macular degeneration (AMD) is the leading cause of severe vision loss in older Americans. It is characterized by atrophy of cells in the central macular region of the retinal pigment epithelium resulting in the loss of central vision. Peripheral vision generally remains intact. AMD is typically classified as early or late, with the late disease being further divided into atrophic (dry) or exudative (wet) forms. The exudative form occurs in only 10% of patients with AMD, but it is responsible for the majority of severe vision loss related to the disease.

Prevention

Multiple risk factors for this disorder have been studied; only increasing age and tobacco abuse have consistently been associated with AMD. Because smoking has been strongly implicated as a risk factor and continued tobacco use is associated with a worse response to laser photocoagulation, tobacco avoidance and smoking cessation should be highly recommended to all patients. Hypertension has also been linked to a worse response to laser therapy; thus, effective blood pressure control is desirable, as well. Finally, antioxidants play a role in tertiary prevention: Patients with intermediate AMD or unilateral advanced AMD had about a 25% reduction of their risk for developing advanced AMD if treated with a high-dose combination of vitamin C, vitamin E, beta-carotene, and zinc. Patients with early or no AMD did not have the same benefit.

Clinical Findings

A. Symptoms and Signs

Patients may report onset of blurred central vision that is either gradual or acute. Wavy or distorted central vision, known as metamorphopsia; intermittent shimmering lights; and central blind spots, termed scotoma, may all occur. Clinical findings include decreased visual acuity, Amsler grid distortion (Figure 44–1), and characteristic abnormalities on dilated funduscopic examination. In early disease, the most common findings are drusen: yellowish-colored deposits deep in the retina. In late disease of the atrophic type, areas of depigmentation are seen in the macula. In the exudative form, abnormal vessels (subretinal neovascularization) leak fluid and blood beneath the macula.

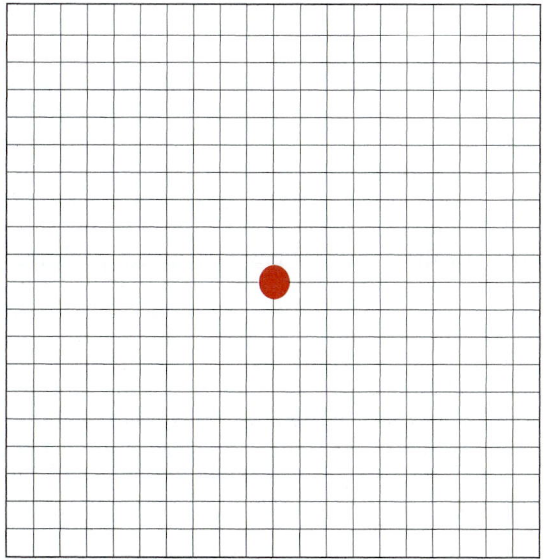

Figure 44–1. Amsler grid for evaluating progression of age-related macular degeneration.

B. Special Examinations

Fluorescein angiography may be used by a specialist to confirm the diagnosis and to help determine if a patient has atrophic or exudative AMD.

Treatment

A. Referral

An ophthalmologist will play a critical role in care of the patient with known or suspected AMD. Urgent referral to an eye specialist should occur if a patient with suspected or known AMD presents with *acute* visual changes. Treatment of exudative AMD is a rapidly advancing field with many ongoing clinical trials of surgical and pharmaceutical interventions. Current treatment options include laser photocoagulation, photodynamic therapy, and antiangiogenesis pharmaceuticals. No effective treatments exist for patient with dry AMD.

Vision rehabilitation is the cornerstone to helping patients maximize their remaining vision and maintain their level of function for as long as possible. Low-vision professionals along with social workers can be of great assistance in recommending optical aids and devices and accessing local, state, and federal resources for the visually impaired. Direct illuminating devices, magnifiers, high-power reading glasses, telescopes, closed-circuit television, large-print publications, and bold-lined paper are some of the many devices that can be employed.

B. Patient Education

Patient education topics include the importance of regular eye examinations, smoking cessation, and routine monitoring for central vision changes. Daily Amsler grid testing is an effective tool for detecting progression. Its use is described at http://www.amd.org.

Prognosis

Many patients with mild dry AMD will not experience significant worsening of their vision. It is difficult to predict which patients will develop advancing disease and further loss of central vision. This condition is generally progressive but is not completely blinding. Peripheral vision should not be affected by AMD.

GLAUCOMA

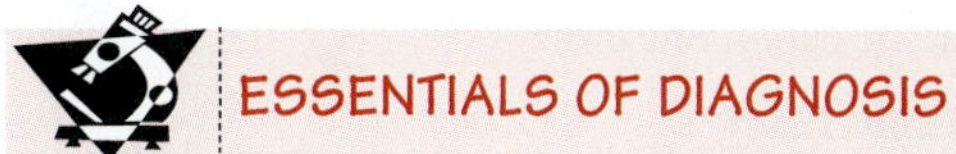

- *Optic neuropathy with variably progressive vision loss.*

- *Intraocular pressure (IOP) is often elevated but may be normal.*

General Considerations

Glaucoma is the second leading cause of blindness in the United States. Although glaucoma is most often associated with elevated IOP, it is the optic neuropathy that defines the disease. Normal IOP is generally accepted to be between 10 and 21 mm Hg. The majority of patients with an IOP greater than 21 mm Hg will not develop glaucoma and 30–50% of patients with glaucoma will have an IOP of less than 21 mm Hg. Despite these facts, it has been clearly shown that as IOP increases, so does the risk of developing glaucoma. Other identified risk factors for glaucoma include family history and advancing age. Additional possible risk factors include diabetes mellitus, hypertension, and myopia.

Prevention

The AAFP and the USPTF do not recommend screening for glaucoma, citing insufficient evidence to recommend for or against routine screening by primary care clinicians for elevated IOP or early glaucoma. The American Academy of Ophthalmology recommends screening for glaucoma by an ophthalmologist every 1–2 years after age 65.

Clinical Findings

A. Symptoms and Signs

Patients with acute angle-closure glaucoma typically present with unilateral intense pain and blurred vision. Patients may report seeing halos around light sources and complain of photophobia, headache, nausea, and vomiting. Physical examination shows a mid-dilated pupil, conjunctival injection, and lid edema. Patients generally have markedly elevated IOP, usually between 60 and 80 mm Hg.

Primary open angle glaucoma is a more insidious disease with a long asymptomatic phase. Patients may notice a gradual loss of peripheral vision. Examination may reveal diminished visual fields, elevated IOP, and abnormalities of the optic disc on direct ophthalmoscopy (symmetrically enlarged cup-to-disc ratio, cup-to-disc ratio asymmetry between the two eyes, or a highly asymmetric cup in one eye).

B. Special Tests

IOP may be measured using a variety of tools. The most readily available tool is the physician's hand. Palpation of the globe through a lightly closed lid can reveal asymmetric hardness or bilaterally firm eyeballs and provide a very gross measure of IOP. More accurate tools include tono-pen, Goldman applanation tonometry, and pneumotonometry (puff test).

Treatment

Patients with significant risk factors or physical findings that raise concern for glaucoma should be referred to an ophthalmologist for further evaluation and confirmation of diagnosis.

A. Acute Angle-Closure Glaucoma

Acute angle-closure glaucoma is a medical emergency that requires immediate referral and treatment.

B. Primary Open-Angle Glaucoma

The treatment of primary open-angle glaucoma consists of pharmacologic and surgical interventions aimed at decreasing the IOP. Although elevated IOP is not required for the diagnosis of glaucoma, it has been shown that reduction of IOP in patients with glaucoma slows the progression of disease. Even patients with normal pressures can benefit from reduction in IOP.

1. Pharmacotherapy—Topical eyedrops or oral medications aimed at decreasing aqueous humor production or increasing outflow are used. Classes of topical agents include β-blockers, α-adrenergic agents, carbonic anhydrase inhibitors, prostaglandin analogs, prostamides, miotics, and epinephrine compounds. Oral medications include carbonic anhydrase inhibitors such as acetazolamide. Topical glaucoma agents have varying degrees of systemic absorption and are capable of producing systemic side effects and drug–drug interactions. Patients should be educated on the importance of routine eye care and of taking medications as prescribed.

2. Surgical intervention—When medical management is unsuccessful, surgical intervention is considered. Laser trabeculoplasty and laser or conventional trabeculectomy are the most commonly performed procedures.

Prognosis

Untreated glaucoma can result in blindness. Rapid treatment of acute angle-closure glaucoma may preserve vision. Treatment of primary open-angle glaucoma can prevent further loss of vision, but typically does not restore lost vision.

Burr J et al: Medical versus surgical interventions for open angle glaucoma. Cochrane Database Syst Rev 2005;(2):CD004399. [PMID: 15846712]

CATARACTS

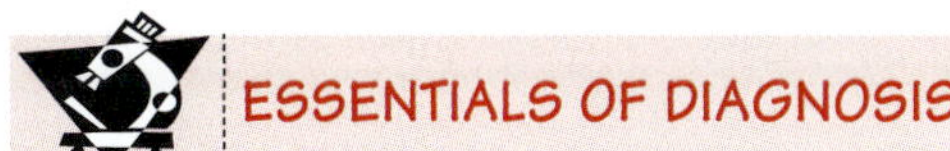

ESSENTIALS OF DIAGNOSIS

- *Opacity or cloudiness of the crystalline lens.*

General Considerations

Any opacification of the lens is termed a *cataract.* Cataract disease is the most common cause of blindness worldwide and the most common eye abnormality in the elderly. Risk factors for cataracts include advancing age, exposure to ultraviolet (UV) B light, glaucoma, smoking, diabetes, and chronic steroid use. Because cataracts tend to develop slowly, the patient may not be fully aware of the degree of vision impairment.

Prevention

Prevention of cataracts is aimed at the modifiable risk factors. Physicians should use steroids at as low a dose as is therapeutic and discontinue them when possible. Patients should be advised on how to minimize UV light exposure as well as the benefits of smoking cessation and control of chronic diseases.

Clinical Findings

Patients may report blurring of vision, "ghosting" of images, difficulty seeing in oncoming lights (glare), and monocular diplopia. The patient may also complain of a decrease in color perception and even note "second sight," which is an improvement in near vision with a nuclear cataract. Examination of the eye reveals the opacification of the lens. Cataracts may be easier to see with dilation of the eye and a direct ophthalmoscope at +5 diopters setting held 6 inches from the patient's eye.

Treatment

The treatment of cataracts is predominantly surgical. Although small cataracts may be treated by an updated eyeglass prescription, most patients with significant symptoms from a cataract benefit from surgical removal and replacement of the lens. Factors influencing the timing of surgery include life expectancy, current level of disability, status of other medical illnesses, family and social situations, and patient expectations.

Family physicians may aid patients in understanding the surgery and in assisting with preoperative management. Routine use of laboratory testing and electrocardiogram screening has not improved surgical outcome. Individuals should receive a history and physical examination prior to undergoing surgery. Additional testing is recommended only if findings are abnormal. Cataract surgery is often accomplished under local anesthesia with minimally invasive techniques. In this case, there is no need to discontinue anticoagulation for the procedure.

Prognosis

Cataracts do not resolve and may progress without treatment. The prognosis with surgical treatment is excellent, and up to 95% of patients obtain improved vision after surgery.

Schein OD et al: The value of routine preoperative medical testing before cataract surgery. Study of Medical Testing for Cataract Surgery. N Engl J Med 2000;342:168. [PMID: 10639542]

DIABETIC RETINOPATHY

ESSENTIALS OF DIAGNOSIS

- *Asymptomatic, gradual vision loss or sudden vision loss in a diabetic patient.*
- *Characteristic funduscopic findings of microaneurysms, flame hemorrhages, exudates, macular edema, and neovascularization.*

General Considerations

Diabetic retinopathy is the leading cause of blindness in adults in the United States. It is important to consider diabetic retinopathy as a disease of the aging eye because prevalence increases with duration of diabetes mellitus. The risk of blindness attributable to this disorder is greatest after 30 years of illness. The disorder has four stages: (1) mild, (2) moderate, and (3) severe nonproliferative retinopathy; and (4) proliferative retinopathy.

Prevention

Patients with diabetes mellitus type 2 should have a comprehensive eye examination by an ophthalmologist shortly after diagnosis to screen for signs of retinopathy. Meticulous glycemic control decreases the risk of development and progression of retinopathy in all patients with diabetes. In addition, tight control of blood pressure also significantly reduces a patient's risk of developing retinopathy.

Clinical Findings

Many patients presenting with diabetic retinopathy are free of symptoms; even those with the severe proliferative form may have 20/20 visual acuity. Others may report decreased vision that has occurred slowly or suddenly, unilaterally or bilaterally. Scotomata or floaters may also be reported. Funduscopic examination reveals any or all of the following: microaneurysms, dot and blot intraretinal hemorrhages, hard exudates, cotton-wool spots, boat-shaped preretinal hemorrhages, neovascularization, and venous beading.

Fluorescein angiography may be performed by an ophthalmologist to further assess the degree of disease.

Treatment

Untreated proliferative retinopathy is relentlessly progressive, leading to significant vision impairment and blindness. In addition to maximizing glucose and blood pressure control, laser photocoagulation surgery (focal and scatter) or vitrectomy is the mainstay of acute and chronic treatment and may preserve vision in certain patients. When vision loss has occurred, vision rehabilitation should be initiated, as described earlier in the discussion of AMD. Topics to review with patients include the importance of an annual, comprehensive eye examination, glycemic control, and hypertension management.

Prognosis

Early diagnosis and treatment, as well as tight glycemic control, improve prognosis.

Jawa A et al: Diabetic nephropathy and retinopathy. Med Clin North Am 2004;88:1001. [PMID: 15308388]

References for Vision Impairment in the Elderly

Goldzweig CL et al. Preventing and managing visual disability in primary care: Clinical applications. JAMA 2004;291:1497. [PMID: 15039417]

Rowe S et al: Preventing Visual loss from chronic eye disease in primary care: Scientific review. JAMA 2004;291:1487. [PMID: 15039416]

WEB SITES

Lighthouse International (health information on vision disorders, treatment, and rehabilitation services):

http://www.lighthouse.org

National Institute on Aging (patient education handout on the aging eye and hearing loss):

http://www.niapublications.org/engagepages/eyes.asp

Oral Health

45

Wanda Gonsalves, MD

Although the nation's oral health is believed to be the best it has ever been, oral diseases remain common in the United States. In May 2000, the first report on oral health from the US Surgeon General, *Oral Health in America: A Report of the Surgeon General,* called attention to a largely overlooked epidemic of oral diseases that is disproportionately shared by Americans: This epidemic strikes in particular the poor, young, and elderly. The report stated that although there are safe and effective measures for preventing oral diseases, these measures are underused. The report called for improved education about oral health, for a renewed understanding of the relationship between oral health and overall health, and for an interdisciplinary approach to oral health that would involve primary care providers.

DENTAL ANATOMY & TOOTH ERUPTION PATTERN

In utero, the 20 primary teeth evolve from the expansion and development of ectodermal and mesodermal tissue at approximately 6 weeks of gestation. The ectoderm forms the dental enamel and the mesoderm forms the pulp and dentin. As the tooth bud evolves, each unit develops a dental lamina that is responsible for the development of the future permanent tooth. The adult dentition is composed of 32 permanent teeth. Figure 45–1 shows the anatomy of the tooth and supporting structures. Table 45–1 outlines the eruption pattern of the teeth.

DENTAL CARIES

General Considerations

Dental caries (tooth decay) is the single most common chronic childhood disease, five times more common than asthma and seven times more common than hayfever among children 5–7 years of age. Minority and low-income children are disproportionately affected. According to the Centers for Disease Control and Prevention (CDC), among children aged 2–11 years, 21% have had untreated tooth decay in primary teeth, and of these, 32% are Mexican American, 27% are African American, and 18% are white. In addition, one third of persons of all ages have untreated decay, 8% of adults older than 20 years of age have lost at least one permanent tooth to dental caries, and many older adults suffer from root caries.

Pathogenesis

Dental caries is a multifactorial, infectious, communicable disease caused by the demineralization of tooth enamel in the presence of a sugar substrate and of acid-forming cariogenic bacteria that are found in the soft gelatinous biofilm plaque; (Figure 45–2). Thus, the development of caries requires a susceptible host, an appropriate substrate (sucrose), and the cariogenic bacteria found in plaque. *Streptococcus mutans* (also known as mutans streptococci [MS]) is considered to be the primary strain causing decay. Additionally, when plaque is not regularly removed, it may calcify to form calculus (tartar) and cause destructive gum disease.

Finally, the development of caries is a dynamic process that involves an imbalance between demineralization and remineralization of enamel. When such an imbalance is caused by environmental factors such as low pH or inadequate formation of saliva, dissolution of enamel occurs and caries result.

Clinical Findings

A. Symptoms and Signs

When enamel is repeatedly exposed to the acid formed by the fermentation of sugars in plaque, demineralized areas develop on the tooth surfaces, between teeth, and on pits and fissures. These areas are painless and appear clinically as opaque or brown spots (Figures 45–3, 45–4, and 45–5). If infection is allowed to progress, a cavity forms that can spread to and through the dentin (the component of the tooth located below the enamel) and to the pulp (composed of nerves and blood vessels; an infection of the pulp is called *pulpitis*), causing pain, necrosis, and, perhaps, an abscess.

B. Diagnosis

Carious lesions progress at various rates and occur at many different locations on the tooth, including the sites of previous restorations. Demineralized lesions (white or brown spots) generally occur at the margins of

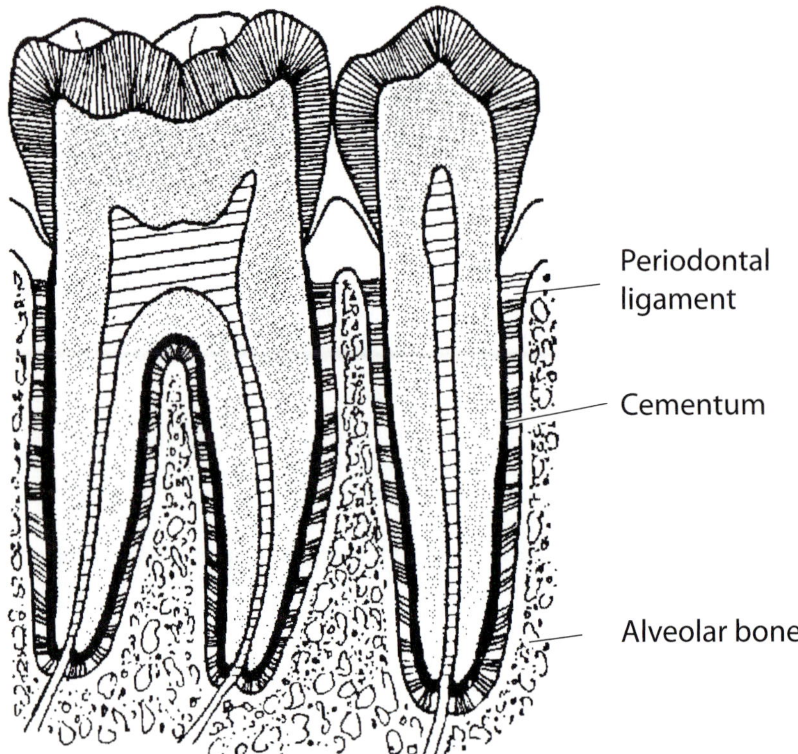

Figure 45–1. Anatomy of the tooth and supporting structures.

the gingiva and can be detected visually; they may not be seen on radiographs. Advanced carious lesions such as those spread through dentin can be detected clinically or, if they occur between the teeth, by radiographs. Root caries, commonly seen in older adults, occur in areas from which the gingiva has receded.

Dental professionals use a dental explorer to detect early caries in the grooves and fissures of posterior teeth. To diagnose secondary caries (caries formed at the site of restorations), dental professionals use digitally acquired and post-processed images.

Risk Assessment

Caries can develop at any time after tooth eruption. Early teeth are principally susceptible to caries caused by the transmission of MS from the mouth of the caregiver to the mouth of the infant or toddler. This type of caries is called *early childhood caries* (ECC) or *baby bottle tooth decay* (BBTD). According to the American Academy of Pediatric Dentistry, ECC "is defined as 'the presence of one or more decayed (noncavitated or cavitated lesions), missing (due to caries), or filled tooth surfaces' in any primary tooth in a child 71 months of age or younger." In children younger than 3 years, any sign of smooth-surface caries is called *severe early childhood caries* (S-ECC). Children with a history of ECC or S-ECC are at a much higher risk of subsequent caries in primary and permanent teeth. Risk factors for caries development are shown in Table 45–2.

ECC contributes to other health problems, including chronic pain, poor nutritional practices, and low self-esteem, which may lead to lack of self-esteem among older children and a great reduction in their ability to succeed in life.

The risk factors for adult caries are similar to those for childhood caries, including those listed in Table 45–2.

Prevention & Treatment

Fluoride, the ionic form of the element fluorine, is widely accepted as a safe and effective practice for the primary prevention of dental caries. Fluoride slows or reverses the progression of existing tooth decay by (1) being incorporated into the enamel before tooth eruption, (2) inhibiting demineralization, (3) enhancing remineralization, and (4) inhibiting bacterial activity in plaque. Unfortunately, only 57% of the US population has access to community water fluoridation, according to the CDC fluoridation census in 2000. Systemic fluoride supplements (tablets,

Table 45–1. Eruption pattern of teeth.

Teeth	Eruption Date
Primary dentition	
Mandibular central incisor	6 mo
Maxillary central incisor	7 mo
Mandibular lateral incisor	7 mo
Maxillary lateral incisor	9 mo
Mandibular first molar	12 mo
Maxillary first molar	14 mo
Mandibular canine	16 mo
Maxillary canine	18 mo
Mandibular second molar	20 mo
Maxillary second molar	24 mo
Permanent dentition	
Mandibular central incisors	6 y
Maxillary first molars	6 y
Mandibular first molars	6 y
Maxillary central incisors	7 y
Mandibular lateral incisors	7 y
Maxillary lateral incisors	8 y
Mandibular canines	9 y
Maxillary first premolars	10 y
Mandibular first premolars	11 y
Maxillary second premolars	11 y
Mandibular second premolars	11 y
Maxillary canines	11 y
Mandibular second molars	12 y
Maxillary second molars	12 y
Mandibular third molars	17–21 y
Maxillary third molars	17–21 y

drops, lozenges) are recommended for children older than 6 months who are at high risk of the development of caries, for infants with ECC, and for adults whose water is not fluoridated or who have diseases that produce a decrease in salivary flow, receding gums, or mental or physical disabilities. A supplemental fluoride dosage schedule is shown in Table 45–3. Topical fluoride supplements such as gels and varnishes are highly concentrated fluoride products that are professionally applied by a dental health provider or a parent (for gels). Varnishes, which are less toxic than gels and more effective than mouth rinses, are applied three times a week, once a year by disposable brushes, cotton-tipped applicators, or cotton pellets.

Before prescribing supplemental fluoride, the primary care provider must determine the fluoride concentration in the child's primary source of drinking water. Natural sources of fluoride include well water exposed to fluorite minerals, certain fruits and vegetables grown in soil irrigated with fluoridated water, and foods such as meats or poultry which may contain 6-7% of total dietary fluoride. Although fluoride supplementation is not recommended for persons who live in communities whose water is optimally fluoridated (0.7–1.2 ppm or > 0.6 mg/L), the bottled water used by many families contains low levels of fluoride. Parents and caregivers should be educated about the benefits of fluoride and the possible side effects of too much fluoride, a condition called fluorosis. Fluorosis results when too much fluoride is obtained from any source when the permanent tooth is forming (Figure 45–6). Thirty-two percent of children and adolescents aged 6–19 years have very mild or greater fluorosis. The benefits and side effects of fluoride use should be weighed against the risk of tooth decay among children at high risk of caries.

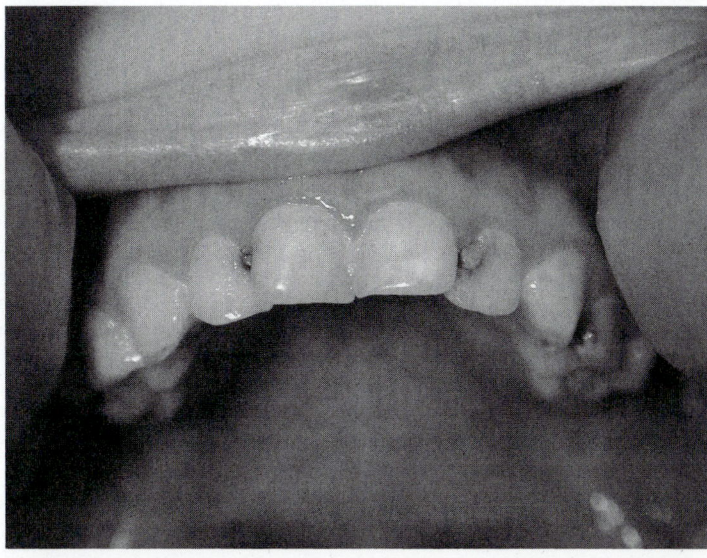

Figure 45–2. Dental caries due to plaque.

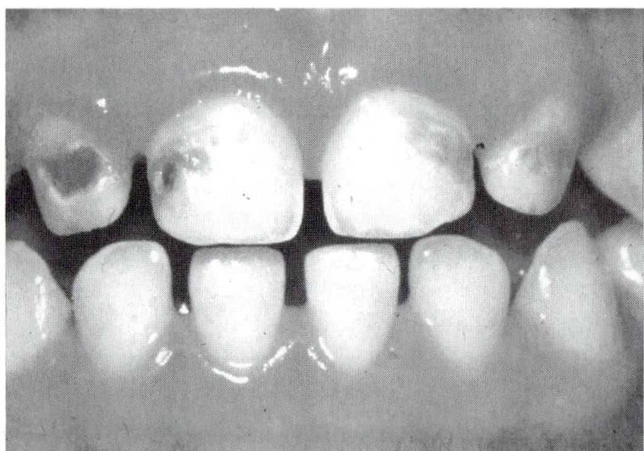

Figure 45–3. Brown spots indicating demineralized areas in enamel.

A second method of preventing dental caries is proper oral hygiene. Before the teeth erupt, a parent may use a washcloth or cotton gauze to clean an infant's mouth and to transition the child to tooth brushing. Parents should supervise brushing and should discourage children younger than 6 years of age from using fluoridated dentifrices because of the risk that toothpaste may be swallowed during brushing. A pea-sized amount of toothpaste is recommended for brushing.

Dental sealants, first introduced in the 1960s, are plastic films that coat the chewing surfaces of primary or permanent teeth. Sealants prevent decay from developing in the pits and fissures of teeth. Dental professionals often use sealants in combination with topical fluorides (Figure 45–7).

Older children and adults should avoid frequent consumption of drinks and snack foods containing sugars. Chewing sugar-free gum or cheese after meals has a saliva buffer effect that may counter plaque acids.

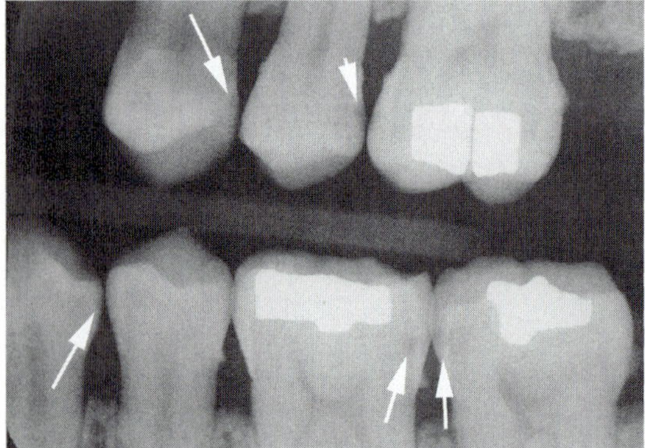

Figure 45–4. Opaque areas indicating demineralized areas in enamel.

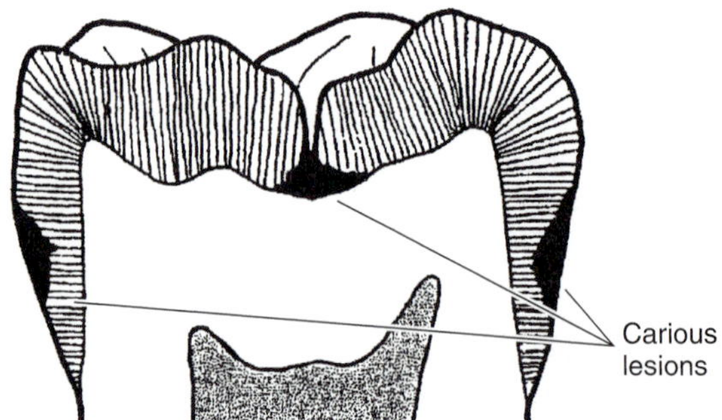

Figure 45–5. Dental caries.

Council on Clinical Affairs, American Academy of Pediatric Dentistry: Clinical guidelines on baby bottle tooth decay/early childhood caries/breastfeeding/: Unique challenges and treatment options. J Am Acad Pediatr Dent (Special Issue: Reference Manual) 2001–02;23:29.

Diagnosis and Management of Dental Caries Throughout Life: NIH Consensus Statement Online 2001 March 26–28;18:1. Available at: http://consensus.nih.gov/cons/115/115_statement.htm.

Holt R et al: ABC of oral health. Dental damage, sequelae, and prevention. Br Med J 2000;320:1717. [PMID: 10864553]

Milgrom P, Reisine S: Oral health in the United States: The post-fluoride generation. Annu Rev Public Health 2000;21:403. [PMID: 10884959]

PERIODONTAL DISEASE

General Considerations

Periodontal disease is the most common oral disease in adults. It is uncommon among young children, affecting less than 1%; however in some studies, up to 25% of Hispanic children between 12 and 17 years of age were affected. Like dental caries, periodontal diseases are caused by bacteria in dental plaque that create an inflammatory response in gingival tissues (gingivitis) or in the soft tissue and bone supporting the teeth (periodontitis). Risk factors that contribute to the development of periodontal disease include poor oral hygiene, environmental factors such as crowded teeth and mouth breathing, steroid hormones, smoking, comorbid conditions such as weakened immune status or diabetes, and low income.

Severe gum disease is defined as a 6-mm loss of attachment of the tooth to the adjacent gum tissue. Severe gum disease affects approximately 14% of adults aged 45–54 years and 23% of those aged 65–74 years. Approximately 25% of adults 65 years of age or older no longer have any natural teeth. The severity of periodontal disease does not increase with age. Rather, the disease is believed to occur in random bursts after periods of quiescence.

Table 45–2. Risk factors for childhood and adult caries.

Risk Factors for Childhood Caries	Risk Factors for Adult Caries
Dietary practices: frequent consumption of foods and beverages containing sugars (juice, milk, formula, soda) and sticky foods	Physical and medical disabilities
Frequent bottle- and breast-feeding on demand	Existing restorations or oral appliances
Maternal or sibling caries	Inadequate salivary flow
Repetitive use of a "sippy cup"	Medications that produce dry mouth
Poor oral hygiene	Radiation therapy
Inadequate fluoridation	Low socioeconomic status
Lack of dental visits	

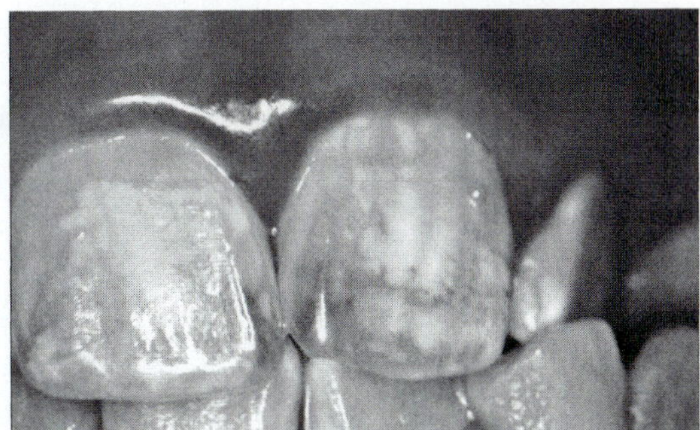

Figure 45–6. Fluorosis.

Pathogenesis

A. Gingivitis

Gingivitis is caused by a reversible inflammatory process that occurs as the result of prolonged exposure of the gingival tissues to plaque. Gingivitis may develop as a result of steroid hormones, which encourage the growth of certain bacteria in plaque during puberty and pregnancy and in women taking oral contraceptive pills.

No special tests are needed to diagnose gingivitis; rather, the disease is diagnosed by clinical assessment. Simple or marginal gingivitis may be painless and is treated by good oral hygiene practices such as tooth brushing and flossing. This type of gingivitis occurs in 50% of the population aged 4 years or older. The inflammation worsens as mineralized plaque forms calculus (tartar) at and below the gum surface (sulcus). Gingivitis may persist for months or years without progressing to periodontitis; this fact suggests that host susceptibility plays an important role in the development of periodontitis. Additionally, gingivitis (Figure 45–8) can be either acute or chronic. A severe form, acute necrotizing ulcerative gingivitis (ANUG), also known as Vincent disease or trench mouth, is associated with anaerobic fusiform bacteria and spirochetes. ANUG (Figure 45–9) is painful, ulcerative, and edematous and produces halitosis and bleeding gingival tissue. Predisposing factors include conditions that contribute to a weakened immune status, such as HIV infection, smoking, malnutrition, viral infections, and, possibly, stress. Chronic gingivitis affects more than 90% of the population and results in gingival enlargement or hyperplasia that resolves when adequate plaque control is instituted. Generalized gingival enlargement or swelling may be caused by drugs such as calcium channel blockers, phenytoin, and cyclosporin (Figure 45–10); by pregnancy; or by systemic diseases such as leukemia, sarcoidosis, and Crohn disease.

B. Periodontitis

Periodontitis is caused by chronic inflammation of gingival soft tissue and supporting structures by plaque microorganisms, specifically gram-negative bacteria that affect gingival

Table 45–3. Supplemental fluoride dosage schedule.

Age	Concentration of Fluoride in Water		
	<0.3 ppm F	0.3–0.6 ppm F	>0.6 ppm F
Birth to 6 months	0	0	0
6 months to 3 years	0.25 mg	0	0
3 to 6 years	0.50 mg	0.25 mg	0
6 to at least 16 years	1.00 mg	0.50 mg	0

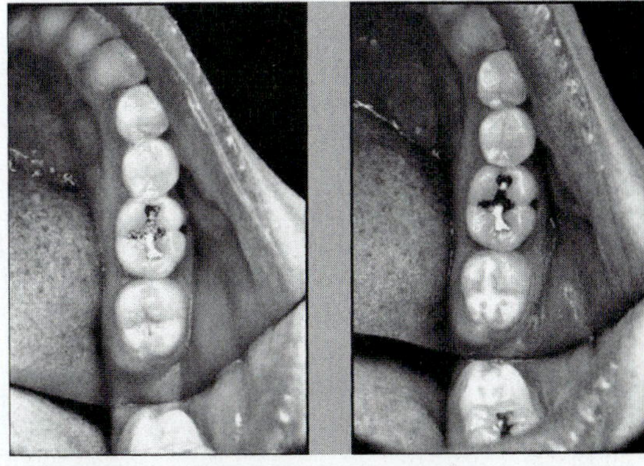

Figure 45–7. Dental sealants.

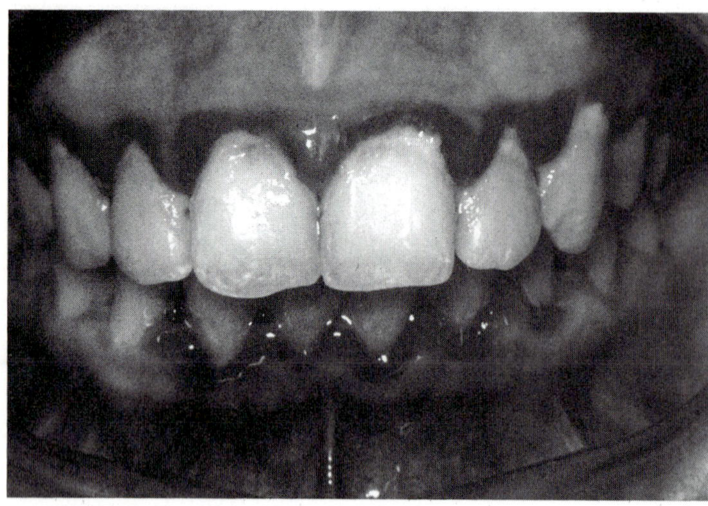

Figure 45–8. Gingivitis.

soft tissues and supporting structures, with resultant loss of periodontal attachment and bony destruction. Periodontitis is common in adults, affecting more than 50% of the population. Adult-onset periodontitis begins in adolescence and is reversible if treated in its early stages, when minimal pockets (gaps) have formed between the tooth and the periodontal attachment. Severe periodontitis is characterized by a 6-mm loss of tooth attachment as detected by the dental health professional by means of dental probes.

If periodontitis is found in children or young adults or if it progresses rapidly, the primary care provider should be alert to the possibility of a systemic cause such as diabetes mellitus, Down syndrome, hypophosphatasia, neutropenia, leukemia, leukocyte adhesion deficiency, or histiocytosis. A less common, rapidly progressing form of adult periodontitis begins in the third or fourth decade of life and is associated with severe gingivitis and rapid bone loss. Several systemic diseases, including diabetes, HIV infection, Down syndrome, and Papillon–Lefèvre syndrome, have been associated with this rare form of periodontitis. Localized juvenile periodontitis (LJP) and localized prepubertal periodontitis (LPP) are forms of early-onset periodontitis seen in teenagers (LJP) and young children (LPP) without evidence of systemic disease. LJP is more common among African-American children. It affects the first molars and incisors, with rapid destruction of bone. Although there is some evidence for autosomal transmission, it is likely heterogenous. Both LJP and LPP are believed to be the result of a bacterial infection (specifically implicated is *Actinobacillus actinomycetemcomitans*) and, possibly, host immunologic deficits.

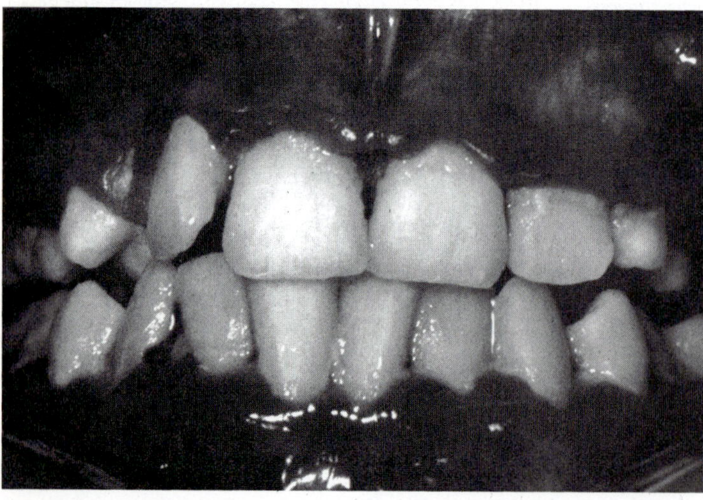

Figure 45–9. Acute necrotizing ulcerative gingivitis (ANUG).

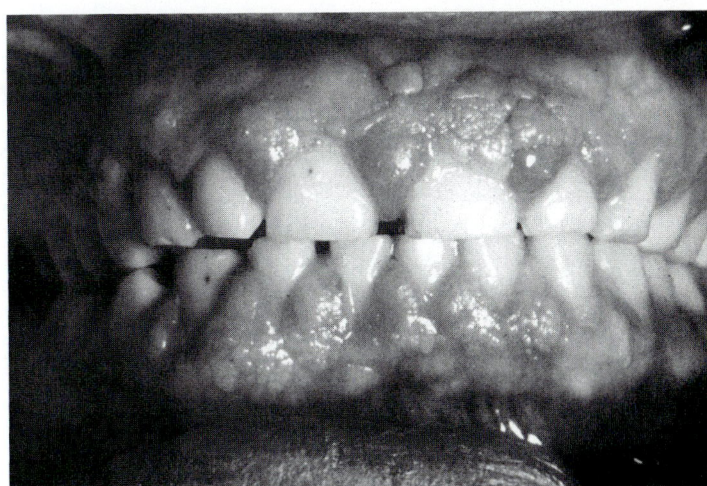

Figure 45–10. Gingival enlargement due to drugs.

Clinical Findings

A. Symptoms and Signs

Clinical signs of gingivitis and periodontitis include interdental papillae edema, erythema, and bleeding on contact during tooth brushing or dental probing (Figure 45–11). The amount of gingival inflammation and bleeding and the probing depth of gingival pockets determine the severity of periodontal disease. Tartar, gum recession, and loose teeth are characteristics of severe periodontal disease. For children younger than 4 years of age, loss of primary teeth may be the first clinical sign of periodontal disease and the systemic manifestation of hypophosphatasia. Dental probing by the dental health professional will detect sulcus depth.

B. Imaging Studies

Bone loss can be detected by radiographs and bone density scans.

Periodontal Health & Systemic Disease

Emerging evidence, particularly from the dental literature, suggests that periodontal disease may be a risk factor for systemic conditions such as cardiovascular disease, diabetes mellitus, and adverse pregnancy outcomes of preterm labor and low birth weight. Current evidence supports a bidirectional relationship between diabetes and periodontal disease. Periodontal disease is a risk factor for poor glycemic control among diabetic patients, and diabetes is associated with increased sever-

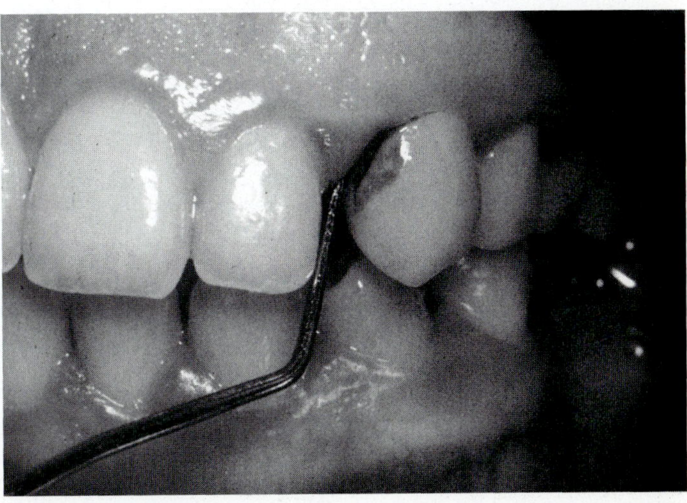

Figure 45–11. Gingival inflammation and bleeding.

ity of periodontal disease. Studies showing the relationship between periodontal disease and cardiovascular disease have proposed that patients with chronic bacterial infection or periodontitis may have (1) a bacteria-induced platelet-aggregation defect that contributes to acute thrombolic events, (2) injury to vascular tissue by bacterial toxins, or (3) vascular injury resulting from a host inflammatory response that predisposes the patient to a systemic disorder such as atherosclerosis. Additionally, the link between periodontal disease and preterm labor has several proposed biological mechanisms, one of which is the infection that is mediated by prostaglandins and cytokines among patients with severe periodontitis. This infection causes decreased fetal growth and premature labor.

Prevention & Treatment

Good oral hygiene is essential for the prevention and control of periodontal diseases. Gingivitis, the mildest form of periodontal disease, is reversible with regular tooth brushing and flossing. An added benefit is provided by over-the-counter and prescription antimicrobial mouth rinses, such as a 0.1–0.2% chlorhexidine gluconate aqueous mouthwash used twice a day. Caution is advised when chlorhexidine is used because it causes superficial staining of the teeth of patients who drink tea, coffee, or red wine. The treatment of periodontitis includes professional care to remove tartar and may require periodontal surgery.

Because tobacco use is an important risk factor for the development and progression of periodontal disease, patients should be counseled about tobacco cessation. Systemic diseases such as diabetes that may contribute to periodontal disease should be well controlled.

Salvi GE et al: Influence of risk factors on the pathogenesis of periodontitis. Periodontal 2000;14:173. [PMID: 9567971]

Teng YT et al: Periodontal health and systemic disorders. J Can Dent Assoc 2002;68:188. [PMID: 11911816]

Zeeman GG et al: Focus on primary care: Periodontal disease: Implications for women's health. Obstet Gynecol Surv 2001; 56:43. [PMID: 11140863]

ORAL & OROPHARYNGEAL CANCERS

General Considerations

In the United States, cancers of the oral cavity and oropharynx comprise approximately 3% of all cancers among men (the ninth most common cancer among men) and 2% of all cancers among women. The prevalence of these cancers increases with age. Since the 1970s, the incidence of these cancers and the death rates associated with them have been slowly decreasing, except among African-American men, for whom the incidence and 5-year mortality estimates are nearly twice as high as for white men.

Table 45–4. Risk factors associated with oral and oropharyngeal cancer.

Tobacco use (smoking or using smokeless tobacco or snuff)
Excessive consumption of alcohol
Viral infections (HSV, HIV, EBV)
Chronic actinic exposure
Betel quid use
Lichen planus
Plummer–Vinson or Paterson–Kelly syndrome
Immunosuppression
Dietary factors (low intake of fruits and vegetables)

HSV, herpes simplex virus; HIV, human immunodeficiency virus; EBV, Epstein–Barr virus.

The overall survival rate for patients with oral and oropharyngeal cancers is only about 51% and has not changed substantially over the past 20 years. However, the 5-year survival estimate for patients with lip carcinoma is more than 90%; this high survival rate is due in part to early detection. Most oral and oropharyngeal cancers are squamous cell carcinomas that arise from the lining of the oral mucosa. These cancers occur most commonly (in order of frequency) on the tongue, the lips, and the floor of the mouth. Sixty percent of oral cancers are advanced by the time they are detected, and about 15% of patients have another cancer in a nearby area such as the larynx, esophagus, or lungs. Early diagnosis, which has been shown to increase survival rates, depends on the discerning clinician who recognizes risk factors and suspicious symptoms and can identify a lesion at an early stage.

Table 45–4 shows the risk factors associated with oral and oropharyngeal cancers. Tobacco use and heavy alcohol consumption are the two principal risk factors responsible for 75% of oral cancers. The incidence of oral cancer is higher among persons who smoke or drink heavily than among those who do not.

Prevention

All forms of tobacco, including cigarette, pipe, chewing, and smokeless, have been shown to be carcinogenic in the susceptible host. Alcohol has been identified as another important risk factor for oral cancer, both independently and synergistically when heavy consumers of alcohol also smoke. Therefore, primary prevention in the form of reducing or eliminating the use of tobacco and alcohol has been strongly recommended. The US Preventive Services Task Force (USPSTF) has not endorsed annual screening (secondary prevention) for asymptomatic patients, stating, "there is insufficient evidence to recommend for or against routine screening" and "clinicians may wish to include an examination for cancerous and precancerous lesions of the oral cavity in the periodic health examination of persons

Table 45–5. Components of an oral cancer examination.[1]

Extraoral Examination
Inspect head and neck
Bimanually palpate lymph nodes and salivary glands
Lips
Inspect and palpate outer surfaces of lip and vermilion border
Inspect and palpate inner labial mucosa
Buccal Mucosa
Inspect and palpate inner cheek lining
Gingiva/Alveolar Ridge
Inspect maxillary/mandibular gingiva and alveolar ridges on both the buccal and lingual aspects
Tongue
Have patient protrude tongue and inspect the dorsal surface
Have patient lift tongue and inspect the ventral surface
Grasping tongue with a piece of gauze and pulling it out to each side, inspect the lateral borders of the tongue from its tip back to the lingual tonsil region
Palpate tongue
Floor of Mouth
Inspect and palpate floor of mouth
Hard Palate
Inspect hard palate
Soft Palate and Oropharynx
Gently depressing the patient's tongue with a mouth mirror or tongue blade, inspect the soft palate and oropharynx

[1]A good oral examination requires an adequate light source, protective gloves, 2 × 2 gauze squares, and a mouth mirror or tongue blade.

who chew or smoke tobacco (or did so previously), older persons who drink regularly, and anyone with suspicious symptoms or lesions detected through self-examination." However, the American Cancer Society and the National Cancer Institute's Dental and Craniofacial Research Group support efforts that promote early detection of oral cancers. The American Cancer Society recommends annual oral cancer examinations for persons aged 40 years or older.

Because primary care providers are more likely than dentists to see patients at high risk of oral and oropharyngeal cancers, providers need to be able to counsel patients about their behaviors and to be knowledgeable about performing oral cancer examinations. The primary screening test for oral cancer is the oral cancer examination, which includes inspection and palpation of extraoral and intraoral tissues (Table 45–5).

Clinical Findings

A. Symptoms and Signs

Early oral cancer and the more common precancerous lesions (leukoplakia) are subtle and asymptomatic. They begin as a white or red patch, progress to a superficial ulceration of the mucosal surface, and later become an endophytic or exophytic growth. Some lesions are solitary lumps. Larger, advanced cancers may be painful and may erode underlying tissue.

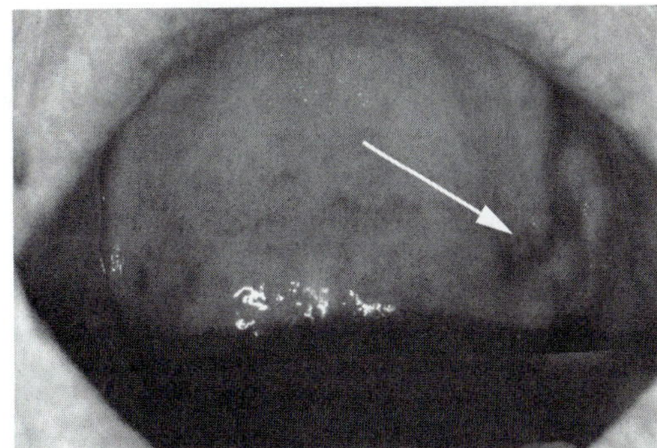

Figure 45–12. Leukoplakia.

According to the definition of the World Health Organization, leukoplakia is "a white patch or plaque that cannot be characterized clinically or pathologically as any other disease." The lesions may be white, red, or a combination of red and white (called *speckled leukoplakia* or *erythroleukoplakia*). Multiple studies have shown that these lesions undergo malignant transformation. Biopsies have shown that erythroplakia and speckled leukoplakia are more likely than other types of leukoplakia to undergo malignant transformation with more severe epithelial dysplasia. Figures 45–12 and 45–13 show leukoplakia.

Oropharyngeal carcinomas can be found in the intraoral cavity, the oral cavity proper, and the oropharyngeal sites. The most common intraoral site is the tongue; lesions frequently develop on its posterior lateral border. Lesions also occur on the floor of the mouth and, less commonly, on the gingiva, buccal mucosa, labial mucosa, or hard palate.

A common cancer of the oral cavity proper is lower lip vermilion carcinoma. These lesions arise from a precancerous lesion called *actinic cheilosis,* which is similar to an actinic keratosis of the skin. Dry, scaly changes appear first and later progress to form a healing ulcer, which is sometimes mistaken for a cold sore or fever blister. Figure 45–14 shows actinic cheilosis.

Oropharyngeal carcinomas commonly arise on the lateral soft palate and the base of the tongue. Presenting symptoms may include dysphagia, painful swallowing (odynophagia), and referred pain to the ear (otalgia). These tumors are often advanced at the time of diagnosis. Oral cancer metastasizes regionally to the contralateral or bilateral cervical and submental lymph nodes. Distant metastases are commonly found in the lungs, but oral cancer may metastasize to any other organ.

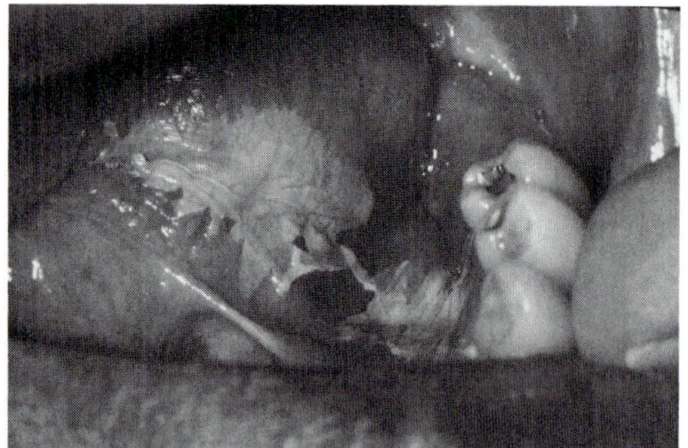

Figure 45–13. Leukoplakia.

B. Diagnosis

All patients whose behaviors put them at risk of oral cancer should undergo a thorough oral examination that involves visual and tactile examination of the mouth, full protrusion of the tongue with the aid of a gauze wipe, and palpation of the tongue, the floor of the mouth, and the lymph nodes in the neck. Because oral cancer and precancerous lesions are asymptomatic, primary care providers need to carefully examine patients who are at risk of oral or oropharyngeal carcinomas. Using a scalpel or small biopsy forceps, the primary care physician should perform a biopsy of any nonhealing white or red lesion that persists for more than 2 weeks. Alternatively, the patient may be referred to a dentist, an oral surgeon, or a head and neck specialist, who can perform the biopsy. Patients with large lesions or advanced disease should undergo a complete head and neck examination, because 15% of these patients will have a second primary cancer at the time of diagnosis. Neck nodules with no identifiable primary tumor may be evaluated by fine-needle aspiration.

C. Imaging Studies

Imaging studies such as computed tomography with contrast and magnetic resonance imaging of the head and neck are used to determine the extent of disease and involvement of the cervical lymph nodes for the purposes of staging.

Treatment

Treatment for oral and lip cancers includes chemotherapy, surgery, radiation, or some combination of these therapies, depending on the extent of the disease. These treatments can cause severe stomatitis (inflammation of the mouth), xerostomia (dry mouth), disfigurement, altered speech and mastication, loss of appetite, and increased susceptibility to oral infection. The management of these complications requires a multidisciplinary team approach by the clinician, oral surgeon, oncologist, and speech therapist. Early diagnosis allows better treatment, cosmetic appearance, and functional outcome and increases the probability of survival. Patients should be encouraged to visit their dental health provider before beginning cancer therapy so that existing health problems can be treated and some complications can be prevented.

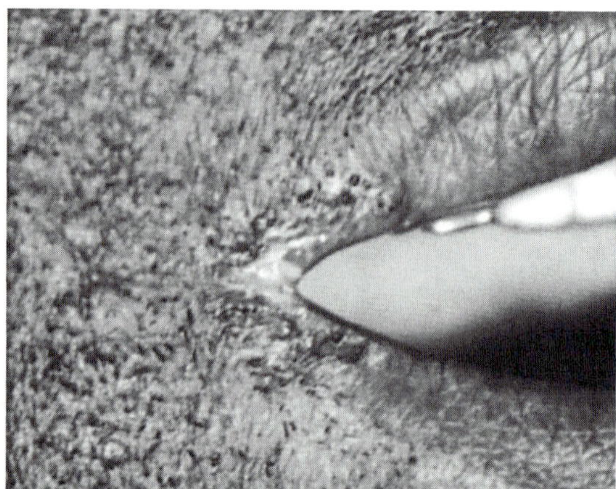

Figure 45–14. Actinic cheilosis.

Mashberg A, Samit A: Early diagnosis of asymptomatic oral and oropharyngeal squamous cancers. CA Cancer J Clin 1995;45: 328. [PMID: 7583906]

Neville BW, Day TA: Oral cancer and precancerous lesions. CA Cancer J Clin 2002;52:195. [PMID: 12139232]

Silverman S Jr: Demographics and occurrence of oral and pharyngeal cancers. The outcomes, the trends, the challenge. J Am Dent Assoc 2001;132;7S. [PMID: 11803655]

Weinberg MA, Estefan DJ: Assessing oral malignancies. Am Fam Physician 2002;65:1379. [PMID: 11996421]

Global References for Oral Health

Beltram-Aguilar ED et al; Centers for Disease Control and Prevention: Surveillance for dental caries, dental sealants, tooth retention, edentulism and enamel fluorosis—United States, 1988–1994 and 1999–2002. MMWR Surveill Summ 2005; 54:1. [PMID: 16121123]

Office of Disease Prevention and Health Promotion, US Department of Health and Human Services: *Healthy People 2010.* Available at: http://www.healthypeople.gov/document/html/objectives/21-08.htm.

US Department of Health and Human Services: *Oral Health in America: A Report of the Surgeon General—Executive Summary.* DHHS, National Institute of Dental and Craniofacial Research, National Institutes of Health, 2000. Available at: http://www.nidr.nih. gov/sgr/execsumm.htm.

Web Sites

Academy of General Dentistry:

http://www.agd.org
American Association of Public Health Dentistry:
http://www.aaphd.org
American Dental Association:
http://www.ada.org
Children's Dental Health Project:
http://www.childent.org
Health Resources and Services Administration (HRSA) Oral Health Initiative:
http://www.hrsa.gov/oralhealth
National Maternal and Child Oral Health Resource Center:
http://www.mchoralhealth.org
US Surgeon General's Report on Children's Oral Health:
http://www.nidcr.nih.gov/sgr/sgr.htm

SECTION V
Therapeutics, Genetics, & Prevention

Pharmacotherapeutics 46

Nicole T. Ansani, PharmD, & Melissa A. Somma, PharmD, CDE[1]

Medication therapy is an integral element of health care interventions. In 2003, approximately 3.2 billion prescriptions were dispensed and this number is expected to increase to 4.5 billion in 2010. Approximately 65% of physician office visits result in a prescription. Although medication use is often supported by "hard science" and evidence, clinical practice often shifts to the "soft science" of medicine, trying to understand patients, their histories, their personalities, their medication adherence, and a way to provide the best possible care.

Of the billions of prescriptions filled each year, it is estimated that approximately half are taken improperly. Therefore, achieving a balance between "hard" and "soft" sciences—by providing evidence-based medication therapy that patients will adhere to—becomes paramount. In selecting medication therapy, physicians must evaluate the evidence, adhere to national guidelines and standards, balance the safety risks and side effects, and incorporate the patient as part of the decision-making process. Figure 46–1 provides a framework for this chapter as it explores provider considerations such as evidence, pharmacokinetics and pharmacodynamics, and safety; health care system factors such as formulary systems and resources; and patient considerations focusing on adherence to medication.

Physicians must continually balance provider considerations, health care system considerations, and patient considerations in promoting optimal medication management. Effective patient-physician communication starts with the physician's confidence in his or her ability to teach and enhance patient skills, as well as the amount of time available to see patients during a typical provider visit. Policies of health care organizations, such as formularies, and evidence-based guidelines can help to improve the efficiency of the system and allow for practice changes and positive patient outcomes. Many factors influence patients' behavior, and it is difficult to predict who will adhere to medication regimens. Therefore, involving patients in the medication decisions, tailoring and simplifying the regimens to meet their needs, and supporting and monitoring of efficacy and safety are essential to providing the best possible care.

TAKING A MEDICATION HISTORY

Discrepancies among documented medication therapy records and actual patient use of medications are common and occur with all classes of medications. Therefore, the first step for the provider in determining optimal medication therapy is to understand what medications patients are actually taking and how they are taking them.

Step 1: Open-Ended Questions

To obtain an accurate medication history, the physician should start by asking open-ended questions; for example, "What medications are you taking?" This approach avoids the common mistake of assuming the patient is taking all medications as prescribed. Although conducting an open-ended medication history may require more time up front, it may ultimately prevent over- or

[1]The authors would like to graciously thank Terry McKaveney for her thoughtful suggestions and review of this chapter.

Patient

- Efficacy of a drug regimen
- Safety of a drug regimen
- Adherence to the drug regimen

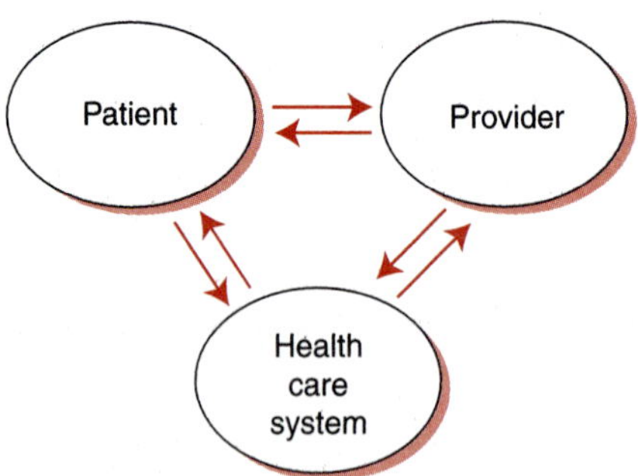

Health care system

- Clinical guidelines
- Formulary choices
- Health care resources

Provider

- Patient medication review
- Evidence-based medicine
- Medication safety

Figure 46–1. Factors in optimal medication therapy.

underprescribing and may also improve patient relationships.

Step 2: Over-the-Counter Medications, Herbal Remedies, & Vitamins

The physician must inquire in a nonjudgmental manner whether patients are taking any over-the-counter (OTC) medications, herbal remedies, or vitamin products. Over 12% of the US population uses herbal remedies on a yearly basis, but only 38.5% report this use to their physicians. Among the reasons cited by consumers for using herbal remedies are feeling a "sense of control," dissatisfaction with traditional medicine, and the belief that conventional medicine has failed them. Partnering with the patient in discussing herbal use may allow for the discovery of untreated indications or patient health concerns, and potentially avoid unwanted adverse effects of drug–drug interactions. Health care professionals have the responsibility to diligently examine the safety and efficacy of herbal remedies in the overall context of patients' medication regimens.

Step 3: Social History

Information about patients' history of alcohol use, smoking, and illicit drug use factors into the overall selection of specific medications. A history of long-term alcohol use resulting in liver function abnormalities, nonadherence, and nutritional deficiencies must be considered in medication selection. Smoking induces the cytochrome P450 (CYP) 3A4 system, speeding up the metabolism of agents such as theophylline.

Follow-up: Assessing the Need for Adherence Aids

A thorough medication history may uncover the need for adherence aids. One of the most useful tools in explaining the proper timing of medication administration is a medication chart. Other adherence aids include medication calendars, medication boxes, and programmable adherence pagers and watches. Written patient education information in the form of handouts or brochures, and proper instructions printed on the written prescription, all increase patient understanding of the medication regimen.

Bedell SE et al: Discrepancies in the use of medications: Their extent and predictors in an outpatient practice. Arch Intern Med 2000;160:2129. [PMID: 10904455]

De Smet PA: Herbal remedies. N Engl J Med 2002;347:2045. [PMID: 12490687]

Editorial. The soft science of medicine. Lancet 2004;363:1247. [PMID: 15094264]

Nichols-English G, Poirier S: Optimizing adherence to pharmaceutical care plans: Nonadherence can be viewed as a behavioral disorder—a condition that is best treated by identifying individual risk factors and designing targeted interventions. J Am Pharm Assoc 2000;40:475. [PMID: 10932456]

Sardesai VM: Herbal medicines: Poisons or potions? J Lab Clin Med 2002;139:343. [PMID: 12066132]

MEDICATION REGIMEN

Polypharmacy

Polypharmacy is defined as the concurrent use of multiple medications or the prescribing of more medications than are clinically indicated. Polypharmacy can be minimized by a thorough medication regimen review. Table 46–1 lists five concise steps to a medication review.

Seemingly simple, a thorough regimen review aids in ensuring that the appropriate medications are prescribed. Consider a diabetic patient with hypertension, hyperlipidemia, and elevated blood glucose not controlled by diet. According to the 2003 American Diabetes Association guidelines, an aspirin, antidiabetic agent, antihypertensive agent, and antihyperlipidemic agent should be prescribed. This amounts to four or five medications, not including medications for any other conditions the patient may have. As in this example, polypharmacy may be unavoidable, but with a good medication regimen review, adverse drug reactions, drug–drug interactions, and duplication of therapy may be avoided. This is also an opportunity to work with a pharmacist to best outline a patient's medication regimen.

Evaluation & Change

A thorough medication history and safety assessment begin to clarify many aspects of a patient's medication regimen, and paired with evidence, can help the clinician make a solid patient-specific decision about a medication regimen. Evidence-based medicine (EBM) is defined as "the conscientious, explicit, and judicious use of the current best evidence in making decisions about the care of individual patients." EBM entails obtaining the best external evidence to support clinical decisions and is, therefore, not restricted solely to randomized trials and meta-analyses.

It is critical to appreciate that EBM does not depend solely on the skills and aptitude of literature evaluation and application of data, but must also incorporate clinical experience. As Shaughnessy and colleagues state, "good clinical practice should be performed like good jazz, with the physician blending the structure of evidence based medicine with the appropriate improvisation of clinical experience." Although EBM is being promoted throughout health care and there is agreement that its practice improves care, physicians may not be familiar with the process of extracting journals, review publications, and databases to help incorporate evidence into practice in an efficient manner. Additionally, the most commonly reported barrier to practicing EBM is a lack of time. However, the goal of EBM is to provide appropriate allocation of effective and efficient care to all patients. As E. J. Huth, MD, has noted, "The strength of a profession lies in its expert generation of information and better management of it than other social groups" (*Annals of Internal Medicine*).

How does a generalist manage to keep up with the wealth of medical information available? Over six million references are estimated to be published in the more than 4000 journals in the National Library of Medicines database, MEDLINE. Slawson and Shaughnessy propose that the practitioner should approach this "information jungle" with a basic equation:

$$\text{Usefulness} = \frac{\text{Relevance} \times \text{Validity}}{\text{Work}}$$

Simple mathematics illustrate that to maximize the usefulness of information, it is necessary to provide the highest level of relevance and validity with the minimum amount of work. Relevance is directly proportional to the relationship and similarities of the information with the patient population most commonly encountered, or its applicability to the physician's practice. Relevance also includes a measure of the impact of change the information creates in the way a physician practices medicine. Validity relates to the intrinsic methodology, study design, and conclusions. Thus, by maximizing the principles of the usefulness equation, the best source of information may be located.

Table 46–1. Reviewing a medication regimen.

1. Match the medication with the diagnosis
2. Review the regimen for duplication of therapy
3. Elicit from patients if they are taking the medicine
4. Review laboratory work and patient history for efficacy/toxicity of the regimen
5. Strive to remove any unnecessary agents from the regimen

Sackett DL: Evidence-based medicine. Spine 1998;23:1085. [PMID: 9615357]

Shaughnessy AF et al: Clinical jazz: Harmonizing clinical experience and evidence-based medicine. J Fam Pract 1998;47:425. [PMID: 9866666]

Slawson DC, Shaughnessy AF: Becoming an information master. Using "medical poetry" to remove the inequities in health care delivery. J Fam Pract 2001;50:51. [PMID: 11195481]

Web Sites

Agency for Healthcare Research and Quality:
http://www.ahrq.gov

Bandolier:
http://www.jr2.ox.ac.uk/Bandolier/index.html

Centre for EBM:
http://www.cebm.jr2.ox.ac.uk/

The Cochrane Library:
http://www.updateusa.com/clibhome/clib.htm

Journal of Family Practice POEMS:
http://www.jfponline.com or http://www.medicalinforetriever.com
Netting the Evidence:
http://www.shef.ac.uk/~scharr/ir/netting

EXPLORING THE EVIDENCE: USE OF GUIDELINES & FORMULARIES

Formulary systems using evidence-based guidelines and principles have been developed by health care systems as a result of the information era in efforts to provide evidence-based, cost-effective medication management. Drug formularies may be defined as "a continuously revised list of medications that are readily available for use within an institution and reflect the current clinical judgment of the medical staff" (*Drug Information: A Guide for Pharmacists,* 2nd ed; McGraw-Hill, 2001). These systems provide an organized, evidence-based approach to care. Guidelines and formulary systems have demonstrated beneficial effects in improving the process of care, improving patient outcomes, and promoting cost containment, cost-effective care, or both, and are recommended by the US President's Advisory Commission on Consumer Protection and Quality.

Evidence-based guidelines are an example of providing high "usefulness" in literature review and application. A guideline is defined by the Institute of Medicine as a "systematically developed statement to assist physicians in patient decisions about appropriate health care for specific clinical circumstances." Four types of evidence-based guidelines exist, and the strength of evidence varies depending on the type of guideline. **Evidence-based clinical practice guidelines** incorporate recent literature regarding the effectiveness of therapy and clinical experience. **Expert consensus guidelines** may be the simplest type of guideline; however, a limitation to this approach is inherent author bias and limited evidence-based sources. **Outcomes-based guidelines** incorporate measures of effectiveness to validate a positive impact on patient care. Lastly, **preference-based guidelines** combine evidence-based and outcomes-based guidelines with patient preferences. These constitute the least common type of guideline, but provide information on patients' values in guiding decisions.

Regardless of the type of guideline format used, it is imperative to test the validity and applicability of the guidelines and, subsequently, the validity of information from which the guideline was developed. To assess these characteristics of guidelines, the physician must consider several factors, as listed in Table 46–2.

Table 46–2. Evaluating the usefulness of clinical guidelines.

1. *Does the guideline clearly define the subject area and clearly state the question to be answered?* This is essential to ensure the applicability of the guideline to practice and to assess the validity of the conclusions.
2. *What criteria were used to determine inclusion of articles/information?* This helps to provide an assessment of methodologic standards that determines whether these standards are similar to the guideline criteria.
3. *How was the search conducted and what criteria were used to assess inclusion of the information?* This ensures completeness of subject material.
4. *Was the level of information to be included assessed?* It is critical to ensure the quality of information reviewed in order to provide a quality recommendation/end point. An assessment of the level of information should include the validity of the study methodology, assessment of the reproducibility of the studies, and the homogeneity of the study results.
5. *What are the results/recommendations?* Are the results statistically and clinically significant, are the results precise, are the recommendations feasible, and will they change practice? Can this recommendation be applied to your specific practice?
6. *When was the guideline updated?* As new evidence is rapidly becoming available, how is this incorporated to ensure the best and most current practice?

Sources: Snaders GD et al: Published web-based guidelines using interactive decision models. J Eval Clin Pract 2001;7:175; Oxman AD et al: Users' guide to the medical literature. VI. How to use an overview. JAMA 1994;272:1367; Siwek J et al: How to write an evidence-based clinical review article. Am Fam Physician 2002;65:251; and Liberati A et al: Which guidelines can we trust? West J Med 2001;174:262.

The Cochrane Collaboration is an example of a system that provides sound clinical practice guidelines. Currently, the Cochrane Collaboration provides systematic reviews, maintains a registry of trials, and is a leading provider of evidence-based guidelines. Cochrane reviews may be located in the Cochrane Library, Cochrane Collaboration, or Cochrane Reviews' Handbook at the following sites: http://www.update-softwarelcom/cochrane/cochrane-frame.html or http://www.cochrane.org. In addition to the Cochrane Collaboration, many medical and professional societies, health maintenance organizations (HMOs), and the Agency for Healthcare Research and Quality (AHRQ) provide practice guidelines and Internet links to these guidelines.

As the demand for published, evidence-based guidelines grows, so does the need for outcomes-focused formulary systems that consider effectiveness, safety, and cost implications to practice. Drug formulary systems are fundamental tools of hospitals, health systems, and managed care organizations to designate preferred products and provide rational, cost-effective prescribing decisions. Traditional formulary decisions are based on comparative efficacy, safety, drug interactions, dosing, pharmacology, pharmacokinetics, and cost.

Pharmacy and Therapeutics (P&T) Committees, composed of physicians, pharmacists, nurses, and administrators and representing all major disciplines of practice, guide the formulary decision process. The goal is to provide high-quality, safe, cost-effective prescribing. By reviewing new medications, drug classes, literature, and safety data, the P&T Committees frame the structure of a formulary system.

Physicians may consider developing a personal formulary as well. A personal formulary includes methodic selection and routine use of one or two drugs for a clinical condition or from a drug class. Selection of agents should be based on the same criteria noted in the P&T Committee review. Rational use of medication requires meeting the patients' clinical needs through appropriate medication selection as well as providing care in the most cost-effective manner. Evidence-based guidelines and formulary systems can optimize patient care when applied appropriately and evaluated, recognizing the needs of the individual patient.

Cesario S et al: Evaluating the level of evidence of qualitative research. J Obstet Gynecol Neonatal Nurs 2002;31:708. [PMID: 12465867]

Johnson N: Creating an outcomes-focused formulary: Resources to assist in determining drugs' values. Formulary 2001;36:807.

Liberati A et al: Which guidelines can we trust? Assessing strength of evidence behind recommendations for clinical practice. West J Med 2001;174:262. [PMID: 11290685]

Robertson J et al: Personal formularies: An index of prescribing quality? Eur J Clin Pharmacol 2001;57:333. [PMID: 11549213]

Scalzitti DA: Evidence-based guidelines: Application to clinical practice. Phys Ther 2001;81:1622. [PMID: 11589640]

Schachtner JM et al: Prevalence and cost savings of therapeutic interchange among US hospital. Am J Health Sust Pharm. 2002 Mar 15;59(6):529. [PMID: 11908245]

Web Sites

Clinical Evidence, BMJ Publishing Group:
http://www.clinicalevidence.org
Health Web:
http://www.uic.edu/depts/lib/health/hw/ebhc
Institute for Clinical Systems Improvement:
http://www.ICSI.org
Medical Matrix:
http://medmatrix.org
National Guideline Clearinghouse:
http://www.guidelines.gov/index.asp
Primary Care Clinical Practice Guidelines:
http://medicine.ucsf.edu/resources/guidelines

BALANCING THE EVIDENCE WITH THE PATIENT

Medication Adherence

"Drugs don't work in patients who don't take them" (C. Everett Coop, MD, former US Surgeon General). Poor adherence to medication therapy is a national concern and a significant barrier in optimal medication management. Medication nonadherence is estimated to result in 125,000 deaths per year in the United States and is responsible for 10% of hospital and 23% of nursing home admissions.

Adherence to medication is defined as the extent to which a person's behavior coincides with his or her medical advice. The term *adherence* is preferred over *compliance* because it implies a patient-centered care model. Despite physicians' best efforts to provide the best care, the average rate of medication adherence is approximately 40–50%. Optimal medication adherence is a key link between process and outcomes in medical care. However, there are no significant predictors of patient nonadherence, and the reasons why patients do not adhere to their medication regimens widely vary among patients and depends on the nature of the illness, patients' involvement in health care decisions, and gender.

Because it is difficult to predict patient adherence behavior, it is critical to identify barriers to adherence that may be controlled or modified. The most common reason for medication nonadherence is that the patient forgot. Other reasons that are cited include other priorities, decision to omit dose, lack of information, and emotional factors. Further, no one intervention has been proven to consistently improve adherence. Common interventions typically result in a 4% to 11% increase in medication adherence rates. Therefore, a combination of interventions is often required to meet the patient's needs. Motivational interviewing techniques are helpful.

Motivational interviewing is a method of engaging the patient to commit to change based on personal motivation. This technique explores the patient's understanding and concerns and evaluates his or her readiness to change. Motivational interviewing is patient centered and requires insight into the patient's views about the proposed medication therapy. When assessing patients' adherence, the simplest method is to nonjudgmentally ask how often they miss doses. Empathizing with patients is important; thus, a physician might ask about medication adherence while providing support, as in the following example: "I know it is difficult to take all of your medications. How often do you miss taking them?" This approach makes the patient comfortable and allows the physician to elicit valuable and truthful information.

Morisky and colleagues developed a validated four-question assessment tool to gauge patient adherence behaviors. Patients are asked:

1. "Do you ever forget to take your medications?"
2. "Are you careless at times about taking your medications?"

3. "When you are feeling better, do you sometimes stop taking your medications?"
4. "Sometimes if you feel worse, do you stop taking your medications?"

Patients who answer "yes" to none or one of these questions are classified as high adherence; those with two to three "yes" responses are classified as medium adherence; and those with four "yes" responses are classified as low adherence.

Motivational interviewing uses an elicit-provide-elicit model whereby the physician can better understand any barriers that exist and provide targeted information when talking with a patient about his or her adherence. The principles of motivational interviewing are encompassed in the acronym READS:

R Roll with resistance
E Express empathy
A Avoid argumentation
D Develop discrepancy
S Support self-efficacy

In addition to using a patient-centered model of interviewing, physicians can incorporate the following 10 steps to improve patient adherence:

1. Convince patients that the treatment plan is necessary and efficacious.
2. Explain exactly what patients should expect. Five key issues that must be addressed are (a) what the drug does, (b) how it should be taken, (c) major side effects, (d) what to do if side effects occur, and (e) how the drug effect will be monitored.
3. Listen carefully.
4. Assess the patient's mental state (depression may be a risk factor for nonadherence).
5. Enlist the help of the patient's family and friends.
6. Keep medication regimens as simple as possible.
7. Troubleshoot potential obstacles (ask patients if they foresee any problems).
8. Build reminders into the treatment plan.
9. Include a plan to monitor adherence.
10. Ask patients how they are doing.

As mentioned earlier, if nonadherence to a medication regimen is identified, physicians can assist patients by helping them create a medication list, use a pill organizer, or develop a medication reminder chart; by providing refill reminders; and, if appropriate, by considering electronic devices and compliance services.

Higgins N, Regan C: A systematic review of the effectiveness of interventions to help older people adhere to medication regimens. Age Ageing 2004;33:224. [PMID: 15082425]

Jaret P: 10 ways to improve patient compliance. Hippocrates 2001;15.

Morisky DE et al: Current and predictive validity of a self-reported measure of medication adherence. Med Care 1986;241:67. [PMID: 3945130]

Osterberg L, Blaschke T: Adherence to medications. N Engl J Med 2005;353:487. [PMID: 16079372]

Possidente CJ et al: Motivational interviewing: A tool to improve medication adherence? Am J Health Syst Pharm 2005;2005:1311. [PMID: 15947131]

Vermeire E et al: Patient adherence to treatment: Three decades of research. A comprehensive review. J Clin Pharm Ther 2001; 26:331. [PMID: 11679023]

Managing Medication Cost

In 2001, the average price of a single prescription was $49.84. In the United States a total of $175.2 billion was spent on drug therapy during that same year. Although the elderly (patients 65 years of age and older) comprise only 13% of the US population, they account for 34% of all prescriptions filled, or 42% of prescription costs. Family physicians, like pharmacists, face the issue of medication cost daily. If the cost of the medication is a factor in nonadherence, several steps can be taken.

First, the physician should determine whether the patient has insurance. If the patient has prescription insurance coverage, the physician should be aware of the prescribing or formulary suggestions. If medically appropriate, an attempt should be made to prescribe within the formulary to aid in decreasing the patient's copayment. Often patients with insurance complain that their copayments are too high, but because they already have insurance, there are few other funding options. In such cases, a thorough medication regimen review with the intention of decreasing numbers of medications, if medically appropriate, can improve safety and decrease cost of medication regimens.

For patients who do not have insurance, a few options can be pursued to help them obtain medications at a reduced cost.

1. If the patient is 65 years of age or older, he or she can apply for drug coverage through Medicare Part D. To determine which plans the patient is eligible for, and associated costs, visit http://www.medicare.gov.
2. Determine if the patient qualifies for any federal, state, or military program. Having a basic understanding of the income requirements can help the physician guide the patient in the right direction.
3. Have contact information available for state Medicaid programs.
4. Consider applying for medication assistance programs sponsored by pharmaceutical manufacturers. In 2002, pharmaceutical manufacturers supplied free or low-cost medications to over 5.5 million people in the United States. Several Internet sites are available to aid in obtaining information on how to use these programs.

Chisholm MA et al: Medication assistance programs for uninsured and indigent patients. Am J Health Syst Pharm 2000;57:1131. [PMID: 10911511]

Web Sites

Helpful sites for locating low-cost drug programs:

http://www.needymeds.com

http://www.rxhope.com

http://www.themedicineprogram.com

ENSURING MEDICATION SAFETY

Lazarou and colleagues reviewed 39 prospective studies of adverse drug reactions (ADRs) and found that the majority were "dose-dependent" and therefore potentially preventable. Other similar reports concur with these findings. With the direct costs of ADRs estimated to be between $1.6 and $4 billion and the estimation of ADRs being the fourth to sixth leading cause of death, there is a significant need for a greater understanding of the mechanisms of these reactions. In a recent cohort study of outpatient Medicare patients, 28% of ADRs were preventable, 42% of which were life-threatening or fatal.

Patients at the highest risk of experiencing ADRs include those on multiple medications (five or more) with various medical conditions, those hospitalized or in nursing home facilities, diabetic patients, cancer patients, and those with renal or hepatic impairment. The classes of drugs most commonly associated with ADRs include nonopioid and opioid analgesics, antibiotics, cardiovascular agents, anticoagulants, and diuretics. Obtaining a thorough patient history, proactive assessment and monitoring of drug safety, assuring proper indication of individual medications, and patient counseling can all help to reduce potential ADRs.

Some basic inquiries, as listed in Table 46–3, can assist the physician in determining if an ADR is truly linked to a particular drug. It is vitally important to report the ADR no matter how minor or major. During premarketing trials, if 1500 patients or more are exposed to a drug, the most common ADRs will be detected. However, more than 30,000 patients must be exposed to the drug in the postmarketing period to detect an ADR in one patient with a power of 0.95 to discover an incidence of 1 in 10,000. There are two simple ways by which physicians can anonymously report ADRs: (1) by logging on to http://www.fda.gov/MEDWATCH or calling 800-FDA-1088, or (2) if in a hospital or nursing home setting, by contacting the pharmacy or local drug information center.

Bates DW et al: The costs of adverse drug events in hospitalized patients. Adverse Drug Events Prevention Study Group. JAMA 1997;277:307. [PMID: 9002493]

Classen D: Medication safety: Moving from illusion to reality. JAMA 2003;289:1154. [PMID: 12622587]

Field TS et al: Risk factors for adverse drug events among nursing home residents. Arch Intern Med 2001;161:1629. [PMID: 11434795]

Table 46–3. Identifying adverse drug reactions (ADRs).

1. Are there any previous reports of an ADR occurring with this agent?
2. Consider the timing of the ADR. Does it match the drug's pharmacokinetic profile for onset of effect?
3. Was there a recent dosage increase or decease?
4. Was a new medication recently added or removed from the regimen?
5. If serum drug levels were available, were they in the toxic range?
6. Has the patient had a similar reaction to medications in the past, especially those of the same class?
7. Are there other drugs or disease conditions that could also cause the symptoms of the event?
8. When the drug was discontinued, did the symptoms resolve?

Source: Stephens M, Talbot J: *The Detection of New Adverse Drug Reactions*, ed 2. Stockton Press, 1998.

Gurwitz JH et al: Incidence and preventability of adverse drug events among older persons in the ambulatory setting. JAMA 2003;289:1107. [PMID: 12622580]

Lazarou J et al: Incidence of adverse drug reactions in hospitalized patients: A meta-analysis of prospective studies. JAMA 1998;279:1200. [PMID: 9555760]

Malhortra S et al: Drug related medical emergencies in the elderly: Role of adverse drug reactions and non-compliance. Postgrad Med 2001;77:703. [PMID: 11677279]

Web Site

Federal Food and Drug Administration (FDA) Safety Information and Adverse Drug Reporting Program:

http://www.fda.gov/MEDWATCH/

MATCHING THE PATIENT & THE DRUG: PHARMACOKINETIC & PHARMACODYNAMIC PRINCIPLES

Although a subset of ADRs is unpredictable, those that are preventable include drug–drug interactions. A grasp of basic pharmacokinetic and pharmacodynamic principles is needed to prevent such interactions. Pharmacokinetics characterizes the rate and extent of absorption, distribution, metabolism, and elimination of a drug. Pharmacodynamics is the study of the relationship between the drug concentration at the site of action and the response of the patient. Where these concepts come together for the physician is at the point of deciding the best drug and dose for a particular patient. In reviewing the patient history, the following patient characteristics should be considered in relation to drug pharmacokinetics:

- **Age:** Most drugs have been studied in adult patients, and recommended dosages may vary in different age groups. Pediatric patients may need a higher dose per kilogram than adult patients, and geriatric patients may need a lower dose per kilogram, due to decreased drug metabolism and elimination.

- **Gender:** Although data are limited, male and female patients can metabolize and eliminate drugs differently, so the optimal drug dosages may differ.
- **Weight:** For patients who are obese or cachectic, changes in drug clearance (rate at which a drug is removed from the body) or volume of distribution (estimated volume a drug occupies in a patient) often necessitate drug dosage adjustments.
- **Disease conditions:** Three disease conditions that must be approached with special caution when prescribing any drug are congestive heart failure (CHF), renal disease, and hepatic failure. As CHF progresses, bodily organ blood flow declines; the ensuing drug clearance decline necessitates lower drug dosages for many agents. As kidney function declines, renal elimination of drugs can decrease, leading to lower drug dosage requirements for renally cleared agents. Finally, as liver function declines, hepatic metabolism and elimination of drugs can decrease, leading to decreased drug dosages of hepatically metabolized and cleared agents.
- **Genetics:** Pharmacogenomics is the study of the relationship of genetics in drug metabolism and ADRs. In a systematic review by Phillips and colleagues, of 27 drugs known to frequently cause ADRs, 59% were known to be influenced by individual patient genetic characteristics. Pharmacogenomics is discussed in detail in Chapter 48.

Erstad BL: Which weight for weight-based dosage regimens in obese patients? Am J Health Syst Pharm 2002;59:2105. [PMID: 12036391]

Meibohm B et al: How important are gender differences in pharmacokinetics? Clin Pharmacokinet 2002;41:329. [PMID: 12036391]

Phillips KA et al: Potential role of pharmacogenomics in reducing adverse drug reactions: A systematic review. JAMA 2001;286: 2270. [PMID: 11710893]

Soldin OP, Soldin SJ: Review: Therapeutic drug monitoring in pediatrics. Ther Drug Monit 2002;24:1. [PMID: 11805714]

DRUG–DRUG INTERACTIONS: UTILIZING PHARMACOKINETIC & PHARMACODYNAMIC PRINCIPLES

Once the patient-specific characteristics noted in the preceding section have been established, the physician can begin to examine drug-specific characteristics. Pharmacokinetic characteristics of a drug can aid in choosing the best drug for the patient and in potentially predicting and understanding ADRs and drug–drug interactions. Table 46–4 summarizes potential pharmacokinetic and pharmacodynamic interactions. The main enzymatic system responsible for drug metabolism is the cytochrome P450 (CYP) system. Metabolism through the CYP system occurs mainly in the liver, but CYP isozymes are also found in the intestines and other organs.

Identifying different CYP isozymes is an area of ongoing research. There are six isozymes for which there is a reasonable amount of knowledge: CYP 1A2, 2C9, 2C19, 2D6, 3A4, and 2E1. Understanding this system allows prediction of drug–drug interactions among many patients. To do this, it is necessary to identify which drugs are metabolized by the CYP 450 system and how they interact with the enzyme system. There are three ways in which a drug can interact with the enzymes:

1. **Substrate:** The drug is metabolized by an enzyme that is specific for an individual CYP receptor.
2. **Inducer:** The drug "revs up" the enzyme system, allowing a greater metabolism capacity.
3. **Inhibitor:** The drug(s) competes with another drug(s) for a specific enzyme binding site, rendering the enzyme inactive.

A review of the patient's medication list can reveal drugs that may compete or use the same enzyme system. A subsequent change in drug selection may prevent a drug interaction. Table 46–5 lists common medications metabolized by the CYP enzyme system.

Identifying patients most at risk for drug–drug interactions and ADRs, carefully monitoring drugs with narrow therapeutic windows (such as warfarin, phenytoin, theophylline, and others), using lower dose therapies when appropriate, and employing systems to identify and prevent drug–drug interactions at the point of patient care all have the potential to reduce ADRs from drug–drug interactions.

Cohen JS: Avoiding adverse reactions. Effective lower-dose drug therapies for older patients. Geriatrics 2000;55:54. [PMID: 10711307]

Committee on Quality of Health Care in America, Institute of Medicine, Kohn L et al, eds: *To Err is Human: Building a Safer Health System.* IOM, 2000.

Flockhart DA, Tanus-Santos JE: Implications of cytochrome P-450 interactions when prescribing medication for hypertension. Arch Intern Med 2002;162:405. [PMID: 11863472]

Gex-Fabry M et al: Therapeutic drug monitoring databases for postmarketing surveillance of drug-drug interactions. Drug Safety 2001;24:947.

Revisions to Joint Commission Standards in Support of Patient Safety and Medical/Health Care Error Reduction. Available at: http://www.jcaho.org/standard/fr_ptsafety.html.

KEEPING UP WITH THE LITERATURE

Subscribing to survey services is one way to stay current with the pertinent literature, while decreasing the amount of work and time required. Survey services pro-

Table 46–4. Classification and examples of mechanisms of drug–drug interactions.

Type of Interaction	Basic Description	Time Course	Example
Absorption	Precipitant drug binds to the object drug Object drug concentration decreases	Hours Rate of concentration of object drug declines dependent on object drug half-life	Antacids taken with digoxin, quinolones, and tetracyclines; antacids absorb drugs in the gastrointestinal tract leading to decreased concentration of those drug entities
Distribution	Precipitant drug *displaces* the object drug from a particular binding site Object drug concentration increases	A day to a week Usually a self-limited interaction; after initial interaction, an equilibrium is reached between object drug concentration in the plasma and at the binding site	Sulfamethoxozole-trimethoprim (SMP/TMX) taken with warfarin; SMP/TMX is more highly protein bound than warfarin and will displace warfarin from its binding sites, leading to an increase in unbound warfarin
Metabolism	Induction Precipitant drug induces (speeds up) the metabolism of the object drug Object drug concentration decreases	Usually within 2 days, but less than 1 week	Some of the most common precipitant agents responsible for induction of hepatic microsomal drug-metabolizing enzymes include carbamazepine, phenytoin, rifampin, and troglitazone; they will induce the hepatic metabolism of agents that require the same hepatic microsomal drug-metabolizing enzymes for metabolism
	Inhibition Precipitant drug inhibits the metabolism of the object drug Object drug concentration increases	Hours	Many exist; some of the most common precipitant agents responsible for inhibition of hepatic microsomal drug-metabolizing enzymes include erythromycin, fluconazole, ketoconazole, nefazadone, and ritonavir; they will inhibit the hepatic metabolism of agents that require the same hepatic microsomal drug-metabolizing enzymes for metabolism
	Competition Precipitant and object drugs compete for metabolic enzymes Both drug concentrations may be altered	Variable	When two drugs use the same hepatic microsomal drug-metabolizing enzymes, competition may occur leading to alterations of either or both serum drug concentrations
Elimination	Precipitant drug competes with the object drug for excretion Both drug concentrations may be altered	Hours	There are three primary methods of renal excretion: glomerular filtration, active tubular secretion, and passive tubular reabsorption; interactions can occur during all three processes; one example is the combination of hydrochlorizide and lithium carbonate; hydrochlorizide causes an increase in sodium reabsorption leading to an increase in lithium reabsorption and thus an increase in the concentration of lithium

(*continued*)

Table 46–4. Classification and examples of mechanisms of drug–drug interactions. *(Continued)*

Type of Interaction	Basic Description	Time Course	Example
Pharmacodynamic	Additive Precipitant drug together with the object drug produce a heightened therapeutic or toxic response	Hours to weeks	There are many; consider two drugs with an adverse effect in common (two sedating agents); together they produce a more pronounced adverse effect (sedation)
	Antagonistic Precipitant drug antagonizes (cancels out) the effect of the object drug		Nonsteroidal anti-inflammatory drugs when given with an antihypertensive agent can cause a rise in the patient's blood pressure over the course of a few weeks, thus antagonizing the desired effect of the blood pressure agent

Sources: Gex-Fabry M et al: Therapeutic drug monitoring databases for postmarketing surveillance of drug-drug interactions. Drug Safety 2001;24:947; and Hansten PD, Horn JR: Pharmacokinetic drug interaction mechanisms and clinical characteristics. In: Hansten and Horn's *Drug Interactions Analysis and Management.* Applied Therapeutics, 1997.

vide an efficient means of reviewing a plethora of medical journals and articles; however, there may be a tendency to overemphasize positive conclusions or draw conclusions that are not fully supported by the data. The conclusions and recommendations presented by such services should be evaluated before incorporating the information into practice. The relevance and validity of the data must be verified.

Three basic categories of survey services exist: (1) abstracting services, (2) review services, and (3) true newsletters. Abstracting services for family medicine practitioners include, but are not limited to, the *ACP Journal Club,* the *Journal of Family Practice,* and *Journal Watch.* **ACP Journal Club** (http://www.acpjc.org) is published by the American College of Physicians–American Society of Internal Medicine. The goal of this service is to provide brief, high-level summaries of current original articles and systematic reviews in a structured abstract format in a timely manner. The ACP Journal Club reviews over 100 journals and uses prestated criteria to select and evaluate data. Pertinent information summaries are provided to subscribers on a bimonthly basis. The **Journal of Family Practice** (http://www.jfponline.com) provides family practice physicians with timely, reliable information supplemented by expert commentary. The goal of this service is to provide evidence-based information on clinically applicable topics in a timely fashion. **Journal Watch Online** (http://www.jwatch.org) is supported by the publishers of the *New England Journal of Medicine.* The goal of this service, similar to the others, is to provide current summaries of the most important research in a timely fashion. An editorial board composed of physicians from many specialty areas reviews, analyzes, and summarizes 55–60 critically important articles. The summaries are published on a bimonthly basis. In addition, this service features Clinical Practice Guidelines Watch and editorials of the year's top medical stories.

Review services provide a concise summary of the specific topic areas, rather than a survey of the literature. One example of a review service is **The Medical Letter** (http://www.medletter.com). *The Medical Letter* is published by an independent nonprofit organization. It provides critical appraisals of new medications or new uses for medications in a clinical context, comparing and contrasting the new medications to similar established agents. This publication is printed bimonthly and provides a concise summary of clinical issues. Its stated goal is to provide "unbiased, reliable, and timely information on new drugs to busy health care professionals." Another example of a review service is **Primary Care Reports** (http://www.ahcpub.com/ahc_root_html/products/newsletters/pcr.html). This service is printed bimonthly and is intended to provide review articles on critical issues in primary care; treatment recommendations are provided with each review.

True newsletters provide concise reviews of current literature with topics from news media and other sources. Examples of this type of newsletter include, but are not limited to, *Drug and Therapeutics Bulletin* and *Therapeutics Letter.* **Drug and Therapeutics Bulletin** (http://www.dtb.org.uk/idtb) is a concise monthly bulletin targeted for physicians and pharmacists that provides evaluations of medications and summarizes randomized, controlled, clinical trials, and consensus statements. The goal of this service is to provide informed and unbiased assessments of medications and their overall place in therapy. The **Therapeutics Letter**

Table 46–5. Drugs metabolized by CYP 450 isozymes.

Isozyme	Substrates	Inducers	Inhibitors
2D6	Antidepressants Amitriptyline Clomipramine Fluoxetine Imipramine Mirtazapine Nortriptyline Paroxetine Trazadone Venlafaxine Antipsychotics Clozapine Fluphenazine Haloperidol Olanzapine Perphenazine Quetiapine Risperidone Thioridazine β-Blockers Bisoprolol Carvedilol Metoprolol Pindolol Propranolol Timolol Pain medications Codeine Fentanyl Hydrocodone Morphine Oxycodone Propoxyphene Tramadol	Antiseizure agents Carbamazepine Phenobarbital Phenytoin Primidone Rifampin Others Ethanol Ritonavir St. John's wort	Antidepressants Proxetine > fluoxetine > sertraline > fluvoxamine Nefazodone Venlafaxine Antipsychotics Haloperidol Perphenazine Thioridazine Other Cimetidine
3A4	Antidepressants Amitriptyline Sertraline Venlafaxine Benzodiazepines Aloprazolan Triazolam Midazolam Calcium blockers Carbamazepine Cisapride Dexamethasone Erythromycin Ethinyl estradiol	Antiseizure agents Carbamazepine Phenobarbital Phenytoin Others Dexamethasone Rifampin	Antibiotics Clarithromycin Erythromycin Antidepressants Nefazodone > fluvoxamine > fluoxetine > sertraline Paroxetine Venlafaxine Antifungals Ketoconazole > itraconazole > fluconazole Others Cimetidine Diltiazem Protease inhibitors

(continued)

Table 46–5. Drugs metabolized by CYP 450 isozymes. *(Continued)*

Isozyme	Substrates	Inducers	Inhibitors

	Glyburide
	Ketoconazole
	Protease inhibitors
	  Ritonavir
	  Saquinavir
	  Indinavir
	  Nelfinavir
	Testosterone
	Theophylline
	Verapamil		

1A2	Amitriptyline
	Clomipramine
	Clozapine
	Imipramine
	Propranolol
	Warfarin
	Theophylline
	Tacrine
		Antiseizure agents
		  Phenobarbital
		  Phenytoin
		Omeprazole
		Rifampin
		Smoking
			Fluvoxamine
			Grapefruit juice
			Quinolone antibiotics
			  Ciprofloxacin
			  Enoxacin > norfloxacin > ofloxacin > lomefloxacin

2E1	Acetaminophen Ethanol	Ethanol Isoniazid	Disulfiram

2C9	Nonsteroidal anti-inflammatory agents
	Phenytoin
	Warfarin
	Torsemide
		Rifampin	Antifungals
			  Fluconazole
			  Ketoconazole
			  Itraconazole
			Others
			  Metronidazole
			  Ritonavir

2C19	Clomipramine
	Diazepam
	Imipramine
	Omeprazole
	Propranolol
		Not known	Antidepressants
			  Fluoxetine
			  Sertraline
			Others
			  Omeprazole
			  Ritonavir

Sources: Hansten PD, Horn JR: Pharmacokinetic drug interaction mechanisms and clinical characteristics. In: *Hansten and Horn's Drug Interactions Analysis and Management.* Applied Therapeutics, 1997; Cupp MJ, Tracy TS: Cytochrome P450: New nomenclature and clinical implications. Am Fam Physician 1998;57:107; Michalets EL: Update: Clinically significant cytochrome P-450 drug interactions. Pharmacotherapy 1998;18:84; and Flockhart DA, Tanus-Santos JE: Implications of cytochrome P-450 interactions with prescribing medication for hypertension. Arch Intern Med 2002;162:405.

(http://www.ti.ubc.ca/pages/letter.html) is a bimonthly newsletter that targets problematic therapeutic issues. This newsletter provides evidence-based reviews written and edited by a team of specialists and working groups of the International Society of Drug Bulletins.

It is recommended that physicians use these services as a scanning system to identify critical articles in the primary literature that should be read in-depth. It is important to note that information alone is not equivalent to working knowledge. Knowledge is gained by interpretation and synthesis of information. Ultimately, the goal of information processing is to gain wisdom, which implies an appropriate application of knowledge to a clinical situation. Survey services provide the information, but it is the clinician's responsibility to analyze, interpret, and apply this information to provide optimal patient care decisions. The goal of information sourcing is to maximize the usefulness score: increase validity and relevance while minimizing the workload.

DRUG INFORMATION & PHARMACOTHERAPY TEXTBOOKS

Textbooks are among the most common sources of information used by medical professionals. Because drug inquiries are frequent topics of clinical questions, it is important to review drug information textbooks. Despite the ease and convenience of use, textbooks have inherent limitations, including the following:

1. Currency of information: in the vastly growing information era, textbooks quickly become dated, primarily due to lag time associated with publishing.
2. Insufficient detail: due to the lack of space and limited literature search, important points may be undervalued.
3. Bias: the author or manufacturer may have conflicts of interest or inherent bias with regard to subject material.
4. Lack of expertise of the author regarding the particular content.
5. Errors in transcription or incorrect interpretation by the author or during the publication process.

Considerations when evaluating the validity of a textbook include the following:

1. Is this the most recent and timely edition?
2. Are statements and facts appropriately referenced?
3. Is the information source likely to contain relevant information? (ie, are you searching for a drug interaction in an adverse drug reaction textbook?)
4. Is the language clear, concise, and appropriate?

Many drug information textbooks and resources are available to address general or specific pharmaceutical categories (eg, ADRs, drug interactions, therapeutic use, dosing, etc). Commonly used drug information resources include, but are not limited to, the *Physicians' Desk Reference*, *American Hospital Formulary Services*, *MICROMEDEX*, *Drug Facts and Comparisons (Facts & Comparisons)*, and the *Drug Information Handbook*.

The most common drug information resource used by family medicine practitioners is the Physicians' Desk Reference (PDR). The *PDR* is a compilation of drug information from manufacturer product information. A survey conducted by the publisher, the Medical Economics Company, reports 82–90% of physicians consider the *PDR* their most useful resource, and it is estimated that the average US physician uses the *PDR* eight times per week. American Hospital Formulary Services (AHFS) contains prescribing drug formulary monographs with information similar to that found in the *PDR*. Additionally, *AHFS* contains detailed therapeutic information, including off-label indications and dosing for those indications. *AHFS* also contains adverse drug reactions summaries, often providing cautionary guidance and recommendations. **MICROMEDEX** is a computerized drug information resource that contains facts from the DRUGDEX Information System. This is a well-referenced, easily searchable, expansive drug information reference, housing information on prescription, nonprescription, and herbal remedies. Facts & Comparisons contains information on prescription and nonprescription medications. Medications are listed by category, with summary sections that provide tables and comparative drug class data. The Drug Information Handbook is a pocket-sized reference that includes referenced drug monographs. The monographs are listed alphabetically and include indications, dosing (including dosing in special populations), ADRs, drug interactions, and monitoring parameters. This reference also contains comparative charts and dosing equivalence tables.

Textbooks focusing on herbal and dietary supplements have also become increasingly important, as the use of these agents is widespread. *The Natural Medicines Comprehensive Database* and the *Natural Pharmacists* are two electronic references that consistently provide valid natural production information.

Cohen JS: Dose discrepancies between the Physicians' Desk Reference and the medical literature, and their possible role in the high incidence of dose-related adverse drug events. Arch Intern Med 2001;16:957. [PMID: 11295958]

Slawson DC et al: Becoming a medical information master: Feeling good about not knowing everything. J Fam Pract 1994;38: 505. [PMID: 8176350]

Sweet BV et al: Usefulness of herbal and dietary supplement references. Ann Pharmacother 2003;37:494. [PMID: 12659602]

Web Sites

Therapeutic Research Faculty, Natural Medicines Comprehensive Database:

http://www.naturaldatabase.com

The Natural Pharmacist:

http://www.tnp.com

UTILIZATION OF DRUG INFORMATION AT HAND: PERSONAL DIGITAL ASSISTANTS

The most common types of questions asked by medical residents relate to treatment or diagnosis of a patient; textbooks and colleagues are utilized as their primary information source. A study that evaluated medical residents' approach to answering 280 clinical questions showed that only 29% of the questions were answered and that lack of time was the most frequent reason (60%) for not answering questions.

Lack of time for pursuing clinical questions reinforces the need for "just-in-time" information, defined as highly filtered information with rapid access and ease of use. Some "delivery" systems have been shown to provide information in under 1 minute. One method of providing "just-in-time" information at the point of care is through handheld technology, or a personal digital assistant (PDA). It is estimated that PDAs are used by 30% of US physicians. A survey of physicians' perspectives on handheld computers in clinical practice reported that these devices increase productivity and improve patient care.

By improving Internet connectivity of handheld systems, improved access to updated evidence-based medication information is possible. For example, the National Library of Medicine has customized *PubMed* for handheld computers, allowing the ease of literature searching at your fingertips. *ePocrates Rx* has been advocated by insurance companies and government agencies to enhance clinical management and decrease medication errors.

In addition to evidence-based systems, benefits of organizer functions such as *PatientKeeper* include keeping track of patient records. This function has helped manage care; however, security issues relating to information storage are a limitation to use of this software. An important feature of handheld technology to the medical professional is the medical/pharmacy-related software, and the flexibility, accessibility, and usability of these systems. Several drug information sources are available. When evaluating these sources, the physician should consider user friendliness, comprehensiveness, accuracy, time interval of updates, freehand writing capabilities, memory requirements, and cost.

A study evaluating the core and supplemental drug information databases available for use with PDAs reviewed 10 core databases, 6 drug interaction analyzers, and 3 dietary supplement databases for scope, completeness, and ease of use. Results reported the best overall performers (in order of total scores) to be *Lexi-Drugs Platnum, Tarascon Pocket Pharmacopeia, ePocrates Rx Pro,* and *Clinical Pharmacology OnHand.*

PDA use is increasing among health care professionals. The multitude of applications and information sources delivered at the point of care provide useful and efficient information resources. In the information era, it is critical to provide evidence-based medicine decisions. Handheld technology allows this to be delivered "just in time."

Al-Ubaydli M: Handheld computers. BMJ 2004;328:1181. [PMID: 15142928]

Classen D: Medication safety: Moving from illusion to reality. 2003;289:1154. [PMID: 12622587]

Enders SJ et al: Drug-information software for palm operating system personal digital assistants: Breadth, clinical dependability, and ease of use. Pharmacotherapy 2002;22:1036. [PMID: 12173788]

Gillespie G: PDAs are willing, but will they be able? Health Data Manage 2002;10:21. [PMID: 12528640]

Green ML et al: Residents' medical information needs in clinic: Are they being met? Am J Med 2000;109:218. [PMID: 10974185]

Information Mastery Working Group: *The Near Future of Medicine: Just-in-Time Information at the Point-of-Care.* University of Virginia School of Medicine, April 2002.

Keplar KE, Urbanski CJ: Personal digital assistant applications for the healthcare provider. Ann Pharmacother 2003;37:287. [PMID: 12549963]

McAlearney AS et al: Doctors' experience with handheld computers in clinical practice: A qualitative study. BMJ 2004;328:1162. [PMID: 15142920]

Web Sites

PubMed:

http://certif.nlm.nih.gov.8080/nlm

ePocrates:

http://www.epocrates.com

Patient Keeper:

http://www.patientkeeper.com

Genetics for Family Physicians 47

Christine M. Mueller, DO, & W. Gregory Feero, MD, PhD

A common misconception in the medical community is that genetic disorders consist of an overwhelming number of complex, extremely rare conditions. However, they collectively comprise a significant proportion of pediatric and adult illnesses. Furthermore, there is now a better understanding of the genetic component of common diseases such as cardiovascular disease, diabetes mellitus, and mental illness.

Primary care physicians are in a unique position to diagnose genetic disorders because they are often the first contact for patients and also provide care for multiple family members. Additionally, burgeoning media attention is leading patients to seek information about genetic testing from their primary caregiver.

In fact, in a recent study, every responding primary care physician reported that he or she had addressed at least one condition with a genetic perspective in the past year. Furthermore, most cases were not referred for genetics consultation; 24% of these physicians felt that genetics consultation was difficult to obtain or not available. Ethical and social dilemmas were also encountered when considering genetic evaluations.

Acheson L et al: Clinical genetics issues encountered by family physicians. Genet Med 2005;7:501. [PMID: 16170242]

GENETIC EVALUATION

Collecting family history information and recognizing key symptoms and signs are the most important components in identifying genetically influenced disorders.

Family History

Most common diseases such as diabetes mellitus, hypertension, and cancer result from a combination of exposure to environmental factors and the effects of variations in multiple genes. However, the inherited variations within these genes can confer individual risks that can be distinguishable from the population-based average. Obtaining a medical family history can help to determine if an individual is at genetic risk of developing common disorders. Most importantly, these diseases often have modifiable risk factors that can be addressed or for which screening interventions can be instituted (Table 47–1).

Family history evaluation can also be useful in identifying rare conditions that may not otherwise be considered in a differential diagnosis. For example, a child with developmental delay may have other family members who have had developmental delays or more severe congenital abnormalities.

Sometimes specific questions will suffice when screening for a particular disease. However, recording family medical history in the form of a pedigree (Figure 47–1) can provide a concise visual tool for recording and interpreting medical information. When obtaining or updating a pedigree, the following general information may be recorded: patient name; date recorded or updated; consanguinity (note relationship); ethnic background of each grandparent, if known; and name and credentials of the person who recorded the pedigree. It is often helpful to include a key that explains symbols used in the pedigree (see Figure 47–1). Specific information such as age, relevant health information, age at diagnosis, age at death (with year, if known), cause of death, infertility (if known), and information about pregnancies (including miscarriages, stillbirths, and pregnancy terminations, along with gestational ages of family members or their partners) is then obtained for each listed family member.

Open-ended questions, such as "describe any medical conditions that affect your mother," provide the most information when obtaining a medical family history. It is often more efficient for patients to begin to generate their own family history at home, and several family history tools have been developed for use by patients. Family medical history may also be confirmed through medical record documentation.

Inheritance Patterns

A pedigree can help to identify a pattern of inheritance for a particular disorder, which can be useful in establishing a diagnosis. For example, if mental retardation is present in more than one generation in a family and only male family members are affected, an X-linked disorder should be considered. Table 47–2 reviews clues to determining patterns of inheritance. Unfortunately, limited collection of family history data, small family size, nonpaternity, delayed age of onset of symptoms, mild expression of disease symptoms, and sex-limited expression of disease symptoms (eg, a

Table 47–1. Disorders for which a positive family history changes screening practices or disease management.

Anemia
Breast cancer
Cardiomyopathy
Colon cancer
Coronary artery disease
Developmental delay
Diabetes mellitus
Dyslipidemia
Emphysema
Gastric cancer
Hearing impairment
Heart failure
Hip dysplasia
Hypertension
Kidney cancer
Liver cancer
Osteoporosis
Pancreatitis
Prostate cancer
Syncope
Thromboembolism
Thyroid cancer
Thyroid disease
Urticaria
Visual impairment

Adapted, courtesy of, Daniel Wattendorf and Alan Guttmacher, National Human Genome Research Institute, National Institutes of Health, Bethesda, MD.

woman with a healthy father whose sisters have breast and ovarian cancer) can complicate the identification of patterns of inheritance.

"Red Flags"

In addition to family history, there are certain clinical clues that should alert a clinician to consider a genetic cause for a medical condition (Table 47–3). Important issues to consider in all age groups are multiple congenital anomalies, earlier-than-usual onset of common conditions, extreme pathology (eg, rare tumors or multiple primary cancers), developmental delay or degeneration, and extreme laboratory values (eg, extremely high cholesterol level).

Bennett R: The family medical history. Prim Care Clin Office Pract 2004;31:479. [PMID: 15331243]

Wattendorf D, Hadley D: Family history: The three generation pedigree. Am Fam Physician 2005;72:441. [PMID: 16100858]

Whelan A et al: Genetic red flags: Clues to thinking genetically in primary care practice. Prim Care Clin Office Pract 2004; 31:497. [PMID: 15331244]

WEB SITE

U.S. Surgeon General's My Family Health Portrait tool: https://familyhistory.hhs.gov/

GENETIC TESTING

Family medical history or clinical clues may lead a clinician to consider genetic testing. Many primary care providers may be unfamiliar with a particular genetic disorder or the availability of genetic testing for a disorder. GeneTests (http://www.genetests.org) is a web-based resource that contains concise reviews and information on genetic testing availability for many genetic disorders. This web site also provides information regarding access to genetic specialists, including medical geneticists (physicians who have residency training in genetics), genetic counselors (individuals with masters degree–level training in genetics), and PhD-qualified individuals with formal clinical genetics training.

Overview of Genetics

Human genetic information is contained in structures called *chromosomes* that are present within virtually every cell nucleus in the body. All somatic cells have 46 chromosomes that are arranged in 23 pairs. The first 22 pairs, called *autosomes,* contain the genetic information for both men and women. The chromosomes that determine sex are XX for females and XY for males. One chromosome from each pair is inherited from the mother and the other from the father. The germ cells or gametes (sperm and egg cells) contain only 23 chromosomes.

Chromosomes contain the thousands of genes that are the basis of inheritance. It is estimated that the entire human genome consists of 25,000 genes. Each gene also comes in pairs; one of each pair is inherited from an individual's father and the other from his or her mother.

Genes are made up of DNA, which consists of two long, paired strands of chemical bases called *nucleotides.* Short strands of DNA along each chromosome comprise each gene, along with intervening sequences of DNA that are likely involved in the control of gene expression. The coding region of each gene specifies the instructions for a particular protein according to the order in which the nucleotides are arranged. Proteins are responsible for the development and functioning of our bodies. During cell replication and division, errors can occur either in the DNA sequence (*mutations*), resulting in a protein that does not function properly, or in the structure of entire chromosomes.

Methods of Genetic Testing

It is difficult to define what constitutes a "genetic" test. A test involving DNA or chromosome studies may be

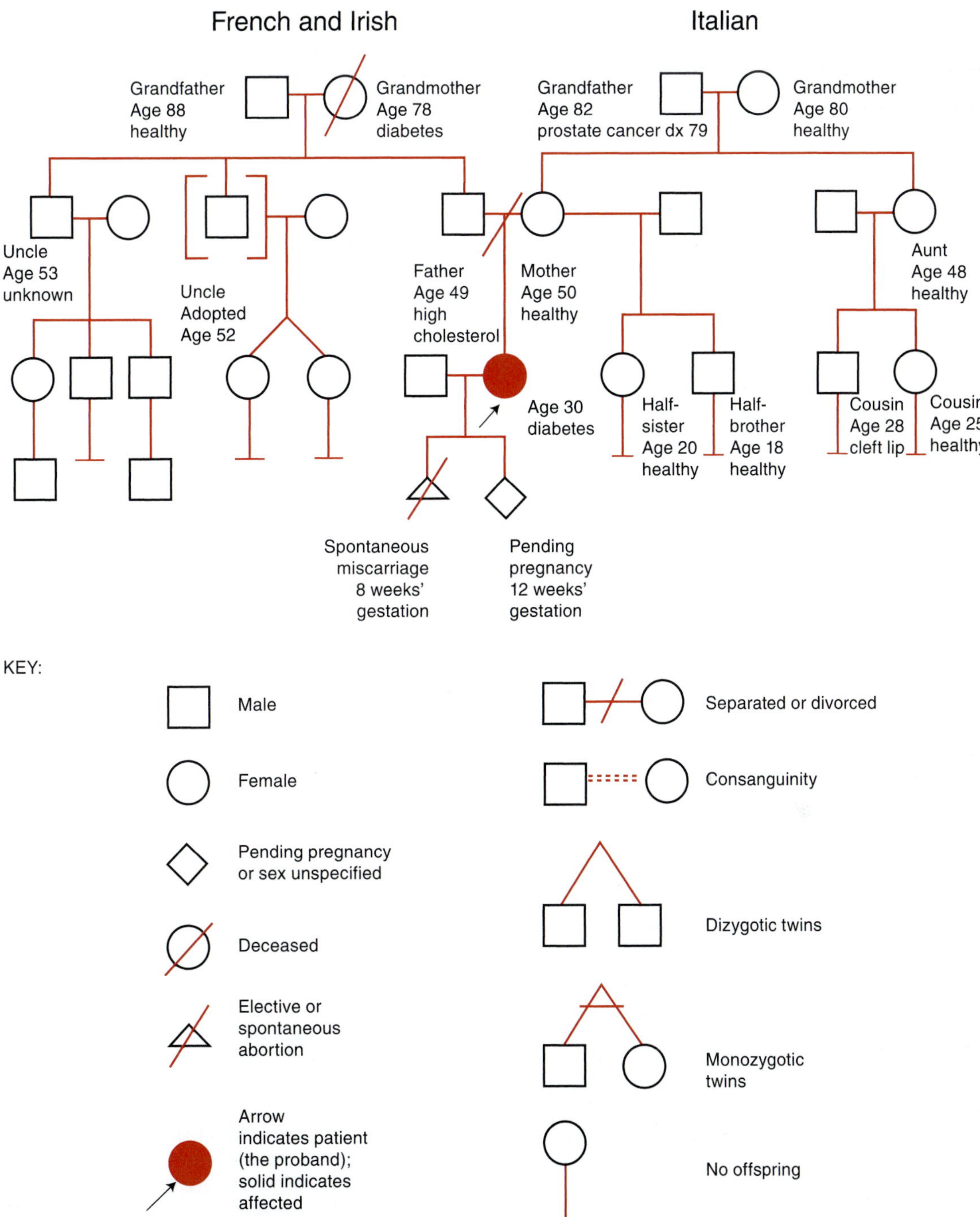

Figure 47–1. Standard pedigree symbols and sample pedigree.

Table 47–2. Clues to determining patterns of inheritance.

Pattern[1]	Diagnostic Clues
Autosomal dominant	Males and females equally affected Transmission passes from one generation to another (vertical inheritance) 50% risk for each offspring to be affected Variable expressivity: affected individuals in the same family may demonstrate varying degrees of phenotypic expression (severity) Reduced penetrance: some individuals who have inherited a genetic mutation may not express the phenotype ("skipped generations" may be seen)
Autosomal recessive	Males and females equally affected Multiple affected offspring and unaffected parents (horizontal inheritance) 25% risk for each offspring to parents with an affected child
X-linked recessive	Affects more males than females Heterozygous females are usually normal or have mild manifestations Inheritance is through maternal side of the family (diagonal inheritance) Female carriers have a 50% risk for each daughter to be a carrier and a 50% risk for each son to be affected All daughters of an affected male are carriers, and none of his sons are affected
X-linked dominant	Affects more females than males Heterozygous females are affected; homozygous females (rare) and males usually have severe or lethal manifestations Heterozygous females have a 50% risk for each offspring to be affected regardless of sex All daughters of an affected male are affected, and none of his sons are affected

[1]For more complex patterns of inheritance, see Korf B: Basic genetics. Prim Care Clin Office Pract 2004;31:461.

considered a genetic test but may not provide information about a person's inherited genetic identity. An example of this type of "genetic" testing is the use of chromosome studies in the subclassification of leukemia. Conversely, tests that are considered routine, and not necessarily "genetic," such as a cholesterol panel, have the potential to reveal genetic information about individuals and their family members (Table 47–4).

Table 47–3. Genetic "red flags."

Preconceptual/Prenatal	Pediatric	Adult
Personal or family history of known or suspected genetic disorder or congenital abnormality Two or more pregnancy losses Unexplained infertility Ethnic predisposition to genetic disorder Mother ≥ age 35 y at time of delivery (increased risk of chromosome abnormalities) Abnormal maternal serum screening Abnormal fetal ultrasound Exposure to teratogen Maternal condition that affects fetal development Parents with close biological relationship	One or more major malformations or dysmorphic features Abnormal newborn screening Abnormal development Congenital hearing loss Congenital blindness or cataracts Constellation of features suggestive of genetic disorder or chromosome abnormality Family history of known or suspected genetic disorder Personal or family history of hereditary cancers Development of degenerative neurologic disorder or unexplained seizures	Family history of known or suspected genetic disorder Diagnosis of common disorder with earlier age of onset than typical, especially if multiple family members are affected (eg, cancer, heart disease, stroke, diabetes mellitus, hearing or vision loss, degenerative neurologic disorder) Pediatric indications that have not yet been evaluated

Table 47–4. Some common adult disorders for which "genetic" testing is available and potentially appropriate for a subset of cases.[1]

Category	Disorder
Hematologic	Anemias Thrombophilias
Oncologic	Breast cancer Colon cancer Leukemia[2] Lymphoma[2] Skin cancer Thyroid cancer
Neurologic	Dementia Headache Movement disorders Seizures Stroke
Psychiatric[2]	Depression Schizophrenia
Endocrinologic	Diabetes mellitus
Rheumatologic	Arthritis
Cardiovascular	Aneurysms Cardiomyopathy Hyperlipidemia Hypertension Sudden death
Pulmonary	Asthma[2] Chronic obstructive pulmonary disease
Gastrointestinal	Cirrhosis
Renal	Renal failure
Ophthalmologic	Glaucoma Sudden vision loss

[1]For some of the listed disorders, only a small proportion of individuals are affected with inherited versions of the disease. Not all of the "genetic" tests for these disorders are DNA based.
[2]Some of the testing for these disorders is related to therapy and not necessarily to disease diagnosis or prognosis, and is not yet widely available clinically.

The test method used to detect a genetic disorder depends on what the genetic change associated with a particular condition primarily affects [eg, in the chromosomes, genes, or proteins (gene products)]. The primary laboratory methods used are cytogenetic analysis, direct DNA testing, biochemical tests, and linkage analysis.

A. Cytogenetic Analysis

Cytogenetic analysis is a microscopic study of chromosomes that is used to identify abnormalities in the number, size, or structure of chromosomes. Chemicals and tissue stains are used to produce a chromosome spread (karyotype).

1. Indications—Cytogenetic analysis is commonly ordered when patients are suspected of having a recognizable chromosome syndrome, in newborns with ambiguous genitalia or multiple malformations of unknown etiology; or after stillbirth of an infant with or without multiple malformations of unknown etiology. Other indications include patients with mental retardation, with or without congenital malformation; those with abnormal or delayed sexual development; couples with more than two unexplained spontaneous miscarriages; relatives of known balanced translocation or inversion carriers; and individuals with acquired chromosome abnormalities such as Philadelphia chromosome in chronic myelogenous leukemia.

Fluorescent in-situ hybridization (FISH) is a cytogenetic technique that uses synthetic DNA probes to evaluate whole chromosomes to rapidly detect missing or extra copies of chromosomes such as X, Y, 13, 18, and 21 in the prenatal setting or to detect submicroscopic deletions or duplications associated with specific genetic syndromes (eg, Prader–Willi, Angelman, DiGeorge).

2. Testable specimens—Suitable specimens for testing may be obtained from blood, fibroblasts, chorionic villi, amniocytes, or the products of conception.

3. Limitations—Cytogenetic testing may fail to identify an abnormality if it is not microscopically visible at the resolution for standard cytogenetic analysis. In addition, in patients with mosaicism, the abnormality may not be present in the cell type being analyzed.

B. Direct DNA Testing

Several methods are used to detect single gene mutations. These include Southern blot analysis, multiplex polymerase chain reaction analysis, allele-specific oligonucleotide hybridization, and direct gene sequencing.

1. Indications—Direct DNA testing may be indicated for patients affected or predisposed to a condition for which the gene change(s) that cause the condition have been identified (eg, cystic fibrosis, myotonic dystrophy, familial adenomatous polyposis).

2. Testable specimens—Specimens may be obtained from blood, fibroblasts, chorionic villi, amniocytes, or the products of conception.

3. Limitations—A negative test result may not rule out the condition. Some disorders are caused by numerous mutations within a gene (allelic heterogeneity), not all of which may be detected by a particular molecular method. Other disorders are caused by more than one gene, all of which may not be known (locus heterogeneity). Likewise, a positive test result does not always mean that the patient will develop the condition (eg, the patient may have reduced penetrance or a mutation of unknown clinical significance).

C. Biochemical Tests

Techniques such as metabolite testing, organic acid analysis, amino acid analysis, and assays of specific enzymes or proteins are used to identify or quantify absent or accumulated metabolites or measure the activity of a specific enzyme.

1. Indications—Biochemical tests are commonly used to help diagnose and monitor disorders such as hemochromatosis, familial hyperlipidemia, and the thrombophilias. Classically, biochemical tests are used to confirm the diagnosis of an inborn error of metabolism (eg, phenylketonuria, Tay–Sachs disease, Hurler syndrome).

2. Testable specimens—Blood, urine, fibroblasts, or specimens from muscle or organ biopsies may be used.

3. Limitations—Specimens for biochemical testing may require special collection, handling, and shipping. These tests are sometimes performed by specialized laboratories and may require expertise for adequate interpretation.

D. Linkage Analysis

Linkage analysis is a process by which differences in genetic sequences that are physically in close proximity ("linked") to a disease gene of interest are analyzed to track the inheritance of a disease gene within a family.

1. Indications—Linkage analysis is generally performed when the location of a gene for a particular disorder is known, but the gene itself is not known; or, alternatively, when the gene is known, but there are too many possible mutations for direct DNA testing to be practical.

2. Testable specimens—Blood, chorionic villi, amniocytes, fibroblasts, and the products of conception may be used.

3. Limitations—Unlike the other types of genetic testing described above, linkage analysis requires multiple samples for analysis, which must be obtained from several family members, including at least one affected relative. However, family members needed for analysis may not be available or may not consent to testing. Furthermore, results are often not available for many weeks, and they may be inconclusive and not 100% accurate.

E. Clinical versus Research Laboratory Testing

Physicians should be aware that US laboratories performing clinical tests are subject to regulation by the Clinical Laboratories Improvement Act (CLIA); however, research laboratories are not. It should also be noted that some research laboratories do not provide test results to patients or their physicians; others provide their results to a clinical laboratory to be confirmed so that a formal report can be issued.

What a Genetic Test Will Reveal

Before ordering testing for heritable disorders, clinicians should carefully consider the relevance of testing and the implications of the testing for their patient. Genetic testing is typically considered to fall into several major categories, which help to determine how the test can be used for clinical decision making for a patient or his or her family members. **Diagnostic testing** is used to confirm or identify a known or suspected genetic disorder in a symptomatic individual. **Predictive testing** is offered to an asymptomatic individual with a family history of a genetic disorder. Patients are further defined as "presymptomatic" if eventual development of symptoms is certain (eg, Huntington disease) or "predispositional" if eventual development of symptoms is likely but not certain (ie, colon cancer). **Carrier testing** is offered to appropriate individuals who have a family member with an autosomal-recessive or X-linked condition (eg, the sister of a boy with Duchenne muscular dystrophy) or individuals in an ethnic group known to have a high carrier rate for a particular disorder (eg, sickle cell anemia in the African-American population).

Prenatal testing is performed during a pregnancy and is offered when there is an increased risk of having a child with a genetic condition. Multiple marker screens, fetal ultrasound, amniocentesis, chorionic villus sampling, and periumbilical blood sampling are all used for prenatal testing. **Preimplantation testing** is performed on early embryos during *in vitro* fertilization, and offered to couples who are at increased risk of having a child with a genetic condition. **Newborn screening** is performed during the newborn period and identifies children who may have an increased risk of a specific genetic disorder so that further evaluation and treatment can be initiated as soon as possible.

Table 47–5 summarizes points to consider with each type of genetic testing.

Genetic Counseling

The current standard of care dictates that genetic counseling be provided to patients prior to initiating DNA-based, clinically driven genetic testing. Depending on the primary care provider's level of comfort with the disorder to be tested for and the testing modality being offered, counseling might best be delivered by that provider or by a genetic specialist. Appropriate counseling, no matter who provides the service, has several key ele-

Table 47–5. Considerations in the use of genetic testing.

Type of Test	Considerations
Diagnostic	Confirming a diagnosis may alter medical management Genetic testing may yield diagnostic information at a lower cost and with less risk than other procedures May have reproductive or psychosocial implications for patient and other family members Negative result requires further testing or follow-up
Predictive	Indicated if early diagnosis allows interventions that reduce morbidity or mortality Identification of the specific genetic mutation should be established in an affected relative first Likelihood of showing disease symptoms is increased but not always 100% Can have psychosocial implications and can influence life Testing of asymptomatic children at risk for adult-onset disorders is strongly discouraged when no medical intervention is available (ACMG policy statement)
Carrier	Identification of the specific genetic mutation in an affected family member may be required May have reproductive or psychosocial implications Can improve risk assessment for members of ethnic groups that are more likely to be carriers for certain genetic disorders
Prenatal	Invasive prenatal diagnostic procedures (eg, amniocentesis, CVS) have an associated risk to the fetus In most cases, a specific genetic mutation must be known in an affected relative (eg, mother with myotonic dystrophy) Prenatal testing for adult-onset disorders is controversial, and parents should receive a complete discussion of the issue
Preimplantation	Only performed at a few centers and available for a limited number of disorders Due to possible errors in preimplantation procedures and DNA analysis, traditional prenatal diagnostic procedures (amniocentesis, CVS) are recommended Cost is very high and may not be covered by insurance
Newborn screening	Usually legally mandated and varies by state Not designed to be diagnostic Further clinical evaluation and patient education is necessary with positive screening results Parents may not realize that testing was done

ACMG, American College of Medical Genetics; CVS, chorionic villus sampling.

ments. Pretest counseling should involve discussion of the mode of inheritance and risk of the condition for the patient and family members; the natural history of the condition; prognosis; presentation of appropriate testing options and interventions, including their risks, benefits, and limitations; discussion of the voluntary nature of genetic testing; and exploration of the social and familial implications of testing. These issues comprise the basis for informed consent, which should be documented before initiating DNA testing.

Post-test counseling involves the proper interpretation of results to the patient, including implications for further testing, management, and risks for other family members. It also may involve continued emotional support and referral to mental health professionals or disease-specific support groups, even for those who have tested negative for a particular disorder that may run in their family, due to feelings of guilt or sadness.

Ethical, Legal, & Social Issues

Many issues can arise when individuals are faced with the diagnosis of or susceptibility to a genetic disorder. Critical issues to consider include, but certainly are not limited to:

- Privacy (the rights of individuals to control access to information about themselves).
- Informed consent (giving permission to do genetic testing with the knowledge of the risks, benefits, effectiveness, and alternatives to testing).
- Confidentiality (acknowledgment that genetic information is sensitive, and that access should be limited to those authorized to receive it).
- Insurance and employment discrimination: Several states have enacted laws to protect individuals from genetic discrimination by insurance companies or in

the workplace. The Health Insurance Portability and Accountability Act (HIPAA) also provides some protection from discrimination. As of the summer of 2007, there is legislation pending before the U.S. Congress that would provide baseline national protections from discrimination on the basis of genetic test results or family history information.

- Nonpaternity or unknown adoption: This information can be unexpectedly revealed through genetic testing.
- Duty to warn (the obligation to disclose information to at-risk relatives if they are in clear and imminent danger): On rare occasions, this duty may require a health care professional to consider breaching patient confidentiality.
- Patient autonomy (the obligation to respect the decision-making capacities of patients who have been fully informed with accurate and unbiased information).
- Professional limitations (the duty of clinicians to realize the extent of their knowledge, skills, attitude, or behavior as they pertain to their practice and the laws, rules, regulations, and standards of care).

Clayton E: Ethical, legal, and social implications of genomic medicine. N Engl J Med 2003;349:562. [PMID: 12904522]

Green M, Botkin J: "Genetic Exceptionalism" in medicine: Clarifying the differences between genetic and nongenetic tests. Ann Intern Med 2003;138:571. [PMID: 126607027]

Korf B: Basic genetics. Prim Care Clin Office Pract 2004;31:461. [PMID: 15331242]

Martin J, Wilikofsky A: Genetic counseling in primary care: Longitudinal, psychosocial issues in genetic diagnosis and counseling. Prim Care Clin Office Pract 2004;31:509. [PMID: 15331245]

WEB SITES

National Human Genome Research Institute: http://www.genome.gov/PolicyEthics/

EXAMPLES IN PRACTICE

Case 1

Ms Smith, a healthy 33-year-old woman, presents to your office for routine health maintenance. On discussing her family history, you discover that her deceased maternal grandfather had colon cancer at age 45, her maternal aunt had colon cancer at age 45, and her mother had a hysterectomy at age 36 for uterine cancer. She asks you if, aside from having her annual Pap smear, she should have any additional cancer screening at her age.

Ms Smith's family history is suggestive of a disorder known as hereditary nonpolyposis colorectal cancer syndrome (HNPCC) or Lynch syndrome. Affecting about 1 in 800 individuals, HNPCC is more prevalent than familial adenomatous polyposis (FAP), and is thought to cause about 5% of all colon cancer cases. Affected individuals have an approximately 80% lifetime risk of colon cancer, as well as increased risks of several other cancers, including uterine, ovarian, urinary, stomach, biliary tract, brain, and small intestine. Unlike individuals with FAP, those with HNPCC have relatively few colon polyps which, when they do occur, tend to be located in the right colon and occur at a slightly older age.

HNPCC is inherited in an autosomal-dominant manner. It results from a mutation in one of at least five different members of a family of genes involved in DNA mismatch repair, with changes in the *MLH1, MSH2,* and *MSH6* genes being the most common. These tumor-suppressor genes are thought to encode for proteins that play a role in DNA repair.

The selection of patients suspected of having HNPCC for germline mutation testing is largely based on clinical criteria that rely on both patient and family history. The most commonly used guidelines include the Amsterdam I and II criteria as well as the Bethesda criteria. Unfortunately, these criteria are a bit cumbersome to recall in the primary care setting. A good general rule would be to think of this diagnosis in families dealing with high burdens of the previously mentioned cancers, or cases of early-onset (age younger than 50 years) colon cancer. Table 47–6 provides clues for determining if individuals are at hereditary risk of cancer.

Given that Ms Smith's family history is suggestive of HNPCC, an appropriate course of action would be to provide her with a referral to either a gastroenterologist familiar with the hereditary colon cancer syndromes or to a genetics clinic for further discussion. If Ms Smith then wished to proceed with testing for HNPCC, contacting her mother or her aunt would be the next step. This is because testing an affected individual is the most infor-

Table 47–6. Indicators of hereditary cancer susceptibility in a family.

Cancer in two or more first-degree relatives
Multiple cancers in multiple generations
Early age of onset (ie, < 50 y for adult-onset cancers)
Multiple cancers in a single individual
Bilateral cancer in a paired organ such as breast, kidney, or ovaries
Recognition of a known association between etiologically related cancers in the family, such as breast and ovarian cancer (HBOC) or adrenocortical carcinoma and breast cancer (Li–Fraumeni syndrome)
Presence of congenital anomalies associated with an increased cancer risk
Presence of precursor lesions known to be associated with cancers (atypical nevi and risk of malignant melanoma)
Recognizable pattern of inheritance

HBOC, hereditary breast-ovarian cancer.

mative approach to determining if a mutation in the *MLH1, MSH2,* or *MSH6* genes is present in the family. If an affected relative is found to have a mutation, and the patient subsequently tests positive for the same gene mutation, she would be a candidate for intense early screening for colon cancer (colonoscopy every 1–2 years starting at age 20–25 years, and annually after age 40), endometrial cancer (by annual endometrial biopsy, starting at 30–35 years), and ovarian cancer (concurrent screening with transvaginal ultrasound and the tumor marker, CA-125). Risk-reducing surgical options might also be considered.

Giardiello F et al: AGA technical review on hereditary colorectal cancer and genetic testing. Gastroenterology 2001;121:198. [PMID: 11438509]

Umar A et al: Revised Bethesda Guidelines for hereditary nonpolyposis colorectal cancer (Lynch syndrome) and microsatellite instability. J Natl Cancer Inst 2004;96:261. [PMID: 14970275]

Guillem J et al: ASCO/SSO review of current role of risk-reducing surgery in common hereditary cancer syndromes. J Clin Oncol 2006;24:4642. [PMID: 17008706]

Case 2

Mr Jones, a 45-year-old man, presented with a 1-year history of gradually worsening fatigue and diffuse arthralgias. His friends frequently compliment him on his healthy tan. Laboratory testing showed mildly elevated liver transaminases, despite his lack of recreational sun exposure. Testing for viral hepatitis was negative, but his ferritin level was elevated. Further testing revealed a markedly elevated fasting transferrin iron saturation. Genetic testing confirmed hereditary hemochromatosis.

Hemochromatosis is a disorder of iron metabolism in which toxic iron overload occurs. It can be inherited or acquired. The most common genetic form has a prevalence of about 1 in 300 in Caucasian populations and is inherited in an autosomal-recessive manner. The disorder becomes symptomatic in the fourth or fifth decade of life in men and about a decade later in women. Typical symptoms and signs include arthralgias, fatigue, abdominal pain, and bronzing of the skin. The classic triad of symptoms includes bronze skin, diabetes, and cirrhosis, but this is probably an uncommon presentation. Untreated, the disease can progress to liver cirrhosis or cardiomyopathy, either of which can be fatal. Diagnosis can be made without gene testing by measuring serum transferrin and iron saturation levels, with confirmatory liver biopsy showing elevated iron stores. Early, repeated phlebotomy to decrease body iron stores is very effective in treating the disease.

In the past decade, a handful of specific mutations in the *HFE* gene have been shown to cause a majority of the genetic cases of hemochromatosis. Most individuals are either homozygous for the C282Y mutation (85%) or compound heterozygotes for the mutations C282Y and H63D (< 10%) in the *HFE* gene. This gene encodes a protein that regulates cellular iron uptake. Although genetic testing is available for this disorder, population screening remains controversial. Many investigators thought that the high prevalence, ease of testing, long presymptomatic state, and simple therapy made this an ideal disorder for screening. However, follow-up population-based studies suggest that many individuals with HFE gene mutations remain completely asymptomatic, a finding that has lessened the enthusiasm for widespread screening programs. Less common forms caused by gene mutations at other loci exist, including a rather severe juvenile form.

Beutler E et al: Penetrance of 845G–> A (C282Y) HFE hereditary haemochromatosis mutation in the USA. Lancet 2002;359: 211. [PMID: 11812557]

Pietrangelo A: Hereditary hemochromatosis—a new look at an old disease. N Engl J Med 2004;350:2383. [PMID: 15175440]

Case 3

Baby Girl Miller had a normal newborn examination in the hospital after birth. A week after discharge, you receive a call from the state newborn screening laboratory reporting that the newborn has a high phenylalanine level suspicious for phenylketonuria (PKU). You immediately call a metabolic specialist in your region and arrange for the newborn to be evaluated at the metabolic clinic the next day.

Metabolic disorders affect 1 in 3500 newborns. They typically are the result of a cell's inability to produce a particular enzyme or metabolize a particular substance. These disorders are almost always inherited in an autosomal-recessive manner, so parents of an affected child are typically carriers (heterozygotes, who have only one copy of the mutant gene) who have no clinical manifestations of the disease. In some cases, the affected offspring does not immediately manifest symptoms. However, unless these disorders are detected and treated early, they can result in mental retardation, physical abnormalities, and, in some individuals, death. For some of these disorders, such as Tay–Sachs disease, there is no specific therapy, and mortality is unavoidable.

Newborn screening programs are an effective public health strategy for the detection and prevention of complications of many genetic diseases. All states in the United States screen newborns for PKU, galactosemia, and hypothyroidism. Tests are available for over 30 disorders, including cystic fibrosis and the more common hemoglobinopathies. Testing varies by state and depends on the availability of funding for screening. Appropriate technology and follow-up, and the lack of treatment for some of these disorders, are important issues for newborn screening programs. Carrier testing is also available for many of these disorders.

Children with congenital abnormalities and developmental delays are also often evaluated initially by primary care physicians. Chromosomal imbalances are involved in approximately 25% of major congenital malformations, single genes in approximately 20%, and known teratogenic exposures in approximately 5%. A genetic cause for developmental delays is estimated to be present in approximately 5–25% of affected individuals. Associated congenital malformations, hearing impairment, growth retardation, and family history increase the likelihood of a genetic etiology. A detailed history, including prenatal, birth, and family history, as well as a thorough physical examination with particular attention to growth parameters, neurologic status, and dysmorphic features or congenital malformations are important in assessing an individual with a congenital malformation or developmental delay.

American College of Medical Genetics Foundation; sponsored by the New York State Department of Health. Evaluation of the Newborn with Single or Multiple Congenital Anomalies: A Clinical Guide. Available at: http://www.health.state.ny.us/nysdoh/dpprd/.

Battaglia A, Carey J: Diagnostic evaluation of developmental delay/mental retardation: An overview. Am J Med Genet C Semin Med Genet 2003;117:3. [PMID: 12561053]

Tandem mass spectrometry in newborn screening. American College of Medical Genetics/American Society of Human Genetics Test and Technology Transfer Committee Working Group. Genet Med 2000;2:267. [PMID: 11252712]

WEB SITE

March of Dimes information on newborn screening by state: http://www.marchofdimes.com/professionals/580.asp

FUTURE DIRECTIONS & CURRENT CHALLENGES

Knowledge of human genetics has improved considerably over the past few decades, and many new single-gene disorders have been identified. Completion of the International Hap Map Project, an extension of the Human Genome Project, has facilitated a large number of recent "genome-wide association studies" that have yeilded a wealth of new data on the genetic underpinnings of many common medical disorders. The International Hap Map Project, an extension of the Genome Project, has set out to create a resource to aid in identifying genetic factors that influence more common medical disorders. It is hoped that this information will lead to the development of diagnostic and screening tests, novel therapies, and strategies for the prevention of these disorders. Some of these rapidly advancing approaches include pharmacogenomics and gene therapy.

Primary care physicians face major challenges in the realm of clinical genetics: (1) they must decide which portion of this new, complex health care delivery process they feel comfortable managing, and identify specialty resources to assist them with patient-care questions or patient referral; (2) they must become familiar with the standard components of the genetic testing process, including pretest counseling, informed consent, proper interpretation of test results, post-test discussion of the implications of test results for their patient and family members, and implementation of appropriate risk reduction and surveillance recommendations; (3) they must keep pace with the new genetic discoveries that are made every year and the most current versions of rapidly evolving disorder-specific evaluation and management recommendations.

The collaborative approach to patient care in the primary care setting is a solid foundation for achieving the maximum benefit of genetic risk assessment and testing for the individual and the family.

ONLINE RESOURCES

Centers for Disease Control and Prevention:
http://www.cdc.gov/node.do/id/0900f3ec8000e2b5

Medline Plus/National Institutes of Health:
http://www.nlm.nih.gov/medlineplus/geneticdisorders.html

National Cancer Institute/National Institutes of Health:
http://www.nci.nih.gov/cancertopics/pdq/genetics

National Coalition of Health Professional Education in Genetics:
http://www.nchpeg.org

Pharmacogenomics 48

Ya'aqov Abrams, MD, & Matthew Krasowski, MD, PhD

The study of pharmacogenomics addresses the interactions of multiple genes and gene products and their impact on drug therapy, with the goal of developing rational means to optimize drug therapy and ensure maximum efficacy with minimal side effects. In a gross way physicians already use pharmacogenomics when choosing cardiac drugs for patients. For example, hypertensive patients of African background and black race tend to respond better to diuretics and worse to angiotensin-converting enzyme inhibitors and β-blockers. A recent study investigating congestive heart failure in blacks was terminated prematurely because of an absolute risk reduction in the death rate of 4%. The Food and Drug Administration (FDA) then approved the combination of two well-known drugs, isosorbide and hydralazine, as an adjunct to standard treatment of heart failure in African Americans.

In practice, however, humans and their genome are much more complicated than a simple classification based on race. For example, hypertension rates in African Americans are higher than in Caucasian Americans, but the same among African Cubans and Caucasian Cubans. Furthermore, studies of human genetic diversity often sample small numbers of members of a racial or ethnic group, and importantly, membership in a particular ethnic group or race is often defined more by the subject's ethnic identification than by objective criteria. Furthermore, genetic studies are not usually designed to assess other important influences on medical phenomena such as environment, social class, poverty, and life-style. Using race to guide prescription of medication is a proxy for understanding the underlying genetic, environmental, social, economic, and life-style causes of illness.

Ordunez P et al: Ethnicity, education, and blood pressure in Cuba. Am J Epidemiol 2005;162:49. [PMID: 15961586]

Rahemtulla T, Bhopal R: Pharmacogenetics and ethnically targeted therapies. BMJ 2005;330:1036. [PMID: 15879369]

Taylor A et al: Combination of isosorbide dinitrate and hydralazine in blacks with heart failure. N Engl J Med 2004;351:2049. [PMID: 15533851]

Wilkinson GR: Drug metabolism and variability among patients in drug response. N Engl J Med 2005;352:2211. [PMID: 15917386]

GENETIC VARIABILITY & ITS EFFECTS ON PHARMACOKINETICS & PHARMACODYNAMICS

The effect of drugs is traditionally divided into pharmacokinetics (how drugs are absorbed, distributed, metabolized, and eliminated) and pharmacodynamics (target or targets underlying the therapeutic effect). In principle, genetic variation can influence either pharmacokinetics or pharmacodynamics, or both. Currently, most clinical application of pharmacogenetics involves pharmacokinetics, but over time more attention will shift to pharmacodynamics. The sequencing of the human genome and intensive research into how genetic variation affects drug response holds the promise of altering the paradigms for medication therapy. However, as will be discussed below, current clinical applications utilizing pharmacogenetics are still rather limited. The coming years should see steady growth in this field that will allow primary care providers and other health professionals to better manage drug therapy.

Evans WE, Relling MV: Moving towards individualized medicine with pharmacogenomics. Nature 2004;429:464. [PMID: 15165072]

Goldstein DB et al: Pharmacogenetics goes genomic. Nat Rev Genet 2003;4:937. [PMID: 14631354]

Genetic Variability

The most common type of genetic variation is single-nucleotide polymorphism (SNP), a situation in which some individuals have one nucleotide at a given position while other individuals have another nucleotide (eg, cytosine versus adenosine, C/A). If this occurs in the coding region of a gene (ie, within coding exons), it may or may not produce a change in the amino acid sequence that results when DNA is transcribed into RNA and RNA is then translated into protein. SNPs that cause a change in amino acid sequence are termed *nonsynonymous* whereas those that do not change amino acid sequence are termed *synonymous*. Typically, synonymous substitutions are thought of as neutral, an assumption that is generally but not always true (an example of this is seen in the gene responsible for cystic fibrosis; see Pagani et al, 2005). Other less common types of genetic variation include insertions or deletions (sometimes referred to collectively as "indels"), partial or total gene deletion, alteration of mRNA splicing (ie, the process of removing introns from genomic DNA sequences that contain exons and introns), variation in gene promoters, and gene duplication or multiplication.

Introduction to some terms and nomenclature used in pharmacogenetics is helpful. In dealing with pharmacogenetic variation of drug-metabolizing enzymes, particularly the cytochrome P450 (CYP) enzymes, *poor metabolizers* represent individuals with little or no enzyme activity, either due to lack of expression of the enzyme or mutations that reduce enzymatic activity (eg, a mutation that alters the active catalytic site). *Extensive metabolizers* are considered the "normal" situation and generally represent individuals with two normal copies of the enzyme gene on each chromosome. *Intermediate metabolizers* have enzyme activity roughly half that of extensive metabolizers. The most common genetic reason underlying intermediate activity is the presence of one copy of the normal gene and one variant copy associated with low activity. *Ultra-rapid metabolizers* have enzyme activity significantly greater than the average population. This is often due to the presence of duplicated or multiplicated copies of a gene (ie, more than the normal two copies of a gene, one on each chromosome). Gene duplication or multiplication is not seen with many genes but can occur with CYP2D6. For example, an individual may have three or more copies of the CYP2D6 gene instead of the normal two copies.

Genetic variants involving drug-metabolizing enzymes are named in a historical but often confusing system to those new to the field. By definition, the normal allele (individual copy of a gene on a chromosome) is defined as *1 (eg, CYP2D6*1). In order of historical discovery, variant alleles were designated *2, *3, *4, and so on, in some cases with subtypes (eg, *3A) added later on. Unfortunately, this nomenclature does not give any clue to the nature of the genetic variation. For instance, *4 and *6 could represent fairly benign genetic variants whereas *5 could signify a variant resulting in complete absence of enzyme activity.

Bertilsson L et al: Molecular genetics of CYP2D6: Clinical relevance with focus on psychotropic drugs. Br J Clin Pharmacol 2002;53:111. [PMID: 11851634]

Pagani F et al: Synonymous mutations in CFTR exon 12 affect splicing and are neutral in evolution. Proc Natl Acad Sci U S A 2005;102:6368. [PMID: 15840711]

Genetic Variation Involving Pharmacokinetics

Although a number of nongenetic factors influence the effects of medications—including disease, organ function, concomitant medications, herbal therapy, age, and gender—there are now many examples in which interindividual differences in medication response are due to variants in genes encoding drug targets, drug-metabolizing enzymes, and drug transporters. Currently, most well-established applications of pharmacogenetics involve pharmacokinetics, specifically drug metabolism.

Several organs can metabolize (biotransform) drug molecules, with the liver being the dominant organ for this purpose in humans and other mammals. The proteins that have been studied in greatest depth are the CYP enzymes, a complicated group of enzymes expressed in liver, intestine, kidney, lung, and some other organs. Several CYP enzymes account for the majority of drug metabolism in humans: CYP3A4/5, CYP2D6, CYP2C9, and CYP2C19. CYP3A4, in particular, has been shown to play a role in the metabolism of over 50% of the prescribed drugs in the United States.

Genetic variation of CYP2D6 was one of the first classic examples of pharmacogenetics. In the 1970s, the experimental (and now obsolete) antihypertensive drug debrisoquine was being tested. For the majority of individuals, this drug provided safe control of hypertension. However, some individuals developed prolonged hypotension lasting for days after receiving the drug. Debrisoquine was later found to be mainly metabolized by CYP2D6, an enzyme found in the liver that is now known to metabolize about 25% of all drugs currently prescribed in the United States. Of the CYP enzymes, CYP2D6 is the most highly genetically polymorphic (ie, it shows the greatest range of genetic variation), with reasonably common genetic variants that include total gene deletion (CYP2D6*5) and gene duplication; rare individuals have been documented who have over 10 functional copies of the CYP2D6 gene. Genetic variation of CYP2D6, as will be discussed below, has clinical importance for psychiatric, cardiac, and opiate medications. CYP2D6 poor metabolizers may experience severe adverse effects to standard doses of certain drugs (debrisoquine being the standard historical example) whereas ultra-rapid metabolizers may degrade a drug so quickly that therapeutic concentrations are not achieved with standard doses.

The CYP enzymes also underlie a number of clinically important drug–drug or drug–food interactions. For example, ketoconazole is a powerful inhibitor of multiple CYP enzymes, including CYP3A4. Ketoconazole thus has potentially dangerous interactions with drugs metabolized by CYP3A4 such as the immunosuppressive drug cyclosporine, if appropriate dose reductions are not made. Conversely, several compounds markedly increase (induce) the expression of CYP enzymes, including rifampin, phenytoin, carbamazepine, phenobarbital, and the herbal antidepressant St John's wort. By increasing the expression of CYP enzymes and other proteins involved in drug metabolism and elimination, inducers such as rifampin can cause not only increased metabolism of other drugs but also of endogenous compounds such as steroid hormones. This is the mechanism underlying unintended pregnancy that can result in women using estrogen-containing oral contraceptives who also receive a CYP inducer such as rifampin. CYP inducers greatly increase the metabolism of the estrogen component of combined oral contraceptives, resulting in therapeutic failure. (For further discussion, see Chapter 46.)

Goldstein DB: Pharmacogenetics in the laboratory and the clinic. N Engl J Med 2003;348:553. [PMID: 12571264]

Kirchheiner J, Brockmoller J: Clinical consequences of cytochrome P450 2C9 polymorphisms. Clin Pharmacol Ther 2005;77:1. [PMID: 15637526]

Weinshilboum R: Inheritance and drug response. N Engl J Med 2003;348:529. [PMID: 12571261]

Genetic Variation Involving Pharmacodynamics

Understanding of genetic variation involving pharmacodynamics has developed more slowly than that of pharmacokinetics. In part, this is because the molecular targets of certain drugs are incompletely understood. A good example of pharmacodynamic genetic variation is for the β_2-adrenergic receptor, the target of β-agonists used in asthma therapy such as albuterol and salmeterol. The importance of understanding pharmacodynamic variation is that it holds the potential of predicting therapeutic efficacy (or lack thereof). This could be especially valuable for disorders such as depression in which weeks or even months may be required to determine effectiveness of a drug.

Flordellis C et al: Pharmacogenomics of adrenoceptors. Pharmacogenomics 2004;5:803. [PMID: 15459404]

Haga SB, Burke W: Using pharmacogenetics to improve drug safety and efficacy. JAMA 2004;291:2869. [PMID: 15199039]

Johnson JA, Evans WE: Molecular diagnostics as a predictive tool: Genetics of drug efficacy and toxicity. Trends Mol Med 2002;8:300. [PMID: 12067617]

SELECTED CLINICAL APPLICATIONS

Although pharmacogenomics is far from fulfilling its promise of developing a patient-specific pharmacologic profile, there are several areas in which genetic testing is routinely used, or is being evaluated for clinical use.

Oncology

Pharmacogenetics began to develop as a distinct discipline beginning in the 1950s, mainly as researchers tried to understand serious adverse effects that occurred in a small number of patients exposed to certain medications. These included prolonged muscle paralysis and apnea in response to the neuromuscular blocker succinylcholine, severe bone marrow toxicity following cancer chemotherapy with azathioprine or 6-mercaptopurine (6-MP) therapy, and the excessive hypotension following administration of the experimental antihypertensive agent debrisoquine, described earlier. These early "classic" cases of pharmacogenetics turned out to be due to genetic variation (polymorphisms) of enzymes that metabolized the particular drugs.

Azathioprine and 6-MP are agents used in the treatment of cancers (eg, acute lymphoblastic leukemia) and, more recently, in disorders with an autoimmune basis such as rheumatoid arthritis and inflammatory bowel disease. Azathioprine is converted to 6-MP in vivo (ie, it is a pro-drug of 6-MP). Although azathioprine and 6-MP both have the potential for bone marrow suppression if used in high doses, about 1 in 300 Caucasians (less in a number of other populations) experience very profound bone marrow toxicity following standard doses of azathioprine and 6-MP, in some cases resulting in death or severe morbidity due to anemia, thrombocytopenia, or leukopenia. Over several years, researchers determined that the enzyme thiopurine methyltransferase (TPMT) converted 6-MP to therapeutically inactive compounds. Certain individuals, however, had very low TPMT enzyme activity (ie, they are TPMT "poor metabolizers"); these individuals are the ones who develop severe toxicity to standard doses of 6-MP and azathioprine. Several clinical laboratory tests can predict upfront whether individuals will have difficulty metabolizing 6-MP and azathioprine.

Due to the significant impact of TPMT polymorphisms on 6-MP and azathioprine, the FDA urged the manufacturers of these drugs to revise the drug label to describe the impact of genetic variation on drug metabolism and of the possible use of genetic testing. Although there is still debate on how to alter dosing in patients with TPMT variants, the package inserts for both 6-MP and azathioprine now include information on pharmacogenetics of TPMT. TPMT poor metabolizers can still receive 6-MP or azathioprine but need markedly reduced dose.

Although genetic variation of TPMT can have a dramatic impact on medication therapy, even individuals completely lacking these enzymes may show no other clinical symptoms. This finding is also seen with absence of other drug-metabolizing enzymes such as butyrylcholinesterase (an enzyme that hydrolyzes succinylcholine) or CYP2D6. Consequently, without laboratory testing or suggestive previous clinical history of unusual medication response, genetic variation of these enzymes cannot be predicted.

TPMT is probably the best-studied pharmacogenetic application; however, newer pharmacogenetics applications in oncology are emerging. A second application involves the drug irinotecan (CPT-11), a chemotherapeutic agent used in the treatment of colorectal cancer. Irinotecan has a complicated metabolism but is inactivated by glucuronidation mediated by UDP-glucuronosyltransferase 1A1 (UGT1A1), an enzyme that also carries out conjugation of bilirubin. A variety of rare, severe mutations in UGT1A1 can result in the Crigler–Najjar syndrome, a devastating disease that can be fatal in childhood unless liver transplantation is performed. A milder mutation, designated UGT1A1*28, is the most common cause of a mostly benign condition called Gilbert syndrome that is often diagnosed incidentally by detection of unconjugated hyperbilirubinemia without associated hepatobiliary pathology. The UGT1A1*28 mutation only causes a partial decrease in enzyme activity, even in individuals possessing two copies of this variant allele. These individuals are, however, at high risk for severe toxicity following irinotecan therapy. With standard doses, such individuals may develop life-threatening neutropenia or diarrhea that is poorly responsive to therapy. A genetic test for UGT1A1*28 became FDA-approved and, similar to 6-MP and azathioprine, the package insert for irinotecan now includes specific information on UGT1A1 genetic variation.

Although the oncology applications for pharmacogenetics do not have widespread importance for primary care, they illustrate the potential of understanding genetic variation. In addition, the FDA has emphasized the importance of including pharmacogenetic information in package inserts for drugs, establishing that physicians at the minimum need to consider pharmacogenetics where applicable in drug therapy.

Dervieux T et al: Pharmacogenetic testing: Proofs of principle and pharmacoeconomic implications. Mutat Res 2005;573:180. [PMID: 15829247]

Marsh S, McLeod H: Pharmacogenetics of irinotecan toxicity. Pharmacogenomics 2004;5:835. [PMID: 15469406]

Mascheretti S, Schreiber S: Genetic testing in Crohn disease: Utility in individualizing patient management. Am J Pharmacogenomics 2005;5:213. [PMID: 16078858]

Wang L, Weinshilboum R: Thiopurine S-methyltransferase pharmacogenetics: Insights, challenges and future directions. Oncogene 2006;25:1629. [PMID: 16550163]

Psychiatry

As previously mentioned, about 25% of medications are metabolized by CYP2D6 or CYP2C19. Psychiatric medications in these categories are currently among the most commonly used (see Table 46–5, in Chapter 46).

Substrates of CYP2D6 can cause significant side effects. For example, fluoxetine can inhibit CYP2D6, and when given with tricyclic antidepressants (TCAs) result in markedly elevated TCA levels, which in turn place a patient at risk for a variety of side effects, among them hypotension, cardiac arrhythmias, and heart block.

A clinical approach to the problem of predicting drug effectiveness and safety is to simply look up drugs in one of the many databases available such as *ePocrates* (http://www.epocrates.com) or *The Medical Letter* (http://www.medicaletter.com). However, as mentioned earlier, drug–drug interactions are not the only variables to consider when anticipating drug safety and efficacy. Psychiatric drugs are usually started at low doses and increased slowly, but a cautious dosing approach may not be ideal in the setting of psychiatric crisis. The need to take drugs that are substrates of the same CYP450 enzymes and unexpected life-threatening reactions to prior use of medications are possible indications for genetic testing. Adding genetic screening for CYP ultra-rapid metabolizers and poor metabolizers would increase the safety of medication prescription. Roche recently released the Amplichip CYP450 test, which is designed to detect polymorphisms of CYP2D6 and CYP2C19.

Anticoagulation

Anticoagulant-related bleeding complications occur in about 3% of patients in the first 3 months of therapy, with the highest risk around the start of anticoagulation. During maintenance therapy there is a risk of bleeding complications of 7.6–16.5 per 100 patient-years. Thus, there is a need to accurately predict both the initial and maintenance doses of warfarin. Polymorphisms in CYP2C9, which metabolizes 80% of the more pharmacologically active *s*-enantiomer of warfarin, account for about 20% of the dose variability of chronic warfarin dosing. Adding another variable, vitamin K epoxide reductase (VKOR), the enzyme that is the final step in the vitamin K recycling cycle (Figure 48–1) and also the target of warfarin—as well as age, height, weight, smoking, and alcohol use—to a pharmacogenomics-based algorithm accounts for 50–55% of the long-term variability in warfarin dosing, depending on the study. At this point, however, this is no better than the standard algorithm in routine use currently.

Focusing on initiation of therapy, in a small study (N = 48), Voora and colleagues showed that a pharmacogenomics-based model led to a stable international normalized ratio (INR) at the same rate as the standard algorithm. However, there was no drop in the risk of over-anticoagulation in the patients at highest risk because of CYP29 polymorphisms.

There has been progress in both areas, but neither application is ready for routine clinical use. There may be a role for pharmacogenetic testing in patients who exhibit extreme sensitivity or resistance to warfarin.

Aquilante CL et al: Influence of coagulation factor, vitamin K epoxide reductase complex subunit 1, and cytochrome P450 2C9 gene polymorphisms on warfarin dose requirements. Clin Pharmacol Ther 2006;79:291. [PMID: 16580898]

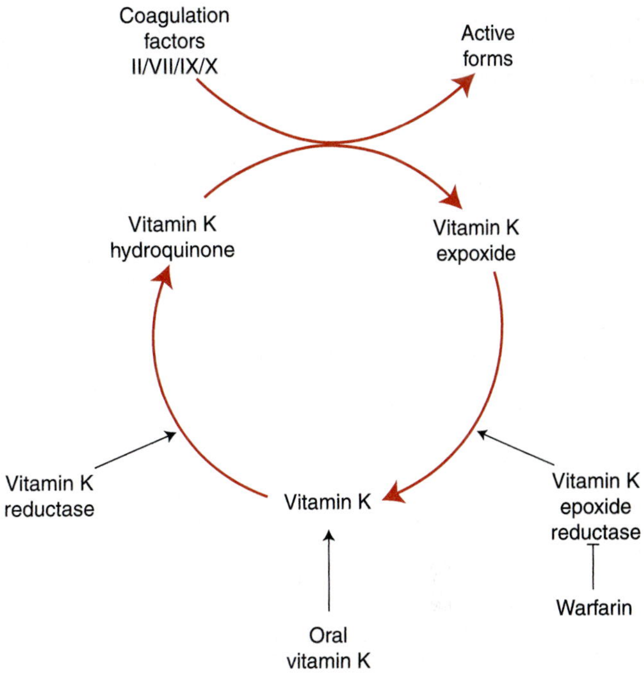

Figure 48–1. Cyclical reduction and oxidation of vitamin K is inhibited by warfarin. Dietary vitamin K is reduced to vitamin K hydroquinone by vitamin K reductase. Vitamin K hydroquinone is then oxidized to vitamin K epoxide in a coupled reaction that results in the activation of coagulation factors II, VII, IX, and X. Vitamin K epoxide is then reduced back to vitamin K by vitamin K epoxide reductase (VKOR). This enzyme is inhibited by warfarin, leading to a block in the cycle, which results in a depletion in activated clotting factors. (Reproduced, with permission, from Hall AM, Wilkins MR: Warfarin: A case history in pharmacogenetics. Heart 2005;91:563.)

Douketis J et al: Clinical risk factors and timing of recurrent venous thromboembolism during the initial 3 months of anticoagulant therapy. Arch Intern Med 2000;160:3431. [PMID: 11112236]

Hall AM, Wilkins MR: Warfarin: A case history in pharmacogenetics. Heart 2005;91:563. [PMID: 15831631]

Sconce E et al: The impact of CYP2C9 and VKORC1 genetic polymorphism and patient characteristics upon warfarin dose requirements: Proposal for a new dosing regimen. Blood 2005;106:2329. [PMID: 15947090]

Voora D et al: Prospective dosing of warfarin based on cytochrome P-450 2C9 genotype. Thromb Haemost 2005;93:700. [PMID: 15841315]

Opiates

Therapeutic and adverse effects of analgesic medications are also influenced by genetic variation. Perhaps the most classic effect is that seen in CYP2D6 poor metabolizers. Codeine (methylmorphine) is demethylated by CYP2D6 to morphine. Codeine is a weak agonist of the μ-opioid receptor responsible for analgesia; consequently, codeine is essentially a prodrug of morphine. CYP2D6 poor metabolizers are unable to convert codeine to morphine and will consequently be "nonresponders" to codeine therapy. CYP2D6 poor metabolizers are also much less likely to abuse codeine (because the active metabolite morphine is not generated), demonstrating that drug metabolism can influence abuse liability. CYP2D6 ultra-rapid metabolizers on the other hand are at risk for life-threatening opiate overdose when small doses of codeine are administered. Gasche and colleagues demonstrated that suppression of CYP3A4 by clarithromycin, which eliminated a secondary pathway for codeine metabolism in the setting of transient renal insufficiency, potentiated the effect of this ultra-rapid metabolism of codeine to morphine. CYP2D6 also plays a role in the metabolism of other analgesics, including methadone, tramadol, hydrocodone, and oxycodone, although CYP2D6 pharmacogenetics has not been systematically studied for these other drugs. The pharmacogenetics of analgesic targets such as the various opioid receptors is an area of active inquiry.

There are no studies that address the overall clinical efficacy and cost-effectiveness of genetic testing to guide pharmacotherapy. In the absence of such an approach Flowers and Veenstra, echoing the standard analysis for screening tests, proposed a framework to address this question (Table 48–1).

At present, the most reasonable approach seems to be heightened awareness of the pitfalls in medication prescription, selected genetic testing in those who have had or seem to be at high risk for preventable side effects, and support of studies designed to ascertain the effectiveness of this technology.

Flowers C, Veenstra D: The role of cost-effectiveness analysis in the era of pharmacogenomics. Pharmacoeconomics 2004;22:481. [PMID: 15217305]

Gasche Y et al: Codeine intoxication associated with ultrarapid CYP2D6 metabolism. N Engl J Med 2004;351:2827. [PMID: 15625333]

Palmer SN et al: Pharmacogenetics of anesthetic and analgesic agents. Anesthesiology 2005;102:665. [PMID: 15731608]

Table 48–1. Considerations in assessing the cost-effectiveness of a pharmacogenomic treatment strategy.

1. What is the frequency of the genetic polymorphism?
2. How closely is the polymorphism linked to a consistent phenotypic drug response?
3. Are there metabolic, environmental, or other significant influences on drug response?
4. What are the sensitivity and specificity of the genomic tests?
5. What alternative tests are available to predict drug response?
6. How prevalent is the disease of interest?
7. What are the characteristic outcomes associated with the disease with and without treatment?
8. How does the pharmacogenomics strategy alter these outcomes?
9. What is the therapeutic range of the drug involved?
10. What alternative treatment options are available?
11. How effective are current monitoring strategies for preventing severe adverse drug reactions and predicting drug response?

Reproduced, with permission, from Flowers C, Veenstra D: The role of cost-effectiveness analysis in the era of pharmacogenomics. Pharmacoeconomics 2004;22:481.

THE FUTURE: CARDIOVASCULAR DISEASE

There has been significant progress in understanding the pharmacogenomics of some medication classes, as previously discussed. The situation in cardiovascular disease is much more complex, perhaps reflecting the multifactorial etiology of hypertension and cardiovascular disease in general. Polymorphisms in the renin-angiotensin, sodium, signal transduction pathways (G-proteins, α- and β-adrenoceptors), and endothelin systems as they pertain to hypertension have been identified. And, as previously noted, patients who have the CYP2D6 poor–metabolizer genotype would seem to be at risk for adverse reactions to β-blockers, but these results were not reproduced in subsequent studies. There have been no studies that consistently link genotype to consistent results from specific medication choices. Thus, at this time genomics cannot be widely used to guide medication choices.

In addition to the preceding considerations, methodologic weaknesses mar many pharmacogenomics studies. These weaknesses include:

1. Failure to control for all causes of treatment response such as compliance with therapy (eg, drug levels, drug–drug interactions).
2. Treatment response: often a single SNP is the variable measured with respect to outcome, whereas the actual gene polymorphism that results in different outcomes may be due to the interaction of several or many SNPs in several loci.
3. Noncoding portions of genes (introns) may regulate the timing or location of gene expression, yet studies often report only the gene product (eg, a receptor) but not the genome.
4. Characterization of the complete metabolic pathway of a drug is often not done. Thus, drug response may be measured with respect to one SNP but differences in responses to a medication may be related to variations in the metabolic pathway (absorption, transport, etc), and not the single SNP being tested.
5. Use of different clinical outcome measures from one study to another.
6. Genetic, social, and environmental differences in populations studied.
7. Lack of placebo control.
8. Different drugs used in studies; in particular, in studies of lipid-lowering agents.
9. Failure to account for linkage disequilibrium.

Despite the preceding reservations, our understanding of the scope of genomics as it pertains to cardiovascular disease is evolving. An intriguing example of this is the observation that genes related to hypertension, hyperlipidemia, diabetes mellitus, and thrombophilia may interact to lead to the metabolic syndrome. Furthermore, some of the characteristics associated with the metabolic syndrome, such as obesity, hypertension, and diabetes, predispose women to preeclampsia. Indeed, one study demonstrated a more than eightfold higher risk of cardiovascular death in women with preeclampsia and a preterm delivery.

As the field of pharmacogenomics develops, we suspect there will be increasing numbers of clinical applications of pharmacogenomic testing. As always, it is the obligation of the practicing physician to order tests and treatments that are based on sound evidence.

Fux R et al: Impact of CYP2D6 genotype on adverse effects during treatment with metoprolol: A prospective clinical study. Clin Pharmacol Ther 2005;78:378. [PMID: 16198657]

Irgens HU et al: Long term mortality of mothers and fathers after pre-eclampsia: Population based cohort study. BMJ 2001;323:1213. [PMID: 11719411]

Marteau JB et al: Genetic determinants of blood pressure regulation. J Hypertens 2005;23:2127. [PMID: 16269952]

Roberts JM, Gammill HS: Preeclampsia, recent insights. Hypertension 2005;46:1243. [PMID: 16230510]

Wuttke H et al: Increased frequency of cytochrome P450 2D6 poor metabolizers among patients with metoprolol-associated adverse effects. Clin Pharmacol Ther 2002;72:429. [PMID: 12386645]

Zineh I et al: Pharmacokinetics and CYP2D6 genotypes do not predict metoprolol adverse events or efficacy in hypertension. Clin Pharmacol Ther 2004;76:536. [PMID: 15592325]

Complementary & Alternative Medicine

49

Wayne B. Jonas, MD, & Ronald A. Chez, MD

BACKGROUND

Practices that lie outside the mainstream of "official" medicine have always been an important part of the public's health care. Recently, these practices—frequently called *complementary and alternative medicine (CAM)*—have become more prominent in the West. In April 1995, a panel of experts convened at the National Institutes of Health (NIH) defined CAM as "a broad domain of healing resources that encompasses all health systems, modalities, practices and their accompanying theories and beliefs, other than those intrinsic to the politically dominant health system of a particular society or culture in a given historical period." Surveys of CAM use have defined it as those practices used for the prevention and treatment of disease that are neither taught widely in medical schools nor generally available in hospitals. CAM is that subset of practices that is not an integral part of conventional care, but is still used by patients in their health care management. Table 49–1 lists some of the categories of CAM defined by the White House Commission on CAM Policy.

Panel on Definition and Description: Defining and describing complementary and alternative medicine. Alt Ther Health Med 1997;3:49.

Patient Use of CAM

Complementary, alternative, and unconventional medicine is becoming increasingly popular in the United States. Two identical surveys of unconventional medicine use in the United States, done in 1990 and 1996, showed a 45% increase in use of CAM by the public. Visits to CAM practitioners increased from 400 million to over 600 million per year. The amount spent on these practices rose from $14 billion to $27 billion—most of it not reimbursed. Professional organizations are now beginning the "integration" of these practices into mainstream medicine. More than 95 of the nation's 125 medical schools require some kind of CAM coursework, many hospitals have developed complementary and integrated medicine programs, and some health management organizations are offering "expanded" benefits packages that include alternative practitioners and services. Biomedical research organizations are also investing more into the investigation of these practices. For example, the budget of the Office of Alternative Medicine at NIH rose from $5 million to the present $123.1 million in 10 years and changed from a coordination office to a National Center for Complementary and Alternative Medicine (NCCAM).

Multiple surveys have been conducted on use of CAM by populations with cancer and HIV infection, as well as by children, minorities, and women. Rates of use are significant in all these populations. Women, for example, are consistently more likely to explore and use CAM. Frequently central in health care decisions for a family, women seek out health care options in a pragmatic way. In the survey by Eisenberg and colleagues, 49% of women used CAM. Emigrant populations often use traditional medicines not commonly used in the West. According to the World Health Organization, between 65% and 80% of the world's health care services are classified as traditional medicine. These become complementary, alternative, or unconventional when used in Western countries. Even in countries in which modern western biomedicine dominates, the public (and more women than men) makes extensive use of unconventional practices. In western Europe and Australia, for example, regular use of complementary and alternative practices ranges from 20% to 70%.

The public uses these practices for both minor and major problems. Surveys show more than 68% of patients with cancer and HIV will use unconventional practices at some point during the course of their illness. Complementary medicine is an area of great public interest and activity, both nationally and worldwide. It appears that CAM has again "come of age" in the West.

Astin JA: Why patients use alternative medicine: Results of a national study. JAMA 1998;279:1548. [PMID: 9605899]

Eisenberg DM et al: Trends in alternative medicine use in the United States 1990–1997: Results of a follow-up national survey. JAMA 1998;280:1569. [PMID: 9820257]

Table 49–1. CAM systems of health care, therapies, or products.[1]

Major Domains of CAM	Examples under Each Domain
Alternative health care systems	Ayurvedic medicine Chiropractic Homeopathic medicine Native American medicine (eg, sweat lodge, medicine wheel) Naturopathic medicine Traditional Chinese medicine (eg, acupuncture, Chinese herbal medicine)
Mind–body interventions	Meditation Hypnosis Guided imagery Dance therapy Music therapy Art therapy Prayer and mental healing
Biological-based therapies	Herbal therapies Special diets (eg, macrobiotics, extremely low-fat or high-carbohydrate diets) Orthomolecular medicine (eg, megavitamin therapy) Individual biological therapies (eg, shark cartilage, bee pollen)
Therapeutic massage, body work, and somatic movement therapies	Massage Feldenkrais Alexander method
Energy therapies	Qigong Reiki Therapeutic touch
Bioelectromagnetics	Magnet therapy

[1]This table was adapted from the major domains of CAM and examples of each developed by the National Center for Complementary and Alternative Medicine, National Institutes of Health.

Physician Use of CAM

Conventional physicians are not only frequently faced with questions about CAM, but also refer patients for CAM treatment and, to a lesser extent, provide CAM services. A review of 25 surveys of conventional physician referral and use of CAM found that 43% of physicians had referred patients for acupuncture, 40% for chiropractic services, and 21% for massage. The majority believed in the efficacy of these three practices. Rates of use of CAM practices ranged from 9% (homeopathy) to 19% (chiropractic and massage). National surveys have confirmed that many physicians refer for and fewer incorporate CAM practices into their health care management.

Risks of CAM

The amount of research on CAM systems and practices is small compared with research on conventional medicine. There are over 1000 times more citations in the National Library of Medicine's bibliographic database, MEDLINE, on conventional cancer treatments than on alternative cancer treatments. With increasing public use of CAM, poor communication between patients and physicians about it, and few studies on the safety and efficacy of most CAM treatments, a situation exists for misuse and harm from these treatments. Many practices, such as acupuncture, homeopathy, and meditation, are low risk but require practitioner competence to avoid inappropriate use. Botanical preparations can be toxic and produce herb–drug interactions. Contamination and poor quality control also exist with these products, especially if shipped from Asia and India.

Potential Benefits of CAM

CAM practices have value for the way physicians manage health and disease. In botanical medicine, for example, there is research showing the benefit of herbal remedies such as ginkgo biloba for improving dementia due to circulation problems and possibly Alzheimer disease, benign prostatic hypertrophy with saw palmetto and other herbal preparations, and the prevention of heart disease with garlic. Several placebo-controlled trials have been done showing that Hypericum (St John's wort) is effective in the treatment of depression, although recent studies in the United States have cast doubt on the generalizability of those studies. Additional studies report that Hypericum is as effective as some conventional antidepressants but produces fewer side effects and costs less. The quality of many of these trials is poor, however, so physicians need to have basic skills in the evaluation of clinical literature.

Le Bars PL et al: A placebo-controlled, double-blind, randomized trial of an extract of Ginkgo biloba for dementia. North American EGb Study Group. JAMA 1997;278:1327. [PMID: 9343463]

ROLE OF THE FAMILY PHYSICIAN

What is the role of the family physician in the management of CAM? The goal is to help patients make informed choices about CAM as they do in conventional medicine. Specifically, physicians can protect, permit, promote, and partner with patients about CAM practices as appropriate.

Protecting Patients from Risks of CAM

Many practices, such as acupuncture, biofeedback, homeopathy, and meditation, are low risk if used by competent practitioners, but if used in place of more effective treatments they can result in harm. Practitioners should be qualified to help patients avoid inappropriate use. Many herbal remedies contain powerful pharmacologic substances with direct toxicity and herb–drug interactions. Contamination and poor quality control occur more often than with conventional drugs, especially if preparations are obtained from overseas.

The family physician can help distinguish between CAM practices with little or no risk of direct toxicity (eg, homeopathy, acupuncture) and those with greater risk of toxicity (eg, megavitamins, herbal remedies). Physicians should be especially cautious about products that can produce toxicity, work with patients so they do not abandon proven care, and alert patients to signs of possible fraud or abuse. "Secret" formulas, cures for multiple conditions, slick advertising for mail-order products, pyramid marketing schemes, and any recommendation to abandon conventional medicine are "red flags" and should be suspect.

Permitting Use of Nonspecific Therapies

Spontaneous healing and placebo effects account for the improvement seen in many illnesses. Science attempts to separate these factors from those that are specific aspects of a therapy. Physicians, however, are interested in how to combine both specific and nonspecific factors for maximum benefit. Many medical systems emphasize high-touch, personalized approaches for the management of chronic disease. The physician can permit the integration of selected CAM approaches that are not harmful or expensive but that may enhance these nonspecific factors.

Promoting CAM Use

Proven therapies that are safe and effective should be available to the public. As research continues, expanded options for managing clinical conditions will arise. Gradually, physicians and patients will have more options for management of disease. In arthritis, for example, there are studies suggesting improvements with homeopathy, acupuncture, vitamin and nutritional supplements, botanical products, diet therapies, mind-body approaches, and manipulation. A similar collection of small studies exists for other conditions such as heart disease, depression, asthma, and addictions. The Cochrane Collaboration conducts systematic reviews of randomized controlled trials on both conventional and complementary medicine and is an excellent source for evidence-based evaluation of such studies. As research accumulates, rational therapeutic options can be developed in these areas.

Partnering with Patients about CAM Use

Over 60% of patients who use CAM practices do not reveal this information to their conventional physicians. Thus, there is a major communication gap between physicians and the public about CAM. Patients use alternative practices for a variety of reasons, among them, because it is part of their social network, because they are not satisfied with the results of their conventional care, or because they have an attraction to CAM philosophies and health beliefs. The overwhelming majority of patients use CAM practices as an adjunct to conventional medicine. Less than 5% use CAM exclusively. Patients who use alternative medicine do not foster antiscience or anticonventional medicine sentiments, or represent a disproportionate number of the uneducated, poor, seriously ill, or neurotic. Often patients do not understand the role of science in medicine and will accept anecdotal evidence or slick marketing as sufficient justification for use. The conventional practitioner can play a role in examining the research base of these medical claims and work with patients to incorporate more evidence into their health care decisions. Quality research on these practices can help to provide this evidence, and the physician can help interpret that evidence with patients.

Other social factors have also influenced the rise in prominence of CAM. These include the prevalence of chronic disease, increasing access to health information, the "consumerization" of medical decision making, a declining faith that scientific breakthroughs will have relevant benefits for personal health, and an increased interest in spirituality. In addition, the public and professionals are increasingly concerned over side effects and escalating costs of conventional health care. Ignorance about CAM practices by physicians and scientists can broaden the communication gap between the public and the profession that serves them. All physicians should learn about these practices and discuss them with patients.

Chez RA, Jonas WB: The challenge of complementary and alternative medicine. Am J Obstet Gynecol 1997;177:1156. [PMID: 9396912]

Lewith G et al: *Clinical Research in Complementary Therapies: Principles, Problems and Solutions.* Churchill Livingston, 2002.

WEB SITES

Cochrane Collaboration:
http://www.cochrane.org

EVIDENCE HIERARCHY OR EVIDENCE HOUSE?

All physicians need good evidence to make medical decisions. Evidence comes in a variety of forms, and

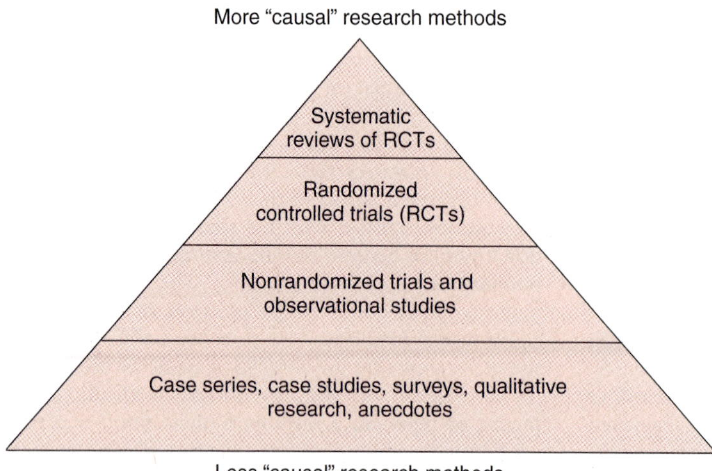

Figure 49–1. The evidence hierarchy.

what may be good for one purpose may not be good for another. The term *evidence-based medicine* has become a synonym for "good" medicine recently, and it is often used to support and deny the value of complementary medicine. Evidence-based medicine uses the "hierarchy of evidence" (Figure 49–1). In this hierarchy, systematic reviews are seen as the "best" evidence, then individual randomized controlled trials (RCTs), then nonrandomized trials, then observational studies, and finally case series. All efforts are focused on approximating evidence at the top of the pyramid, and lower levels are considered inferior. Clinical experiments on causal links between an intervention and outcomes become the gold standard when this model is used.

All family physicians have seen patients who recover from disease because of complex factors, many of which are not additive and cannot be isolated in controlled experiments. Under these circumstances, observational data from clinical practice may offer the best evidence rather than controlled trials. Patients' illnesses are complex, and holistic phenomena cannot be reduced to single, objective measures. Often highly subjective judgments about life quality may be the best information with which to make a decision. Such experiences may be captured only with qualitative research, not with scans or blood tests. In that case the meaning patients have of their illness and recovery is the "best" evidence for medical decisions. Sometimes the "best" evidence comes from laboratory tests. For example, the most crucial evidence for management of St John's wort in patients on immunosuppressive medications comes from a laboratory finding that it accelerates drug metabolism via cytochrome P450. Arranging evidence in a "hierarchy" obscures the fact that the "best" evidence may not be about cause and effect, may not be objective, and may not be clinical.

We suggest that family physicians not use an evidence hierarchy, rather that they build an evidence "house" (Figure 49–2). On the left side of this house is evidence for causal attributions, for mechanisms of action, and for "proof." However, if physicians confine themselves to the left side of the house they will never know about the relevance of a treatment for patients or what happens in the real world of clinical practice. They will also not know if proven treatments can be generalized to populations such as the ones they see or the health care delivery system in which they practice. The "rooms" on the right side of the house provide evidence about patient relevance and usefulness, in practices both proven and unproven.

How evidence is approached has ethical implications. Different groups prefer different types of evidence. Regulatory authorities are most interested in RCTs or systematic reviews (left side), which may never be done. Health care practitioners usually want to know the likelihood of benefit or harm from a treatment (right side). Patients are intensely interested in stories and descriptions of cures (right side). Rationalists want to know how things work and so need laboratory evidence (left side). If one type of evidence is selected to the exclusion of others, science will not allow for full public input into clinical decisions. A livable house needs both a kitchen and a bathroom, a place to sleep and play. Each type of evidence has different functions and all need to be of high quality.

Jonas WB: Evidence, ethics and evaluation of global medicine. In Callahan D, ed: *Ethical Issues in Complementary and Alternative Medicine.* Hastings Center Report, 2001.

Kelner M, Wellman B: *Complementary and Alternative Medicine: Challenge and Change.* Gordon & Breach, 2000.

Linde K, Jonas WB: Evaluating complementary and alternative medicine: The balance of rigor and relevance. In Jonas WB,

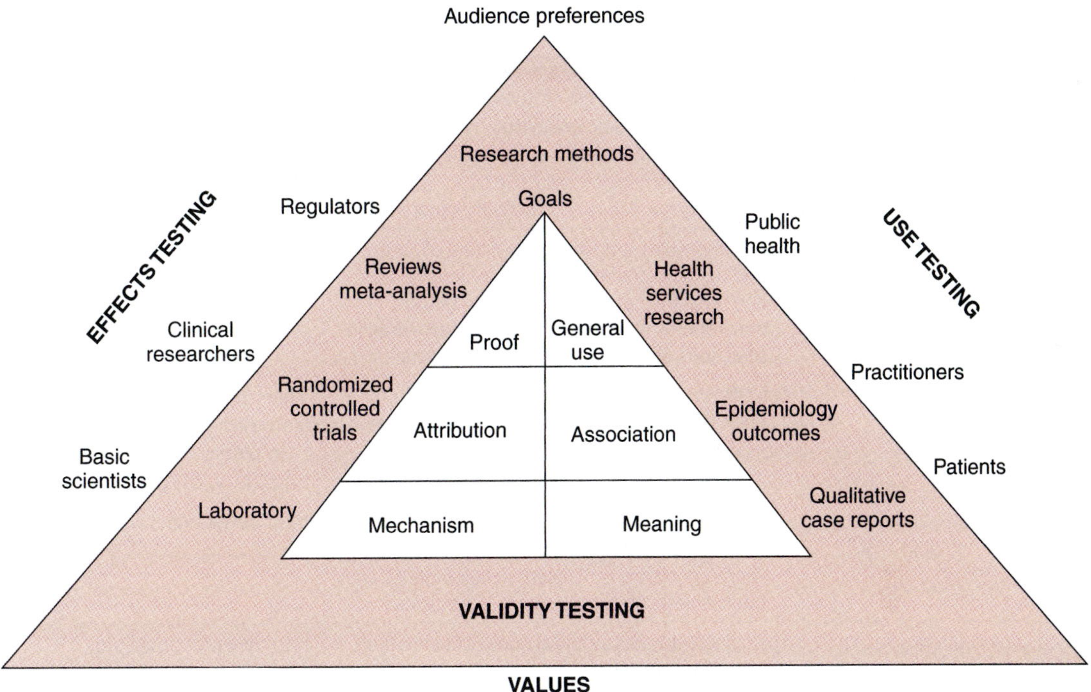

Figure 49–2. The evidence house.

Levin J, eds: *Essentials of Complementary and Alternative Medicine.* Lippincott Williams & Wilkins, 1999.

AN EVIDENCE-BASED APPROACH

Most treatment decisions require information about whether a practice has a specific effect, and about the magnitude of that effect in practice. This evidence is provided by RCTs and outcomes research, respectively. An evidence-based practice, then, would involve clinical expertise, informed patient communication, and quality research. This presumes that the physician has good clinical and communication skills. Medical training and experience address these prerequisites, but evaluation of the research evidence may not be something physicians feel fully prepared for in CAM. Obtaining research, selecting appropriate research for clinical situations, and then evaluating the quality of that research in CAM are essential for a fully evidence-based practice that addresses these topics.

Finding & Selecting Good Information

Where can the family physician obtain research on CAM? Several groups have collated and produced CAM-specific databases, although central, comprehensive, and easily accessed sources for quality CAM literature are not yet available. Table 49–2 lists useful sources of clinical information on CAM and what they provide. When searching these databases physicians should look for the following key terms: (1) *meta-analyses and systematic reviews,* (2) *randomized controlled trials,* and (3) *observational* or *prospective outcomes data.* Although there are many other types of studies, physicians must be cautious about using these for problem-oriented decision making in practice. If no research information is found in the databases listed, there is likely to be little relevant practice-oriented evidence for that clinical condition. A search for this information need not be time consuming; in fact, a trained office assistant can often do the search, streamlining time spent on this process. After completing a literature search the physician can be confident, knowing the quantity of evidence on the therapy. Patients are usually grateful for this effort, because many come to their physician in the hopes of obtaining science-based information they can trust.

Risks & Types of Evidence for Practice

If there are studies on a specific type of CAM practice, then the risk of toxicity and the cost of the therapy indicate which types of data are needed. Low-risk practices include over-the-counter homeopathic medications, acupuncture, gentle massage or manipulation, meditation, relaxation and biofeedback, other mind–body methods, and vitamin and mineral supplementa-

Table 49–2. Sources of CAM information for health care practitioners.

Source of CAM Information	Description	Where to Go
Cochrane Library	Database of Systematic Reviews: systematic reviews of RCTs of CAM and conventional therapies Controlled Trials Register: extensive bibliographic listing of controlled trials and conference proceedings	http://www.cochrane.org http://gateway.ovid.com
Natural Medicines Comprehensive Database	Comprehensive listing and cross-listing of natural and herbal therapies, separate "all known uses" and "effectiveness" sections, safety ratings, mechanisms of action, side effects, herb–drug interactions, and review of available evidence	http://www.naturaldatabase.com
National Library of Medicine	Powerful search engine that allows searches of PubMed and all government guidelines combined Includes "synonym and related terms" option	Search engine: hstat.nlm.nih.gov Individual guidelines at: http://www.guideline.gov http://www.cdc.gov/publications
Focus on Alternative and Complementary Therapies (FACT)	Quarterly review journal of CAM therapies Contains evidence-based reviews, focus articles, short reports, news of recent developments, and book reviews on complementary medicine	http://www.exeter.ac.uk/FACT
PubMed Clinical Queries Search Engine	The old standby has a clinical queries filter to limit your search results Click on "Clinical Queries" on the left blue banner to access the filter For the most comprehensive search, use the key words "complementary medicine"	http://www.pubmed.org
National Center for Complementary and Alternative Medicine (NCCAM)	Clinical Trials Section: listing of clinical trials indexed by treatment or by condition Cross-linked to http://www.clinicaltrials.gov and PubMed	http://www.nccam.nih.gov
Agency for Healthcare Research and Quality (AHRQ)	For information on the quality, safety, efficiency, and effectiveness of health care for all Americans	http://www.ahrq.gov
Clinical Evidence	Promotes informed decision making by summarizing what is known, and not known, about > 200 medical conditions and > 2000 treatments	http://www.clinicalevidence.com/ceweb/condition/index.jsp
TRIP	Allows health professionals to easily find the highest-quality material available on the Internet	http://www.tripdatabase.com
Family Physicians Inquiry Network	Provides clinicians with answers to 80% of their clinical questions in 60 seconds	http://www.fpin.org/

CAM, complementary and alternative medicine; RCT, randomized controlled trial.
Reproduced, with permission, from Beutler AI, Jonas WB: Complementary and alternative medicine for the sports medicine physician. In: Birrer RB, O'Connor FG, eds: *Sports Medicine for the Primary Care Physician.* CRC Press, 2004:315.

tion below toxic doses. Low-cost therapies involving self-care are also often low risk. High-risk practices include herbal therapies, high-dosage vitamins and minerals, vaccine products, colonics, and intravenous administration of substances. Some otherwise harmless therapies can result in considerable cost if they require major life-style changes. Herbal therapies can produce serious adverse effects. Because patients frequently use herbal remedies along with prescription medications, physicians should specifically inquire about their use. High-risk or high-cost practices and products require RCT data.

Under some circumstances observational (outcomes) data are more important, and in other circumstances RCT data are more important. Outcomes research provides the probability of an effect and the absolute magnitude of effects in the context of normal clinical care. It is more similar to clinical practice and usually involves a wide variety of patients and variations of care to fit the patient's circumstances. It does not provide information on whether a treatment is specific or better than another treatment. With low-risk practices, the physician wants to know the probability of benefit from the therapy. Quality outcomes data from practices are preferable to RCT data if the data are collected from actual practice populations similar to the practitioner's patient. This may be sufficient evidence for making clinical decisions. Often it will be the only useful information available for chronic conditions. For example, if quality outcomes studies report a 75% probability of improving allergic rhinitis using a nontoxic, low-cost, homeopathic remedy, this information can assist in deciding on its use.

For high-risk, high-cost interventions, the physician should use RCTs (or meta-analyses of those trials). RCTs address the relative benefit of one therapy over another (or no therapy). RCTs can determine if the treatment is the cause of improvement, and how much the treatment adds to either no treatment or placebo treatment. RCTs provide relative (not absolute) information effects between a CAM and a control practice. They are difficult to do properly for more than short periods and difficult if the therapy being tested is complex and individualized or if there are marked patient preferences. In addition, RCTs remove any choice about therapy and, if blinded, blunt expectations—both of which exist in clinical practice. They are largely dependent on the control group, which requires careful selection and management. Strong patient preference for CAM, differing cultural groups, and informed consent may also alter RCT results. The importance of RCTs increases the more we need to know about specific benefit–harm comparisons, such as with high-risk, high-cost interventions.

The more a CAM practice addresses chronic disease and depends on self-care (eg, meditation, yoga, biofeedback), or involves a complex system (eg, classical homeopathy, traditional Chinese medicine, Unani–Tibb), the more outcomes data are important. The more a CAM practice involves high-risk or high-cost interventions, the more essential RCT data become.

Evaluating Study Quality

Once data are found and the preferred type of study is selected, the practitioner should apply some minimum quality criteria to these studies (Table 49–3). Three items can be quickly checked: (1) blind and random allocation of subjects to comparison groups (in RCTs) or blind outcome assessments (in outcomes research), (2) the clinical relevance and reliability of the outcome measures, and (3) the number of subjects that could be fully analyzed at the end of the study compared with the number entered. These same minimum quality criteria apply to RCTs or observational studies, except that blinded, random allocation to treatment and comparison groups does not apply in the latter. However, evaluation of effects before and after treatment can be blinded to the treatment given in any study. Detailed descriptions of patients, interventions, and drop-outs are hallmarks of a quality outcomes trial.

Table 49–3. Minimum guidelines for assessment of study quality.

Study Type	Guidelines			
Randomized controlled trials	Was there concealed random allocation to comparison groups?	Were outcome measures of known or probable clinical importance?	Were there few lost to follow-up compared with the number of bad outcomes (< 20%)?	
Observational and outcomes studies	Were outcome measures assessed blind to patient treatment?	Were outcome measures of known or probable clinical importance?	Were there few lost to follow-up compared with the number of bad outcomes (< 20%)?	Were confidence intervals reported and were they narrow or broad?
Reviews	Were explicit criteria for selecting articles and rating their quality used?	Was there a comprehensive search for all relevant articles?	Were negative and unpublished articles found?	

Adapted, with permission, from Haynes RB et al: Transferring evidence from research into practice: 2. getting the evidence straight. ACP J Club 1997;126:A14.

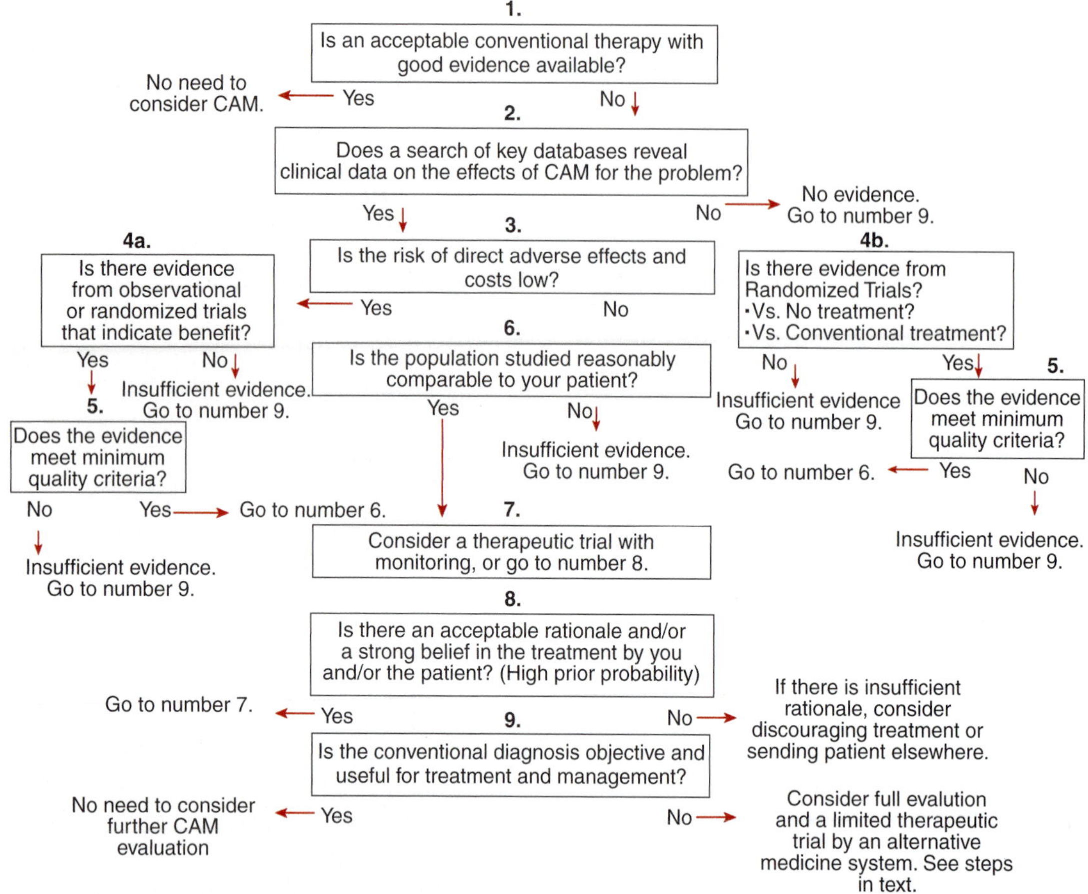

Figure 49–3. Decision tree for evidence-based complementary and alternative medicine.

Finally, one can ask if the probability of benefits reported in the outcomes study is worth the inconvenience, risk of side effects, and costs of the treatment and, in addition, whether confidence intervals were reported. Confidence intervals are the range of minimum to maximum benefit expected in 95% of similar studies. If confidence intervals are narrow, the physician can be confident that similar benefits will occur with other patients. If confidence intervals are broad, the chance of benefits from treatment in other patients will be unpredictable.

Quality screening questions that show there are marked quality flaws in the studies retrieved indicate that the evidence in the study is insufficient and so should not be used as a basis for clinical decisions.

Population Studied

Even if good evidence is found for a practice, physicians should determine whether the population in the studies is similar to the patient being seen. Although this matching is largely subjective, physicians can compare five areas. Specifically, they should determine if the study was done (1) in a primary, secondary, or tertiary referral center; (2) in a western, eastern, developing, or industrialized country; and (3) with diagnostic criteria similar to the patient (eg, the same criteria were used to diagnose osteoarthritis or congestive heart failure); and should determine if (4) the age and (5) the gender of the study population were similar. If the study population is not similar to the patient being seen, then the data, even though valid, cannot be applied to the situation. The study country may be especially important for some CAM practices. For example, data on use of acupuncture to treat chronic pain derives largely from China. Pain perception may be different in China than in the United States. Results from a study done in one country may not be applicable in another. If the study and clinic population match, an appropriate body of evidence for moving forward with a therapeutic trial exists.

Balancing Beliefs

Belief in the treatment by the physician and the patient needs to be explicitly considered in CAM. In conventional medicine, both patient and physician accept the plausibility of treatment. Belief has long been known to affect outcome. Strong belief enhances positive outcomes and weak belief interferes with them. A physician may feel that a CAM practice has incredibly low plausibility although the patient may have a strong belief in the therapy. This so-called "prior probability" (or belief) by the physician and patient should be considered in the decision to allow or not allow the patient to use a treatment. If physician and patient have similar beliefs, then a decision is easily made. Sometimes, however, the patient has a strong belief in the therapy but the physician finds it unbelievable. In such situations, the physician should work with the patient to decide the best action—including referral elsewhere as an option.

Alternative Diagnoses

Some diagnoses are not very useful for management of a patient's illness. If the family physician's conventional diagnosis is not helping a patient, the clinician may want to consider an evaluation by an alternative system. Chinese medicine uses energy diagnosis, for example, and homeopathy has a remedy classification system. Sometimes obtaining an assessment from a CAM system may prove useful. For example, a 51-year-old woman with several years of idiopathic urticaria had obtained no relief from several conventional physicians. A homeopathic assessment showed that she might benefit from the remedy Mercurius. She was given several small doses and the urticaria cleared.

The physician should also be alert to practitioners who pursue CAM diagnoses that are not useful. In such situations, a complicated CAM evaluation and treatment with little effect might be managed simply and effectively by conventional medicine. For example, a 57-year-old man with cardiovascular disease and recurrent bouts of angina was treated by a CAM practitioner for 3 years with special diets and nutritional supplements without help. Consultation with a conventional practitioner showed that he had myxedema. A thyroid supplement cleared his angina rapidly.

In cases in which the diagnostic approach of the medical system fails, a professional consultation may be needed. In situations in which the alternative system's diagnostic and treatment approach is clear, a limited therapeutic trial with specific treatment goals and follow-up can be attempted. Of course, quality products and qualified practitioners must be located. In situations of serious disease, such as cancer, anxiety-ridden patients may seek out CAM treatments. Under these circumstances, good training and clinical experience and protection of patients from harm (even from themselves) should prevail.

Evidence-based medicine can be applied to CAM. Figure 49–3 summarizes the steps involved, and Table 49–4 summarizes questions for CAM management. Although evidence-based CAM may initially seem like a large task, appropriate data-driven clinical decisions can be made with CAM as with all medical care.

Table 49–4. Questions for evidence-based CAMT management.

A patient is using a complementary and alternative medicine therapy (CAMT) or an alternative treatment is sought. The following questions should be answered.

1. Has the patient received proper conventional medical care?
2. Is the CAMT likely to produce direct toxic or adverse effects or is it high cost?
3. Are there clinical data from randomized trials or outcomes research on the CAMT?
4. Do the studies meet minimum quality criteria? (Table 49–3)
5. Is the study population similar to the patient using or seeking the CAMT?
6. Is the plausibility of the therapy acceptable to both patient and physician?
7. Can a quality product or a qualified practitioner be accessed?
8. Can the patient be monitored while undergoing the CAMT?
9. Is a full diagnostic assessment by a conventional or CAM system in order?

Eisenberg DM: Advising patients who seek alternative medical therapies. Ann Intern Med 1997;127:61. [PMID: 9214254]

Gatchel RJ, Maddrey AM: Clinical outcome research in complementary and alternative medicine: An overview of experimental design and analysis. Altern Ther Health Med 1998;4:36. [PMID: 9737030]

Jonas WB: Clinical trials for chronic disease: Randomized, controlled clinical trials are essential. J NIH Res 1997;9:33.

Kirsch I: *How Expectancies Shape Experience.* American Psychological Association, 1999.

WEB SITES

Clinical Pearls News: Current Research in Nutrition and Integrative Medicine:

http://www.clinicalpearls.com

National Center for Complementary and Alternative Medicine (NCCAM):

http://nccam.nih.gov

Chronic Pain Management 50

Ronald M. Glick, MD, & Dawn A. Marcus, MD

General Considerations

Pain is defined by the International Association for the Study of Pain as "an unpleasant sensory or emotional experience associated with actual or potential tissue damage or described in terms of such damage." This definition emphasizes that the pain experience is multidimensional and may include sensory, cognitive, and emotional components. Additionally, the latter part of the definition allows for the possibility, as in chronic pain states, that the overt tissue damage may no longer be present. Pain persisting longer than 3–6 months is defined as chronic pain. Pain persisting for 3 months, however, is unlikely to resolve spontaneously and will continue to be reported by patients after 12 months. In addition, many of the secondary problems associated with chronic pain, such as deconditioning, depression, sleep disturbance, and disability, begin within the first few months of the onset of symptoms of pain. Studies indicate that early patient identification and treatment are essential to reduce pain chronicity and prevent further disability.

Chronic pain is one of the most common complaints seen in primary care. A survey of 89 general practices in Italy showed pain as a complaint for 3 of every 10 patients seen. Among these patients, pain was chronic for over half (53%). Women were more likely than men to report both acute (1.2:1) and chronic pain (1.8:1). The most common type of pain was musculoskeletal (63%). Similarly, a survey of over 10,000 women attending general practices identified a chronic pain complaint in 38% of women, with over 80% consulting their physician for their chronic pain complaint. The most common site for chronic pain was the back (54%).

Costs related to chronic pain are high. A survey of an employer claims' database showed annual direct plus indirect costs for employees with painful conditions were 1.5–3.5 times greater than for the average employee ($7088–16,874 vs $4849; $P < .01$). Of the costs, about 60% were attributed to direct health care expenses. Among patients with low back pain, there is an estimated direct cost for medical expenses of $357 per month.

Koleva D et al: Pain in primary care: An Italian survey. Eur J Public Health 2005;15:475. [PMID: 16150816]

Ritzwoller DP et al: The association of comorbidities, utilization and costs for patients identified with low back pain. BMC Musculoskelet Disord 2006;7:72. [PMID: 16982001]

Smith BH et al; Royal College of General Practitioners' Oral Contraception Study: Is chronic pain a distinct diagnosis in primary care? Evidence arising from the Royal College of General Practitioners' Oral Contraception Study. Fam Pract 2004;21:66. [PMID: 14760048]

White AG et al: Economic burden of illness for employees with painful conditions. J Occup Environ Med 2005;47:884-892. [PMID: 16155473]

Pathogenesis

Acute pain occurs following some form of tissue injury (eg, ankle sprain), and is treated with RICE (rest, immobilization, compression, and elevation) and pain-soothing treatments, such as heat, ice, and massage. During the acute period of tissue injury and healing, patients appropriately limit activity to reduce risks of further injury (eg, development of a Charcot joint in a patient with neuropathy who risks aggravation of the injury because of impaired sensation). Studies show that patients improve best after acute injury when they reduce activities to what can be tolerated and allow healing to occur, in contrast to patients treated with either bed rest or acute physical therapy.

Chronic pain occurs after the acute healing period has been completed or in the context of chronic degenerative changes (eg, neuropathy or arthritis). Restriction of activity in patients with chronic pain leads to deconditioning, with muscle and bone loss that increases pain and the risk for reinjury, and also promotes psychological sluggishness, if not depression. Consequently, the RICE approach will actually aggravate the symptoms of chronic pain. The natural response of restricting activities when experiencing pain is appropriate for acute injury pain but aggravates chronic pain. Patients with chronic pain require an active, progressive exercise program. They must learn appropriate strategies for treating pain, must avoid a tendency to restrict activity excessively, and must resume more normal activity levels through a stepwise, progressive activity program.

Clinical Findings

The most common chronic pain conditions in young and middle adulthood are low back pain, neck pain, and headaches. Musculoskeletal diseases rank fifth in

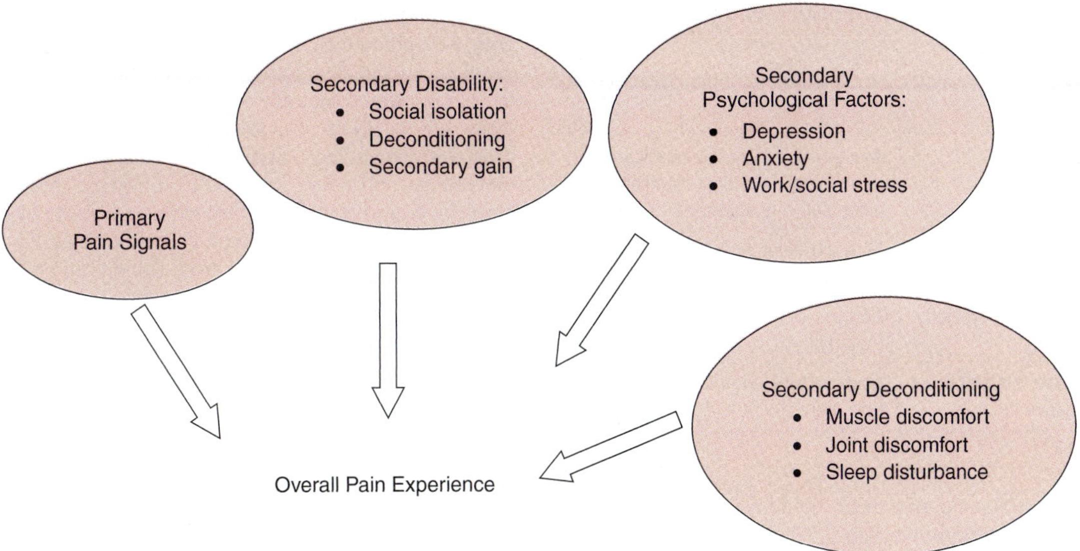

Figure 50–1. Primary and secondary features of chronic pain.

generating hospital expenses and first in generating expenses related to work absenteeism and disability. The most common cause of chronic pain in older adults is degenerative joint and disc diseases, with arthritis causing chronic pain in over 80% of elderly patients with pain. Other causes of chronic pain that occur more frequently with increasing age are pain related to cancer, vascular disease, and neuropathy (eg, postherpetic neuralgia). Throughout the life cycle, pain can be associated with a variety of general medical conditions, such as Crohn's disease or sickle cell anemia.

The overall pain experience includes primary pain-generating signals, along with common secondary problems that develop regardless of pain etiology and that complicate pain management (Figure 50–1). Both physical (eg, joint restrictions and deconditioning) and psychological (eg, depression and anxiety) changes frequently accompany chronic pain. Psychological distress is common. In one survey, psychological disorders occurred in 55% of patients with chronic pain versus 24% of controls. General anxiety was reported in 40% of chronic pain patients and in 14% of controls. Major depression occurred in 22% of pain patients and in only 4% of controls. Psychosocial stress may result from difficulties related to school or work, family relationships, social isolation, and legal and financial areas. Although the possibility of secondary gain (eg, litigation) may increase pain complaints, true malingering and factitious disorders are uncommon, occurring in only 1–10% of patients. The *Diagnostic and Statistical Manual of Mental Disorders,* Fourth Edition, Text Revision (*DSM-IV-TR*), appropriately recognizes the ability of psychological variables to influence complaints of pain and offers the designation of a Pain Disorder, reflecting the coexistence of both physical dysfunction and psychological factors, both of which affect patients' overall presentation and function. The family physician is in a unique position to identify and treat the physical and psychosocial factors influencing complaints of pain.

Manchikanti L et al: Comparison of psychological status of chronic pain patients and the general population. Pain Physician 2002;5:40. [PMID: 16902665]

Treatment

Chronic pain management focuses on reduction in symptoms and improvement of function rather than on disease cure. Both medication and nonmedication treatment modalities effectively decrease primary and secondary symptoms of chronic pain (Table 50–1). However, physicians and patients must accept that complete resolution of complaints of pain may not be possible. Thus they need to work toward rehabilitative goals of reducing symptoms and minimizing disability. Although modern medicine and rehabilitation techniques can be beneficial, the patient's mindset must shift from the search for a medical cure to engaging in collaborative rehabilitation, geared toward decreasing pain and optimizing function. Goals of chronic pain rehabilitation are improvement in both pain and secondary symptoms, including deconditioning, depression, and disability (Table 50–2). Early

Table 50–1. Comprehensive treatment of chronic pain.

Specialist	Treatment Modalities
Physician	Analgesics, adjunctive medications, nerve blocks, medical counseling to foster self-management
Physical/occupational therapist	Musculoskeletal dysfunction, deconditioning, work simplification
Psychology/psychiatry	Address locus of control, depression therapy, anxiety therapy
Complementary/alternative therapist	Acupuncture, yoga/tai chi, meditation, chiropractic therapy

identification and treatment should reduce the severity of secondary symptoms.

A. Psychological Approaches

Cognitive-behavioral therapy (CBT) is an effective psychological treatment technique that challenges a dysfunctional perception of pain ("My pain must be cured. I can't do anything if I have pain.") and replaces it with one that is more conducive to change ("Pain limits me from lifting 25 pounds, but I can still carry a bag of groceries."). CBT helps change patients' perceptions or locus of control from external control (believing pain is not controllable by the patient) to internal control (believing the patient can positively influence symptoms). When patients endorse an external locus of control, they see themselves as victims of the pain and as powerless to improve their situation. This results in the expectation that only fate or the physician can help when pain becomes severe. When expectations are not met, these patients seek alternative evaluations and treatments (eg, another physician, a different diagnostic test, or surgical procedures) that may not be in their best interest. The clinician must help patients to move into a pain self-management, internal locus of control belief system, in which patients see themselves as the agent for change. Greater perceived self-control of pain decreases both pain and secondary symptoms. Although CBT is typically the purview of psychologists, the family physician can reinforce these concepts through interactions with the patient. Mind–body approaches can be very helpful and are often integrated with CBT in a self-management program (see later discussion).

Jensen MP et al: Changes in beliefs, catastrophizing, and coping are associated with improvement in multidisciplinary pain treatment. J Consult Clin Psychol 2001;69:655. [PMID: 11550731]

B. Physical and Occupational Therapy

Identification and treatment of musculoskeletal dysfunctions and decisions concerning limitations on activity often require consultation with physical or occupational therapists. Reconditioning, active stretching and strengthening exercises, and graded activity programs are effective for managing chronic pain. Physical therapists should instruct patients in a daily exercise routine as well as flare management techniques (eg, trigger point massage, oscillatory movements, and use of heat and ice). Exercise therapy is most effective when initiated through a supervised physical therapy program rather than through self-exercise. Occupational therapists will address work simplification, body mechanics, and pacing skills.

As noted, secondary problems can develop rapidly after a problem with pain starts and should be addressed early in the course of treatment of pain. The most important intervention is reinforcing the need to resume more normal activity schedules (eg, returning to work or school), even on a modified basis. Prolonged absence from normal activities increases the difficulty of reducing disability. Return to normal activity as soon as possible, however, should be the primary goal of pain management and the physician should work to expedite that return, with modifications if needed. Conflicts with an employer, fear of losing a job and benefits, or other intervening factors need to be identified and addressed to facilitate a successful return to work. In addition, the longer the patient with pain has avoided employment or school, the more difficult and emotionally stressful a return to work or school becomes. In the case of a child or adolescent, anxiety around return to school may actually increase complaints of pain. Migraines and abdominal pain, for example, are particularly reactive to anxiety and the associated avoidant behavior, creating a vicious cycle.

Table 50–2. Appropriate treatment goals.

General Goal	Specific Treatment Target
Decreased pain	Pain reduction to moderate levels; reduced frequency and duration of flares
Improved function	Return to school/work; increased number of household chores; increased participation in leisure activities
Improved sleep	Reduced number of wake-ups; improved overall sleep to 5 h per night
Improved mood	Increased participation in social activities; reduced time in bed/inactive; improved nutrition intake
Reduced use of medical resources	Reduced emergency department visits; reduced use of excessive analgesics; decreased repeat consultations or studies

Table 50–3. Medication management of chronic pain.

Symptom Treated	Medication Class	Examples
Pain	Analgesics	Acetaminophen NSAIDs Tramadol
	Long-acting opioids	Sustained-release morphine, oxycodone, or transdermal fentanyl
Neuropathic pain	Antidepressants Anticonvulsants	Duloxetine, 30–60 mg twice daily Gabapentin, 300–1200 mg three times daily Pregabalin, 75–200 mg three times daily
Muscle spasm	Muscle relaxants	Tizanidine, 2–8 mg at bedtime to three times daily
Sleep disturbance	Antidepressants	Nortriptyline, 25–75 mg at bedtime
Depression	Antidepressants	Bupropion, sustained release, 75–150 mg twice daily Escitalopram, 5–20 mg daily

NSAIDs, nonsteroidal anti-inflammatory drugs.

Additionally, counseling should be directed toward issues concerning mood, sleep, and other psychosocial factors. Severe symptoms of depression or anxiety or significant psychosocial stressors may necessitate a psychiatric referral.

Faas A: Exercises: Which ones are worth trying, for which patients, and when? Spine 1996;21:2877. [PMID: 9112711]

Torstensen TA et al: Efficiency and costs of medical exercise therapy, conventional physiotherapy, and self-exercise in patients with chronic low back pain. A pragmatic, randomized, single-blinded, controlled trial with 1-year follow-up. Spine 1998; 23:2616. [PMID: 9854761]

C. Pharmacotherapy

Medications are prescribed to treat an underlying medical condition (eg, disease-modifying medications in rheumatoid arthritis), relieve symptoms of pain, and relieve secondary symptoms (eg, depression, anxiety, or sleep disturbance). Most medications used to treat chronic pain address the latter two factors (Table 50–3).

1. Pain relievers—Analgesics rarely eliminate pain entirely, and may result in either significant adverse effects or habituation. Treatment should begin with simple analgesics, such as acetaminophen or nonsteroidal anti-inflammatory drugs (NSAIDs). Daily doses of acetaminophen should not exceed 4 g, and patients need to consider the cumulative dosage from both over-the-counter and prescription pain relievers. Acetaminophen should be restricted in patients with significant alcohol intake or liver disease. A variety of available NSAIDs share similar efficacy and tolerability. Patients with gastrointestinal disease may tolerate cyclooxygenase-2 (COX-2) inhibitors better than standard NSAIDs; however, as noted below, these agents have been associated with increased risk of heart disease and stroke.

Tramadol is a novel analgesic that has weak serotonergic and noradrenergic properties as well as weak μ opioid activation. Despite the opioid agonist effect, in the absence of a history of opioid dependence, tramadol does not pose the same level of concern regarding abuse potential, physical tolerance, and psychological dependence as the true opioids. It thus offers an option falling between first-tier of agents (ie, acetaminophen and NSAIDs) and the stronger opioid medications. Common side effects include sedation, dizziness, and nausea. Although the full dosage is 100 mg four times daily, a lower dosage (eg, 50 mg three times daily) is commonly prescribed, with extra dosing on an as-needed basis. The 400-mg maximum dose should be strictly adhered to given the potential for seizures at higher doses. For older adults or those taking other centrally acting agents, a maximum of 200–300 mg/day is a more reasonable maximum. As noted below, there is great concern regarding risk for falls and impaired cognition with these medications in older adults. Finally, the potential exists for inducing a serotonin syndrome when tramadol is used in combination with antidepressants or other serotonergic agents (eg, selective serotonin reuptake inhibitors [SSRIs] such as paroxetine or escitalopram; tricyclic antidepressants [TCAs] such as amitriptyline or nortriptyline; or novel agents such as trazodone or mirtazapine). This syndrome can be seen as a paradoxic excitation associated with excessive activation of central nervous system serotonin, with psychological effects that include hyperarousal, irritability, and agitation; neuromotor effects that include tremor, jitteriness, rigidity, and (at an extreme) seizures; and cardiac effects that include tachycardia and hypertension.

The use of opioids for management of chronic pain is controversial. Although isolated treatment with opioids is not effective for managing chronic pain, opioids can provide a safe, cost-effective adjunctive pain therapy because

Table 50–4. Opioid conversion chart.[1]

	Oral Dose (mg)	Transdermal Dose (mcg/h)	Intravenous Dose (mg)	Brand Names
Morphine sulfate	15		5	MSContin, Kadian, Oramorph
Hydromorphone	4		0.8	Dilaudid
Oxycodone	10			Percocet, Roxicet, Oxycontin
Hydrocodone	15			Vicodin, Lorcet, Norco
Meperidine[2]	150		35	Demerol
Fentanyl		6.25		Duragesic

[1]Dose conversions are approximate, with variation based on both individual patients and drug preparations.
[2]Should be avoided (see text).

of reduced morbidity and cost associated with organ toxicity from analgesics. Chronic opioid use has been shown to reduce both pain and disability. Opioids may be considered in patients with severe, disabling chronic pain that is unrelieved with simple analgesics and is associated with significant impairment in daily functioning and quality of life. Relative contraindications include a history of substance abuse, serious psychopathology, and lack of motivation to engage in an appropriate therapy program or to improve functioning. Patients with no history of substance abuse are at low risk for abuse with prescribed medications. Patients with current addiction problems should be referred to a drug rehabilitation facility before pain management is initiated. Patients with recent substance abuse or addiction problems should be managed by a pain specialist, ideally in conjunction with a counselor specializing in treating patients with these types of problems.

Patients who have severe chronic pain that is constantly present are best managed with long-acting medication rather than frequent dosing with immediate-release agents. Short-acting medications are best used infrequently for intermittent, short-lived pain flares. Long-acting opioids include sustained-release morphine sulfate, sustained-release oxycodone, transdermal fentanyl, and methadone. Methadone is the least expensive (about one tenth the cost of brand-name opioids); however, titration is difficult because of individual variability in metabolism. Opioid equivalence charts may be helpful when converting patients from one medication to another (Table 50–4). For example, the amount of opioid administered from a 100-mcg/h fentanyl patch is roughly equivalent to an oral dose of 240 mg morphine sulfate daily. In general, musculoskeletal pain is more responsive to opioids than neuropathic pain or chronic headache. Opioids may be a useful adjunctive treatment to other neuropathic medications in patients with neuropathic pain and, due to the high cost of gastrointestinal and renal effects of chronic analgesic therapy, can provide a cost-effective alternative for patients with chronic pain when properly monitored. Meperidine should be avoided given the potential for adverse effects related to accumulation of normeperidine and a somewhat greater addictive potential.

Attal N et al: Effects of IV morphine in central pain: A randomized placebo-controlled study. Neurology 2002;26:554. [PMID: 11865132]

Cepeda MS et al: Tramadol for osteoarthritis. Cochrane Database Syst Rev 2006;(3):CD005522. [PMID: 16856101]

Marcus DA: Pharmacoeconomics of opioid therapy for chronic non-malignant pain. Expert Opin Pharmacother 2002;3:229. [PMID: 11866673]

Sloan P, Babul N: Extended-release opioids for the management of chronic non-malignant pain. Expert Opin Drug Deliv 2006;3:489. [PMID: 16822224]

Stillman M: Clinical approach to patients with neuropathic pain. Cleve Clin J Med 2006;73:726. [PMID: 16913197]

2. Adjunctive medications—Adjunctive medications supplement the benefits from analgesics, treat neuropathic or central pain, and treat secondary complaints. In addition, effective use of adjunctive agents often reduces the need for analgesic medications. Adjunctive agents interact with the mechanism of neuropathic or central pain and chronic headache by reducing nervous system wind-up, the process by which the nervous system amplifies and eventually perpetuates pain signals in the absence of ongoing nociceptive input from the periphery.

The two primary categories of adjunctive analgesics are antidepressants and anticonvulsants. Among the antidepressants, the greatest analgesia is achieved by dual serotonin- and norepinephrine-activating agents. Traditionally, this has meant prescribing TCAs. Agents such as nortriptyline have shown efficacy for neuropathic pain, fibromyalgia, and migraines, and their advantages include once-daily dosing, help for sleep, and modest cost. However, TCAs are associated with anticholinergic effects, orthostasis, and the potential for cardiac arrhythmia, the latter being a concern particularly in prepubertal children.

Two newer agents have dual norepinephrine and serotonin reuptake inhibition and have been used for chronic pain states. Venlafaxine is an energizing antidepressant with some utility for chronic pain states; the greatest concern as far as adverse effects is the potential to increase blood pressure at higher doses. Duloxetine, a newer dual-action agent, is the only antidepressant to come onto the market with an indication for pain associated with diabetic peripheral neuropathy, in contrast to the preceding agents, which are used off label; research also supports its use in patients with fibromyalgia.

Comorbid depression, anxiety symptoms, sleep disturbance, and loss of energy are commonly seen in individuals with chronic pain. Many patients do not tolerate antidepressant medications or experience adverse effects (eg, sexual dysfunction with SSRIs). For such individuals, it may be preferable to find a tolerated agent that will help with mood and associated symptoms. For example, an anergic overweight woman with fibromyalgia may benefit from treatment with bupropion; alternatives to TCAs for a patient with depression and a sleep disturbance would include mirtazapine or trazodone.

Anticonvulsants, particularly gabapentin, have become a mainstay in the treatment of neuropathic pain. They are also beneficial for treating chronic headaches and may be beneficial for treating fibromyalgia. Newer anticonvulsant drugs that show promise in the treatment of neuropathic pain include topiramate, oxcarbazepine, and zonisamide. Some have multiple mechanisms of action, including membrane stabilization involving sodium and calcium channels, *N*-methyl-D-aspartate blockade, and GABAergic effects. Newly available is pregabalin, which pharmacologically resembles gabapentin. Both agents are the only drugs in this class with an indication for pain associated with diabetic peripheral neuropathy and postherpetic neuralgia. Pregabalin was recently approved for fibromyalgia.

Most muscle relaxants (eg, carisoprodol and cyclobenzaprine) used to treat acute musculoskeletal pain are associated with significant sedation, reducing their usefulness as a treatment for chronic pain, for which the primary focus is reducing disability and time spent in bed. Tizanidine, a unique muscle relaxant with both antispasticity and α-adrenergic effects, results in reduced spasticity and reduced pain perception with both acute and chronic use. In addition to reducing spasticity related to neurologic conditions (eg, multiple sclerosis, stroke, or spinal cord injury), tizanidine can also reduce symptoms associated with myofascial pain, fibromyalgia, and headaches, with some evidence of benefit for neuropathic pain. Tizanidine is often used in low doses (2–8 mg daily) given at bedtime or divided into three daily doses. Tizanidine is mildly sedating, which can assist with associated sleep disturbance.

Regarding dosing, medical mythology suggested that low doses of adjunctive agents were analgesic. The older agent, gabapentin, has nonlinear pharmacokinetics, making optimal dosage selection difficult. Dose-response studies with both duloxetine and pregabalin have demonstrated a fairly linear response, indicating that efficacy may be found at higher doses among patients with a limited initial response to a low dose. The clinical applicability of this linear response with duloxetine and pregabalin has been confirmed in controlled clinical trials.

Ansari A: The efficacy of newer antidepressants in the treatment of chronic pain: A review of current literature. Harv Rev Psychiatry 2000;7:257. [PMID: 10689591]

Ben-Menachem E: Pregabalin pharmacology and its relevance to clinical practice. Epilepsia 2004;45(Suppl 6):13.

Crofford LJ et al: Pregabalin for the treatment of fibromyalgia syndrome: Results of a randomized, double-blind, placebo-controlled trial. Arthritis Rheum 2005;52:1264. [PMID: 15818684]

Goldstein DJ et al: Duloxetine vs. placebo in patients with painful diabetic neuropathy. Pain 2005;116:109. [PMID: 15927394]

Hunziker ME et al: Duloxetine hydrochloride: A new dual-acting medication for the treatment of major depressive disorder. Clin Ther 2005;27:1126. [PMID: 16199241]

Mathew NT: Antiepileptic drugs in migraine prevention. Headache 2001;41(Suppl 1):18. [PMID: 11903536]

Sabatowski R et al: Pregabalin reduces pain and improves sleep and mood disturbances in patients with post-herpetic neuralgia: Results of a randomized, placebo-controlled clinical trial. Pain 2004;109:26. [PMID: 15082123]

3. Adverse events with chronic pain medications— The annual costs associated with toxicity from nonopioid analgesics approach $1.9 billion, with $1.35 billion caused by NSAID toxicity. Gastric ulcers occur in 15–30% of chronic NSAID users. In addition, renal impairment occurs in 24% and renal papillary necrosis in 12% of arthritic patients using chronic NSAIDs. Fortunately, renal insufficiency is often improved when the drugs are discontinued. NSAIDs must be used with particular caution in the elderly, as their use reduces the effectiveness of diuretics and doubles the risk for hospitalization from congestive heart failure.

COX-2 inhibitors were initially widely used in patients with chronic pain to minimize costs from gastric toxicity. COX-2 inhibitor analgesics now have limited use, especially in elderly patients, due to postmarketing identification of increased risk for myocardial infarction and stroke. Some of this increased risk may have resulted from inappropriate use of these medications. For example, a review of community-dwelling Medicaid recipients aged 50–84 years in Tennessee showed no increased occurrence of serious coronary heart disease in rofecoxib users prescribed daily dosages of 25 mg or less. Those prescribed more than 25 mg daily, however, had a 1.7 times greater risk of serious heart disease occurrence. Interestingly, a survey of chronic users of rofecoxib in 2001 showed that nearly one fifth were prescribed more than 25 mg daily, with most using this high dosage chronically. A recent, large, observational study of Medicaid enrollees found no difference in cardiovascular event occurrence between patients using a COX-2 selective inhibitor versus a non-naproxen NSAID. Conversely, a Canadian retrospective analysis showed a higher risk of death and recurrent congestive heart failure in elderly patients with preexisting congestive heart failure prescribed rofecoxib or NSAIDs compared with celecoxib. These data suggest that significant toxicity may occur with both NSAIDs and selective COX-2 inhibitors.

Opioids are not associated with organ toxicity. Practitioners must monitor for evidence of the development of tolerance (reduced effectiveness of the medication over time) or abuse (failure to identify prescribed opioids on random urine testing or repeated lost or overused medications). In either circumstance, patients will likely need a change in treatment.

Newer anticonvulsants used to treat neuropathic pain do not require the frequent laboratory monitoring that is common with older anticonvulsants (eg, carbamazepine and sodium valproate). Gabapentin is cleared by the kidneys, requiring dose adjustment or reduced frequency of administration in patients with renal insufficiency. Dialysis patients receive gabapentin dosing after each treatment with hemodialysis.

TCAs, typically prescribed in low to moderate doses to treat neuropathic pain, are still associated with a small risk for cardiac arrhythmia. All prepubertal children treated with TCAs should receive a baseline electrocardiogram (ECG), followed by regular assessments of heart rate and blood pressure, periodic testing of antidepressant drug levels, and repeat ECGs. Similarly, older adults or individuals with a history of cardiac disease should also be monitored with blood tests and ECGs when TCA doses approach the low therapeutic range. SSRIs and bupropion have been associated with seizures in higher doses and should be used with caution in individuals with tendencies to seizure. Venlafaxine can have a cardiac stimulatory effect at higher doses and blood pressure should be watched. Antidepressants, particularly those with a prominent serotoninergic effect, have been associated with the potential for suicidality and should be monitored closely in patients at risk and in children or adolescents.

Tizanidine and duloxetine have been associated with hepatotoxicity and should be avoided in individuals with a history of liver problems. Periodic liver enzyme screening should be obtained in patients taking these agents chronically.

Griffin MR et al: High frequency of use of rofecoxib at greater than recommended doses: Cause for concern. Pharmacoepidemiol Drug Saf 2004;13:339. [PMID: 15170762]

Hudson M et al: Differences in outcomes of patients with congestive heart failure prescribed celecoxib, rofecoxib, or non-steroidal anti-inflammatory drugs: Population based study. BMJ 2005;330:1370. [PMID: 15947399]

Ray WA et al: COX-2 selective non-steroidal anti-inflammatory drugs and risk of serious coronary heart disease. Lancet 2002;360:1071. [PMID: 12383990]

Shaya FT et al: Selective cyclooxygenase-2 inhibition and cardiovascular effects. An observational study of a Medicaid population. Arch Intern Med 2005;165:181. [PMID: 15668364]

4. Medication management in pediatric patients and in older patients—Chronically administered opioids are generally avoided in pediatric patients, although there are certainly exceptions with chronic disease states such as hemophilia and sickle cell disease. Acetaminophen and NSAIDs should be considered first-line therapy for pediatric patients with pain. TCAs and gabapentin have been extensively utilized for neuropathic pain in pediatric patients, and pediatric dosing guidelines are available. As noted, caution must be taken regarding the potential for cardiac conduction disturbance with the use of TCAs in prepubertal children.

When selecting medication for older adults, physicians need to strongly consider the side-effect profiles, particularly for agents that have central nervous system effects—including opioids, antidepressants, and anticonvulsants. As opposed to the mild sedation or dizziness experienced by younger individuals, geriatric patients may experience more profound drowsiness, confusion, delirium, and increased risk for falls. Medical comorbidities and medications for these conditions increase the risk for adverse events in geriatric patients. The potential for activation or inhibition of cytochrome P450 pathways is problematic in patients taking multiple medications, particularly agents with a narrow therapeutic index, such as digoxin and warfarin. With the exception of gabapentin, the dosing of adjunctive analgesics typically is lower for older adults.

Low to modest doses of opioids may be a very useful part of the treatment regimen for geriatric patients with pain, particularly because of good tolerability at low doses. It is common to see older patients with arthritis who are unable to tolerate even the COX-2 agents. Additionally, as the degree of degenerative disease progresses, benefits from NSAIDs may be limited, necessitating stronger analgesia. When used judiciously, opioids typically are well tolerated and can allow individuals to retain a level of functioning sufficient to maintain their independence.

D. Interventional Pain Management

Interventional techniques are considered for patients failing conservative therapy or when specific nervous system pathology has been identified. Lumbar epidural steroid injections are effective for treating herniated discs or spinal stenosis. Sympathetic blocks reduce the burning pain of complex regional pain syndrome or reflex sympathetic dystrophy that may develop after acute extremity injury or surgery. Trigger point injections are useful for localized muscle pain. The benefit from injections is often transient, so these techniques are generally used in conjunction with physical therapy and medication management. Radiofrequency ablation

(RFA) may be considered for recalcitrant symptoms of facet, disc, sympathetic, or neural pain; pulsed RFA appears to have the same beneficial effect with reduced risk of deafferentation pain.

Implantable devices, including intrathecal pumps and dorsal column stimulators, can be used to treat individuals with cancer-related pain or severe incapacitating pain resulting from nonmalignant conditions. Intrathecal medications are considered for patients requiring high medication doses when side effects from oral medications become intolerable. Dorsal column stimulators are considered when pain is limited to a single extremity. For the treatment of pain resulting from nonmalignant conditions, it is essential to obtain psychological consultation prior to the surgery.

Nerve blocks may be particularly beneficial for postherpetic neuralgia, which can be quite difficult to treat. The early use of antiviral agents (eg, valacyclovir) is important in attenuating the initial infection and decreasing the acute pain as well as chronic symptoms. In addition, early treatment of zoster with TCAs (25 mg of amitriptyline daily for 90 days) reduces chronicity of symptoms of postherpetic neuralgia. Nerve blocks, particularly thoracic epidural local anesthetics or intercostal blocks, can be used in the acute or chronic stage. Early use of nerve blocks, especially within the first 2 months of onset of symptoms, greatly decreases the incidence and severity of postherpetic neuralgia.

Bowsher D: The effects of pre-emptive treatment of postherpetic neuralgia with amitriptyline: A randomized, double-blind, placebo-controlled trial. J Pain Symptom Manage 1997;13: 327. [PMID: 9204652]

Kapural L, Mekhail N: Radiofrequency ablation for chronic pain control. Curr Pain Headache Rep 2001;5:517. [PMID: 11676886]

Rainov NG et al: Long-term intrathecal infusion of drug combinations for chronic back and leg pain. J Pain Symptom Manage 2001;22:862. [PMID: 11576803]

E. Complementary and Alternative Therapies

Complementary and alternative treatments are used by 40% of chronic pain sufferers. Acupuncture reduces pain for a variety of painful musculoskeletal conditions, including fibromyalgia, and recent studies have shown efficacy in osteoarthritis. Chiropractic treatment is recommended for acute pain. There is no clear consensus on the effectiveness of chiropractic manipulation for chronic pain, and controlled studies are needed to provide efficacy data. Exercise therapy effectively reduces pain in elderly patients with osteoarthritis. Mind–body approaches (eg, meditation, guided imagery, and yoga) engage the patient actively in treatment, changing the locus of control and encouraging use of health-promoting behaviors. Mind–body techniques are also effective in reducing pain. Among biologically based treatments, the nutritional supplement glucosamine has been well studied and appears to have a pain-relieving and possibly joint–preserving effect. Glucosamine does not provide an antirheumatic effect on joints; however, its use is associated with significant pain reduction.

Dias RC et al: Impact of an exercise and walking protocol on quality of life for elderly people with OA of the knee. Physiother Res Int 2003;8:121-130. [PMID: 14533368]

Gouze JN et al: Exogenous glucosmine effectively protects chondrocytes from the arthritogenic effects of IL-1beta. Arthritis Res Ther 2006;8:R173. [PMID: 17109745]

Gray CM et al: Complementary and alternative medicine use among health plan members. A cross-sectional survey. Eff Clin Pract 2002;5:17. [PMID: 11878283]

Hameline MT: Symptomatic outcomes and perceived satisfaction levels of chiropractic patients with a primary diagnosis involving acute neck pain. J Manipulative Physiol Ther 2006;29: 288-296. [PMID: 16690383]

Linde K et al: Acupuncture for osteoarthritic pain: An observational study in routine care. Rheumatology (Oxford) 2006;45:222. [PMID: 16368731]

Martin K et al: Weight loss and exercise walking reduce pain and improve physical functioning in overweight postmenopausal women with knee osteoarthritis. J Clin Rheumatol 2001; 7:219. [PMID: 17039138]

Messier SP et al: Exercise and weight loss in obese older adults with knee osteoarthritis: A preliminary study. J Am Geriatr Soc 2000;48:1062. [PMID: 10983905]

Santilli V et al: Chiropractic manipulation in the treatment of acute back pain and sciatica with disc protrusion: A randomized double-blind clinical trial of active and simulated spinal manipulations. Spine J 2006;6:131. [PMID: 16517383]

White P: A background to acupuncture and its use in chronic painful musculoskeletal conditions. J R Soc Health 2006;126:219. [PMID: 17004405]

Travel Medicine 51

William H. Markle, MD, FAAFD, DTM&H, & Calvin L. Wilson, MD

The number of people traveling around the globe increases annually. Of about 50 million international travelers from the United States and Canada each year, about 35 million travel to parts of the developing world. Many travelers are business people going to large cities where health risks are few; increasingly, however, travelers are seeking out exotic locations as tourist destinations. Pretravel health advice is often an afterthought for these travelers.

Only a small percentage of travelers consult a specialized travel clinic before leaving on a trip. Many people ask their family physician for recommendations, and at times the advice they receive is either uninformed or out of date. It is important for all primary care physicians to be prepared to give accurate advice to travelers about both pretravel preparation and how to deal with illnesses contracted abroad. Sometimes there is not enough time to obtain the required immunizations and priorities must be established. The goal of this chapter is to enable the family physician to provide guidance to patients wishing to be prepared for illnesses and emergencies related to travel.

Steffen R et al: *Manual of Travel Medicine and Health,* 2nd ed. BC Decker, 2003.

Zuckerman JN: Recent developments: Travel medicine. BMJ 2002;325:260. [PMID: 12153925]

PRETRAVEL PREPARATION & CONCERNS

Case Illustration

A 28-year-old man in good health is planning a 2-month trip to Kenya. He will be working in Nairobi but also plans to visit game parks and participate in outdoor activities.

- What history must be obtained?
- What specific advice should the patient be given?
- What immunizations are needed?
- What malaria prophylaxis is recommended?
- Where can the physician find the answers to these questions?

The first step is to obtain a thorough history—including any preexisting medical conditions and use of medications that may have side effects or may interact with other drugs that will be prescribed—and to perform a thorough physical examination. What is the patient's exact itinerary, what countries will he visit en route, in what order? What accommodations will he have? Will he remain in urban areas or visit some rural regions? What is his immunization history? This information will help determine necessary immunizations and prophylaxis. The physician can also help the traveler ensure he has items such as insect repellent that may be essential. If the patient has a chronic illness, he should be given pertinent portions of his medical record and a list of allergies to take along in case he must seek medical care abroad.

Several web sites provide helpful information about travel and health requirements. (See listing at the end of this chapter.) After reviewing these requirements, the physician would find that this patient faces several risks that should be discussed. These include:

- Malaria, especially at lower elevations such as in game parks.
- Diarrhea, caused by parasites or bacteria such as *Escherichia coli* or *Shigella.*
- Typhoid fever and other salmonelloses.
- Hepatitis A, B, or C.
- Schistosomiasis, especially if swimming or wading in local bodies of water.
- Violence and petty thievery, especially in urban areas such as Nairobi.
- HIV/AIDS and other sexually transmitted diseases.
- Poor infrastructure for dealing with serious emergencies, such as motor vehicle accidents, especially outside of urban areas.

Travelers who monitor the most common risks found at their destination can better prepare in advance and equip themselves with resources to ensure a smooth, safe trip.

Travelers' Medical Kit

Every traveler should carry a medical kit that addresses basic care for common illnesses and injuries. The components of such a kit are listed in Table 51–1, but it must be adjusted depending on individual needs. If a patient uses a medication that is taken regularly, he or she should be advised to carry along enough to last for the entire trip, a small supply should also be kept in carry-on bags, in case luggage is lost or delayed. The traveler should carry a letter from a physician if he or she plans to take along any controlled substance. This letter will help answer questions from immigration officials and other authorities. Travelers should not forget to bring spare eyeglasses or contact lenses, contact lens solution, and their ophthalmologic prescription, in case of loss or breakage.

If the traveler is planning a long stay, the physician may be asked to supply a prescribed medication on a regular basis from the United States, particularly if the drug in question is not available abroad. Increasingly, however, medications prescribed in the United States are available abroad (often much more cheaply) and can be obtained without difficulty by a knowledgeable traveler. Travelers should be cautioned to carefully examine any medications bought overseas, because ingredients may differ from those used in US products, and some ingredients may not be considered safe by US standards.

Table 51–1. Medical kit for travelers.

Insect repellent with up to 30% DEET, Picaridin, or oil of lemon eucalyptus
Permethrin spray for clothing and mosquito nets, if traveling to the tropics
Sunscreen (minimum SPF 15)
Dressings, gauze pads, adhesive tape, adhesive bandages, small bottle of disinfectant, elastic bandage (eg, Ace), scissors, tweezers
Moleskin, if extensive hiking is planned
Hand wipes, liquid soap, hand sanitizer, facial tissues
Aspirin, acetaminophen, or other analgesic drug
Antidiarrheal (eg, Lomotil, Imodium, Pepto-Bismol)
Antacid (eg, Tums), antihistamine (H_2 blocker)
Eye drops (for allergy and infection)
Ear drops (if risk of external otitis)
Dimenhydrinate or scopolamine, if motion sickness is a problem with air or water travel
Sleep aid
Laxative
Antihistamines (preferably nonsedating agents such as loratadine, but diphenhydramine is often useful as a sleep aid in addition to its antihistamine activity)
Cold and cough medications
Asthma medications and inhalers, if needed
Topical antibiotics, antifungals, steroids, and vaginal antifungal drugs
Antibiotics (eg, ciprofloxacin, sulfamethoxazole-trimethoprim, amoxicillin, doxycycline)[1]
Malaria prophylaxis (see text)
Water purification kit or filter (see text)
Acetazolamide, if travel is contemplated to elevations > 8000 ft (2500 m) above sea level
Syringes and needles (3–5-mL syringes, 21–25-gauge needles), if traveling in underdeveloped countries where instrument sterilization may be uncertain
Injectable epinephrine (eg, Epi-Pen), if traveler has a history of anaphylactic reactions to foods or insect bites

SPF, sun protection factor.

[1]Inclusion of antibiotics depends on familiarity of the traveler with these medications and the likelihood they will be needed, based on the itinerary.

Jong E, McMullen R: *The Travel and Tropical Medicine Handbook*, 3rd ed. Saunders, 2002.

Insurance

Travelers should check their health insurance policies to determine whether they include coverage for medical expenses incurred abroad. If coverage is provided, they should bring a blank insurance form in case it is needed or it becomes necessary to contact the insurance company. Term travel health insurance policies are also available. Evacuation insurance is essential in the event of a serious accident or medical problem. Some policies will return travelers to their home cities; others will evacuate them to the nearest location where they can receive medical care comparable to that available in their home country. Among the more well-known companies offering evacuation insurance and emergency travel insurance are CSA Travel Protection (http://www.csatravelprotection.com), Global Alert (http://www.globalalerttravel.info), International SOS (http://www.internationalsos.com), Medjet Assist (http://www.medjetassistance.com), and Multi-National (http://www.mnui.com/europrivacy.asp). Policies can also be obtained through travel agencies. Finally, the traveler may wish to purchase trip insurance. This type of insurance ensures reimbursement in case a trip must be canceled for medical or other reasons beyond the traveler's control. (It should be noted that most trip insurance policies do not cover cancellation for personal reasons, such as a change in plans.) This insurance is especially attractive for older travelers, who are more likely to have a medical emergency that prevents them from traveling.

Air Travel Concerns

Some medical conditions require special attention during air travel. These include any severe, common illness; anemia; clotting disorders; disfiguring dermatoses; dyspnea

Table 51–2. Contraindications to air travel.

Unstable angina
Myocardial infarction in past 2 wk (or 6 wk, if complicated)
Active bronchospasm
Neurosurgery or skull fracture in past 2 wk
Uncontrolled cardiac disease (congestive heart failure or arrhythmia)
Percutaneous coronary intervention in past 5 days (or 2 wk, if complicated)
Cerebral infarction in past 2 wk.
Pneumothorax in past 2–3 wk
Colonoscopy with polypectomy in past 24 h
Late pregnancy (long flights)
Highly contagious diseases, including active tuberculosis
Major uncontrolled psychiatric disorders
Cyanosis
Pulmonary hypertension
Recent middle ear surgery
Scuba diving in past 24 h
Hemoglobin < 7.5 g
Heart, lung, or gastrointestinal surgery in past 3 wk
Noncommunicating lung cysts

at rest; incontinence; otitis media; pulmonary or acute upper respiratory infections; and sickle cell hemoglobinopathies. Medical contraindications to air travel are listed in Table 51–2. Ill or handicapped travelers must notify the airline 72 hours before departure to be sure the plane is properly equipped. Services such as a wheelchair, oxygen, stretcher, and other necessary equipment can usually be provided with advance notice.

Jong E, McMullen R: *The Travel and Tropical Medicine Handbook,* 3rd ed. Saunders, 2002.

Sohail MR, Fischer PR: Health risks to air travelers. Infect Dis Clin North Am 2005;19:67. [PMID: 15701547]

Food & Water Sanitation

Many infectious diseases can be prevented by attention to food and water sanitation. These include intestinal viral, bacterial, and parasitic diseases. The guidelines that follow can help travelers prevent many food- and water-borne illnesses.

Travelers should be advised to avoid eating food that has not been cooked adequately or peeled by them. Cooking must be thorough, not just warming, and a clean knife must be used for peeling. If fish are eaten, they should be fresh, not dried or old-looking. Cans should be inspected for bulging or gas formation. Only dairy products that have been pasteurized should be consumed, and products that have been ultrapasteurized by the UHT method are preferred. Raw vegetables and fruits should be cleaned with a brush, soap, and water, and then ideally sterilized with boiling water or by soaking in a bleach solution (approximately 2 teaspoons or 10 mL of chlorine bleach in 1 liter of clean water). Hands should be kept clean and fingernails trimmed. Clean silverware and plates should be used; these can be rinsed in boiling water or bleach rinse to sterilize them.

Travelers should be advised that bottled or canned drinks are safe as long as the seal is intact. Iced and lukewarm drinks should not be trusted, but hot drinks such as coffee or tea are generally safe if prepared recently and still hot when served. Tap water can be purified either by boiling and treating with iodine or chlorine or by filtering with a reliable ultra–filter water purification system, as described below:

- Bring water to a rolling boil for 1 minute at sea level or 3 minutes if over 2000 m (6500 ft) elevation. Treat with iodine (10 drops of tincture per liter) and let stand for 30 minutes; or treat with chlorine (1–2 drops of chlorine bleach per liter of water) and let stand for 30 minutes. Although chlorine may not kill all parasitic cysts or viruses, water treated with chlorine has a better taste than iodized water; furthermore, chlorine does not affect thyroid function over long periods of use.
- Reliable water purification systems are available through various sources. (For example, Campmor [http://www.campmor.com] includes information on several systems.) A pore size of 0.2 microns is needed to filter out all enteric bacteria and parasites. If the water is cloudy or especially dirty-looking, some gross filtration or sedimentation must be done first before using a small-pore filter. Adding iodine resins to the filter will kill viruses if contact is sufficient.

Backer H: Water disinfection for international and wilderness travelers. Clin Infect Dis 2002;34:355. [PMID: 11774083]

Injury Prevention

The leading cause of mortality and morbidity in travelers is motor vehicle accidents. Other common accidents that occur during travel include drowning, carbon monoxide poisoning, electric shock, and drug reactions. Travelers should be aware that jet lag and other causes of drowsiness while traveling (eg, medications to alleviate motion sickness) may heighten the risk of injury. If a traumatic injury occurs, travelers should be cautioned not to agree to blood transfusions unless absolutely necessary.

Although the risks to personal security in many parts of the world may be similar to those encountered in many urban areas of the United States, a traveler may be at greater risk in areas where he or she is an obvious foreigner or tourist. Most commonly, the risks to personal security are related to theft of personal belongings and the occasional violent methods used, especially in the urban areas of Africa and Latin America. Women, especially those traveling alone, are at greatest risk of personal assault, often because the sexualized image of western women portrayed by American media has given men of many cultures a mistaken impression of their willingness and availability.

Another rarely discussed but important area of personal security is that of sexual activity while traveling. The incidence of sexually transmitted diseases, especially HIV, is quite high in many popular tourist destinations, including much of Africa, the Caribbean, Thailand, and some parts of Latin America. Travelers should be cautioned to use good judgment (especially in situations involving alcohol use), barrier protection such as condoms, and caution with oral-genital contact.

McInnes RJ et al: Unintentional injury during foreign travel: A review. J Travel Med 2002;9:297. [PMID: 12962584]

Obtaining Medical Care Abroad

Obtaining reliable medical care abroad can be difficult. Frequent travelers may wish to become members of the International Association for Medical Assistance to Travelers (IAMAT), which provides up-to-date advice on where to seek competent medical care for virtually any area of the world. (Contact information: 417 Center St, Lewiston, NY 14092; 716-754-4883; info@iamat.org; http://www.iamat.org.) The International Society for Travel Medicine (http://www.istm.org) and the American Society of Tropical Medicine and Hygiene (www.astmh.org) are also excellent resources for those seeking to find travel clinics anywhere in the world.

Immunizations

Up-to-date immunization information can be obtained from the Centers for Disease Control and Prevention (CDC) web site, http://www.cdc.gov/travel, which contains a wealth of information.

No vaccines are currently *required* for travel, with the exception of yellow fever vaccine if travel is planned to an endemic area. However, travelers from the United States should be up to date on all routine immunizations, including diphtheria, tetanus, measles, mumps, varicella, rubella, influenza, pneumonia, and, for children, pertussis and *Haemophilus influenzae* type b (Hib; see Chapter 7). For previously immunized adults, a single dose of polio vaccine is recommended if traveling to an area with a risk of polio. Europe and the western hemisphere have been certified polio free.

Typhoid and hepatitis A vaccines are recommended for travelers to most areas of the world. Two typhoid vaccines are currently available: Ty21a and Vi. Efficacy of both vaccines is about 70%. Ty21a is a live oral vaccine that conveys protection for 5 years. It is taken as a series of four tablets, one every other day. The tablets must be kept refrigerated until taken. Vi is a parenteral vaccine that provides protection for 2 years. Persons receiving this vaccine have a higher incidence of systemic reactions such as fever or malaise for the first 2–3 days after administration than those who receive the oral vaccine, and they may also develop injection-site soreness.

Meningococcal vaccine is indicated for travelers to areas of sub-Saharan Africa where meningococcal disease is endemic or epidemic. Japanese B encephalitis vaccine is recommended for travelers to endemic areas of rural Asia, especially if the traveler plans to stay longer than 30 days. Cholera vaccine is no longer available in the United States; however, an oral vaccine is available abroad and may be useful in certain situations. Rabies vaccine is recommended for travelers to high-risk developing countries, especially long-term travelers or those who may have extensive outdoor or nighttime exposure.

Hepatitis B vaccine is recommended for travelers to high-risk areas, especially long-term travelers and those engaging in high-risk sexual behaviors. Medical workers must be vaccinated, as should the future adoptive parents of children from a developing country.

Table 51–3 summarizes information for these and other vaccines. For additional information, refer to the CDC web site listed earlier.

Centers for Disease Control and Prevention, Kozarsky P et al: *Health Information for International Travel 2005-06.* US Department of Health and Human Services, CDC, Elsevier, 2005.

Ryan ET, Kain KC: Health advice and immunizations for travelers. N Engl J Med 2000;342:1716. [PMID: 10841875]

TREATMENT OF TRAVEL-RELATED ILLNESSES

TRAVELER'S DIARRHEA

ESSENTIALS OF DIAGNOSIS

- *Twofold increase in frequency of unformed bowel movements, usually more than four to five stools per day.*
- *Abrupt onset while traveling or soon after returning home.*
- *Abdominal cramps, bloating, and malaise.*
- *Generally self-limiting after 3–4 days.*

Table 51–3. Vaccines that may be administered to travelers.

Vaccine	Efficacy (%)	Partial Protection Begins	Duration of Protection
Live Vaccines			
Cholera (oral)	62–80	After 8 days	At least 6 mo
MMR	> 95	28 days after first dose	Life-long
Tuberculosis (bCG)	Variable	After 6–8 wk	Variable
Typhoid Ty21a (oral)	63–71	After third dose	5 y
Varicella	97	After 4–6 wk	At least 10 y
Yellow fever	> 99	After 10–14 days	At least 10 y
Inactive Vaccines			
Diphtheria	95	After second dose	5–10 y
Hepatitis A	95–100	2 wk after first dose	6–12 y
Hepatitis B	> 95	4 wk after second dose	At least 15 y
Influenza	86–87	Variable	1 y
Japanese B encephalitis	80–91	10 days after second dose	2–4 y
Meningococcal	75–100	After 14 days	3 y or more
Pertussis	80–85	After second dose	At least 2 y
Pneumococcal PCV7	> 90	After second dose	Unknown
Pneumococcal 23	56–81	Variable	5–10 y
Polio (injectable)	> 95	After third dose	Probably life-long
Rabies	> 99	7 days after second dose	> 2 y
Tetanus	> 99	After second dose	10 y
Typhoid Vi	55–75	After 7 days	2 y

MMR, measles, mumps, rubella; bCG, bacillus Calmette–Guérin.

General Considerations

Traveler's diarrhea is caused by fecal-oral contamination of food or water by bacteria, parasites, and viruses. It is a risk in developing countries, and the best chance for prevention involves strict attention to hygiene, sanitation, and food preparation, as outlined earlier. It is, however, extremely difficult to avoid all dangers in food and drink. Multiple studies have shown no correlation between personal hygiene measures and traveler's diarrhea, and simply eating in restaurants can be hazardous. Nevertheless it is prudent to follow basic hygiene measures while abroad. In contrast to the developed world, where viruses are the most common cause of diarrhea, enterotoxigenic *E coli* and other bacteria are the most common causes of diarrhea in most parts of the developing world.

Prevention

Although prophylaxis is generally discouraged, it may be indicated in patients with active inflammatory bowel disease, diabetes mellitus type 1, heart disease (elderly patients), AIDS and other immunosuppressive disorders, as well as those on proton pump inhibitor therapy. Travelers planning an exceptionally important short trip may also wish to use prophylactic medications.

Prophylaxis can be obtained using either the fluoroquinolone antibiotics (90% protection) or Pepto-Bismol (65% protection) at the following dosages: ciprofloxacin, 500 mg daily; levofloxacin, 500 mg daily; norfloxacin, 400 mg daily; ofloxacin, 300 mg daily; or Pepto-Bismol, 2 tablets four times daily.

Clinical Findings

Traveler's diarrhea is characterized by the abrupt onset of at least a twofold increase in loose stools, usually four to five stools per day, while traveling or soon after returning home. Other common symptoms include abdominal cramps, bloating, urgency, malaise, and nausea. Symptoms usually resolve in 3–4 days if not treated but can last longer. Depending on the cause, fever or bloody stools may occur, but these symptoms are not common. Physical findings include a benign abdomen with diffuse tenderness but no rigidity and increased bowel sounds. Patients may appear dehydrated. Although stool examination and culture may yield a cause, in 20–50% of cases no pathogen is identified.

Treatment

Treatment for traveler's diarrhea always includes fluid replacement and usually includes fluoroquinolone antibiotics (or, in children, azithromycin or trimethoprim-sulfamethoxazole). Imodium may be used for adults but must be combined with the antibiotic. Rifaximin is a newer antibiotic indicated only for *E coli*–induced traveler's diarrhea. The dosage is 200 mg three times daily for 3 days. It is especially useful in patients who develop traveler's diarrhea after visiting Mexico or Latin America and is less useful when *Campylobacter* is the causative pathogen. There is some early evidence that rifaximin is useful for prophylaxis of diarrhea, but these data are still preliminary. In many countries, particularly Thailand, *Campylobacter* infections are now frequently resistant to fluoroquinolones; thus, azithromycin or other antibiotics are often needed. Although a 3- to 5–day course of antibiotics is usually recommended, there is evidence that 1–2 days of treatment may be sufficient.

Fluid replacement is best accomplished using the World Health Organization (WHO) ORS salts, available in most countries, according to the following formula: 3.5 g of sodium chloride (NaCl), 2.9 g of trisodium citrate dehydrate, 1.5 g of potassium chloride (KCl), and 20 g of glucose in 1 L of water. (In the United States, these salts can be obtained through Cera Products, Jessup, MD; 888-237-2598). ORS can be home–made, if necessary, using the following formula: 1 level teaspoon of table salt, $^3/_4$ teaspoon of baking soda, and 4 tablespoons of sugar in 1 L of water; orange juice can be added, if available, to provide potassium. Adults should drink one 8-ounce glass after every diarrheal stool. Children younger than 2 years of age should be given 2–4 ounces, and those between 2 and 10 years, 4–7 ounces.

Women who are breast-feeding should be instructed to continue to do so. Patients can be advised to eat boiled rice, which often leads to faster resolution of diarrhea.

Casburn-Jones AC, Farthing MJ: Traveler's diarrhea. J Gastroenterol Hepatol 2004;19:610. [PMID: 15151613]

Shlim DR: Update in traveler's diarrhea. Infect Dis Clin North Am 2005;19:137. [PMID: 15701551]

MALARIA

ESSENTIALS OF DIAGNOSIS

- *Abrupt onset of fever, headache, chills, myalgias, and malaise during or after returning from an area in which malaria is endemic.*
- *Recurrence of symptoms every 1–2 days (highly variable).*
- *Thick and thin Giemsa-stained blood smears showing* Plasmodium *(diagnostic gold standard), or confirmation by rapid diagnostic testing for malaria.*

General Considerations

At least 40% of the world's population live in areas in which malaria is endemic, and about 5% are infected at any one time. Although 90% of cases occur in sub-Saharan Africa, the disease is found throughout the tropics. In most countries the distribution is spotty. Nonetheless, malaria causes an estimated two to three million deaths a year.

Malaria results from infection with *Plasmodium falciparum, P vivax, P malariae,* or *P ovale.* The first two species account for the majority of infections. The vector for transmission to humans is the female *Anopheles* mosquito. With the exception of Central America and parts of the Middle East, most *P falciparum* infections are resistant to chloroquine, and some strains of *P vivax,* mainly in Southeast Asia, are also resistant. Travelers to the tropics should receive prophylaxis based on the CDC recommendations.

Incubation periods differ among the *Plasmodium* species (Table 51–4), and at times may be much longer than those usually reported. *P falciparum* and *P malariae* do not form hypnozoites nor do they produce chronic liver infection. Thus, infected patients do not relapse if treatment is adequate. This is not the case for *P vivax* and *P ovale.* Reactivation of dormant hypnozoites in the liver can occur—sometimes decades after the original infection—in patients infected with these species, leading to relapse. Most cases of severe and cerebral malaria are caused by *P falciparum.*

Prevention

A. General Measures

To prevent malaria, travelers to endemic areas should be advised about basic measures to prevent mosquito bites, including wearing long sleeves, long pants, and light-colored clothing; avoiding perfumes that might attract mosquitoes; using a mosquito repellent containing 30% DEET, Picaridin, or oil of lemon eucalyptus; and treating bed nets with permethrin.

B. Malaria Prophylaxis

Four medications are currently available in the United States for malaria prophylaxis: chloroquine, mefloquine, doxycycline, and atovaquone-proguanil (Malarone). Primaquine has been used as a prophylactic medication, but this is not yet an approved indication.

1. Chloroquine—As previously noted, most strains of *P falciparum* worldwide have developed resistance to

Table 51–4. *Plasmodium* species causing human malaria.

Species	Average Incubation Period	Duration of Untreated Infection (max)
P falciparum	13.1 days; no earlier than 8 days	2 y
P vivax	13.4 days	4 y
P malariae	13–28 days	40 y
P ovale	14.1 days	4 y

chloroquine, but the drug is still effective in Central America above the Panama Canal and in some areas of the Middle East. It should not be used for prophylaxis of travelers to other areas. It has few serious side effects and is safe to use in pregnancy. Side effects include pruritus, headache, myalgia, alopecia, and spotty depigmentation of hair. Because it can cause exacerbations of psoriasis, eczema, and dermatitis, caution should be used if it is prescribed to people with these disorders. Retinal injury may occur with lifetime doses over 100 g. Dosages for prophylaxis in adults and children are listed in Table 51–5. Prophylaxis should begin 1–2 weeks before the traveler's planned arrival in a malaria-

Table 51–5. Prophylaxis and treatment dosages for malaria.

Drug	Dosage	
	Adults	Children
Malaria Prophylaxis		
Chloroquine	300 mg base (500 mg salt) per wk	5 mg base/kg/wk to max of adult dose
Mefloquine[1]	250 mg/wk	5 mg/kg/wk or the equivalent in divided adult tablets, based on child's weight: 15–19 kg: 1/4 tab/wk 20–30 kg: 1/2 tab/wk 31–45 kg: 3/4 tab/wk > 45 kg: use adult dose
Atovaquone-proguanil (Malarone)[2]	250 mg atovaquone/100 mg proguanil tablet per day	Pediatric tablets contain 62.5 mg atovaquone/25 mg proguanil; dosages are based on child's weight: 11–20 kg: 1 pediatric tab/day 21–30 kg: 2 pediatric tab/day 31–40 kg: 3 pediatric tab/day > 40 kg: 1 adult tab/day
Doxycycline[3]	100 mg/day	Children > 8 y: 2 mg/kg/day up to max of the adult dose
Treatment of Malarial Disease		
Mefloquine[1]	1250 mg once	25 mg/kg once, up to max of adult dose[4]
Atovaquone-proguanil (Malarone)[2]	4 tab once daily for 3 days	Using adult tablets, based on child's weight: 11–20 kg: 1 tab/day for 3 days 21–30 kg: 2 tab/day for 3 days 31–40 kg: 3 tab/day for 3 days > 40 kg: use adult dose
Sulfadoxine-pyrimethamine (Fansidar)	3 tab once	Children < 1 y: 1/4 tab 1–3 y: 1/2 tab 4–8 y: 1 tab 9–14 y: 2 tab given all at once

tab, tablet.
[1]Cautious use in pregnancy.
[2]Not for use in pregnant or breast-feeding women.
[3]Contraindicated in pregnant or breast-feeding women and in children younger than 8 years of age.
[4]This regimen tends to cause considerable gastrointestinal upset.

endemic area and should continue for 4 weeks after return home.

2. Mefloquine—Mefloquine is effective for prophylaxis in most areas of the world except the border area between Thailand and Myanmar. *P falciparum* shows a patchy resistance to the drug in some areas. Although it is safe to use in pregnancy, many physicians do not prescribe it for pregnant patients in the first trimester. The most serious side effects are neuropsychiatric, such as bad dreams, paresthesias, hallucinations, and even psychotic reactions. Other side effects include vertigo, headache, gastrointestinal upset, pruritus, confusion, seizures, hepatotoxicity, and depression. Caution is advised in patients with cardiac conduction abnormalities. Dosages for prophylaxis are listed in Table 51–5. As with chloroquine, prophylaxis should begin 1–2 weeks before arrival in a malaria-endemic area and continue for 4 weeks after return.

3. Atovaquone-proguanil—The combination drug atovaquone-proguanil (Malarone) is effective and safe for children but is not recommended for use in women who are pregnant or breast-feeding. Side effects include abdominal pain, vomiting, and headache, and the drug is contraindicated in patients with severe renal insufficiency. Prophylaxis should begin 1–2 days before arrival in a malaria-endemic area and continue for 7 days after return (see Table 51–5).

4. Doxycycline—Doxycycline is efficacious and safe and the most inexpensive choice for prophylaxis. Its use is contraindicated in pregnancy, in breast-feeding women, and in children younger than 8 years old. Side effects include gastrointestinal upset, vaginal yeast infections, phototoxicity, hepatic toxicity, pseudomembranous colitis, and increased intracranial pressure. Prophylaxis should begin 1 day before arrival in the malarial area and continue for 4 weeks after return (see Table 51–5).

Clinical Findings

A. Symptoms and Signs

Classic symptoms of malaria in a nonimmune person include chills, headache, and aching. Abdominal pain, vomiting, and diarrhea can also occur. Physical findings include fever, tachycardia, and flushed skin; mental confusion and jaundice may also be present. The spleen and liver are often palpable, especially in persons who have had repeated infections. Severe malarial infection, usually due to *P falciparum,* causes a range of complications that include renal failure, hemoglobinuria, hemolytic anemia, acute respiratory failure, shock, hypoglycemia, and cerebral malaria, with seizures, coma, and death. Long-term complications include hypersplenism, nephrotic syndrome, and seizure disorder.

B. Laboratory Findings

The gold standard for diagnosis remains thick and thin blood smears stained with Giemsa stain. The thick films are more sensitive and the thin smear more accurate for identifying the species of malaria. The smears must be prepared and evaluated in a reputable laboratory, which may not always be available to a traveler when symptoms develop abroad.

Rapid diagnostic "dipstick" tests are available and in selected cases travelers may be given special training in how to use them. The tests should only be considered for travelers to distant malaria-endemic areas without adequate medical facilities and are not generally recommended for travelers. Numerous tests are available, including First Response, NOW Malaria, and One Step. Information on rapid diagnostic tests for malaria available in the United States may be obtained from the following web sites: http://www.binax.com, http://www.bio-quant.com, http://www.rapidtest.com, http://www.globalemed.com, and http://www.premieremed-corp.com. Complete information about these diagnostic tests is also available from the WHO web site, at http://www.wpro.who.int.rdt.

Differential Diagnosis

The differential diagnosis of malaria includes most febrile tropical illnesses prevalent in the area the traveler has visited (see Fever in a Returning Traveler, later). The illnesses most often confused with malaria include influenza and viral infections, dengue fever, babesiosis, relapsing fever, yellow fever, hepatitis, typhoid fever, kala-azar, urinary tract infections, tuberculosis, endocarditis, and meningitis (especially in patients with cerebral symptoms).

Treatment

If the traveler plans to visit a remote area without adequate medical facilities, he or she may wish to take along medication for presumptive treatment if symptoms of malaria develop. Presumptive treatment should not take the place of being evaluated at a medical facility; however, it could be lifesaving if help is not nearby.

Medications that are currently recommended for treatment of malaria include mefloquine and atovaquone-proguanil, but only if these agents are not being used as prophylaxis (see Table 51–5). Sulfadoxine-pyrimethamine (Fansidar) is a popular choice, especially in Africa; however, there is widespread resistance to this agent in many areas of the world. Allergic reactions are a problem, and sulfadoxine-pyrimethamine can cause Stephens–Johnson syndrome, toxic epidermal necrolysis, anemia, thrombocytopenia, seizures, gastrointestinal upset, headaches, tremor, and kernicterus in newborns.

Artemisinin-based combination therapies (ACT) are available abroad but not in the United States. Artemisinin is derived from the plant *Artemisia annua* (sweet wormwood), which has been used for centuries in China for medicinal purposes. Artemisinin derivatives such as artemether and artesunate are well tolerated and are given in combination with another drug such as amodiaquine, sulfadoxine-pyrimethamine, mefloquine, or lumefantrine. Combination therapy has the advantage of slowing the development of drug resistance and reducing the length of required treatment, and it is more effective than monotherapy with any single agent.

More information about ACT, and malaria in general, is available at the Roll Back Malaria web site: http://www.rbm.who.int.

Baird JK: Effectiveness of antimalarial drugs. N Engl J Med 2005;352:1565. [PMID: 15829537]

Chen LH, Keystone JS: New strategies for the prevention of malaria in travelers. Infect Dis Clin North Am 2005;19:185. [PMID: 15701554]

TREATMENT OF THE RETURNING TRAVELER

Despite the best preparations, many travelers become sick while abroad or are ill upon their return home. This section describes three common problems—fever, diarrhea, and eosinophilia—with the goal of assisting the family physician to make a final diagnosis and provide appropriate treatment to the returning traveler. The differential diagnosis depends on the traveler's itinerary, and all possibilities cannot be covered here. Fever and eosinophilia, in particular, may occur as symptoms in a wide range of infections and inflammatory conditions.

Fever in a Returning Traveler

Fever in a returning traveler requires a thorough history (including immunizations and any use of prophylactic medications) and physical examination. Often, localized symptoms or signs (eg, respiratory symptoms, jaundice) help narrow the diagnosis. If the diagnosis is not immediately obvious, consideration must be given to diseases that are endemic in the areas visited. Stable patients may be safely observed for a few days, and most fevers will resolve spontaneously. No definite cause is found in up to 25% of returning travelers with a fever. Fever may have a noninfectious cause, and occult malignancies, systemic lupus erythematosus, and other rheumatologic diseases should be considered in the differential diagnosis.

If illness persists or the patient is unstable, laboratory evaluation becomes the key to the diagnosis. Laboratory studies that may be appropriate include a complete blood count; malaria smear; typhoid culture or antigen test; urinalysis; liver function tests; cultures of blood, urine, and possibly cerebrospinal fluid; stool examination; hepatitis serology; and other serologies, depending on the patient's possible exposure. Acute and convalescent sera are useful in making a final diagnosis. A bone marrow aspirate may be helpful.

If tuberculosis is suspected, the patient should have a chest radiograph and purified protein derivative (PPD) testing for tuberculosis. Seriously ill patients must be hospitalized, and any patient suspected of having a highly contagious condition must be isolated. This is especially true of travelers returning from Africa with hemorrhagic fever. Any suspected case of viral hemorrhagic fever must be reported to the local health department and to the CDC.

Differential diagnoses to consider in a traveler returning with fever are listed in Table 51–6. It is important to remember that "the common is still common" and, in fact, the most common causes of fever in returned travelers are illnesses such as upper and lower respiratory tract infections, sinusitis, urinary tract infections, and influ-

Table 51–6. Selected causes of fever in a returning traveler (not in order of frequency).

Short Incubation (< 28 days)	Long Incubation (> 28 days)
Babesiosis	Brucellosis (some cases)
Bartonellosis	Filariasis
Brucellosis (some cases)	Fungal diseases
Borreliosis	Hepatitis B and C
Cytomegalovirus and other viruses	Acute HIV infection
Dengue fever, yellow fever, and hemorrhagic fever viruses	Leishmaniasis
Endocarditis	Liver abscess (amoebic)
Hepatitis A	Malaria (some cases)
Histoplasmosis and other fungal diseases	Melioidosis
Leptospirosis	Syphilis
Listeriosis	Trypanosomiasis (American and African)
Malaria (some cases)	Tuberculosis
Meningococcemia	
Plague	
Rickettsial diseases	
Sepsis	
Toxoplasmosis	
Traveler's diarrhea	
Typhoid or paratyphoid fever	

enza. Thus, the conditions in Table 51–6 should be considered only if a more common cause is not readily apparent.

Malaria is one of the more common and worrisome causes of fever in a returning traveler, and most cases of serious fevers requiring hospitalization in travelers are due to malaria. Infections, especially with *P falciparum*, often occur within 2 weeks of the mosquito bite but may occur up to 5 years after exposure (especially if caused by *P vivax* or *P ovale*). In a seriously ill febrile traveler for whom no cause can be found, it is wise to include empiric treatment for malaria, even if the results of the blood smear are negative. (Refer to the earlier discussion of malaria.)

Blair JE: Evaluation of fever in the international traveler: Unwanted "souvenir" can have many causes. Postgrad Med 2004:116:13. [PMID: 15274285]

Diarrhea in a Returning Traveler

As discussed earlier, traveler's diarrhea is an acute condition that usually resolves within 2 weeks. Most bacterial infections can be treated successfully with ciprofloxacin. Some travelers, however, develop a persistent diarrhea that can be difficult to diagnose and treat. Among the causes are those related to diet, such as lactase deficiency (which can be treated with lactose restriction for 7–10 days) or transient small bowel bacterial overgrowth (which may require antibiotic treatment). In some travelers, a change from the person's usual diet or consumption of treated water or unpasteurized milk causes a lingering diarrhea termed *Brainerd diarrhea.*

Causes of persistent diarrhea in a returning traveler are listed in Table 51–7. If the patient's response to antibiotic treatment is inadequate or the diarrhea has persisted for at least 14 days, a stool examination should be performed. Two or three stools must be examined. In addition to checking for ova and parasites, evaluation for *Giardia* antigen and bacterial culture should also be performed. If symptoms of rectal disease are present, sigmoidoscopic examination should be done. If the results of all these tests are negative, the physician should consider an empiric trial of metronidazole for treatment of possible *Giardia* infection. Irritable bowel syndrome and, less commonly, inflammatory bowel disease may develop after travel in those who experience a bout of bacterial or viral diarrhea.

Yates J: Traveler's diarrhea. Am Fam Physician 2005;71:2095.

Table 51–7. Selected causes of persistent diarrhea (> 14 days) in a returning traveler.

Parasites, especially *Giardia, Entamoeba histolytica, Cyclospora, Cryptosporidium, Microsporidium*
Bacteria, such as *Campylobacter, Escherichia coli* spp (enteropathogenic or toxin-producing strains), *Shigella, Salmonella, Aeromonas,* noncholera *Vibrios, Yersinia, Clostridium difficile*
Lactase deficiency
Bacterial overgrowth
Irritable bowel disease
Inflammatory bowel syndrome
Idiopathic (Brainerd diarrhea)

Reproduced, with permission, from Yates J: Traveler's diarrhea. Am Fam Physician 2005;71:2095

Eosinophilia in a Returning Traveler

High levels of eosinophilia (> 450 eosinophils per microliter) almost always indicates a parasitic infection. High levels of eosinophilia are a characteristic finding in helminthic infections, especially for those that have an extraintestinal migration phase and produce tissue infection. Strongyloides and lymphatic and tissue filariasis cause some of the highest levels, and infection in humans can persist for many years if not treated. Protozoa such as *Giardia* and *Plasmodium* species do not generally cause eosinophilia, with the exceptions noted in Table 51–8. Schistosomiasis has become a serious problem for people swimming or rafting in freshwater in Africa. Allergic disorders, such as allergic rhinitis and asthma, can also cause eosinophilia. In a study by Schulte and colleagues, a definitive diagnosis could be made in only 36% of 689 returning travelers with eosinophilia.

The workup for a traveler with eosinophilia must include multiple stool examinations, including stool concentration if schistosomiasis is suspected. Biopsy specimens of skin lesions (onchocerciasis) or swollen lymph nodes (filariasis) can be examined for definitive diagnosis. Several serologic tests are available from the CDC or special laboratories. These include tests for toxocariasis, strongyloidiasis, lymphatic filariasis, trichinosis, schistosomiasis, cysticercosis, and paragonimiasis.

Cook GC, Zumla AI: *Manson's Tropical Diseases,* 21st ed. Saunders, 2003.

DuPont HL, Steffen R: *Textbook of Travel Medicine and Health,* 2nd ed. BC Decker, 2001.

Gyawali P, Whitty CJM: Investigating eosinophilia in patients returned from the tropics. Hosp Med 2001;62:25. [PMID: 11211457]

Schulte C et al: Diagnostic significance of blood eosinophilia in returning travelers. Clin Infect Dis 2002;34:407. [PMID: 11753824]

OTHER RESOURCES

Hill DR et al: The practice of travel medicine: Guidelines by the Infectious Diseases Society of America. Clin Infect Dis 2006;43:1499. [PMID: 17109284]

Hunter GW et al: *Hunter's Tropical Medicine and Emerging Infectious Diseases,* 8th ed. Saunders, 2000.

Table 51–8. Selected causes of eosinophilia in a traveler.

Infectious Causes	Noninfectious Causes
Helminthic: Angiostrongyliasis, ascariasis, capillariasis, clonorchiasis, cutaneous larva migrans, echinococcosis, enterobiasis, fasciolopsiasis, filariasis, gnathostomiasis, hookworm, loiasis, onchocerciasis, paragonimiasis, schistosomiasis, strongyloidiasis, toxocariasis, trichinosis Protozoal: *Blastocystis hominis, Dientamoeba fragilis, Isospora belli* Fungal: Bronchopulmonary aspergillosis Viral: Hepatitis B, HIV Ectoparasitic: Scabies Other: Tropical pulmonary eosinophilia (related to tissue filarial infections)	Allergic disorders: Atopic eczema, urticaria, asthma, allergic rhinitis, drug reaction Inflammatory bowel disease Malignancy Vasculitis

Keystone J et al: *Travel Medicine.* Mosby, 2003.

Steffen R et al: *Manual of Travel Medicine and Health,* 2nd ed. BC Decker, 2003.

Zuckerman JN: *Principles & Practice of Travel Medicine.* Wiley, 2001.

WEB SITES

Centers for Disease Control and Prevention:

http://www.cdc.gov/travel (includes advice regarding children, the elderly, and pets; also evaluates cruise ships)

http://www.cdc.gov/travel/outbreaks.htm (to determine if recent outbreaks have occurred in a particular area)

Pan American Health Organization (information on countries in the western hemisphere):

http://www.paho.org

Promed (Program for Monitoring Emerging Diseases; includes a listserve):

http://www.promedmail.org.

Travel Medicine (general travel health information with links to many other sites):

https://www.travmed.com

World Health Organization (worldwide disease surveillance information):

http://www.who.int/

SECTION VI
Psychosocial Disorders

Depression in Diverse Populations 52

Annelle B. Primm, MD, MPH, & Marisela Gomez, MD, PhD, MPH

General Considerations

The Surgeon General's *Report on Mental Health,* issued by former Surgeon General David Satcher, MD, called the nation's attention to the importance of mental health in overall health. The report cited the commonality of mental illness and the fact that undertreatment of mental illness is a huge problem fueled by stigma and barriers to access such as uninsurance and discriminatory insurance coverage. Several demographic groups were identified as being at particularly high risk for having unmet mental health needs: children and youth, older adults, and members of medically underserved ethnic and racial groups. Because these demographic groups rely primarily on the primary care setting for their mental health needs, the report made strong recommendations for an expanded role for primary care physicians and allied health practitioners in the provision of mental health services.

The leading causes of disability (counting lost years of healthy life) in western countries at ages 15–44 years is depression. Depression is estimated to cost the US economy $43 billion annually due to expenses related to care, absenteeism, and reduced productivity on the job, as well as premature death and suicide. In the United States, the point prevalence and lifetime prevalence of depression are 6.6% and 16.6%, respectively. Typical age of onset of major depression is 27–35 years, although depression can occur at any time during the life cycle from childhood to late life. Depression in adolescence and adulthood is more common among women: adult women with depression outnumber men approximately 2:1, and female adolescents outnumber male adolescents approximately 2.5:1. Medical illness and disability—more common in the elderly—are risk factors for depression. (Depression in older patients is discussed in detail in Chapter 41.)

Kessler RC et al: The epidemiology of major depressive disorder: Results from the National Comorbidity Survey Replication (NCS-R). JAMA 2003;289:3095. [PMID: 12813115]

US Department of Health and Human Services: *Mental Health: A Report of the Surgeon General.* National Institute of Mental Health, 2000. Available at: http://www.surgeongeneral.gov/library/mentalhealth/home.html.

Etiology & Pathogenesis of Depression

Potentially lethal, depression is associated with abnormal functioning of the brain and can cause prolonged suffering. Depression often has a genetic basis, and clusters of affected individuals may occur within families. In the absence of a family history of depression, neurodegenerative disorders, stroke, thyroid disorders, epilepsy, metabolic disorders, cancer, and infection (eg, HIV/AIDS) are just some of the conditions that may involve or cause a depressed state. Additionally, acute and chronic socioenvironmental stimuli, negative life events, and stressful situations may lead to depression.

There is a spectrum of type and level of severity of depression, ranging from subclinical varieties to major depression. The type of depression relates to the number and intensity of the following symptoms: sadness, anxiety, or irritability; low self-esteem; and a diminished sense of well-being with negative effects on sleep, appetite, motivation, energy, and intellectual functioning.

Major depression typically occurs in episodes, with a clear beginning and end. An individual with major depression exhibits symptoms that represent a change

Table 52–1. Incidence of depression co-occurring with other medical illnesses.

Medical Condition	Patients with Depression (%)
Myocardial infarction (MI)	40–65
Coronary artery disease (without MI)	18–20
Parkinson disease	40
Multiple sclerosis	40
Stroke	10–27
Cancer	25
Diabetes mellitus	25

from his or her usual level of functioning. After an episode of major depression, the person returns to his or her baseline, but there is a high likelihood of additional episodes. Fifty percent of those who have one episode will have a second episode, and with each additional episode, the risk of relapse is greater. The propensity for relapse is the reason why major depression is often regarded as a chronic disease.

Prevention

The American Academy of Family Physicians states that mental health services are an integral component of the continuum of care in the primary care setting. However, the reluctance of individuals to seek care for mental health problems along with a likelihood of somatization of emotional issues pose giant obstacles for mental health care in these settings. Studies report that approximately 40% of patients with major depression do not want or perceive the need for treatment. Only 20–30% of patients with emotional or psychological issues report these to their primary care physicians, and 80% of patients with depression present initially with physical symptoms such as pain or fatigue or worsening symptoms of a chronic medical illness. Table 52–1 lists common medical conditions that may lead to or co-occur with depression.

A. Depression and Other Chronic Illnesses

Depression is an independent risk factor in the development of cardiovascular diseases (heart disease, stroke), commonly co-occurring with hypertension and congestive heart failure. Stroke, a frequent complication of heart disease and diabetes, is also independently associated with depression. Other chronic conditions that frequently co-occur with depression include HIV/AIDS, arthritis and chronic pain syndromes, sickle cell disease, and cancer. Depression has an impact on a person's ability to follow a treatment plan, including adherence to medication or other therapies, diet, and exercise. Depression commonly co-occurs with chronic diseases, complicating treatment, threatening chronic disease outcome, and contributing to high health care costs.

Chronic diseases, such as cardiovascular diseases (stroke and heart disease), diabetes mellitus, and cancer are among the most prevalent, costly, and preventable of all health problems, accounting for one third of the years of potential life lost before age 65. Meanwhile, the top three risk factors causing death are tobacco use, physical inactivity and poor diet, and alcohol use. These risk factors correlate closely with the leading causes of death mentioned above. Interestingly, depression has been linked to all three of these risk factors. Hence, screening, diagnosis, and treatment of depression could have an impact on the course and management of chronic diseases and could serve as a preventive measure in helping to reduce an individual's risk for multiple chronic diseases.

Depression is one of the most common complications of chronic diseases and medical conditions. Individuals with chronic diseases must cope with the stress of their illness and any treatment they are undertaking. Their self-perception ("sick" role) along with disease-related limitations can lead to psychological and physical challenges, resulting in depression. In addition, some chronic diseases (eg, HIV/AIDS, multiple sclerosis, systemic lupus erythematosus) may cause depression through direct or indirect effects on brain chemistry. Although approximately one third of individuals with chronic medical conditions may experience symptoms of depression (see Table 52–1), individuals with chronic illnesses often overlook symptoms and signs of depression, assuming that feeling "down" or depressed is normal while living with a serious, chronic illness. In addition, because symptoms and signs of depression are frequently masked by other medical conditions, health care providers treating individuals with chronic diseases may not recognize that the underlying cause of depressed mood, decreased energy, sleep changes, or appetite changes is depression. Therefore, a high index of suspicion should be maintained when treating patients who present with symptoms and signs of physical chronic conditions, multiple somatic complaints, or chronic pain complaints, and screening should be utilized in these populations with consistent systems in place for diagnosis, treatment, and follow-up.

B. Impact of Health Disparities

The prevalence of depression among racial and ethnic groups is very similar when adjusted for other social and health-related factors. However, when adjusted for these factors, disparities exist by race and ethnicity in the diagnosis and treatment of depression. African Americans and Hispanics with depression are less likely than whites to have their condition diagnosed or treated properly, or to receive treatment from mental health sectors (eg, psychiatrists). In addition, individuals with less than 16 years of education are more likely than those with postsecondary education to receive mental health care from general medical services. Despite increases in the rate of antidepressant medication use over the past 12 years among all racial and ethnic groups, this increase has been disproportionately higher in whites compared with non-Hispanic blacks.

Over the past decade, the discrepancy between receipt of treatment for mental disorders for whites and non-Hispanic blacks increased by more than 100%. Overall, studies show that racial and ethnic disparities exist in mental health status in general, utilization of mental health services, quality of care and outcome regardless of socioeconomic status in the four major underserved ethnic and racial groups: African Americans, American Indians, Asian Americans, and Hispanics. For nonwhite populations, the chronic stress of discrimination and subsequent effects on immune regulation of living as a member of a marginalized racial and ethnic group can lead to depression. The increased risk of living in poverty with inadequate access to health care and inadequate treatment, more prevalent in populations of color, may multiply this stress and result in persistent and recurring episodes of depression.

Risk of mental illness and poor mental health outcomes in African American and other underserved populations is also increased due to nonfamilial factors associated with depression (eg, socioeconomic status, environmental factors, access to health care, cultural incompetence in the health care system, and higher rates of health disorders). Because of the independent increased risk of chronic diseases and mental illness in minority racial and ethnic populations, the impact of mental illness on chronic diseases is increased substantially, if not exponentially. Combining the social determinants of depression with the stigma of mental illness experienced by most racial and ethnic groups, the risk that depression will co-occur with and complicate the course, management, and outcome of chronic diseases is further increased. For these reasons, primary care practitioners must be vigilant in screening for depression all populations presenting with chronic illnesses. This standard of care would serve to minimize and prevent the historic and potential disparate care for minority groups at greater risk for both depression and other chronic medical conditions. These practices would also assure an equal playing field in primary care settings for access, diagnosis, and treatment for all populations at risk for the co-occurrence of depression and chronic illnesses.

Applied Research Center and Northwest Federation of Community Organizations. Closing the Gap: Solutions to Race-Based Health Disparities, 2005. Available at: http://www.arc.org/Pages/pubs/closinggap_b.html.

Centers for Disease Control and Prevention (CDC): Racial/ethnic disparities in prevalence, treatment, and control of hypertension—United States, 1999–2002. MMWR Morb Mortal Wkly Rep 2005;54:7. [PMID: 15647724]

Corson K et al: Screening for depression and suicidality in a VA primary care setting: 2 items are better than 1 item. Am J Manag Care 2004;10(Pt 2):839. [PMID: 15609737]

Kessler RC et al: Prevalence and treatment of mental disorders, 1990 to 2003. N Engl J Med 2005;352:2515. [PMID: 15958807]

Smedley BD et al, eds: *Unequal Treatment: Confronting Racial and Ethnic Disparities in Health Care.* National Academy Press, 2003.

Turner RJ et al: Personal resources and depression in the transition to adulthood: Ethnic comparisons. J Health Soc Behav 2004; 45:34. [PMID: 15179906]

US Department of Health and Human Services: *Mental Health: Culture, Race and Ethnicity—A Supplement to Mental Health: A Report of the Surgeon General.* DHHS, 2001.

US National Healthcare Disparities Report, 2004. Agency for Healthcare Research and Quality (AHRQ), 2005. Available at: http://www.qualitytools.ahrq.gov/disparitiesreport/.

US Preventive Services Task Force: Screening for depression: Recommendations and rationale. Ann Intern Med 2002;136:760. [PMID: 12020145]

Wells K et al: Impact of disseminating quality improvement programs for depression in managed primary care: A randomized controlled trial. JAMA 2000;283:212. [PMID: 10634337]

Clinical Findings

A. Symptoms and Signs

The *Diagnostic and Statistical Manual of Mental Disorders,* Fourth Edition, Text Revision (*DSM-IV-TR*) classifies depressive disorders into three categories: major depressive disorder, dysthymic disorder, and depressive disorder not otherwise specified. Specific features associated with these disorders are described below.

1. Major depressive disorder—The nine features typical of a major depressive episode are:

- **Depressed mood:** Feeling sad, low, empty, hopeless, gloomy, or down in the dumps; different from a normal sense of sadness or grief.
- **Anhedonia:** Inability to enjoy usual activities (eg, sex, hobbies, daily routines).
- **Change in appetite or weight:** A decrease in appetite (most patients) or an increase in appetite associated with craving specific foods.
- **Change in sleep pattern:** Insomnia (difficulty falling asleep, staying asleep, or waking early) in most patients; hypersomnia in some.
- **Change in activity:** Retardation of psychomotor activities (speech, thinking, movement) or increased or agitated psychomotor activities (cannot sit still, pacing, hand wringing).
- **Loss of energy:** Decreased energy, tiredness, fatigue.
- **Cognitive changes:** Inability to think, concentrate, or make decisions.
- **Sense of worthlessness or guilt:** Excessive feelings of low self-esteem, self-blame, and lack of self-worth.

- **Thoughts of death or suicide** (including suicidal ideation, suicidal attempts).

In more than 90% of patients diagnosed with a major depressive disorder (characterized by several major depressive episodes), two of these nine features are present: depressed mood or anhedonia (the loss of interest or pleasure) that predominates for at least 2 weeks and causes significant distress or impairment in the individual's social, occupational, or other important areas of functioning. Four additional features must be present during this same 2-week period for the patient to be diagnosed with the disorder.

2. Dysthymic disorder—Dysthymic disorder is distinguished by a chronically depressed mood that occurs for most of the day more days than not for at least 2 years. Individuals described their mood as sad or "down in the dumps." Periods of depressed moods often include at least two of the following: poor appetite or overeating, insomnia or hypersomnia, low energy or fatigue, low self-esteem, poor concentration or difficulty making decisions, and feelings of hopelessness.

3. Depressive disorders not otherwise specified—This *DSM-IV-TR* category encompasses four distinct presentations. Symptoms of *premenstrual dysphoric disorder* (markedly depressed mood, marked anxiety, marked affective lability, decreased interest in activities) regularly occur during the last week of the luteal phase and resolve a few days after onset of menses. *Depression due to a medical condition* is suspected when the history, physical examination, or laboratory findings indicate that a prominent and persistent depressed mood or markedly diminished interest or pleasure in all or almost all activities is the direct physiologic consequence of a general medical condition. *Seasonal affective disorder (SAD)* is characterized by episodes of hypersomnia, anergia, and a craving for sweets associated with a particular time of the year. It usually occurs in the winter months and resolves in the spring. *Substance-induced mood disorder* refers to prominent and persistent depressed mood that is due to the direct physiologic effects of a substance (drug of abuse, medication, toxin).

B. Screening Measures

1. Depression—The US Preventive Services Task Force (USPSTF) 2005 guidelines and the American Academy of Family Physicians recommend screening for depression in the primary care setting using a two-question initial screening test to detect the presence of depressed mood and anhedonia ("Over the past 2 weeks, have you felt down, depressed or hopeless?" and "Over the past 2 weeks, have you felt little interest or pleasure in doing things?"). These are the first two questions of the nine–question Patient Health Questionnaire (PHQ-9), a screening tool for depression developed and validated in mental health and primary care settings and based on the *DSM-IV-TR*. A positive response to either question requires a more detailed clinical interview or a more specific tool that uses standard diagnostic criteria (ie, *DSM-IV-TR*) to determine the presence or absence of specific depressive disorders, such as major depression or dysthymia, and severity of depression. The presence and severity of depression and co-occurring psychological problems (eg, anxiety, panic attacks, or substance abuse) also should be identified.

Table 52–2. Depression screening instruments commonly used in primary care settings.

Beck Depression Inventory
Center for Epidemiologic Studies Depression Screen (CES-D)
General Health Questionnaire
Medical Outcomes Study Depression Screen
Patient Health Questionnaire (PHQ-9)
Primary Care Evaluation of Mental Disorders
Symptom-Driven Diagnostic System–Primary Care
Zung Self-Assessment Depression Scale

Table 52–2 lists several screening instruments for depression and suicide. The PHQ-9 appears to perform as well as longer instruments. Positive findings from an instrument and clinical interview, resulting in a diagnosis of major depression, must be followed up with appropriate treatment and monitoring. Studies show that when compared with usual care, screening for depression can improve outcomes, particularly when screening is coupled with system changes that help ensure adequate treatment and follow-up.

2. Suicide—Risk factors for attempted suicide include mood disorders or other mental disorders, comorbid substance abuse disorders, history of deliberate self-harm, and history of suicide attempts. Suicide risk is determined along a continuum ranging from suicidal ideation alone (relatively less severe) to suicidal ideation with a plan (more severe, associated with a significant risk for attempted suicide). Currently, the most commonly used screening instruments to determine risk for suicide (ie, the Scale for Suicide Ideation [SSI], Scale for Suicide Ideation-Worst [SSI-W], and the Suicidal Ideation Questionnaire [SIQ)]) have not been validated in primary care settings. However, some instruments for detecting risk of depression (eg, PHQ-9) identify the presence of suicidal ideation. Once a risk of suicide is established, referral to specialty mental health services is indicated.

American Psychiatric Association: *Diagnostic and Statistical Manual*, 4th ed, text revision. APA, 2000.

Kroenke K et al: The patient health questionnaire-2: Validity of a two-item depression screener. Med Care 2003;41:1284. [PMID: 14583691]

Pignone MP et al: Screening for depression in adults: A summary of the evidence for the U.S. Preventive Services Task Force. Ann Intern Med 2002;136:765. [PMID: 12020146]

Schulberg HC et al: Preventing suicide in primary care patients: The primary care physician's role. Gen Hosp Psychiatry 2004;26:337. [PMID: 15474633]

US Preventive Medicine Task Force: *The Guide to Clinical Preventive Services 2005. Screening for Depression.* Available at: http://www.ahrq.gov/clinic/pocketgd.pdf.

WEB SITE

PHQ-9 is available online from the MacArthur Foundation at: http://www.depression-primarycare.org/clinicians/toolkits.

Treatment

Primary care providers are the sole contacts for more than 50% of patients with mental illness and therefore become an important determinant in assuring recognition and treatment of depression. Treatment of mental disorders has increased substantially over the past decades, and since the early 1990s, an increase of more than 150% in the rate of treatment in the sector of general medical services has occurred. Despite this increased rate of treatment, the majority of adults with mental disorders do not receive treatment. Additionally, many patients receiving treatment in this sector of services did not receive a complete clinical assessment or receive treatment or appropriate ongoing monitoring in accordance with accepted standards of care. Predictors of receiving guideline-concordant care include being white, female, severely ill, and having mental health insurance coverage.

Effective treatments—including psychopharmacologic, psychotherapeutic (behavioral or counseling), and complementary and alternative therapies—and combinations of these are available for depressed patients identified in primary care settings. Treatment guidelines of the American Psychiatric Association (APA), as well as multiple research studies, confirm differential effectiveness of these therapies in individuals diagnosed with depression. Selection of an initial treatment modality should be influenced by both clinical (eg, severity of symptoms) and other factors (eg, patient preference). In general, evidence-based recommendation for treatment of moderate to severe depression in the primary care setting involves a combination of pharmacotherapy and psychotherapy, and for the treatment of mild to moderate depression, psychotherapy alone.

A. Psychotherapeutic Interventions (Behavioral Therapy or Counseling)

Effective psychotherapy alone as an initial treatment modality may be considered for patients with mild to moderate major depressive disorder. Cognitive-behavioral therapy (CBT) and interpersonal therapy are psychotherapeutic approaches used in the treatment of patients with major depressive disorder, with documented beneficial outcomes. The physician should consider multiple factors when determining the frequency for individual patients, including the specific type and goals of psychotherapy, the frequency necessary to create and maintain a therapeutic relationship, the frequency of visits required to ensure treatment adherence, and the frequency necessary to monitor and address suicidality. If the regimen needed to address these parameters cannot be met in the primary care setting, referral for specialty mental health services may be indicated (to psychiatric nurses, counselors, psychologists, or psychiatrists either attached to the practice or in other organizations). However the service is provided, every physician has an obligation to ensure that patients are made aware of psychotherapy as an option and are assisted in accessing it.

B. Pharmacotherapy

Antidepressant medications may be provided as an initial primary treatment for patients with mild symptoms of major depressive disorder, and these medications should be provided for all patients with moderate to severe symptoms. Improved outcome should be noted within 6–8 weeks of initiating therapy. The most commonly used antidepressant medications are listed in Table 52–3.

The APA guidelines for treatment of depression state that the "initial selection of an antidepressant medication will largely be based on the anticipated side effects, the safety or tolerability of these side effects for individual patients, patient preference, quantity and quality of clinical trial data regarding the medication, and its cost." The following medications are likely to be optimal for most patients: selective serotonin reuptake inhibitors (SSRIs), desipramine, nortriptyline, bupropion, and venlafaxine. Because of their potential to cause serious side effects and the need for dietary restrictions, monoamine oxidase inhibitors (MAOIs) typically are reserved for patients who do not respond to other treatments. SSRIs are usually first-line of therapy due to their less problematic side effects. Patients prescribed antidepressant medication should be monitored to assess their response to pharmacotherapy as well as the emergence of side effects, clinical condition, and safety. If no response is seen within the initial 6- to 8-week period of pharmacologic therapy, referral for specialty mental health care may be needed.

C. Complementary and Alternative Therapies

Increasing evidence in the medical literature supports the beneficial role of spirituality in the health of patients. Some studies show a beneficial effect of exercise programs in treatment of depression, in comparison to antidepressant medication alone. Meditation-based cognitive therapy has been shown to be effective for treatment of and decreasing recurrence of major depressive disorder.

Table 52–3. Pharmacologic agents used in treatment of depression.

Drug Class and Agents	Starting Dose (mg/day)	Usual Dose (mg/day)
Dopamine-Norepinephrine Reuptake Inhibitors		
Bupropion[1]	150	300
Bupropion, sustained release	150	300
MAOIs		
Irreversible, nonselective		
Phenelzine	15	15–90
Tranylcypromine	10	30–60
Reversible MAOI-A		
Moclobemide	150	300–600
Norepinephrine-Serotonin Modulator		
Mirtazapine	15	15–45
Serotonin Modulators		
Nefazodone	50	150–300
Trazodone	50	75–300
Serotonin-Norepinephrine Reuptake Inhibitors		
Duloxetine	40	40–120
Venlafaxine	37.5	75–225
Venlafaxine, extended release	37.5	75–225
SSRIs[1]		
Citalopram	20	20–60
Escitalopram[2]	10	10
Fluoxetine	20	20–60
Fluvoxamine	50	50–300
Paroxetine	20	20–60
Sertraline	50	50–200
Tricyclics and Tetracyclics		
Tertiary amine tricyclics		
Amitriptyline	25–50	100–300
Clomipramine	25	100–250
Doxepin	25–50	100–300
Imipramine	25–50	100–300
Trimipramine	25–50	100–300
Secondary amine tricyclics		
Desipramine[1]	25–50	100–300
Nortriptyline[1]	25	50–150
Protriptyline	10	15–60
Tetracyclics		
Amoxapine	50	100–400
Maprotiline	50	100–225

MAOI, monoamine oxidase inhibitor; SSRI, selective serotonin reuptake inhibitor.

[1]Optimal medications in terms of the patient's acceptance of side effects, safety.

[2]New medications recently approved based on premarketing research. Caution should be used until long-term outcomes are reported.

D. Combination Therapy

The combination of a specific effective psychotherapy and medication is recommended for patients with moderate to severe depression associated with psychosocial issues and interpersonal problems. Patients who have had a history of only partial response to adequate trials of either treatment alone may benefit from combined treatment. Patients with poor adherence to individual treatments may also benefit from combined treatment of any form. Most studies of CBT support its use either alone or in addition to pharmacotherapy in decreasing depressive recurrence. Incorporating spirituality into different forms of psychotherapy has been shown to be effective in improving other modalities of treatment, reducing relapse rates, and enhancing functional recovery for depression.

E. Quality Improvement Programs

Increasingly, studies have shown that several resources should be incorporated into primary care settings to enhance diagnosis and treatment outcomes for individuals with depression in these settings. The general constituents of these programs are assessment, diagnosis, treatment, and follow-up. Several intervention programs, which have shown improved outcomes for patients with depression for up to 5 years in primary care settings across the United States, delineate an emphasis on quality improvement that includes provider training (in counseling, psychotherapy, medication management), nurse assessment, patient education, resources to support medication management or evidence-based psychotherapy, and consistent follow-up at set intervals. Primary care settings instituting variations of these basic criteria or interventions show consistent improvement in outcomes across different cultural groups (race and ethnicity, gender, age, urban vs rural) compared with regular care (without interventions).

F. Cultural Competence

Lack of cultural competence may result in underdiagnosis and misdiagnosis of depression. Studies have shown that different racial and ethnic groups, as well as age and gender groups, experience and communicate symptoms of depression differently and prefer different forms of treatment. For example, among Latinos, depression is often expressed largely in somatic terms (eg, "nerves" or headaches). Asian patients may present similarly with somatic complaints during a depressive episode highlighting feelings of weakness, tiredness, or "imbalance." Consequently, physicians responding to different cultural populations must recognize and consider this diversity if they are to provide the most effective care (Table 52–4).

Table 52–4. Prerequisites for cultural competence in assessment, diagnosis, and treatment of depression.

Recognition of:
Language differences
Health literacy barriers
Somatic presentations
Use of cultural idioms of distress
Treatment preference
Nonwestern context of mental illness and care (eg, spirituality and balance, herbs, nature, relational, circular, mind/body/spirit, present oriented)

Underrecognition of depression among immigrant populations and Latinos may be related to language differences, health literacy barriers, somatic presentations, and use of culturally based idioms of distress. In addition, among African American, American Indian, and Alaska Native people and Latinos, negative stigma still exist around depression and other forms of mental illness, creating obstacles to affected individuals identifying and seeking appropriate medical care. For example, the Latino population, as a group, appears more receptive to psychotherapy or combined counseling and medication than to pharmacotherapy alone, although both may be efficacious.

Such barriers can be overcome. Recent studies have shown that Chinese Americans report symptoms of depression in response to a Chinese language version of the Beck Depression Inventory. Once providers develop sensitivity for discerning differing presentations of depression, assessment and treatment can proceed. Reports show that various cultural minority groups, including elderly blacks and Latinos, adult Asians, Latinos, and African Americans, respond similarly to whites in depression treatment and follow up, once identified.

Agency for Health Care Policy and Research: *Depression in Primary Care, Vol 2: Treatment of Major Depression.* US Department of Health and Human Services, 1993.

American Academy of Family Physicians: *Mental Health Care Services by Family Physicians.* Available at: http://www.aafp.org.

American Psychiatric Association: *Practice Guideline for the Treatment of Patients With Major Depressive Disorder,* 2nd ed. Available at: http://www.psych.org/psych_pract/treatg/pg/Depression2e.book-7.cfm#ai.

Arean PA et al: Improving depression care for older, minority patients in primary care. Med Care 2005;43:381. [PMID: 15778641]

D'Souza RF et al: Spiritually augmented cognitive behavioural therapy. Australas Psychiatry 2004;12:148. [PMID: 15715760]

Grandbois D: Stigma of mental illness among American Indian and Alaska Native nations: Historical and contemporary perspectives. Issues Ment Health Nurs 2005;26:1001. [PMID: 16283996]

Katon W et al: Long-term effects of a collaborative care intervention in persistently depressed primary care patients. J Gen Intern Med 2002;17:741. [PMID: 12390549]

Lewis-Fernandez R et al: Depression in US Hispanics: Diagnostic and management considerations in family practice. J Am Board Fam Pract 2005;18:282. [PMID: 15994474]

Mason O et al: A qualitative study of mindfulness-based cognitive therapy for depression. Br J Med Psychol 2001;74:197. [PMID: 11802836]

Primm A et al: The acceptability of a culturally-tailored depression education videotape to African Americans. J Natl Med Assoc 2002;94:1007. [PMID: 12443007]

Robinson WD et al: Depression treatment in primary care. J Am Board Fam Pract 2005;18:79. [PMID: 15798136]

Smith JL et al: A primary care intervention for depression. J Rural Health 2001;16:313. [PMID: 11218319]

Wells K et al: Five-year impact of quality improvement for depression: Results of a group-level randomized controlled trial. Arch Gen Psychiatry 2004;61:378. [PMID: 15066896]

Wells K et al: Quality improvement for depression in primary care: Do patients with subthreshold depression benefit in the long run? Am J Psychiatry 2005;162:1149. [PMID: 15930064]

Yeung A et al: Use of the Chinese version of the Beck Depression Inventory for screening depression in primary care. J Nerv Ment Dis 2002;190:94. [PMID: 11889362]

Anxiety Disorders

53

Philip J. Michels, PhD, Jamee H. Lucas, MD, & Sharm Steadman, PharmD

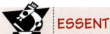

ESSENTIALS OF DIAGNOSIS

- *Feelings of apprehension, anxiety, or panic in situations that do not call for fear or to a degree that is excessive for the situation.*
- *Diagnosis is usually a process of exclusion and is based on patient history.*

General Considerations

Anxiety is a diffuse, unpleasant, and often vague subjective feeling of apprehension accompanied by objective symptoms of autonomic nervous system arousal. The experience of anxiety is associated with a sense of danger or a lack of control over events. The psychological component varies from individual to individual and is strongly influenced by personality and coping mechanisms.

Many factors contribute to the experience of anxiety by individuals in our society. We live in a rapidly changing culture characterized by continuous technologic advancements, proliferation of ever more refined information, and a mass media and entertainment industry saturated with violence and sexuality, all of which promote feelings of insecurity. In the workplace, downsizing, restructuring, mergers, and specialization are commonplace; transient work relationships and the elimination of benefits such as health insurance and retirement provisions increase the sense of insecurity.

Anxiety is pathologic when it occurs in situations that do not call for fear or when the degree of anxiety is excessive for the situation. Anxiety may occur as a result of life events, as a symptom of a primary anxiety disorder, as a secondary response to another psychiatric disorder or medical illness, or as a side effect of a medication.

The majority of individuals with mental disorders receive psychiatric care from primary care settings, whereas less than 20% receive care in specialized mental health settings. Among mental disorders, anxiety disorders have the highest overall prevalence rate, yet only 23% of anxious patients receive treatment. Patients with anxiety disorders are at increased risk of other medical comorbidities, longer hospital stays, more procedures, higher overall health care costs, failure in school or at work, low-paying jobs, and financial dependence in the form of welfare or other government subsidies.

Mendlowicz MV, Stein MB: Quality of life in individuals with anxiety disorders. Am J Psychiatry 2000;157:669. [PMID: 10784456]

Pathogenesis

A. Biomedical Influences

Because the symptoms of anxiety are so varied and prevalent, several etiologies exist to explain them. A recent meta-analysis revealed a significant genetic component, especially for panic disorder, generalized anxiety, and phobias. Temperament, which has genetic roots, is a broad vulnerability factor for anxiety disorders.

The inhibitory transmitter γ-aminobutyric acid (GABA) occupies about 40% of all synapses and is clearly implicated in the anxiety disorders, as is the endocrine system. Exposure to a stressor activates the release of an endogenous opioid, β-endorphin, which is co-released with adrenocorticotropic hormone.

B. Psychological Influences

Family dysfunction and parental psychopathology are involved in the development and maintenance of anxiety. Families of anxious children are more involved, controlling, and rejecting, and less intimate than are families who do not manifest anxiety. Parents of anxious children promote cautious and avoidant child behavior.

Behavioral and cognitive explanations define anxiety as a learned response. Anxiety develops in response to neutral or positive stimuli that become associated with a noxious or aversive event. Fearful associations develop from the situational context and the physical sensations present at the time. The patient may generalize (ie, classify objects and events based on a common characteristic) and thereby establish new cues to trigger anxiety. Previously neutral situations become feared and avoided. By avoiding anxiety-arousing stimuli, anxiety is diminished.

As panic and avoidance become more chronic, the behaviors involved become more habitual and awareness of one's thoughts in relation to these anxiety states diminishes. Information-processing prejudices such as selectively attending to threatening stimuli become involuntary and unconscious. A person's appraisal of an event, rather than intrinsic characteristics of that event, defines stress, evokes anxiety, and influences the ability to cope. Failure to cope elicits fear and vulnerability.

Kagan J, Snidman N: Early childhood predictors of adult anxiety disorders. Biol Psychiatry 1999;46:1536. [PMID: 10599481]

Prevention

Training in stress inoculation, relaxation training, and cognitive-behavioral therapy can be implemented through an integrated curriculum in public education during the early and middle years. School settings provide furtive environments for group modeling and an opportunity to reach large numbers of people. The work of Dr Martin Seligman (see Gillham et al) demonstrates the sizable advantages of such school-based programs.

Gillham JR et al: Prevention of depressive symptoms in schoolchildren: Two-year follow-up. Psychol Sci 1995;6:343.

Clinical Findings

A. Symptoms and Signs

Examination of the patient usually yields few clues to assist in establishing the diagnosis of an anxiety disorder. Diagnosis is complicated by the amount of symptoms and their overlap with other disease states; thus anxiety often becomes a diagnosis of exclusion. Table 53–1 lists various symptoms of anxiety by organ system.

Despite the variety and diffuse nature of many of these symptoms, anxiety disorders can often be identified by exploration of the patient's history, along with a few laboratory values. The symptoms of each anxiety disorder are sufficiently specific to arrive at the diagnosis by taking a thorough history from the patient, including pertinent past, social, and family information. Recognition of anxiety subtypes is often made on the basis of history alone.

B. Diagnostic Criteria

The *Diagnostic and Statistical Manual of Mental Disorders,* Fourth Edition, Text Revision *(DSM-IV-TR)* differentiates several anxiety disorders. Diagnostic criteria for each disorder are presented below.

1. Panic disorder—A **panic attack** involves a discrete period of intense fear or discomfort that has a sudden onset, rapidly builds to a peak, usually in 10 minutes or less, and is often accompanied by a sense of imminent danger or impending doom and an urge to escape. About 33–50% of panic-stricken people from community samples have **agoraphobia,** a fear of being in places or situations from which escape might be difficult or embarrassing or in which help may not be available. Individuals suffering from panic disorder without agoraphobia have higher success rates than those with agoraphobia.

2. Simple phobias—A **phobia** refers to significant, provoked, and irrational anxiety that a person experiences when near a specific object or situation that is feared. Patients with simple phobias do not usually seek treatment. They avoid the particular object or situation that evokes anxiety.

3. Social phobia—A social phobia involves clinically significant anxiety that occurs when an individual is exposed to certain types of social or performance situations. The lifetime prevalence of social phobia is estimated to be as high as 13%. Social phobia affects most areas of life, particularly education, career, and romantic relationships.

4. Obsessive-compulsive disorder (OCD)—OCD involves intrusive thoughts that cause marked anxiety or distress. Compulsions (compelling acts) neutralize anxiety. The disorder typically stages as Obsession → Anxiety → Compulsion → Relief. Onset is usually gradual and the course is typically chronic. Up to 80% of patients with OCD evidence depression, anxiety, substance abuse, work disability, or all of these findings.

5. Post-traumatic stress disorder (PTSD)—PTSD involves the patient reexperiencing an extremely traumatic event accompanied by symptoms of increased arousal and avoidance of stimuli associated with the trauma. Rape, war-related stress, assault, and accidents commonly precipitate PTSD. The traumatizing effect is linked to the fact that these events are unexpected, uncontrollable, or inescapable. Optimally, new experiences are assimilated and

Table 53–1. Somatic symptoms of anxiety.

System	Symptoms
Musculoskeletal	Muscle tightness, spasms, back pain, headache, weakness, tremors, fatigue, restlessness, exaggerated startle response, jitters
Cardiovascular	Palpitations, rapid heartbeat, hot and cold spells, flushing, pallor
Gastrointestinal	Dry mouth, diarrhea, upset stomach, lump in throat, nausea, vomiting
Bladder	Frequent urination
Central nervous	Dizziness, paresthesias, light-headedness
Respiratory	Hyperventilation, shortness of breath, constriction in chest
Miscellaneous	Sweating, clammy hands

Source: Sharma R, et al: Anxiety states. In: Flauherty et al, eds: Psychiatry: *Diagnosis and Treatment.* Appleton & Lange, 1993.

expressed. Acute stress disorder entails the same PTSD-type symptoms, which occur immediately in the aftermath of a traumatic event but resolve within 4 weeks.

6. Generalized anxiety disorder (GAD)—GAD involves at least 6 months of persistent and excessive anxiety and worry with an inability to stop worrying. These chronic worriers commonly display insomnia; feel irritable, tense, and tired; and have difficulty concentrating. The degree of comorbidity between GAD and other psychiatric disorders is high. Patients with GAD show higher general medical utilization than patients with depression.

7. Substance-induced anxiety disorder—In this disorder, anxiety is a direct physiologic consequence of a drug of abuse, medication, or exposure to a toxin.

8. Adjustment disorder with anxious mood—In patients with this disorder, clinically significant symptoms of anxiety occur in response to an identifiable stressor within 3 months after the onset of the stressor and resolve within 6 months after the termination of the stressor. However, symptoms may persist longer if they occur in response to a chronic stressor (eg, a disabling chronic medical condition) or to a stressor that has enduring consequences (eg, financial effects of a divorce).

9. Anxiety disorder due to a general medical condition—In this disorder, prominent symptoms of anxiety are judged to be a direct physiologic consequence of a general medical condition. It is estimated that up to 20% of medical patients experience anxiety during the course of their medical illness.

When organic etiology is ruled out of a **somatizing** presentation, the patients involved usually are less educated, have psychiatric disorders, and belong to a culture that deemphasizes emotional displays while focusing on bodily concerns. Many of these patients lack social support and have suffered trauma.

C. Laboratory Findings

There are no gold standard laboratory studies to diagnose anxiety disorders. It is reasonable to perform a limited empiric evaluation to identify the etiology of the symptoms as well as evaluate for comorbid medical problems that may complicate the treatment. This evaluation may include a complete blood count, electrolyte, glucose, creatinine, calcium, liver panel, and thyroid function test. Further testing should be tailored on an individual basis, depending on the clinical circumstances. Urine drug screening should be considered, because illicit drug use and withdrawal may be a possible differential diagnosis and patients with anxiety may self-medicate with drugs of abuse.

Fricchione G: Clinical practice. Generalized anxiety disorder. N Engl J Med 2004;351:675. [PMID: 15306669]

D. Imaging Studies

Although functional magnetic resonance imaging may eventually allow identification of the specific neural events underlying symptom reports, there are no imaging studies that diagnose anxiety disorder. Imaging studies are completed only to preclude any laboratory abnormalities or organic disease that may mimic anxiety or panic. Such studies include but are not limited to thyroid scan and cardiac diagnostics.

E. Special Tests

Psychological tests resort to self-report of symptoms and are major assessment tools for anxiety. This is unfortunate given that most other medical diagnoses (eg, diabetes mellitus) rely on both symptom self-report and systematic biomedical measurements (eg, the glucose tolerance test).

The State-Trait Anxiety Inventory measures the frequency and intensity of transient anxiety processes and anxiety proneness as a character trait. Other validated measures are the Anxiety Sensitivity Inventory, Agoraphobic Cognitions and Body Sensations Questionnaires, and the Panic Belief Questionnaire.

Comorbidity can comprehensively be assessed by the Minnesota Multiphasic Personality Inventory-II (MMPI-2), a test composed of 567 true–false test items that can be completed in about 2 hours. The Profile of Mood States (POMS) primarily measures mood states in psychiatric outpatients. Its advantage over the MMPI-2 is a completion time of about 10 minutes.

Chambless DL et al: The assessment of fear in agoraphobics: The Body Sensations Questionnaire and the agoraphobic cognitions questionnaire. J Consult Clin Psychol 1984;52:1090. [PMID: 6520279]

Hathaway SR, McKinley C: *Minnesota Multiphasic Personality Inventory-2.* National Computer Systems, University of Minnesota, 1989.

McNair DM et al: *Profile of Mood States, Revised.* Educational and Industrial Testing Service, 1992.

Peterson RA, Reiss S: *Manual for the Anxiety Sensitivity Index,* 2nd ed. International Diagnostic Services, 1992.

Spielberger CD: *State-Trait Anxiety Inventory.* Consulting Psychologists Press, 1983.

Differential Diagnosis

Because anxiety is an ubiquitous symptom of numerous conditions, family physicians must be alert to the possibility of alternative medical causes. A thorough evaluation and workup is essential to alleviate patients' concerns that their symptoms are due to other chronic or severe medical conditions.

The first step in planning a diagnostic evaluation is to perform a thorough history and physical examination. Table 53–2 presents the differential diagnosis of other medical conditions that may present with anxi-

Table 53–2. Differential diagnosis of anxiety disorders.

Cardiovascular
Acute coronary syndrome, congestive heart failure, mitral valve prolapse, dysrhythmia, syncope, hypertension
Drugs
β-Agonists, caffeine, digoxin toxicity, levodopa, nicotinic acid, pseudoephedrine, selective serotonin reuptake inhibitors, steroids, stimulants (methylphenidate, dextroamphetamine), theophylline preparations, thyroid preparations
Endocrine disorders
Hyper/hypothyroidism, hyperadrenalism
Neoplastic
Carcinoid syndrome, pheochromocytoma, insulinoma
Neurologic disorders
Parkinsonism, encephalopathy, restless leg syndrome, seizure, vertigo, brain tumor
Pulmonary
Asthma (acute), chronic obstructive pulmonary disease, hyperventilation, pneumonia, pneumothorax, pulmonary edema, pulmonary embolus
Psychiatric
Affective disorders, drug abuse and dependence/withdrawal syndromes
Other conditions
Anaphylaxis, anemia, electrolyte abnormalities, porphyria, menopause

ety-like symptoms. The clinician must rule out psychiatric disorders and ascertain if symptoms of anxiety are secondary to a medical illness or to a side effect of a medication. If anxiety did not predate a medical illness, subsequent anxiety may represent an adjustment disorder with anxious mood. The most likely organic cause of anxiety is alcohol and drug use (withdrawal or intoxication). Caffeine toxicity and increased sensitivity to caffeine also commonly mimic symptoms of anxiety.

Symptoms of cardiovascular abnormalities such as chest discomfort, shortness of breath, and palpitations are also cardinal symptoms of anxiety. Many anxious patients function poorly because they believe that they have heart disease. The electrocardiogram can be a useful tool to differentiate anxiety from a significant cardiac abnormality. Further evaluation should be considered based on the patient's symptoms and risk profile. When further cardiac evaluation yields normal results, the anxious patient is more effectively reassured.

A careful auscultatory examination of the heart may reveal evidence of mitral valve prolapse, the most common valvular abnormality in adults. Long-term studies have shown that complications from mitral valve prolapse are rare, but often these patients present with palpitations and a generalized sense of being unwell that may mimic anxiety.

The primary care physician must be alert to acute medical conditions that can present with hyperventilation or dyspnea such as pulmonary conditions. The differentiation between these entities can be as simple as checking a pulse oxygen saturation but will often require more advanced diagnostic studies such as chest radiography, computed tomography (CT), or pulmonary angiography.

Musculoskeletal pain syndromes, psychological problems, and esophageal disorders, including esophageal motility disorders and gastroesophageal reflux disease, are the most common noncardiac explanations of chest pain. Most patients with chronic unexplained chest pain have concomitant psychiatric diagnoses, especially anxiety.

Hyperthyroidism and hypoglycemia may be mistaken for anxiety. Hypoparathyroidism, hyperkalemia, hyperthermia, hyponatremia, hypothyroidism, menopause, porphyria, and carcinoid tumors are less common causes of organic anxiety syndromes.

Anxiety exacerbates gastrointestinal conditions such as colitis, ulcers, and irritable bowel syndrome. Treating anxiety often resolves or improves gastrointestinal symptoms. Anxiety, hyperventilation, and dyspnea may accompany recurrent pulmonary emboli with few reliable physical signs.

Depression is the most common psychiatric disorder associated with anxiety. Symptoms that discriminate clinical depression from anxiety include depressed mood, lack of energy, and loss of interest and pleasure.

Ingested substances such as medications or alcohol can elicit anxiety symptoms. Patients with anxiety disorders commonly drink to excess. Alcohol and drug problems involving dependence rather than abuse are most strongly associated with problems involving anxiety. Anxiety disorder and alcohol disorder can each initiate the other, especially in cases of alcohol dependence. Although many alcoholic patients present with anxiety, these symptoms decrease rapidly when the patient stops drinking. Only a small percentage (perhaps 10%) have persistent symptoms of anxiety.

Kushner MG et al: The relationship between anxiety disorders and alcohol use disorders: A review of major perspectives and findings. Clin Psychol Rev 2000;20:149. [PMID: 10721495]

Treatment

The continuity of care and established physician–patient relationship characteristic of the primary care setting offer treatment advantages for patients with an anxiety disorder. However, physicians often miss signs of psychiatric problems in their patients because of a biomedical orientation. The result is excessive diagnostic testing, increased costs, frustrated patients, and cynical physicians.

Positive patient expectations and trust have a formidable impact on prognosis. By increasing their familiarity with standard cognitive-behavioral techniques and psychotropic medications, family physicians can enhance outcomes for patients with anxiety disorders. Several of the cognitive-behavioral techniques described below can easily be implemented by a busy family physician as supplemental treatment to psychopharmacology. Seeing patients more frequently while maintaining the time constraints of a 15-minute office visit can improve patient functioning without punishing the busy family physician. Other interventions can be offered through referral to mental health specialists. If after several 15-minute office visits the patient remains unimproved or nonadherent, referral or consultation may also be appropriate.

A. Pharmacotherapy

Medications provide symptomatic relief but do not cure the underlying anxiety disorder for which they are prescribed. The decision to prescribe medication should be based on the patient's degree of emotional distress, the level of functional disability, and the side effects of the medication. Table 53–3 provides a summary of the dosage range, indications, and financial costs associated with psychotherapeutic agents commonly used in the treatment of anxiety disorders.

1. Selective serotonin reuptake inhibitors (SSRIs)— SSRIs are now considered the first line of medication treatment for most anxiety disorders, with the exception of situ-

Table 53–3. Pharmacotherapy for anxiety disorders.

Drug Name	Usual Dosage Range	FDA Approved Indications	Comments
Benzodiazepines[1]			
Alprazolam[2] (Xanax, Xanax XR, Niravam)	0.5–4 mg (3–6 mg, up to 10 mg daily for panic) divided into 3 doses	Short-term relief of anxiety Panic disorder	XR dosed once daily Reduce doses for elderly or patients with hepatic disease Physical dependence can occur with relatively short-term use Abrupt discontinuation can result in rebound anxiety or withdrawal symptoms Rapid-dissolve tablet available
Chlorazepate[2] (Tranxene)	15–60 mg in divided doses	Short-term relief of anxiety	Reduce doses for elderly or patients with hepatic disease Physical dependence can occur with relatively short-term use
Clonazepam[2] (Klonopin)	0.25–0.5 mg twice daily (max dose 4 mg/day)	Panic disorder	Long duration of effect results in smoother control Rapid-dissolve tablet available
Diazepam[2] (Valium)	2–10 mg 2–4 times daily (max dose 40 mg/day)	Anxiety disorders Short term relief of anxiety	Reduce doses for elderly or patients with hepatic disease Physical and psychological dependence can occur with continuous use
Lorazepam[2] (Ativan)	2–6 mg in divided doses	Short-term relief of anxiety Anxiety associated with depression	Effective when given orally or by IM/IV injection Preferred in patients with hepatic insufficiency because of no active metabolites
Selective Serotonin Reuptake Inhibitors (SSRIs)			
Escitalopram (Lexapro)	10 mg once daily	Generalized anxiety disorder	No significant additional benefit if dose increased to 20 mg
Fluoxetine[2] (Prozac)	10–60 mg once daily	GAD Panic disorder OCD PMDD	Doses should be taken in morning Start with low dose and titrate to effective dose

(*continued*)

Table 53–3. Pharmacotherapy for anxiety disorders. *(Continued)*

Drug Name	Usual Dosage Range	FDA Approved Indications	Comments
Selective Serotonin Reuptake Inhibitors (SSRIs) *(cont.)*			
Paroxetine[2] (Paxil, Paxil CR)	10–60 mg (12.5–62.5 mg CR) once daily	Panic disorder Social anxiety disorder GAD PTSD OCD PMDD	Start with low dose and titrate to effective dose Abrupt discontinuation can result in rebound anxiety or withdrawal symptoms CR formulation has lower gastric intolerance
Sertraline (Zoloft)	25–200 mg once daily	Panic disorder Social anxiety disorder OCD PTSD Pediatric OCD	Start with low dose and titrate to effective dose Abrupt discontinuation can result in rebound anxiety or withdrawal symptoms
Miscellaneous			
Venlafaxine (Effexor, Effexor XR)	75–225 mg in 2–3 divided doses	GAD Social anxiety disorder	Initiate with 37.5 mg daily and titrate up to effective dose XR formulation dosed once daily Taper dose upon discontinuation to avoid rebound or withdrawal symptoms
Buspirone[2] (BuSpar)	10–60 mg in divided doses	GAD	Not for situational anxiety; therapeutic benefit may not be achieved for up to 1 mo No risk of physical or psychological dependence Avoid in patients with severe renal or hepatic impairment

XR, extended release; IM, intramuscular; IV, intravenous; GAD, generalized anxiety disorder; OCD, obsessive-compulsive disorder; PMDD, premenstrual dysphoric disorder; CR, controlled release; PTSD, post-traumatic stress disorder.
[1]All benzodiazepines are Schedule IV controlled substances.
[2]Generic formulations are available.

ational anxiety. SSRIs are well tolerated, have low potential for overdose, and are not associated with psychological or physical dependence.

Recommendations on dosing have been to start low and titrate slowly upward to therapeutic levels in order to minimize jitteriness and insomnia that may occur with higher initial doses. An exception would be the treatment of OCD, which often requires higher than usual dosing. When a patient exhibits both depression and anxiety, SSRIs are strongly recommended. Common side effects include nausea, diarrhea, headache, and sexual dysfunction.

2. Benzodiazepines—These agents remain the treatment of choice for panic attacks, anticipatory anxiety, phobic avoidance, and transient situational stress reactions. They may be used as short-term therapy of panic disorder until concurrent SSRIs become effective. Use of benzodiazepines should be limited to 2–4 months of continuous therapy to limit the potential for psychological or physical dependence. Common side effects include anterograde amnesia, difficulty in balance, impairment of driving ability, and additive effects with alcohol. Use in elderly patients has been associated with paradoxical excitement and an increased risk of falls and hip fractures.

Tolerance to the antianxiety effects is uncommon. The abrupt discontinuation of benzodiazepines, especially those with short half-lives, is associated with withdrawal syndromes of relatively rapid onset. A rebound syndrome similar to but more transiently intense than the original disorder may begin over a few days. Abrupt discontinuation of high doses of alprazolam may result in psychotic behaviors or seizures; a slow taper is essential.

3. Buspirone (BuSpar)—Buspirone has an unknown mechanism of action but appears to affect neurotransmitters in a manner different than benzodiazepines. Because of delayed onset of action of at least 2 weeks, it is indicated only in the treatment of GAD. Although studies have found buspirone to be as effective as benzodiazepines for GAD, many patients who previously received benzodiazepines do not perceive it to be as effective because they do not experience the "buzz" they had with benzodiazepines. Buspirone does not impair driving or cognition and is not additive with alcohol. The most common side effects are restlessness, dizziness, and headache.

4. Tricyclic antidepressants (TCAs)—TCAs may be considered after failed trials of SSRIs, when other agents are not an option because of side effects or concerns of addiction or dependence. They are more commonly used as adjunctive therapy when the patient also has insomnia or chronic pain. Adherence is low secondary to the high incidence of unacceptable side effects.

5. β-Blockers—β-Blockers are primarily used to reduce the autonomic symptoms (rapid heart rate, flushing, sweating) associated with performance anxiety. The medication is usually taken only when needed about one-half hour before an anxiety-inducing situation. Dizziness, drowsiness, and light-headedness are the most common side effects.

6. Atypical anticonvulsants—These agents are being used frequently as adjunctive therapy to augment the activity of SSRIs in patients with refractory symptoms of anxiety. Gabapentin (Neurontin) has been shown to augment SSRI activity in the treatment of panic disorder and OCD and to reduce anxiety associated with chronic pain syndrome. Clinical studies have also demonstrated the effectiveness of other atypical anticonvulsants such as carbamazepine, valproic acid, and lamotrigine.

B. Psychotherapeutic Interventions

1. Behavioral therapy—Behavioral therapy focuses on overt behavior, with an emphasis on "how to" improve rather than "why" the problem exists. Several forms of behavioral therapy are available to assist patients in managing anxiety. The family physician's role involves explaining a behavioral procedure and prescribing homework. Time management need not suffer; 15-minute office visits sequenced about 1–2 weeks apart are usually adequate to provide therapy.

During **exposure therapy** the patient is repeatedly brought into contact with what is feared until discomfort subsides. The longer the exposure interval and the more intensive the exposure experience (massed trials) are, the better. To enhance adherence initially, often a significant other is present, or a benzodiazepine is used; as therapy proceeds, both are gradually eliminated.

Although few people are formally educated in stress management, a large repertoire of **coping skills** is available. Table 53–4 offers a partial list of such strategies that can be given as a patient handout.

Table 53–4. Effective coping strategies.

Talk or write about stressful problems
Do enjoyable activities
Get enough rest and relaxation
Exercise regularly
Eat properly (beware of caffeine, chocolate, and alcohol)
Plan your time and set priorities
Accept responsibility for your role in a problem
Make expectations realistic
Get involved with others
Build in self-rewards
Utilize a sense of humor
Learn assertiveness
Attend support groups

Numerous types of **relaxation training** are useful in the treatment of all anxiety disorders and also have been shown to assist in anger management. Learning to relax is an inexpensive and easily accessible strategy. Reduction in the body's consumption of oxygen, blood lactate level (associated with muscle tension), metabolism, and heart and respiration rates occurs during practice. Home practice for 20 minutes or more twice each day in a quiet place produces significant effects. Commercialized relaxation tapes are available for eidetic imagery and progressive muscle relaxation.

Panic attacks can be mediated by a highly effective technique, **breathing retraining,** which involves slow, deep (diaphragmatic) breathing. Slow inhalation, holding the breath, and slow exhalation are repeated for 10 or more sequences. During slow, deep breathing the patient is told to substitute realistic thoughts ("I'm having a panic attack and I'm not in any danger") for panic-inducing thoughts ("I'm having a heart attack and I'll die soon"). This provides a sense of self-mastery and restores oxygen-carbon dioxide balance to the body. **Interoceptive exposure,** in which patients go through the symptoms of a panic attack (elevated heart rate, hot flashes, sweating, etc) in a controlled setting, can also be beneficial, by reinforcing for patients that these symptoms need not develop into a full-blown attack.

In the **worry exposure technique,** the patient is asked to do the following:

1. Identify (perhaps write down) and distinguish worrisome thoughts from pleasant thoughts.
2. Establish a 30-minute worry period at the same place and time each day.
3. Use the 30-minute period to worry about concerns and to engage in problem solving.
4. Postpone worries outside the 30-minute worry period with reminders that they can be considered during the next worry period (the patient may

choose to write down new worries to avoid worrying about forgetting them).

5. During intrusions replace worries with attention to present moment experiences, activities, or pleasant memories.

This strategy challenges dysfunctional beliefs about the uncontrollability of thoughts and the dangerous consequences of failing to worry. Delusional jealousy also can be mediated by this approach.

In **mismatch strategy,** the physician asks the patient to write a detailed account of the content of the worry (eg, exposure to a particular situation normally avoided) and then asks the patient to worry about what could happen in that situation. Finally, the patient is instructed to enter the situation and observe what really happens to assess the validity of the worry thoughts.

Lastly, the family physician can ask the patient to practice alternative endings for worry sequences. Rather than rehearsing catastrophic outcomes, the patient contemplates positive scenarios in response to worry triggers.

2. Cognitive therapy—Cognitive therapy is behavioral therapy of the mind. Based on the theory that thoughts, images, and assumptions usually account for the onset and persistence of anxiety, cognitive therapy assumes that the way patients perceive and appraise events and interpret arousal-related bodily sensations as dangerous (anxiety sensitivity) provokes symptoms of anxiety. Cognitive changes are the best predictors of treatment outcome for the anxiety disorders.

Achieving thought control is of central importance to mental health. Patients with OCD and GAD are especially prone to poor thought control. These patients devalue their ability to adequately deal with threats. Homework involving "self-talk" must be believed by the patient to be useful.

Because alternative interpretations and explanations (cognitive restructuring) are always available for upsetting events, patients can assume more control of and accept more responsibility for their adaptation. Acceptance of these assumptions empowers the patient. Documented durable improvement results from **cognitive restructuring** (substituting rational assumptions and perspectives and transforming the meaning of events and physiologic arousal cues).

Although it is not possible to control all outside events, it is possible to control one's reaction to any event. Patients are advised that as soon as they are aware of being upset, they should pause and reflect on:

1. The event.
2. Thoughts about the event.
3. Associated feelings.
4. Another way to perceive the event (another meaning) that is also true and makes sense.

When time permits, patients may enter this information in a small notebook for review with the family physician at a subsequent office visit.

Brown TA, Barlow DH: Long-term outcome in cognitive-behavioral treatment of panic disorder: Clinical predictors and alternative strategies for assessment. J Consult Clin Psychol 1995;63:754. [PMID: 7593868]

C. Complementary and Alternative Therapies

Use of alternative therapies is more common among people with psychiatric problems and especially people with self-defined anxiety than among the rest of the population. Most alternative therapies are used without supervision. Because there are so few data on the relative effectiveness of these therapies, most people tend to try a therapist who has been recommended and, by trial and error, find a preferred therapy.

Massage therapies can be classified as energy methods, manipulative therapies, and combinations of each. Swedish massage is the most common form of massage and is usually given with oil. Movements called *effleurage* (smooth stroking) and *pétrissage* (kneading-type movements) are done up and down the back and across many tissues of the body. The Trager method, similar to many other types of massage therapy, involves gentle holding and rocking of different body parts. **Reflexology,** an energy method, could be called a massage therapy because it involves kneading, stroking, rubbing, and other massage procedures. These procedures are centered on particular points of the feet, hands, or ears. Although few controlled studies exist utilizing massage therapy, most people report anxiety-reduction benefits. There are no empiric data on the efficacy of reflexology.

Herbal therapies for anxiety include kava-kava, valerian, St John's wort, and melatonin. Several clinical studies have demonstrated the effectiveness of kava-kava which has a mechanism of action similar to that of the benzodiazepines. However, long-term use or high doses are associated with development of peripheral neuropathy. A recent Food and Drug Administration (FDA) warning was issued regarding the potential for kava-kava to cause hepatotoxicity, and this product has been removed from the market in several European countries. Limited data support the role of valerian in relieving anxiety and insomnia, but it has additive effects with other central nervous system depressants and alcohol. Melatonin has been primarily promoted to reduce the symptoms of jet lag and sleep-cycle disturbances. **Acupuncture** has been demonstrated to reduce anxiety across a variety of populations and presenting problems. However, additional double-blind, placebo-controlled studies are needed.

Research indicates the benefits of **yoga** to quality of life and improved health. Yoga, which involves body postures and *asanas* (body maneuvers), appears to exercise various tissues, organs, and organ systems and provide an avenue to address character armors, attitudes, and tensions. Specific application to stress management is widespread with generally significant positive results. As is the case with acupuncture, however, better controlled research is needed.

Kessler RC et al: The use of complementary and alternative therapies to treat anxiety and depression in the United States. Am J Psychiatry 2001;158:289. [PMID: 11156813]

D. Consultation or Referral

Attempting the previously discussed treatment recommendations during multiple 15-minute continuity office visits often renders referral unnecessary. However, referral may be necessary when symptoms reoccur or when tapering a medication is difficult. Referral is appropriate when the family physician is uncomfortable with an indicated therapy, when patients are potentially suicidal or are actively abusing drugs, when noncompliance is suspected, or when psychopathology is severe. Referral of patients with OCD and PTSD is mandatory. Given the expected need to individualize treatment and provide novel treatment options, the busy family physician has neither the time nor the expertise to engage in the comprehensive interventions required.

If psychotherapy is the preferred method of managing symptoms, the specialized training of a clinical or a counseling psychologist is recommended. When psychopharmacology is warranted, the expertise of a psychiatrist is unmatched. Sound treatment is based on specific and accurate diagnosis and relies on empirically validated procedures that take into account the personality of the patient.

Table 53–5 provides several referral treatments and their indications for the effective nonpharmacologic management of anxiety disorders.

E. Management of Specific Anxiety Disorders

1. Panic disorder—Recommended treatment includes breathing retraining, cognitive restructuring, interoceptive exposure, and relaxation training. If anxiety is short term, benzodiazepines should be used; if anxiety is chronic, paroxetine, fluvoxamine, citalopram, fluoxetine, sertraline, nefazodone, or imipramine should be used.

Although current treatments allow control of panic disorder, full recovery is questionable. Psychological treatments involve lower relapse rates, higher levels of acceptability, lower attrition rates and are better tolerated than many pharmacologic treatments. Exposure and deep breathing are especially effective for patients with panic attacks and agoraphobia.

The percentage of patients who become free of panic attacks from medication is generally 50–80% in acute pharmacologic trials, and this percentage rises with longer treatment. SSRIs reduced panic attack frequency to zero in 36–86% of patients and were well tolerated over long-term administration. Additionally, because of the high rate of depression comorbidity associated with panic attacks, SSRIs are the pharmacologic treatment of choice.

Benzodiazepines are best used for acute management. In most studies relapse after discontinuation of

Table 53–5. Referral interventions and indications for use.

Type of Intervention	Description	Indications
Psychotherapy		
Individual	Insight, empowerment, support	Privacy, complicated patient
Group	Interactive, common interest	Social skills, support, vicarious learning
Family	Therapeutic environment and patient	Enabling, dysfunctional family
Eye movement desensitization and reprocessing (EMDR)	Follow oscillation movement of object (pencil) thinking of trauma Mixed results	Post-traumatic stress disorder
Hypnosis	Relaxation induction; suggestions	Suggestible patient
Biofeedback	EMG, EKG, EEG monitoring of physiologic parameters to alter activity; cost is a limiting factor	Headaches, tension, blood flow, etc
Stress innoculation/anxiety management	Multifaceted, comprehensive cognitive–behavioral therapy	All anxiety disorders
Assertiveness training	Learn skills to be firm, not nasty	Dependent, unassertive, aggressive patients
Transcranial magnetic stimulation (TMS)	Noninvasive, painless method of brain stimulation via electrical current using changing magnetic fields	Applications are in their infancy

EMG, electromyogram; ECG, electrocardiogram; EEG, electroencephalogram.

medications has been relatively high, ranging from one third to three fourths of patients, suggesting the need to be on the medications for at least 6 months.

2. Simple phobias—Recommended treatment includes exposure therapy, deep breathing, relaxation training, and cognitive restructuring, as well as short-term use of benzodiazepines.

3. Social phobia—Recommended treatment includes exposure therapy, cognitive restructuring, relaxation training, social skills training, and group therapy; medications that may be helpful include paroxetine, sertraline, clonazepam, and β-blockers.

When fearing negative evaluation, patients narrow their attention to social threat cues. Cognitive therapy corrects these distortions whereas exposure therapy reduces anticipatory fear. In cognitive-behavioral group settings, 81% of patients had significant improvement that was maintained 5.5 years later.

The SSRIs sertraline and paroxetine are both approved by the FDA for treatment of social anxiety disorder. β-Blockers on an as-needed basis may be helpful in patients who experience performance anxiety, even though published data supporting their benefit are limited. These agents can reduce hand tremor and tachycardia symptoms without causing cognitive impairment.

4. OCD—Recommended treatment includes referral as well as exposure therapy, response prevention, cognitive restructuring, and pharmacotherapy with fluoxetine, fluvoxamine, sertraline, or clomipramine Behavior therapy and SSRIs are primarily recommended. Homework assignments expose patients to stimuli associated with their obsessions. During **response prevention,** patients refrain from rituals (fixed behaviors that reduce anxiety) for progressively longer intervals until discomfort diminishes.

Pharmacologic options can at best reduce OCD symptoms by 50%, which may improve the patient's quality of life. Effective dosages are usually significantly higher than those required for depression or other anxiety disorders (eg, fluoxetine, up to 80 mg/day). TCAs other than clomipramine do not appear to be effective in patients with OCD. Sertraline is the only SSRI approved for treatment of OCD in children.

5. PTSD—Recommended treatment includes referral as well as individual or group psychotherapy, relaxation training, or cognitive restructuring; eye movement desensitization and reprocessing also can be considered. Pharmacotherapy with sertraline, paroxetine, or benzodiazepines is based on symptom severity and history of substance abuse. Like OCD, PTSD is especially hard to treat. Early intervention reduces tendencies for substance abuse, secondary gain, litigation, and malingering. Referral is mandatory.

Some form of exposure or desensitization is essential. Patients put frightening memories into words while receiving new and incompatible information. Systematic exposure to the traumatic memory in a safe environment allows a reevaluation of and habituation to threat cues.

Although there is no established pharmacotherapy for PTSD, about 70% of patients seem to benefit from pharmacotherapy with moderate to marked effects. Sertraline, paroxetine, and fluoxetine have been shown to produce acute improvement and decreased relapse rates in patients with PTSD.

SSRIs, especially fluoxetine, appear to have the greatest efficacy of any single class of medications. Clonazepam and buspirone may be helpful in suppressing hyperarousal symptoms. The anticonvulsant carbamazepine has been shown to decrease flashbacks, hyperarousal, and impulsivity. Carbamazepine, lithium, and β-blockers may be helpful in patients with poor impulse control.

6. GAD—Recommended treatment includes worry exposure, thought control techniques (mismatch, cognitive restructuring), and relaxation training. Pharmacotherapy may include venlafaxine, sertraline, escitalopram, paroxetine, buspirone, and benzodiazepines.

No treatment is convincingly effective for GAD. Although cognitive-behavioral therapy appears to produce superior results, effects remain variable. Cognitive psychotherapy addresses probability overestimation (ie, overestimating the likelihood of negative events) and catastrophic thinking and has been shown to improve sleep.

Nonvalidated coping strategies such as physical action, thought replacement, analysis, counterpropaganda, and talking to a friend have been used, with varying success, but no one strategy is more efficient and none is rated "very efficient" by patients. Talking to a friend may be more efficient when thoughts are intense, whereas thought replacement may work well when intensity is low.

Antidepressants are often considered first-line therapy for GAD, in part because of the frequent association of GAD with depression. Although the TCAs are effective for GAD, the SSRIs are more frequently prescribed because of a more favorable side-effect profile. The SSRIs are well-demonstrated medications of choice for most anxiety disorders; however, although the SSRIs, notably citalopram, paroxetine, and venlafaxine, have shown promise in the treatment of GAD, their role in this treatment is still under investigation. Response to benzodiazepines is variable. When conspicuous worry, apprehension, irritability, and depression exist, buspirone has been especially effective and has been shown to be comparable to benzodiazepines in multiple studies of GAD.

7. Other anxiety disorders—Treatment of patients with substance-induced anxiety disorder consists of eliminating the drug of abuse, medication, or toxin exposure that is the cause of the disorder. In patients with persistent symptoms of adjustment disorder with anxious mood, referral for psychotherapy is recommended.

Culpepper L: Generalized anxiety disorder in primary care: Emerging issues in management and treatment. J Clin Psychiatry 2002;63:35. [PMID: 12044106]

Raj BA, Sheehan DV: Social anxiety disorder. Med Clin North Am 2001;85:712. [PMID: 11349481]

Shalev AY: Acute stress reactions in adults. Biol Psychiatry 2002;51:532. [PMID: 11950455]

Stewart SH, Kushner MG: Introduction to the Special Issue on "Anxiety Sensitivity and Addictive Behaviors." Addict Behav 2001;26:775. [PMID: 1168544]

F. Special Populations

1. Children and youth—Transient fears are common in children of all ages and represent part of the normal developmental process. Normal fears need to be distinguished from the anxiety disorders of adulthood, which are more prevalent among children and adolescents than any other mental problem. Children with anxiety disorders exhibit a high rate of comorbidity, especially with other, secondary anxiety disorders.

Anxiety is often manifested among children by avoidance behavior, distorted thinking, or subjective distress. The *DSM-IV-TR* anxiety designations of childhood and adolescence include **separation anxiety disorder** (excessive anxiety concerning separation from home or from those to whom the child is attached) and **overanxious disorder** (at least 6 months of persistent and excessive anxiety and worry). Separation anxiety disorder is treated by exposure to the feared event (eg, the child attends school despite discomfort). Psychotherapy is the treatment of choice for overanxious disorder.

Cognitive-behavioral treatment for children with anxiety disorders is the first-line treatment recommended. Similar approaches to those described for adults are utilized, with emphasis on exposure paradigms. Response rates for children have ranged from 70% to 80%.

Caution remains in effect regarding the prominent prescribing of medication for the treatment of childhood anxiety disorders. Few data are available on the impact of age on absorption, metabolism, therapeutic levels, or possible drug interactions. It is expected that to achieve the same serum levels in children compared with adults the relative dose would be higher.

Despite this caution, FDA indications for adults with anxiety disorders are often used in children and adolescents. Approximately 50–70% of children with these disorders respond to SSRIs.

2. The elderly—Although the most common form of psychiatric condition in the elderly, anxiety disorders are still underdiagnosed. Polypharmacy is often present. Altered pharmacokinetics and pharmacodynamics in the geriatric population lead to greater sensitivity to and prolonged half-life of the medication due to decreased clearance of the drugs. Because of these drug complications, psychotherapy is attractive.

G. Patients with Related Conditions

1. Personality disorders—Personality disorders are life-long characterologic problems that significantly complicate treatment and outcome. Poor compliance, medication abuse, interpersonal agitation, and poor insight characterize patients with personality disorders. These patients suffer more from anxiety than patients without personality disorders. Prescribing of benzodiazepines is contraindicated. (For further discussion of personality disorders, see Chapter 54.)

2. Hyperventilation—During hyperventilation excessive rate and depth of breathing produce a marked drop in carbon dioxide and blood alkalinity. These changes can be subtle. A person may slightly overbreathe for a long time. Even a yawn may trigger symptoms, accounting for the sudden nature of panic attacks during sleep. Breathing retraining is recommended.

3. Insomnia—Patients with anxiety disorders commonly have sleep problems that worsen anxiety. Sympathomimetic amines may cause sleep-onset insomnia, whereas alcohol abuse produces sleep-termination insomnia. Benzodiazepines are frequently prescribed as sedative-hypnotics. For sleep-onset insomnia, triazolam and zolpidem are rapidly acting compounds with short half-lives. For sleep maintenance, longer acting drugs such as flurazepam and quazepam are more effective. Tolerance for the sedative effects, alteration of sleep topography, suppression of rapid eye movement (REM; dream sleep), impaired cognitive function, the occurrence of falls, and REM rebound following discontinuation are contraindications to the use of benzodiazepines in treatment of chronic insomnia.

Sleep hygiene suggestions provide an effective initial treatment option. Patients are asked to review and alter life-style patterns that interfere with sleep. Table 53–6 outlines these suggestions for patient use. Adherence with recommendations and shift work are limiting factors.

Labellarte MJ et al: The treatment of anxiety disorders in children and adolescents. Biol Psychiatry 1999;46:1567. [PMID: 10599484]

Lichstein KL et al: Relaxation and sleep compression for late-life insomnia: A placebo-controlled trial. J Consult Clin Psychol 2001;69:227. [PMID: 11393600]

Sheikh JI, Cassidy EL: Treatment of anxiety disorders in the elderly: Issues and strategies. J Anxiety Disord 2000;14:173. [PMID: 10864384]

Prognosis

Just 30 years ago, most estimates were that 80% of patients with anxiety disorders would not significantly

Table 53–6. Sleep hygiene recommendations.

Keep a sleep diary for a few weeks and monitor sleep-related activities
Establish a regular sleep–wake cycle (go to bed at about the same time and get up at about the same time)
Get regular exercise
Reduce noise
Avoid all naps
Eat dinner at a reasonable hour to allow time to digest food
Avoid excessive amounts of caffeine (chocolates, soft drinks, coffee, tea), especially before bedtime
Avoid excessive fluid intake before bed
Avoid in-bed activities such as reading, eating, or watching TV
Avoid clock watching while trying to sleep
If not asleep within 10–15 min after going to bed, get up:
If you still want to lie down, do so in another room
When sleepy, go back to bed
If not asleep in 10–15 min, repeat these steps

benefit from available treatment. Today the opposite is true. For the majority of patients with anxiety disorders—especially panic disorder, specific phobias, and social phobia—treatment with a combination of cognitive-behavioral therapy and an SSRI carries an excellent prognosis Although these treatments show promise in the treatment of OCD, GAD, and PTSD, efficacy is more variable.

WEB SITES

Anxiety Disorders of America:
http://www.adaa.org/

Anxiety/Panic Internet Resource:
http://www.algy.com/anxiety

Internet Mental Health:
http://www.mentalhealth.com/

National Institute of Mental Health:
http://www.nimh.nih.gov/anxiety/anxeitymenu.cfm

Personality Disorders 54

William Elder, PhD

ESSENTIALS OF DIAGNOSIS

- *Enduring pattern of behavior that deviates from cultural expectations and leads to clinically significant distress or functional impairment.*
- *Pattern is inflexible, pervasive, stable, of long duration, and traceable at least to adolescence or early adulthood.*
- *Pattern is not a manifestation or consequence of another mental disorder or due to direct physiologic effects of substances or general medical conditions.*
- *Medical crises or transfers of care may produce symptoms that mimic personality disorders.*

General Considerations

Personality disorders (PDs) are a heterogeneous group of deeply ingrained and enduring behavioral patterns characterized by inflexible and extreme responses to a broad range of situations, manifesting in cognition (ways of perceiving and interpreting self, others, and events), affectivity (range, intensity, lability, and appropriateness of response), interpersonal functioning, and impulse control. PDs impinge on medical practice in multiple ways, including self-destructive behaviors, interpersonal disturbances, and nonadherence. Appropriate physician responses and effective treatments exist for many PDs. Borderline personality disorder (BPD) is an extremely debilitating and notoriously difficult to treat disorder. BPD may be misattributed to other PDs, and behaviors of patients in crises may also misleadingly suggest BPD. Correct diagnosis of PDs and proper intervention will help to improve patient outcomes.

Ten PDs are currently distinguished clinically. They are often grouped into three clusters: odd or eccentric (cluster A); dramatic, emotional, or erratic (cluster B); and anxious or fearful (cluster C). These groupings are helpful in broadly categorizing PD difficulties but are limited in their usefulness because they do not signify similarities in etiologies and treatment response. Table 54–1 summarizes the 10 PDs.

PDs are relatively common, with a prevalence of 10–18% in the general population. Patients with PDs may seek help from family physicians for physical complaints, rather than psychiatric help. Higher rates for all types of PDs are found in medical settings. Prevalence of BPD in the general community is 1.2%.

PDs have a pervasive impact because they are central to who the person is. They are major sources of long-term disability and are associated with greatly increased mortality. Patients with PDs have fewer coping skills and during stressful situations may have greater difficulties, which are worsened by poor social competency, impulse control, and social support. Patients with BPD are frequently maltreated in the forms of sexual, physical, and emotional abuse; physical neglect; and witnessing violence. PDs are identified in 70–85% of persons identified as criminal, 60–70% of persons with alcohol dependence, and 70–90% of persons who are drug dependent.

Borderline, schizoid, schizotypal, and dependent PDs are associated with high degrees of functional impairments and greater risk for depression and alcohol abuse. Obsessive-compulsive and narcissistic PDs may not result in appreciable degrees of impairment. Dependent PD is associated with a marked increase in health care utilization.

Pathogenesis

A. PD

PDs are syndromes rather than diseases. Avoidant, dependent, and schizoid PDs appear to be heritable. Similarly, schizotypal disorder is considered to be heritable, as one end of a schizotypal-schizophrenia spectrum. Twin and adoption studies suggest a genetic predisposition for antisocial PD, as well as environmental influences, via poor parenting and role modeling. Histrionic PD may be related to indulged tendencies toward emotional expressiveness.

B. BPD

BPD may result from both constitutional and environmental factors. Genetically, BPD is five times more common among first-degree relatives of those with the disorder but to say to what degree BPD is heritable is difficult given the reciprocity between family and child that occurs during development. BPD symptoms have been attributed to highly pathologic and conflicted interactions between

Table 54–1. Clinical features and clusters of 10 *DSM-IV-TR* personality disorders.

Cluster	Personality Disorder	Clinical Features
Cluster A: odd, eccentric	Paranoid	Suspicious; overly sensitive; misinterpretations
	Schizotypal	Detached; perceptual and cognitive distortions; eccentric behavior
	Schizoid	Detached; introverted, constricted affect
Cluster B: dramatic, emotional, erratic	Antisocial	Manipulative; selfish, lacks empathy; explosive anger; legal problems since adolescence
	Borderline	Dependent and demanding; unstable interpersonal relationships, self-image, and affects; impulsivity; micropsychotic symptoms
	Histrionic	Dramatic; attention seeking and emotionality; superficial, ie, vague and focused on appearances
	Narcissistic	Self-important; arrogance and grandiosity; need for admiration; lacks empathy; rages
Cluster C: anxious, fearful	Avoidant	Anxiously detached; feels inadequate; hypersensitive to negative evaluation
	Dependent	Clinging, submissive, and self-sacrificing; needs to be taken care of; hypersensitive to negative evaluation
	Obsessive-compulsive	Preoccupied with orderliness, perfectionism, and control

mother and child. The conflict brings great ambivalence about relationships and interferes with the child's ability to regulate affect. (Additional discussion of this process appears later, under "Termination of Care.") Child sexual abuse has been thought causal in BPD, but a recent meta-analysis did not support this hypothesis. It is certainly the case that traumatic childhood experiences are common in patients with BPD. As a group, patients with antisocial and borderline PDs report higher frequencies of perinatal brain injury, head trauma, and encephalitis.

C. Common Comorbid Conditions

Substance abuse disorders frequently co-occur in community and clinical populations, particularly with antisocial, borderline, avoidant, and paranoid PDs. Anorexia nervosa, bulimia nervosa, and binge eating may be seen in patients who are obsessional, borderline, and avoidant, respectively. Self-injurious skin picking can be conceptualized as an impulse control disorder and has been found with significant frequency in patients with obsessive-compulsive PD and BPD. Up to 50% of patients with BPD have major depressive disorders or bipolar disorders.

Prevention

Except for efforts to address the roots of criminal behaviors that are common in antisocial PD, there is no literature on prevention of PDs. Primary prevention could consist of better treatment of parental mental illnesses that have a negative impact on parent–child interactions and public health interventions to reduce prenatal brain insults. Both primary and secondary prevention could occur with increased interventions in family functioning and parenting skills.

Clinical Findings

PDs were once referred to as character disorders. Various descriptive labels have appeared in the literature, such as the oral fixated character, the impulsive personality, and the introverted personality type. Each of these represents a theory of personality (psychoanalytic, developmental, and analytical, respectively) that has been applied clinically.

Currently, there are few points of correspondence between personality theory and diagnosis of PDs. A relatively atheoretical, categorical perspective dominates clinical practice in the United States. In the categorical perspective, PDs represent qualitatively distinct clinical syndromes.

The *Diagnostic and Statistical Manual of Mental Disorders,* Fourth Edition, Text Revision (*DSM-IV-TR*) exemplifies the categorical perspective. PDs appear as "Axis II disorders," which does not imply that PDs are conditions that are less severe than clinical disorders such as depression, which appear on Axis I. Instead, the additional axis provides a place where pervasive, persisting disorders may be differentially recorded. Mental retardation, similarly pervasive and persistent, is also an Axis II disorder.

A. Symptoms and Signs

1. PD—Clinical lore about appearance and presentations of PDs exists. Anything extreme in appearance that is not ethnically appropriate or currently fashionable may suggest a PD. Examples include flamboyant jewelry, particularly in men, tattoos and piercing in older men and women, steel-toed boots in men, and excessive cosmetics and large hair ribbons in women.

The patient's style of interacting with the physician can be revealing about personality difficulties. For example, the dependent patient will seek much advice and be unable to make an independent decision. The patient with antisocial PD may be "smooth talking" or threatening. Interactions with patients with BPD can be very difficult. The patient will switch from extreme idealization to devaluation of the physician. The patient may cause "splitting" among staff, with some people siding with the patient and others extremely angry with the patient. Table 54–2 describes problem behaviors associated with various PDs, as well as helpful responses and management strategies.

Physician countertransference may be a sign of a PD. Reactions such as anger, guilt, desire to punish, desire to reject, desire to please, sexual fantasies, and a sense that the physician is the "one person" capable of helping the patient are all examples of physician countertransference responses to patient PDs. Self-reflection about the encounter is recommended for managing the strong feelings and interpersonal conflict encountered in medical care.

2. BPD—Physicians may overattribute or underattribute patient difficulties to BPD; therefore, it is important to be sensitive to BPD phenomena and to ascertain whether patient difficulties and symptoms represent BPD. BPD diagnostic criteria call for a pervasive pattern of instability in interpersonal relationships, self-image, and affect, and marked impulsivity beginning by early adulthood and present in a variety of contexts as indicated by at least five of the following:

1. Frantic efforts to avoid real or imagined abandonment (not including suicidal behaviors).
2. A pattern of unstable and intense interpersonal relationships characterized by alternating extremes of idealization and devaluation.
3. Identity disturbance: a markedly and persistently unstable self-image or sense of self.
4. Impulsivity in at least two areas that are potentially self-damaging (not including suicidal behaviors).
5. Recurrent suicidal behavior, gestures, threats, or self-mutilating behavior.
6. Affective instability due to a marked reactivity of mood (eg, intense episodic dysphoria, irritability, or anxiety usually lasting a few hours and only rarely more than a few days).
7. Chronic feelings of emptiness.
8. Inappropriate intense anger or difficulty controlling anger.
9. Transient, stress-related paranoid ideation or severe dissociative symptoms.

BPDs make up a heterogeneous group with subgroups consisting of patients differing in affective, impulsive, and micropsychotic symptom clusters. These differences can suggest different treatments, discussed later. Patients with BPD have significantly higher rates of suicidal ideation and 70–80% exhibit self-harming behavior at least once. Suicide attempts are often regarded as manipulative gestures, but suicide rates are very high in this population: 3–9.5% of patients with BPD receiving inpatient care eventually kill themselves. Self-harming behaviors in the form of self-mutilation, such as wrist scratching, are symptomatic of BPD. Nausea and vomiting may be a primary care analogue of self-mutilation in some patients with BPD, and a common chief complaint. Obtaining a history suggesting BPD may mitigate the need for extensive and invasive gastrointestinal symptom evaluations and may suggest more effective treatment strategies directed to personality functioning.

B. Special Tests

No laboratory tests exist for PDs. Structured clinical interviews and personality inventories may be helpful in differentiating PDs and tracking treatment response. Interpretation by a psychologist enhances the value of the results. A consult should be considered in cases of diagnostic uncertainty.

American Psychiatric Association: *Diagnostic and Statistical Manual of Mental Disorders,* 4th ed, text revision. APA, 2000.

Beck AT et al: Dysfunctional beliefs discriminate personality disorders. Behav Res Ther 2001;39:1213. [PMID: 11579990]

Gross R et al: Borderline personality disorder in primary care. Arch Intern Med 2002;162:53. [PMID: 11996618]

Sansone RA et al: Borderline personality symptomatology, experience of multiple types of trauma and health care utilization among women in a primary care setting. J Clin Psychiatry 1998;59:108. [PMID: 9541152]

Skodol A et al: Functional impairment in patients with schizotypal, borderline, avoidant, or obsessive-compulsive personality disorder. Am J Psychiatry 2002;159:276. [PMID: 11823271]

Differential Diagnosis

A. PD

Accurate diagnosis is essential for proper response to and treatment of PDs.

- Histrionic PD patients are dramatic and manipulative, but lack the affective instability of BPD. Impulsivity, when seen, is related to attention seeking and sexual acting out.

Table 54–2. Problem behaviors associated with personality disorders.

	Personality Disorder				
	Paranoid	**Schizotypal**	**Schizoid**	**Antisocial**	**Borderline**
Patient's perspective	People are malevolent. Situation is dangerous.	Understanding of care may be odd or near delusional.	Illness will bring too much attention and invade privacy.	Threatened if unable to feel "on top." Illness presents opportunity for crime.	Fears abandonment. Overreacts to symptoms and situation.
Problem behaviors	Fearful. Misconstrues events and explanations. Irrational. Argumentative.	Odd health beliefs and behaviors. Poor hygiene. Avoids care.	Unresponsive to kindness. Difficult to motivate. Avoids care.	Acts out to gain control. Malingering. Uses staff and physicians. Superficially charming. Drug seeking.	Idealizes, then devalues care. Self-destructive acts. Splits staff.
Helpful physician responses and management strategies	Be empathic toward patient's fears, even when they seem irrational. Carefully explain care plan. Provide advance information about risks. Protect patient's independence.	Communicate directly. Avoid misinterpreting patient as intentionally noncompliant. Do not reject patient for oddness. Honor patient's beliefs.	Manage personal frustration at feeling unappreciated. Maintain a low-key approach. Appreciate patient's need for privacy.	Do not succumb to patient's anger and manipulation. Avoid punitive reactions to patients. Motivate by addressing patient's self-interest. Set clear limits that interventions must be medically indicated.	Manage feelings of hopelessness about patient. Avoid getting too close emotionally. Schedule frequent periodic check-ups. Tolerate periodic angry outbursts, but set limits. Monitor for self-destructive behavior. Discuss feelings with co-workers.

- Dependent PD patients fear abandonment, but patients with BPD have more affective instability and impulsivity.
- Schizotypal PD patients have the micropsychotic symptoms of BPD, but are odder and lack the affective instability of BPD.
- Paranoid PD patients have volatile anger, but lack the impulsivity, self-destructiveness, and abandonment issues of the BPD patient.
- Narcissistic PD patients have rages and reactive mood, but have a stable, idealized self-image in contrast to the patient with BPD, who has an unstable identity.
- Antisocial PD patients are often less impulsive than intentionally aggressive for materialistic gains. Patients with BPD act out when needy and to gain support.

B. Other Mental Disorders

A PD is not diagnosed if symptoms are explained by an Axis I condition or substance use. Although PDs may share impulsivity, raging, and grandiosity with bipolar disorder, they seldom have the same intensity and rate of speech or irrationality of thought that a manic episode brings. Substance use disorders differ from antisocial PD when illegal behaviors are restricted to substance use and procurement. Dissociative identity disorder, formerly known as multiple personality disorder, may have a more traumatic etiology similar to BPD. Obsessive-compulsive PD is not on the same spectrum as obsessive-compulsive disorder. Although patients with both disorders are quite orderly and inflexible, patients with obsessive-compulsive PD are comfortable with their behavior whereas patients with obsessive-compulsive disorder recognize that their behavior and thoughts are irrational. A diagnosis of PD does not apply when changes in behavior result from changes in brain function. For example, although personality changes are expected in dementia, a diagnosis of PD is not indicated. An Axis I diagnosis "personality change due to a...[general medical condition]" is available when a change in personality characteristics is the direct physiologic consequence of a general medical condition. Because transient changes in personality are common in children and adolescents, diagnosis of a PD is not appropriate for a patient younger than 18 years of

Histrionic	Narcissistic	Avoidant	Dependent	Obsessive-Compulsive
Illness results in feeling unattractive or presents an opportunity to receive attention.	Illness results in feeling inadequate or is an opportunity to receive admiration.	Illness is personal. Fears exposure.	Fears abandonment. Intensifies feelings of helplessness.	Fears losing control of body and emotions. Feels shame.
Overly dramatic, attention-seeking. Excessively familiar relationship. Not objective—overemphasis on feeling states.	Demanding and entitled attitude. Will overly praise or devalue care providers to maintain sense of superiority.	Missed appointments. Delay seeking care. Extremely non-assertive.	Dramatic and urgent demands for medical attention. May contribute to or prolong illness to get attention.	Unable to relinquish control to health care team. Great difficulty and anger at any change. Excessive attention to detail.
Avoid frustration with patient vagueness. Show respectful and professional concern for feelings, with emphasis on objective issues. Avoid excessive familiarity.	Avoid rejecting the patient for being too demanding. Avoid seeking patient's approval. Generously validate patient's concerns, with attentive but factual response to questions. Protect self-esteem of patients by giving them a role in their care.	Provide empathic response to inadequacy. Be patient with timidity. Work toward clear treatment plans—must obtain patient's view. Treat anxiety disorder.	When exhausted by patient needs, avoid hostile rejection of patient. Give reassurance and consistency. Set limits to availability—schedule regular visits. Help patient obtain outside support.	Avoid impatience. Thorough history taking and careful diagnostic workups are reassuring. Give clear and thorough explanations. Avoid control battles; treat patient as a partner; encourage self-monitoring.

age unless the behavioral pattern has been present for at least 1 year.

C. Cultural Considerations

Culturally related characteristics may erroneously suggest PDs. Promiscuity, suspiciousness, and recklessness have different norms in different cultures. The degree of physical or emotional closeness sought and the intensity of emotional expression also differ. Manner of dress and health beliefs may seem strange to the conventional western physician. Passivity, especially with one's elders, is not a sign of dependency in most recently immigrated individuals. Constricted affect is a normal response when entering a new environment. Asking someone from the culture if the behavior is extreme can be helpful, as can evaluating for significant interpersonal difficulties.

Treatment

Miller has described how experienced family physicians differentially and efficiently respond to visits that can be categorized as routine, ceremony, or drama. In some cases, good application of family medicine's care principles may be beneficial psychotherapeutically. (Compare the psychotherapy of PDs described below with the patient-centered method of family practice.) Suggestions for helping patients with PDs in a nonpsychiatric medical setting appear in Table 54–2. Table 54–3 offers suggestions for helping patients who present with BPD.

Common wisdom has held that personality cannot be changed. However, increasingly specific psychopharmacologic and psychotherapeutic interventions have brought improved outcomes and some cures. The most effective treatments are multidisciplinary, combining medications, individual and group psychotherapies, and a high level of communication among providers. Comorbid substance dependence, violent acting out toward others, or severely self-harming behaviors must be addressed first, via inpatient care.

Miller WL: Routine, ceremony, or drama: An exploratory field study of the primary care clinical encounter. J Fam Pract 1992;34:289. [PMID: 1541955]

A. Risk Management

Physicians should acknowledge the threats and challenges associated with PDs. General risk management considerations include:

Table 54–3. Working with patients with BPD in medical settings.

1. Recognize the characteristics. The patient fears abandonment and increases demands on the physician. May be noncompliant, manipulative, somatasize, or "split" the health care team.
2. Behavior is need driven. Demands may be overt or covert. Identify needs and motivations. Patient has little insight into problems. Externalization is symptomatic.
3. Tolerate patient's behaviors. Speaking "harshly or strictly" will activate abandonment fears and worsen the situation. Use a nonconfrontational and an educational approach.
4. A long-term plan provides stability for the patient. Follow continuity of care principles. This may be curative for the patient.
5. Titrate closeness and visit frequency. Avoid extremes of constant availability.
6. Set limits. Make clear agreements about call and office visits. Point out to patients that you are almost always involved in solving some type of problem and are unable to give full attention to their problems without an appointment. Suggest that patients schedule fairly frequent visits so that a regular time is available to discuss the problems they are experiencing.
7. Foresee problems related to abandonment fears such as when the social situation is disturbed, when the patient is referred, or when there are changes in physician or staff.
8. Use a multidisciplinary approach. Involve a highly skilled clinical psychologist or clinical social worker in the care. Encourage communication and cooperation among the care team.
9. Monitor your and the staff's reactions. Frustration and anger may be expected. Discuss the situation. Help the staff to recognize the etiology of the frustration might originate in the patient's personality not in the crisis of the moment. Coordinate responses to patients.
10. Set personal limits for the number of these challenging patients that you accept into your practice.

- Having good collaboration and communication with a qualified mental health professional.
- Attention to documentation of communications and risk assessments.
- Attention to transference and countertransference issues described earlier.
- Consultation with a colleague regarding high-risk situations.
- Careful management of termination of care, even when it is the patient's decision.
- Informed consent from the patient and, if appropriate, family members, regarding the risks inherent in the disorder and uncertainties in the treatment outcome.

B. Consultation or Referral

Consultation or referral should be considered when the following exist:

- The patient has several psychiatric diagnoses.
- The patient is experiencing depressive or anhedonic symptoms even if subthreshold (risk for suicide).
- The patient has significant problems with self-regulation.
- The patient has moderate to severe substance use disorder(s).
- The diagnosis is uncertain or the presentation is puzzling.
- Initial treatment by the family physician is ineffective.
- The physician or staff are unable to compensate for and are overwhelmed by the patient's personality problems.

Patient acceptance of treatment can be difficult. The patient may disagree about what is wrong. Symptomatically, patients with PD may externalize blame for their problems. PD behavioral patterns also tend to be ego-syntonic. That is, even patients who agree that their behavior is excessive may believe that the excess is reasonable, given their perception of the circumstances. Treatment may also be difficult if it is perceived as an attempt to control the patient; referral may be experienced as devaluing or as abandonment. Thus treatment and referral suggestions should be offered with an understanding of how patients with various PDs may perceive them. Table 54–2 describes patient perspectives on care common to different PDs.

C. Pharmacotherapy

In many cases, medications are effective only as a means to manage stress-exacerbated symptoms. For example, under stress, paranoid, schizoid, or schizotypal patients may experience delusions, distress, and hallucinations, which can be helped with antipsychotic medications. When not stressed, the odd behavior and beliefs of these patients remain unresponsive to treatment. Patients with narcissistic, antisocial, or histrionic PDs are not helped with current medications, including antidepressants, unless a mood disorder coexists.

Some PDs may be successfully treated with medications. Avoidant PD appears to be an alternative conceptualization of social phobia. It can be treated with selective serotonin reuptake inhibitors (SSRIs) and selective serotonin and norepinephrine reuptake inhibitors (SNRIs). Patients with obsessive-compulsive PD may become less irritable and compulsive with SSRIs. Rejection sensitivity seen in patients with dependent PD may be helped by SSRIs.

Soloff has proposed three symptom-specific pharmacotherapy algorithms for PDs. They are based on differential medication effects on cognitive disturbances, behavioral dyscontrol, and affective dysregulation. Soloff's first algorithm is for treatment of PDs in which cognitive-perceptual symptoms are most significant (ie, patients with suspiciousness, paranoid ideation, and micropsychotic symptoms). The second algorithm is for treatment of affective dysregulation (ie, patients with a depressed, angry, anxious, labile mood). The third algorithm is for treatment of impulsive-behavioral symptoms (ie, patients with impulsive aggression, binging, or self-injuring behaviors). Practice guidelines for treatment of BPD were published by the American Psychiatric Association (APA) in October 2001, with rerecommendation by the APA in 2005. The guidelines are largely in accord with Soloff's recommendations. Recommendations that follow are based on the APA guidelines. It should be noted that current guidelines are based on a small database that lacks sufficient randomized controlled trials. Therefore, each treatment should be approached as an empirical trial, with the patient as a coinvestigator. Side effects, risk–benefit ratios, conjoint medications, and patient preferences should be considered carefully. Pharmacotherapy is an adjuvant to psychotherapy; medications do not cure character and will never be a substitute for the work of a therapist.

SSRIs and SNRIs are effective with affective dysregulation. Tricyclic antidepressants are no more effective than SSRIs and should not be used, given their cardiotoxic effects with overdose and a possibility of paradoxical worsening of symptoms. Monoamine oxidase inhibitors (MAOIs) were proven useful in treating BPD prior to the advent of SSRIs and offer a second treatment option for affective dysregulation, including rejection sensitivity. Mood stabilizers offer an additional level of treatment. Lithium should be used in conjunction with an antidepressant, whereas valproate and carbamazepine may be offered alone. Although patients with BPD often complain of anxiety, benzodiazepines are contraindicated, having been shown to cause increased impulsivity. Clonazepam, a benzodiazepine with anticonvulsant and antimanic properties, is associated with increased serotonin levels and may be useful adjunctively for anxiety, anger, and dysphoric mood.

Antipsychotics are the most researched medications for the treatment of BPDs and should be the first-line treatment when cognitive-perceptual symptoms are significant. Low doses should be tried first. There is no evidence that antipsychotics are helpful for BPD cognitive-perceptual symptoms in the long term. Antipsychotics may also be used adjuvantly with antidepressants for affective dysregulation, particularly with anger. Antipsychotics such as risperidone may exacerbate or induce manic symptoms, although they produce symptom improvement in bipolar disorder when used in conjunction with mood-stabilizing medications. When the recent guidelines were written, there was insufficient evidence that third-generation antipsychotics (eg, risperidone or olanzapine) would be effective with cognitive-perceptual symptoms in BPD, but given the side-effect profiles of conventional versus third-generation antipsychotics, the newer drugs are being used increasingly, empirically. The atypical antipsychotic clozapine is effective in personality disturbances that are cognitive-perceptual and impulsive but, given its risk for agranulocytosis, should be reserved until several trials of other medications have failed.

Risperidone appears superior to conventional antipsychotics in treatment of impulsivity and aggression, especially in BPD. However, SSRIs at low to moderately high doses should be tried first. If needed, low-dose antipsychotics may then be added to SSRIs, or used more aggressively as a last line of treatment. Mood-stabilizing medications are indicated as midlevel treatment for impulsivity. Lithium is effective, perhaps because of its impact on serotonin levels. The anticonvulsant divalproex sodium has been used to treat irritability and impulsivity in patients with BPD who have not responded to SSRI therapy, apparently independent of the presence of abnormal electroencephalographic findings. Carbamazepine is also effective as a mood stabilizer. Use of mood stabilizers requires various laboratory tests to monitor metabolic functioning. Various antipsychotic medications carry risks for extrapyramidal symptoms, tardive dyskinesia, weight gain, diabetes mellitus, extended Q-T intervals, and other problems.

American Psychiatric Association: *Practice Guideline for the Treatment of Patients with Borderline Personality Disorder.* APA, 2001.

Oldham JM: *Guideline Watch: Practice Guideline for the Treatment of Patients with Borderline Personality Disorder.* American Psychiatric Association, 2005. Available at: http://www.psych.org/psych_pract/treatg/g/BPD_watch_031505.pdf.

Soloff PH: Psychopharmacology of borderline personality disorder. Psychiatr Clin North Am 2000;23:169. [PMID: 10729938]

D. Psychotherapeutic Interventions

Some PDs are amenable to some forms of psychotherapy. Treatments of less than 1 year duration probably represent crisis interventions or treatments of concurrent Axis I disorders rather than attempts to address core PD psychopathology. Psychotherapy for borderline and narcissistic personalities tends to take significantly longer. Even with extended duration, treatment goals tend to be for functional improvement such as decreased symptom severity and decreased acting out, rather than complete remission of symptoms. Anxiety-related PDs, such as avoidant and dependent PDs, are most amenable to psychotherapy, followed by BPD, followed by schizotypal PD. Cognitive-behavioral psychotherapy, which challenges irrational beliefs, may be effective with avoidant, dependent, obsessive-compulsive, narcissistic, and paranoid PDs. Because individuals with antisocial PD are manipulative and seldom take responsibility for their behavior, psychotherapy is difficult and relatively rare, unless court-ordered interventions are counted as psychotherapy, which is questionable.

Successful treatment of borderline and narcissistic PDs requires high levels of therapist experience. Skills in managing the therapeutic alliance and creating a stable, trusting relationship are crucial. Insight is less of a focus. Psychotherapy for narcissistic PDs may be highly specialized wherein the patient's hypersensitivity to slights is confronted only after much trust building and attainment of positive transference.

Group therapy and partial hospitalization are effective for patients with schizotypal and borderline PDs. Dialectical behavior therapy is a unique form of psychotherapy that is effective for BPD. During individual and group therapies the patient's beliefs, contradictions, and acting out are empathically accepted. That is, the patient's personhood is responded to positively, and dysfunctional behaviors are responded to matter-of-factly, neither sympathizing with, nor punishing, the patient. Sessions focus on learning to solve problems, control emotions, manage anxiety, and improve interpersonal relationships. After many months of this consistent and intensive treatment, limits are set on the patient's behavior.

E. Transfer and End-of-Care Separation Strategies

Patients with certain PDs may have great difficulty separating from their family physician. Separation is also difficult for patients with chronic illnesses and other psychiatric disorders or those who are socially isolated. Responses to termination can be understood in the context of attachment and loss. According to attachment theory, humans form strong bonds that serve basic biological functions by ensuring that the very young are protected. Separation of the young from their object of attachment results in crying, clinging, increased anxiety, and a possibility of depression or anger upon rapprochement. Even for patients without mental disorders, attachment-related behaviors can resurface during times of stress as panic and anxiety, particularly with the helplessness and dependence that accompany illness and hospitalization or loss of the powerful figure that the physician may represent.

Developmentally oriented theorists have suggested that BPD pathology originates in a disturbed attachment process. Abandonment is extremely traumatic for children. Depression and difficulty forming new relationships result. The notion in BPD is that during the critical period of ages 2–3 when the child typically practices separation from the mother, the parent of the borderline progeny is unable to accept the child's distancing from the parent and is inconsistent upon the child's return, alternatively rejecting or indulging the child. This pattern repeats through childhood and is replicated in adulthood, where there is great ambivalence about relationships. BPD relational patterns seem to approximate the practicing phase of childhood where there is highly emotional approaching and distancing from the pseudoparental object. Tenuous relationships may be formed and abandonment fears are strong. This interpersonal pattern applies to the physician–patient relationship, as well. The patient, fearing abandonment, alternates between extremes of overvaluing and devaluing the physician. During times away from the physician, the patient may be preoccupied with thoughts of the physician and may experience physical distress.

The following suggestions may help to avoid serious problems for patients undergoing separation:

- Inform patients in advance of upcoming separations.
- Review with patients their responses to previous losses. This will give some prediction about how the patient will react to the termination as well as help the physician–patient team identify strengths on which to capitalize and weaknesses to address.
- Take the pending separation as an opportunity to review the patient's health care and the role of the physician-patient relationship in the process of care.
- Have patients express how the relationship has been beneficial, what they may have learned about themselves in that relationship, and how that could be helpful in future relationships.
- Resist a desire to not say goodbye to patients. This may happen for a number of reasons, including fear of hurting patients, reluctance to cause "clinging" behaviors, or anger at noncompliant yet demanding patients.
- Understand the patient's reaction to the news. Some patients may be cool or otherwise noncommittal to the physician's leaving. A patient who does not want to speak about an upcoming separation can be offered the opportunity to speak about it at a future visit. The patient should know that any and all emotional responses are acceptable. Issues of trust and feelings of abandonment warrant explicit discussion.
- Initiate the discussion with a brief statement that the physician is leaving. Follow this with a brief silence that allows patients to understand and respond. If the silence persists, ask patients what they are thinking or feeling. Body language may provide clues. They can be asked to elaborate on their feelings or, if not responding, gently confronted with a question like, "I am wondering what this news is like for you."
- When possible, introduce patients to their new care provider. This meeting facilitates information transfer and symbolizes a turning over of the relationship with the patient.
- Ask new patients how they feel about their previous physician.

F. Termination of Care

Despite the physician's best efforts, it is sometimes necessary to terminate care against the patient's wishes. The following steps and policies should be considered:

- Have a clear policy about what circumstances will produce care termination, such as repeated drug abuse, violent acting out including threatening, repeatedly missed appointments, physician's opinion that care has reached maximal therapeutic benefit, and so on.
- Try contracting with the patient to stop these behaviors first.
- Give patients written, advanced warning that care is being terminated. Thirty days warning is typical. The physician may need to provide care in the interim unless circumstances argue otherwise. If not, patients should be given directions on where they may receive care.
- Ethical practice includes physician freedom to choose whom they will serve. However, termination of a patient with a mental disorder requires consideration of patient competency and emotional status, or else abandonment is possible. Consulting with a colleague is an appropriate means to ensure that consideration is given to patient needs.
- Be aware of any specific policies or actions required by state laws and regulations.

Prognosis

Perhaps half of all patients with PDs never receive treatment. Several of the PDs, although pervasive in their negative effects, are perhaps not sufficiently impairing or distressing to warrant treatment. Treatment outcomes are improving for the PDs that are extremely debilitating, such as BPD. PDs with anxiety components have good potential for improvement. Debate remains as to whether any treatment other than incarceration can be effective for individuals with antisocial PD, and with this, whether effect seen comes with age (ie, the person becomes less disruptive as age 40 is approached). Patients with BPD appear to improve by age 40, as well. Patients with BPD who are in treatment improve at a rate seven times their natural course.

Somatoform Disorders, Factitious Disorder, & Malingering

55

William Elder, PhD

ESSENTIALS OF DIAGNOSIS

- *Unexplained physical symptoms or irrational anxiety about illness or appearance, for which biomedical findings are not consistent with a general medical condition.*
- *While somatoform disorders are unintentional, factitious disorder and malingering are intentional.*
- *Often associated with comorbid or primary mental disorders.*

General Considerations

Somatoform disorders involve unexplained physical symptoms that bring significant distress and functional impairment. They present one of the more common and most difficult problems in primary care. They are seldom "cured" and should be approached as a chronic disease. Recognition, a patient-centered approach, and specific treatments may help alleviate symptoms and distress.

Essential features of somatoform disorders include the following:

- Physical symptoms or irrational anxiety about illness or appearance, for which biomedical findings are not consistent with a general medical condition. Somatoform disorders have specific courses, symptoms, and complaints (Table 55–1).
- Symptoms develop with or are worsened by psychological stress and are not intentional.
- Symptoms that vary along a spectrum of seriousness. Somatic expression of psychological distress is normal. Comorbid or primary mental disorders are common with somatoform symptoms.
- Extensive utilization of medical care. Paradoxically, treatment and attempts to reassure patients can be counterproductive.
- Feelings of frustration on the part of the physician. Patients are often seen as "difficult patients."

Ten percent of all medical services are provided to patients with no organic disease. Twenty-six percent of primary care patients meet criteria for somatic "preoccupation": 19% of patients have medically unexplainable symptoms and 25–50% of visits involve symptoms that have no serious cause. Most patients with medically unexplained symptoms do not have somatoform disorders, but where somatoform disorders are present, symptoms persists much longer and the cost of ambulatory care is 9–14 times greater than in controls. With appropriate recognition and treatment, costs of care may be reduced by 50%. Individuals with somatoform disorders undergo numerous medical examinations, diagnostic procedures, surgeries, and hospitalizations. They risk increased morbidity from these procedures. Eighty-two percent stop working at some point because of their difficulties.

Pathogenesis

To some degree, somatoform symptoms should be considered normal. Bodily experiences of emotions are common. Examples include anger in the jaw, tension in the shoulders, loss in the chest, disappointment in the gut, shame in the reddening face, fear in the bowels, and so on. Children quickly feel ill when they learn that a friend is sick or when family stress is high. So-called student's syndrome, experienced by medical students in their first pathology class, is an example of nonpathologic fear of having a disease.

Regarding somatoform disorders, some individuals are susceptible to overexperiencing sensations, apparently through a difference in gating, which is worsened by anxiety or psychological stress. Other individuals demonstrate obsessive tendencies. Fears of disease may form. A vicious process of symptom amplification has been demonstrated in hypochondriasis whereby obsession about the body focuses attention on sensations, which when misinterpreted cause anxiety, increasing sensations and further worsening obsessiveness. Perceptual disturbances and

Table 55–1. Somatoform disorders, Factitous Disorder, and Malingering.

	Symptom Presentation	Type of Symptoms	Prevalence and Gender Ratios	Voluntary Control over Symptoms	Symptom Duration	Age of Onset
Somatization disorder	Sees self as sickly; frequent medical care	Multiple systems or functions of several types, including pain and pseudoneurologic	0.2–2% in females; < 0.2% in males	No	Chronic, recurring and/or stable	Adolescence or early 20s; rare in aged
Undifferentiated somatoform disorder	Sees self as ill; frequent medical care	Single system of symptom	Common	No	More than 6 months	Early 20s
Conversion disorder	Onset after acute stress	Single, pseudoneurologic	0.01–0.1%; females much more common	No	Sudden onset; short duration	Adolescence
Pain disorder	Focus solely on pain; pain behaviors	Pain; low back, neck, pelvic; emotional changes	Common	No	Sudden onset; worsens with time	All ages; 30s–40s most common
Hypochondriasis	Fearful of disease; preoccupied with symptoms; not reassured	Multiple; normal bodily sensations; may be vague	4–9% of medical practices; equal	No	Long history, worsens after actual illness	Any, but typically early adulthood; concerns without fears not abnormal in elderly
Body dysmorphic disorder	Excessive concern about imagined defect in appearance	Specific complaints of defect	?	No	Usually several years	Adolescence; early 20s
Factitious disorder with physical symptoms	Multiple operations; infections	Nonhealing and unremitting	Rare	Yes	Chronic; multiple admissions; remits with confrontation	Early adulthood
Malingering	Protest; demand for medical help	Vague pain and/or paralysis common	?	Yes	Multiple episodes of same problem	Early adulthood

bodily concerns apparent in body dysmorphic disorder are similar to obsessive-compulsive disorders but when extreme may suggest a mild thought disorder. Genetic factors, demonstrated in adoption studies, appear to play a role in the development of somatic sensitivities and obsessive tendencies. Traumatic experiences in the form of sexual, physical, and emotional abuse and witnessing violence are predictive of somatoform disorders and demonstrate the role of anxiety in development of somatic symptoms.

Because families differ in how they respond to symptoms and illnesses, individual differences in health beliefs and illness-related behaviors are to be expected. Families also shape the tendency to experience, display, and magnify somatic symptoms; thus, somatoform disorders or malingering may be modeled or reinforced by adults. Social factors include single parenthood, living alone, unemployment, and marital and job difficulties.

Gender ratios and prevalence of somatoform disorders differ across cultures. In North America, somatization, conversion, and pain disorders are more frequent in women whereas hypochondriasis and body dysmorphic disorder involve men and women equally. Somatoform symptoms are more prevalent among Chinese-American, Asian, and South American patients.

Cultures have different explanatory models for physical functioning and disease processes. Disorders with somatoform characteristics specific to certain cultures include the *dhat* syndrome in India, which is a concern about semen loss, and *koro* in Southeast Asia, a preoccupation that the penis will disappear into the abdomen, resulting in death. A nondelusional sense of having worms in the head or burning hands is sometimes reported by people in Africa and Southeast Asia. Cultures influence illness behaviors, such as whether a medical clinician or traditional healer is sought first, or how emotions should be expressed. Cultures also sanction religious and healing rituals that promote behaviors that may appear conversion-like. Thus, somatoform-like symptoms should be evaluated for appropriateness to the patient's social context. Behaviors sanctioned by the culture are typically not considered pathologic.

Western medicine's dominant conceptualization of the mechanism of somatoform symptoms is that of somatization, a process in which mental phenomena such as emotions manifest as physical symptoms. As a concept, somatization assumes psychopathology. It originated in psychoanalytic theory, where it was considered a primitive, psychological defense against unconscious conflicts, needs, and desires that the individual was too weak to express. The notion of somatization as a defense has some clinical utility and constitutes an improvement over beliefs that some feminine physical complaints reflect a uterus loose in the body, hence the term *hysterical*, derived from the Greek word for uterus. However, the notion of somatization as pathologic ignores the normalcy of physical expression of emotions and the social construction of illness behaviors, including the belief that conventional medical treatments such as medication and surgery can solve most problems.

Clinical Findings

A. Symptoms and Signs

Somatoform symptoms can suggest a large number of general medical conditions. However, in addition to ruling out general medical conditions, diagnosis may also be made by inclusion. The following features should increase suspicion of a somatoform presentation:

- Unexplained symptoms that are chronic or constantly change.
- Multiple symptoms. Four symptoms in men and six in women suggest somatic preoccupation. Fainting, menstrual problems, headache, chest pain, dizziness, and palpitations are the symptoms most likely to be somatoform.
- Vague or highly personalized, idiosyncratic complaints.
- Inability of more than three physicians to make a diagnosis.
- Presence of another mental disorder, especially depressive, anxiety, or substance use disorders.
- Distrust toward the physician.
- Physician experience of frustration.
- Paradoxic worsening of symptoms with treatment.
- High utilization, including repeated visits, frequent telephone calls, multiple medications, and repeated subspecialty referrals.
- Disproportionate disability and role impairment.

B. Diagnostic Criteria

Somatoform disorders are mental disorders that involve physical symptoms or irrational anxiety about illness or appearance, and for which biomedical findings are not consistent with a general medical condition. Diagnosis requires a finding that the symptoms have brought unneeded medical treatment or that there is significant impairment in social, occupational, or other important areas of functioning. Somatoform disorders cannot be caused by another mental condition or by direct effects of substances. If the disorder occurs in the presence of a general medical condition, complaints or impairment must be in excess of what would be expected from the physical findings and history.

1. Somatization disorder—This persistent pattern of recurring, multiple somatic complaints begins before age 30. Patients view themselves as "sickly." Historically, somatization disorder was referred to as *hysteria* or Briquet syndrome, a fluctuating mental disorder in young women characterized by frequent complaints of physical illness involving multiple organ systems. Current diagnostic criteria are more extensive, requiring a history of pain related to at least four different sites or functions, two gastrointestinal symptoms other than pain, one sexual symptom other than pain, and one pseudoneurologic symptom other than pain. Common sites of pain include the head, abdomen, back, joints, extremities, chest, and rectum and common functions include pain during menstruation, during sexual intercourse, or during urination. Common gastrointestinal symptoms include nausea, bloating, diarrhea, or multiple food intolerances. Sexual symptoms include sexual indifference, sexual dysfunction, and menstrual problems. Pseudoneurologic symptoms can be motor related (eg, impaired coordination or balance, paralysis or localized weakness, difficulty swallowing including "lump in throat," aphonia, and urinary retention) or sensory-perceptual (eg, minor hallucinations, loss of touch or pain sensation, double vision, blindness, and deafness). Seizures, amnesia, and loss of consciousness are also possible.

2. Undifferentiated somatoform disorder—This is a residual diagnosis for clinically significant, somatoform complaints persisting for more than 6 months. Examples include chronic fatigue, weakness, and anorexia as well as the symptoms described with regard to somatization disorder, when insufficient in number to meet diagnostic criteria for somatization disorder.

3. Conversion disorder (formerly hysterical conversion disorder)—This consists solely of pseudoneurologic symptoms such as those described with somatization disorder (ie, deficits affecting the central nervous system, voluntary motor or sensory functions). Psychological factors in the form of stressors or emotional conflicts are expected and precede the symptoms. Depending on the medical naivete of the patient, symptoms are often quite implausible, not conforming to anatomic pathways or physiologic mechanisms. Symptoms may symbolically represent emotional conflicts, such as arm immobility, as an expression of anger and impotence. Other clues indicating that the symptoms are pseudoneurologic include worsening in the presence of others; noninjuries despite dramatic falls; normal reflexes, muscle tone, and pupillary reactions; and striking inconsistencies on repeated examinations. Symptoms may be experienced with a relative lack of concern (so-called *la belle indifference*) but dramatic or histrionic presentations are more common. Course is an important consideration. Conversion disorder is rare before age 10 or after age 35 years. Symptoms are transient, rarely lasting beyond 2 weeks, and respond to reassurance, suggestion, and psychological support. Secondary gain, seen in malingering, may be apparent but is not primary in conversion disorders.

4. Pain disorder associated with psychological factors—This disorder is the psychiatric equivalent of chronic nonmalignant pain syndrome, except that no minimum duration of symptoms is required. Psychological factors play a significant role in the pain picture, including its onset, severity, exacerbation, and maintenance. Physical pathologies are possible and frequent but organic findings are insufficient to explain the severity of the pain. Common sites for pain include the lower back, neck, pelvis, and head. Patients with this disorder may follow a downward spiral of poor functioning, especially if they lack adequate skills to adaptively cope with their losses of physical functioning and situational changes. The experience of pain will severely disrupt patients' lives; thus functional deficits are common, including disability, increased use of the health care system, abuse of medications, and relational and vocational disruptions. Depression or anxiety may be secondary or may also be primary or comorbid, predisposing the patient to an increased experience of pain as well as a deficient ability to cope with the illness situation. Patients with severe depression or with terminal conditions are at increased risk of suicide. Insomnia is frequently associated with pain complaints.

5. Hypochondriasis—The individual with hypochondriasis is preoccupied with fears of having a serious disease. The preoccupation may originate in an overfocus on and misinterpretation of normal physiologic sensations (eg, orthostatic dizziness), erroneous attributions about the body (eg, "aching veins"), or obsession about minor physical abnormalities. Patients are easily alarmed when hearing of new diseases or knowing someone who is sick. Fears persist despite medical reassurance. Hypochondriacal concerns (ie, attention to symptoms and fear of death) are common in panic disorders. In the case of concerns about physical abnormalities, the individual must believe that the abnormality indicates the presence of a disease; otherwise a diagnosis of body dysmorphic disorder is more appropriate.

6. Body dysmorphic disorder—This disorder involves excessive preoccupation with a minor or imagined defect of one or more body parts. Concern may not focus exclusively on a false belief one is obese, which would indicate an eating disorder. Although many people are concerned about their appearance, the concerns and behaviors associated with this disorder are extreme, distressing, time consuming, and debilitating. Self-consciousness is significant, and avoidance of public exposure, hiding of defects, and nondisclosure to the physician are common. Medical, dental, and surgical treatments are sought but may only worsen preoccupations. Concerns about appropriateness of sexual characteristics may be better represented in a diagnosis of gender identity disorder. Concerns about appearance are common during major depressive episodes. Patients who insist that an imagined defect is real and hideous will meet the criteria for delusional disorder, somatic type.

7. Malingering, factitious disorder, and factitious disorder by proxy—These are not somatoform disorders; symptoms are voluntary and deceptive. Deception is obtained by feigning or self-inducing symptoms or by falsifying histories or laboratory findings. Common symptoms include fever, self-mutilation, hemorrhage, and seizures. Malingering and factitious disorder differ by whether symptom gain is primary or secondary. In malingering, symptoms are produced to gain rewards or avoid punishments (secondary gains). Factitious disorder involves production of symptoms in order to assume the sick role (primary gain). Unlike malingering, factitious disorder is considered a mental disorder principally because the need to be in the sick role is abnormal. Factitious disorder by proxy occurs when illness is caused by a caregiver, typically to meet a need for drama and to be a rescuer of the patient. Direct evidence, such as inconsistent laboratory or physical findings or observations (eg, injection of bacteria), may be the first sign that symptoms are intentional. Earlier signs of factitious disorder include patients who are migratory or have no visitors, are comfortable with more aggressive treatments including extended hospitalization, are connected in some manner with the health professions, or whose presentation is exaggerated and quite dramatic (Munchausen syndrome).

C. Screening and Diagnostic Measures

Valid diagnostic and screening questionnaires exist, but often lack clinical utility in comparison to an interview. Where doubts remain, a referral for evaluation is probably in order. Asking questions about depressed mood and hopelessness or loss of interest has great sensitivity for depressive disorder, if the depression is not occult. Questions should address cognitive symptoms, such as guilt and lowered self-esteem, endorsement of which may suggest depression even in the absence of sad mood. Questions should also evaluate patients suspected of having body dysmorphic disorder (Table 55–2).

Differential Diagnosis

Diagnosis should be considered tentative and provisional until there is considerable external support. General medical conditions characterized by multiple and confusing somatic symptoms (eg, hyperparathyroidism, porphyria, multiple sclerosis, and systemic lupus erythematosus) should be considered. Conversion disorder, in particular, is often misdiagnosed, with medical diagnoses eventually replacing up to 50% of conversion diagnoses. Shaibani and Sabbagh have described several clinical tests that may reveal whether conversion symptoms are pseudoneurologic. Onset of multiple physical symptoms in early adulthood suggests somatization disorder but in the elderly suggests a general medical condition. Primary or secondary depression should be considered in any patient suspected of having somatoform disorder. Other mental disorders, including anxiety disorders and substance-related disorders, are frequently seen with somatoform disorders and in some cases may better explain symptoms and thus constitute the better diagnosis. Personality disorders (eg, histrionic, borderline, or antisocial personality disorder) are also frequently associated with somatoform disorders.

Table 55–2. Questions to evaluate body dysmorphic disorder.

1. Do you worry about the appearance of your face or body? If so, what is your concern?
2. How bad do you think your (face or body part) appears?
3. How much time do you spend worrying about your (face or body part)?
4. Have you done anything to hide or rid yourself of the problem?
5. How does this concern with your appearance affect your life?

Source: Adapted, with permission, from Phillips KA: Body dysmorphic disorder: diagnosis and treatment of the imagined ugliness. J Clin Psychiatry 1996;57(suppl 8):61.

Shaibani A, Sabbagh MN: Pseudoneurologic syndromes: Recognition and diagnosis. Am Fam Physician 1998;57:2485. [PMID: 9614416]

Complications

Failure to recognize and properly treat somatoform complaints can lead to excessive diagnostic procedures and treatments, which perpetuate patient preoccupations and place the patient at risk for iatrogenic disorders. Use of unidentified, unconventional, or alternative treatments by patients with somatoform disorders may interact negatively with prescribed medications. Dependencies on sedative, analgesic, or narcotic agents are common iatrogenic complications.

Treatment

Characterizing medically unexplained symptoms as pathologic may lead physicians to misconstrue patients as solely suffering from a psychiatric disorder. In reality, primary care patients are usually quite different from those seen in specialty psychiatric care. The notion and usefulness of discrete disease entities are problematic to begin with. Primary care patients present with undifferentiated symptoms that are best addressed with a comprehensive approach that includes continuity of care and attention to the physician–patient relationship. "Pathologizing" makes patients feel illegitimate, in itself a major source of distress, and produces stereotypes of patients as "crocks, whiners, or difficult." If this happens, the relevance of the patient's experience and the potential of partnership between patient and physician are both obviated. A patient-centered method, so important to family practice, becomes impossible. Patients who consider their physicians as patient centered are more satisfied with care, are referred less, and receive fewer diagnostic tests.

Even without attributions of a mental disorder, somatoform symptoms present one of the most difficult challenges in primary care. Patient characteristics considered as difficult include extensive or exaggerated complaints, nonadherence with treatment recommendations, and behaviors that raise suspicion of seeking drugs. Uncertainties associated with the diagnosis, the sense that the focus is not medical and therefore the interaction is inappropriate, patient symptom amplification, and the sense that services are being overused inappropriately contribute to the perception that the patient is difficult. Furthermore, most physicians sought their career in order to cure people; treatment of people with these chronic conditions conflicts with that goal.

A. General Recommendations

Somatoform symptoms exist on a continuum and should rarely indicate that the patient's difficulties are to be attributed solely to a mental disorder. Comprehensive, continuous, patient-centered care appropriately addresses most primary care patient presentations. The following general recommendations apply to such an approach.

1. First visits—A therapeutic alliance should be built by a thorough history and physical examination and by a review of the patient's records. The physician should show curiosity and interest in the patient's complaints and validate the patient's suffering. Psychogenic attributions should be avoided. To appear puzzled initially is a good strategy. Delivery of a diagnosis is a key treatment step with somatoform disorders. Different disorders require different types of information. Suggestions for statements to be made to the patient appear in Table 55–3.

2. Management—The disorder should be treated as a chronic illness, with the focus on functioning rather than symptom cure. Gradual change should be expected, with periods of improvement and relapse. Physicians should practice secondary prevention, especially of iatrogenic harm. When new symptoms arise, at least a limited physical examination should be performed. However, invasive diagnostic and therapeutic procedures should be permitted only on the basis of objective evidence, not subjective complaints. The need for unnecessary tests and procedures can be avoided by having the patient feel "known" by the physician.

3. Patient-centered care—Feelings of illegitimacy by patients and common physician attitudes toward patients contribute to power differentials and struggles. These can be avoided by practicing the relational behaviors patients prefer from their providers. Physicians should speak with patients as equals, listen well, ask lots of questions, answer lots of questions, explain things understandably, and allow patients to make decisions about their care. A collaborative relationship should be developed in which the physician works together with the patient to understand and manage patient problems. The "common ground" shared by the physician and the patient should be monitored and differences discussed.

4. Office visits—Regular, brief appointments should be scheduled, thus avoiding "as-needed" medications and office visits that make medical attention contingent on symptoms. Practical time-related strategies include negotiating and setting the agenda early in the visit, paying attention to the emotional agenda, listening actively rather than in a controlling manner, soliciting the patient's attributions for the problems, and communicating empathetically.

5. Psychosocial issues—Reassurance should be provided to the patient, but not too soon. Psychosocial questions should be interspersed with biomedical ones to explore all issues: physiologic, anatomic, social, family, and psychological. The physician should inquire about trauma and abuse. As trust builds, the patient should be encouraged to explore psychological issues that may be related to symptoms. In this way, symptoms can be linked to the patient's life and feelings. The term *stress* should not be overused. Eventually and subtly, patients are likely to reveal their personal side and concerns.

6. Family involvement—Family members should be invited to participate in patients' visits. An occasional family conference can be valuable. Each person's opinion about the illness and treatment can be solicited, and family members can be asked how family life would be different if the patient were without symptoms. Physicians should solicit and constantly return to the patient's and family's strengths and areas of competence.

B. Pharmacotherapy

Because these patients may be extremely sensitive to side effects, psychopharmacologic agents generally should not be used unless the patient has a demonstrated pharmacologically responsive mental disorder such as major depression, generalized anxiety disorder, panic disorder, or obsessive-compulsive disorder. (For further discussion of these disorders, see Chapters 52–54.) Selective serotonin reuptake inhibitors (SSRIs), other nontricyclic antidepressants, and benzodiazepines are the medications most frequently used for coexisting psychiatric conditions. Treatment should be initiated at subtherapeutic doses and increased very gradually, as described elsewhere (see Chapters 52–54).

Contrary to standard placebo effect-enhancing practice (ie, enthusiastic recommendation of a medication), psychopharmacologic agents should be recommended

Table 55–3. Delivering the diagnosis in somatoform and related disorders.

Disorder	Statements
Somatization disorder	1. I know that you are experiencing much discomfort and feeling very ill. 2. You have a medical disorder called somatization disorder. 3. This disorder runs in families and has a unique pattern of symptoms. It does not cause physical deterioration or shorten life. 4. It is not curable, but manageable. A specific treatment plan is required.
Conversion disorder	1. Avoid terms "conversion disorder" and "psychogenic." 2. After thorough evaluation, the (symptom name, eg, blindness) will resolve very quickly. 3. It is, in fact, starting to improve at this time.
Pain disorder	1. I have reviewed your records and thoroughly evaluated you. 2. All appropriate interventions have been tried. 3. You have a medical condition called somatoform pain disorder. 4. Your disorder is not life-threatening but I know that you are experiencing much discomfort and (specific function, eg, moving) quite poorly. 5. Our goal must be rehabilitation, not necessarily being pain free. 6. A specific treatment plan is required.
Hypochondriasis	1. Reassurance of nonpathology is unlikely to be helpful. A diagnostic label will be helpful. 2. You have a syndrome of neurologic amplification of body sensations. 3. The syndrome is not life-threatening but requires careful monitoring. 4. We need to schedule regular appointments. I want you to discuss your concerns at these appointments and I'll examine you thoroughly.
Body dysmorphic disorder	1. I can see that you are very concerned about this sense that your (body part, eg, nose) is ugly. 2. You get very anxious when you think about people seeing it and want to hide it. You even want to stay away from others because you are so anxious. 3. What I suggest we do for now is try these measures to treat your anxiety so that your suffering is less and you function better, not missing out on things that you would otherwise like to do.
Factitious disorder	1. The physician may decide to directly confront a patient. However, if family or other social situation is available to promote the patient's need to save face, a therapeutic double bind is suggested. A thorough physical examination and attempt to build a therapeutic alliance must be performed before delivering the diagnosis. 2. Sometimes people do things to make themselves ill. We call this problem factitious disorder. 3. You have an unusual problem. I believe it will respond to one more attempt to treat it. If, however, the problem does not respond to this attempt, a diagnosis of factitious disorder will be established.
Malingering	1. Informing the patient that his or her deception has been detected can be dangerous and should be handled carefully. In some cases it may be better to deprive the patient of any benefits of the sick role, which will extinguish the behavior. 2. I guess I am wondering if there might be some reason for you to be sick right now. 3. Have you thought about what might happen if you continue to do this?

Source: Adapted, with permission, from McCahill ME: Somatoform and related disorders: delivery of diagnosis as first step. Am Fam Physician 1995;52(1):193.

with a degree of pessimism, with the notion that it is unlikely to be very beneficial but may be worth a try. Hypochondriasis and body dysmorphic disorders are similar to obsessive-compulsive disorder and patients with these disorders may benefit directly from higher doses of SSRIs, if side effects are tolerated. Those with transitorily extreme dysmorphic concerns may benefit from temporary treatment with an atypical antipsychotic medication.

C. Consultation or Referral

Involvement of a mental health clinician may be helpful to diagnose comorbid mental conditions, offer suggestions for psychotropic medications, and engage some patients in psychotherapy. However, patients are unlikely to see the value of consultation or may experience referral as an accusation that their symptoms are not authentic. Pressuring the patient to accept a consultation is unlikely to be effective and may render the consultant encounter unproductive. Trust must first be established and psychological issues must be made a legitimate subject for discussion. The idea of referral can be reintroduced later. When possible, it can be more effective to see the patient along with the mental health clinician so that a comprehensive approach continues to be emphasized, the patient does not feel abandoned, and doubts that the patient's concerns are not taken seriously are alleviated. Extreme distress or preoccupations worsening to delusional levels may require inpatient hospitalization.

D. Psychotherapeutic Interventions

Standardized group or individual cognitive-behavioral therapies can be an effective treatment for chronic somatoform disorders, reducing somatic symptoms, distress, impairment, and medical care utilization and costs. Cognitive interventions train the patient to identify and restructure dysfunctional beliefs and assumptions about health. Behaviorally, the patient is encouraged to experiment with activities that are counter to usual practices, such as avoidance, "doctor shopping," or excess seeking of reassurance. In addition, patients learn relaxation and meditation techniques to manage symptoms of anxiety. Patients with high emotional distress respond more rapidly to psychotherapy and patients able to at least partially attribute symptoms to psychological factors show better therapeutic outcomes than patients who firmly believe that their physical symptoms have a physical cause.

E. Complementary and Alternative Therapies

It is to be expected that patients with somatoform symptoms often try alternative treatments such as herbal remedies, mind–body interventions, and other nonwestern medical approaches. In these patients, conventional treatments appear to have failed, distrust of physicians may be high, and distress is great. Federal regulations require that label claims and instructions on herbal products and supplements address symptoms only; therefore, there are no specific herbal agents for somatoform disorders, per se. Given the plethora of symptoms that can exist in patients with somatoform disorders, it is not surprising that there are numerous alternative medications that patients may try.

Patients with pain disorder or primary or comorbid anxiety may benefit from body and mind–body interventions such as massage, movement therapies, manipulations, relaxation, guided imagery, and hypnosis. The placebo effect of various remedies may be helpful, particularly if the agents are largely inert, as bothersome side effects seen in conventional medicines will be favorably avoided. Alternative therapies often include "nonspecific therapeutic effects" that go beyond the placebo effect and can be beneficial. Nonspecific effects include warmth and listening skills of the practitioner, empowerment that comes from legitimization of the patient's problem, and an egalitarian approach to care. These may be recognized as important constituents of the patient-centered approach. Physicians may wish to recommend alternative treatments and collaborate with alternative practitioners but should also be prepared to protect the patient by cautioning against treatments that are potentially harmful, excessively expensive, or that circumvent conventional treatments that are needed for demonstrated medical conditions.

F. Patient Education

The American Academy of Family Physicians has developed a patient education handout for somatoform disorders. Information is similar to and expands on the key statements for somatization disorder appearing in Table 55–3. The web address for the handout is http://www.familydoctor.org/handouts/162.html.

Epstein RM, Quill TE, McWhinney IR: Somatization reconsidered: Incorporating the patient's experience of illness. Arch Intern Med 1999;159:215. [PMID: 9989533]

Jackson JL, Passamonti M: The outcomes among patients presenting in primary care with a psychical symptom at 5 years. J Gen Intern Med 2005;20:1032. [PMID: 16307629]

Righter EL, Sansone RA: Managing somatic preoccupation. Am Fam Physician 1999;59:3113. [PMID: 10392593]

Schweickhardt A et al: Differentiation of somatizing patients in primary care: Why the effects of treatment are always moderate. J Nerv Ment Dis 2005;193:813. [PMID: 16319704]

Substance Use Disorders

56

Robert Mallin, MD

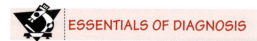

- *Screening positive (answering yes to two or more questions) on the CAGE questionnaire.*
- *A pattern of substance misuse during which the patient maintains control over use (abuse) or during which control over use is lost (dependence).*
- *Presence of a withdrawal syndrome.*
- *Medical history of addiction to drugs or alcohol.*

General Considerations

The prevalence of alcohol and drug disorders in primary care outpatients is between 23% and 37%. The cost to society of these disorders is staggering. Each year in the United States substance use disorders are associated with 100,000 deaths and costs of approximately $100 billion. The high prevalence of these disorders in primary care outpatients suggests that family physicians are confronted with these problems daily. However, these disorders rarely present overtly. Patients in denial about the connection between their substance use and the consequences caused by it frequently minimize the amount of their use and often do not seek assistance for their substance use problem.

The epidemiology of alcohol and drug disorders has been well studied and is most often reported from data of the National Institute of Mental Health Epidemiologic Catchment Area Program (ECA). Lifetime prevalence rates for alcohol disorders from the ECA survey data were 13.5%. For men, the lifetime prevalence was found to be 23.8%, and for women, 4.7%. The National Comorbidity Survey revealed lifetime prevalence of alcohol abuse without dependence to be 12.5% for men and 6.4% for women. For alcohol dependence, the lifetime prevalence was 20.1% in men and 8.2% in women. The ECA data yield an overall prevalence of drug use disorders of 6.2%. As with alcohol use disorders, drug use disorders occur more frequently in men (lifetime prevalence 7.7%) than in women (4.8%). Characteristics known to influence the epidemiology of substance use disorders include gender, age, race, family history, marital status, employment status, and educational status.

Crum RM et al: The association of depression and problem drinking: Analyses from the Baltimore ECA follow-up study. Epidemiologic Catchment Area. Addict Behav 2001;26:765. [PMID: 11676386]

Regier DA et al: Prevalence of anxiety disorders and their comorbidity with mood and addictive disorders. Br J Psychiatry Suppl 1998;(34):24. [PMID: 9829013]

Pathogenesis

The difference between abuse and dependence is an important one. With substance abuse, patients retain control of their use. This control may be affected by poor judgment and social and environmental factors, and mitigated by the consequences of the patient's use. Patients who become dependent (addicted) no longer have full control of their drug use. The brain has been "hijacked" by a substance that affects the mechanism of control over the use of that substance. This addiction is far more than physical dependence. The need to use the drug becomes as powerful as the drives of thirst and hunger. Evidence that the brains of addicted individuals are different from those of nonaddicted persons is enormous. Many of these abnormalities predate the use of the substance and are thought to be inherited. In genetically predisposed individuals, substances of abuse cause changes in the dopaminergic mesolimbic system that result in a loss of control over substance use. These changes are mediated by several neurotransmitters: dopamine, γ-aminobutyric acid (GABA), glutamate, serotonin, and endorphins. The different classes of substances of abuse act through one or more of these neurotransmitters, ultimately affecting the level of dopamine in the mesolimbic system (otherwise known as the reward pathway). These changes in the brain are permanent and are the primary reason for relapse in the addicted patient trying to maintain abstinence or control of use.

Prevention

Although neurobiology plays a large role in addiction, the precursors of substance abuse are also environmental

Table 56–1. Environmental risk factors for substance abuse.

Family factors
Sexual or physical abuse
Parental or sibling substance abuse
Parental approval or tacit approval of child's substance use
Disruptive family conflict
Poor communication
Poor discipline
Poor supervision
Parental rejection
School factors
Lack of involvement in school activities
Poor school climate
Norms that condone substance use
Unfair rules
School failure
Community factors
Poor community bonding
Disorganized neighborhoods
Crime
Drug use
Poverty
Low employment
Community norms that condone substance use
Peer factors
Bonding to peer group that engages in substance use or other antisocial behaviors

and include family, school, community, and peer factors (Table 56–1). These multiple factors make the design of effective prevention very difficult. Primary prevention is designed to prevent the use of substances, thereby making abuse impossible. These programs are designed primarily for the young. Secondary prevention consists of screening programs to identify abuse early and to redirect the patient's behavior before addiction becomes overt. In tertiary prevention, the focus is on the treatment of addictive behavior in an effort to prevent the consequences of compulsive use. Prevention programs can be divided into those that address the four environmental areas of risk: family, school, peers, and community. Family physicians can support these efforts by including the following behaviors in their practice:

- Supporting efforts to strengthen parenting skills, family support, and communication.
- Providing patient and community education about drug and alcohol use, abuse, and treatment.
- Screening and assessing patients of all ages for substance use disorders in the office and hospital.
- Supporting community efforts in substance abuse prevention.
- Endorsing and promoting public policy that supports prevention, early detection, and treatment of substance use disorders.

Botvin GJ, Griffin KW: Life skills training as a primary prevention approach for adolescent drug abuse and other problem behaviors. Int J Emerg Ment Health 2002;4:41. [PMID: 12014292]

Kodjo CM, Klein JD: Prevention and risk of adolescent substance abuse. The role of adolescents, families, and communities. Pediatr Clin North Am 2002;49:257. [PMID: 11993282]

Clinical Findings

A. Symptoms and Signs

The signs and symptoms of substance abuse are varied and often subtle. This is complicated by the fact that most patients do not recognize their substance use as the cause of their problems and are often quite resistant to that interpretation. Consequently the family physician must have a high index of suspicion, recognizing that the prevalence of substance use disorders in outpatient primary care is high. A perspective that recognizes the prevalence of these disorders will enable physicians to interpret potential clues to substance use (Table 56–2).

The diagnosis of substance abuse or dependence is made primarily on the basis of a careful history. However, substance-disordered patients may be deliberately less than truthful in their history, and often the patient's denial prevents the physician from seeing the connection between substance use and its consequences. Signs of sedative hypnotic or alcohol withdrawal may be misinterpreted as an anxiety disorder. Chronic use of stimulants may present as a psychotic disorder. In fact, in the face of active substance abuse, other psychiatric diagnoses often must wait for detoxification before they can be accurately assessed.

B. Screening Measures

The diagnosis of substance use disorders is most typically begun with a screening test that identifies a user at risk. The CAGE questionnaire (Table 55–3) is perhaps the most widely used screening tool for the identification of patients at risk for substance use disorders. When a patient answers yes to two or more questions of the CAGE, the sensitivity is 60–90% and the specificity 40–60% for substance use disorders. Because a screening test is more predictive when applied to a population more likely to have a disease, clinical clues to substance use disorders may be useful indicators to determine who to screen (see Table 56–2).

C. Methods to Differentiate Abuse from Dependence

1. Diagnostic criteria—Once a patient with a substance use problem is identified, it becomes necessary to

Table 56–2. Clinical clues of alcohol and drug problems.

Social history
- Arrest for driving under the influence of alcohol once (75% association with alcoholism) or twice (95% association)
- Loss of job or sent home from work for alcohol or drug reasons
- Domestic violence
- Child abuse/neglect
- Family instability (divorce, separation)
- Frequent, unplanned absences
- Personal isolation
- Problems at work/school
- Mood swings and psychological problems

Medical history
- History of addiction to any drug
- Withdrawal syndrome
- Depression
- Anxiety disorder
- Recurrent pancreatitis
- Recurrent hepatitis
- Hepatomegaly
- Peripheral neuropathy
- Myocardial infarction < age 30 (cocaine)
- Blood alcohol level > 300 or > 100 without impairment
- Alcohol on breath or intoxicated at office visit
- Tremor
- Mild hypertension
- Estrogen-mediated signs (telangectasias, spider angiomas, palmer erythema, muscle atrophy)
- Gastrointestinal complaints
- Sleep disturbances
- Eating disorders
- Sexual dysfunction

determine whether the disorder involves abuse or dependence. Substance abuse is a pattern of misuse during which the patient maintains control, whereas in substance dependence, control over use is lost. Physiologic dependence, evidenced by a withdrawal syndrome, may exist in either state. The *Diagnostic and Statistical Manual of Mental Disorders,* Fourth Edition, Text Revision (*DSM-IV-TR*) diagnostic criteria for substance abuse and dependence are listed in Tables 56–4 and 56–5.

2. Withdrawal syndromes—Although not always seen with substance abuse, physiologic dependence suggests abuse unless the patient is on long-term prescribed addictive medicines. Table 56–6 contrasts signs and symptoms of withdrawal from alcohol and other sedative-hypnotic drugs, opiates, and cocaine and other stimulant drugs. Alcohol withdrawal may be life threatening, if not properly treated. Opiate withdrawal is not life threatening and neither is withdrawal from cocaine or other stimulants, although they both may be associated with morbidity and relapse to substance abuse.

Table 56–3. CAGE questions adapted to include drugs.[1]

1. Have you felt you ought to **C**ut down on your drinking or drug use?
2. Have people **A**nnoyed you by criticizing your drinking or drug use?
3. Have you felt **G**uilty about your drinking or drug use?
4. Have you ever had a drink or used drugs first thing in the morning to steady your nerves or to get rid of a hangover or to get the day started? (**E**ye-opener)

[1]Two or more yes answers indicates a need for a more in-depth assessment. Even one positive response should raise a red flag about problem drinking or drug use.
Source: Adapted, with permission, from Schulz JE, Parran T Jr: Principles of identification and intervention. In: Graham AW, Shultz TK, eds: *Principles of Addiction Medicine*, 2nd ed. American Society of Addiction Medicine, 1998.

In dealing with sedative-hypnotic, alcohol, or opiate withdrawal, assessment of the degree of withdrawal is important to determine appropriate use and dose of medication to reduce symptoms and, in the case of sedative hypnotic drugs or alcohol, prevent seizures and mortality. The Clinical Institute Withdrawal Assess-

Table 56–4. *DSM-IV-TR* criteria for substance abuse.

A maladaptive pattern of substance use, leading to clinically significant impairment or distress, as manifested by two (or more) of the following occurring at any time within a 12-month period:

1. Recurrent substance use resulting in failure to fulfill major role obligations at work, school, or home (eg, repeated absences or poor work performance related to substance use; substance-related absences, suspensions, or expulsions from school; neglect of children or household).
2. Recurrent substance use in situations in which it is physically hazardous (eg, driving an automobile or operating a machine when impaired by substance use).
3. Recurrent substance-related legal problems (eg, arrests for substance-related disorderly conduct).
4. Continued substance use despite having persistent social or interpersonal problems caused or exacerbated by the effects of the substance (eg, arguments with spouse about consequences of intoxication, physical fights).

The symptoms have never met the criteria for Substance Dependence for this class of substance.

Modified, with permission, from American Psychiatric Association: *Diagnostic and Statistical Manual of Mental Disorders,* 4th ed, text revision. American Psychiatric Press, 2000.

Table 56–5. *DSM-IV-TR* criteria for substance dependence.

A maladaptive pattern of substance use, leading to clinically significant impairment or distress, as manifested by three (or more) of the following occurring at any time in the same 12-month period:

1. Tolerance as defined by either of the following:
   a. A need for markedly increased amounts of the substance to achieve intoxication or the desired effect.
   b. Markedly diminished effect with continued use of the same amount of the substance.
2. Withdrawal, as manifested by either of the following:
   a. The characteristic withdrawal syndrome for the substance.
   b. The same (or closely related) substance is taken to relieve or avoid withdrawal symptoms.
3. The substance is often taken in larger amounts or over a longer period than was intended.
4. There is a persistent desire or unsuccessful efforts to cut down or control substance use.
5. A great deal of time is spent in activities necessary to obtain the substance, use the substance, or recover from its effects.
6. Important social, occupational, or recreational activities are given up or reduced because of substance use.
7. The substance use is continued despite knowledge of having a persistant or recurrent physical or psychological problem that is likely to have been caused or exacerbated by the substance.

Modified, with permission, from American Psychiatric Association: *Diagnostic and Statistical Manual of Mental Disorders,* 4th ed, text revision. American Psychiatric Press, 2000.

ment of Alcohol Scale, Revised (CIWA-AR) allows quantification of the signs and symptoms of withdrawal in a predictable fashion that allows clinicians to discuss the severity of withdrawal for a given patient and thus choose intervention strategies that are effective and safe. This tool is available online and can be downloaded from the American Society of Addiction Medicine (ASAM) web site (http://asam.org).

D. Laboratory Findings

Biochemical markers may help support the diagnostic criteria gathered in the history, or can be used as a screening mechanism to consider patients for further evaluation (Table 56–7).

American Psychiatric Association: *Diagnostic and Statistical Manual of Mental Disorders,* 4th ed, text revision. APA, 2000.

Reynaud M et al: Objective diagnosis of alcohol abuse: Compared values of carbohydrate-deficient transferrin (CDT), gamma-glutamyl transferase (GGT), and mean corpuscular volume (MCV). Alcohol Clin Exp Res 2000;24:1414. [PMID: 11003208]

Staab JP et al: Detection and diagnosis of psychiatric disorders in primary medical care settings. Med Clin North Am 2001; 85:579. [PMID: 11349474]

Differential Diagnosis

Because substance abuse is a behavioral disorder, when considering a differential diagnosis, psychiatric disorders often come to mind. Indeed, there is a high comorbidity between substance use disorders and psychiatric disorders. Approximately 50% of psychiatric patients have a substance use disorder. For patients with addictions, however, the rates of psychiatric disorders are similar to the general population. Problems such as substance-induced mood disorders (frequently noted in alcohol, opiate, and stimulant abuse) and substance-induced psychotic disorders (most frequently associated with stimulant abuse) complicate differentiation of primary psychiatric disorders from those that are primarily substance use disorders. Most clinicians agree that psychiatric disorders cannot be reliably assessed in patients who are currently or recently intoxicated. Thus detoxification and a period of abstinence are necessary before evaluation for other psychiatric disorders may effectively be done.

Other than the dilemma of determining whether a substance-induced or comorbid psychiatric disorder is present, differential diagnosis in substance abuse revolves around the issues of abuse versus dependence (see earlier discussion). The essential difference is a loss of control over use in dependence that is not present in abuse. This distinction is complicated, however, by the chronic and waxing and waning nature of substance use disorders. As a result, it is necessary to examine a patient's behavior over an extended period of time, looking for evidence of past loss of control of use that may not currently be present. Usually in addiction a pattern of progressively increasing loss of control becomes evident as the consequences of chronic substance abuse unfold.

Complications

The medical complications of substance abuse are legion and profoundly affect the health of our population (Table 56–8). The number of deaths attributed to the abuse of substances exceeds 500,000 yearly, with tobacco use accounting for 380,000 of these deaths. (For discussion of tobacco use, see Chapter 57.) Cardiovascular disease and cancer lead this list. Alcohol causes approximately 100,000 deaths yearly and is associated with motor vehicle accidents, other accidents, homicides, cirrhosis of the liver, and suicide. Injection drug use is responsible for the fastest growing population of HIV infection. In addition to medical complications, substance abuse causes considerable neuropsychiatric morbidity, both as a primary cause (Table 56–9) and by exacerbating existing psychiatric disorders.

Table 56–6. Symptoms and signs of withdrawal from alcohol, opioids, and cocaine.

Substance of Abuse	Manifestations of Withdrawal
Alcohol	Autonomic hyperactivity: diaphoresis, tachycardia, elevated blood pressure Tremor Insomnia Nausea or vomiting Transient visual, tactile, or auditory hallucinations or illusions Psychomotor agitation Anxiety Generalized seizure activity
Opioids	Mild elevation of pulse rate, respiratory rate, blood pressure, and temperature Piloerection (gooseflesh) Dysphoric mood, drug craving Lacrimation or rhinorrhea Mydriasis, yawning, diaphoresis Anorexia, abdominal cramps, vomiting, diarrhea Insomnia Weakness
Cocaine	Dysphoric mood Fatigue, malaise Vivid, unpleasant dreams Sleep disturbance Increased appetite Psychomotor retardation or agitation

Acute substance-induced psychosis is often indistinguishable from a primary psychotic disorder such as schizophrenia in the setting of substance abuse. Neurocognitive states such as dementia may be substance induced and result in permanent brain damage. Depression, commonly diagnosed and treated in the primary care setting, may often be complicated by a substance-induced mood disorder. Often what appears to be treatment-resistant depression is actually the result of persistent substance abuse. Withdrawal syndromes often present as episodes of anxiety, sleep disorders, mood disorders, or seizure disorders.

Mallin R et al: Detection of substance use disorders in patients presenting with depression. Subst Abus 2002;23:115. [PMID: 1244356]

Treatment

Many substance use disorders resolve spontaneously or with brief interventions on the part of physicians or other authority figures in the workplace, legal system, family, or society. This occurs because patients with substance abuse disorders continue to maintain control over their use, and when the consequences of that use outweigh the benefits of the drug, they choose to quit. Patients with substance dependence disorders, on the other hand, have impaired control by definition. They rarely improve without assistance.

Substance use disorders can be treated successfully. Brief interventions and outpatient, inpatient, and residen-

Table 56–7. Biochemical markers of substance use disorders.

Marker	Substance	Sensitivity (%)	Specificity (%)	Predictive Value (%)
Mean corpuscular volume (MCV)	Alcohol	24	96	63
γ-Glutamyltransferase (GGT)	Alcohol	42	76	61
Carbohydrate-deficient transferrin (CDT)	Alcohol	67	97	84

Table 56–8. Medical complications of substance abuse.

Drug	Medical Complication
Alcohol	Trauma
	Hypertension
	Cardiomyopathy
	Dysrhythmias
	Ischemic heart disease
	Hemorrhagic stroke
	Esophageal reflux
	Barret esophagus
	Mallory–Weiss tears
	Esophageal cancer
	Acute gastritis
	Pancreatitis
	Chronic diarrhea, malabsorption
	Alcoholic hepatitis
	Cirrhosis
	Hepatic failure
	Hepatic carcinoma
	Nasopharyngeal cancer
	Headache
	Sleep disorders
	Memory impairment
	Dementia
	Peripheral neuropathy
	Fetal alcohol syndrome
	Sexual dysfunction
	Substance-induced mood disorders
	Substance-induced psychotic disorders
	Immune dysfunction
Cocaine (other stimulants)	Chest pain
	Congestive heart failure
	Cardiac dysrhythmias
	Cardiovascular collapse
	Seizures
	Cerebrovascular accidents
	Headache
	Spontaneous pneumothorax
	Noncardiogenic pulmonary edema
	Nasal septal perforations
Injection drug use	Hepatitis C, B
	HIV infection
	Subacute endocarditis
	Soft tissue abscesses

tial treatment programs reduce morbidity and mortality associated with substance abuse and dependence. Determining the type and intensity of treatment that is best for a given patient may be difficult. ASAM has developed guidelines for clinicians to help determine the level and intensity of treatment for patients (Table 56–10). Once patients have been adequately assessed treatment can begin. Detoxification, patient education, identification of defenses, overcoming denial, relapse prevention, orientation to 12-step recovery programs, and family services are the goals of substance abuse treatment.

Table 56–9. Neuropsychiatric complications of substance abuse.

Substance-induced mood disorder, depressed/elevated
Substance-induced anxiety disorder
Substance-induced psychotic disorder
Substance-induced personality change
Substance intoxication
Substance withdrawal
Delirium
Wernicke disease
Korsakoff syndrome (alcohol-induced persisting amnestic disorder)
Transient amnestic states (blackouts)
Substance-induced persisting dementia

A. Intervention

Once screening and diagnosis are complete, it is time for the physician to share the assessment with the patient. Because of the nature of substance abuse, patients rarely choose to seek help for their alcohol or drug problem until the consequences far outweigh the positive aspects of treatment. Intervention may be seen as a means of bringing these consequences to the attention of the patient. It can be accomplished by a wide range of approaches, some quite informal, others carefully orchestrated and executed. Physicians or family members can often intervene simply by giving the patient feedback about his or her behavior, describing the feelings that behavior generates, avoiding enabling behavior, and offering help.

The traditional intervention for alcohol or drug addiction, is a formal process, best accomplished by an addictions specialist trained in this process. This approach is often effective, resulting in positive results in about 80% of cases. Although effective, the traditional, formal model of intervention is often less than ideal for the family physician. Specialist involvement and orchestration of significant relationships of the patient are sometimes difficult to achieve. In addition, if the intervention fails, it may be difficult if not impossible for the physician to continue a relationship with the patient. Another approach to consider is that of the brief intervention. This highly effective approach to intervention is based on motivational interviewing and the stages of change model (also known as the transtheoretical model).

Table 56–10. American Society of Addiction Medicine placement criteria.

Levels of service

Level 0.5:	Early intervention
Level I:	Outpatient services
Level II:	Intensive outpatient/partial hospitalization services
Level III:	Resident/inpatient services
Level IV:	Medically managed intensive inpatient services

Assessment dimensions

1. Acute intoxication and/or withdrawal potential
2. Biomedical conditions and complications
3. Emotional/behavioral conditions and complications (eg, psychiatric conditions, psychological or emotional/behavioral complications of known or unknown origin, poor impulse control, changes in mental status, transient neuropsychiatric complications)
4. Treatment acceptance/resistance
5. Relapse/continued use potential
6. Recovery/living environment

Reproduced, with permission, from Mee-Lee D et al: *Patient Placement Criteria for the Treatment of Substance-Related Disorders*, 2nd ed. American Society of Addiction Medicine, 1996.

Table 56–11. DEATH glossary: pitfalls to avoid when presenting the diagnosis.

Drinking or drug use details are not relevant; talking with a drunk is not useful. Patients will often give long and complex explanations for their drug or alcohol use and why they do not have a problem with it. It may be necessary to interrupt these explanations and move on. In addition, patients who are intoxicated cannot process the information given to them and it is appropriate to reschedule them and ask them not to drink prior to that visit.

Etiology: Patients may try to elicit or provide an explanation for their addiction. It is unlikely that this will be useful. Just as when treating other chronic illnesses without clear etiologies, it is important to focus on the evidence for the diagnosis and the plan for treatment, and not be distracted by theoretical discussions of etiology.

Arguments: Arguments can seriously damage the patient–physician relationship and should be avoided at all costs. Respect, sympathy, and support are your best defenses against arguments.

Threats: Threats are a serious cause of damage to the therapeutic relationship; threats, guilt, and shame do not promote recovery.

Hedging: Although arguments are detrimental, there should be no hedging on the diagnosis. If the patient appears unable to accept the diagnosis, an agreement to disagree should be made as well as another appointment to continue the discussion.

Modified, with permission, from Schulz JE, Parran T Jr: Principles of identification and intervention. In: Graham AW, Shultz TK, eds: *Principles of Addiction Medicine*, 2nd ed. American Society of Addiction Medicine, 1998.

1. Stages of change—Underlying the strategy of the brief intervention is the stages of change model, developed by Prochascka and DiClementi. In this model, behavioral change is viewed as a process that evolves over time through a series of stages: precontemplation, contemplation, preparation, action, maintenance, and termination. The individual must progress through each of these stages to reach the next and cannot leap past one to get to another.

Individuals in the **precontemplation** stage are not planning to take any action in the foreseeable future. This is the stage most often described as denial. Patients in this stage do not perceive their behavior as problematic. In the **contemplation** stage, people perceive they have a problem and believe they should do something about it. Many addicted patients who do not appear to be ready for traditional treatment programs are in this stage. They recognize that they have a substance problem, believe they should stop using the addictive substance, but seem unable to do so. In the **preparation** stage, patients have made a decision to change and plan to do so soon, usually within the next month. These patients are ready to enter action-oriented treatment programs. **Action** refers to the stage of change during which patients make specific changes in their behavior. In the case of addiction, abstinence is the generally agreed upon behavior that signifies action. **Maintenance** is the period after action during which the changed behavior persists and patients work toward preventing relapse. Maintenance often requires a longer sustained effort than patients anticipate, and failure to continue with maintenance behavior is a common cause of relapse. **Termination** describes the stage in which there is no temptation, and there is no risk of returning to old habits. In the case of addiction, most patients must work toward a lifetime of maintenance rather than termination. The risk of relapse is such that few truly reach this final stage for the disease of addiction.

2. Brief interventions—Presenting the diagnosis of a substance use disorder by itself may be viewed as a brief intervention. Most physicians who have worked with these patients will not be surprised to hear that as many as 70% of patients are in the precontemplation or contemplation stage when presented with the diagnosis. The resistance associated with these stages tends to force clinicians into one of two modalities—either avoiding the diagnosis or confronting and arguing with the patient. Both of these approaches are futile. One approach in presenting the diagnosis is to use the DEATH glossary (Table 56–11), a list of pitfalls to avoid when presenting the diagnosis of addiction. On a more positive note, the SOAPE glossary

Table 56–12. SOAPE glossary for presenting the diagnosis.

Support: Use phrases such as "we need to work together on this," "I am concerned about you and will follow up closely with you," and "As with all medical illnesses the more people you work with, the better you will feel." These words reinforce the physician–patient relationship, strengthen the collaborative model of chronic illness management, and help convince the patient that the physician will not just present the diagnosis and leave.

Optimism: Most patients have controlled their alcohol or drug use at times and may have quit for periods of time. They may expect failure. By giving a strong optimistic message such as "You can get well," "Treatment works," and "You can expect to see improvements in many areas of your life," the physican can motivate the patient.

Absolution: By describing addiction as a disease and telling patients that they are not responsible for having an illness, but that now only they can take responsibility for their recovery, the physician can lessen the burden of guilt and shame that is often a barrier to recovery.

Plan: Having a plan is important to the acceptance of the illness. Using readiness to change categories can help in designing a plan that uses the patient's willingness to move ahead. Indicating that abstinence is desirable, but recognizing that all patients will not be able to commit to that goal immediately can help prevent a sense of failure early in the process. Ask "What do you think you will be able to do at this point?"

Explanatory model: Understanding the patient's beliefs about addiction may be important. Many patients believe this is a moral weakness and that they lack willpower. An explanation that willpower cannot resolve illnesses such as diabetes or alcoholism may go a long way to reassure the patient that recovery is possible.

Modified, with permission, from Clark WD: Alcoholism: Blocks to diagnosis and treatment. Am J Med 1981;71:285.

(Table 56–12) describes suggestions to use when talking to patients about their addiction.

Even for patients in the precontemplative stage at presentation of the diagnosis, continued use of the brief intervention strategy will ultimately reduce the amount of drug use if not result in abstinence.

Brief interventions should include some of the elements of motivational interviewing. These elements include offering empathetic, objective feedback of data; meeting patient expectations; working with ambivalence; assessing barriers and strengths; reinterpreting past experience in light of current medical consequences; negotiating a follow-up plan; and providing hope.

B. Detoxification

Detoxification and treatment of withdrawal, and any medical complications, must have first priority. Alcohol and other sedative-hypnotic drugs share the same neurobiologic withdrawal process. Chronic use of this class of drugs results in downregulation of the GABA receptors throughout the central nervous system. GABA is an inhibitory neurotransmitter and is uniformly depressed during sedative-hypnotic use. Abrupt cessation of sedative-hypnotic drug use results in upregulation of GABA receptors and a relative paucity of GABA for inhibition. The result is stimulation of the autonomic nervous system and the appearance of the signs and symptoms listed in Table 56–6. Withdrawal seizures are a common manifestation of sedative-hypnotic withdrawal, occurring in 11–33% of patients withdrawing from alcohol.

Alcohol withdrawal seizures are best treated with benzodiazepines and by addressing the withdrawal process itself. Long-term treatment of alcohol withdrawal seizures is not recommended, and phenytoin should not be used to treat seizures associated with alcohol withdrawal. The cornerstones of treatment for alcohol withdrawal syndrome are the benzodiazepines. All drugs that provide cross-tolerance with alcohol are effective in reducing the symptoms and sequelae of alcohol withdrawal, but none has the safety profile and evidence of efficacy of the benzodiazepines. Table 56–13 summarizes recommendations in the treatment of alcohol withdrawal. Opiate withdrawal may not be life threatening, but the symptoms are significant enough that without supportive treatment, most patients will not remain in treatment. Table 56–14 outlines recommendations for the treatment of opiate withdrawal. The symptoms of cocaine and other stimulant withdrawal are somewhat less predictable and much harder to improve. Despite multiple studies with many different drug classes,

Table 56–13. Treatment regimens for alcohol withdrawal.

Use the Clinical Institute Withdrawal Assessment of Alcohol Scale, Revised (CIWA-AR) for monitoring
- Assess the patient using the CIWA-AR scale every 4 h until the score is below 8 for 24 h
- For CIWA-AR >10
  - Give chlordiazepoxide, 50–100 mg, or diazepam, 10–20 mg, or oxazepam, 30–60 mg, or lorazepam, 2–4 mg
- Repeat the CIWA-AR 1 h after the dose to assess the need for further medication

Non–symptom-driven regimens
- For patients likely to experience withdrawal use chlordiazepoxide, 50 mg, every 6 h for four doses followed by 50 mg every 8 h for three doses, followed by 50 mg every 12 h for two doses, and finally by 50 mg at bedtime for one dose
- Other benzodiazepines may be substituted at equivalent doses

Patients on a predetermined dosing schedule should be monitored frequently both for breakthrough withdrawal symptoms as well as for excessive sedation

Table 56–14. Treatment for opioid withdrawal.

Methadone: A pure opioid agonist restricted by federal legislation to inpatient treatment or specialized outpatient drug treatment programs. Initial dosage is 15–20 mg for 2–3 days, then tapered with a 10–15% reduction in dose daily guided by patient's symptoms and clinical findings.

Clonidine: An α-adrenergic blocker, 0.2 mg every 4 h to relieve symptoms of withdrawal, may be effective. Hypotension is a risk and sometimes limits the dose. It can be continued for 10–14 days and tapered by the third day by 0.2 mg daily.

Buprenorphine: This partial μ receptor agonist can be administered sublingually in doses of 2, 4, or 8 mg every 4 h for the management of opioid withdrawal symptoms.

Naltrexone/clonidine: A rapid form of opioid detoxification involves pretreatment with 0.2–0.3 mg of clonidine followed by 12.5 mg of naltrexone (a pure opioid antagonist). Naltrexone is increased to 25 mg on the second day, 50 mg on day 3, and 100 mg on day 4, with clonidine given at 0.1–0.3 mg three times daily.

no medications have been shown to reliably reduce the symptoms and craving associated with cocaine withdrawal.

C. Patient Education

Patients' knowledge and understanding of the nature of substance use disorders are the key to their recovery. For patients still in control of their use, education about appropriate substance use will help them to choose responsibly if they continue to use. For patients who meet the criteria for substance dependence (addiction), abstinence is the only safe recommendation. Once having made the transition to addiction, patients can never use addictive substances reliably again. The neurobiologic changes in the brain are permanent, and loss of control may occur at any time when the brain is presented with an addictive substance. The occurrence of loss of control can be unpredictable; consequently addicted patients may find that they can use for a variable period of time with control, which gives them the false impression that they were never addicted in the first place or perhaps that they have been cured. Invariably if they continue to use addictive substances they will lose control of their use and begin to experience consequences at or above the level they did before. Understanding that the problem of addiction is a chronic disorder for which there is remission but not cure becomes essential. The question then becomes not whether to remain abstinent but rather how to remain abstinent.

D. Identification of Defenses and Overcoming Denial

During this phase of treatment patients typically work in a group therapy setting and are encouraged to look at the defenses that have prevented them from seeking help sooner. Denial can best be defined as the inability to see the causal relationship between drug use and its consequences. For example, a patient who believes he drank because he lost his job may be encouraged to consider that he lost his job because he drank.

E. Relapse Prevention

Once patients are educated to the nature of their disease and have identified destructive defense mechanisms, relapse prevention becomes the primary goal. Identification of triggers for alcohol and drug use, plans to prevent opportunities to relapse, and new ways to deal with problems help patients to maintain their abstinence. In most treatment programs a relapse prevention plan is developed and individualized for each patient.

F. Twelve-Step Recovery Programs

It would be difficult to overstate the contribution 12-step programs make to recovery. Despite millions of dollars in research and the efforts of a large segment of the scientific community, no treatment, medication, or psychotherapy has taken the place of the 12 steps.

Twelve-step recovery has its roots in Alcoholics Anonymous (AA), founded in 1935. Today over 200 recovery organizations use the 12 steps with some modifications for patients with substance use disorders. These programs include Al-Anon, for friends and family of alcoholics; Narcotics Anonymous (NA), for those with drug problems other than alcohol; and Cocaine Anonymous, for those with cocaine addiction. At the heart of each of these fellowships is the program of recovery outlined in the 12 steps (Table 56–15). AA and related 12-step programs are spiritual, not religious in nature. No one is told they must believe in anything, including God. Agnostics and atheists are welcome in AA, and are not asked to convert to any religious belief. Newcomers in AA are encouraged to go to meetings regularly (daily is wise initially), get a sponsor, and begin work on the 12 steps. A sponsor is usually someone of the same sex, who is in stable recovery, and has successfully negotiated the steps. The sponsor helps guide the newcomer through the steps and provides a source of information, and encouragement. At meetings members share their experiences, relaying information about strategies for recovery. AA meetings vary in their composition and structure; consequently if a patient feels uncomfortable at one meeting another may be more acceptable. There are meetings for women or men only, those for young people, physicians, lawyers, and for virtually any special interest group in most large cities. There is often a great deal of confusion about what AA does and does not do. AA is not treatment. Despite the close connection many treatment programs have with 12-step recovery fellowships, these fellowships are

Table 56–15. The 12 Steps of Alcoholics Anonymous.

We:

1. Admitted we were powerless over alcohol—that our lives had become unmanageable;
2. Came to believe that a Power greater than ourselves could restore us to sanity;
3. Made a decision to turn our will and our lives over to the care of God *as we understood Him;*
4. Made a searching and fearless moral inventory of ourselves;
5. Admitted to ourselves, and to another human being the exact nature of our wrongs;
6. Were entirely ready to have God remove all these defects of character;
7. Humbly asked Him to remove our shortcomings;
8. Made a list of all persons we had harmed, and became willing to make amends to them all;
9. Made direct amends to such people wherever possible, except when to do so would injure them or others;
10. Continued to take personal inventory and when we were wrong promptly admitted it;
11. Sought through prayer and meditation to improve our conscious contact with God *as we understand Him,* praying only for knowledge of His will for us and the power to carry that out;
12. Having had a spiritual awakening as the result of these steps, we tried to carry this message to alcoholics, and to practice these principles in all our affairs.

Source: Alcoholics Anonymous World Service.

not affiliated with treatment centers by design. Table 56–16 lists some of the self-described limitations of AA and other 12-step groups.

From multiple sources, it appears clear that AA and other 12-step recovery programs are among the most effective tools to combat substance disorders. About 6–10% of the population have been to an AA meeting during their lives. This number doubles for those with alcohol problems. Although 50% of those who come to AA leave, of those who stay for a year, 67% stay sober; of those who stay for 2 years, 85% stay sober; and of those who stay sober for 5 years, 90% remain sober indefinitely. Outcome studies of 8087 patients treated in 57 different inpatient and outpatient treatment programs showed that those attending AA at 1-year follow up were 50% more likely to be abstinent than those not attending. Adolescents studied were found to be four times more likely to be abstinent if they attended AA/NA when compared with those who did not. Finally, in an effort to identify which groups in AA did better than others, studies of involvement in AA (defined as service work, having a sponsor, leading meetings, etc) found that those who were involved maintained abstinence better than those who just attended meetings.

Table 56–16. Limitations of 12-step groups.

AA does not solicit members; it will only reach out to people who ask for help.

AA does not keep records of membership (although some AA groups will provide phone lists for group members).

AA does not engage in research.

There is no formal control or follow-up on members by AA.

AA does not make medical or psychiatric diagnoses. Each member needs to decide if he or she is an addict.

AA as a whole does not provide housing, food, clothing, jobs, or money to newcomers (although individual members may do this).

AA is self-supporting through its own members' contributions; it does not accept money from outside sources.

Source: *A Brief Guide to Alcoholics Anonymous*. Alcoholics Anonymous World Service Inc., 1972.

Having a list of AA members willing to escort potential new members to meetings is a powerful tool for physicians to help patients into recovery. Generally in every AA district, there is a person identified as the chair of the Cooperation with Professional Community Committee who can help physicians identify people willing to perform this service. Al-Anon and NA have similar contacts. These contacts can often supply physicians with relevant literature to help dispel some of the myths patients may hold regarding 12-step recovery. Patients often use these myths as excuses for why AA will not work for them, and understanding this as resistance and ambivalence about entering a life of recovery is important for the physician. Family physicians are in a unique position to encourage patients to invest in 12-step recovery. Recovering persons are keenly aware of this fact and physicians are encouraged and welcomed at open AA and other 12-step meetings to become more familiar with the way they work.

G. Pharmacotherapeutic Treatment of Addiction

Agents useful in the treatment of withdrawal were discussed earlier (see Detoxification). The agents discussed here are used to help prevent relapse into alcohol or other drug use. These drugs attempt to influence drug use by one of several mechanisms:

1. Sensitizing the body's response to result in a negative reaction to ingesting the drug, causing an aversion reaction such as with disulfiram and alcohol.
2. Reducing the reinforcing effects of a drug, such as the use of naltrexone in alcoholism.
3. Blocking the effects of a drug by binding to the receptor site, such as naltrexone for opiates.
4. Saturating the receptor sites by agonists, such as the use of methadone in opioid maintenance therapy.

5. Unique approaches, such as the creation of an immunization to cocaine.

Drug therapy for addiction holds promise. As our understanding of the neurobiology of addiction improves, so does the chance that we can intervene at a molecular level to prevent relapse. At the current level, however, pharmacotherapy to prevent relapse must be relegated to an adjunctive position. No drug alone has provided sufficient power to prevent relapse to addictive behavior. Still in some patients the use of appropriate medication may give them the edge necessary to move closer to recovery.

1. Pharmacotherapy for alcoholism—Disulfiram, naltrexone, possibly other opioid antagonists, selective serotonin reuptake inhibitors (SSRIs), and acamprosate are currently used in the prevention of relapse in alcoholism. Acamprosate appears to be the most promising of these medications. Although the goal of abstinence for patients addicted to alcohol cannot be met by medication alone at this time, in selected patients it may improve their chances for stable recovery.

a. Disulfiram—Disulfiram inhibits aldehyde dehydrogenase, the enzyme that catalyzes the oxidation of acetaldehyde to acetic acid. Thus, if a patient taking disulfiram ingests alcohol, the acetaldehyde levels rise. The result is referred to as the disulfiram-ethanol reaction. This manifests as flushing of the skin, palpitations, decreased blood pressure, nausea, vomiting, shortness of breath, blurred vision, and confusion. The reactions are usually related to the dose of both disulfiram and alcohol. This reaction can be severe and with doses of disulfiram over 500 mg and 2 ounces of alcohol death has been reported. Common side effects of disulfiram include drowsiness, lethargy, peripheral neuropathy, hepatotoxicity, and hypertension.

In the United States, doses of 250–500 mg are most commonly used. Because of individual variability in the disulfiram-ethanol reaction, often these doses do not produce a sufficient reaction to deter the patient from drinking. In the United Kingdom, it is common to perform an ethanol challenge test to determine the appropriate dose to produce an aversion effect. Whether disulfiram is actually effective in preventing relapse is the subject of some debate. Most studies have failed to show a statistically significant result. On closer examination, it appears that compliance with the medication appears to be the most important factor. In a large Veterans Administration multicenter study, a direct relationship was found between compliance with drug therapy and abstinence. In addition, the involvement of a patient's spouse in observing the patient's consumption of disulfiram results in considerable improvement on outcome. It appears that disulfiram can be a useful adjunct for patients who have a history of sudden relapse and who have a social situation in which compliance may be adequately monitored.

b. Naltrexone—Naltrexone, an opioid antagonist, has been shown to reduce drinking in animal studies and in human alcoholics. Initial optimism over the potential of this discovery was tempered by several studies indicating that the effects of reducing drinking and preventing relapse diminished over time and overall failed to reduce relapse to heavy drinking. Still, the effect of naltrexone on alcohol craving is promising in that it suggests that the opioid system is involved in the craving for alcohol in alcoholism; this may open the door to the development of other opioid-active drugs that will have an impact on drinking.

c. Serotonergic drugs—Animal studies have consistently shown that SSRIs reduce alcohol intake in animal models. The data with respect to humans are less clear or consistent. It appears that the SSRIs reduce drinking in heavily drinking, nondepressed alcoholics, but probably only about 15–20% from pretreatment levels. When abstinence is the outcome studied, the results are not promising. However, the SSRIs may eventually find a place in concert with other anticraving medication. SSRIs appear to reduce drinking in a more robust fashion in alcoholics with comorbid depression.

d. Acamprosate (calcium acetylhomotaurinate)—Acamprosate has been shown to reduce craving for alcohol in alcoholics. It appears to effect both GABA and glutamine neurotransmission, both important in alcohol's effect in the brain. Unlike naltrexone, the effects of acamprosate on relapse appear to be greater and longer lasting. Twice as many alcoholics remained abstinent in a 12-month period while taking acamprosate compared with those who took placebo. The addition of disulfiram to the regimen appears to increase the effectiveness of acamprosate. Acamprosate has a very benign side-effect profile and appears to be free of any effects on mood, concentration, attention, or psychomotor performance. Acamprosate has been studied extensively in Europe with good results. It has been approved for use in the United States and is intended to be part of a comprehensive recovery program.

2. Pharmacotherapy for cocaine addiction—The state of the art in the pharmacologic treatment of cocaine addiction makes it difficult to recommend any medication-based treatment with any confidence. Despite great interest and much activity devoted to finding an effective pharmacologic intervention for cocaine and other stimulant addiction, none has withstood the test of rigorous study. Heterocyclic antidepressants such as desipramine, SSRIs, monoamine oxidase inhibitors, dopamine agonists such as bromocriptine, neuroleptics, anticonvulsants, and calcium channel blockers have all been tried in cocaine addiction. Variable results, often positive in animal studies, have led to attempts to treat cocaine addicts with these drugs. As each potentially effective drug is studied more rigorously, however, little in the way of positive results is found. These drugs are used to try to ameliorate the craving for cocaine or to mediate the withdrawal symptoms of anhedonia and fatigue. An attempt to use stimulants such as methylphenidate or amphetamine for cocaine dependence in a way analogous to that of methadone maintenance for opiate addiction has produced disappointing results. One of the more interesting approaches to a pharmacologic answer to cocaine addiction, has been the development of a "vaccine" for cocaine. In this approach, a cocaine-like hapten linked to a foreign protein produces antibodies that attach to cocaine molecules, preventing them from crossing the blood–brain barrier. This approach has had some success in animal models but has yet to be tested on humans.

3. Pharmacotherapy for opiate addiction—Agonist maintenance treatment with methadone is the primary pharmacologic treatment for opioid treatment. The rationale for the use of methadone and its longer acting relative, levo-α-acetylmethadol (LAAM), is to saturate the opiate receptors, thus blocking euphoria and preventing the abstinence syndrome. Methadone and LAAM treatment programs are highly regulated by the federal government; therefore, the average family physician would not be prescribing this drug, although certainly he or she might see patients who are on a maintenance program. Methadone programs are frequently referred to as "harm reduction programs" because the primary beneficiary of these programs is society. Reductions in crime and in the costs of active intravenous heroin abuse are clearly demonstrated as a result of these programs. The addict also benefits with a dramatic decrease in the risk of death due to addiction or contraction of HIV disease. There is social stabilization in the addict's life as well, especially when appropriate social services are provided by the maintenance program.

Antagonist maintenance with naltrexone was initially thought to be ideal given its essentially complete blockade of opioid-reinforcing properties. Unfortunately, only 10–20% of patients remained in treatment when this approach is used. The most important use of naltrexone at this time appears to be in the management of health care professionals with opioid dependence. Compliance with a naltrexone regimen ensures abstinence and allows health care professionals to work in an environment where opioids may be accessible. Doses of 350 mg weekly divided into 3 days, will provide complete protection from the effects of opioids.

Buprenorphine, a partial opioid agonist with κ antagonist effects, is currently being tested as an alternative to methadone maintenance treatment. Dosing of this medication is problematic, with 65% of patients remaining abstinent at 16 mg/day compared with 28% abstinence at 4 mg/day. Buprenorphine may decrease the use of cocaine in opioid-dependent patients. It also has less potential for diversion, making it an attractive alternative to methadone. New federal regulations allowing maintenance treatment of opioid dependence by primary care physicians have been approved. Primary care physicians who have received training and are certified by the Drug Enforcement Agency may now prescribe buprenorphine for maintenance therapy for opioid addicts.

Anton RF: Pharmacologic approaches to the management of alcoholism. J Clin Psychiatry 2001;62(suppl 20):11.[PMID: 11584870]

Chang PH, Steinberg MB: Alcohol withdrawal. Med Clin North Am 2001;85:1191. [PMID: 11565494]

Kosanke N et al: Feasibility of matching alcohol patients to ASAM levels of care. Am J Addict 2002;11:124. [PMID: 12028742]

Krambeer LL: Methadone therapy for opioid dependence. Am Fam Physician 2001;63:2404. [PMID: 11430455]

Moyer A et al: Brief interventions for alcohol problems: A meta-analytic review of controlled investigations in treatment-seeking and non-treatment-seeking populations. Addiction 2002;97: 279. [PMID: 11964101]

Weisner C, Matzger H: A prospective study of the factors influencing entry to alcohol and drug treatment. J Behav Health Serv Res 2002;29:126. [PMID: 12032970]

Tobacco Cessation 57

Martin C. Mahoney, MD, PhD, FAAFP, & Andrew Hyland, PhD

General Considerations

Nicotine dependence results in an immense burden to patients, their families, and the health care system. Increased efforts to promote smoking cessation are a key element in decreasing the tobacco-related disease burden over the next 20 years. Brief interventions to encourage cessation, along with supportive counseling and the use of pharmacotherapies for nicotine dependence currently available (and under development), represent promising opportunities for clinicians to promote cessation and decrease tobacco-attributable morbidity and mortality among their patients.

The primary goals of Healthy People 2010 are to increase quality and years of healthy life and eliminate health disparities (http://www.health.gov/healthypeople). Because tobacco use varies by income and race and ethnicity, increased smoking cessation will play a key role in realizing these goals. Toward this end, two of the Healthy People 2010 objectives are to reduce the prevalence of cigarette smoking among adults from 24% to 12% and to increase the number of yearly cessation attempts among smokers from 41% to 75%.

Food and Drug Administration (FDA)–approved pharmacotherapies (nicotine gum, patch, inhaler, spray, lozenges, and bupropion) can double the likelihood of smoking cessation, even when used without psychosocial therapy. However, individuals with lower incomes are less likely to report prior use of such therapies. Increased access to these effective therapies can increase the number of quit attempts.

Fiore C et al: *Treating Tobacco Use and Dependence. Clinical Practice Guideline.* US Department of Health and Human Services, Public Health Service, 2000. Available at http://www.surgeongeneral.gov/tobacco.

Brief Interventions

Smoking cessation treatment often begins with a brief intervention, in which a physician or other health care provider advises smokers to quit and may recommend methods for quitting. For many smokers, the only contact with the health care system may be through their family physician, and office visits often provide the impetus for smokers to attempt to stop smoking.

Meta-analyses report that brief interventions have significant potential to reduce smoking rates, with even minimal brief interventions conferring an estimated 30% increased likelihood of cessation. A recent Cochrane review of brief smoking cessation advice from a physician compared with no advice (or usual care) identified a significant increase in the odds of quitting. Although previous studies have examined the effect of brief interventions in controlled settings, little research has been conducted to examine their effects in nonexperimental settings over an extended period of time.

A. Use of Brief Interventions to Promote Smoking Cessation

The updated smoking treatment guidelines from the Agency for Healthcare Research and Quality (AHRQ) recommend that health care workers screen all patients for tobacco use and provide advice and follow-up behavioral treatments to all tobacco users. Current users are advised to quit; those who are willing to make a quit attempt are given appropriate assistance, along with arrangements for a follow-up visit; those who are identified as former smokers are given advice to prevent relapse; and primary prevention is engaged for persons who have never used tobacco. The aim of these guidelines is to increase smoking cessation through improved understanding of the health consequences of smoking, better information about the availability and proper use of treatments, and the provision of encouragement and support.

Controlled studies have found that physician involvement, especially more extensive interventions, increases quit rates. This approach has also been found to be cost effective. Overall, the interventions recommended by AHRQ cost about $2500 per year of life saved, whereas mammography screening costs about $50,000 per year of life saved.

Although studies find that physician interventions are an efficacious and cost-effective way to increase quit rates, patient reports indicate that much of the smoking population does not receive them. The Centers for Disease Control and Prevention (CDC) found that only 70% of smokers had seen a physician in the past year, and only 37% of these reported they were advised to stop smoking, which represents about 25% of all smokers. In another study, 91% of participating physicians indicated that providing advice regarding smoking cessation was important, but only 47% of smokers reported that their physicians had advised them to quit. Although higher rates have been reported by patients in recent years, less than 65% of smokers seeing a physician were advised to quit.

Estimates of the prevalence of brief interventions vary. The CDC found that the rate at which smokers had ever received physician advice increased from 26.4% in 1976 to 56.1% in 1991. However, a 1995 study of population-based settings found that while physicians asked about two thirds of patients if they smoked, they provided counseling to only 21%. A 1997 survey of physicians found that only 8% reported that they provided follow-up advice to smokers, and less than 50% were planning on increasing their rate of interventions in the next 6 months. In a study of smokers in California in 1998, 49% reported receiving advice from a physician to quit smoking in the past year, but of these only 12% reported that their physician suggested a quit date, only 7% received a prescription for nicotine replacement therapy, and only 10% were offered suggestions concerning other assistance. Furthermore, physicians who advise their patients who smoke to quit once may fail to provide additional advice if these patients do not demonstrate any initiative to quit. More recent data from the 1996 and 1999 Current Population Survey of Tobacco Use Supplements indicate the rate of physician advice increased from 56% in 1996 to 63% in 1999. The discrepancies in these surveys can be attributed in part to methodologic differences, the time period examined, whether the survey was based on physician or patient report, how long after the visit the survey was conducted, sample size, and smoker and demographic variations.

B. Characteristics of Those Who Receive a Brief Intervention

Limited attention has been directed to examining differences in rates of brief interventions by gender, age, and racial and ethnic group. Reports indicate that in Australia physicians were more likely to offer advice to men, whereas in the United States advice was more likely to be given to women. The CDC found that only 25% of adolescents reported that their physicians had provided advice on smoking. Older patients (50–74 years old) were about five times as likely to receive brief interventions as younger patients, with those aged 65 and above about 1.5 times as likely to receive advice as those aged 18–24. One study found whites more likely than nonwhites to receive advice, whereas another found whites less likely than blacks and Asians, but more likely than Hispanics and others to receive advice. Recent studies indicate that younger, less educated, black or Hispanic men are less likely to receive brief interventions than other demographic groups.

C. Effectiveness of Brief Interventions

Many studies have examined the effectiveness of brief interventions. Based on a meta-analysis of seven studies, AHRQ reported that physician advice increased 6-month quit rates by 2.3% (10.2% vs 7.9% for controls). Another meta-analysis of four randomized clinical trials reported that brief interventions increased 1-year quit rates by 2.7%. Pooled data from 17 studies included in a Cochrane review of brief smoking cessation advice from a physician compared with no advice (or usual care) identified an increase in the odds of being smoke-free after 6 months (OR = 1.74, 95% CI = 1.48–2.05); simple advice yielded an absolute difference of 2.5% in the rate of smoking cessation. Studies also find that more intensive interventions are more successful. One-year quit rates were found to be higher when physicians offered advice plus follow-up (15.8%) than advice only (12.7%). The most recent AHRQ tobacco treatment guidelines support these findings.

A population-based study of brief interventions using the 1990 California Tobacco Survey surveyed 9796 current smokers and found that those who had been advised to stop smoking in their most recent physician visit were significantly more likely to attempt to quit (OR = 1.61, 95% CI = 1.31–1.98). There was no significant difference in the number of quit attempts by smokers who had been previously advised to quit but not in their most recent physician visit and quit attempts by smokers who had never received such advice. Only the intention or attempt to quit was considered and not whether quits were successful. Physician advice to quit was reported to increase the likelihood of making a future quit attempt by 50–100%, with stronger effects among those who received repeated brief interventions over time.

Although these results generally indicate that even minimal brief interventions increased quit rates by an estimated 30%, little is known about the effects on specific demographic groups. Few studies have looked at both quitting and quit attempts, and no studies have considered other outcomes such as switching to low-tar cigarettes, decreasing the amount smoked, changes in motivation to stop smoking, or changes in the use of stop-smoking pharmacotherapies.

D. Attempts to Encourage Brief Interventions

Interventions designed to increase rates of physician advice and counseling have been shown to be effective. In a study based on the 1993 Community Intervention Trial for Smoking Cessation (COMMIT) survey, it was found that physicians in intervention communities were more likely than those in control communities to advise patients to stop smoking, encourage patients to set a quit date, and recommend use of nicotine replacement therapy. Thus, studies indicate the potential to increase brief interventions, which has important implications for developing mechanisms to promote physician interventions as a clinical stop-smoking intervention.

Repeated advice with follow-up may be necessary to encourage smokers, particularly heavy smokers, to quit. Smokers generally try to quit repeatedly before they are successful. Nevertheless, the incremental effect of advice given a second time may be less than the first time; the percentage of those previously advised to quit who have not yet stopped smoking increases, and smokers may become frustrated after trying and failing multiple times. In that case, interventions, especially those that are less extensive, become less effective over time. In these patients, more extensive interventions may be necessary.

Centers for Disease Control and Prevention (CDC): Use of clinical preventive services by adults aged < 65 years enrolled in health-maintenance organizations—United States, 1996. MMWR Morb Mortal Wkly Rep 1998;47:613. [PMID: 9699811]

A clinical practice guideline for treating tobacco use and dependence: A US Public Health Service report. The Tobacco Use and Dependence Clinical Practice Guideline Panel, Staff, and Consortium Representatives. JAMA 2000;283:3244. [PMID: 10866874]

Cromwell J et al: Cost-effectiveness of the clinical practice recommendations in the AHCPR guideline for smoking cessation. Agency for Health Care Policy and Research. JAMA 1997;278:1759. [PMID: 9388153]

Goldstein MG et al: A population-based survey of physician smoking cessation counseling practices. Prev Med 1998;27(Pt 1):720. [PMID: 9808804]

Hyland A et al: Effect of physician clinical interventions on indicators of cessation. Nicotine Tobacco Res 2003;5:781.

Kottke TE et al: Delivery rates for preventive services in 44 midwestern clinics. Mayo Clin Proc 1997;72:515. [PMID: 9179135]

Lancaster T, Stead L: Physician advice for smoking cessation. Cochrane Database Syst Rev 2004(4):CD000165. [PMID: 15494989]

Ockene JK et al: Tobacco control activities of primary-care physicians in the Community Intervention Trial for Smoking Cessation. COMMIT Research Group. Tob Control 1997;6 (suppl 2):S49. [PMID: 9583653]

Thorndike AN et al: National patterns in the treatment of smokers by physicians. JAMA 1998;279:604. [PMID: 9486755]

Diagnosis & Treatment

The Tobacco Use and Dependence Clinical Practice Guideline Panel recommends five specific actions ("the 5 A's"—Ask about tobacco use, Advise all tobacco users to quit, Assess interest in quitting, Assist in developing a quit plan, and Arrange for follow-up to assess progress) for integration into all clinical practice settings. These systematic approaches to tobacco dependence require less than 3 minutes to deliver, but the potential yield is enormous. Recently, the American Academy of Family Physicians has promoted the use of a more basic model focused on "Ask and Act." Physicians are encouraged to *ask* about the tobacco use habits of all patients, including interest in quitting, and then to *act* on that information by working with the patient to set a quit date, assuring access to behavioral counseling (through quitlines or local programs), addressing the need for pharmacotherapy, and assuring follow-up (Table 57–1). An online toolkit is available that includes posters, quitline wallet cards, patient education materials, and information on reimbursement for tobacco cessation counseling services (http://www.aafp.org/x40868.xml). Family physicians are encouraged to have patients contact the National Network of Tobacco Cessation Quitlines at (800) QUIT-NOW, or (800) 784-8669. Callers are automatically routed to a state-run quitline or the National Cancer Institute quitline and receive immediate advice on quitting, referrals to other sources, and an offer to have educational materials mailed to them.

Table 57–1. Simplified model for addressing tobacco use and dependence: Ask and act.

Ask:
Do you smoke?
How much do you want to quit? (1–10 scale)
How confident are you in your ability to quit? (1–10 scale)
Act:
Have you set a quit date?
Provide quit advice or referral
Provide pharmacotherapy prescription
Arrange for follow-up

From http://www.askandact.org.

The tobacco dependence guidelines recommend that all smokers receive at least a brief intervention. Although intensive interventions are more effective, they are not likely to be attended by the majority of smokers interested in quitting. Therefore, policies that restrict access to treatment by requiring attendance at intensive smoking cessation clinics are likely to be detrimental to smokers because they discourage quit attempts.

A. Pharmacotherapy

Tobacco users have a physical dependence on nicotine, in addition to a variety of reinforced psychological and social behaviors. The Fagerstrom nicotine dependence scale was developed to aid in quantifying the magnitude of addiction and to aid in selecting pharmacotherapy. Alternatives to the Fagerstrom scale include a modified CAGE questionnaire and an abbreviated version of the Fagerstrom scale. The revision to the Fagerstrom Tolerance Scale, the Fagerstrom Test for Nicotine Dependence (FTND), suggests that the time to first daily cigarette represents the single best indicator of nicotine dependence.

Pharmacotherapy doubles the effect of any tobacco cessation intervention. Patients who are willing and able to participate in counseling programs in addition to receiving pharmacotherapy should be encouraged to do so. Use of adjunctive pharmacotherapy should be strongly considered for all persons, including hospitalized patients, given the distinct health benefits associated with cessation.

The US Public Health Service guideline on management of tobacco dependence recommends sustained-release bupropion and all forms of nicotine replacement (eg, resin or gum, inhaler, nasal spray, lozenges, and patch) as first-line agents. Varenicline (Chantix), available since June 2006, represents another first-line agent. A medical chart form to facilitate both patient discussion and documentation relating to use of first-line adjunctive pharmacotherapy for the treatment of tobacco dependence is given in Table 57–2. It lists the first-line agents for smoking cessation pharmacotherapy along with recommended starting doses. Patients should be queried about prior use of these agents and their experiences and asked if they are interested in a particular agent. Clinicians are encouraged to apply appropriate clinical judgment when assessing contraindications to the use of a particular agent. This chart can be used to document the prescription, any discussion of possible side effects, and other instructions given to the patient.

1. Bupropion—Sustained-release bupropion is started at a dose of 150 mg daily for 3 days before increasing to 150 mg twice daily on day 4. Treatment with bupropion is begun 1–2 weeks before the anticipated quit date; its use is contraindicated among patients with a history of seizure disorders, current substance abuse, or other conditions that may lower the seizure threshold. Bupropion can be used in combination with nicotine replacement.

2. Varenicline—A selective $\alpha_4\beta_2$ nicotinic receptor partial agonist, varenicline was developed specifically for smoking cessation—and is the first new pharmacotherapy for tobacco cessation since bupropion became available in 1997. It appears to work by moderating symptoms of nicotine withdrawal, including reduced craving and decreased smoking satisfaction and psychological reward.

Varenicline is distributed in monthly dose packs and is stated 1 week prior to the identified quit date. Continuous abstinence rates during weeks 9–12 with varenicline are 44%. The starting month package titrates the dose from 0.5 mg daily for 3 days, to 0.5 mg twice daily for days 4–7, and then to 1 mg twice daily beginning on day 8. A full treatment course of 12 weeks is recommended, and patients who are abstinent at 12 weeks may continue with another 12 weeks of treatment.

The most commonly encountered side effects are nausea, insomnia, and abnormal dreams; these are generally rated as mild and often resolve within several days or may be managed with a dose reduction. Varenicline is minimally metabolized and is largely excreted in urine. There are no known drug interactions. Dose modification is necessary with severe renal disease.

3. Nicotine replacement therapy (NRT)—Patients should be counseled to stop smoking completely prior to initiating NRT. Nicotine patches, lozenges, and resin are available over the counter, whereas nicotine nasal sprays and the nicotine inhaler systems both require prescriptions. Reduced dose regimens of nicotine replacement might be considered for patients consuming fewer than 10 cigarettes daily or those weighing less than 100 pounds. Using two forms of nicotine replacement (eg, patch and resin) results in higher quit rates and should be recommended if other forms of nicotine replacement are not effective alone.

Clonidine and nortriptyline both represent second-line pharmacotherapy for use among patients in whom first-line agents have been judged to be inappropriate or ineffective. (Therefore, neither of these products is included in Table 57–1.) Although neither clonidine nor nortriptyline is approved by the FDA as adjunctive therapy for smoking cessation, several studies have demonstrated an approximate doubling in abstinence rates. Studies of clonidine have reported a variety of doses. It should be noted that the abrupt discontinuation of clonidine can result in rebound hypertension and other symptoms. Only a limited number of studies have examined the use of nortriptyline as a cessation aid and its use is tempered by concerns about potential side effects. Use of either of these agents for smoking cessation requires a clear discussion of risks and benefits with the patient and close monitoring by the treating physician.

Nicotine-containing products are not associated with the occurrence of acute cardiac events. This finding is consistent with the observation that NRT is rarely able to achieve blood levels of nicotine associated with smoking. Nonetheless, NRT should be approached cautiously among patients who are within 2 weeks of an acute myocardial infarction, are known to have significant arrhythmias, and have significant or worsening symptoms of angina.

Clinical experience with use of these adjunctive agents in pregnant women and adolescents is generally limited. Smokers with concurrent or prior depression may benefit from use of bupropion. Clinical judgment is advised regarding a comprehensive assessment of the risks and benefits associated with use of adjunctive pharmacotherapy in each of these settings.

Use of adjunctive pharmacotherapy may be continued for up to 6 months or longer. Patients should be encouraged to wean themselves off nicotine replacements after about 6–12 weeks of treatment; however, some patients elect to continue nicotine-containing therapy long term.

4. Emerging pharmacotherapies for cessation—Rimonabant (Acomplia) is a cannabinoid receptor antagonist developed as an antiobesity medication. Rimonabant has been shown to affect lipid and glucose metabolism,

Table 57–2. Chart aid for use of first-line adjunctive pharmacotherapy in smoking cessation.

Stop Smoking Medication	Used in Past	Patient Would Like to Use?	Contraindications	Side Effects	Rx Given (Dose/Frequency/Number)	Other Instructions Given
Nicotine patch (7, 14, or 21 mg/24 h for 4 weeks, then taper 2 weeks and 2 weeks)	Yes—Rx/OTC No	Yes No	Concurrent smoking	Local skin reaction Insomnia	7/14/21 mg patch every 24 h for 4 weeks then taper every 2 weeks	Dosing, side effects reviewed Behavioral counseling &/or quitline referral Set quit date:_____ F/U appt:_____
Nicotine gum (1–24 cigs/day—2 mg gum *or* 25+ cigs/day—4 mg gum; max 24 pieces/day for up to 12 weeks)	Yes—Rx/OTC No	Yes No	Concurrent smoking	Mouth soreness Dyspepsia	2 mg gum 4 mg gum Max 24 pieces/day for up to 12 weeks	Dosing, side effects reviewed Behavioral counseling &/or quitline referral Set quit date:_____ F/U appt:_____
Nicotine nasal spray (8–40 doses/day for 3–6 months)	Yes—Rx No	Yes No	Concurrent smoking	Nasal irritation	_____doses/day for 3–6 months	Dosing, side effects reviewed Behavioral counseling &/or quitline referral Set quit date:_____ F/U appt:_____
Nicotine inhaler (6–16 cartridges/day for up to 6 months)	Yes—Rx/OTC No	Yes No	Concurrent smoking	Local irritation of mouth and throat	_____Cartridges/day for_____months	Dosing, side effects reviewed Behavioral counseling &/or quitline referral Set quit date:_____ F/U appt:_____
Nicotine lozenges (if first cig smoked within 30 min of arising—4 mg lozenge; if first cig after 30 min of arising—2-mg lozenge; max 5 loz/6 h or 20 loz/day for up to 12 weeks)	Yes—Rx/OTC No	Yes No	Concurrent smoking Contains phenylalanine	Mouth soreness Dyspepsia	2-mg lozenge 4-mg lozenge Maximum 20 loz/day for up to 12 weeks	Dosing, side effects reviewed Behavioral counseling &/or quitline referral Set quit date:_____ F/U appt:_____

Zyban/bupropion SR	Yes—Rx No	Yes No	History of seizures History of eating disorder Currently treated for depression Used MAO inhibitor within past 14 days	Local skin reaction Insomnia	150 mg orally every day for 3 days, then 150 mg twice a day	Dosing, side effects reviewed Quit on day #8 Behavioral counseling &/or quitline referral Set quit date:_____ F/U appt:______
Chantix/varenicline	Yes—Rx No	Yes No	Severe renal disease	Nausea Insomnia, abnormal dreams GI symptoms	0.5 mg orally for 3 days, then 0.5 mg twice daily for 4 days, then 1.0 mg twice daily for 12 wk	Dosing, side effects reviewed Quit on day #8 Behavioral counseling &/or quitline referral Set quit date: _________ F/U appt: _________

Rx, prescription; OTC, over-the-counter; F/U, follow-up; MAO, monoamine oxidase; GI, gastrointestinal.

decease insulin resistance, and reduce intra-abdominal adiposity. Clinical trials using rimonabant have demonstrated significant weight loss, as well as reductions in weight circumference. In addition, this drug has been demonstrated to aid in smoking cessation (28% cessation with rimonabant vs 16% placebo), although the mechanism of action for its efficacy is unknown. It is anticipated that a new application will be submitted in the future.

A nicotine conjugate vaccine (NicVAX) is also under investigation. This vaccine contains a modified nicotine molecule that stimulates the immune system to produce antibodies that bind to nicotine, preventing it from entering the brain. This action blocks the positive reward stimulus associated with smoking and is thought to contribute to extinction. Results of a phase II study show marked increases in nicotine antibody levels across all vaccine dose groups, as well as differences by dose level. Subjects, who continued to smoke during this study, did not report any changes in symptoms of withdrawal or numbers of cigarettes smoked; cotinine levels were unchanged. The vaccine appeared be well tolerated with few adverse events attributed to its use. Follow-up studies are under way.

Fagerstrom KO: Measuring degree of physical dependence to tobacco smoking with reference to individualization of treatment. Addict Behav 1978;3:235. [PMID: 735910]

Gonzales D et al: Varenicline, an alpha4beta2 nicotinic acetylcholine receptor partial agonist, vs sustained-release bupropion and placebo for smoking cessation: A randomized controlled trial. JAMA 2006;296:47. [PMID: 16820546]

Hatsukami DK et al: Safety and immunogenicity of nicotine conjugate vaccine in current smokers. Clin Pharmacol Ther 2005;78:456. [PMID: 16321612]

Henningfield JE et al: Pharmacotherapy for nicotine dependence. CA Cancer J Clin 2005;55:281. [PMID: 16166074]

Jorenby DE et al: Efficacy of varenicline, an alpha4beta2 nicotinic acetylcholine receptor partial agonist, vs placebo or sustained-release bupropion for smoking cessation: A randomized controlled trial. JAMA 2006;296:56. [PMID: 16820547]

Mallin R: Smoking cessation: Integration of behavioral and drug therapies. Am Fam Physician 2002;65:1107. [PMID: 11925087]

Okuyemi KS et al: Pharmacotherapy of smoking cessation. Arch Fam Med 2000;9:270. [PMID: 10728115]

Pi-Sunyer FX et al: Effect of rimonabant, a cannabinoid-1 receptor blocker, on weight and cardiometabolic risk factors in overweight or obese patients: RIO-North America: A randomized controlled trial. JAMA 2006;295:761. [PMID: 16478899]

Tonstad S et al: Effect of maintenance therapy with varenicline on smoking cessation: A randomized controlled trial. JAMA 2006;296:64. [PMID: 16820548]

Youth tobacco surveillance—United States, 1998–1999. MMWR CDC Surveill Summ 2000;49:1. [PMID: 11057729]

B. Counseling Patients at the Precontemplation Stage of Quitting

For patients who are currently unwilling to make a quit attempt, clinicians should present a brief motivation intervention structured around "the 5 R's":

1. *Relevance*—make tobacco cessation personally relevant (personal medical history, family composition).
2. *Risk*—review the negative effects of quitting (include both immediate and long-term risks).
3. *Rewards*—identify the benefits of quitting (improved sense of taste and smell, personal sense of accomplishment, money saved, health benefits).
4. *Roadblocks*—identify perceived barriers to quitting and ways of overcoming these impediments (symptoms of withdrawal, weight gain, lack of social supports).
5. *Repetition*—repeat this intervention at all office visits.

C. Relapse

Although risk of relapse is greatest immediately following the quit attempt, it can occur months or even years following cessation. Because tobacco use status will be determined for all patients at each visit, physicians should encourage all former tobacco users to remain abstinent and encourage these patients to express specific concerns or difficulties. These topics can be addressed briefly during the scheduled office visit or explored more fully during a subsequent appointment. Approaches can include reassurance, motivational counseling, extended pharmacotherapy, recommendations for exercise, or referral to supportive or behavioral therapy.

Future Directions & Current Challenges

All clinicians should implement a systematic approach for the identification and assessment of smoking status among all patients. This must include *asking* about tobacco use and *acting* to provide office-based or off-site counseling, as well as arranging linkages to quitlines, print and Internet-based educational materials, community-based cessation classes, and access to pharmacotherapy. Two questions are critical: "Do you smoke?" and "Do you want to quit?" Clinicians can offer interventions during an office visit that can facilitate a quit attempt, ultimately saving a patient's life and reducing comorbidity. Physicians are reminded that Medicare programs cover pharmacotherapies.

Most health plans provide some coverage for pharmacotherapy and tobacco cessation counseling or classes. Since early 2005, Medicare has provided tobacco cessation counseling for smokers who have a tobacco-related health condition or whose therapy is affected by tobacco use. Also, beginning in 2006, the Medicare prescription drug benefit covers prescribed smoking cessation treatments.

Although the Medicaid program covers smoking cessation drugs, federal law allows for state exclusions. As a result, during 2000, some form of pharmacotherapy coverage was offered by 67% of states (n = 34/51), with over-the-counter NRT coverage by 43–45% and coverage of prescription pharmacotherapy by 45–61%; counseling was covered by 23% of the states.

Because the majority of smokers cycle through multiple periods of relapse and remission, nicotine dependence should be viewed as a chronic disease. In this way clinicians will better understand the requirement for ongoing and continuous attention rather than just acute care. Clinicians should also recognize that despite the potential for relapse, numerous effective treatments for cessation are currently available, including the approval of a new prescription agent during 2006 and the possible addition of other therapies in the future.

Smoking cessation treatments delivered by clinicians, whether physicians or non-physicians (eg, psychologist, nurse, dentist, or counselor), can increase abstinence. Therefore all members of the health care system should be empowered to provide smoking cessation interventions. Finally, it is important to emphasize that the combination of pharmacotherapy and behavioral counseling for each smoker will help to maximize the likelihood of achieving long term abstinence.

Borland R et al: The effectiveness of callback counseling for smoking cessation: A randomized trial. Addiction 2001;96:881. [PMID: 11399219]

Centers for Disease Control and Prevention (CDC): State Medicaid coverage for tobacco-dependence treatments–United States, 1994–2002. MMWR Morb Mortal Wkly Rep 2004;53:54. [PMID: 14749613]

Mahoney MC, Jaen CR: Counseling for tobacco cessation. Am Fam Physician 2001;64:1881. [PMID: 11764866]

Interpersonal Violence 58

Robert W. Smith, MD, MBA

General Considerations

Interpersonal violence is endemic in the United States. There has been growing public awareness through the media, community advocacy groups, and education in the schools to address this family-based problem. Inextricably tied to social, financial, cultural, racial, and behavioral factors, these conflicts require a multidisciplinary approach by the physician that addresses prevention, detection, intervention, and resolution.

Family physicians must maintain a high index of suspicion for interpersonal violence in their patient populations. Subtle presentations in patient behavior are often difficult to detect, and cultural and social factors may limit the manner and nature of presentation to the physician. Although challenges and opportunities for prevention and intervention are available on a societal level, the family physician is in a unique position to make a meaningful impact before violence escalates.

Interpersonal violence encompasses a wide variety of circumstances. These include:

- Rape.
- Attempted rape.
- Sexual violence and predatory behaviors.
- Psychological abuse.
- Stalking.
- Physical abuse.
- Financial abuse.
- Neglect (of dependent person).
- Homicide.

These manifestations can be further characterized by the status of the individual vulnerable to such acts. Those at great risk include children, the elderly, pregnant women, persons who are physically or mentally challenged, immigrants, and members of racial or cultural minorities.

Definitions

Neglect is the chronic failure of one person who is responsible for the physical and emotional needs of another person to provide for those needs. This form of abuse most often occurs in family relationships and is directed at elders, children, or disabled family members. However, caregivers in other societal settings, including child and adult day care, schools, group homes, nursing facilities, and hospitals, may be involved in neglect of a dependent person.

Physical violence, as defined by the Centers for Disease Control and Prevention (CDC), is the "intentional use of physical force with the potential for causing death, disability, injury, or harm." This includes, but is not limited to, the following acts: scratching, pushing, shoving, throwing, grabbing, biting, choking, shaking, slapping, punching, burning, use of a weapon, and use of restraints or one's body, size, or strength against another person.

The CDC definition of **sexual violence** includes the following actions:

- "The use of physical force to compel a person to engage in a sexual act against his or her will, whether or not the act is completed."
- "An attempted or completed sex act involving a person who is unable to understand the nature or condition of the act, to decline participation, or to communicate unwillingness to engage in the sexual act."
- "Abusive sexual contact."

Violence need not always be physical in nature. Humiliation, controlling behavior, repeated verbal assaults, isolation, and public harassment can all produce psychological trauma. Emotional violence can coexist with physical violence, or stand alone. Techniques such as withholding money, withholding transportation, and limiting freedom of movement or association are often employed in abusive relationships. Financial abuse most often involves the inappropriate transfer or use of an elder's funds for the caregiver's purposes.

WEB SITE

Centers for Disease Control and Prevention fact sheet on interpersonal violence:

http://www.cdc.gov/ncipc/factsheets/ipvoverview.htm.

Epidemiology

Numerous studies have revealed disturbing evidence about the magnitude of interpersonal violence in US society as well as opportunities for intervention. An estimated 25% of women and 7.9% of men are victimized at some point in their lives by a former spouse, cohabiting partner, or date. In one survey, 7.7% of women and 0.3% of men reported having been raped, and 22.1% of women and 7.4% of men had been physically assaulted. A typical respondent male victim averaged 4.4 physical assaults while women averaged 6.9 physical assaults. Thus, repeat victimization offers an opportunity for physicians to identify and intervene with persons at risk.

The annual incidence of all interpersonal violence has been estimated at 47 assaults per 1000 women and 32 assaults per 1000 men. Other estimates suggest that as a result of the 1.3 million women and 800,000 men who are physically abused in the United States each year, there are over two million injuries and 1300 deaths. Of particular concern is the finding that persons living in homes in which violent acts occur are more than four times likely to be involved in additional violent acts than are those living in homes that are violence free.

Children, the elderly, and pregnant women are particularly vulnerable groups. Each year approximately one million children in the United States are identified as victims of family violence, and more than 500,000 elders are abused or neglected in domestic settings. Half of homeless women and children report fleeing domestic violence. Pregnant women are far more likely to suffer physical abuse. It is a sobering fact that homicide is the leading cause of maternal death in the United States.

In mixed-sex domestic violence, the female partner is 30% more likely to be killed than the male partner, and most of these murders are committed with firearms. Although 28% of female homicide victims were killed by their current or former male partners, only 3% of men were murdered by current or former female partners.

African-American, Native-American, and Alaskan Native women and men report higher rates of domestic violence than the population as a whole, but socioeconomic factors confound the interpretation of such data. African Americans have a spousal homicide rate 8.4 times that of whites, whereas partners in interracial marriages have similar rates.

Other studies indicate a higher number of unreported incidents of physical and sexual abuse. More difficult to measure is psychological abuse or neglect, which is often insidious and difficult to detect.

Centers for Disease Control and Prevention (CDC): *Costs of Intimate Partner Violence Against Women in the United States.* CDC, National Center for Injury Prevention and Control, 2003. Available at: http://www.cdc.gov/ncipc/pub-res/ipv_cost/ipv.htm.

Riggs DS et al: Risk for domestic violence: Factors associated with perpetration and victimization. J Clin Psychol 2000;56:1289. [PMID: 11051060]

Tjaden P, Thoennes N: *Extent, Nature, and Consequences of Intimate Partner Violence: Findings from the National Violence Against Women Survey.* Publication No. NCJ 181867. US Department of Justice, 2000. Available at: http://www.ncjrs.org/pdffiles1/nij/181867.pdf.

Natural History of Interpersonal Violence in Adults

Interpersonal violence among known partners occurs in cycles. Although there are clear steps to the cycle of violence, this should not imply that there is no escalation. In fact, with each cycle the victim is exposed to additional risk. Similar cycles can be adapted to elder and child abuse and sexual predatory behavior. The steps in known partner abuse are outlined in Figure 58–1.

Detection & Intervention

Refer to Chapter 42 for more detailed information about abuse in the elderly.

A. Adults

1. Identification and screening—To identify cases of interpersonal violence, it is essential that family physicians maintain a high index of suspicion at all times. Victims of abuse often feel ashamed, have low self-esteem, or are unable to share their circumstances readily. Creating an atmosphere that promotes a welcoming, frank, and professional discussion will allow patients the opportunity to bring their concerns forward to the physician.

Screening tools have been advocated; however, the value of these tools for domestic violence has not been clearly demonstrated. Because of a lack of specific studies, the US Preventive Services Task Force has issued an "I" recommendation on methodologies of screening for family and intimate partner violence, indicating that there is insufficient evidence for or against the use of such tools.

The American Medical Association and American College of Obstetricians and Gynecologists recommend specific direct questioning of patients, when appropriate, in a nonthreatening manner. The policy of the American Academy of Family Physicians regarding family violence can be found at the association's web site (http://www.aafp.org/x16506.xml). Several simple screening questions may of value in the patient interview and should be incorporated by the physician when taking a relevant history, at the time of the well visit, or when screening for other diseases. Much like screening for alcohol abuse or depression, low-threat questions can be incorporated to ascertain the possibility of abuse in the home situation (Table 58–1). Often, these questions can be incorporated into a history or review of systems questionnaire with little difficulty. Periodic rescreening of patients is advised.

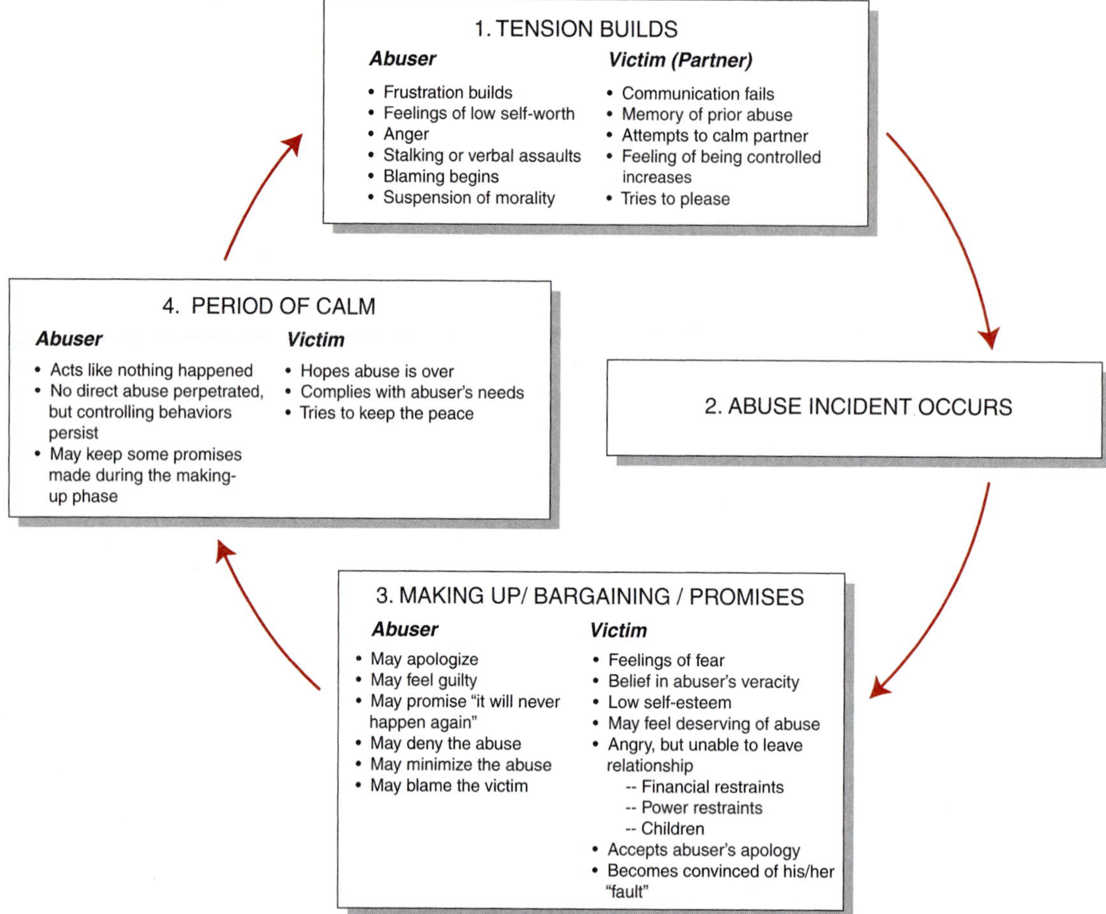

Figure 58–1. Steps in the cycle of interpersonal violence. With each new cycle the level of violence usually escalates.

The use of prompts in electronic medical records is an interesting area of development. Certain complexes, complaints, and findings could trigger a reminder for the physician to ask a question about violence in the home or workplace. Much research remains to be done to ascertain the value of such prompting.

Additional questions have been proposed by various advocacy groups. Screening questions suggested for attorneys can be adapted by the family physician; these can be obtained from the American Bar Association web site at http://www.abanet.org/domviol/mrdv/identify.html. Family physicians should endeavor to become familiar with a wide range of potential questions in order to utilize an appropriate approach from a wide repertoire.

Ebell MH: Routine screening for depression, alcohol problems, and domestic violence. Am Fam Physician 2004;69:2421. [PMID: 15168964]

US Preventive Services Task Force: Screening for family and intimate partner violence: Recommendation statement. Ann Intern Med 2004;140:382. [PMID: 14996680]

2. Interventions—The abusive spouse or family member often accompanies the patient to the office visit to

Table 58–1. Screening questions for interpersonal violence in adults.

1. Do you feel safe in your current relationship?
2. Do you perceive any threats to your safety on a regular basis?
3. Have you been hit or hurt by someone in the past?
4. Would you care to share any concerns you might have regarding interpersonal violence in your home or among your friends?
5. Have you ever been or are you currently concerned about harming your partner or someone close to you?
6. Would you like information about interpersonal violence or substance abuse programs in our community?

monitor the information being delivered and the manner in which it is portrayed by the victim. Although it is not abnormal for a spouse or significant other to attend a physician visit, the physician should be alert to cues, including nonverbal behaviors that might signal an abusive situation. In particular, physicians should carefully evaluate situations in which someone else does all the talking for a competent and able patient.

Perpetrators of abuse often have a history of interpersonal violence in their family of origin or were victims of nonfamily interpersonal violence at one point in their lives. It is often difficult to identify the inciting event, because frank communication with those who perpetrate violence is usually difficult. Insecurity, anger, a need to control, power needs, and moral issues are often complicated by defensiveness, shame, embarrassment, low self-esteem, and fear on the part of the abuser. Often, abusive individuals have no viable model of behavior in which to contextualize the intervention of a physician; to avoid being the victims of a confrontation, they may revert to controlling behavior in the office or become aggressive. Physicians must consider the safety of their staff when confronting such individuals.

Intensive therapy is often required for both the abuser and the victim. A period of physical separation is often required initially for the safety of the victim. Referral to an appropriate safe house in the community and obtaining a personal protective order from a judge are important first steps, and the patient should be encouraged to take these steps, if appropriate. The use of an advocate, volunteer or paid, is of great value in assisting the victim to follow through with these initial steps. Legal advice is often necessary, and family physicians should have a list of resources available for patients to seek legal advice early in the process.

During this period, therapy for the victim is aimed at improving objective decision making, reestablishing self-esteem, reversing the cycle of self-blaming, and addressing the reality of the situation. Reality-oriented interventions complement insight-based approaches. Objective testing of victim hypotheses of what happened often results in greater fear, so a supportive, encouraging therapist and environment are required. Eventually, group therapy can be utilized, once the victim has reorganized his or her thoughts and is able to share experiences in a productive way with others.

The abuser also requires therapy. Depending on the circumstance, this may occur in the penal system. Therapy is aimed at reordering the emotional responses of the abuser and improving self-esteem. Developing a new world view and set of behaviors is very difficult and takes a great deal of effort on the part of the therapist and the abuser.

Family therapy may have a place in the early stages of the cycle of violence. If both the abuser and the victim recognize the maladaptive pattern of behavior in their arguments prior to the onset of physical or severe emotional abuse, couple's counseling may be successful in ending the cycle of violence. However, communications skills training alone may not be enough to create a change in behaviors.

Consideration needs to be given to the patient's spiritual, ethnic, and cultural background in order to place any intervention into a context that will maximize its success. "One size fits all" therapies may not have lasting benefit. It is critical that the family physician be supportive of the therapist and encourage the victim to continue in therapy. "Relapse" rates (ie, returning to the abusive relationship) are high; physicians should not become judgmental about such reconciliations but rather should remain supportive of victims.

B. Children

Specific and direct questioning about childhood injuries is advocated by emergency physicians and pediatricians. Direct questioning of parents should be done in private to maximize value, maintain confidence, and reassure family members of the physician's intent to help, not hurt, the child or the family.

The Virtual Hospital (http://www.vh.org/pediatric/provider/pediatrics/domesticviolence/screening.html) lists specific cues that should heighten the physician's index of suspicion regarding domestic violence and child abuse. "Red flags" should be raised when:

- One partner insists on accompanying the other parent and child, and speaks for them.
- A parent is reluctant to talk with the other partner present.
- The child's history does not fit the injury or illness.
- A parent makes frequent appointments for vague, poorly defined complaints.
- Medical attention for injuries is sought later than would be expected.
- The family uses emergency department services more often than is usual.
- A parent attempts to hide the child's injuries with clothing.
- A parent or child has several injuries, at various stages of healing.

Family physicians should be alert to the symptoms and signs of potential child abuse or neglect listed in Table 58–2.

C. Special Populations

Several groups within the US population are especially vulnerable to interpersonal violence. These groups

Table 58–2. Symptoms and signs of potential abuse and neglect in children.

Physical Abuse	Neglect	Emotional Abuse	Sexual Abuse
Burns	Malnutrition	Self-injury	Self-injury
School problems	Lack of supervision	Anger	Inappropriate sexuality for age
Self-destructive or suicidal behavior	Poor dental hygiene	Depression	Seductiveness
Unexplained cuts, bruises, or welts	Inappropriate clothing	Apathy	Eating disorders
Inappropriate fear of adults	Poor hygiene	Eating disorders	Poor hygiene
Early-onset depression, alcohol or drug use	Extreme hunger	Anxiety	Sleep disorders
Bruises in the shape of objects		Anger	Excessive aggression
Injuries in uncommon locations			Fear of a particular person
Bite marks			Withdrawal
			Suicidal behavior

include recent immigrants, ethnic and racial minorities, the homeless, and people with disabilities, and gays and lesbians.

Vulnerable populations, including those with physical or mental challenges, may find it difficult to contextualize their experience or communicate it in a manner the physician can understand. Patience and time are warranted. Followers of some religious and cultural traditions may tolerate levels of behavior that are not accepted by the mainstream culture in the Untied States. This is not to say that some cultural paradigms are inherently more violent than others; rather, the norms of acceptable or expected behaviors, including the sharing of intimate family details, create additional challenges to discovery of aberrant and abusive relationships for the physician. These challenges may apply to a wide variety of behaviors, including child rearing, depression screening, and sexuality concerns.

The key to identification of abuse in these situations is an understanding of cultural influences. To this end, enlisting the collaboration of an advocate who has proper training and connection with the culture is essential. This person may also play an important role in supporting the patient's decision making when seeking appropriate interventions.

Open-ended questions about a patient's cultural norms may provide an appropriate avenue and manner for inquiry into the presence or absence of interpersonal violence in the patient's life. An inherent lack of trust in law enforcement may be a specific challenge in poor minority communities and among the homeless. Misunderstanding of interpersonal violence and the stigma associated with it may inhibit the reporting or seeking of assistance. Additional information can be obtained from specific resources such as the University of Michigan Program for Multicultural Health, available at http://www.med.umich.edu/multicultural/ccp/cdv.htm. An additional resource for the African-American community is available at http://www.dvinstitute.org/.

The possibility that partners in same-sex relationships may be victims of interpersonal violence is sometimes overlooked. A wide range of social factors may contribute to underreporting of abuse in this population, and frequency of physical and sexual abuse may be higher than most physicians would expect. Gay and lesbian patients should be questioned, as all patients are, in a safe environment and in a nonthreatening manner.

Regan KV et al: Measuring physical violence in male same-sex relationships. J Interpers Violence 2002;17:235.

Waldner-Haugrud L, Gratch LV: Sexual coercion in gay/lesbian relationships: Descriptives and gender differences. Violence Vict 1997;12:87. [PMID: 9360290]

Prevention

Given the pervasiveness of interpersonal violence, and the inherent difficulties of detection and intervention, methods of primary prevention are of critical importance in addressing this problem. The effectiveness of prevention programs remains an ongoing topic of study.

Family physicians should consider a routine discussion of interpersonal violence as part of the normal health maintenance routine. This can be part of the usual discussion of safety issues, including seat belt use, gun safety, and smoke protectors. In a matter-of-fact manner, the physician can introduce discussion of interpersonal violence in a wide variety of contexts, including well woman care, routine "physicals," and other health maintenance visits.

A routine discussion of parenting techniques, referral to appropriate parenting classes, and provision of printed information have all been shown to have a positive effect on families at risk for child abuse or neglect. A plan for abuse identification, prevention, and training can be part of the individual education plan and the transition plan for children with developmental and physical disabilities.

Living situations of elderly patients should be well documented and understood, especially if the caregivers are not well known or are not part of the physician's personal practice. Information obtained and communication established during times of calm may be useful later should an incident occur.

Safety Instructions for Patients

The American Bar Association provides a domestic violence safety plan on its web site at http://www.abanet.org/tips/dvsafety.html. Adult patients can be referred to this resource for updated recommendations on how to protect themselves in situations in which interpersonal violence is an imminent threat. Family physicians should also be aware of local resources, and update contacts with them annually, to assure a readily available system of referral for safe houses, ongoing care, and legal intervention. Although these options vary from community to community, local resources can usually provide assistance to physicians, particularly when dealing with complicated cases.

Reporting

Readers should familiarize themselves with the laws of their state regarding the required reporting of violent crimes involving adults. In general, acts of violence that involve lethal force or firearms and rape must be reported to the local police agency. Adequate and complete documentation of all encounter details—including quotations, details, and time requirements—is an important medicolegal requirement. Family physicians working in emergency departments should follow the policies and procedures of their institution in the management and reporting a such violent crimes.

The reporting of an individual's confidentially expressed intent to harm another person places the physician in a far more difficult ethical and legal position that may require legal advice. In emergencies, particularly when a patient is believed to be in danger, the patient should be told to call 911.

Elder abuse is also covered by state laws, and physicians should report in accordance with the local law at the time of the suspected abuse. In general, APS should be notified of suspected neglect or abuse. Other agencies that may require notification, depending on the state, include the Area Agency on Aging and the County Department of Social Services.

The reporting of child abuse to Child Protective Services is a requirement in all 50 states. Some states require reporting to the local police agency as well. Most states have established toll-free numbers for reporting suspected child abuse. The National Child Abuse Hotline, at 1-800-4-A-CHILD (1-800-422-4453), is another avenue for reporting suspected abuse, neglect, or sexual assault of a child.

Ahmad M, Lachs MS: Elder abuse and neglect: What physicians can and should do. Cleve Clin J Med 2002;69:801. [PMID: 12371803]

Web Sites

American Bar Association Commission on Domestic Violence: http://www.abanet.org/domviol/mrdv/

Feminist Majority Foundation fact sheet on domestic violence: http://www.feminist.org/other/dv/dvfact.html

SECTION VII
Physician–Patient Issues

Communication 59

Nancy Levine, MD, & Marian Block, MD

PHYSICIAN–PATIENT COMMUNICATION

The Therapeutic Alliance

It is within the context of communication that the therapeutic alliance between physician and patient is formed. When communication with a patient is nonjudgmental, respectful, and genuine, the stage is set for a successful therapeutic alliance. Medical knowledge is vitally necessary, but alone it is insufficient to accomplish the tasks of caring for a patient. It is the ability of the physician to translate medical knowledge for the patient and to enlist the trust of the patient that will ultimately lead to good health care for the patient.

Good communication has several beneficial effects on the relationship between the physician and the patient. It improves patient satisfaction, adherence,[1] and health. It also improves physicians' satisfaction with their work and the accuracy of information they obtain from patients and decreases the likelihood that physicians will be sued for malpractice.

Patient Satisfaction

The impact of good communication on patient satisfaction is the best studied of these benefits. Ware and colleagues extensively reviewed the evidence for the validity of using patient satisfaction and other patient rating scales, concluding that patients' ratings of interpersonal aspects of care provide not only useful and valid information for quality assessment but also the best source of data on the interpersonal aspects of care.

Patients generally want more information than their physicians give them. The amount of information given to the patient strongly correlates with patient satisfaction. Physicians spend a small fraction of their time giving information, 1 minute out of 20, and believe that they spend more time than they actually do. Thus the correlation between the amount of information patients receive and their satisfaction with the visit is a strong and consistent observation in the medical literature.

Many other physician behaviors also correlate with satisfaction. These include courtesy, attention, listening, empathy, and sympathy. Patients whose physicians communicate and interpret emotions well and are friendly, concerned, take time to answer questions, and give explanations are more satisfied. Patients rate their physicians positively if they are encouraging, open, and attentive and negatively if they dominate the encounter.

Physicians' personal qualities are rated highly if the encounter centers on the patient rather than on the physician's concerns. Physicians who ask many directive questions and keep tight control over the interaction tend to have patients who feel that their physicians do not listen to them.

Buller MK, Buller DB: Physicians' communication style and patient satisfaction. J Health Soc Behav 1987;28:375. [PMID: 3429807]

Ware JE Jr, Hays RD: Methods for measuring patient satisfaction with specific medical encounters. Med Care 1988;26:393. [PMID: 3352332]

Physician Satisfaction

Physician satisfaction, although not as well studied as patient satisfaction, is very important for physicians' per-

[1]The term *adherence* is used throughout this chapter in preference to *compliance.*

sonal and professional lives. Physicians find reward and meaning in their interpersonal relationships with patients. The quality of those relationships is directly related to physician satisfaction with their work. Good communication with patients will improve the quality of the relationship and thus improve physician satisfaction.

Accuracy of Information Obtained

In 1988 George Engel said, "The interview is the most powerful, encompassing, sensitive, and versatile instrument available to the physician." In a 1984 study, Beckman and Frankel discovered that physicians frequently interrupted patients before they completely expressed their concerns, and rarely returned to patients' initial concerns. They found that physicians controlled the interview with directive questions and they postulated that these interviewing tactics resulted in a loss of relevant information. They also found that these behaviors resulted in an incomplete clinical picture and disorganized care, thus leading to the collection of inaccurate information. Accurate information is lost when physicians use medical jargon. In one study, 50% of physician–patient interactions were adversely affected by the physicians' use of medical jargon. Patients frequently believed they understood the jargon, but actually did not.

Other behaviors by the physician interfere with accurate data collection. Excessive control of the interview by the physician limits patients' ability to communicate all of their concerns; hence the patient database is flawed. The way a question is asked has an important impact on the information received. Patients who are asked "What concerns you about this problem?" give better information than patients who are asked "What worries you about this problem?" The use of closed-ended questions (questions that have yes/no answers) limits the ability of patients to describe symptoms in their own words. In summary, physicians can improve the accuracy of their medical interviews if they use open-ended questions, allow patients to fully answer a question before interrupting, and avoid the use of medical jargon.

Beckman HB, Frankel RM: The effect of physician behavior on the collection of data. Ann Intern Med 1984;101:692. [PMID: 6486600]

Engel GL: In White KL, ed: *The Task of Medicine: Dialogue at Wickenburg*. Kaiser Family Foundation, 1988.

Health Outcomes

The relationship between improved health and good communication is more difficult to study than the correlation between patient satisfaction and good communication. Outcomes are influenced by many more variables and are temporally more distant. However, evidence indicates that good communication between physicians and patients correlates with good health outcomes. Patients with peptic ulcer disease who are involved in their own care through shared decision making with their physicians have less functional impairment due to their illness. When there is agreement between physicians and patients about the nature and severity of the patient's health problem, improvement in or resolution of the problem occurs more often. Physicians who are less controlling, give more information, and show more emotion have patients with fewer functional limitations, lower blood pressure, and lower blood glucose levels. Patients who can express their emotions, both positive and negative, have improved health outcomes; in addition, when the ratio of patient to physician talk is high, patients are healthier. Open-ended questions are superior to directive questions. Patients who are allowed to tell their story in their own words have lower blood pressures. In a study in which anesthesiologists were trained to give patients more detailed information about what to expect during their hospitalization, the patients required less pain medicine and left the hospital earlier.

Malpractice Suits

Physicians who communicate well are less likely to be named in a lawsuit. Patients of frequently sued physicians are more likely to say they were rushed, never received explanations, felt ignored, and felt their physicians did not communicate with them. There was no correlation between quality of care and adverse outcomes and malpractice claims in one study. These studies and others suggest that physicians are sued because patients are unhappy with their care and not because of poor quality of care.

Adherence

There is ample evidence that good communication leads to better adherence to a physician's advice. Francis and colleagues found a strong association between patient satisfaction and adherence: poor adherence results when parents of young patients have unmet expectations from the visit, when there is a lack of warmth on the part of the physician, and when parents fail to receive an explanation for their child's illness. A number of communication techniques are associated with improved adherence. Patients are more likely to be adherent if they have the opportunity to explain their understanding of their problem and ask questions. When patients are coached to ask more questions they are more likely to keep future appointments. Physicians who recognize nonverbal cues have patients who keep appointments more often.

COMMUNICATION SKILLS

All the communication techniques described so far can be easily learned and used in the standard medical interview. Several excellent textbooks are available for thorough review of these (see Coulehan and Block, and Cole and Bird). The following techniques are especially important.

1. A statement such as "How did you hope I might help you at this visit?" will elicit important concerns that patients might not otherwise express.
2. Expressing empathy is an important basic skill. Empathy has three components in the physician–patient relationship. The first component is knowing how the patient views a problem, the second is understanding that point of view, and the third is acknowledging to the patient that the physician understands his or her point of view. To be genuinely empathetic the physician needs to accomplish all three of these.
3. Patients should be allowed to completely express their concerns and should be asked if they have any specific requests.
4. Patients' explanation of their problem should be elicited and a mutual understanding of that problem negotiated. A question such as "What do you think is the cause of your problem?" is often helpful.
5. Patients should be encouraged to express feelings about their illness by asking "How are you feeling about this illness?" It is important for physicians to be aware that they do not need to resolve patients' negative feelings. Simply expressing negative emotions is a relief for patients.
6. Patients should be given specific information about their health condition.
7. Physicians should involve patients in their treatment plan. Patients who are collaborators in their care will feel in control of their illness; this will lead to an improved ability to cope with the illness. Patients who are passive will feel that the illness controls them and may give up working to improve their health. Physicians can accomplish this by asking questions about how patients feel the proposed treatment plan might work and by giving them choices about the plan.
8. Reassurance is a powerful communication tool. At its best it can allay anxiety and enable patients to cope with difficult health problems. When offered prematurely, however, it can seem insincere and worsen anxiety. It is important for the physician to truly understand the patient's concerns and perform a thorough medical evaluation of the problem before offering reassurance.

Cole S, Bird J: *The Medical Interview: The Three-Function Approach,* 3rd ed. Mosby, 2000.

Coulehan J, Block M: *The Medical Interview: Mastering Skills for Clinical Practice,* 5th ed. F.A. Davis, 2005.

SPECIAL COMMUNICATION CHALLENGES

There are a number of situations that physicians find especially challenging. Many of these topics are reviewed in detail in other chapters of this book. The focus here is mainly on the communication issues that these special situations pose for clinicians and their patients.

The Angry Patient

Although other emotional responses of patients toward their illness are difficult for physicians to deal with, none poses a greater challenge than the patient who is angry. Anxiety and sadness can be difficult responses to address, but physicians usually find it easier to be sympathetic or empathetic. The natural reaction to anger is defensiveness, not empathy. It requires considerable communication skills to develop empathy with a patient who is angry.

The clinician must first recognize anger, then acknowledge it, understand it, and respond to it. Recognizing it is easy if patients state that they are angry, but often they do not. Recognizing anger in a patient often requires that the physician recognize defensiveness in him- or herself. If a physician is feeling defensive, it is likely that the patient is angry. There may be other cues such as patient voice tone or agitation. If a physician senses that the patient is angry, and the patient has not volunteered this, it is important for the physician to explore the anger. An observation such as "You seem upset" may be helpful in encouraging the patient to share his or her feelings. It is important that the physician's language match what he or she sees in the patient. If the patient seems furious and the physician says "You seem a little upset," the patient is likely to become angrier. Conversely, if the physician says "You seem furious" and the patient is a little piqued, the patient will deny it.

Once the patient has shared that he or she is angry, the physician is in a position to explore why. Patients may be angry for a myriad of reasons, most of which have little to do with the physician. Until a physician understands why the patient is angry, he or she will be unable to address the anger in a constructive way. Often patients state the reason for their anger in response to the initial reflection "you seem upset." If they do not, the physician will need to acknowledge the anger and ask specifically about it. "I see that you are upset; are you willing to share with me what it is about?" The answer to this question will determine how the physician proceeds. The patient's anger may be directed at the physician justifiably and may require an apology. It is more likely to be directed at someone or something else over which the physician has no control. The task is then to empathize with the patient. Once the patient feels understood, the physician will be able to move the conversation to other areas.

It is important to understand that anger is often displaced, especially when a patient is ill. The sadness and loss of control patients feel about their illness are directed in the form of anger at those caring for them. The anger is really directed at the illness, not the physician. If the patient seems angry with the physician or another member of the health care team and the physician genuinely feels that the team has provided good care, the patient may be manifesting displaced anger. This anger also needs to be explored and understood but may not be resolved as easily as other forms of anger. Awareness that the anger is displaced may, however, prevent an automatic defensive response on the part of the physician, which typically encourages the patient to feel justified in his or her anger. In such situations, it is important after exploring the anger to redirect the conversation to the difficulties and frustrations of the patient's illness.

Adherence

Adherence is a complex problem for physicians and their patients. Negotiation is one of the key concepts when addressing problems with adherence. The physician and the patient need to agree about the nature of the problem at hand and agree about the evaluation and treatment of it. Without this agreement, there is no reason for the patient to follow the advice of the physician. Patients come to their physicians with certain beliefs about their illness and expectations about its evaluation and treatment. They will follow their physician's advice if the advice is consistent with these beliefs. Various communication strategies set the stage for successful negotiation.

Eliciting accurate information about patient adherence is the first step in dealing with nonadherence. If a physician does not know that the patient is not following medical advice, he or she cannot intervene to help. Several methods are suggested in the medical literature to elicit information about adherence. The physician can count medication, measure drug levels, look at outcomes, or ask the patient. The most effective method is to ask. With a well-framed question, patients will give accurate information about their adherence 80% of the time. Asking a patient "Are you taking your medication?" is unlikely to yield accurate information. The answer to this type of question is an automatic yes. Physicians who ask specific questions about medication names, dosages, and times elicit more accurate information about adherence. Giving patients permission to be nonadherent with a question such as "Some of my patients have difficulty remembering to take their blood pressure medicine every day; I wonder if you have found this also?" is often fruitful. Patients are relieved to hear that their problem is common and assume from the tone of the question that the physician is likely to be forgiving.

Once it has been established that the patient is not following medical advice, the next task is to determine the reason(s). Because these usually have to do with patients' beliefs, goals, and expectations, questions to elucidate these will be important. Patients' beliefs are varied and it is impossible to predict them without asking. A patient might have had a father who took the same medicine the physician is prescribing and who died of complications of the disease anyway. A patient might believe that she can tell when her blood pressure is high and therefore takes her medicine only on these days. A patient might believe that he has no control over his illness and therefore the treatment will not work. Useful questions to elicit patients' beliefs, goals, and expectations include the following: "Do you know anyone with your condition?" and if so, "How was he or she treated?" "What happened to him or her?" "Have you read anything about your condition?" "What have you read?" "What do you think caused what you have?" "How do you think you should be treated?" "What kinds of tests do you think you should have?" "What might prevent you from following my advice?"

These types of questions will quickly demonstrate where the physician and patient disagree. The next step is to come to some common agreement with the patient about how to proceed. The nature of the disagreement will determine how the problem is resolved. It is important to realize that it needs to be resolved in such a way that the physician feels he or she is providing good medical care and the patient feels he or she is receiving good medical care. To accomplish this, the physician and patient will need to influence each other. There are some common useful strategies for negotiation. The physician can correct misperceptions, refer the patient to a trusted source (friend, family member, article, organization, etc), explore options with the patient, suggest alternatives that are consistent with the patient's beliefs or goals, or compromise.

A word about the use of fear as a motivating tactic is important. It is commonly used by physicians and is usually unsuccessful for a variety of reasons. It greatly increases anxiety, which often encourages the behavior physicians are trying to stop. For example, the typical response to "If you don't stop smoking you are going to get lung cancer!" is to smoke more in response to the increased anxiety. Fear can make an illness seem more overwhelming and a common response to reduce anxiety is to deny the problem exists; thus adherence is worsened, not improved. Fear tactics are not only ineffective, but are often counterproductive.

Patients are much more likely to adhere with treatment recommendations if physicians point out the positive results of following the advice rather than the negative results of not following it. "If you stop smoking you will reduce your chances of lung cancer" is a more powerful motivator than "If you don't stop smoking you might get lung cancer." Physicians should focus on patients' successes, even if they are small, rather than on their failures; encourage patients' strengths, attitudes, and actions; and offer hope. When patients are hopeful about their condition they are more likely to be able to make changes in their lives to accomplish the task at hand. When physicians are hopeful they are more effective clinicians.

Patients' behavior is strongly influenced by their social context; thus it is important to explore this. What is their cultural background and do they share the same cultural beliefs about their condition as this group? They might subscribe to a belief that holds that illness is a punishment for bad behavior. They might come from a culture in which herbal remedies are used for their condition. Friends and family are also important: A patient might believe that a weight-loss diet will help his heart condition, but he has a wife who does the cooking and who believes that the main way to express her love is to feed her loved ones. Another patient may be unable to quit smoking because all of her friends smoke.

In summary, effective communication is the main tool a physician has to assess adherence to advice and to intervene for the good of the patient if the patient is not following that advice. The key principles of good communication concerning adherence include a nonjudgmental exploration of the problem, information giving, encouraging the patient to share beliefs and asking questions, asking about the social context of the problem, and focusing on the positive results of the advice being given to patients.

Communicating with Patients Who Have a Terminal Illness

Much of caring for patients at the end of life involves communicating with them and their families. Communication revolves around two main areas: giving bad or sad news and discussing goals and wishes for medical care. Certainly all the general rules for communication are important in these circumstances. There are unique and predictable difficulties for patients and physicians when discussing end-of-life care. The discussion here focuses on "the bad-news consultation."

The first communication problem a clinician typically encounters is how much to tell the patient about his or her illness. Physicians often assume that patients desire full information about their illness and this is usually a correct assumption. However, some patients do not want to know a bad prognosis; thus the physician needs to be skilled at assessing the patient's desire for information. A question such as "If it is bad news, do you want to know?" might be helpful to begin this discussion. If the patient does not want to be given bad news, there are two further areas for discussion. The first is to determine if there is someone else that the patient wants to receive the news and the second is to explore the reasons that the patient does not want to know.

Once the physician has determined the patient does want to hear the bad news, it is important to set up the interview carefully. When patients are satisfied with this initial interview they are less likely to be depressed later in their illness. Does the patient want anyone else to be present? Is the setting private and free of interruptions? Does the physician have enough time? The physician's attitude should be to convey understanding and reassurance. The main goal of the session is to give the news. Any further discussion of treatment goals and choices may overwhelm the patient and should be deferred to a future visit.

The next task is to give the news. A "warning" such as "I'm afraid I have some bad news" will help the patient prepare for the information. The news should then be delivered in a simple, direct, and straightforward manner. The physician should pause to give the patient time to react and assess the patient's reaction before proceeding. Often the reaction is obvious: the patient may cry or become angry. The patient may, however, be silent, and the physician may need to ask "How are you feeling about this news?" At this point the patient's reaction will direct the rest of the interview. Regardless of where the discussion goes from this point, the clinician should continuously monitor and respond to the patient's emotions, understanding, and desire for information.

Attention to the end of this interview is important for future care. The physician should inquire about the patient's understanding of his or her illness: "Can you tell me what you understand about your illness?" The physician should communicate continued support ("I'm going to do everything I can to help you through this") and should offer hope, but be realistic ("Let's hope for the best and prepare for the worst"). Finally, the patient will need a follow-up visit within a short period of time to discuss options and goals of treatment.

Patient Education & Counseling

Effective patient education serves a number of important purposes in the clinical encounter. It satisfies the patient's desire to know about his or her condition, it improves patient satisfaction and adherence, and it relieves the patient's anxiety. It also improves health outcomes and reduces health risks. Physicians must be acutely aware that patients misunderstand and forget much of what they hear from their physician.

The ultimate goal in patient education is to change behavior in order to improve the health of the patient. To accomplish this goal patients need to understand their illness, recognize behaviors that put them at risk, make decisions about treatment options, and adhere to their physician's advice.

Studies show that patients commonly believe their physician does not give them enough information. Other studies show that patients commonly misunderstand or do not remember the information their physician gives them and that high levels of interpersonal skill on the part of the physician correlate with the amount of information a physician gives to a patient and the amount the patient recalls. Some situations are predictably associated with poor recall. These include discussion of many medical problems at one visit, patient anxiety, prescription of more than one medication, and relaying of new or bad news. Techniques that can be used to improve a patient's recall of information include simplification, repetition, giving specific information, checking the patient's understanding, discussing fewer problems, and limiting new medications. Physicians should also negotiate an agreement with the patient about the nature of and solution to the problem and explore patients' ideas about the problem. More nonverbal immediacy such as closer interpersonal distance, more eye contact, and leaning toward the patient is beneficial. It is also important to assess what a patient wants to know.

These interventions target information giving and recall and are critical. Behavior change, however, is more complicated than simply giving information that the patient can understand and remember. Physicians need to assess patients' understanding of the problem and assess and understand their motivation to change. Questions targeted toward the patient's understanding of the disease such as "What do you know about your condition?" and questions directed at motivation to change such as "What are you willing to do about your condition?" are also useful.

Physicians need to present options and help patients make choices. Patients are more likely to make behavior changes successfully if they have several choices. Too many options, however, may be overwhelming. Statements such as "Your options are..." and questions such as "Which option will you choose?" or "How will you go about it?" are helpful. Some additional important areas of communication include continued offers of support from the physician, encouragement of small successes by the physician, and continued reassessment of the problem.

Cultural Competence 60

Kathleen A. Culhane-Pera, MD, MA, & Sonia Patten, PhD

Family practitioners have long recognized the importance of cultural competence in health care. Increasingly, such knowledge and skills are being recognized as important elements of medical care by other medical professions (ie, American Medical Association, American College of Emergency Physicians, and College of Obstetricians and Gynecologists), accrediting bodies (ie, Joint Commission on Accreditation of Healthcare Organizations), and medical educational organizations (ie, Association of American Medical Colleges, Accreditation Council on Graduate Medical Education, and Licensed Committee on Medical Education).

Government agencies are promoting culturally competent health care. Healthy People 2010, the US Department of Health and Human Services' (DHHS) 10-year program to improve health, has two goals: (1) to increase quality and years of healthy life, and (2) to eliminate health disparities. As part of the Initiative to Eliminate Racial and Ethnic Disparities in Health, the DHHS approved the National Standards for Culturally and Linguistically Appropriate Services in December 2000. Title VI of the 1964 Civil Rights Act guarantees the right to equal access to federally funded services regardless of gender, age, race, ethnicity, religion, or national origin, including people of limited English proficiency. The Centers for Medicare and Medicaid Services requires that Medicare+Choice Organizations provide culturally and linguistically appropriate care. The state of New Jersey requires that all licensed physicians receive culturally competent training, and other states are considering similar legislation.

The Institute of Medicine's (IOM) 2001 report, *Crossing the Quality Chasm,* documents the failures of the US medical system and asserts that the system must become equitable and patient centered, as well as safe, timely, efficient, and effective. The following year, the IOM released *Unequal Treatment,* a powerful critique of how health care providers' prejudices, biases, and stereotyping contribute to unequal treatment of racial and ethnic minorities. Two subsequent IOM reports highlight how health care providers must consider patients' cultural and social backgrounds in order to effectively communicate, particularly in working with people with limited health literacy. These reports list specific recommendations that are relevant for family physicians as they provide primary care to a diverse US population.

Given these requirements and recommendations, this chapter addresses three topics. Why is cultural competence important? What about culture is important in medicine? And how can physicians provide culturally competent care in clinical settings?

Gilbert MJ: *Principles and Recommended Standards for Cultural Competence Education of Healthcare Professionals.* California Endowment, 2003. Available at www.calendow.org

Institute of Medicine: *Crossing the Quality Chasm: A New Health System for the 21st Century.* Committee on Quality of Health Care in America, 2001.

Smedley BD et al: *Unequal Treatment: Confronting Racial and Ethnic Disparities in Health Care.* Institute of Medicine, Committee on Understanding and Eliminating Racial and Ethnic Disparities in Health Care, 2003. Available at www.iom.org

US Department of Health and Human Services: Healthy People 2010. DHHS, 2000. Available at: http://www.health.gov/healthypeople/Document/html/uih/uih_2.htm.

US Department of Health and Human Services: National Standards on Culturally and Linguistically Appropriate Services in Health Care. Available at: http://www.omhrc.gov/omh/programs/2pgprograms/finalreport.pdf.

WHY IS CULTURAL COMPETENCE IMPORTANT?

Culture Influences People's Views of Health, Illness, & Treatment

Health, illness, and treatment are strongly influenced by cultural contexts. It may seem strange to practitioners of scientifically based biomedicine that the cultures of providers and patients are major factors in clinical encounters. It is the case, however, that all humans have been socialized from childhood to define and experience the world in ways that are shared with other members of their group.

Culture provides concepts, rules, behaviors, and meanings that are basic to and are expressed in the ways people relate to other people, to the supernatural, and to the environment. A person's culture is like a pair of glasses with just the "right prescription" that is created by socialization and life experiences. Through these cultural lenses, people interpret and categorize the events of the world, rendering the world understandable, orderly, and predictable. Culture is learned, and no single individual is a repository for his or her entire culture. Not all members of a cultural group believe, think, or act in the same manner. This point is very important for health care providers, who must avoid presuppositions about patients based on their participation in particular cultures.

The Diverse US Population

The changing demographics of the United States provide compelling reasons for health care providers to consider the impact of cultural factors on health, disease, and health care. The population is diverse; according to the 2000 census, non-Hispanic whites comprise 69.1% of the population, non-Hispanic blacks 12.1%, Hispanics 12.5%, Asians 3.6%, and American Indians 0.7%. The population as a whole will grow more slowly than it has in the past but subgroups within it will have different trajectories, such that the aggregated current ethnic minority populations will eventually outnumber the historic majority of European Americans. Projecting to the year 2060, non-Hispanic whites will comprise less than half of the population, while Hispanic whites and blacks will have increased to 26.6%, non-Hispanic blacks to 13.3%, Asians to 9.4%, and American Indians to 0.8%. Differential birth and immigration rates influence the changing composition of US society. In the 2000 census, foreign-born individuals comprised 13.3% of the total population, up from 8% in 1990. In some US cities, more than half of the residents are foreign born. This rate of growth among immigrants, refugees, and undocumented foreign-born residents is a highly politicized issue. For providers, it means that cultural differences are in the foreground of the health care arena.

Racial and ethnic categories are now widely recognized as social categories that humans create for a variety of purposes (eg, to describe, influence, or control human behavior; to impact policy and law). In the 2000 census, for the first time people could choose to indicate membership in more than one category; 97.6% of respondents described themselves as belonging to one racial or ethnic category, and 2.4% identified themselves as belonging to two to six racial or ethnic categories. Presently the terms *race* and *ethnic group* are used in ways that make them virtually interchangeable, and recently the targeting of pharmaceuticals to a specific race means that race is being used as a surrogate marker for genetics.

Racial & Ethnic Health Disparities

People from ethnic and racial minority groups have worse health care statistics than people from majority populations. For instance, African Americans, Native Americans, and Hispanics have worse health care outcomes for diabetes mellitus, cancer, and cardiovascular disease; experience more delays in receiving antibiotics for pneumonia and thrombolytic therapy for heart attacks; have higher rates of postoperative pulmonary embolism and septicemia; have more hospitalizations for uncontrolled diabetes; and report receiving less health care information from health care providers.

These ethnic and racial disparities in health are due to a complex interaction of many factors, from those that increase exposure to disease to those that decrease access to health care. One socioeconomic factor is that people without health insurance and economic resources have worse health status than people with insurance and economic resources. Another factor is that people with limited English proficiency and poor literacy skills have access to poor-quality health care services. However, even after controlling for socioeconomic class, ethnic minority groups still have worse health status than majority peoples. Institutional discrimination and individual discriminatory practices in health care settings have been cited as contributing causes, which must be addressed. Engaging in culturally competent care is an important remedy in redressing discriminatory practices in medical care.

Patient-Centered Care Includes Culturally Competent Care

An anthropological perspective makes the distinction between disease and illness, with physicians focusing on the biological processes of disease and patients focusing on the experience of the illness. A movement toward patient-centered medical care with emphases on improved communication and patient–provider satisfaction (and hence, improved health care outcomes) has built upon Engel's bio-psycho-social model to keep patients' human dimension in the center of medical interactions. Addressing patients' cultural beliefs, values, and expectations and incorporating their family and community in the therapeutic process improves health care outcomes.

The patient-centered care approach requires that physicians elicit and respectfully respond to patients' beliefs, concerns, and experiences with their illnesses—all culturally influenced dimensions. Patient-centered care is culturally competent care.

Eisenberg L: Disease and illness. Distinctions between professional and popular ideas of sickness. Cult Med Psychiatry 1977;1:9. [PMID: 756356]

Engel G: The need for a new medical model: A challenge for biomedicine. Science 1977;196:129. [PMID: 847460]

Smedley A, Smedley BD: Race as biology is fiction, racism as a social problem is real: Anthropological and historical perspectives on the social construction of race. Am Psychol 2005;60:16. [PMID: 15641918]

Stewart M et al: *Patient-centered Medicine: Transforming the Clinical Method*, 2nd ed. Radcliffe Medical Press, 2003.

US Department of Health and Human Services: *2005 National Healthcare Disparities Report.* AHRQ Publication No. 06-0017. Agency for Healthcare Research and Quality, December 2005. Available at: http://www.ahrq.gov/qual/nhdr05/nhdr05.htm.

WHAT ABOUT CULTURE IS IMPORTANT?

MT was a 72-year-old Hmong woman with a severe headache, blurred vision, and gait instability. A computed tomography scan revealed intracerebellar hemorrhage and evidence for early pontine herniation. Neurologists and neurosurgeons recommended a craniotomy to evacuate the clot, reduce the pressure, and save her life. The family refused an operation and left the hospital against medical advice to perform traditional Hmong treatments.

In this situation, and similar situations when patients and physicians have different perspectives about appropriate responses to illness, exploring the cultural issues can be enlightening. This section describes seven concepts about the influence of culture on patients and physicians that are pertinent to providing medical care in cross-cultural settings. Throughout this discussion, the preceding case study will be used to illustrate major points. After the description of each concept, the information is applied to MT's case.

A word of caution: Readers need to consider the following descriptions of general cultural beliefs and practices as information that illustrates the significance of culture in diagnosing and treating disease and illness. The information should *not* be interpreted as stereotypical statements about all people from any specific cultural group. Cultural beliefs and practices can vary considerably among members of any one group.

Concepts of Bodily Functions

All cultures have an internally consistent system of beliefs about how the body functions normally, how and why it can be influenced by factors that cause it to function abnormally, and how it can be restored to health. Human beings have created many systems of thought about bodily functions and malfunctions: the Chinese system of balance between *yin* and *yang*; the Ayurvedic concept of balance in nature; western systems of biomedicine, homeopathy, and naturopathy; as well as systems indigenous to many ethnic groups.

Each ethnic group's beliefs about the functioning of the natural, social, and supernatural worlds are germane to its ideas about health, illness, and healing. The natural realm includes ideas about the connections between people and the earth's elements of soil, water, air, plants, animals, and so on. The social realm connotes ideas about individuals and the appropriate interaction between people of different ages, genders, lineages, and ethnic groups. And the supernatural realm includes the religious beliefs about birth, death, afterlife, reincarnation, souls, spirits, and interactions between the spiritual world and the human world.

Application to the case: Hmong people originated in China and migrated into Southeast Asia where they were involved in the United States' secret war in Laos in the 1960s and 1970s. Refugees from the war, they fled into Thailand and were resettled in western countries. Their kinship system is patrilineal, the residence pattern is patrilocal, and the system of political power is patriarchal. Hmong religion is animistic, including beliefs of reincarnation, multiple souls, and ongoing relationships between the living and the spirits of ancestors. Hmong concepts of health and disease are influenced by animism and are similar to the Chinese humoral theory of balance between *yin* and *yang*.

Classification of Diseases

Each ethnic group has its own classification system of diseases. Although each ethnic group may recognize diarrhea or fevers, for example, the categories for classifying them vary from group to group and do not necessarily correspond with one another. This presents problems for translation of words and of ideas between systems of disease. For example, whereas physicians may be concerned about dehydration in all types of diarrhea, Pakistani mothers may be more likely to use oral rehydration solution for some types of diarrhea and less likely to use it for other types.

Entities that are recognized by certain ethnic groups and not others have been studied as folk illnesses or culture-bound syndromes. These entities are ailments with coherent concepts of etiologies, pathophysiologies, and treatments, but they may also be expressions of mental or social distress that have social and symbolic meanings. Examples include Latino *empacho, nervios, mollera caida, mal de ojo,* and *susto;* Malaysian *amok;* Laotian *latah;* African American "high blood"; and English "colds." Some entities, such as premenstrual syndrome, bulimia, and anorexia nervosa, have moved from folk illness to biomedical diagnosis. Culture-bound syndromes are part of the *Diagnostic and Statistical Manual of Mental Disorders IV*, but can also be considered as disease entities in their own right, rather than subsumed under psychiatric categories.

Application to the case: The Hmong disease classification system for headache seems straightforward, as there is only one word for headache (*mob taub hau*), but there are multiple types of headaches based on etiology. One recognized type of headache is associated with stroke. Strokes are described by the neurologic defect (*tuag tes tuag taw* means dead hand dead foot) as well as by multiple etiologies. Contact with biomedicine has altered the concept of stroke for some Hmong people in the United States.

Theories of Disease Causation

Every system of health and disease considers causation, linking events in the social, natural, and supernatural realms with recognized sicknesses. The finding of a cause can guide therapy prospectively, confirm actions retrospectively, and give an explanation for illnesses, thus giving solace and meaning to human suffering.

Delineating etiologies can be a complex process dependent on the interpretation of many factors. Multiple etiologies may surface during a sickness episode, and multiple etiologies, even seemingly contradictory etiologies, may remain after the event. In any given ethnic group there is likely to be overlap amongst four etiologic categories: individual, natural, social, and supernatural.

Application to the case: The Hmong concepts of etiology include all four types, with natural causes being the most common, particularly for everyday nonserious illnesses. Chronic persistent sicknesses, serious illnesses, and problems occurring after social conflicts or around spiritual events may also have social and supernatural etiologies. Supernatural and social etiologies can be discovered with various divination procedures, or during shaman's ceremonies. Multiple etiologies can be speculated upon, can be investigated concurrently, and can coexist to cause a person's problem.

Treatment Options

Multiple treatment options are available throughout the world, including in the United States, where allopathic medicine is well established, alternative and complementary healing methods are growing, and traditional healing approaches of many people from around the globe are available. Kleinman has divided types of healers into three sectors that are overlapping and interconnected rather than mutually exclusive: a popular or lay sector, a folk sector, and a professional sector. These three sectors operate continuously and concurrently. The vast majority of illnesses are treated in the lay sector, as self therapy and home therapy deal with all ailments; often it is only when this sector is unable to respond adequately to a sickness that help is sought from the folk or professional sectors. All three sectors are active in the United States. One national telephone survey estimated that one third of all Americans use some kind of complementary medicine in the lay or folk sector, whether massage, herbs, acupuncture, vitamins, or traditional ethnic medical systems.

Application to the case: In Laos, the Hmong traditional system of healing included well-developed lay and folk sectors. In extended families there were men and women who knew about diseases and treatments, grandparents who knew about maintaining health and preventing disease, and heads of households who had the responsibility to maintain relationships with the spirits. In villages there were experts in diagnosis, herbal remedies, rituals, and shamanic ceremonies. Access to professionals (Chinese, Laotian, or western) was limited due to their physical distance from other peoples. People had contact with biomedical personnel at refugee camps in Thailand.

Interpretation of Bodily Signs & Symptoms

The four preceding discussions have focused on an ethnic group's general understanding of health and disease. The two that follow focus on how individual patients and families in such a group may deal with particular sickness within the context of their cultural beliefs and behaviors.

Initially, individuals sense a symptom or other people perceive a sign. Questions arise. Is this normal or abnormal? If it is abnormal, what does it signify? Is it serious or mild? What has caused it? What should be done about it? The answers to these questions are influenced by people's understandings of their culture's general approach to bodily functions and malfunctions, disease classification, etiology, and seriousness, but also may be influenced by other individual factors. Together the answers constitute what Kleinman has called an "explanatory model."

Kleinman has described individuals' explanatory models of their sickness as having five aspects: the etiology of the condition, timing and mode of onset of symptoms, pathophysiologic processes, natural history and severity of illness, and appropriate treatments. The sick person, family members, social network, and providers have their own explanatory models about the sickness event, and these may be complementary or contradictory. The more agreement there is between the explanatory models, the smoother the interactions among people may be, while the more disagreement between the concepts, the more conflict there may be.

Application to the case: At home, MT had had a severe headache for which her husband gave her Tylenol, a Thai pharmaceutical preparation (probably aspirin or acetaminophen), and a Hmong herbal remedy. As the headache worsened, the husband called her sons. The whole family became alarmed as her gait became unstable. As their actions were not helpful, they sought assistance from the hospital. Her husband and sons believed the physicians' interpretation of bleeding in the brain, but they were concerned about the invasive and potentially harmful nature of the proposed operation. A shaman discovered that one of her souls had left her body and was going to be reincarnated. They knew a shamanic ritual at home was necessary to return her soul to her body. During the ceremony, the shaman discovered a long-standing intrafamilial conflict that had contributed to the soul loss.

Medical Decision Making

Once sick individuals have interpreted their signs or symptoms, they have to decide whom to consult. Given the lay, folk, and professional sectors, how do they select a healer? The decision-making process is complex and includes cultural and social influences.

Cultural beliefs about health, sickness, and etiology influence which healers are deemed appropriate to treat the problem. After the healer has been chosen and the healing method completed, cultural factors continue to influence the healing process as sick individuals and family members evaluate the method's effectiveness, discern the etiologies, learn from the experience, and consider need for further assistance.

Social factors also influence the process, as sick individuals' social networks express their approval or disapproval for certain healers and healing methods. The greater the social dissonance between a healer and patient (resulting from differences in socioeconomic class, language abilities, geographic location, income level, religion, etc), the less likely it is the patient will chose that healer.

Ethnic identity, the extent to which individuals and families identify with a particular ethnic group, also influences their choice of healers. Although ethnic identity may be strong when people initially arrive in another country, that identity changes over time by the process of acculturation. Acculturation is an irregular, dynamic, bidirectional process that results in considerable variation for individuals, families, and communities.

People can utilize multiple healing methods without accepting a given method's theoretical underpinnings or without wholeheartedly choosing the system as their preferred healing system. For instance, Chinese people who believe that health results from a balance of *yin* and *yang* may obtain vaccinations without accepting concepts of immunology or epidemiology and without embracing allopathic medicine. Likewise, mainstream Americans may use acupuncture without embracing the traditional Chinese concepts of *qi* (*chi*), meridians, and balance, and without rejecting allopathic medicine.

Application to the case: The traditional spiritual beliefs were extremely important to the couple and to their sons. They knew that the shaman's ceremony was necessary to retrieve MT's soul and return her to spiritual health, if she were to survive an operation. In the hospital, the family decision-making process included a discussion of the pros and cons, with the younger more acculturated members wanting the surgery and the older sons and her husband choosing the traditional ceremony. In the morning, after the shaman ceremony, the family met again, assessed that her physical condition had not improved but her souls were intact, and decided she could survive an operation.

Healer–Sick Person Relations

Every cultural system has expectations about the healer–sick person-family relationship. The rules of this relationship—the preferred styles of communication, the appropriate approach to relevant topics, and the amount of power that the healer exerts over the patient and family—are culturally influenced. Physicians in the United States learn a preferred manner of physician–patient relationships, which some patients may experience as foreign, rude, mean, or unacceptable (see later discussion).

Cultural values are always present in the clinical encounter. Physicians' biomedical and western values may conflict with values of patients from other cultures. For instance, physicians may believe in their ability to conquer problems and exert control over nature, whereas patients may trust their ability to live in harmony with nature; or physicians may focus on physical and psychological issues whereas patients expect to pursue social and spiritual issues.

There is a power differential between healers and patients that can be both helpful and harmful to patients. Biomedical physicians generally are from middle and upper socioeconomic classes, have high incomes, often are from the dominant social group, and have privileged knowledge. People have long expressed their feelings of powerlessness in relationships with health care providers in biomedical institutions. Add the dimensions of different languages, different expectations of healer–sick person and extended family relations, and verbal and nonverbal language barriers and the situation is ripe for patients from various ethnic groups to feel disempowered in their encounters with biomedical health care providers.

Application to the case: When the family had decided to take MT home, they felt the neurologists' frustration and anger at their decision, which perplexed them. "Why should they be angry with our taking care of our mother? After all, it is up to us, her family, to make the appropriate decisions for her." However, they felt support from the neurosurgeon; his accepting attitude that there was more at stake than the physical body and his respectful attitude towards their beliefs made it easier for them to return for the operation. And they felt the support of the shaman, who after his ceremony said that the woman was spiritually strong enough to survive the operation. Indeed, she survived the operation and went home a week later, with some residual hemiparesis.

Culhane-Pera KA et al: *Healing by Heart: Clinical and Ethical Case Stories of Hmong Families and Western Providers.* Vanderbilt University Press, 2003.

Ember CR, Ember E, eds: *Encyclopedia of Medical Anthropology: Health and Illness in the World's Cultures. Volume 1: Topics. Volume II: Cultures. Human Relations Area File.* Kluwer/Plenum, 2004.

Helman CG: *Culture, Health and Illness: An Introduction for Health Professionals,* 4th ed. Butterworth-Heinemann, 2000.

Kleinman A: *Patients and Healers in the Context of Culture: An Exploration of the Borderland Between Anthropology, Medicine, and Psychiatry.* University of California Press, 1980.

HOW CAN PHYSICIANS PROVIDE CULTURALLY COMPETENT MEDICAL CARE?

Learn about Oneself as a Cultural Being

"Culture" isn't just a factor for "others," "ethnic groups," or "minority peoples"; culture is an important aspect of every human being. Physicians need to know how their personal cultural backgrounds influence their views and values about health, disease, and treatment and their reactions to others, as well as how their biomedical training influences them. Biomedicine is a cultural system influenced by historical, social, economic, political, religious, and scientific events, with its own language and its own values that can clash with providers' personal beliefs and with patients' cultural beliefs and values.

Learn about Patients as Cultural Beings

Physicians need to familiarize themselves with the communities they serve. This includes important historical events, such as migration or refugee movement; social structure and function, such as which family members have more influence in making medical decisions; various religious beliefs and practices, such as a dominant religion or conflicting religious factions; prevailing health beliefs about health, disease, and treatments; use of complementary and alternative healing practices, such as herbalists, masseuses, or spiritual healers; and expectations of life-cycle events, such as birth, child development, puberty, old age, and death.

Kleinman notes that all individuals—patients, family members, and healers—create cognitive explanatory models of an illness event that change over time. The five components of explanatory models are etiology, pathophysiology, symptom, projected course, and expected treatment. Providers need to know prevailing cultural concepts of health, disease, and treatment; prevailing medical decision-making patterns; and prevailing values and ethical frameworks, so they can understand the context of patients' explanatory models.

Learn Culturally Appropriate Communication Skills

For optimal communication, physicians must adapt their standard interviewing techniques to fit patients' communication styles, rather than assuming that one style of communication fits all and rather than expecting patients to adjust to their preferred style. Difficulties delivering health care in multicultural settings may arise from patients' and providers' differences in health beliefs, expectations of life-cycle events, moral values, or ethical principles. Knowing what communication style to use is a challenge. Providers cannot assume that because a patient is from one ethnic group he or she will prefer a specific approach. However, physicians can learn general approaches from community experts, such as bilingual-bicultural colleagues, and be attuned to patients' verbal and nonverbal cues. Physicians also have to be proficient in multiple languages or learn to work with interpreters (Table 60–1).

Table 60–1. Recommendations for working with interpreters.

1. Greet patients in their language.
2. Introduce yourself and everyone present.
3. Arrange seats in a triad and address the patient.
4. Speak clearly in a normal voice.
5. Use common terms and simple language structure.
6. Express one idea at a time, and pause for interpretation.
7. Expect the interpreter to use the first person singular, verbatim translation approach.
8. Consider multiple meanings to nonverbal gestures.
9. Ask the same questions in different ways if you get inconsistent or unconnected responses.
10. Ask the interpreter to explain issues, but do not place the interpreter in the middle of conflicts.

Apply Cultural Information & Skills in Clinical Interactions

Understanding general information about the communities with which they work, physicians are ready to apply that cultural information to specific medical encounters. One multicultural patient-centered approach to the clinical encounter is Berlin and Fowkes's LEARN model.

1. *Listen* to patients' perspectives—The important first step is to listen to patients' and families' stories about their illness experiences. Physicians must ask and display genuine desire to hear patients' perspectives. To elicit their perspective of their illness (or "dis-ease") or their explanatory models, physicians can try Kleinman's questions or modifications thereof (Table 60–2).

2. *Explain* medical views—After they have completed gathering information from the patient's story and physical findings, physicians need to explain their views of the patients' conditions. Physicians can explain the biomedical assessment by building upon patients' ideas, beliefs, and values, and by addressing their fears and concerns.

Table 60–2. Kleinman's questions for exploring explanatory models.

1. What do you call your problem?
2. What do you think has caused your problem?
3. Why do you think it started when it did?
4. What does your sickness do to you?
5. How severe is it? Will it have a long or short course?
6. What do you fear most about your sickness?
7. What chief problems has your sickness caused for you?
8. What kind of treatment do you think you should receive?

Five alternative questions:

1. What do you think is wrong?
2. What are you afraid of?
3. What do you think has caused the problem?
4. What have you tried to relieve the problem?
5. What do you think would help you?

3. *Acknowledge* similarities and differences—Physicians can acknowledge where patients', families', and providers' perspectives about the illness etiology, projected course, or treatment options are similar and different.

4. *Recommend* a course of action—While explaining recommendations for diagnostic or therapeutic plans, physicians must ask permission, explain options, and ask what approaches patients want.

5. *Negotiate* plans—Depending on how much disagreement there is between patients' desires and medical recommendations, physicians may need to negotiate a plan and work with patients' perspectives about their bodies, illnesses, and desired treatments.

Provide Linguistically & Culturally Appropriate Patient Education

Providing patient education for diverse patient populations requires that providers first assess patients' language preferences and literacy skills (both in English and in other languages), and then target education to be compatible with patients' language abilities, literacy levels, and cultural concepts. Multicultural and multilingual resources—from written pamphlets to audiotapes and videotapes, community agencies, internet sites, and bilingual-bicultural patient educators and advocates—are invaluable assets to support patient empowerment.

Deal with Cultural Conflicts

Difficulties delivering health care in multicultural settings may arise from different patient and provider health beliefs, expectations of life-cycle events, moral values, or ethical principles. Cross-cultural ethical conflicts can challenge providers' personal beliefs, personal morals, and professional integrity. When physicians encounter conflicting beliefs and values, it is very tempting to protect and preserve their own models by ignoring, rejecting, or disparaging other viewpoints. The costs of doing so can be the loss of patients to other providers, decreased patient satisfaction, increased nonadherence, worse patient outcomes, as well as diminished provider satisfaction and competence—all of which increase health disparities. Understanding how patients' and providers' different cultural beliefs and values contribute to the situation is a first step in responding to specific patients in clinical encounters. Then solutions can be found, whether by compromising, negotiating alternative approaches, consulting ethics committees or community members, or referring patients to other providers.

Do Not Abuse Power

In the context of multicultural care, physicians have to recognize power differences between patients and providers, be aware of power struggles that can arise, and avoid abuse of power. To these ends, physicians need to know about their personal and professional biases and prejudices, and need to monitor their actions and emotional reactions to patients. Balint groups, physician support groups, ethics committees, and faith communities are ways to examine personal struggles. Physicians can consider "caring-in-relation" and "power-in-relation" as ways to avoid abuse of power.

Create & Work within Culturally Competent Institutions

Physicians need to be active members in clinics, hospitals, and medical societies so as to create culturally competent institutions. Physicians can be powerful advocates for hiring bilingual-bicultural workers, employing trained interpreters, creating health education approaches for patients with limited English proficiency, and engaging institutions in caring for diverse patients. The more systems are constructed to empower patients and avoid prejudices and biases, the more physicians can provide culturally competent care and improve the health of all patients.

Berlin EA, Fowkes WC: A teaching framework for cross-cultural health care. Application in family practice. West J Med 1983;39:934. [PMID: 6666112]

Candib L: *Medicine and the Family: a Feminist Perspective.* Basic Books, 1995.

Institute of Medicine: *Speaking of Health: Assessing Health Communication Strategies for Diverse Populations.* IOM, Committee on Communication for Behavior Change in the 21st Century: Improving the Health of Diverse Populations, 2002.

Kleinman A et al: Culture, illness, and care: Clinical lessons from anthropologic and cross-cultural research. Ann Intern Med 1978;88:251. [PMID: 626456]

Nielsen-Bohlman L et al, eds: *Health Literacy: A Prescription to End Confusion.* Institute of Medicine, Committee on Health Literacy, 2004.

Vawter DE et al: A model for culturally responsive health care. In Culhane-Pera KA et al, eds: *Healing by Heart: Clinical and Ethical Case Stories of Hmong Families and Western Providers.* Vanderbilt University Press, 2003:297.

Web Sites

Asian and Pacific Islander American Health Forum:

http://www.apiahf.org

Asian American Network for Cancer Awareness, Research, and Training:

http://www.aancart.org/

Association for Asian Pacific Community Health Organizations:

http://www.aapcho.org

Bayer Institute for Health Care Communication:

http://www.bayerinstitute.org

Center for Cross-cultural Health:

http://www.crosshealth.com

Country Studies, Library of Congress:

http://lcweb2.loc.gov/frd/cs

Cross Cultural Health Care Program:

http://www.xculture.org

Cultural Profiles, Center for Applied Linguistics:

http://www.culturalorientation.net/fact.html

Ethnomed:

http://www.ethnomed.org

Islamic Health and Human Services:

http://hammoude.com/Ihhs.html

National Health Law Program:

http://www.healthlaw.org

National Hispanic Medical Association:

http://www.nhmamd.org/

Provider's Guide to Quality and Culture:

http://erc.msh.org

Resources for Cross-cultural Health:

http://www.diversityrx.org

US Department of Health and Human Services Culturally and Linguistically Appropriate Services (CLAS) guidelines:

http://www.omhrc.gov/clas/guide2a.asp

Vietnamese Community Health Promotion Project:

http://www.suckhoelavang.org/

World Education; Culture, Health and Literacy:

http://www.worlded.org/us/health/docs/culture/about.html

Health & Health Care Disparities 61

Jeannette E. South-Paul, MD, & Evelyn L. Lewis, MD, MA

BACKGROUND & DEFINITIONS

Ethnic and racial minorities manifest significantly poorer health status than their white counterparts. Factors that can explain these disparities include limited access to health care, poor socioeconomic status, and a variety of environmental influences. Other documented reasons for health disparities include discrimination, overdependence on publicly funded facilities, and logistical barriers to health care such as insufficient transportation, medically underserved geographic areas, and cost of services. Although these disparities have existed for more than two centuries, defining and characterizing disparities in health and health care are necessary beginnings to understanding the problem and seeking effective solutions to the problem of unequal health status.

Health disparities are defined by the National Institutes of Health as "differences in the incidence, prevalence, mortality, and burden of diseases and other adverse health conditions that exist among specific population groups in the United States." Cardiovascular disease, cancer, and diabetes mellitus are the most commonly reported health disparities followed by cerebrovascular diseases, unintentional injuries, and HIV/AIDS. Assessing these differences requires that a variety of factors including age, gender, nationality, family of origin, education, income, geographic location, race or ethnicity, sexual orientation, and disability be considered.

Health care disparities are defined by the Institute of Medicine (IOM) as "differences in the quality of health care that are not due to access-related factors or clinical needs, preferences and appropriateness of intervention." Causes of health care disparities most often relate to quality and include provider–patient relationships, provider bias and discrimination, and patient variables such as mistrust of the health care system and refusal of treatment. Although disparities in health and health care can be inextricably tied to one another, distinguishing between them increases our understanding of the complexity of the problem.

Concerns regarding health and health care disparities are amplified when the dramatic changes in the population served during the last two decades of the 20th century are considered. Between 1980 and 2000 the white non-Hispanic population of the United States increased 7.9% compared with an 88% increase in the aggregated minority (people of races other than white or of Hispanic ethnicity) population. An estimated 1 in 4 Americans (almost 70 million persons) is classified as a member of one of the four major racial or ethnic minority groups: African American, Latino/Hispanic, Native American, and Asian/Pacific Islander. By the year 2050, the US census estimates that people of color will represent 1 in 3 Americans. These populations bear a disproportionate burden of illness and disease relative to their percentage distribution in the population. Understanding the factors that contribute to inequities in health among these populations and the strategies that have resulted in improved health can inform and promote the delivery of quality health care.

Marmot M: Inequalities in health. N Engl J Med 2001;345:134 [PMID: 11450663]

Smedley BD et al: *Unequal Treatment: Confronting Racial and Ethnic Disparities in Health Care.* Institute of Medicine, Committee on Understanding and Eliminating Racial and Ethnic Disparities in Health Care, 2002.

US Department of Health and Human Services: Healthy People 2010: National Health Promotion and Disease Prevention Objectives; conference ed in 2 vols. DHHS, 2000.

Wong MD et al: Contribution of major diseases to disparities in mortality. N Engl J Med 2002;347:1585. [PMID: 12432046]

HEALTH CARE DISPARITIES & THE LITERATURE

Institute of Medicine (IOM) Reports

In 1999, a report from the IOM entitled *Unequal Treatment: Confronting Racial and Ethnic Disparities in Health Care* was written in response to a request from Congress to the IOM to address the extent of racial and ethnic disparities in health care. Following review of more than 100 publications, the IOM study committee concluded that research findings consistently indicated that minorities were less likely than whites to receive needed services, including lifesaving procedures. The most commonly reported health care disparities were seen in cardiovascular disease, cancer, and diabetes. Other illnesses included cerebrovascular diseases, mental illness, and HIV/AIDS.

The IOM committee outlined three sets of factors that likely contributed to the complex problem of health care disparities. The first set of factors relates to minority patients' attitudes toward health care, preferences for treatment and subtle differences in the ways that racial and ethnic groups respond to treatment, particularly pharmaceutical interventions. The second group relates to the operation of health care systems and the legal and regulatory environment in which they function. These factors include lack of translation services for those with limited English proficiency, lack of resources for those with limited health literacy, where care is received, and how it is delivered. The third set of factors is derived from the clinical encounter. The committee's review suggested that provider bias, clinical uncertainty, and stereotyping or beliefs about the behavior of minorities may have a negative impact on the health outcomes of minorities. On the other side of the clinical encounter is the patient; his or her reaction to the provider's biased or stereotyped behaviors may also contribute to disparities.

National Healthcare Disparities Report

With a directive from the Healthcare Research and Quality Act of 1999 (Public Law 106-129) and guidance from the IOM, the Agency for Healthcare Research and Quality (AHRQ) developed and produced two reports. The first of these, the *National Healthcare Disparities Report* (NHDR), was the first national comprehensive effort to measure differences in access and use of health care services by various populations. It incorporated a broad set of performance measures through which the data on differences in the use of services, access to health care, differences in use of services by priority populations, and impressions of quality for seven clinical conditions could be viewed and assessed. The second report, the *National Healthcare Quality Report* (NHQR), focused on safety, effectiveness, patient centeredness, and timeliness, with equity as a cross-cutting dimension. The two reports were released simultaneously in 2003 to provide a more comprehensive view of the performance of the health care system, its strengths, and areas that should serve as a focal point for future improvement. The performance measures underlying the two reports will be used to monitor the nation's progress toward improved health care delivery.

The NHQR sought to analyze national disparities as both a function of health care access and quality. This includes an analysis of disparities related to socioeconomic position as well as to race and ethnicity, and attempts to capture the relationship between race/ethnicity and socioeconomic position. The NHQR's key findings were that inequality in quality persists, disparities come at a personal and societal price, differential access may lead to disparities in quality, opportunities to provide preventive care are frequently missed, knowledge of why disparities exist is limited, improvement is possible, and data limitations hinder targeted improvement efforts to provide the level of baseline data that may be used to measure the effect of national initiatives to reduce disparities.

In 2005, a third NHQR was released. It highlights four key themes: disparities are pervasive and still exist, some disparities are diminishing, opportunities for improvement remain, and information about disparities is improving. New databases and measures have been added to provide a more comprehensive assessment of disparities and new methods developed for tracking changes in disparities in a standardized fashion. This allows for the identification of specific disparities that are improving and disparities that are worsening.

Web Site

Agency for Healthcare Research and Quality, 2005 National Healthcare Disparities Report:

http://www.qualitytoolsahrq.gov/qualityreport/2005/browse/browse.aspx.

Healthy People 2010

Healthy People 2010 was launched in January of 2000. The program is a set of comprehensive health objectives for the nation that can be used by many different people, states, communities, professional organizations, and others to help them develop programs to improve health. The Healthy People 2010 objectives build on the 1979 Surgeon General's report, *Healthy People,* and the Healthy People 2000: National Health Promotion and Disease Prevention Objectives, which established national health objectives and served as the basis for the development of state and community plans. All three initiatives were developed through broad consultation, backed by the best scientific knowledge available, and were designed to measure programs over time.

The two overarching goals of Healthy People 2010—to increase quality and years of healthy life and eliminate health disparities—served as a guide for developing the 467 objectives, designed to serve as a roadmap to measure progress. The achievement of these national objectives is dependent in part on the ability of health agencies at all levels of government and on nongovernmental organizations to assess objective progress.

Web Sites

More information about Healthy People 2010 is available from:

http://www.healthypeople.gov and http://www.cdc.gov/nchs/about/otheract/hpdata2010/abouthp.htm.

HISTORICAL FACTORS

Original American citizens of color bear a historical legacy that affects all aspects of their integration into society today. American Indians make up a fraction of today's citizens (0.7% in the 2000 census) but have significant health disparities. The prevalence of diabetes mellitus, obesity, alcoholism, and suicide is substantially greater in this population than in other US population groups. They are the one population with a health system that was established to help meet their medical needs. The availability of these services, however, is limited by distance for the many American Indians living in rural areas, and they may be completely inaccessible to those living in urban areas.

African Americans encompass several groups who came to the United States at different times. The impact of slavery on the original Africans cannot be minimized. Residual effects of this historical tragedy have been associated with discriminatory residential practices, educational disadvantage, and treatment practices in separate but unequal health care facilities. Later immigrants of African origin came to the United States from the West Indies. These islands also received many slaves during the early to mid 19th century but abolished slavery before the Emancipation Proclamation did so in the United States in 1865. These differing experiences have influenced the views of Caribbean Americans and result in differences between them and African Americans who descended directly from slaves on the North American continent. The final group of immigrants from African countries chose to come to the United States in recent years for educational, economic, and political reasons. Cultural differences often exist among these three groups and include differences in customs, family roles, religious preferences, and their definition and experience of illness and disease.

Despite the fact that the foundation of the United States was a union of indigenous groups and immigrants, the preceding groups along with new immigrants bear much of the burden of disease in the nation today. The number of immigrants entering the United States during the past 15 years has increased dramatically compared with the numbers seen in the previous four decades. Political crises, natural disasters, poverty, and hunger have forced population groups of significant size to leave their homes. These migrations have resulted in loss of homes and support systems, overcrowding and overexposure, decreased access to food and medical services, and contact with new infectious agents and other toxins.

Lillie-Blanton M, Laveist T: Race/ethnicity, the social environment, and health. Soc Sci Med 1996;43:83. [PPMID: 8816013]

IMMIGRANTS & REFUGEES

The term *immigrant* has been applied to legal and illegal (undocumented) refugees and children adopted from other countries. Most immigrants reside in linguistically isolated households (those in which no one over the age of 14 speaks English), which were identified for the first time in the 1990 census). Four percent of US households are in this category. This figure includes 30% of Asian households, 23% of Hispanic households, and 28% of all immigrant households with school-age children.

Fewer health care and preventive services are available for a population whose first language is not English. Furthermore, significant migrations and population shifts have severely taxed the municipal, educational, and health care resources of many American communities, especially those in the most affected states: California, Texas, and Florida.

Immigrants enter the United States from many countries, but those coming from Mexico represent the largest group. Many Mexican immigrants arrive in the United States healthier than their white counterparts. However, their health deteriorates the longer they live here, possibly as a result of life-style changes (years of difficult labor, poverty, smoking, poor diet, and lack of attention to prevention) and a lack of health insurance. One study found that 2.6% of recent Mexican immigrants had diabetes mellitus, compared with 7.7% of Mexican immigrants who had lived in the United States for 15 years. More than two thirds of recent Mexican immigrants and 44.8% of "long-term immigrants" have no health insurance, compared with 22.5% of Mexican-born Americans and 12.3% of US-born whites. Fewer than 10% of recent Mexican immigrants reported using emergency departments in 2000. Furthermore, more than 33% of Mexican women aged 18–64 years who were recent immigrants had not had a Pap smear in 3 years. About 37% of recent Mexican immigrants visited a health clinic instead of a physician for health care, compared with about 15% of US-born whites.

Some immigrants, especially those from non-European countries, have a longer life expectancy and more years of life free of disability and dependency than do native-born citizens. This longevity is likely related to the "healthy immigrant effect" (ie, that those who migrate abroad represent a healthier and more motivated segment of the population of origin). However, life-style in the country of origin may continue to influence immigrant health in negative ways. Life expectancy and infant mortality rates among new refugees from the former Soviet Union compare poorly with those of the general population in the United States. In spite of reported universal health care coverage in the Soviet bloc, there were wide variations between communities, access to care was dependent on Communist party membership, and there was little emphasis on promoting a healthy life-style. Heavy cigarette use, high alcohol intake, poor dietary intake, little attention to physical fitness, and crowded living conditions contributed to poor health in this population.

Pregnant women are of major concern because of risk for poor pregnancy outcomes. In spite of these concerns, evidence suggests that infants of Mexican immigrants have favorable birth outcomes despite their high socioeconomic risks. These favorable outcomes have been associated with a protective sociocultural orientation among this immigrant group, including a strong family unit. Yet, one fourth of infants of immigrants in predominantly Spanish-speaking households are at high risk for serious infectious disease despite using preventive care. As these children mature beyond the neonatal period, factors predisposing to illness are large households, poor access to care, and maternal characteristics, including smoking, pregnancy complications, and employment.

Lack of understanding by health care providers of traditional remedies for common ailments can result in negative interactions between patients and clinicians and in misdiagnosis, both of which hinder health care utilization. The special problems of unemployment, depression, surviving torture, and obtaining assistance are all made more difficult for refugees living in small communities that lack sufficiently large ethnic populations to facilitate culturally sensitive provision of health care.

Refugees tend to settle in communities where fellow immigrants already live. In recent years East African refugees have gravitated toward the north central United States, specifically Minnesota; Afghan refugees have settled in the San Francisco Bay Area; and citizens of the former Yugoslavia have migrated to specific areas of the United Kingdom and the United States, to name just a few examples.

With the exception of Southeast Asian refugees, there are few clinical studies on the health problems of refugees after arrival in the United States. Tuberculosis, nutritional deficiencies, intestinal parasites, chronic hepatitis B infection, lack of immunization, and depression are major problems in many groups. The great variation in health and psychosocial issues, as well as cultural beliefs, among refugees requires careful attention during the medical encounter. In addition to a complete history and physical examination, tests for tuberculosis, hepatitis B surface antigen, ova and parasites, as well as hemoglobin measurement, are advised for most groups.

Health care for children of immigrant families. American Academy of Pediatrics. Committee on Community Health Services. Pediatrics 1997;100:153. [PMID: 9229707]

Hjern A et al: Political violence, family stress and mental health of refugee children in exile. Scand J Soc Med 1998;26:18. [PMID: 9526760]

Mollica RF et al: Effects of war trauma on Cambodian refugee adolescents' functional health and mental health status. J Am Acad Child Adolesc Psychiatry 1997;36:1098. [PMID: 9256589]

Pernice R, Brook J: Refugees' and immigrants' mental health: Association of demographic and post-immigration factors. J Soc Psychol 1996;136:511. [PMID: 8855381]

Wallace S, Zuniga E: Mexican immigrants' health status worsens after living in US. October 14, 2005. Available at: http://www.kaisernetwork.org/daily_reports/re-index.

POVERTY

A greater percentage of African Americans and Latinos are below 200% of the federal poverty line than are non-Hispanic white Americans across the lifespan (53%, 59%, and 25%, respectively). Financial disadvantage has an impact on health in that mortality rates around the world decline with increasing social class, a concept most easily associated with access to financial resources.

Poor, minority, and uninsured children are twice as likely as other children to lack usual sources of care, nearly twice as likely to wait 60 minutes or more at their sites of care, and use only about half as many physician services after adjusting for health status. Poverty, minority status, and absence of insurance exert independent effects on access to and use of primary care. Homelessness results in poor health status and high service use among children. Homeless children were reported to experience a higher number of acute illness symptoms, including fever, ear infection, diarrhea, and asthma. Emergency department and outpatient medical visits are also higher among the homeless group.

Newacheck PW et al: Children's access to primary care: Differences by race, income, and insurance status. Pediatrics 1996;97:26. [PMID: 8545220]

Nickens HW: The role of race/ethnicity and social class in minority health status. Health Serv Res 1995;30(Pt 2):151. [PMID: 7721589]

Weinreb L et al: Determinants of health and service use patterns in homeless and low-income housed children. Pediatrics 1998; 102:554. [PMID: 9738176]

UNINSURANCE & UNDERINSURANCE

A substantial portion of the US population is medically uninsured or underinsured. A greater percentage of racial and ethnic minorities and immigrants are in this category. These numbers increase if individuals who have been without health insurance for 3 or more months in a given year are included. Underinsurance is the inability to pay out-of-pocket expenses despite having insurance and usually implies inability to use preventive services as well. The underinsured category includes unemployed persons aged 55–64 years and those not provided health insurance coverage through their jobs. These individuals are not eligible for Medicare and must pay high individual health premiums when they can obtain some form of group coverage. Lack of health insurance is associated with delayed health care and increased mortality. Underinsurance also may result in adverse health consequences. An estimated eight million children from diverse groups in the United States are uninsured. Substantial differences in both sources of care and utilization of medical services exist between insured and uninsured children.

In 2003, 35% of all nonelderly adult Hispanics living in the United States lacked health insurance coverage (either private or public), compared with 20% of African-American, 19% of Asian or Pacific Islander, 27% of American Indian, and 12% of non-Hispanic white nonelderly citizens. Because Hispanics are more likely to be uninsured than any other ethnic group and because they are the fastest growing minority group in the United States, it is likely that the number of uninsured in the US population will steadily increase.

Persons with Medicare and Medicaid have twice the mortality of those with employer-provided insurance, and the working uninsured show greater mortality than the working insured. The higher mortality in those with public insurance (Medicaid) or with no insurance probably reflects a combined effect of existing health status; exposure to illness, trauma, and disease; and access to medical care. Although the general health and mental health of the uninsured are slightly worse in comparison with the privately insured, the uninsured have fewer chronic health problems. (This may reflect the fact that the majority of the uninsured are working poor. If they become so sick that they are unable to work, these individuals often qualify for disability or medical assistance and no longer fall into the category of "uninsured.")

There are marked discrepancies in access to and utilization of medical services, including preventive services, between uninsured and insured children, although both groups have similar rates of chronic health conditions and limitations of activity (evidence of the general health of the children being seen). The 2002 IOM report, *Unequal Treatment,* documented the widespread evidence of racial and ethnic disparities in health care. Only 5 of the 103 published studies cited in this report addressed health disparities in children, yet disparities of equivalent magnitude and persistence to those seen in adults appear to exist in children. Substantial gaps in insurance coverage exist such that 37% of Hispanic, 23% of African-American, and 20% of non-Hispanic white children have no health insurance. When they have health insurance, children of color are more likely to be insured through public programs such as Medicaid and the State Children's Health Insurance Program (SCHIP) than to have private insurance.

Children who are eligible for Medicaid but remain unenrolled are often younger than 6 years of age, live in female-headed single-parent families, or are African American or Hispanic. Not only do uninsured children lack routine medical care and sick care, they also lack appropriate well-child care compared with insured children. Children who have a chronic disease, such as asthma, face difficulties of access to care and utilize substantially fewer outpatient and inpatient services.

Parents' utilization of health care services has a large impact on the service use of their children. Even if all children were universally insured, parental health care access and utilization would remain a key determinant in children's use of services. Neglecting financial access to care for adults who serve as caregivers for children may have the unintended effect of diminishing the impact of targeted health insurance programs for children.

The uninsured can manifest similar psychopathology as is seen in refugees. Rates of current psychiatric disorders (including major depression, anxiety disorders, and history of sexual trauma) are extremely high in ethnically diverse women who are receiving public medical assistance or are uninsured. These women also report behaviors that pose serious health risks, including smoking (23%) and illicit drug use (2%). Fewer than half have access to comprehensive primary medical care. Young, poor women who seek care in public-sector clinics would benefit from comprehensive medical care addressing their psychosocial needs.

In the United States, the cost of health care services is a major barrier to health care access. In addition, three fourths of persons in the United States who have difficulty paying their medical bills have some type of health insurance. Although the affordability of health care among persons without health insurance has been described, few details regarding affordability among persons who are underinsured exist.

Investigators who looked at state programs offering subsidized coverage in commercial managed care organizations to low-income and previously uninsured people found no evidence of pent-up demand or an unusual level of chronic illness between people enrolled through large employer-benefit plans and previously uninsured patients. Similarly, there was little evidence of underutilization, although dissatisfaction and reported barriers to service were more frequent among nonwhite enrollees. In another study, undocumented immigrants had more complicated and serious diagnoses on admission but a lower adjusted average length of stay than native-born populations and those with permanent residency status (insured by Medicaid or of uninsured status) admitted to the same hospital.

Although generalist physicians appear to be more likely than specialists to provide care for poor adult patients, they may still perceive financial and nonfinancial barriers to caring for these patients. Nonwhite physicians were more likely to care for uninsured and Medicaid patients than were white physicians. In addition to reimbursement, nonfinancial factors played an important role in physicians' decisions not to care for Medicaid or uninsured patients. For example, perceived risks of litigation and poor reimbursement were cited by 60–90% of physicians as important in the decision not to care for Medicaid and uninsured patients.

Beal AC: Policies to reduce racial and ethnic disparities in child health and health care. Health Aff (Millwood) 2004;23:171. [PMID: 15371383]

Hanson KL: Is insurance for children enough? The link between parents' and children's health care use revisited. Inquiry 1998;35:294. [PMID: 9809057]

Kilbreth EH et al: State-sponsored programs for the uninsured: Is there adverse selection? Inquiry 1998;35:250. [PMID: 9809054]

Thamer M et al: Health insurance coverage among foreign-born US residents: The impact of race, ethnicity, and length of residence. Am J Publ Health 1997;87:96. [PMID: 9065235]

HOUSING & GEOGRAPHIC FACTORS

Racial residential segregation has been suggested as a fundamental cause of racial disparities in health. Although legislation exists to eliminate discrimination in housing, the degree of residential segregation remains extremely high for most African Americans in the United States. Williams and Collins argue that segregation is a primary cause of racial differences in socioeconomic status by determining access to education and employment opportunities. Furthermore, segregation creates conditions that hamper a healthy social and physical environment. Levels of racial residential segregation grew dramatically from 1860 to 1940 and have been maintained since then.

Recent research has linked racial segregation to higher cancer risk; the risk increases as the degree of segregation increases. Minorities living in highly segregated metropolitan areas are more than 2.5 times more likely to develop cancer from air pollutants when compared with whites. Hispanics who live in highly segregated areas are affected the most, with a risk 6.4 times that of whites. When neighborhood poverty indicators and population density are controlled, the disparities in cancer risk persist, although at lower levels.

A study by Skinner and colleagues noted the contribution of community of residence to health disparities. The investigators suggested that black patients are concentrated in a small number of poorly performing hospitals. In this study, nearly 70% of black patients with myocardial infarctions were treated at only about 20% of regional medical centers. When more than one million Medicare recipients from 1997 to 2001 were examined, death rates for patients presenting with acute myocardial infarction were 19% higher at these hospitals than at facilities that saw only white patients. Because the factors contributing to health disparities are so complex, there is no one solution. However, these findings suggest that spending must be increased and quality improved at medical centers that primarily treat minorities and the poor.

Young to middle-aged residents of impoverished urban areas manifest excess mortality from several causes, both acute and chronic. African-American youth in some urban areas face lower probabilities of surviving to 45 years of age than white youths nationwide face of surviving to 65 years. Minorities comprise 80% of residents of high-poverty, urban areas in the United States and more than 90% in the largest metropolitan areas. The lower the socioeconomic position held, the less ability the person has to gain access to information, services, or technologies that could provide protection from or modify risks.

For most Americans, housing equity is a major source of wealth. Residential segregation in such a fashion, therefore, directly influences socioeconomic status. Income predicts variation in health for both white and African Americans, but African Americans report poorer health than whites at all levels of income. People residing in disadvantaged neighborhoods have a higher incidence of heart disease than people who live in more advantaged neighborhoods. The quality of housing is also likely to be worse in highly segregated areas, and poor housing conditions adversely affect health. For example, research reveals that a lack of residential facilities and concerns about personal safety can discourage leisure-time physical exercise.

Geronimus A: To mitigate, resist, or undo: Addressing structural influences on the health of urban populations. Am J Public Health 2000;90:867. [PMID: 10846503]

Link BG et al: Social epidemiology and the fundamental cause concept: On the structuring of effective cancer screens by socioeconomic status. Milbank Q 1998;76:375. [PMID: 9738168]

Morello-Frosch R, Jesdale BM: Separate and unequal: Residential segregation and estimated cancer risks associated with ambient air toxics in U.S. metropolitan areas. Environ Health Perspect 2006;114:386. [PMID: 16507462]

Skinner J et al: Mortality after acute myocardial infarction in hospitals that disproportionately treat Black patients. Circulation 2005;112:2634. [PMID: 16246963]

Williams DR, Collins C: Racial residential segregation: A fundamental cause of racial disparities in health. Public Health Rep 2001;116:404. [PMID: 12042604]

MENTAL HEALTH ISSUES

Disparities in mental health services have been known to exist among diverse communities for decades. Among these disparities are a high rate of misdiagnosis, lack of linguistically competent therapists, culturally insensitive diagnostic measures, and increased exposure to abuse.

The practice of psychiatry is heavily influenced by culture. The cultural identity of patients as well as providers, their perceptions of mental illness and appropriate treatment, their background, and their current environment potentially all have an impact on the psychiatric diagnosis made, the therapy selected, and the therapeutic outcome. Mental illness has been diagnosed more frequently in African Americans and Hispanics than in non-Hispanic white Americans for more than 100 years. Many of the studies reporting these data have been criticized for faulty methodology, cultural bias, and suspect racial theories.

There is some evidence that appropriate research and mental health care delivery for these populations are influenced by factors such as poor cultural validation of the *Diagnostic and Statistical Manual of Mental Disorders*, misdiagnosis of minority patients, and the unwillingness of many psychiatrists to acknowledge culturally defined syndromes and folk-healing systems.

General mental health screening is difficult in part because assessment of psychological health in non–English-speaking populations is impeded by lack of instruments that are language and population specific. Patients whose first language is not English most often undergo psychiatric evaluation and treatment in English. Cultural nuances are encoded in language in ways that are often not readily conveyed in translation, even when equivalent words in the second language are used. An appropriately trained interpreter will routinely identify these nuances for the monolingual clinician. When such an interpreter is not available, these nuances can be clarified through consultation with a clinician who shares the patient's first language and culture to maximize delivery of quality health care.

Kirmayer LJ, Groleau D: Affective disorders in cultural context. Psychiatr Clin North Am 2001;24:465. [PMID: 11593857]

DISCRIMINATION

In addition to cost, there are significant differences in how physicians make therapeutic decisions with respect to the minority status of the patient. Women, ethnic minorities, and uninsured persons receive fewer procedures than do affluent white male patients. Furthermore, the race and sex of a patient independently influence how physicians manage acute conditions such as chest pain. For example, women and minorities are less likely to be diagnosed with angina when presenting with comparable risk factors and the same symptoms as white men.

Illegal immigrants underutilize health services, especially preventive services such as prenatal care, dental care, and immunizations due to cost, language, cultural barriers, and fear of apprehension by immigration authorities. Further complicating efforts to provide access to health care for this group is fear for the well-being of family members who may be undocumented, even when the patient is here legally. The increasing number of immigrants entering the United States in recent years has resulted in more legislation seeking to restrict access of various refugee and immigrant groups to public services. Legislation such as Proposition 187, passed in California in 1994, prohibits people lacking legal residency status from obtaining all but emergency medical care at any health care facility receiving public funds.

This legislation has encouraged further obstacles to health care access for countless other people residing in the United States. For example, minorities who were born in the United States find that they are pressured to produce immigration documentation to receive care. Family physicians seeking to care for immigrants and refugees must recognize and effectively deal with problems in communication, establish trust regarding immigration concerns, understand cultural mores influencing the encounter, find the resources to provide necessary services, make an accurate diagnosis, and negotiate a treatment. Unfortunately, fear of these restrictive immigration laws and socioeconomic hardships combine to delay both seeking and obtaining curative care for these populations.

Title VI of the federal Civil Rights Act states that "no person in the United States shall, on the ground of race, color, or national origin, be excluded from participation in, be denied the benefits of, or be subjected to discrimination under any program or activity receiving Federal financial assistance." Current federal mandates assuring access to emergency medical services and new restrictions on financing of health care for immigrants under federal programs such as Medicaid and Medicare appear to be in direct conflict. The Personal Responsibility and Work Opportunity Reconciliation Act and the Illegal Immigration Reform and Immigrant Responsibility Act specifically reaffirm federal law on delivery of emergency services without addressing the financing of that care. Unfunded mandates in an era of diminished ability to shift costs onto insured patients create a major dilemma for the institutions that provide uncompensated care. Medicaid is considered one form of insurance, although the level of reimbursement of providers has been so low that many providers will not treat patients with that coverage.

Leape LL et al: Underuse of cardiac procedures: Do women, ethnic minorities, and the uninsured fail to receive needed revascularization? Ann Intern Med 1999;130:183. [PMID: 10049196]

Schulman KA et al: The effect of race and sex on physicians' recommendations for cardiac catheterization. N Engl J Med 1999;340:618. [PMID: 10029647]

Williams DR: Race, socioeconomic status, and health. The added effects of racism and discrimination. Ann N Y Acad Sci 1999; 896:173. [PMID: 10681897]

LANGUAGE & LANGUAGE LITERACY

The physician–patient relationship is grounded in communication and the effective use of language. One of the first principles taught in medical school is the importance of the patient's history. Along with clinical reasoning, observations, and nonverbal cues, skillful use of language establishes the clinical interview as the clinician's most powerful tool.

The 2000 census found that more than 46 million Americans speak a language different than that of their clinician. In the United States, the primary "other language" is Spanish. Approximately 25% of Hispanics were born outside of the United States and Puerto Rico, but more than 77% of them note speaking Spanish as their primary language at home. Contributing to the discrepancy, the demographic profiles of the nation's health care providers does not mirror population trends. In California, although 32% of the population is Latino, only 4% of nurses, 4% of physicians, and 6% of dentists are Latino.

Cultural competence is not necessarily associated with language fluency. The effectiveness of communication between a clinician and patient is influenced by the cultural exposure that fosters command of the meaning of the words and phrases. A patient and clinician who do not share a common language face more challenges to quality care than those who share this foundation of communication. Such language differences can have a negative impact on the clinical encounter. Parents, providers, hospital staff, and quality improvement professionals agree that language and cultural differences lead to communication issues that can have a pervasive, negative impact on the quality and safety of care children receive. Disagreement remains, however, regarding changes that are needed to improve health care delivery in the language-discordant environment.

Linguistic competence refers to the capacity of an organization and its personnel to communicate effectively and convey information in a manner that is easily understood by diverse audiences, including persons of limited English proficiency, those who have low literacy skills or are not literate, and individuals with disabilities. Linguistic competency requires organizational and provider capacity to respond effectively to the health literacy needs of populations served. The organization must have policy, structures, practices, procedures, and dedicated resources to support this capacity (Table 61–1). Federal standards have been established for clinical practice when language discordance is present. To maintain quality of care and adhere to the federal guidelines for culturally and linguistically appropriate services (CLAS), clinicians must provide accommodation for patients in their chosen language.

Table 61–1. Linguistic resources for health care.

Bilingual-bicultural staff
Cultural brokers
Foreign language interpretation services, including distance technologies
Sign language interpretation services
TTY (teletypewriter) services
Assistive technology devices
Computer-assisted real-time translation (CART) or viable real-time transcription
Print materials in easy-to-read, low-literacy, picture and symbol formats
Materials in alternative formats (audiotape, Braille, enlarged print)
Translation services
Ethnic media in languages other than English (eg, radio, television, Internet, newspapers, periodicals)

Courtesy of Goode TD, Jones W: National Center for Cultural Competence, Georgetown University Center for Child & Human Development, modified 2004. http://gucchd.georgetown.edu/nccc.

Bethell C et al. Quality and safety of hospital care for children from Spanish-speaking families with limited English proficiency. J Healthcare Quality 2006;28(3):W3-2.

Duran DG, Pacheco G, eds: *Quality Health Services for Hispanics: The Cultural Competency Component.* DHHS Publication No. 99-21. National Alliance for Hispanic Health, 2000.

Morales LS et al: The impact of interpreters on parents' experiences with ambulatory care for their children. Med Care Res Rev 2006;63:110. [PMID: 16686075]

Woloshin S et al. Language barriers in medicine in the United States. JAMA 1995;273:724. [PMID: 7853631]

Web Site

National Standards for Culturally and Linguistically Appropriate Services (CLAS) in Health Care, Office of Minority Health Resource Center:

http://www.omhrc.gov/CLAS

HEALTH CARE FOR THE DISABLED

Americans with disabilities are more than twice as likely to postpone needed health care because they cannot afford it. In addition, the National Organization on Disability has determined that people with disabilities are four times more likely to have special needs that are not covered by health insurance. Many nonelderly adults (46%) with disabilities note that they go without equipment and other items due to cost. More than a third postpone care because of cost, skip doses or split pills due to medication costs, and spend less on basics such as food, heat, and other services in order to pay for health care. Those with Medicare alone (no supplemental coverage) report the highest rates of serious cost-related problems due to gaps in Medicare's benefit package. Those receiving Medicaid fare better due to the broad scope of benefits and relatively low cost-sharing requirements of Medicaid. However, more than 20% of adults with disabilities on Medicaid reported that physicians would not accept their insurance—more than twice the percentage of patients having private insurance or Medicare.

Current data suggest that health disparities between people with and without disabilities are as pervasive as those recognized between ethnic minority groups. People with disabilities were included in the Healthy People plan to provide a broad look at the health of this population. Of the 467 objectives listed in Healthy People 2010, 207 subobjectives address people with disabilities. Some of the subobjectives focus on areas outside of the usual scope of health care or health care services, such as education, employment, transportation, and housing—all of which have a direct impact on wellness and quality of life.

In addition to examining the health of all citizens with disabilities, particular focus is directed to evaluating the health status of women with disabilities. Regardless of age, women with functional limitations were consistently less likely to have received a Pap test during the past 3 years than women without functional limitations.

The National Survey of SSI Children and Families (July 2001 to June 2002) examined children with disabilities who were receiving SSI and their families. Children receiving SSI are more likely to live in a family headed by a single mother, and approximately 50% live in a household with at least one other individual reported to have had a disability. SSI support was the most important source of family income, accounting for nearly half of the income for the children's families, and earnings accounting for almost 40%.

Although the Americans With Disabilities Act was enacted 15 years ago in an effort to improve access of people with disabilities to a broad range of services, women with physical disabilities continue to receive less preventive health screening than women without disabilities and less than is recommended. Significant disparities exist in medical care utilization for breast and cervical cancer screening as well as for oral health care. Furthermore, women with more severe disabilities undergo less screening than those with mild or moderate disability.

Adults with developmental disabilities are more likely to lead sedentary lifestyles and seven times as likely to report inadequate emotional support, compared with nondisabled adults. Adults with both physical and developmental disabilities were significantly more likely to report being in fair or poor health than adults without disabilities. Similar rates of tobacco use and overweight or obesity were reported. Adults with developmental disabilities had a similar or greater risk of having four of five chronic health conditions compared with nondisabled adults. Women with disabilities had 40% greater odds of violence in the 5 years preceding the interview, and these women appeared to be at particular risk for severe violence.

US Surgeon General Richard H. Carmona, MD, MPH, released "The Surgeon General's Call to Action to Improve the Health and Wellness of Persons with Disabilities" on the 15th anniversary of the Americans with Disabilities Act in July 2005. The four goals of the Call to Action are to:

1. Increase understanding nationwide that people with disabilities can lead long, healthy, and productive lives.
2. Increase knowledge among health care professionals and provide then with tools to screen, diagnose, and treat the whole person with a disability with dignity.
3. Increase awareness among people with disabilities of the steps they can take to develop and maintain a healthy life-style.
4. Increase accessible health care and support services to promote independence for people with disabilities.

FUTURE DIRECTIONS & CURRENT CHALLENGES

Multiple factors contribute to the persistence of health and health care disparities in the United States today. These factors originate in the patients, in the clinicians providing care, and in the systems in which they must interact. Equitable, quality health care for all is achievable in an environment that values cultural competence. Cultural competence is necessary in multiple domains: values and attitudes; communication styles; community and consumer participation; physical environment, materials, and resources; policies and procedures; population-based clinical practice; and training and professional development. Only by assuming responsibility and accountability for this global problem at all levels of the health care system will there be any hope of narrowing the gap and ensuring health for all.

Brownridge DA: Partner violence against women with disabilities: prevalence, risk, and explanations. Violence Against Women 2006;12:805. [PMID: 16905674]

Havercamp SM et al: Health disparities among adults with developmental disabilities, adults with other disabilities, and adults not reporting disability in North Carolina. Public Health Rep 2004;119:418. [PMID: 15219799]

Smeltzer SC: Preventive health screening for breast and cervical cancer and osteoporosis in women with physical disabilities. Fam Community Health 2006;29:35S. [PMID: 16344635]

Stephens DL et al: A longitudinal study of employment and skill acquisition among individuals with developmental disabilities. Res Dev Disabil 2005;26:469. [PMID: 16168884]

Caring for Gay, Lesbian, Bisexual, & Transgender Patients

62

Peter J Katsufrakis, MD, MBA

BACKGROUND

Who Is Gay? What Is "Bisexual"?

The complexity of human sexual behavior defies simple categorization. Sexual orientation manifests as fantasies, desires, actual behavior, and self- or other-identified labels. For example, a man could think of himself and describe himself as heterosexual, engage in sex with men and women in equal numbers, and in his sexual fantasies focus almost exclusively on male images; a simple label fails to capture the reality of his sexuality. Even when considering only sexual behaviors, differences may exist between actual versus desired, past versus present, admitted versus practiced, and consensual versus forced.

In the medical setting, asking about a patient's label (eg, "Are you gay or bisexual?") importantly assesses her or his self perception, but may fail to identify medically significant information. Many individuals who engage in same-gender high-risk sexual behaviors do not self-identify as gay or bisexual. Men who have sex with men (MSM) may be at increased risk for sexually transmitted diseases (STDs) compared with men who have sex with women only. Women who have sex with men and women (WSMW) may have an increased risk for STDs and substance abuse compared with either women who have sex with women (WSW) or women who have sex with men only. Differentiation would not be possible by asking a patient only if she identifies herself as lesbian, as both WSMW and WSW may identify themselves as lesbian.

Little specific literature exists describing the characteristics of bisexual men and women separate from either strictly heterosexual or homosexual persons. Research studies that include bisexual-identified individuals typically group them with homosexual patients during statistical analysis, limiting information about bisexuality as distinct from heterosexuality or homosexuality.

Historically, research focusing on gay, lesbian, bisexual, and transgender (GLBT) patients frequently suffers from definitional differences that limit cross-study comparisons, small sample size, population sampling bias, and other shortcomings. Changing societal attitudes, improved research methodology, and increased resources are improving our knowledge gaps.

Kinsey's original reports that 10% of men were predominantly gay and 6% of women were lesbians have been supplanted by more recent studies using probability sampling methods that estimate 5–9% of men are gay and 3–4% of women are lesbians. For the purposes of this chapter and in the interest of simplicity, we will refer to gay men and lesbians as if they were single populations. However, this is a gross oversimplification of very complex and diverse human behavior.

Homophobia, Heterosexism, & Sexual Prejudice

Homophobia is defined as an irrational fear of, aversion to, or discrimination against homosexuality or homosexuals. Heterosexism is the belief that heterosexuality is the natural, normal, acceptable, or superior form of sexuality. Sexual prejudice encompasses negative attitudes toward an individual because of her or his sexual orientation. In their most extreme manifestation, homophobia and sexual prejudice result in physical violence and murder.

Homophobia is pervasive: in one survey of students attending a US medical school, 25% of students reported believing homosexuality is immoral and dangerous to the institution of the family, and 9% believed that homosexuality was a mental disorder. Similarly, 543 internal medicine house staff surveyed in Canada reported witnessing homophobic remarks directed toward lesbians or gay men by more than 50% of all attending physicians, peers, patients, nurses, or other health care workers. Lesbian physicians are four times more likely to experience sexual orientation–based harassment than heterosexual physicians, and one third of lesbian physicians report sexual orientation harassment in the work setting after medical school.

Homophobia is also dangerous: one survey of physicians found that 52% had observed colleagues providing substandard care to patients because of sexual orientation. In another study, 37% of young gay men reported antigay harassment in the previous 6 months, resulting in increased suicidal ideation and diminished self-esteem. In

HIV-seropositive gay men who were otherwise healthy, HIV infection advanced more rapidly, exhibiting a dose-response relationship, in participants who concealed their homosexual identity. A study of 1067 lesbians and gay men found that feelings of victimization that resulted from perceived social stigma were a significant contributor to depression. And a study of 912 Latino men found that experiences of social discrimination were strong predictors of suicidal ideation, anxiety, and depressed mood.

Overcoming entrenched prejudices and eliminating discriminatory practices are fundamental to the provision of effective health care to all patients. Bias against LGBT individuals seems to respond more effectively to experiential interventions (eg, interaction with LGBT individuals) than to rational interventions (eg, information dissemination). In a clinical setting, physicians can help communicate tolerance via posters including diverse same-sex couples, stickers depicting a rainbow flag or pink triangle, and a visible nondiscrimination statement stating that equal care will be provided to all patients, regardless of age, race, ethnicity, physical ability or attributes, religion, sexual identity, and gender identity. Modeling tolerance and speaking out against bias are also ways in which physicians can help combat antihomosexual prejudice.

Web Sites

Gay and Lesbian Medical Association (GLMA):
http://www.glma.org

"Creating a Safe Clinical Environment for Men Who Have Sex With Men," available at:
http://www.glma.org/medical/clinical/msm_safe_clinical.pdf

"Guidelines for Care of Lesbian, Gay, Bisexual and Transgender Patients," developed by the GLMA:
http://www.glma.org/medical/clinical/lgbti_clinical_guidelines.pdf

Parents, Families and Friends of Lesbians and Gays (PFLAG):
http://www.pflag.org/

DIAGNOSTIC & MANAGEMENT CONSIDERATIONS

The willingness of LGBT patients to disclose sexual orientation and details of their personal lives is strongly influenced by the perceived tolerance (or intolerance) of their physician. Because a patient's sexual practices will modify risk for various diseases and can thus influence disease screening and the diagnostic evaluation, honest discussion of the patient's sexual and social life is vital to promote optimal health. Failure to identify an LGBT patient may cause the treating physician to fail in counseling a patient and in considering a diagnosis, thus risking the patient's life and the physician's reputation. Incorrect assumptions about patients can have similar adverse outcomes (Table 62–1). Using simple conversational techniques, and mastering a very manageable amount of medical information, will allow family physicians to provide superior care to LGBT patients.

Table 62–1. Pitfalls in caring for gay and lesbian patients.

Assumption	Solution
Assumption about sexual orientation: Many patients are neither exclusively heterosexual nor exclusively homosexual.	Learn to inquire about sexual orientation in a nonjudgmental manner that recognizes the range of human diversity and apply this learning to all patients.
Assumptions about sexual activity: Lesbian and gay male patients may have numerous different sexual partners, be in a monogamous relationship, be celibate, or vary in patterns of activity over time.	Take a specific, sensitive sexual history from all patients.
Assumptions about contraception: The need for contraception arises from a wish to prevent pregnancy from heterosexual intercourse, *regardless* of the patient's gender identity, sexual orientation, or label.	Inquire about need (rather than assuming need) or lack of need for all patients. Tailor recommendations to patient's needs.
Assumptions about marriage: Lesbians and gay men may have been, and may still be, married to persons of the opposite sex. Additionally, individuals in same-sex relationships may refer to themselves as married, and physicians doing otherwise risk alienating their patients.	Inquire about significant relationships for all patients. Use the terminology that your patients choose.
Assumptions about parenting: Lesbian and gay male couples are often interested in and choose to bear and raise children.	Inquire about parenting wishes and choices, and be prepared to discuss options.

HIV/AIDS

ESSENTIALS OF DIAGNOSIS

- *Not all gay men are at risk for HIV, but testing for HIV is recommended for all patients aged 13–64 years seen in health care settings after the patient is notified that testing will be performed unless the patient declines.*
- *Periodic screening (HIV blood tests) is recommended for all persons who are sexually active outside a mutually monogamous relationship.*
- *Blood tests for HIV antibodies have sensitivity and specificity greater than 99%.*
- *HIV viral load tests (eg, HIV polymerase chain reaction) should not be used for HIV screening due to the high false-positive rate.*

General Considerations

Any publication on GLBT health that omitted mention of HIV would be incomplete, but thorough coverage of the topic is beyond the scope of this chapter. References included at the end of this discussion can assist physicians in the management of HIV-infected individuals.

Gay men comprise the largest number of AIDS cases in the United States. Young gay men and those with substance abuse problems are at greater risk. Increasingly, African-American and Latino men are disproportionately affected. Increased stigma associated with homosexuality in ethnic minority communities often drives individuals at risk to hide, complicating efforts at diagnosis and treatment.

Prevention

Until an effective vaccine is available (estimated to be at least 5–10 years hence) behavioral interventions are the best means to stop the spread of HIV. Physicians should screen all patients for risk behaviors (unprotected intercourse, multiple partners, concurrent sex and substance use, injection drug use, etc) and should intervene to reduce risk and test for HIV in patients with a positive risk history. A "harm reduction" strategy should be pursued if it is impossible to eliminate all risk (eg, stopping needle sharing until drug abuse can be stopped, keeping condoms available when sex with a new partner is possible, etc). Because patients engaging in risky behaviors often will not seek counseling, physicians must proactively assess each patient's risk and intervene when needed.

Clinical Findings

Physicians should consider and test for HIV in individuals presenting with routine viral infection symptoms. Patients with acute HIV infection present with symptoms that are generally indistinguishable from common viral infections, including fever (96%), adenopathy (74%), pharyngitis (70%), rash (70%), and other nonspecific symptoms. HIV viral load tests (eg, polymerase chain reaction) become positive 1–2 weeks before routine (antibody-based) HIV tests and may be useful in diagnosis (as distinct from screening).

Latent HIV infection may be essentially asymptomatic for years. Generalized lymphadenopathy may persist for years; its disappearance may herald clinically significant immune system decline, marked by nonspecific symptoms such as fevers, weight loss, and diarrhea. Early immune dysfunction results in diseases such as herpes zoster or persistent vaginal candidiasis. Without effective antiretroviral treatment almost all patients will progress to one or more AIDS-defining illnesses.

Treatment

Patients infected with HIV require a comprehensive care plan that involves skilled physicians, ancillary health services, pharmacologic therapy, and access to social and other support services. Excellent resources exist to guide physicians in the detailed management and care of patients with HIV/AIDS (see below). The family physician's role in HIV care will be determined by the knowledge, skill, comfort level, and personal preferences of the physician, as well as the accessibility of referral physicians. Family physicians may serve primarily in case finding, by testing and referring patients found to be HIV positive, or may assume full responsibility for comprehensive management of HIV and its complications.

Bartlett JG: *The Johns Hopkins Hospital 2005–06 Guide To Medical Care Of Patients With HIV Infection,* 12th ed. Lippincott Williams & Wilkins, 2005.

Web Sites

AIDS Education and Training Centers (AETCs):

http://www.aids-ed.org/

AETC Warmline/Pepline, a national HIV patient management and postexposure prophylaxis telephone consultation service:

http://www.ucsf.edu/hivcntr/

InSite Knowledge Base, a comprehensive, on-line textbook of HIV disease from the University of California San Francisco and San Francisco General Hospital:

http://hivinsite.ucsf.edu/InSite?page=KB

National Institutes of Health treatment guidelines:

http://www.aidsinfo.nih.gov/guidelines

US Department of Health and Human Services' AIDSinfo:

http://www.aidsinfo.nih.gov/

Patient Education Resources

AIDS Education Global Information System:

http://www.aegis.com/

Bartlett JG, Finkbeiner AK: *The Guide to Living with HIV Infection: Developed at the Johns Hopkins AIDS Clinic,* 6th ed. Johns Hopkins University Press, 2006.

The Body (HIV prevention, state-of-the-art treatment issues, forums, humor):

http://www.thebody.com/

Gay Men's Health Crisis:

http://www.gmhc.org

Project Inform:

http://www.projectinform.org

SEXUALLY TRANSMITTED DISEASES

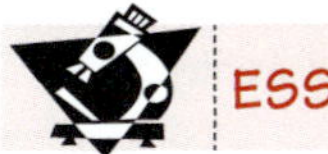

ESSENTIALS OF DIAGNOSIS

- *Many sexually active gay men are at increased risk for most STDs, requiring routine periodic screening.*
- *Suspicion or diagnosis of one STD should routinely lead to testing for concomitant HIV and syphilis.*
- *Although generally at lower risk for STDs, lesbians have a higher incidence of bacterial vaginosis than heterosexual women.*

General Considerations

In the United States, causes of genital ulcer disease (GUD) in heterosexual and homosexual men are most commonly due to herpes simplex and syphilis. Other causes of GUD are less common, although epidemiology may be changing; an outbreak of lymphogranuloma venereum in MSM first reported in the Netherlands has produced cases of GUD and proctocolitis in MSM throughout Europe and the United States.

Gonorrhea, chlamydia, and nonchlamydial nongonococcal urethritis (NGU) are common problems in sexually active gay men. As each of these may cause asymptomatic infection, periodic screening may be useful to detect clinically silent disease. Organisms that commonly cause enteritis and proctocolitis may be sexually transmitted, and even organisms not commonly thought to be pathogenic, such as *Endolimax nana* and *Blastocystis hominis,* should be treated in the symptomatic patient lacking other causes of abdominal symptoms.

Kaposi sarcoma (KS) poses another health risk for gay men. Although generally associated with HIV infection, KS seems to be the result of infection with a separate herpesvirus, KSHV/HHV-8, and can occur in the absence of HIV. It appears that this virus is sexually transmitted, probably by receptive anal intercourse, and may be carried in saliva. Although cases of KS among gay men in the absence of coexisting HIV infection are rare and even in HIV-infected patients the incidence has decreased significantly from the early period of the AIDS epidemic, physicians should be suspicious of red or purple patches or nodules on the skin or mucous membranes, and should evaluate or refer patients for treatment when indicated.

Fellatio, commonly thought to be a "safe" sexual practice, may be an independent risk factor for urethral gonorrhea and for nonchlamydial NGU; has been implicated in HIV transmission; and has been recently associated with localized syphilis epidemics in gay men. Syphilis epidemics have also been associated with high-risk sexual activity among HIV-positive men.

Some researchers have shown comparable rates of STDs between lesbians and heterosexual women, though the types of infections varied; genital herpes and genital warts were more common in the heterosexual women, and bacterial vaginosis (BV) was more common in lesbians. Other investigators have replicated observed different prevalence of BV and warts, but not herpes, although the nature of the inner-city population studied may preclude generalizing these findings to all lesbians.

Fethers K et al: Sexually transmitted infections and risk behaviours in women who have sex with women. Sex Transm Infect 2000;76:345. [PMID: 11141849]

Prevention

Counseling has been shown to reduce risk behaviors, and patients reporting high-risk behaviors or those diagnosed with an STD should receive or be referred for individual or group counseling. Additionally, MSM patients engaging in sex outside a mutually monogamous relationship should receive periodic STD screening, as should women having sex with men and women (see Chapter 14 for screening recommendations and other information about STDs). If not immune, gay men should be vaccinated against hepatitis A and hepatitis B.

Patient Education

All patients in whom a STD is suspected or diagnosed should receive information about routes of transmission and how to reduce infection risk. Information about specific treatment, if any, as well as potential coinfection with other sexually transmissible agents should also be provided. Patients should be counseled to contact sex partners; in lieu of this, the physician or health department may notify partners.

Centers for Disease Control and Prevention; Workowski KA, Berman SM: Sexually transmitted disease treatment guidelines, 2006. MMWR Recomm Rep 2006;55(RR-11):1. [PMID: 16888612]

Johnson WD et al: Interventions to modify sexual risk behaviors for preventing HIV infection in men who have sex with men. Cochrane Database Syst Rev 2003;(1)CD001230. [PMID: 12535405]

HUMAN PAPILLOMAVIRUS INFECTION

ESSENTIALS OF DIAGNOSIS

- *Human papillomavirus (HPV) causes cervical cancer in both heterosexual and lesbian women; lesbians should be offered Papanicolaou (Pap) smear screening according to the same guidelines used for heterosexual women.*
- *Some investigators recommend that men who have engaged in receptive anal intercourse receive anal Pap smears.*

General Considerations

HPV is a pervasive infection throughout the population, manifesting in more than 100 types that infect various parts of the human body. HPV types that infect the genitalia carry varying risk for dysplasia and neoplasia. Ironically, the types that cause the most visually apparent warts are usually the types with least risk for dysplasia; conversely, the types causing clinically inapparent disease carry high dysplastic risk.

Prevention

Secondary prevention via Pap smear remains the cornerstone of screening. One study of lesbians revealed that 25% of respondents had not had a Pap test within the past 3 years, and 7.6% had never had a Pap test. Lesbian patients may mistakenly believe themselves to be less susceptible to cervical cancer than heterosexuals or bisexuals, even though one study showed 79% reported previous sexual intercourse with a man. Even in women reporting no prior sex with men, HPV DNA and squamous intraepithelial lesions (SILs) may be found in up to 20% of patients. Thus cervical Pap smears should be performed routinely, supplemented by HPV DNA testing if and when indicated. Individuals with abnormal screening tests should receive colposcopy or anoscopy and subsequent follow-up as indicated by findings.

A gay man's risk of anal squamous cell carcinoma is equivalent to the historical risk of cervical cancer that women faced prior to the advent of Pap screening. Anal HPV DNA is very prevalent in gay men; in one study it was detected in 91.6% of HIV-positive and 65.9% of HIV-negative men. HIV exacerbates HPV effects, and is associated with more prevalent HPV infection and higher-grade SILs. Screening HIV-positive homosexual and bisexual men for anal SILs and anal squamous cell carcinomas with anal Pap tests offers quality-adjusted life expectancy benefits at a cost comparable with other accepted clinical preventive interventions. Because the observed increased incidence of anal cancer does not appear to be solely due to HIV infection, high-resolution anoscopy and cytologic screening of all MSM with anal condyloma and other benign noncondylomatous anal disorders is supported by current knowledge.

Experimental vaccination has been shown to prevent infection with some types of HPV commonly associated with cancer development. A quadrivalent vaccine against HPV is available and licensed for females aged 9–26 years, and studies of HPV vaccine use in MSM are ongoing. Additional discussion of HPV appears in Chapter 14.

SUBSTANCE ABUSE

General Considerations

Alcohol, psychoactive drug, and tobacco use appear more widespread in gay men and lesbians than in the general heterosexual population. Several studies suggest that lesbians consume more alcohol and use other psychoactive substances more than heterosexual women. A recent review of tobacco use found that smoking rates among adolescent and adult lesbians, gays, and bisexuals are higher than in the general population.

Alcohol use has been associated with high-risk sexual behavior (ie, unprotected anal and oral intercourse). Gay men who have unprotected anal intercourse are more likely to have a drinking problem and to drink more than gay men who do not have unprotected intercourse, and unprotected intercourse after drinking is more common with nonsteady sexual partners. Drug use is also associated with increased high-risk sexual behaviors. Drugs for which this association has been demonstrated include hallucinogens, nitrate inhalants, and cocaine and other stimulants. Drug use during high-risk sex is common. However, associations between drug use and high-risk sexual behavior exist only for current use, not past drug or alcohol use. Thus, efforts to provide adequate treatment to patients with substance abuse problems can diminish their subsequent risk of acquiring HIV and other STDs.

In some venues the prevalence of illicit drug use and associated high-risk sexual activity is dramatic, with use of substances such as methylenedioxymethamphetamine (MDMA or ecstasy) approaching 80% of the population. Men who attend "circuit parties"—a series of dances or parties held over a weekend that are attended by hundreds to thousands of gay and bisexual men—should be considered at high risk for concurrent illicit substance use and should be counseled accordingly.

Anabolic steroid use is a problem among a subset of gay men. One British study of over 1000 gay men recruited from five gymnasiums found that 13.5% of the study population used anabolic steroids, and users were more likely than never users (21% vs 13%) to report engaging in unprotected anal intercourse, increasing their risk for HIV infection.

Pathogenesis

Several theories have been proposed to explain the increased substance use seen in GLBT patients. The observed behavior has been variously explained as a maladaptive coping strategy to deal with societal bias against homosexuality; a consequence of bars serving as a primary social gathering place for lesbians and gay men; due to a genetic predisposition to substance abuse linked to genes coding for same-sex attraction; a coping method for dealing with stresses such as fear of HIV infection, lack of social supports, fear of discrimination in housing or employment, and rejection by family or friends on the basis of sexual orientation; or something else. Research to date has not explained causation.

Reasons for steroid use are more straightforward: to modify the patient's musculature to conform more closely with an idealized male form. Significant social pressures may cause patients to resort to steroids as a means to achieve an idealized masculine physique, and for these patients substantial support and counseling may be required to overcome steroid abuse.

Prevention & Treatment

By and large, prevention, clinical findings, complications, and treatment of substance abuse in LGBT populations are similar to these management considerations in heterosexual populations (see Chapter 56 for further discussion). However, modification of standard treatment approaches to reflect GLBT culture may enhance treatment effectiveness. Differences to consider with this population include:

- The prevalence of methamphetamine use, and its association with high-risk sexual behavior among some groups of gay men.
- Concomitant use of sildenafil (Viagra) or other treatments for erectile dysfunction, and "club drugs" (eg, methylenedioxymethamphetamine [MDMA] or ecstasy, amphetamines, gamma hydroxybutyrate, ketamine). Erectile dysfunction treatments, either with or without other substance use, are associated with high-risk sexual behavior.

Center for Substance Abuse Treatment of the Substance Abuse and Mental Health Services Administation: *A Provider's Introduction to Substance Abuse Treatment for Lesbian, Gay, Bisexual, and Transgender Individuals,* DHHS Publication No. (SMA) 01–3498. US Department of Health and Human Services, 2001.

Cochran SD et al: Estimates of alcohol use and clinical treatment needs among homosexually active men and women in the U.S. population. J Consult Clin Psychol 2000;68:1062. [PMID: 11142540]

Shoptaw S et al: Behavioral treatment approaches for methamphetamine dependence and HIV-related sexual risk behaviors among urban gay and bisexual men. Drug Alcohol Depend 2005;78:125. [PMID: 15845315]

DEPRESSION

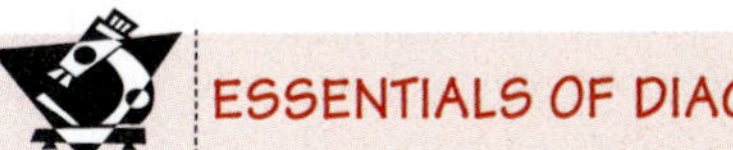

ESSENTIALS OF DIAGNOSIS

- *Depression and anxiety are more prevalent in lesbians and gay men than in the general population.*
- *Suicidal ideation, attempts at suicide, and completed acts of suicide are more common in gay, lesbian, and bisexual youth than in their heterosexual counterparts.*
- *Suicide risk seems to be increased around the time an individual "comes out" (reveals his or her gay or lesbian identity to others).*
- *Lack of social supports, lack of family support, and poor relationship quality are significant predictors of depression.*

General Considerations

Feelings of being stigmatized, internalized homophobia (the direction of society's negative attitudes toward the self), and actual experiences of discrimination or violence contribute to gay men's distress. In a study of HIV-infected men that may have relevance for all gay men, it was found that men who did not demonstrate traditional gender identity were more likely to have current symptoms of anxiety and depression and to have had a lifetime history of depression. Depression has also been linked to the AIDS epidemic, and particularly to being a caregiver for someone with AIDS, regardless of whether the caregiver is infected with HIV or not.

Well-designed studies with valid sampling techniques have demonstrated that suicidal ideation, attempts at suicide, and completed acts of suicide are more common in gay, lesbian, and bisexual youth than in their heterosexual counterparts. Population-based research demonstrates significantly higher rates of suicidal symptoms and suicide attempts among men who reported same-sex partners than among men who reported exclusively opposite-sex partners. Other investigators have demonstrated similar findings (eg, in a study of twins in which one brother reported same-sex partners after age 18 and the other did not). Suicidality has been linked to the process of "coming out," or revealing one's homosexual orientation to others. Thus, physicians caring for gay adolescents or adults disclosing their sexual orientation to others should be especially sensitive to symptoms or signs suggesting any increase in suicide risk.

Research on the mental health of lesbians is limited. One study considered predictors of depression and looked at relationship status, relationship satisfaction, social support from friends, social support from family, "outness" (degree to which the woman publicly shared her sexual orientation), and relationship satisfaction. Lack of social support from friends, poor relationship satisfaction, and lack of perceived social support from family were significant predictors of depression.

Prevention

Well-being is enhanced during later stages of gay identity development, suggesting that helping to facilitate an individual's synthesis of his or her gay identity may alleviate depressive symptoms. Conversely, in HIV-positive men, concealment of homosexuality is associated with lower CD4 counts and depressive symptoms, lending further support to the idea that facilitating gay identity development may alleviate or prevent depression in some patients.

Clinical Findings

Symptoms and signs of depression in lesbian and gay male patients are very similar to those in heterosexual populations (see Chapter 52). Although depression is often associated with decreased sexual activity, one study of gay men revealed 16% had heightened sexual interest while depressed. Predictors of depression in lesbians (eg, social support from friends, relationship status satisfaction, and perceived social support from family) are similar to predictors for heterosexual women.

Bancroft J et al: The relation between mood and sexuality in gay men. Arch Sex Behav 2003;32:231. [PMID: 12807295]

Halpin SA, Allen MW: Changes in psychosocial well-being during stages of gay identity development. J Homosex 2004;47:109. [PMID: 15271626]

Oetjen H, Rothblum ED: When lesbians aren't gay: Factors affecting depression among lesbians. J Homosex 2000;39:49. [PMID: 1864377]

Ullrich PM et al: Concealment of homosexual identity, social support and CD4 cell count among HIV-seropositive gay men. J Psychosom Res 2003;54:205. [PMID: 12614830]

OTHER HEALTH CONCERNS

Breast Cancer

Breast cancer may be more common in nulliparous or uniparous women and thus may be more common in lesbians, but well-designed, prospective studies are lacking. One study compiling survey data from almost 12,000 women found lesbians had greater prevalence rates of obesity and alcohol and tobacco use, and lower rates of parity and birth control pill use. Another study confirmed higher prevalence of nulliparity, and also found higher prevalence of other health risk factors, including high daily alcohol intake, higher body mass index, and higher prevalence of current smoking.

Case P et al: Sexual orientation, health risk factors, and physical functioning in the Nurses' Health Study II. J Womens Health (Larchmt) 2004;13:1033. [PMID: 15665660]

Erectile Dysfunction

Studies have demonstrated that erectile dysfunction is more common in homosexual than in heterosexual men, although overall prevalence was still less than 4%. Associated with this observation, gay men also report higher levels of performance anxiety (eg, are more likely to agree with the statement "If I feel I'm expected to respond sexually, I have difficulty getting aroused") than do heterosexual men; this was true even when men reporting erectile dysfunction were excluded from analysis.

Erectile dysfunction is more common in HIV-positive homosexual men than in HIV-negative homosexual men. Declines in serum testosterone have been associated with HIV infection, suggesting one possible etiology for this difference.

Bancroft J et al: Erectile and ejaculatory problems in gay and heterosexual men. Arch Sex Behav 2005;34:285. [PMID: 15971011]

Contraception & Reproductive Health

Physicians who assume that all women of reproductive age need contraception risk alienating lesbian patients, who may consequently decline to disclose their sexual orientation. However, lesbians who are sexually active with men may be interested in obtaining contraceptives.

Lesbian patients may also be, or wish to become, mothers and so may welcome a discussion of reproductive options. Parenthood options available to lesbians and gay men include adoption, artificial insemination, surrogacy, or heterosexual intercourse. Existing evidence suggests that gay men and lesbians have parenting skills comparable to heterosexual parents. When compared with children of heterosexual parents, children of gay men and lesbians seem to be no different in significant variables measured, including their sexual or gender identity, personality traits, and intelligence. Despite this, gay men and lesbians may face unjustified barriers in their attempts to become foster and adoptive parents. Issues that warrant physician awareness include parental legal rights and durable power of attorney; gestation and pregnancy; choice of surrogate, sperm, or egg donor; possible HIV risk; and routine preconception and prenatal care. Physicians caring for lesbians and gay men wishing to become parents should maintain information about appropriate referrals to facilitate this process.

Boivin J et al: Guidelines for counselling in infertility: Outline version. Hum Reprod 2001;16:1301. [PMID: 11387309]

Garcia TC: Primary care of the lesbian/gay/bisexual/transgendered woman patient. Int J Fertil Womens Med 2003;48:246. [PMID: 15646394]

SPECIAL POPULATIONS WITHIN THE GAY & LESBIAN COMMUNITY

Transgender Patients

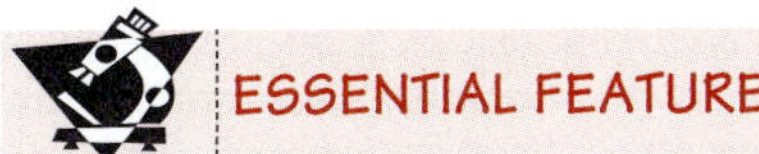

ESSENTIAL FEATURES

- *Rather than assume, physicians should determine how patients wish to be addressed and understand how they conceptualize their gender.*
- *Sex reassignment in adolescence may be indicated for carefully selected patients.*
- *Sex reassignment should be managed by multispecialty teams with experience caring for this population.*

The *Diagnostic and Statistical Manual of Mental Disorders,* Fourth Edition, Text Revision (*DSM-IV-TR*) diagnoses for gender identity disorder, transvestic fetishism, and gender identity disorder not otherwise specified describe conditions in which an individual may experience discordance between his or her perceived and observed gender; however, the descriptions fail to capture the full spectrum of experiences of individuals who do not fit traditional gender roles. The *DSM-IV-TR* characterization considers transgender individuals as suffering pathology, in a manner similar to the characterization of homosexuality prior to the American Psychiatric Association's 1973 revision of the *DSM.* Increased knowledge and changing societal attitudes may alter this characterization at some future time, as well.

Prevalence varies from country to country, with the ratio of male(-to-female) to female(-to-male) patients consistently showing a male preponderance ranging from approximately 2:1 to more than 4:1. Culture influences these patients' experiences, as some cultures do not recognize a transsexual identity and may assign a mystical or religious significance to transgender individuals.

A. Terminology

Terminology can be problematic when describing transgender individuals, reflecting evolving knowledge. *Transgender* can be used as an umbrella term for a diverse group of individuals who cross or transcend culturally defined categories of gender in some way. *Transsexual* often refers to an individual who has undergone partial or complete sex reassignment surgery (SRS). *Intersex* individuals are born with both male and female sexual characteristics and organs, such that unambiguous assignment of male or female sex at birth is not possible.

Considering gender-discordant individuals born with male genitalia, one classification system characterizes *transvestites* as men who never wished to change their sex and become a woman, had never taken female hormones, and had never seriously considered sex change surgery. This classification is consistent with the *DSM-IV-TR* diagnostic criteria of transvestic fetishism, which occurs only in heterosexual males.

Transsexuals, who differ from transvestites, wish to change their sex and become a woman, have taken female hormones, and have seriously considered (or undertaken) SRS. *Transgender* individuals have been described as men who generally cross-dress more frequently, possibly daily, and often have a more stable sense of feminine identification than transvestites, although not necessarily to the point that they desire SRS. In this schema, "transgender" falls on a continuum between transvestite and transsexual. In other usage, the term *transgender* serves as an umbrella for patients experiencing discordance between their physical gender and their gender identity.

The term *male-to-female* (MTF) describes individuals born with male genitalia who may undergo treatment to create a female-appearing body; the reverse is true for *female-to-male* (FTM) individuals. Additional ways to characterize the biological, social, psychological, and legal identity of transgender individuals have been described. In caring for an individual patient, the best approach for physicians is to determine how patients wish to be addressed and to understand how they conceptualize their gender.

In the spectrum of gender identity disorder, individuals who experience the strongest feelings of dissonance between their gender identity and their physical appearance believe the quest for full hormonal and surgical sex reassignment is vital because they actually feel "trapped" in an anatomically wrong body. Currently, the transgender movement includes cross-dressers, female and male impersonators, transgenderists and bigender persons (who identify as both man and woman), as well as transsexuals who have undergone or desire to undergo sex reassignment therapy. Limited research into the etiology of gender identity disorder suggests that it may be multifactorial; there may be anatomic brain differences between transsexual and nontranssexual individuals, as well as differences in parental rearing. Regardless of the etiology or classification, the needs of transgender patients are increasingly recognized as valid, authentic, and deserving of attention from health care educators, researchers, policy makers, and clinicians of all types.

B. Treatment

Some patients choose partial medical or surgical treatment of their gender dysphoria, finding that a physical existence with components of both genders best addresses the emotional dysphoria caused by their birth physiognomy. Others wish to use surgery and hormonal treatment to manifest physically their "internal" gender as fully as possible. The literature describing the health needs of transgender patients focuses principally upon psychological and psychiatric evaluation and treatment, surgical modification or SRS, and hormonal therapy. Although common practice is to delay initiating sex reassignment therapy until the patient is at least 18 or 21 years of age, treatment in adolescence is well tolerated for carefully selected individuals, does not lead to postoperative regret, and may forestall psychopathology seen in transgender individuals forced to delay therapy.

The psychiatric literature historically has indicated that transsexual patients suffer from increased Axis I psychopathology. Transsexual men have been reported to experience less sexual drive, more psychiatric symptoms, and a greater feminine gender role than transvestite or transgender men. However, a population of transvestite, transgender, and transsexual men not seen for clinical reasons was virtually indistinguishable from non–cross-dressing men using a measure of personality traits, a sexual functioning inventory, and measures of psychological distress. Another study of 137 transsexual individuals completing the Minnesota Multiphasic Personality Inventory found that transsexualism is usually an isolated diagnosis and is not part of any general psychopathologic disorder. Initial treatment of a patient considering SRS should include a complete psychological evaluation by a therapist experienced in working with this population.

Intensive psychological counseling, hormonal treatment, and living in the role of the desired gender for a period of at least 1 year should precede surgical treatment. Surgical treatment can involve the breasts, genitalia, and larynx. Breast surgery includes reduction, removal, and implant placement. One survey of MTF transsexual patients found that 75% were satisfied with breast surgery results, although 15% opted to undergo additional mammaplasty. Genital surgery may include penile skin inversion or sigmoidocolpoplasty for male-to-female transsexuals and meta-idioplasties and neophalloplasties for female-to-male transsexuals; careful attention to technique can result in greater than 90% patient satisfaction with cosmetic and functional results that endures years after surgery. Cricothyroid approximation surgery has been employed to raise the vocal pitch of MTF patients. Interestingly, even in health systems funded by government support, courts have found that transsexuals have the right to SRS. Because of individual psychological and anatomic variations, surgical approaches must be tailored to individual patients, and patients seeking SRS should be referred to teams experienced with these procedures.

Hormonal treatment is often employed in both genders. Hormones induce feminization or virilization and suppress the hypothalamic-pituitary-gonadal axis. Cross-sex hormonal treatment may have substantial medical side effects, so the smallest doses needed to achieve the desired result should be used. Treatment with ethinyl estradiol in MTF transsexuals causes an increase in subcutaneous and visceral fat and a decrease in the thigh muscle area, whereas administration of testosterone in FTM transsexuals markedly increases the thigh muscle area, reduces subcutaneous fat at all levels measured, but slightly increases the visceral fat area. Outcome studies suggest that known complications of hormonal therapy such as galactorrhea and thromboembolic events occur, but that the incidence of complications can be held to acceptable levels with careful attention to regimens used. Extensive experience with hormonal therapies in transsexual patients indicates that hormonal therapy, particularly if transdermal formulations are used, does not cause increased morbidity or mortality; monitoring luteinizing hormone levels in MTF transsexuals may increase the benefit-to-risk ratio by limiting hormone-related bone loss.

American Psychiatric Association: *Diagnostic and Statistical Manual of Mental Disorders,* 4th ed, text revision. APA, 2000.

Lombardi E: Enhancing transgender health care. Am J Public Health 2001;91:869. [PMID: 11392924]

Lombardi EL et al: Gender violence: Transgender experiences with violence and discrimination. J Homosex 2001;42:89. [PMID: 11991568]

Thyen U et al: Deciding on gender in children with intersex conditions: Considerations and controversies. Treat Endocrinol 2005;4:1. [PMID: 15649096]

Warne GL et al: Hormonal therapies for individuals with intersex conditions: Protocol for use. Treat Endocrinol 2005;4:19. [PMID: 15649098]

Adolescents

Lesbian and gay adolescents are vulnerable to parental wrath and withdrawal of support upon disclosure or suspicion of their homosexual orientation. This can initiate a chain of events that leaves the youth homeless and vulnerable. Lacking employable skills, homeless gay youths may resort to prostitution or "survival sex" to support themselves.

Gay youths have an increased risk for suicide compared with their heterosexual peers, and gender nonconformity may be particularly detrimental to boys. Despite this, homosexual adolescents are generally more similar to than different from their heterosexual peers, face many of the same challenges, and mostly grow up healthy and happy.

Physicians caring for families need to be aware of the possibility that the normal adolescent struggle to establish identity may be compounded when a teen recognizes his or her gay or lesbian identity, particularly when this occurs in a potentially hostile environment. Physicians can play a vital role in helping the adolescent—and his or her family—accept the patient's sexual orientation. Parental acceptance and support can dramatically reduce the adverse effects of "coming out" and the potential risk for suicide, and can increase the likelihood of healthy psychological development and maturation.

Garofalo R, Katz E: Health care issues of gay and lesbian youth. Curr Opin Pediatr 2001;13:298. [PMID: 11717552]

Perrin EC et al: Gay and lesbian issues in pediatric health care. Curr Probl Pediatr Adolesc Health Care 2004;34:355. [PMID: 15570222]

Older Lesbians & Gay Men

Older lesbians and gay men developed and matured in a different social milieu, when society was less tolerant of homosexuality and the consequences of being gay or lesbian included even greater threats to the individual's social and family relationships, housing, and livelihood than exist today. Thus, older patients may be even less willing to disclose their homosexual orientation to physicians, and may have special health care needs.

Although not extensive, research suggests that many lesbians and gay men successfully navigate the aging process and remain connected and involved in life. In fact, the demands of being gay may cause individuals to face the challenges associated with aging more successfully than their heterosexual counterparts.

McMahon E: The older homosexual: Current concepts of lesbian, gay, bisexual, and transgender older Americans. Clin Geriatr Med 2003;19:587. [PMID: 14567010]

Family & Community

One aspect of being gay or lesbian that may be overlooked in caring for a patient's medical needs is the role of family and social networks in providing support and sustenance to the GLBT patient. In this context, family often includes individuals unrelated by biological ties. A sometimes useful concept is that of "family of origin," which consists of parents, siblings, and others with whom one shares a blood relation, contrasted with "family of choice," which includes those close friendship relationships that endure over time and incorporate the same types of support and emotions often associated with idealized views of the traditional family. The family of a lesbian or gay patient, just as with heterosexual patients, is a vital part of the individual's health and can serve as a source of both stress and support. Physicians caring for gay men and lesbians need to assess the resources and stressors that exist within the family, as defined by the patient.

Hospice & Palliative Medicine 63

Terence L. Gutgsell, MD, Kenneth L. Kirsh, PhD, Bonnie Meyer, DMin, Steven D. Passik, PhD, Hahn X. Pham, MD, & Sherri Weisenfluh, LCSW

BACKGROUND

Homes for the dying or, as they were soon to be called, *hospices,* were established in Ireland and France in the 19th century. But it was not until 1967 that the first truly modern hospice, Saint Christopher's, was founded in London. There, Dr Cicely Saunders, a former nurse and social worker who had earned a medical degree, helped to establish the underlying philosophy of hospice and palliative medicine. She emphasized excellence in pain and symptom management; care of the whole person, including physical, emotional, social, and spiritual needs; and the need for research in this newly developing field of medicine. Interdisciplinary team care became the norm, as it became clear that no one physician, nurse, social worker, or chaplain could address all the needs of the terminally ill person. Further, although the focus of care was clearly on the dying individual, the needs of the family were also addressed.

Florence Wald, RN, PhD, Dean of the Yale School of Nursing, invited Dr Saunders to lecture to medical, nursing, and social work students at Yale in 1963 on care of the terminally ill. Dr Wald spent 1968 at Saint Christopher's on sabbatical and after her return to the United States helped to establish the Connecticut Hospice, the first hospice in the United States, in 1974. In 1982, the Congress created the Medicare Hospice Benefit (MHB), and in 1986, the benefit was made permanent. By 2004, 3650 hospice programs were providing health care services to the terminally ill and their families throughout the United States.

Eligibility criteria for hospice enrollment through the MHB require that patients waive traditional Medicare coverage for curative and life-prolonging care related to the terminal diagnosis and be certified by their physician and the hospice medical director as having a life expectancy of 6 months or less if the disease runs its usual course. Recertification periods within the MHB allow for reexamination of hospice eligibility. If the hospice medical director believes the patient has a prognosis of 6 months or less if the disease runs its usual course, the patient may be recertified as eligible for the MHB even if the patient has already been receiving the benefit for 6 months or longer.

The goal of hospice care is to relieve suffering and improve the patient's and family's quality of daily life. To achieve those goals, hospice care has come to be defined as holistic, person, and family centered rather than disease centered. Hospice provides a team composed of members trained to care for problems in a holistic manner: physician, nurse, social worker, chaplain, bereavement counselor, nursing assistant, and volunteer. The hospice team meets weekly, under the direction of the hospice medical director, to review the care plans of all patients. The hospice program is charged with providing medications for the relief of physical distress, durable medical equipment, supplies, a multidisciplinary team to provide care, and bereavement support before and after the patient's death.

Palliative medicine has been developing as a medical subspecialty in the United States over the past 15 years, with the purpose of bringing a "hospice-like" approach to patients with terminal or life-limiting illnesses who have a prognosis of more than 6 months or to those pursuing aggressive life-prolonging treatments. The goals of palliative care programs are similar to hospice: pain and symptom control; emotional, social, and spiritual support of patients and families; and facilitation of clear and compassionate communication regarding goals of treatment.

Many models of palliative care are under development. There are palliative care consultation teams in hospitals, nursing home, and in clinics. The growth of palliative care consultation programs over the past 10 years has been significant and mirrors the growth of hospice since 1974. The number of hospital-based palliative care consultation programs has increased linearly from 632 (15%) in 2000 to 1027 (25%) in 2003.

Palliative medicine fellowships are undergoing rapid development as well. In the early 1990s, the first US palliative medicine fellowship was initiated. By June 2006, 49 programs offered 119 fellowships for advanced training. In September 2006, the field of palliative medicine was officially recognized as a subspecialty by the American Board of Medical Specialties.

PAIN & SYMPTOM MANAGEMENT

Good symptom control is the cornerstone of palliative medicine. Distressing symptoms can consume patients and rob them of their will to live. Uncontrolled symptoms detract from patients' quality of life, their interactions with loved ones, and their ability to attend to important issues at the end of life. Many studies have documented the high frequency of symptoms and the tendency for symptoms to

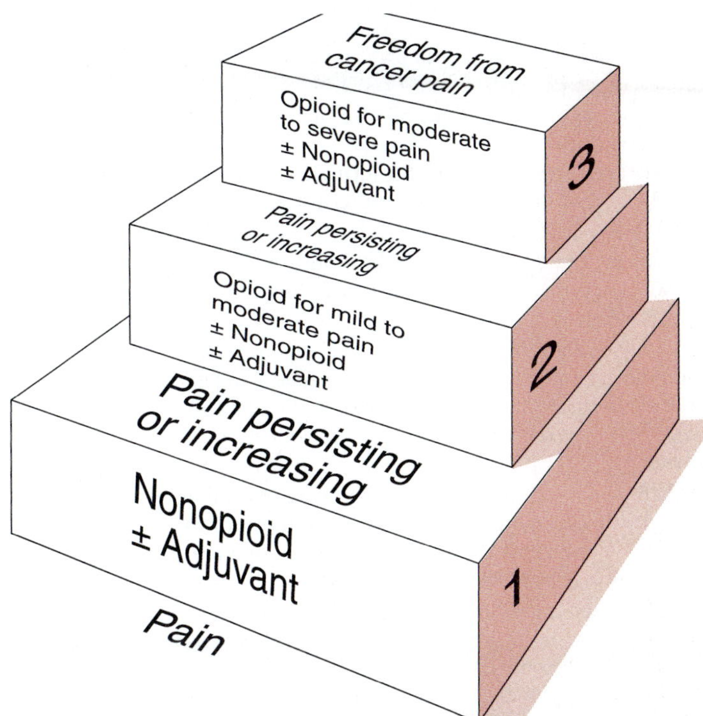

Figure 63–1. WHO three-step pain control guidelines.

increase in intensity as a disease progresses. The following discussion reviews management of some common symptoms. As with most medical problems, successful management of symptoms starts with a careful history and physical examination, with therapy directed at the underlying cause, if possible.

Pain

Pain can be classified physiologically as somatic, visceral, neuropathic, or of mixed type. Pain can occur from direct tumor involvement, as a consequence of cancer therapy, or from unrelated pathology. It is important to remember that pain is a subjective experience that can be influenced by psychosocial and spiritual issues.

The World Health Organization (WHO) published guidelines on pain control in 1996 (Figure 63–1). These guidelines have proven effective in large-scale studies in cancer patients, and for the majority of patients their application will lead to effective pain control. Based initially on the severity of the patient's pain, different medications can be used and adjustments made depending on the patient's response.

General principles of opioid administration include the following:

- Equianalgesic tables for opioids are available in most general pharmacology texts; these tables may differ slightly.
- Morphine is the most commonly used opioid and is the most versatile in terms of available formulations.
- Opioid-naive patients should be started on morphine sulfate, 5 mg immediate-release formulation, given orally every 4 hours (scheduled), and every 2 hours as needed. This regimen can then be converted to the sustained-release formulation based on the previous 24-hour dose, and titrated based on pain control.
- Chronic pain deserves around-the-clock pain medication, not just as-needed dosing.
- As needed medications should always be provided for breakthrough pain.
- Breakthrough doses are generally 10–15% of the 24-hour dose.
- Breakthrough medications can be given as frequently as the time to peak onset of action: 1–2 hours for oral immediate-release formulations and 10–15 minutes for intravenous formulations.
- When pain control is inadequate, the scheduled dose should be increased by 30–50% after 24 hours (after 48 hours for fentanyl patches). The amount of breakthrough medication used must be considered in calculating the additional amount of drug patients can tolerate—usually being able to tolerate an additional dose equivalent to the amount of breakthrough medication.

- There is no specific limit to the opioid dose; these agents should be titrated until pain control is achieved or side effects develop.
- Fentanyl patches should not be used alone for acute severe pain. Because of the delayed onset of effect (12 hours) and long half-life of this formulation, it cannot be titrated quickly for rapid pain control.
- The lowest available fentanyl patch may be excessive in patients who are opioid naive (a 12 mcg/h fentanyl patch is approximately equivalent to 25 mg of morphine sulfate).
- Morphine sulfate, hydromorphone, and fentanyl can be administered subcutaneously for patients unable to take oral formulations and who do not have intravenous access. Subcutaneous doses are equivalent to intravenous doses.
- When pain is severe, parenteral opioids are preferable because of their quicker onset of action and ease of titration. Conversion to oral formulations can occur after pain is controlled.
- With patient-controlled analgesia (PCA), opioids can be infused at a continuous basal rate and patients control the administration of bolus doses. The total hourly dose and lockout interval between boluses are preprogrammed. PCA can be administered intravenously or subcutaneously at home with specialized syringe drivers or infusion pumps.
- With most opioids, oral and parenteral doses are not equal—parenteral morphine sulfate supplies one third the oral morphine sulfate dose, and parenteral hydromorphone one quarter the oral hydromorphone dose. Care must therefore be taken when converting from the oral to the parenteral form.
- When side effects develop and are not easily controlled, options include decreasing the opioid dose if pain is well controlled, opioid rotation, or decreasing the opioid dose and adding adjuvant pain medication.
- Because nausea and vomiting are common transient side effects of opioid therapy, metoclopramide or haloperidol is sometimes started prophylactically for the first several days of opioid therapy.
- Tolerance to the respiratory depressant effects occurs rapidly; thus, opioids can be used safely when titrated to pain control.
- Constipation is a side effect of opioids to which patients do not become tolerant; laxatives should be included whenever patients are receiving opioids.
- Methadone has a biphasic and variable half-life; therefore, administration can be difficult and should be attempted carefully and probably by those experienced in its use.
- Psychostimulants, such as methylphenidate and amphetamine, can be prescribed for some patients troubled by persistent opioid induced sedation.

Unlike opioids, nonsteroidal anti-inflammatory drugs (NSAIDs) and acetaminophen have a ceiling effect to their analgesia. The use of opioid-nonopioid combinations therefore is limited by the dose of the NSAIDs or acetaminophen. Despite this fact, NSAIDs are effective pain medication, especially for inflammatory conditions. Their use can decrease the amount of opioids required and hence decrease the incidence of opioid side effects. Unless contraindicated, all pain protocols should include NSAIDs.

Neuropathic pain results from nerve injury. Often described as sharp, electric shocklike, or burning in nature, neuropathic pain generally occurs along specific dermatomes. Patients with neuropathic pain occasionally respond to opioids alone; however, many require the addition of adjuvant pain medications. Commonly used adjuvants for neuropathic pain include tricyclic antidepressants, anticonvulsants, and antiarrhythmics. The choice of an adjuvant is usually dictated by the individual drug side-effect profile, the potential for drug interactions, and the previous drug therapy. The secondary amines, nortriptyline and desipramine, are generally better tolerated than amitriptyline. The analgesic effects of tricyclic antidepressants occur at lower doses and usually within several days, as compared with the antidepressant effects. Data on use of selective serotonin reuptake inhibitors (SSRIs) for neuropathic pain are not convincing; however, recent studies suggest that serotonin and norepinephrine reuptake inhibitors (SNRIs) may be as beneficial at tricyclic agents for pain control. Of the anticonvulsants, gabapentin, pregabalin, carbamazepine, and valproic acid are commonly used for neuropathic pain. Carbamazepine and valproic acid are cost-effective but have a higher risk of drug interactions and toxicity compared with gabapentin and pregabalin. Gabapentin requires more frequent dosing, slower titration secondary to sedation, and dose adjustments for renal insufficiency. Antiarrhythmics, topical lidocaine, and oral mexiletine have also been used successfully for neuropathic pain. For adjuvant pain medications, standard initial dosing and titration guidelines should be followed, although lower than usual doses have been effective for pain control. In elderly patients, it is generally safer to start at low doses and titrate at a slower rate.

Corticosteroids, benzodiazepines, and anticholinergics are also used as adjuvant pain medication. Corticosteroids, by decreasing tumor-associated edema and by their anti-inflammatory effects, are useful for pain due to multiple pathologies, including bone metastasis, liver capsule distention from metastasis, and conditions in which the tumor is compressing sensitive structures. Benzodiazepines and baclofen are indicated for pain from spasticity. Anticholinergics can relieve colic due to intestinal obstruction.

In addition to drug therapy for pain control, interventions such as palliative radiation therapy for bone metastasis, nerve blocks (eg,, celiac plexus block for pancreatic cancer), palliative surgical resection, or immobilization of fractures should be considered. Before under-

Table 63–1. Complementary modalities used in palliative medicine.

Therapy	Brief Description	Recommendations
Acupuncture	Stimulation of defined points on the skin using a needle, electrical current (electroacupuncture), or pressure (acupressure). These points correspond to meridians, or pathways of energy flow with the intent to correct energy imbalances and restore a normal, healthy flow of energy in the body.	1. Acupuncture may provide pain relief in terminally ill patients with cancer pain. 2. Acupuncture may provide relief from breathlessness. 3. Acupressure may reduce chemotherapy- and radiation-induced nausea and vomiting.
Aromatherapy	Therapeutic use of essential oils, which are applied to the skin or inhaled. The impact on the emotional and psychological state is mediated through the olfactory nerve and the limbic system in the brain.	1. Aromatherapy may be used in conjunction with other complementary therapies, such as massage. 2. Aromatherapy may provide reduction in anxiety.
Massage therapy	Manipulation of the muscles and soft tissues of the body for therapeutic purposes.	1. Massage might provide short-term reduction in cancer pain. 2. Massage has been shown to reduce stress and anxiety and enhance feelings of relaxation.
Hypnosis	A state of increased receptivity of suggestion and direction.	1. Hypnotherapy may reduce nausea and vomiting in persons receiving chemotherapy. 2. Hypnotherapy can enhance pain relief.
Relaxation	The use of muscular relaxation techniques to release tension. These techniques are often used in conjunction with meditation, biofeedback, and guided imagery techniques.	1. Relaxation can reduce stress and tension. 2. Relaxation techniques can improve pain control in advanced cancer patients.
Therapeutic touch	A technique performed by physical touch and/or the use of hand movements to balance any disturbances in a person's energy flow.	1. Therapeutic touch may increase hemoglobin levels. 2. Therapeutic touch may relieve anxiety and tension and reduce the effects of stress on the immune system.
Music therapy	The use of music as a therapy to influence mental, behavioral, or physiologic disorders.	1. Music therapy may assist in the reduction of pain perception. 2. Music therapy may reduce anxiety and help persons cope with grief and loss.
Support group	The use of groups and psychosocial interventions to help persons learn how to cope better with their disease.	1. Support groups can enhance the quality of life. 2. Support group therapy can improve pain management and coping skills. 3. Support group therapy can reduce anxiety and depression.

taking such interventions, the patient's overall prognosis and the effectiveness of less invasive measures should be taken into consideration. Complementary therapies are often used in hospice and palliative care for treatment of pain and other symptoms. Some of these therapies are described in Table 63–1.

Fear of addiction should not hinder the use opioids for pain control. Addiction is a rare occurrence in patients with terminal illness and in patients without a prior history of drug abuse. Psychological addiction should be differentiated from physical dependence. Patients with physical dependence develop withdrawal symptoms with the abrupt cessation of a drug or significant reduction of dosage. If the need arises for a rapid decrease in the opioid dose, administering 25% of the stable dose can prevent withdrawal symptoms. In patients previously receiving steady opioid doses, dose escalation portends disease progression rather than tolerance to opioid analgesic effects. Analgesic tolerance, like addiction, is rarely seen.

Nausea & Vomiting

Nausea and vomiting entail a complex physiologic process. Several discrete afferent neural pathways terminate

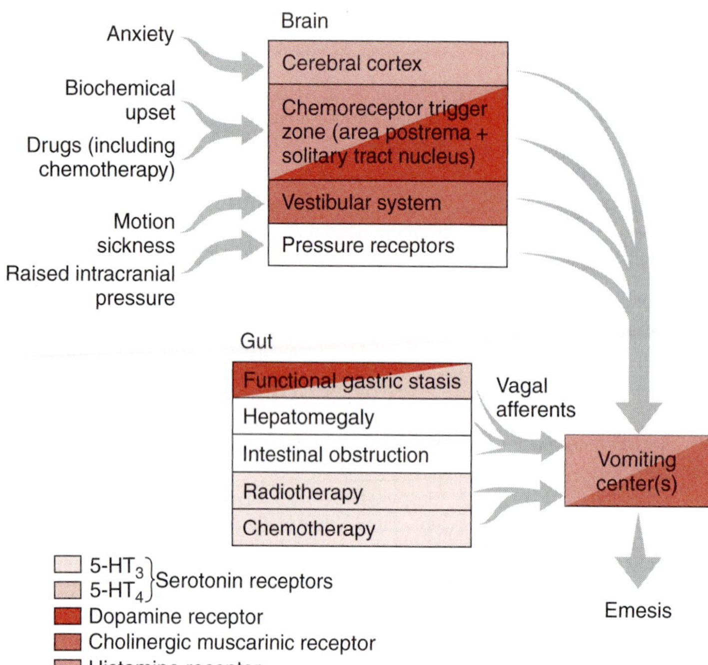

Figure 63–2. Vomiting pathways. (Reproduced, with permission, from Baines MJ: ABC of palliative care. Nausea, vomiting, and intestinal obstruction. BJM 1997;315:1148.)

at the "vomiting center" (Figure 63–2). Stimulation of this center leads to the efferent emetic reflex; however, because multiple receptors and neurotransmitters are involved with each pathway, patients can experience nausea without vomiting and vice versa.

The list of possible etiologies of nausea and vomiting is extensive. Treatment should be directed at correcting the underlying pathology when possible. The choice of antiemetics is based primarily on the suspected afferent pathway involved. Other factors to consider include route of administration, patient's previous antiemetic drug experience, drug side-effect profile, and cost of therapy.

Classes of antiemetics include the following:

- Butyrophenones: haloperidol and droperidol (narrow-spectrum dopamine-2 antagonists).
- Phenothiazines: promethazine, prochlorperazine, and chlorpromazine (broad-spectrum anticholinergic, antihistamine, and antidopaminergic).
- Benzamide: metoclopramide (antidopaminergic, cholinergic, and at high doses 5-hydroxytryptamine-3 [$5\text{-}HT_3$] antagonist).
- $5\text{-}HT_3$ receptor antagonists: ondansetron, granisetron, and dolasetron.
- Anticholinergics: scopolamine, hyoscyamine, and glycopyrrolate.
- Antihistamines: meclizine and diphenhydramine.
- Cannabinoids: dronabinol.
- Corticosteroids: dexamethasone.

Drug therapy for specific causes of nausea and vomiting includes the following:

- Vestibular dysfunction (motion induced): antihistamines, anticholinergics, or both.
- Delayed gastric emptying or squashed stomach syndrome (hepatomegaly, ascites): metoclopramide.
- Drug-induced and metabolic causes (hypercalcemia, uremia): selective antidopaminergic agents, haloperidol or dronabinol.
- Increased intracranial pressure: steroids, specifically dexamethasone.
- Chemotherapy and radiation induced: $5\text{-}HT_3$ receptor antagonists.
- Anticipatory nausea associated with chemotherapy: benzodiazepines.

Caveat: Dronabinol has an unknown antiemetic mechanism, and its psychomimetic effects limit its use to refractory nausea.

About one third of patients require more than one antiemetic for symptom control. A combination of high-potency specific receptor antagonists is recommended before reverting to broad-spectrum, low-affinity drugs. Antiemetics that can be administered by several different routes, including the subcutaneous route, can prove extremely useful. Such versatile drugs include haloperidol, metoclopramide, glycopyrrolate, ondansetron, and dexamethasone.

Nausea and vomiting may be presenting symptoms of malignant gastrointestinal obstruction. If the patient's situation is not amendable to invasive procedures such as venting gastrostomy, intraluminal stent, or surgical diversion, palliative medications can help relieve symptoms. With partial obstruction, the use of metoclopramide and dexamethasone along with a low-fiber diet can provide significant symptom relief for several weeks or longer. When obstruction becomes complete, therapy is geared at decreasing intestinal motility and decreasing secretions. Anticholinergics and somatostatin analogs are both effective for this purpose. The combination of haloperidol, an anticholinergic, and octreotide can preclude the use of nasogastric tube decompression for many patients with complete intestinal obstruction.

DYSPNEA

Dyspnea can be present with or without hypoxia and, like pain, is a subjective experience. With a broad differential existing for dyspnea, reversible causes should always be considered first. The optimal therapy is aimed at the presumed etiology. Palliative therapy can involve chemotherapy, radiotherapy, thoracentesis, pericardiocentesis, and bronchial stent placement. Minor adjustments in the environment, such as providing a fan and keeping the room temperature cool, or a careful trial of supplemental oxygen can help dyspneic patients. Available palliative drug therapies include steroids, opioids, bronchodilators, diuretics, anxiolytics, antibiotics, and anticoagulants. All these drugs can be used in combination, depending on the etiology of dyspnea.

Opioids can relieve breathlessness associated with advanced cancer. The mechanism is unclear. Opioid administration, dose, frequency, and titration are the same as for pain control. The use of nebulized morphine sulfate is not more effective than placebo. Opioids can increase exercise tolerance and reduce dyspnea in patients with chronic obstructive airways. Fear of addiction or fear of respiratory depression should not preclude a trial of opioids in this population. Starting at low doses, carefully titrating the dose to achieve symptom control, and close monitoring allow for safe and effective use.

Steroids are useful for dyspnea from bronchospasm and tumor-associated edema. Specific indications include malignant bronchial obstruction, carcinomatous lymphangitis, and superior vena cava syndrome. Dexamethasone can be started at 8 mg twice daily and subsequently reduced to the lowest effective dose. Dexamethasone is more potent and has lower mineralocorticoid activity than other steroids, resulting in less fluid retention.

Some patients with dyspnea express disturbing fears of suffocation and choking. Understandably, anxiety often coexists with chronic dyspnea. Anxiety can heighten breathlessness, making symptom control more difficult. The use of anxiolytics such as benzodiazepines and phenothiazines can help treat dyspnea associated with a high component of anxiety. Lorazepam, 0.5–1 mg, can be tried initially. If patients show benefit, long-acting diazepam or clonazepam can then be prescribed. Low-dose chlorpromazine has also shown benefit in relieving both dyspnea and anxiety.

Anorexia & Cachexia

Anorexia (poor appetite) and cachexia (severe weight loss) are prevalent distressing symptoms in patients with advanced cancer. Factors released either by the tumor or by the host response appear to produce the anorexia–cachexia syndrome. Cytokines implicated include tumor necrosis factor, interferon-γ, and interleukins-1 and -6. The syndrome is characterized by impaired metabolism of carbohydrates, protein, and lipids. A perpetual catabolic state ensues, with loss of protein and lipid stores. Patients lose weight and appear malnourished despite adequate nutrient intake. There is an abundant amount of research in this field, but little effective drug therapy available. Medications prescribed for the anorexia-cachexia syndrome include megestrol acetate, corticosteroids, dronabinol, and anabolic steroids. Megestrol acetate, a progestin, has been shown to increase appetite and result in weight gain; doses start at 160 mg/day and can be titrated to 800 mg/day if required. Corticosteroids, such as dexamethasone, can be prescribed as an appetite stimulant for patients in whom side effects of long-term steroid use are of less concern. Beneficial effects tend to be limited to several weeks. Significant weight gain is not seen with corticosteroids in this population. Dexamethasone can be started at 2–4 mg daily, with titration to 16 mg daily as needed. The lowest effective steroid dose should always be used. Androgens and dronabinol have been effective for patients with AIDS-associated anorexia and cachexia. Investigations are ongoing with respect to the use of omega-3 fatty acids and melatonin.

Anorexia can be provoked by conditions such as delayed gastric emptying, constipation, mucositis, or thrush, or even ill-fitting dentures. Metoclopramide, a prokinetic agent, can improve anorexia associated with early satiety or nausea. It is important not to overlook reversible causes of anorexia.

Nutritional support, parenteral and enteral, has not been shown to prolong survival in patients with advanced cancer who are not candidates for disease-specific therapy. Regardless, a role for palliative nutritional support exists. Patients who suffer from concurrent malnutrition—for example, patients with dysphagia from head and neck cancer or patients with gastrointestinal dysfunction from radiation toxicity or neuromuscular disorders—can potentially benefit from nutritional support. Consideration of artificial nutrition should be on an individual basis.

Asthenia

Asthenia is generally described as excessive fatigue. Patients with asthenia feel tired after minimal activity or lack the energy to perform daily activities. Patients become increasingly dependent on others for basic needs. Feelings of helplessness can lead to mood disturbances and depression, symptoms that often accompany asthenia. Asthenia is pervasive in advanced disease and may result from direct tumor effects (eg, cancer cachexia, paraneoplastic neuropathy or myopathy, and tumor involvement of the central nervous system [CNS] or spine) or be a consequence of therapy (eg, steroid myopathy, chemotherapy, radiation, or drug toxicity). Unfortunately, when disease-specific therapy is not effective, asthenia is difficult to palliate.

Nondrug therapies include a trial of transfusion for anemia; optimizing fluid and nutritional status; aggressive treatment of nausea, vomiting, and constipation; oxygen supplementation for hypoxia; moderate physical therapy to improve mobility; providing appropriate assistive devices; and providing psychosocial support. Symptomatic drug therapy includes corticosteroids and psychostimulants. A short course of dexamethasone or methylphenidate can increase patients' energy levels and improve their mood. The usual starting dose of dexamethasone is 2–4 mg once or twice daily and of methylphenidate, 2.5–5 mg twice daily. To lessen potential insomnia at night, these drugs should be administered early in the day (ie, 0800 and 1200 hours).

Key Considerations in Symptom Management

Physicians caring for patients with terminal illnesses must consider carefully the risks and benefits of all interventions in the context of the patient's quality of life and prognosis. Whenever possible, the patient and loved ones should be included in the decision-making process. The appropriateness of interventions should be reevaluated as disease progresses.

Physicians should pay special attention to details of drug prescribing, written instructions, side-effect profile, potential drug interactions, and cost of therapy. Any of these factors can easily affect treatment outcome. The patient's response to therapy should be assessed frequently, and trials of drug therapy discontinued if ineffective. Knowing when to consult specialists is a basic and essential part of care; as a general rule, a consult should be considered whenever a patient's symptoms are difficult to control.

PSYCHIATRIC DIMENSIONS IN PALLIATIVE CARE

Depression

There is a common assumption that all patients with terminal illnesses are and should be depressed. This thought promotes the underdiagnosis of depression and in turn its undertreatment. Depressive states exist on a continuum from normal sadness that accompanies life-limiting disease to major affective disorders. It is important that physicians differentiate among these levels of distress. Studies have suggested that physicians and nurses do not recognize levels of depressive symptoms and that failure to do this is worse when such symptoms are more severe.

Diagnosing depression in physically healthy patients depends heavily on the presence of somatic symptoms such as decreased appetite, loss of energy, insomnia, loss of sexual drive, and psychomotor retardation. These neurovegetative symptoms of depression are very compelling when present in the absence of physical illness but are less reliable for diagnosing depression in patients with advanced disease, in whom loss of appetite can be due to chemotherapy, fatigue can be due to cancer, and lack of sleep can be due to unrelieved pain. It is often difficult to determine whether somatic symptoms in patients with advanced disease are a result of depression or other medical causes.

Persistently depressed mood and sadness can be an appropriate response for a patient with a life-threatening disease, so the diagnosis of depression in patients with advanced cancer relies more on the other psychologic or "cognitive symptoms." Anhedonia is a useful, if not the most reliable, depressive symptom to monitor. Cancer patients who are not depressed, although periodically sad, maintain the capacity for experiencing pleasure, and there is nothing inherent to the disease or treatment process that robs them of the ability to feel pleasure. Such patients react positively to opportunities to engage in the activities that they enjoy, even though the range of activities available to them may be diminished. Indeed, some patients with far advanced disease experience exhilaration in things such as intimacies with family or friends knowing that the experiences are among the last they might have. Feelings of hopelessness, worthlessness, excessive guilt, loss of self-esteem, and wishes to die are also among the most diagnostically reliable symptoms of depression in cancer patients.

The interpretation of even these more reliable symptoms can be difficult. Hopelessness that is pervasive and accompanied by a sense of despair or despondency is likely to present as a symptom of a depressive disorder. Suicidal ideation, even rather mild and passive forms, is very likely associated with significant degrees of depression in patients with advanced disease. Several groups, recognizing the difficulties in applying traditional diagnoses of depression from the *Diagnostic and Statistical Manual of Mental Disorders* in these settings, have tried to define a group of more relevant variables responsive to a range of interventions. These variables include loss of meaning, hopelessness, loss of dignity, boredom, and demoralization.

Anxiety

Patients with advanced disease may present with a complex mixture of physical and psychological symptoms in the context of their frightening reality. Thus, recognizing anxiety symptoms that require treatment can be challenging. Patients with anxiety complain of tension or restlessness, or they exhibit jitteriness, autonomic hyperactivity, vigilance, insomnia, distractibility, shortness of breath, numbness, apprehension, worry, or rumination. Often the physical or somatic manifestations of anxiety overshadow the psychological or cognitive ones. These symptoms are a cue to further inquiry about the patient's psychological state, which is commonly one of fear, worry, or apprehension. In deciding whether to treat anxiety, the patient's subjective level of distress is the primary impetus for the initiation of treatment rather than qualifying for a psychiatric diagnosis. Other considerations include problematic patient behavior such as nonadherence, family and staff reactions to the patient's distress, and the balancing of the risks and benefits of treatment.

In this population anxiety is a symptom that can have many etiologies. It may be encountered as a component of an adjustment disorder, panic disorder, generalized anxiety disorder, phobia, or agitated depression. Additionally, in patients with advanced disease, symptoms of anxiety are most likely to arise from some medical complication of the illness or treatment such as organic anxiety disorder, delirium, or other organic mental disorders. Hypoxia, sepsis, poorly controlled pain, and adverse drug reactions such as akathisia, or withdrawal states are specific entities that often present as anxiety. Withdrawal from benzodiazepines, for example, can present first as agitation or anxiety, although the diagnosis is often missed in cancer patients with advanced disease, and especially the elderly, in whom physiologic dependence on these medications is often unrecognized.

Although anxiety in patients with advanced disease commonly results from medical complications, psychological factors related to existential issues equally as often cause anxiety, particularly in patients who are alert and not confused. Patients frequently fear isolation and estrangement from others, and may have a general sense of feeling like an outcast. Financial burdens and family role changes are common stressors.

Delirium & Dementia

Delirium has been characterized as an etiologically nonspecific, global, cerebral dysfunction, characterized by concurrent disturbances of level of consciousness, attention, thinking, perception, memory, psychomotor behavior, emotion, and the sleep-wake cycle. Disorientation, fluctuation, or waxing and waning of symptoms, as well as acute or abrupt onset of such disturbances, are other critical features of delirium. Delirium is also conceptualized as a reversible process, in contrast to dementia. At times it is difficult to differentiate delirium from dementia because they frequently share such common clinical features as impaired memory, thinking, judgment, and disorientation.

Dementia appears in relatively alert individuals with little or no clouding of consciousness. The temporal onset of symptoms in dementia is more insidious or chronically progressive, and the patient's sleep-wake cycle is generally not impaired. Most prominent in dementia are difficulties in short- and long-term memory, impaired judgment, and abstract thinking as well as disturbed higher cortical functions (ie, aphasia, apraxia, etc). Occasionally delirium is superimposed on an underlying dementia, as in the case of an elderly patient, a patient with AIDS, or a patient with a paraneoplastic syndrome.

Delirium is most common in patients with far advanced disease. Between 15% and 20% of hospitalized cancer patients have organic mental disorders. In one study, more than 75% of terminally ill cancer patients were found to have delirium. Delirium can be due either to the direct effects of cancer on the CNS, or to indirect CNS effects of the disease or treatments (medications, electrolyte imbalance, failure of a vital organ or system, infection, vascular complications, and preexisting cognitive impairment or dementia). Early symptoms of delirium can be misdiagnosed as anxiety, anger, depression, psychosis, or unreasonable or uncooperative attitudes toward rehabilitative efforts or other treatments. In any patient showing acute onset of agitation, impaired cognitive function, altered attention span, or a fluctuating level of consciousness, a diagnosis of delirium should be considered.

A common error among medical and nursing staff is to conclude that a new psychological symptom is functional without completely ruling out all possible organic etiologies. For example, given the large numbers of drugs patients with advanced disease require, and the fragile state of their physiologic functioning, even routinely ordered hypnotics are enough to create an organic mental syndrome. Opioid analgesics such as levorphanol, morphine sulfate, and meperidine are common causes of confusional states, particularly in the elderly and in patients with advanced disease. Except for steroids and biological response modifiers, most patients receiving these agents will not develop prominent CNS effects.

The spectrum of mental disturbances related to steroids includes minor mood lability, affective disorders (mania or depression), cognitive impairment (reversible dementia), and delirium (steroid psychosis). The incidence of these disorders ranges from 3% to 57% in noncancer populations, and they occur most commonly on higher doses. Symptoms usually develop within the first 2 weeks of treatment, but in fact can occur at any time and on any dose, even during the tapering phase. Prior psychiatric illness or prior disturbance on steroids is a poor to fair predictor of susceptibility to, or the nature of, mental disturbances during subsequent steroid treatments. These disorders are often rapidly reversible upon dose reduction or discontinuation.

Breitbart W: Spirituality and meaning in supportive care: Spirituality- and meaning-centered group psychotherapy interventions in advanced cancer. Support Care Cancer 2002;10:272. [PMID: 12029426]

Chochinov HM: Dignity-conserving care—a new model for palliative care: Helping the patient feel valued. JAMA 2002;287:2253. [PMID: 11980525]

Kissane DW: Demoralisation: Its impact on informed consent and medical care. Med J Aust 2001;175:537. [PMID: 11795544]

CARE OF THE DYING PATIENT

At some point in a person's illness, whether it be progressive cancer or an end-stage medical illness, it becomes clear that further attempts to treat the underlying condition are not only futile but harmful in that they expose the patient to treatments that do more harm than good, delay the important conversations that must occur around the issues of death and dying, and reduce the likelihood of good symptom control because of the focus on disease management. Family practitioners and general internists, because of their long-term patient-centered relationships, are in the best position to have conversations about the status of the illness, treatment options with attendant benefits and burdens, prognosis issues, goals of care, and the use of hospice or palliative care services.

Carey interviewed 84 terminally ill patients to understand what factors predict who best will cope with dying and what can be done by physicians and other professionals to make life more meaningful. His findings were as follows:

1. Most people want to hear the truth from their physicians. Patients with a limited life expectancy prefer to be told in person, with time allowed to express feelings and ask questions.
2. Patients want to be assured that their physician will not abandon them.
3. If the physician feels that he or she does not have the time or training to provide effective counseling for the patient or family, it is best to refer the patient elsewhere for care.
4. The proper administration of pain medication is a major factor in emotional adjustment to the terminal illness. Patients have greater peace if they know that suffering will be kept at a minimum.
5. Because of the patient's many needs, physicians should be willing to seek and accept the help of other professionals, including clergy, social workers, and nurses.

An essential first step in facilitating the shift from the curative to the palliative mode is in communicating the terminal diagnosis. Buckman describes a six-step protocol for such a conversation:

1. Getting started: The patient and his or her support person should attend. Ensure a comfortable environment. Allot adequate time, and prevent interruptions. Know the facts of the illness and treatment to date.
2. Ask what the patient knows and assess the ability to comprehend the information.
3. Find out how much the patient wants to know, taking into account cultural, religious, social, and personal issues.
4. Share the information in small bits using simple language. Avoid technical terms, jargon, and euphemisms. Pause frequently. Check for understanding.
5. Respond to feelings. Listen. Empathize. Reflect. Be aware of nonverbal communication.
6. Next steps: treat symptoms, make referrals, plan for support, and schedule a timely follow-up visit.

Similarly, predicting the course of the illness and the patient's life expectancy is an essential component of good end-of-life care. Most patients and family members want to have this information for emotional, spiritual, and practical reasons. Loprinzi suggests that these discussions should contain the following elements:

1. Acknowledge uncertainty.
2. Foretell a general, realistic time frame.
3. Recommend "doing the things that should be done."
4. Provide realistic assurance that the physician will be available to help the patient through the dying process.
5. Refer the patient to other professionals for emotional and spiritual support in "dying well."
6. Ask the patients what he or she wants to accomplish.
7. Encourage additional questions.

As death approaches the patient will develop a series of signs that predict its closeness (Table 63–2). It is important to recognize that death is approaching and share this information compassionately with the patient, if desired, and family. Medical care should be simplified as much as possible. Laboratory tests, radiologic procedures, and other interventions should be done only if they will result in improvement of the patient's comfort. Nonessential medications should be discontinued. Blood pressure medicines, for example, may be safely reduced in dosage or stopped as the

Table 63–2. Signs of impending death.

1. Bed bound
2. Confusion
3. Cool/mottled extremities
4. Death rattle
5. Decreased hearing and vision
6. Decreased urinary output
7. Difficulty swallowing
8. Diminished interest in conversation
9. Diminished interest in oral intake
10. Disoriented to time
11. Drowsiness progressing to extended periods of somnolence
12. Dry mouth
13. Hallucination
14. Increasing distancing from all but a few intimate others
15. Limited attention span
16. Profound weakness

patient becomes bed bound, reduces his or her activity, and reduces oral intake. Artificially provided hydration and nutrition are seldom necessary or helpful for the dying person. More often than not, administration of fluids results in progressive edema, lung congestion, oral secretions, and frequent urination with attendant discomfort and distress. Experienced hospice professionals note no increase in discomfort or suffering with the naturally occurring dehydration that accompanies the dying process. However, some authorities suggest that modest intravenous or subcutaneous fluids may be helpful for the delirious dying patient who is not responding to neuroleptics. A brief trial of fluids in this circumstance may be warranted. Family members frequently are concerned that not providing food by some route will result in increased suffering and "starvation" of their loved one. Confronting this misconception with care and compassion but directly usually provides reassurance for the concerned family that food is not necessary at the "time of dying."

Certain medications are important to manage the symptoms that may occur during the dying process (Table 63–3). Additionally, of great importance are the following nursing interventions, which should not be forgotten:

1. Daily bathing with application of a lubricating lotion or talcum powder to the entire body.
2. Frequent cleaning of the mouth with application of lip balm.
3. Application of artificial tears and lubricating ointment to the eyes.
4. Comfortable positioning in the bed with pillows placed under the calves or for other areas of support.
5. An open window for fresh air if possible; if not, then a fan at the bedside.
6. A calm and peaceful environment.

Family members may be instructed in these nursing interventions and participate in the care of their loved one. This often is very meaningful and comforting to both the patient and family member. As the patient

Table 63–3. Drugs used to control symptoms in the dying process.

Symptom	Drug Class	Drug	Route[1]	Dose
Pain	Nonopioid NSAID	Ketorolac	IV/SC	15–30 mg every 6 h
	Opioid	Morphine	IV/SC	4 mg every 4 h
			PR	15 mg every 4 h
"Death rattle"	Anticholinergic	Scopolamine	TD	1 patch every 3 days
		Atropine	IV/SC	0.2–0.4 mg every 2 h
		Glycopyrrolate	IV/SC	0.2 mg every 4 h
		Hyoscyamine	SL	0.125–0.25 mg every 4 h
Dyspnea	Opioid	Morphine	IV/SC	4 mg every 4 h
			PR	15 mg every 4 h
Restlessness/anxiety	Benzodiazepine	Midazolam	SC	2–5 mg every 2 h
		Lorazepam	IV/SC/SL	0.5–1.0 mg every 4 h
Agitation/hallucinations	Antipsychotic	Haloperidol	IV/SC	5–10 mg every 30 min to effect
		Thorazine	IV	12.5–25 mg every 6 h
			PR	25–50 mg every 6 h

NSAID, nonsteroidal anti-inflammatory drug; IV, intravenous; SC, subcutaneous; PR, rectal; SL, sublingual; TD, transdermal.
[1]The oral route is not listed as it is often not a viable choice in the last 48 h.

becomes minimally responsive or nonresponsive, family members are encouraged to gently talk to and touch their loved one.

Buckman R: *How to Break Bad News: A Guide for Health Care Professionals*. University of Toronto Press, 1992.

Cary RG: Living until death: A program of service and research for the terminally ill. In Kubler-Ross E, ed: *Death: The Final Stages of Growth*. Simon and Schuster, 1975.

Loprinzi CL et al: Doc, how much time do I have? J Clin Oncol 2000;18:699. [PMID: 10653888]

Nelson A et al: The dying cancer patient. Semin Oncol 2000; 27:84. [PMID: 10697024]

ADVANCE CARE PLANNING

Advance directives are legal documents that allow patients to make their health care choices known. Terms for advance directive documents are not standardized from state to state but usually encompass one or more of the following options:

1. Patients appoint someone (surrogate or proxy) to make health care decisions for them.
2. Patients specify their own choices regarding various life-sustaining treatments (often called a Living Will).
3. Patients sign a form alerting emergency medical workers (EMS) that they have signed an advance directive.

Advance directive documents go into effect when a patient loses decision-making capability. Most states, through law, require the document to be witnessed and or notarized. The American Bar Association Commission on Legal Problems of the Elderly (http://www.abanet.org) suggests that patients are best served by selecting a trusted individual to serve as a surrogate and executing a Living Will to provide guidance on treatment choices. The National Hospice and Palliative Care Organization web site (http://www.caringinfo.org) urges all family members regardless of age to have meaningful discussions about end-of-life decisions.

Patients, families, and the health care system benefit from advance directives and from the decision-making process patients and their families go through to create a written document. Advance care planning (the process of arriving at an end-of-life care decision) is important to patients because they can "direct" and inform the health care system when they are no longer able to speak for themselves. Families benefit from advance directives, because they are relieved from making extremely difficult decisions that often lead to family disagreements over the patient's wishes. Advance care planning is important to physicians because they can be assured they are following the patient's wishes.

In 2005 this issue received national attention when the case of Terri Schiavo, a young woman who had suffered severe brain damage 15 years earlier, became front-page news throughout the United States. Schiavo's husband Michael had requested that her gastric feeding tube be removed; her parents opposed this action. Legal battles ensued, but in the end the courts supported the right to refuse treatment based on Michael Schiavo's argument that his wife had previously communicated her desire not to be kept alive by artificial means. The strong feelings that surrounded this case illustrate the importance of conversations relating to advance directives and the anguish and conflict that can beset families involved in such weighty decisions.

How to Start the Process

The advance care planning process should begin with physicians educating themselves about legal statutes that exist for advance directive documents and where to direct patients for further education. Hospices, senior citizen centers, and hospital social service or spiritual care departments are all good resources for obtaining documents and educational materials.

The ideal time to discuss an advance care directive is when a patient is still healthy. Such discussions should become a part of routine health care. Although advance directive documents are important, advance care planning is a process that allows for adequate time to reflect, educate, and involve family members. A physician can initiate an end-of-life care discussion with a patient, direct the patient on where to obtain information, and encourage the patient to seek additional guidance from religious or legal advisors. Patients should also be encouraged to have a discussion with their family members so that family can be made aware of their loved ones' health care preferences. Ideally, the physician should follow up with the patient at a later date to address questions or concerns and obtain a copy of a signed advance directive document for inclusion in the patient's medical record. Physicians who follow a patient for several years may want to have further discussions periodically to ensure that any documents on file still reflect the patient's choices. States may or may not outline specific processes for changing an advance directive.

Numerous articles and studies have shown that the avoidance of planning for end-of-life care results in families agonizing over difficult health care decisions, costly futile care, and time-consuming lawsuits to sort out the results. Hammes and Briggs give the following common reasons why health care professionals avoid having end-of-life conversations:

1. A belief that the person is not sick enough, may become upset, is not capable enough to understand, and will be robbed of hope.

2. Lack of confidence in their own skills related to delivering bad news.
3. A perceived lack of time.
4. A belief that there are simply too many contingencies for individuals to have to consider regarding their future potential medical conditions.

Patients may also wish to avoid end-of-life conversations. Fear and a lack of understanding of medical technology prevent patients from initiating discussions with their physicians. A study conducted in 2000 by the National Hospice and Palliative Care Organization found that adult children would have an easier time discussing sex or drugs with their teenage children than having end-of-life care discussions with their aging parents. That so few individuals have signed advance care directives may in large part be a result of a combination of health care professional and patient avoidance. The need for conversation, however, could not be more critical.

Hammes BJ, Briggs L: *Respecting Choices.* Gundersen Lutheran Medical Foundation, 2001.

National Hospice Foundation: *Baby Boomers Fear Talking to Parents About Death.* National Hospice Foundation, 1999.

Talking to the Palliative Care Patient

As the change from curative care to palliative care begins, opportunities to engage in meaningful compassionate discussions with patients will appear. Asking patients what they understand about their disease can inform physicians of patients' perceptions and possible gaps in knowledge about the disease progression. When discussing new palliative care options, the discussion should include the goal of each treatment. Patients and their families should have a clear understanding of the benefits and the burdens of any proposed treatment.

Patients, when asked about end-of-life care choices, often use vague phrases such as "I don't want to be a vegetable" or "I don't want to be hooked up to machines" to convey their wishes. Such phrases, although descriptive, leave gaps in a loved one's ability to make concrete treatment decisions if not further explored. End-of-life care discussions are often difficult because the conversation is based on patients' and their family members' values and beliefs. Some individuals believe that removing a loved one from a ventilator constitutes murder. Others, when asked about feeding tubes, wonder about "starving their loved one to death." Such beliefs are often difficult to address and are clearly emotionally laden. Additionally, when the patient dies, the loved one, having felt forced to make a difficult decision may face a longer and more complicated bereavement period.

One approach to helping patients with advance directives is to guide the conversation to what would constitute a "good day" for the patient. By focusing on living each day to the best extent possible the physician can learn what is important to the patient and can help the patient weigh treatment options against the patient's measure of a good day. Several documents exist to help patients think about what is important to them. *Five Wishes,* produced by Aging with Dignity, and Caring Connections, the web site maintained by the National Hospice and Palliative Care Organization, are designed to assist patients and their families by leading them through a series of questions designed to stimulate thought and conversation about quality of life issues.

Sabatino CF: End-of-life care legal trends. Internal memorandum. American Bar Association Commission on Legal Problems of the Elderly, 2000. Available at: http://www.abanet.org.

Sabatino CF: *10 Legal Myths About Advance Medical Directives.* American Bar Association Commission on Legal Problems of the Elderly, 2002. Available at: http://www.abanet.org.

Web Sites

Aging with Dignity (Five Wishes):

http://www.agingwithdignity.org.

American Association of Retired Persons (state-by-state guidebooks for advance directives):

http://www.aarp.org.

Caring Connections, maintained by the National Hospice and Palliative Care Association (free, state-specific forms; an advance directive checklist, and additional information):

http://www.caringinfo.org.

SPIRITUAL DIMENSIONS IN PALLIATIVE CARE

Palliative care physicians have observed that their patients have needs that transcend physical pain, social disruptions, and psychiatric disorders. Chochinov notes, "More ubiquitous aspects of suffering—including psychological, existential, or spiritual distress—are not necessarily well understood or researched, nor do they necessarily engender a well-considered response."

The spiritual dimensions in palliative care include consideration of the patient's religious practices (eg, prayer, sacraments, and rituals) but also attend to what may be called the existential concerns of the patient. Chochinov lists these as "an overwhelming sense of hopelessness, existential or spiritual angst; loss of sense of dignity; sensing oneself a burden to others; or a waning of one's will to live and a growing desire for death...." To this list can be added concerns such as the loss of a sense of meaning, a paralyzing sense of guilt and regret, broken relationships with loved ones, difficulties with one's concept of divinity or a sense of difficulty in a relationship with a personalized deity, feelings of anger, feelings of grief, and feelings of despair. Unmet religious needs and unresolved existential concerns cause spiritual distress and can also result in psychiatric disorders such as depression or anxiety, as well as an increased sense of physical pain for the patient.

Recent studies have examined the importance of spirituality to physicians and to patients who are seriously or terminally ill, and whether and how physicians should address the spiritual concerns of these patients. (For a brief summary see Astrow and Sulmasy, 2004). Holmes and colleagues considered the results of some of these studies, conducted a study of their own, and came to the following conclusions:

> *It seems patients tend to desire a sophisticated and somewhat controlled relationship with PCPs [primary care providers] around spirituality: They want their concerns cared about but not discussed or talked about, and they want to be prayed for but not with. These results indicate that, instead of discussing spiritual issues, PCPs may more appropriately "care" for the spiritual concerns of their patients by simply asking and listening... and leave the more active roles to others who have specific training in this area....*

A study conducted by MacLean and colleagues concludes that patients' "desire for spiritual interaction increased with increasing severity of illness setting and decreased with referring to more-intense spiritual interactions."

Although intense intervention such as praying for a patient may not be welcome, being present, attentive, and supportive invites patients to share the physical, emotional, and spiritual aspects of their suffering. For the physician who is comfortable going a step further with a patient who presents spiritual concerns, Puchalski and Sandoval offer a simple assessment tool, known by its acronym, FICA:

F: Faith, belief, meaning. Ask: "Do you consider yourself spiritual or religious?" "Do you have spiritual beliefs that help you cope with stress?" If the patient answers no, the physician might ask, "What gives your life meaning?"

I: Importance and influence. Ask: "What importance does your faith or belief have in your life?" "Have your beliefs influenced you in how you handle stress?" "Do you have specific beliefs that might influence your health care decisions?"

C: Community. Ask: "Are you a part of a spiritual or religious community? Is this of support to you and how?" "Is there a group of people you really love or who are important to you?"

A: Address/action in care. Ask: "How should the health care provider address these issues in your health care?" Appropriate action might involve referral to chaplains, clergy, and other spiritual care providers.

Often the presence of spiritual suffering will emerge as patients tell their stories. To attend to this suffering requires that the health care professional be aware of and attentive to his or her own spirituality. The decision to share personal insights, experiences, and resources must be done with sensitivity and compassion, and with respect for the patient's faith tradition and practice.

Consultation with and referral to a chaplain or other faith-based community leader is often appropriate. Professional chaplains are trained to understand and respect religious and cultural diversity and to assist patients and families in dealing with a wide variety of spiritual issues. Meador notes that "the clergy member of the team brings an interpretive, liturgical, and communal sense of spiritual care from her or his pastoral formation unique to that vocational formation."

Victor Frankl, a psychiatrist whose writings were based on his experience in a Nazi concentration camp, observed: "Man is not destroyed by suffering; he is destroyed by suffering without meaning." Palliative care therefore extends beyond the physical dimensions of suffering to attend to the spiritual suffering that may be present. A physician can attend to this dimension of healing by offering a listening ear, a word of kindness, and a referral to a professional spiritual caregiver.

Astrow AB, Sulmasy DP: Spirituality and the patient-physician relationship. JAMA 2004;291:2884. [PMID: 15199045]

Chochinov H: Dying, dignity, and new horizons in palliative end-of-life care. CA Cancer J Clin 2006;56:84. [PMID: 16514136]

Frankl VE: *Man's Search for Meaning.* Simon and Schuster, 1984.

Holmes SM et al: Screening the soul: Communication regarding spiritual concerns among primary care physicians and seriously ill patients approaching the end of life. Am J Hosp Palliat Med 2006;23:25. [PMID: 16450660]

MacLean CD et al. Patient preference for physician discussion and practice of spirituality. J Gen Intern Med 2003;18:38. [PMID: 12534762]

Meador KG: Spiritual care at the end of life: What is it and who does it? N C Med J 2004;65:226. [PMID: 15481492]

Puchalski C, Sandoval C. Spiritual care. In O'Neill JF et al, eds: *A Clinical Guide to Supportive & Palliative Care for HIV/AIDS.* Health Resources and Services Administration, 2003. Available at: http://hab.hrsa.gov/tools/palliative/chap13.html.

RESOURCES

Books

Dickerson E et al: *Palliative Care Pocket Consultant, A Reference Guide for Symptom Management in Palliative Care,* 2nd ed. Kendal/Hunt, 2001.

Doka K: *Living with Life-Threatening Illness: A Guide for Patients, their Families, and Caregivers.* Jossey-Bass, 1998.

Doyle D et al, eds: *Oxford Textbook of Palliative Medicine,* 3rd ed. Oxford University Press, 2004.

Lynn J, Harrold J: *Handbook for Mortals: Guidance for People Facing Serious Illness.* Oxford University Press, 1999.

Participant's Handbook and Trainer's Guide for Education for Physicians on End-of-Life Care (EPEC). American Medical Association; available at: http://www.ama-assn.org/catalog/.

Twycross R, Wilcock A, eds: *Hospice and Palliative Care Formulary, USA.* Palliativedrugs.com Ltd, 2006.

Journals

American Journal of Hospice & Palliative Care. Enck RE, ed. Prime National Publishing Corporation, Weston, MA.

Hospice Journal. Lind DL, ed. The Haworth Press Inc, Binghamton, NY.

Journal of Pain and Symptom Management. Portenoy RK, ed. Elsevier Science Publishers, New York.

Journal of Palliative Medicine. Weissman DE, ed. Mary Ann Liebert, Inc, Larchmont, NY.

Supportive Care in Cancer. Senn HJ, ed. Springer-Verlag, Heidelburg, Germany.

Web Sites

ACP-ASIM End-of-Life Care Consensus Panel:
http://www.acponline.org/ethics/eolc.htm.

Alliance of State Pain Initiatives (ASPI):
http://aspi.wisc.edu/.

AMA: Education for Physicians in End-of-Life Care:
http://www.epec.net/EPEC/webpages/index.cfm.

American Academy of Hospice and Palliative Medicine:
http://www.aahpm.org.

American Alliance of Cancer Pain Initiatives:
http://www.aacpi.org.

American Board of Hospice and Palliative Medicine:
http://www.abhpm.org.

End-of-Life Physician Education Resource Center (EPERC):
http://www.eperc.mcw.edu/.

Growth House:
http://www.growthhouse.org

Last Acts:
http://www.lastacts.org.

National Hospice and Palliative Care Organization (NHPCO):
http://www.nhpco.org.

Supportive Care of the Dying:
http://www.careofdying.org.

Index

Note: A 't' following a page number indicates a table. An 'f' indicates a figure.

I

V